SPORTS MEDICINE
PRINCIPLES OF PRIMARY CARE

SPORTS MEDICINE
PRINCIPLES OF PRIMARY CARE

Editors

Giles R. Scuderi, M.D.
Insall Scott Kelly Institute
for Orthopaedics and Sports Medicine
Beth Israel Medical Center—North Division
New York, NY

Peter D. McCann, M.D.
Insall Scott Kelly Institute
for Orthopaedics and Sports Medicine
Beth Israel Medical Center—North Division
New York, NY

Peter J. Bruno, M.D.
Beth Israel Medical Center—North Division
New York, NY

Medical Illustrator

Lydia V. Kibiuk

with 874 illustrations

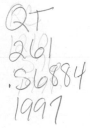 **Mosby**

St. Louis Baltimore Boston Carlsbad Chicago Naples New York Philadelphia Portland
London Madrid Mexico City Singapore Sydney Tokyo Toronto Wiesbaden

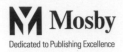

A Times Mirror
Company

Vice President and Publisher: Anne S. Patterson
Editor: Robert Hurley
Developmental Editor: Lauranne Billus
Project Manager: Christopher J. Baumle
Project Specialist: David Orzechowski
Manufacturing Manager: William Winneberger
Design Manager: Nancy McDonald
Cover Illustrations: Heidi Merscher
Cover Photos: Tony Stone Images, Custom Medical & PhotoDisk, Inc.

1st EDITION

Printed in the United States of America
Composition by Digitype
Printing/binding by Quebecor Printing

Mosby–Year Book, Inc.
11830 Westline Industrial Drive
St. Louis, Missouri 63146

Library of Congress Cataloging-in-Publication Data
Sports medicine : principles of primary care / editors, Giles R.
   Scuderi, Peter D. McCann, Peter J. Bruno ; medical illustrator,
   Lydia V. Kibiuk. — 1st ed.
       p.   cm.
   Includes bibliographical references and index.
   ISBN 0-8151-7771-2
   1. Sports medicine.   I. Scuderi, Giles R.   II. McCann, Peter D.
III. Bruno, Peter J.
   [DNLM: 1. Sports Medicine.   2. Athletic Injuries.   QT 261 S7655
1996]
RC1210.S76   1996
617.1'027 — dc20
DNLM/DLC
for Library of Congress   96-28208
                                                              CIP

97 98 99 00 01 / 9 8 7 6 5 4 3 2 1

This book is dedicated to our families who continue to support us through all our endeavors.

Giles R. Scuderi, M.D.
Peter D. McCann, M.D.
Peter R. Bruno, M.D.

PREFACE

Three factors have contributed to our interest in writing this book. In the past 20 years there has been a virtual explosion in the public's interest and participation in organized recreational sports. Consequently, a great interest has developed in the management and prevention of sports-related injuries. Concomitant with this increased interest and demand in the management of sports injuries has been an enormous increase in the capability of successful management of sports-related injuries. Finally, in the past decade we have seen an enormous change in the practice of medicine with the advent of managed care. With this new system, greater responsibility is placed on primary care physicians not only to direct referral to specialists, but also to diagnose and manage the more straightforward medical and surgical problems. For this reason, the primary care physician is often called on to diagnose and manage sports-related injuries, and it is to this group of health care providers that we direct our efforts in this book.

Our objective in this book is to provide a reference, comprehensive in scope, that will help the primary care provider manage virtually all aspects of sports medicine. The text can be used as a practical guide for the initial diagnosis and management of sports-related injuries and serve as a source for specific parameters to determine appropriate referrals to orthopaedic specialists.

We gratefully acknowledge the tremendous efforts of the authors who contributed to this textbook as well as the helpful guidance of our editors. We hope that this text will be a helpful guide for the primary care health providers in the treatment of patients with sports-related injuries.

Giles R. Scuderi, MD
Peter D. McCann, MD
Peter R. Bruno, MD

CONTRIBUTORS

Peter J. Bruno, M.D.
Clinical Instructor in Medicine
New York University School of Medicine
Assistant Attending Physician
Beth Israel Medical Center—North Division
Attending Physician
Lenox Hill Hospital
New York, New York

Joe H. Camp, D.D.S., M.S.D.
Adjunct Assistant Professor
University of North Carolina
School of Dentistry
Trauma Dentist to Charlotte Hornets & Carolina Panthers
Private Practice of Endodontics
Charlotte, North Carolina

Gail Chorney, M.D.
Assistant Professor Orthopedic Surgery
New York University School of Medicine
Associate Chief, Pediatric Orthopedics
Hospital for Joint Diseases
New York, New York

Seth A. Cohen, M.D.
Assistant Clinical Professor
Columbia University
Attending Physician
Beth Israel Medical Center
St. Luke's Roosevelt Hospital Center
New York, New York

Fred D. Cushner, M.D.
Greater Washington Orthopaedic Group
Silver Spring, Maryland

Gilbert B. Cushner, M.D., F.A.C.B.
Assistant Clinical Professor of Medicine
George Washington University School of Medicine
Attending Physician
Holy Cross Hospital
Silver Spring, Maryland

David Abramson, M.D.
Clinical Professor of Ophthalmology
Cornell University Medical Center
Attending Ophthalmologist
New York Hospital
New York, New York

J.O. Andreasen, D.D.S., Odont. Dr. HC, F.R.C.S.
Department of Oral and Maxillofacial Surgery
University Hospital
Copenhagen, Denmark

John A. Bergfeld, M.D.
Head-Section of Sports Medicine
Cleveland Clinic Foundation
Team Physician for Cleveland Cavaliers
Consultant to Baltimore Ravens
Physician for Cleveland Ballet
Cleveland, Ohio

Jacqueline R. Berning, Ph.D., R.D.
Assistant Professor
University of Colorado—Colorado Springs
Nutrition Consultant
Denver Broncos
University of Colorado Athletic Department
Cleveland Indians Minor League Teams
Colorado Springs, Colorado

Louis U. Bigliani, M.D.
Professor of Orthopaedic Surgery
College of Physicians and Surgeons, Columbia University
Chief, The Shoulder Service
New York Orthopaedic Hospital
Columbia Presbyterian Medical Center
New York, New York

Jeffrey E. Deckey, M.D.
Post-Doctorate Resident Fellow
The New York Orthopaedic Hospital
Columbia Presbyterian Medical Center
New York, New York

David R. Diduch, M.S., M.D.
Assistant Professor
University of Virginia
Department of Orthopaedic Surgery
University of Virginia Health Science Center
Charlottesville, Virginia

Cherise M. Dyal, M.D.
Assistant Professor of Orthopaedic Surgery
Albert Einstein College of Medicine
Assistant Attending Physician of Orthopaedic Surgery
Montefiore Medical Center
Bronx, New York

Michael S. Ferrara, Ph.D., A.T.C.
Director of Athletic Training
Associate Professor
Ball State University
Muncie, Indiana

Matthew E. Fink, M.D.
Professor of Neurology
Albert Einstein College of Medicine
Chairman, Department of Neurology
Beth Israel Medical Center
New York, New York

Laura L. Forese, M.D., M.P.H.
Assistant Professor of Orthopaedic Surgery
Columbia University
New York, New York

Stephen Paul Geary, M.D.
Director of Sports Medicine
Department of Orthopaedic Surgery
Ochsner Clinic
New Orleans, Louisiana

Peter G. Gerbino II, M.D.
Harvard Medical School
Fellow in Sports Medicine
Children's Hospital
Boston, Massachusetts

Dennis J. Gleason, B.S.
Prevention and Education Coordinator
Alcoholism Council in Niagara County, Inc.
State University of New York at Buffalo
Niagara Falls, New York

David A. Gold, M.D.
Associate Attending
Department of Orthopedic Surgery
Chilton Memorial Hospital
Orthopedic Surgery and Sports Medicine Center
Wayne, New Jersey

Robert T. Goldman, M.D.
Fellow
Insall Scott Kelly Institute for
Orthopaedics and Sports Medicine
New York, New York

Robert S. Gotlin, D.O.
Assistant Professor
Physical Medicine and Rehabilitation
Mount Sinai School of Medicine
Assistant Chairman
Department of Physical Medicine and Rehabilitation
Physician-in-Charge
Orthopaedic, Sports, and Spine Section
Beth Israel Medical Center—North Division
New York, New York

Alex M. Greenberg, D.D.S.
Assistant Clinical Professor
Division of Oral and Maxillofacial Surgery
Columbia University School of Dental and Oral Surgery
Clinical Instructor, Oral and Maxillofacial Surgery
The Mount Sinai School of Medicine
Columbia Presbyterian Medical Center
Assistant Attending Physician
Beth Israel Medical Center
Mount Sinai Medical Center
New York, New York

Letha Y. Griffin, M.D., Ph.D.
Staff Physician
Peachtree Orthopaedic Clinic, P.A.
Team Physician
Georgia State University
Agnes Scott College
Piedmont Hospital
Atlanta, Georgia

Steven F. Harwin, M.D., F.A.C.S.
Assistant Clinical Professor
Department of Orthopaedic Surgery
Albert Einstein College of Medicine
Physician-in-Charge
Adult Reconstructive Surgery
Beth Israel Medical Center
New York, New York

Richard H. Haug, D.D.S.
Associate Professor of Surgery
Case Reserve University
Director, Oral and Maxillofacial Surgery
Department of Surgery
MetroHealth Medical Center
Cleveland, Ohio

David C. Helfgott, M.D.
Clinical Assistant Professor of Medicine
Cornell University Medical College
Assistant Attending Physician
The New York Hospital
The Beth Israel Medical Center
New York, New York

David L. Herbert, J.D.
Senior Partner
Herbert, Benson and Scott
Canton, Ohio

Gordon Huie, P.A.
Senior Physician Assistant
Insall Scott Kelly Institute for Sports Medicine
Supervising Physician Assistant
Beth Israel Medical Center—North Division
New York, New York

Paul M. Juris, Ed.D.
Adjunct Assistant Professor
Teachers College, Columbia University
Research Coordinator
Beth Israel Medical Center
New York, New York

Barbara Kahn, R.N., O.N.C.
Hospital for Special Surgery
New York, New York

Susan M. Kaschalk, B.S.
Exercise Physiologist
Program Director
Center for Functional Rehabilitation
St. Joseph Mercy Hospital
Pontiac, Michigan

Daniel J. Kane, M.D.
Attending Physician
Department of Physical Medicine and Rehabilitation
Beth Israel Medical Center
New York, New York

Michael A. Kelly, M.D.
Director
Insall Scott Kelly Institute for
Orthopaedics and Sports Medicine
Attending Orthopaedic Surgeon
Department of Orthopaedic Surgery
Beth Israel Medical Center
New York, New York

Gwen S. Korovin, M.D.
Attending Physician
Lenox Hill Hospital
Consultant
Ames Vocal Dynamics Laboratory
New York, New York

Michael D. Kurtz, D.D.S.
Special Lecturer in Sports Dentistry
Columbia University
School of Dental and Oral Surgery
New York, New York

Gregory M. Lieberman, M.D.
Fellow
Insall Scott Kelly Institute for
Orthopaedics and Sports Medicine
Beth Israel Medical Center—North Division
New York, New York

Ulla Kristiina Laakso, M.D.
Clinical Instructor
Department of Psychiatry
Albert Einstein College of Medicine
New York, New York
Attending Psychiatrist
Beth Israel Medical Center
Lenox Hill Hospital
New York, New York

Richard A. Marder, M.D.
Associate Professor
Chief, Sports Medicine Service
Department of Orthopaedic Surgery
University of California, Davis
School of Medicine
Sacramento, California

Nino D. Marino, Ph.D.
Physician-in-Charge
Echocardiography Laboratory
Lenox Hill Hospital
Consultant in Cardiology
New York Knicks
New York, New York

Peter D. McCann, M.D.
Director
Insall Scott Kelly Institute for
Orthopaedics and Sports Medicine
Assistant Chairman
Department of Orthopaedic Surgery
Beth Israel Medical Center—North Division
New York, New York

Mary Mendelsohn, M.D.
Ophthalmology Fellow
New York Hospital—Cornell Medical Center
Attending Physician
Bellevue Medical Center
New York, New York

Lyle J. Micheli, M.D.
Associate Clinical Professor of Orthopaedic Surgery
Harvard Medical School
Director, Division of Sports Medicine
Children's Hospital
Boston, Massachusetts

Harris M. Nagler, M.D.
Professor of Urology
The Albert Einstein College of
Medicine of Yeshiva University
Chairman, Department of Urology
Beth Israel Medical Center
New York, New York

Michael A. Palmer, M.D., M.A.
Fellow in Orthopaedics and
Sports Medicine and Rehabilitation
Beth Israel Hospital—North Division
New York City, New York

Andrew H. Patterson, M.D.
Director, Orthopaedic Surgery
St. Luke's—Roosevelt Hospital Center
New York, New York

Stuart M. Popowitz, M.D.
Senior Resident
Department of Urology
Beth Israel Medical Center
New York, New York

Martin A. Posner, M.D.
Associate Clinical Professor of Orthopaedic Surgery
Mt. Sinai School of Medicine
Chief of Hand Services
Hospital for Joint Diseases
Lenox Hill Hospital
Mount Sinai Hospital
New York, New York

Kenneth J. Richter, D.O.
Clinical Associate Professor
Michigan State University
Associate Professor
Wayne State University
Medical Director
Rehabilitation Programming & Services
St. Joseph Mercy Hospital
Medical Director
United States Cerebral Palsy Athletic Association
Pontiac, Michigan

Melvin P. Rosenwasser, M.D.
Associate Professor of Orthopaedic Surgery
Columbia University College of Physicians and Surgeons
Attending Orthopaedic Surgeon
Columbia Presbyterian Medical Center
New York, New York

Michael Saunders, RPT, ATC
Trainer for New York Knicks
Faculty at Insall Scott Kelly Institute for Sports Medicine
Beth Israel Hospital—North
New York, New York

Robert S. Scheinberg, M.D.
Clinical Professor, Division of Dermatology
University of California at San Diego Medical Center
Dermatologist
Medical Group of North County, Inc.
Oceanside, California

Susan Craig Scott, M.D.
Assistant Professor
Mount Sinai School of Medicine
Clinical Assistant Professor Surgery
Beth Israel North Division Hospital
New York, New York

W. Norman Scott, M.D.
Director
Insall Scott Kelly Institute for
Orthopaedics & Sports Medicine
Chairman
Department of Orthopaedic Surgery
Beth Israel Medical Center
New York, New York

Giles R. Scuderi, M.D.
Director
Insall Scott Kelly Institute for
Orthopaedics and Sports Medicine
Attending Orthopaedic Surgeon
Department of Orthopaedic Surgery
Beth Israel Medical Center—North Division
New York, New York

Jerome H. Siegel, M.D., F.A.C.P., F.A.C.G.
Associate Clinical Professor Medicine
Mount Sinai School of Medicine
Chief of Endoscopy
Attending Physician
Beth Israel Medical Center—North Division
New York, New York

Francesca M. Thompson, M.D.
Assistant Professor of Clinical Orthopaedics
Columbia University College of Physicians & Surgeons
Chief, Adult Orthopaedic Foot Clinic
St. Luke's—Roosevelt Hospital Center
New York, New York

Joseph S. Torg, M.D.
Professor of Orthopaedic Surgery
Hospital of the University of Pennsylvania
Director, University of Pennsylvania Sports Medicine Center
University of Pennsylvania Sports Medicine Center
Philadelphia, Pennsylvania

Andrew M. Tucker, M.D.
Assistant Professor
Department of Family Medicine
University of Maryland
Director Primary Care Sports Medicine
Kernan Hospital
Baltimore, Maryland

Mark Weidenbaum, M.D.
Associate Professor Orthopaedic Surgery
College of Physicians & Surgeons, Columbia University
Assistant Attending Surgeon
New York Orthopaedic Hospital
Columbia Presbyterian Medical Center
New York, New York
Helen Hayes Hospital
West Haverstraw, New York

Robert H. Wilson, M.D.
Instructor
Howard University College of Medicine
Instructor
Division of Orthopaedic Surgery
Howard University Hospital
Washington, D.C.

Ira Wolfe, B.A.
Consultant, Shoulder Service
Columbia Presbyterian Medical Center
New York, New York

Ken Yamaguchi, M.D.
Assistant Professor
Department of Orthopaedic Surgery
Washington University School of Medicine
Chief, Shoulder and Elbow Service
Barnes-Jewish Hospital at
Washington University Medical Center
St. Louis, Missouri

CONTENTS

Section I General Principles of Sports Medicine

1 • Why Sports Medicine 3

Barbara A. Kahn
Giles R. Scuderi
Peter D. McCann

2 • Muscle and Exercise Physiology 8

Paul Juris

3 • Cardiopulmonary Conditions 18

Nino D. Marino
Peter J. Bruno

4 • Head Trauma 35

Matthew E. Fink

5 • Gastrointestinal System 39

Seth A. Cohen
Jerome H. Siegel

6 • Genitourinary Injuries 46

Stuart M. Popowitz
Harris N. Nagler

7 • Preparticipation Evaluation 61

Andrew M. Tucker
John A. Bergfeld

8 • On-Field Emergencies 74

Richard A. Marder

9 • Women in Sports 86

Letha Y. Griffin

Section II Common Sports Injuries

10 • Wound Healing 99

Susan Craig Scott

11 • Dermatologic Conditions 104

Robert S. Scheinberg

12 • Eye Injuries 115

Mary Mendelsohn
David Abramson

13 • Craniofacial Injuries 129

Alex M. Greenberg
Richard H. Haug

14 • Dental Injuries 149

Michael D. Kurtz
Joe H. Camp
J.O. Andreasen

15 • Otorhinolaryngology 175

Gwen S. Korovin

16 • The Cervical Spine, Spinal Cord, and Brachial Plexus 186

Joseph S. Torg

17 • The Thoracic and Lumbar Spine 202

Jeffrey E. Deckey
Mark Weidenbaum

18 • The Shoulder 220

Ken Yamaguchi
Ira Wolfe
Louis U. Bigliani

19 • The Elbow and Forearm 242

Robert T. Goldman
Peter D. McCann

20 • The Wrist 265

Melvin P. Rosenwasser
Robert H. Wilson

21 • The Hand 287

Martin A. Posne

22 • Pelvis, Hip, and Thigh 306

Gregory M. Lieberman
Steven F. Harwin

23 • Knee Injuries 336

David Diduch
Giles R. Scuderi
W. Norman Scott

24 • The Leg   375

Stephen P. Geary
Michael A. Kelly

25 • The Foot and Ankle   386

Cherise M. Dyal
Francesca M. Thompson

Section III   The Pediatric Athlete

26 • The Lower Extremity   413

Peter G. Gerbino, II
Lyle J. Micheli

27 • The Upper Extremity   433

Laura Forese

28 • The Spine   441

Gail S. Chorney

Section IV   Rehabilitation

29 • Rehabilitation Techniques and Therapeutic
    Modalities   449

David A. Gold
Michael Saunders
Gordon Huie

30 • The Lower Extremity   463

Robert S. Gotlin

31 • The Upper Extremity   507

Daniel J. Kane
Robert S. Gotlin

32 • The Spine   534

Robert S. Gotlin
Michael A. Palmer

Section V   Other Factors and Perspectives

33 • Nutrition   557

Jacqueline R. Berning

34 • Fluid Balance   568

Gilbert B. Cushner
Fred D. Cushner

35 • Substance Abuse   578

Dennis J. Gleason

36 • Infectious Diseases   581

David C. Helfgott

37 • Sports Psychology   587

Ulla Kristiina Laasko

38 • Sport for the Athlete with a Physical
    Disability   598

Michael S. Ferrara
Kenneth J. Richter
Susan M. Kaschalk

39 • Medicolegal Issues   609

Andrew H. Patterson

40 • Legal Issues in Sports Medicine   611

David L. Herbert

SPORTS MEDICINE
PRINCIPLES OF PRIMARY CARE

GENERAL PRINCIPLES OF SPORTS MEDICINE

CHAPTER 1

WHY SPORTS MEDICINE

Barbara A. Kahn
Giles R. Scuderi
Peter D. McCann

The increased understanding of the relationship between physical fitness and health among the current growing population has led to a reevaluation of the importance of sports and physical activity in our daily lives. While this has led to a decrease in certain medical conditions such as heart disease, it has also increased sports related injuries. Consequently, this has created the need for improved and specialized medical care. Advances in the field of sports medicine have provided the techniques necessary to prevent, cure, and recover from injuries which detract and often terminate participation in physical activity and athletics.

HISTORY

Throughout history, man's ability to survive and take care of his family has depended on his physical capabilities. Speed, strength, and skill were essential survival tools during early civilization. Progression led to the transformation of these physical attributes to organized contests where highly trained members began competing in a team-like fashion.

Therapeutic exercise has been in existence as far back as 1000 B.C. Milo, an Olympic wrestler in ancient Greece, used to lift a calf every day until it reached adulthood. This marked the beginning of strength training using progressive resistance exercises. Herodicus became known as the first sports physician to treat injuries with therapeutic diet and exercise. Although his methods were criticized at first, other physicians came to observe and utilize his techniques leading to the specialization of sports medicine. In the second century A.D. Galen became the first appointed team physician. His purpose was to cure injured gladiators so that they could return to battle. Galen was followed by Oribasius of Pergamum, who claimed that the body's organs had greater function while being physically stressed. Aurilianus in the fifth century was the

first physician to institute postoperative exercise programs to promote healing.

Physical education in the United States started at Amherst College in Massachusetts with the appointment of Edward Hitchcock Jr. as professor of physical education and hygiene in 1854. He developed a program incorporating the Swedish and German methods of gymnastics and running with the American games of football, basketball, and track. Dr. Hitchcock also served as the school physician for Amherst College, enabling him to record the prevalence of injury and disease among the student population. He published several books on athletics which earned him the titles of America's first team physician and founder of physical education in the United States.

In 1885 the American Alliance of Health, Physical Education, and Recreation (AAHPER) was founded. Dance was added in 1977 and the organization became known as AAHPERD, which it remains to this day. Its purpose was to promote research in exercise and maintain high standards for physical education. After President John F. Kennedy was inaugurated, he took an interest in promoting physical education and formed the President's Council on Physical Fitness. This ensured the standardization of the school system to promote and educate youngsters about the advantages of regular physical exercise.

The evolution of athletic training and sports medicine occurred from the expansion of intercollegiate athletics. The National Collegiate Athletic Association (NCAA), founded in 1906, standardized team sports among colleges and universities. Its purpose back then and now is to promote intercollegiate athletics, govern national championships, and enforce rules for sport safety and competitiveness.

As the number of participating athletes grew during the 1950s the demand for clinicians to care for medical needs and athletic injuries increased. Physicians were called upon to provide immediate treatment to otherwise young, health individuals. Aggressive treatment with a rapid return to competition created the need for a highly specialized and challenging field of medical care.

WOMEN IN SPORTS

The acceptance of female athletes, both professionally and recreationally, added a new dimension to both sports medicine and sports in general. During the 1800s women were forbidden to engage in any type of physical activity. Frailty and pallor were symbols of a woman's status in society, for only poor, working-class females showed any signs of physical well-being or strength. Doctors in the late 1800s felt that females were an inherently ill species due to their reproductive cycles and felt that most diseases, regardless of origin, were diseases of the womb.[10]

The Women's Suffrage Movement of the 1870s introduced women into the collegiate system, which was a cause for major concern for many physicians. It was believed that the stress brought about by studying would cause infertility and uterine atrophy because the brain was in direct competition with the uterus.[10] To prevent this from happening, women were encouraged to engage in noncontact activities such as walking, swimming, tennis, and golf. In 1896 the bicycle was invented. Women abandoned all sense of morals and sexual taboos that had been bestowed on them to participate in bicycle riding.

World Wars I and II forced women to enter the work force to support the war effort. They worked long hours mostly in factories. To compensate for poor working conditions recreational and team sports were organized by factory owners to alleviate stress. In the 1940s Philip Wrigley, owner of the Chicago Cubs, formed a professional female baseball league to fill the void left by the absence of men's professional baseball. It was tremendously popular, but no further advancement in women's athletics came about once the men returned after the war ended.

In 1972 Title IX was enacted, which prohibited discrimination on the basis of sex in any educational institution receiving federal funding. Under Title IX women were to receive a percentage of funding high enough to give them equivalent uniforms, playing fields, coaches, and budgets to that of their male counterparts. Title IX opened the door for women to enter competitive sports at the high school and college levels. This had a major impact on the field of sports medicine for young women.

DISABLED ATHLETES IN SPORTS

Women were not the only group experiencing exclusion from recreational and competitive sports. Until the late 1950s persons with either physical or mental disabilities were unable to become involved in physical activity at all. At present, it is estimated that 2 to 3 million people with disabilities participate in sports each year in the United States.[5] Part of the reason for this is due to the ad-

vancement in special equipment needed for the disabled to participate in a wide variety of activities. Disabled athletes now compete in basketball, skiing, swimming, and many other sports. The advent of sport-specific wheelchairs became the catalyst for competitive sports for the disabled about 35 years ago. In the late 1970s special committees were formed to represent disabled athletic participants. This included organizations on the national and international level to include the deaf, blind, wheelchair bound, dwarfed, and cerebral palsied among many others. Health care personnel realize the benefits of physical activity for individuals with disabilities and are developing ways to treat and prevent injuries incurred by these athletes. Burnham et al.[2a] in 1991 found that injuries sustained during the 1988 Canadian Paralympics occurred most often in the musculoskeletal, general medical, and disability related groups. Richter and his colleagues studied injury patterns of athletes with cerebral palsy at the same paralympic games and found that 60% of the athletes with cerebral palsy reported an injury or illness, as compared with 75% of participants from the 1988 Olympic Games.[12] The study also found that of these reported injuries the most commonly traumatized region was the shoulder and respiratory tract in the disabled athlete.

Sports medicine physicians have needed to adapt their practice to treat disabled athletes differently than other groups because they are prone to specific injuries. For example, athletes who are blind tend to injure their lower extremities most often. Those athletes with cerebral palsy and spinal cord injuries have a tendency toward urinary retention, infections, and dehydration. Because prolonged immobilization leads to bone loss, wheelchair athletes are at an extreme risk for sustaining fractures. In addition these athletes are prone to developing pressure sores or ulcers due to increased friction and loss of sensation.[12] It is apparent then how the field of sports medicine has needed to advance and become more specialized over the past 40 years.

SPORTS AND THE ELDERLY POPULATION

In 1989 there were 25 million Americans above the age of 65. It is expected that this number will rise to 65 million in the year 2030, which will equal approximately 20% of the population.[4] In 1900 the average life expectancy was only 48.2 years for males and 51.1 years for females. By 1987 these numbers increased to 72.2 years and 78.9 years respectively, with individuals over 85 years of age becoming the largest growing portion of the American population.[14] Researchers have found that moderate-intensity physical activity such as walking, stair-climbing, cycling, and gardening convey health benefits. Epidemiologic studies have shown a decrease in cardiovascular morbidity/mortality and increased longevity in people who participate in moderate activity on a regular basis. It is estimated that at least 6 million Americans have coronary artery disease and that 500,000 patients will undergo coronary artery bypass grafting or angioplasty each year.[6] Even with these findings, there has been a 30% decrease in coronary artery disease in the United States since

1960.[6] This decrease can be attributed to a change in the lifestyles of middle-age and elderly people. The United States Masters Swimming Association (USMS) serves as the national governing body for aquatic athletes competing in organized events over the age of 20. In 1989, there were 28,600 athletes registered in the USMS. Of these, 34% were between the ages of 30 and 39, and 23% were between 40 and 49.[13] Other moderate intensity cardiovascular activities done by middle-age and elderly athletes include cycling, jogging, golfing, rock climbing, and tennis. Bicycling is an excellent sport for athletes of any age. It offers cardiovascular benefits comparable with those of jogging yet relies on smooth motion, which does not overstress the muscles and joints. Eighty-six million Americans will ride a bicycle this year, with 30% of these being above 30 years of age.[11]

In 1975 the United States Tennis Association (USTA) established a seniors division to include athletes desiring to play tennis competitively up through age 85.[9] This was in response to the growing number of senior athletes wanting to play competitive tennis. It has been shown that senior athletes who play tennis regularly suffer less injuries than the intermittent recreational athlete of the same age. The same is true for the jogger, rock climber, bicycler, etc. All mature athletes need to be involved in a proper conditioning program to include stretching, warm up, endurance, and strength training to avoid injury. Since this is not always possible or done properly, it is important for the sports medicine physician to be able to recognize and treat mature athletes. Physiologic changes such as osteoporosis, decreased elasticity of articular cartilage, and spinal disc degeneration need to be addressed when treating an older person but should not be considered factors that necessarily end an individual's athletic career.

EFFECTS OF EXERCISE ON PSYCHOLOGIC WELL-BEING

In today's society sports and physical fitness play an important role in physical well-being. Great emphasis has been placed on living longer, disease prevention, and holistic treatment through diet and exercise. Over the past several years, more and more studies have been conducted in the area of exercise and physical health. As we will discuss later in this chapter, many serious health problems can be controlled or obliterated through moderate, consistent physical activity. We have not as yet addressed psychologic well-being in regard to physical activity. There is a growing amount of evidence to support the fact that exercising regularly can heighten intellectual acuity and self-concept while decreasing anxiety and levels of depression. Exercise promotes release of serotonins and endorphins, which are natural pain killers and antidepressants inherently produced by the brain. Release of these substances into the blood produces a euphoric sense intrinsically. Hilyer and Mitchell[6a] studied three groups of college students in regard to self-concept and found that the group which was most positively affected had both exercise and mental counseling as opposed to counseling alone. To support these results a study was conducted by Eickhoff et al.,[3a] which proved that young women with low self-concept who became involved in a 10-week aerobic dance program showed greater improvement in self-concept and self-esteem than any other group involved. Additional studies have been conducted in the area of mental acuity Bowers et al. showed that reaction time in a mental task involving memory could be significantly reduced following a 10-week aerobic exercise program in middle-aged adults.[2] Similarly, it has been demonstrated that cognition was improved either during or immediately after physical activity in both the younger adult and geriatric patient.

In terms of anxiety, there is a direct correlation between stress levels and high blood pressure, heart attack, and stroke. Reducing the stress level of a "type A personality" would greatly decrease the risk of severe health ailments. Many studies have been conducted on this subject. Of those which included physical activity as a parameter, anxiety levels have been shown to decrease significantly in the groups engaging in exercise programs.

For many years it has been noted that chronic psychologic and emotional disturbances are associated with deterioration of one's health status. Therefore, it appears that the converse must also be true; improving one's physical health can improve psychologic wellness. Depression affects thousands of people in the United States alone and accounts for the majority of cases seen by psychotherapists daily. It has been proven that exercise of any type helps alleviate depression, with the longest programs having the greatest effect. When comparing exercise programs with relaxation techniques and psychotherapy, exercise was proven to be more effective at decreasing depression than relaxation techniques and equally as effective as psychotherapy.[2] We can therefore conclude that moderate, consistent physical activity can promote physiologic as well as psychologic health.

CONDITIONING

DeLorme[2b] in 1940 introduced a way to increase muscular strength using cables and pulleys systematically while gradually increasing resistance. This method of conditioning became known as progressive resistance exercise. In 1978 the American College of Sports Medicine (ACSM) updated their recommendations for exercise in adults to include muscular strengthening and endurance exercises.[3] They defined physical fitness as being composed of cardiorespiratory fitness, body composition, muscular strength, endurance, and flexibility.

Flexibility can be defined as the range of motion of a joint or a series of joints that are influenced by muscles, tendons, ligaments, bones, and bony structures.[1] Flexibility varies in accordance with several intrinsic and extrinsic factors. Aging causes a decrease in flexibility, with the only increase being seen from birth to adolescence. Males are, in general, less flexible than females. The level and type of activity performed, the rest intervals between activities, temperature, and specific joint involvement all have strong influences on flexibility. Adequate flexibility helps to prevent soft tissue injuries. As tendons and ligaments are stretched repeatedly lengthening occurs, giving way to free movement with less stiffness. Because sprains, strains, and tears of both muscle and connective tissue are common sports related injuries, it is important to present proper stretching and conditioning techniques to the recreational and professional athlete. These injuries generally respond well to a therapeutic program of rest with stretching and nonsteroidal anti-inflammatory medications. When patient compliance to this regime is poor or when athletes ignore symptoms of overuse injuries, more serious injuries can occur.

Conditioning for sports is no longer restricted to those athletes playing team sports. Participants at all levels in every sport should be engaged in a conditioning program to help reduce the risk of injury during sporting activity. Maximum performance in athletic activity can best be obtained by conditioning the body with a sport-specific series of exercises designed to maximize the body's ability to withstand the demands inherent within a sport.[8] The role of conditioning to modify sports injuries and risk of injury is still being researched at present. Injuries of the skeletal muscle and musculoskeletal junction are common causes of pain and disability. Improved understanding of normal physiologic mechanisms, as well as pathologies, will lead to new strategies for injury prevention and treatment. For example, resistive training strengthens the structures surrounding a joint. This is a positive influence since it spares the joint which is most susceptible to injury, prevents osteoporosis, improves posture, assists in weight control, and rehabilitates and prevents injury.

ADVANCES IN SPORTS MEDICINE

The field of sports medicine grew rapidly during the 1970s with increased numbers of participants in both recreational and competitive athletics. Family practitioners and internists contributed to the welfare of the athlete by conducting physicals and treating medical conditions in conjunction with the orthopaedist. Additionally, orthopaedic surgeons were being required to attend many organized sporting events to treat injuries on the field or sidelines. The foundation of the American Orthopaedic Society for Sports Medicine (AOSSM) in 1972 confirmed the existence of sports medicine as its own medical specialty. The American Medical Society for Sports Medicine (AMSSM) arose as more nonorthopaedic physicians who were interested in sports medicine saw the benefits of the AOSSM. These primary care physicians found that the ACSM was too heterogeneous and research oriented to satisfy their needs. Members of the AMSSM are board certified physicians in primary care who have completed a fellowship in sports medicine or meet certain practice requirements and have passed a standardized exam that leads to a Certification of Qualifications. The interaction between the AOSSM and the AMSSM is instrumental in maintaining the excellence of sports medicine care.

Current research is also going beyond evaluation of specific injuries and various treatment measures. Epidemiologic studies are now directed at surveying the injury patterns of the athlete, the sporting activity, and the environment in which the event occurs. These studies shift some investigations from treatment modalities to possible preventive measures. In fact, this type of investigation can be undertaken as a multicenter study with a single epidemiologic team, which establishes a single protocol and uniform definitions. With this common interest, multicenter studies can acquire larger amounts of more diverse information. As more information is gathered, changes or modifications in a specific sports venue may reduce the injury rate.

CURRENT ISSUES

Over the last decade the concept of team physician has evolved from the original model of an orthopaedic surgeon taking complete responsibility for the medical needs of a sports team. Many nonorthopaedic physicians, including family practitioners, internists, and pediatricians, are now actively involved in many sports medicine programs. The ideal team physician is a combination of a primary care physician and an orthpaedic surgeon. This permits complete care of the athlete, dealing with all the aspects of medical care as well as traumatic injuries. Since many sports injuries do not necessarily require surgery, primary care physicians are at the forefront of prevention and treatment. The AMSSM, in recognizing this fact, has qualified sports medicine primary care physicians. Working closely with consulting orthopaedic surgeons, the athlete will receive the optimal care.

One of the most challenging problems that is arising in the current state of health care is the role of the team physician in the managed care environment. Many find it difficult to care for players because the player's coverage is not a plan with which the physician participates. Prompt diagnosis and treatment remain the most cost effective means of returning the athlete to competition. It is for this reason that as health care changes, health care providers and legislators realize that the best treatment for sports related injuries is provided by team physicians with an expertise in sports medicine. This will maintain the continuity of care with these athletes, enable the team physician to make decisions regarding return to competition, and is probably the most cost-effective means of delivering health care to these athletes.

In this time of health care reform it appears that the primary care physician will have the initial responsibility of administering treatment to the injured athlete. Following recommended treatment plans or algorithms, these physicians should be able to manage many of the injuries. However, it behooves them to refer the athlete to a specialist as soon as it becomes apparent that the injury is not improving or is beyond the scope of their expertise.

REFERENCES

1. Anderson B, Burke ER: Scientific, medical and practical aspects of stretching, *Clin Sports Med* 10(1):63–86, 1991.
2. Anthony J: Psychologic aspects of exercise, *Clin Sports Med* 10(1):171–180, 1991.
2a. Burnham R, Newell E, Steadward R: Spartle medicine for the physically disabled: The Canadian team experience at the 1988 Seoul Paralympics games, *Clin J Sports Med* 1(3):193–196, 1991.
2b. DeLorme T, Watkins A: Techniques of progressive resistance exercise. *Arch Phys Med* 29:263, 1948.
3. DiNubile NA: Strength training, *Clin Sports Med* 10(1): 33–62, 1991.
3a. Eickoff J, Thorland W, Ansorge C: Selected physiological and psychological effects of aerobic dancing among young adult women, *Sports Med Phys Fitness* 23:278, 1983.
4. Elia, EA: Exercise in the elderly, *Clin Sports Med* 10(1): 141–155, 1991.
5. Ferrara MS et al: The injury experience of the competitive athlete with a disability: Prevention implications, *Med Sci Sport Ex* 24(2):184–188, 1994.
6. Gordon NF, Scott CB: The role of exercise in the primary and secondary prevention of coronary artery disease, *Clin Sports Med* 10(1):87–103, 1991.
6a. Hilyer J, Mitchell W: Effect of systematic physical fitness training combined with counseling on the self-concept of college students, *Counsel Psychol* 26:427–436, 1979.
7. Kibler WB: Clinical implications of exercise: Injury and performance. In M Schafer, ed: American Academy of Orthopaedic Surgeons 43:17–24, 1994.
8. Kibler WB, Chandler TJ, Reuter BH: Advances in conditioning. In LY Griffen, ed: *Orthopaedic Knowledge Update Sports Medicine*, American Academy of Orthopaedic Surgeons 1:65–72, 1994.
9. Leach RE, Abramowitz A: The senior tennis player, *Clin Sports Med* 10(2):283–290, 1991.
10. Lutter MJ: History of women in sports, *Clin Sports Med* 13(2):263–279, 1994.
11. McLennan JG, McLennan JC: Cycling and the older athlete, *Clin Sports Med* 10(2):291–299, 1991.
12. Peck DM, McKeag DB: Athletes with disabilities, *Phys Sports Med* 22(4):59–62, 1994.
13. Richardson AB, Miller JW: Swimming and the older athlete, *Clin Sports Med* 10(2):301–318, 1991.
14. Seto JL, Brewster CE: Musculoskeletal conditioning of the older athlete, *Clin Sports Med* 10(2):401–429, 1991.

CHAPTER 2

MUSCLE AND EXERCISE PHYSIOLOGY

Paul M. Juris

Tradition, or perhaps convention, has it that a discourse on exercise physiology would focus on the subject of muscle ultrastructure and the various energy producing systems that allow for muscle contraction. The importance of such a discussion cannot be overstated, yet a slightly different perspective might be more appropriate when addressing the issues of sports medicine and rehabilitation.

From a more global approach, one might consider that the essential role of muscle is to either move or fixate the skeleton so that purposeful behavior can occur. This broad concept has led to numerous discussions of the musculoskeletal system and the interaction between muscle and bone. Absent from this model, however, is the nervous system, which is primarily responsible for the coordination of muscular activity.

Conventionally, neural and muscular behavior have been treated separately as either muscle physiology or neurophysiology. This scientific dichotomy is problematic in that one system does not function appropriately without the other. While muscles act directly on the skeleton, they cannot do so unless there is neural input instructing them on how to function. On the other hand, although the nervous system provides the primary impetus for muscles to contract, its activity would be immaterial without intact musculature. Thus, the discussion of physiology from this perspective will explore the intact neuromuscular system, focusing on the essential functional element of this system, the motor unit.

THE MOTOR UNIT

The principle component of the neuromuscular system, as seen in Fig. 2-1, is the motor unit. The motor unit is defined as the cell body and dendrites of a motor neuron, its axon and branches, and all of the muscle fibers which it innervates. Motor units can generally be classified as either fast twitch or slow twitch, referring to their twitch characteristics. Likewise, they can be characterized according to their resistance to fatigue, in which case they are referred to as fast-fatigable (FF), fast-fatigue resistant (FR), or slow-fatigue resistant (S). In all cases, the linkage between the motor neuron and the muscle cell is closely related to the character of the motor unit.

Cell diameter, for example, relates directly to the type of motor unit and is consistent with both neural and muscular components. In general, FF type units have larger axon diameters than S units, and the muscle cells tend to be larger as well.[6] Motor axon diameter bears a direct relationship to nerve conduction velocity. This is simply because the larger the area of the axonal cylinder, the less resistance there is to the flow of electrons. Thus, fast twitch motor neurons tend to have higher conduction velocities than slow twitch nerve cells. These findings have been reported in studies of cat hindlimb alpha motoneurons wherein the conduction velocities of FF nerve cells were more than 15 m/s faster than those of S neurons.[7,8]

Another contributor to conduction velocity is the nature of conduction along the nerve cell. Motor neurons are covered in an insulating sheath called myelin (refer to Fig. 2-2). The myelin is interrupted periodically along the axon by nodes, which cause the depolarized signal to jump from one node to the next in wavelike fashion. This form of signal conduction is referred to as "saltatory conduction" after the Latin *saltare*, meaning "to leap." The wider the nodal spacing, the more rapidly the signal jumps from node to node, and consequently, the faster the rate of transmission. Fast twitch motor units have greater internodal distances than slow twitch units, contributing to their faster conduction velocity.

In addition to their signal transmission characteristics, motor units can be separated into groups with different excitatory potentials. In other words, the strength of the input required to evoke an action potential along the

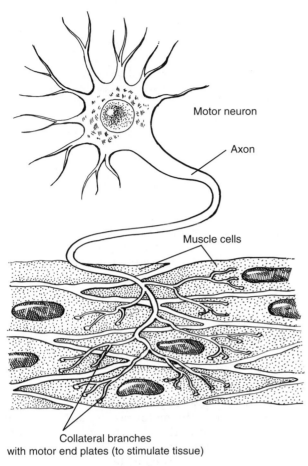

Fig. 2-1. Motor unit.

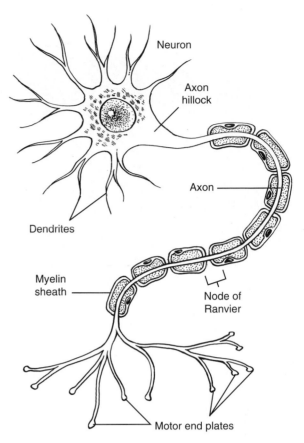

Fig. 2-2. Myelination/nodes of Ranvier.

nerve cell varies between fast and slow twitch motor units. While slow twitch neurons are more readily excited (have a lower firing threshold), fast twitch neurons require more input in order to overcome a higher excitatory threshold.

Muscle fiber characteristics in motor units closely parallel their associated nerve cells. Muscle fibers can be categorized histochemically according to the level of myosin-ATPase associated with the cell. Myosin-ATPase is bound to the myosin heads and is related to twitch speed. Fast twitch muscle fibers have higher levels of myosin-ATPase and consequently, stain darkly in slide preparations. Slow twitch fibers, on the other hand, have low levels of myosin-ATPase and thus appear very light under stain (refer to Fig. 2-3).

Muscle twitch responses are also clearly distinguishable between FF, FR, and S motor unit types. Enoka[13] describes three such motor units from the medial gastrocnemius of the cat. Muscle fibers from the FF motor unit produce nearly 50 grams of force with a twitch time of less than 100 ms. Twitch tension from FR fibers was recorded at less than 20 gm, with a twitch duration of greater than 100 ms. Fibers from the S motor unit achieved a tension of less than 10 gm over a period of more than 200 ms. Thus, the diversity of motor unit types provides the neuromuscular system with a fairly precise means of controlling contractile activity, thus influencing the nature of motor coordination.

MOTOR-UNIT RECRUITMENT

The gradation of muscle contraction is necessary in order for purposeful movement to occur. The force required to hold a 12-pound bowling ball, for example, is greater than that needed to hold a crystal goblet. The higher force may serve both conditions, but in the latter case is unnecessary and may result in damage or injury. Through a diverse motor-unit pool, the neuromuscular system has a means of controlling not only the amplitude of muscle activity, but the rate of change in tension as well. These are accomplished through motor unit recruitment strategies.

It is first necessary to understand that motor-unit activity adheres to the "all-or-none" principle. That is, once the firing threshold of a motor unit is reached, depolarization of the nerve cell proceeds, resulting in the stimulation of all of the associated muscle fibers. Those fibers will respond by contracting fully, meaning that they will produce the maximal amount of force that they are capable of producing. Thus, a motor unit can be viewed as either quiescent or fully contracting; there are no other possibilities.

The gradation of muscle contraction, therefore, must account for this phenomenon, and accordingly, there are two essential means by which force modulation is accomplished. These are sometimes referred to as recruitment or frequency strategies. Under a recruitment strategy, the nervous system recruits a progressive number of motor units

Cross sections of muscle

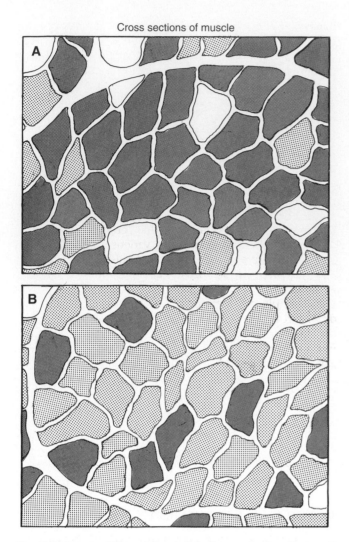

Fig. 2-3. Myosin ATPase stains dark in the predominantly type II muscle (**a**). Type I muscle (**b**) shows little staining.

until the appropriate level of force output is achieved. Frequency strategies involve the repeated stimulation of a fixed number of motor units, contributing to tension development with each successive twitch response.

Either an isolated or combined application of these strategies will result in graded muscle tension. It is gener-

ally reported, however, that recruitment is the predominant strategy for a step-wise or gross increase in muscle force, while smooth changes or minor fluctuations in twitch tension emanate from frequency control schemes.[10,26,35] Milner-Brown and Stein[29] suggest that recruitment occurs under low-level muscular contractions, while the manipulation of firing rate becomes more critical at higher force levels. Regardless of their specific manner of activation, the presence of these two strategies and the associated variety of muscle torque profiles that can be generated suggest that a high degree of variability exists in the recruitment of motor units. Yet, evidence exists suggesting that the recruitment of motor units follows a quite orderly pattern.

Henneman's Size Principle

Through decades of research in the area of motor control, many hypotheses have emerged explaining the nature of motor activity and the systematic activation of motor units. One theory presented over 35 years ago, however, remains relatively unchallenged in its explanation of the governing of muscle force output. Henneman's size principle[15] states that the activation of motor units at the spinal cord level follows an orderly progression from the low threshold, slow twitch nerve cells, to the higher threshold, fast twitch motor neurons.

Low force contractions, therefore, will involve only slow twitch motor units, while high force muscle activity will result from the sequential activation of first slow then fast twitch nerve cells. More specifically, Komi and Viitasalo[26] suggest that the contribution of fast twitch motor units begins when force output reaches 60% of an individual's maximal volitional contraction (MVC). Thus, for contractions below this level, recruitment strategies may be employed exclusively to the low threshold motor units. Tension requirements above 60% MVC, on the other hand, will be met by applying combined recruitment and frequency schemes to the entire available motor unit pool (this scheme is presented graphically in Fig. 2-4).

This model of motor unit activation offers a logical interpretation of the dynamic control of muscle force output. It is not, however, the solitary explanation, and may only partially explain the diverse mechanisms controlling motor outflow. For example, 20 years ago Milner-Brown, Stein, and Lee[30] introduced the notion

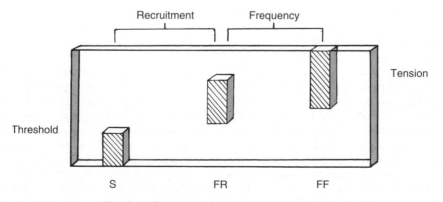

Fig. 2-4. Illustration of recruitment strategies.

of motor unit synchronization, wherein individuals demonstrated a propensity to group discharges from different motor units. Most of the subjects falling into this category were either weight lifters or were involved in manual jobs requiring the exertion of large, briefly applied forces. Ostensibly, synchronization is an efficient strategy by which one can develop high forces through the combined output of various motor unit pools.

Although motor unit synchronization offers an alternative explanation to the control of motor outflow, it does not necessarily conflict with Henneman's premise. It is quite possible that the clustering of motor units follows a similar progression along the threshold hierarchy, wherein low threshold units are grouped first and high threshold units enter the cluster in response to greater force demands. In this sense, synchronization is not an alternative strategy, but rather a different method of employing the size principle. Instead of recruiting individual motor units in a specified sequence, the nervous system can engage groups of motor units simultaneously in order to achieve high force levels more efficiently. This concept is supported by De Luca,[10] whose notion of a "common drive" suggests that individual motor units are not individually controlled but that motoneuron pools are controlled as a whole.

In essence, the synchronized output of a set of clustered slow twitch motor units may equal the force generated by single fast twitch motor units. It follows then, that the combined force output of synchronized motor unit pools may exceed the sum force generated by sequentially activated individual motor units. The result is not only an extension of the potential range of muscle force output, but a more finite degree of control over the development and disposition of muscle force.

It is worth repeating that Henneman's size principle has been largely unchallenged during the past 4 decades. There is evidence, however, suggesting that additional recruitment schemes exist, not necessarily as replacements for the size principle but perhaps as coexisting strategies for the control of motor neurons. Person,[34] for example, examined the activity of motoneuron pools during submaximal isometric contractions when individuals were either in a "fixed body" position or in a "free posture." The author reports that while subjects were "fixed" the recruitment of motor units followed an orderly sequence, as described by Henneman. Under "free posture" conditions, on the other hand, subjects demonstrated significant variability in the recruitment and deactivation of motor units.

This variability in the pattern of muscle activation is apparently related to the nature of the neuromuscular activity. Person argues that under normal movement conditions the recruitment of motor units and their differential control are coordinated by the combination of afferent and supraspinal structures. In other words, the process of neuromuscular coordination is generated from higher levels in the central nervous system (CNS) from which a choice of inputs to independent motoneurons or motoneuron pools can be made. Consequently, the CNS may be capable of selective recruitment resulting in movement-specific motor-unit firing patterns.

The method by which selective recruitment occurs has been partially explained by Burke et al.,[7] who postulated that during voluntary contractions a neural switching mechanism can redirect the excitation of motor units towards high threshold neurons, while simultaneously depressing slow twitch units. Basmajian[1] also discusses the selective inhibition of superfluous motor pathways, resulting in the excitation of only those motor-unit pools that will yield the appropriate muscle activity for specific tasks. Both of these authors support Person's notion of high level control mechanisms. Belanger and McComas,[3] however, in addressing Burke's hypothesis, failed to detect evidence of selective control of motor units under conditions of isometric ankle plantar and dorsiflexion. So the evidence associated with selective recruitment is not altogether certain.

The lack of consistency in the various findings may relate to the nature of the experimental task rather than the absolute presence or absence of recruitment selectivity. Much of the work focusing on motor-unit recruitment involves simple tasks performed under highly regulated conditions. It is quite possible that under these circumstances the innervation of motor units follows a tightly regulated linear pattern, as described by Henneman. Person's investigation, on the other hand, compared a simplistic condition in which coordinated muscle activity for postural control was not required, to one which involved the dual task of having to perform muscular contractions while simultaneously maintaining posture and equilibrium. In this case, the difference in task complexity might explain the varied findings. The implication, although somewhat speculative, is that the CNS has the ability to vary the strategy by which motor units are recruited, adhering to a regulatory pattern under more simple movement conditions and switching to a more adaptable combination of linear recruitment, synchronization, and selective recruitment as movement complexity increases (Fig. 2-5 on page 12).

The Extent of Motor Unit Activation

The nature of the movement may also influence the extent to which motor units can be recruited. To pose this as a question, one may ask under what conditions can motor units be maximally recruited? It is often suggested, for instance, that moderate-level prolonged contractions will involve the complete recruitment of available motor units. This assumption, however, is flawed in its logic and is not supported scientifically.

In essence, the activation of motor units is influenced by three principle factors. The first involves the force levels inherent in the muscular contractions. Second is the contraction rate, or velocity of shortening. Last is the type of contraction itself, that is, whether the muscle is developing tension isometrically, concentrically, or eccentrically.

As discussed previously, in relating Henneman's size principle, the contribution or innervation of high threshold, fast twitch motor units is associated with increased force levels. Prolonged contractions that involve moderate loads may not possess the characteristic force requirements that would elicit a response from fast twitch motor units, and there is little scientific evidence to suggest that such muscular activity would involve the activation of high threshold units. To the contrary, there

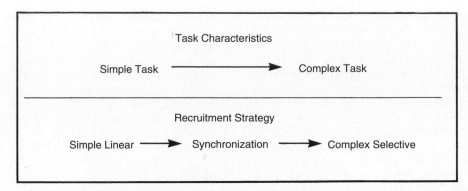

Fig. 2-5. Change in recruitment strategy with task complexity.

is ample evidence to indicate a direct relationship between the type of motor-unit activity witnessed during a contraction and the velocity, force, and shortening characteristic of that contraction.

Moritani and Muro,[33] for example, have demonstrated a linear relationship between EMG amplitudes, mean power frequencies, and the level of muscular contraction. This suggests that higher threshold motor units are activated only when enhanced levels of force production are attempted.

Motor-unit recruitment associated with various force levels has also been investigated by Hannerz.[21] Motor units recruited at 15% MVC fired at a rate of 10/sec. At 60% MVC, the rate increased to 20/sec, and at 90% MVC, firing rate reached 35/sec. These findings represent the gradual change from slow twitch to fast twitch motor units as the level of contraction rises. Hannerz also discovered an interesting alteration in firing behavior when comparing isometric and isotonic contractions. During a 20% static contraction, low frequency motor units fired continuously. When the level of muscular work was increased to 25%, new motor units were recruited. During a low-level twitch contraction involving a higher velocity of shortening, only the new motor units were activated, indicating a direct relationship between the speed of the muscle contraction and the recruitment of high threshold motor units.

Further comparisons between the two contraction types were performed by Grimby and Hannerz[17] in 1977. Using wire electrodes the authors distinguished between two types of motor units. The first was labeled *continuously firing long interval motor units* (CLMUS) and could discharge at long intervals. During maximum sustained efforts, CLMUS fired at 30 to 50 msec intervals. With twitch contractions, the intervals decreased, reducing to 10 msec during maximum twitches. Alternating movements were characterized by intervals of 15 to 20 msec.

The second motor unit type isolated by Grimby and Hannerz was an *intermittently firing short interval motor unit* (ISMUS). These units were inactive during weak or moderately sustained efforts and only fired occasionally during maximal isometric contractions. During rapid alternating movements, however, these motor units fired in high frequency bursts with intervals between 20 and 40 msec. Both CLMUS and ISMUS were then recorded simultaneously. Prolonged sustained contractions involved only CLMUS, while during rapid accelerations both fired. These results indicate that there is a clear difference in the way that motor units are recruited when one develops tension either isometrically, isotonically, or at different rates of shortening. It is only in the rapid moving condition that both types of motor units fired.

Finally, Enoka and Fuglevand[15] have demonstrated that isometric contractions will not involve maximal motor-unit recruitment. Their subjects were instructed to produce a maximal volitional contraction (MVC) on top of which was introduced an electrical stimulus. The authors discovered that muscle force output increased with added stimulation. Arguably, the MVC could not have involved maximal motor-unit recruitment because under those conditions no additional stimulus would have increased force output. The inability of the system to recruit high threshold motor units during isometric contractions has been explained by Tax and colleagues,[39] who demonstrated that recruitment thresholds were lower during isotonic contractions than they were under isometric conditions.

From the combined scientific evidence then, it can be argued that the maximal recruitment of motor units cannot be achieved under conditions of sustained maximal isometric or prolonged moderate-level isotonic contractions. Rather, it is only when rapid, forceful movements are attempted that motor-unit populations are fully recruited.

Strength Development

It is noteworthy that exercise physiology chapters exploring strength development focus primarily on changes at the muscular level. In context with this discussion, however, adaptations in strength will be examined from the neuromuscular level. A change in strength implies that not only has the muscle improved its contractile capability, but the motor drive has evolved as well. This notion is supported by studies utilizing an electromyograph (EMG) as an instrument by which nervous system activity can be explored. Häkkinen and Komi,[18] for example, show that EMG amplitude rises linearly with muscle tension. By itself, this only shows an immediate change in neural drive in order to increase muscle output. But there is evidence depicting a more lasting change in the integrated EMG (IEMG) over the course of training programs.[18,25,32,41] These studies demonstrate training induced changes not only in maximal tension development, but in maximal IEMG as well. These results do depict learning at the nervous system level. The role of the neuromuscular system in learning becomes more evident in examining the time course of strength development.

Several authors have demonstrated strength improvement within a relatively short period of time. Ishida, Moritani, and Itoh,[22] for example, documented a 31% increase in maximal volitional contraction (MVC) in their training subjects. All but 1% of this change occurred within the first 4 weeks of training. Moritani and deVries[32] demonstrated an average strength gain of 17% within 7 weeks, while others showed maximal strength increases within 4 weeks.[18,25] These results are significant, not by virtue of the fact that subjects experienced a gain in strength but because their strength improvement came in the absence of muscular hypertrophy. Thus, the enhanced muscle tension experienced by their subjects could not be related to increased contractility. Rather, a change in the pattern of muscle activation was most likely the impetus for improved strength.

The phenomenon of "neural learning" has also been demonstrated in studies in which the effects of training on one limb are seen in the contralateral untrained limb. Such bilateral transfer was noticed, for example, by Komi et al.,[27] whose subjects experienced a 20% increase in isometric knee extension strength in their trained limbs and an 11% increase in MVC in their nontrained limbs. Moritani and deVries[32] found similar results in comparisons of elbow flexor strength, but remarkably, increases in MVC on the untrained side were greater than that of the trained side (21% v. 17%). Once again, these results can hardly be attributed to muscle hypertrophy. It is more likely that subjects experienced a reorganization of the efferent systems that are responsible for the muscle activity under investigation.

Besides increased strength as an end product of weight training, changes in the actual patterns of neuromotor behavior have been documented. In the previously discussed study by Milner-Brown, Stein, and Lee,[30] for example, 2 out of 10 subjects who exercised their first dorsal interosseous muscle showed a tendency for the synchronization of discharges. It is quite possible that the firing of motor units had become synchronized as a function of resistance training. Synchronization, therefore, may be one means by which the nervous system can effect a permanent increase in muscle tension without a concomitant change in muscle mass.

This is not to suggest that muscle hypertrophy bears no significance to strength development. Strength training studies have clearly demonstrated muscle mass changes as a consequence of the strengthening paradigms. The role of the central nervous system, however, cannot be overlooked and may in fact be the most critical determinant of the nature of hypertrophic gains at the muscle level.

Morphologic Adaptation and Neural Drive

Traditional theory suggests that the types of loads employed during training dictate the nature of the muscular response. For instance, light loads and high repetitions create muscle "tone," while heavy loads lifted with few repetitions would induce increases in muscle "mass." This very simplistic view overlooks key factors, such as the recruitment of motor units that would contribute to specific morphologic adaptation. In addition, it fails to consider the difference in training responses among slow twitch and fast twitch muscle fibers. On a more scientific level, one might suggest that any exercise which invokes motor-unit recruitment throughout the threshold scale would result in hypertrophy of all of the muscle fibers recruited. In other words, if all of the motor units are recruited in the manner described by Henneman, then both slow twitch and fast twitch muscle cells should experience equal levels of hypertrophy. Although this concept might address the issue of total muscular development, it does not distinguish between different characteristics of adaptation, such as "tone" or "mass." Furthermore, it has not been supported scientifically, as evidenced in the findings of studies involving strength or power training.

One should begin with an operational definition of strength and power. Power is defined as force applied over a given distance for a specific period of time. More simply stated, power is force times velocity. It follows that exercises involving high, rapidly achieved force levels would constitute power training exercises. An example of such an exercise is weighted jumping.

Strength, on the other hand, is not so easily defined, and in fact, is somewhat nebulous because of the variety of measures used for its assessment. For instance, strength is often measured as one's maximal volitional isometric contraction (MVC) or as a one-repetition maximum (1 RM). Strength can also be characterized as isokinetic peak torque. All of these make the exact meaning of strength unclear because they yield different results. An interesting interpretation of strength was issued by Bohannon,[5] who claimed that strength was simply "one's ability to bring force to bear on the environment." This is an attractive definition because it places strength into a task specific context. In theory then, any exercise that improves one's ability to apply force in a task specific context can be considered a strength developing exercise (this includes, of course, power training exercises). In order to distinguish between strength and power exercises, strength training exercises will be limited to loaded movements that do not involve high velocities, such as a leg press done at a relatively slow, consistent pace.

Two strength training studies warrant mention, not so much for their demonstration of strength gains, but for the absence of morphologic adaptation despite the demonstrated strength gains. Dons and colleagues[11] in 1979 examined strength changes in subjects performing controlled squat exercises over a 7-week interval. In addition, they monitored the number and size of slow and fast twitch fibers before and after training. Subjects exercising at 80% of their 1 RM experienced a 42% increase in strength after 7 weeks. Interestingly, there was no change in the relative number of fast or slow twitch fibers, nor did the area of those fibers or the ratio between fast twitch and slow twitch fibers change.

The results of this study mirrored those of Moritani and deVries[32] and serve to reinforce the notion that early strength gains are most likely the end product of adaptation within the central nervous system. It is possible that with training beyond 7 weeks the subjects of both studies would have experienced changes in the area and ratio of fast twitch and slow twitch fibers. Häkkinen and others[20] addressed this issue by investigating strength and muscle changes in various groups engaged in "high intensity" strength training programs over a 12-month period. Curiously, none of the subjects demonstrated a change in fast twitch or slow twitch fiber area. Perhaps it is not the duration of exercise but the nature of the exercise that contributes most significantly to changes at the muscle level. Several studies, in fact, support this contention.

Thorstensson et al.,[41] for instance, investigated the effects of 8 weeks of squat and jump training. Their subjects demonstrated an increase in FT/ST area ratio from 1.20 to 1.37 over the training period. Although the training interval of 8 weeks was similar to those of the previously mentioned strength studies, clearly the nature of the activity was different. Likewise, Häkkinen et al.[19] examined the effects of 24 weeks of "explosive" jumping and noticed an increase in the area of fast twitch muscle fibers and a decrease in the area of slow twitch cells. The result was an increase in FT/ST area ratio. Again, the principle difference between this study and their 1987 work was the nature of the training involved.

Similar results have been reported in isokinetic training studies. Costill et al.[9] witnessed a decrease in the percent of ST area and an increase in the percent of FT area after 7 weeks of isokinetic training at 180°/sec. More recently, Bell and colleagues[4] detected a 5% increase in FT cross-sectional area and a 10% increase in myosin-ATPase activity after a course of "high velocity" isokinetic training.

The findings of these studies clearly suggest that the type of training in which one engages has a marked influence on the muscular response. Specifically, it has been demonstrated that power training results in an increase in FT/ST area ratio or a selectively greater increase in the area of fast twitch muscle fibers. Strength training, on the other hand, does not seem to affect this ratio. This is a curious phenomenon. If Henneman's size principle holds true, then clearly there ought to be equal development of both ST and FT fiber populations, since the recruitment of these fibers progresses systematically along the motor unit scale. Assuming, for instance, that power training involves more fast twitch muscle fibers than strength training, one might expect more hypertrophy among the fast twitch muscle cells in power trained subjects. Slow twitch fibers, however, should also experience some growth, since they are presumably recruited first. Yet, these do not seem to change.

Two theories may explain this behavior. First, the neuromuscular system might actually experience a form of selective recruitment during power training exercises. This concept was presented by Schmidtbleicher and Haralambie[38] in a study in which the push-off time of the upper extremity was studied in low- and high-intensity training groups. The high-intensity group experienced a significant reduction in push-off time, while the low-intensity group did not improve, prompting the authors to suggest that high-intensity training involved only fast twitch motor units, while low-intensity training employed both ST and FT units. In this case, the selective activation of type II motor units would lead to the hypertrophy of only fast twitch muscle fibers.

Although this theory does provide an explanation for selective hypertrophy, it is somewhat problematic. The assumption that only FT motor units, and hence fibers, would be recruited during an ongoing exercise is not, in itself, without fault. In light of the fact that fast twitch muscle cells are easily fatigued, it is arguable that the selective recruitment of these cells would be impossible, since they would fatigue rapidly and leave the neuromuscular system with no force generating mechanism. If they were selectively recruited and subsequently fatigue, then the system would, out of necessity, be forced to employ slow twitch units in order to maintain some level of motor activity. In that case, ST muscle cells should experience some growth.

The second explanation behind selective hypertrophy is not only interesting but is also quite possibly the driving mechanism behind muscle growth. Studies comparing strength training to power training, or isotonic training to isometric training, have yielded a very fascinating result. Referring to the study by Häkkinen and others,[19] the authors noted a 24% increase in the rate at which tension was developed in the power-trained group. This increase correlated positively with the detected increase in FT fiber area in that population of subjects. Peak isometric torque, on the other hand, experienced only a 10% improvement, which was deemed not significant by the authors.

A study conducted by Duchateau and Hainaut[12] reported similar findings. Subjects who trained isometrically experienced an increase in peak torque, while those undergoing isotonic training increased their rate of tension development. Rate of tension development may actually be the single most significant factor in the production of strength and power. It may also be the most significant contributor to the selective hypertrophy of muscle fibers. Komi[25] suggests that "the degree of hypertrophy may follow the effects of the motor input," citing rate of tension development as the primary factor. The mechanism behind the rate of tension development is clearly elucidated.

The time course of tension development is depicted in Fig. 2-6. On the left is a slowly developing muscle tension curve with its associated IEMG activity. It can be seen that peak EMG activity precedes peak muscle tension. This occurs naturally, as the muscle responds to the neural drive with a slight delay. To the right is a tension curve that is increasing at a faster rate. Notice that the IEMG activity has shifted in time, and like the tension curve, has a markedly increased slope. This phenomenon was presented in Komi's work in 1986, depicting the change in rate of tension development and the shift in IEMG activity that accompanies power training.

It has been suggested that the characteristic shape of the EMG profile, and hence the nature of the neural drive to the muscle, is actually responsible for creating the hy-

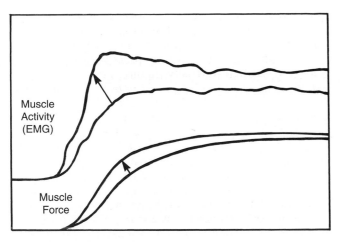

Fig. 2-6. Increase in slope of neural drive, as seen in EMG profile, is reflected by an increase in rate of tension development, producing strength increases.

pertrophic muscular response. More simply stated, if the pattern of neural drive to the muscle follows a gradual rise to peak, then training in this fashion might produce a general hypertrophy of ST and FT fibers, regardless of the level of tension developed. If, however, neural input rises rapidly, as depicted in an EMG trace with a high slope, then the musculature might experience a selective recruitment of FT muscle cells following training.

Speed Specificity

A quarter century ago Moffroid and Whipple[31] presented a study examining the effects of exercise speed on increases in isokinetic torque. The authors noted that torque increases were specific at and below the speed of exercise, which touched off a flurry of research activity leading to one of the more controversial issues involving strength development. How specifically are strength gains related to the speed at which exercises are performed? The answer to this question has been elusive at best, given the contradictory scientific literature.

Moffroid and Whipple's study provides evidence that strength gains do not occur at speeds above those employed during training and thus are speed specific. One should note, however, that their training speeds of 6 and 18 revolutions/min are comparable to 36 and 108°/sec, neither of which could truly be considered a high velocity. Thus, it is difficult to determine from this study whether similar training responses would exist if exercises were performed at higher speeds. This issue was addressed in a study by Ewing and colleagues,[16] who trained their subjects at 60 and 240°/sec. When tested at the slow speed, only the slowly trained group exhibited torque increases. At the fast speed, on the other hand, torque improvements were noted only in the fast-trained group, indicating a speed specific response.

These results, however, are hardly consistent throughout the literature. Bell at al.,[4] for example, trained their subjects at 180°/sec but found strength improvements at test speeds ranging from 90°/s to 240°/s. Contrary to Moffroid and Whipple, this study does indicate that strength gains can transcend training speeds, particularly

when training is slow and testing is fast. Other studies have presented similar findings after evaluating a variety of movement speeds. For example, subjects who trained at either 60°/s or 180°/s demonstrated strength gains at all testing speeds from 60°/s to 300°/s, while those whose training was performed at 300°/s experienced gains only at higher angular velocities.[24,36] Evidently, speed specificity is related only to high training velocities, at least as indicated by these works. Still, the issue of specificity of velocity is somewhat obscured.

Perhaps the most significant work to emerge during the last decade is the 1993 study presented by Behm and Sale.[2] In this investigation subjects trained one limb by attempting rapid contractions at resistances that prevented motion entirely (isometric), and the other limb at resistances that allowed movement to occur at a high rate of speed (300°/s). At the conclusion of the 16-week training period, both limbs experienced the same high-velocity-specific training response. The authors concluded that the stimulus for a high-velocity training response was the repeated attempt to produce a high-speed movement, rather than the actual movement speed. The results of this study have far-reaching implications.

Because of the difficulty involved in the control of limb pacing, the majority of the studies examining speed specificity have employed isokinetic devices. Such devices allow the experimenter to apply an external regulatory constraint on movement speed by the selection of a preset velocity which can not be exceeded by the performer. It is here that Behm and Sale's findings have their greatest impact. During isokinetic exercise or testing, one is instructed to exert as much force as possible against the machine, which in turn will constrain the movement to its preset speed of 60°/s, for example. One can well imagine, however, that in the absence of such constraints, an attempt to move a limb with maximal force would produce a motion far in excess of 60°/s. In essence, the intention on a isokinetic device is to move as rapidly as possible while the actual motion occurs at a slower rate.

This would explain the common finding among isokinetic studies that training at a slow speed can lead to increased strength at fast testing velocities. Because the intention at all training speeds is to move as rapidly as possible, a carry over in strength from one rate of motion to another is clearly feasible. Unfortunately, the most important implication to emerge from Behm and Sale's work is lost in isokinetic testing. Strength gains are specific to the speeds at which training occurs. If one desires to move quickly with maximum force production, then one should adopt a training regime that requires such motion.

RECOMMENDATIONS FOR STRENGTH TRAINING

In 1957 Rasch and Morehouse[37] conducted a study that would eventually become a landmark in strength training literature. In this investigation 49 subjects trained their biceps for a period of six weeks. At the end of the training period the subjects were evaluated for strength under familiar and unfamiliar positions. The subjects demonstrated strength gains in the familiar position, but not when the position was unfamiliar. These results indicate that isolated muscle training does not necessarily lead to strength gains, but that strength really involves the acquisition of skill in a movement specific manner.

The mechanism underlying this phenomenon of task-specific strength changes appears to be related to the recruitment of motor units. It has been demonstrated, for example, that in multifunctional muscles the order of recruitment can be varied continuously by changing the task and consequently the direction of movement and the mechanical properties acting on the joints and limbs.[40] This results in a "directional programming" of muscle forces, than when done repeatedly, results in strength gains specific to that movement and body position.

This theory has been advanced by Loeb,[28] who not only addresses the recruitment of motor units, but suggests that the physical composition of the neuromuscular system is influenced by movement dependency. Referring once again to the discussion of motor-unit activation, one can infer that the recruitment of motor units is influenced by the desired speed of movement and the force requirements of the task. Loeb, on the other hand, in following ter har Romeny and colleagues,[40] suggests that motor units are recruited in a manner that befits the task at hand. In fact, he goes further to suggest that motor units are organized into "task groups" that may comprise a combination of slow twitch, fast twitch, and intermediate units. These motor unit groupings are developed as one's movement repertoire grows.

Indeed, Loeb argues that not only are motor units grouped according to task, but that the physical orientation of muscle fibers is also task related, rather than simply organized according to motor unit type. For instance, it is generally accepted that muscle fibers are bundled into homogeneous groupings so that motor units of similar type will occupy a common region within the muscle. Loeb, on the other hand, suggests that the grouping of motor units is task related, and that fibers from motor units may actually traverse several areas within a single muscle. It is also possible, Loeb argues, that fibers from motor unit task groups may actually span different muscles as well. The development of strength, therefore, may well require the activation of various motor-unit task groups involving several muscles, with specifically applied movement patterns.

Strength development, therefore, requires considerably more than the simple repeated contractions of isolated muscle groups. If we return to the original premise of this chapter, that the functions of muscle are to stabilize or move the skeleton, then strength development should involve one or both of these functions. Stabilization and movement, however, are also task dependent. Thus the activation of motor units or task groups will also depend upon the nature of the movements. In essence, strength enhancement can be achieved through the application of various natural resisted movements that incorporate different speeds and loading conditions. In this way the subject will most likely activate all of the appropriate motor units for those given tasks, not only developing isolated muscle strength but coordination and skill as well. A concern for skill, rather than muscle tone or mass, will lead to more effective functional strength gains that translate from the gym or rehabilitation center to the real world.

REFERENCES

1. Basmajian JV: Motor learning and control: a working hypothesis, *Arch Phys Med Rehabil* 58:38–41, 1977.
2. Behm DG, Sale DG: Intended rather than actual movement velocity determines the velocity-specific training response, *J App Physiol* 74(1):359–368, 1993.
3. Belanger AY, McComas AJ: Extent of motor unit activation during effort, *J App Physiol* 51(5):1131–1135, 1981.
4. Bell GH et al: Effect of high velocity resistance training on peak torque, cross sectional area and myofibrillar ATPase activity, *J Sports Med Phys Fit* 32:10–18, 1992.
5. Bohannon RW: The clinical measurement of strength, *Clin Rehab* 1:5–17, 1987.
6. Burke RE: On the central nervous system control of fast and slow twitch motor units. In Desmedt JE (ed): *New Developments in Electromyography and Clinical Neurophysiology,* 3:69–94, Basel, 1973, Karger.
7. Burke RE et al: Physiological types and histochemical profiles in motor units of the cat gastrocnemius, *J Physiol* 234:723–748, 1973.
8. Burke RE, Rymer WZ, Walsh JV: Relative strength of synaptic input from short-latency pathways to motor units of defined type in cat medial gastrocnemius, *J Neurophysiol* 39:447–458, 1976.
9. Costill DL et al: Adaptations in skeletal muscle following strength training, *J App Physiol* 46(1):96–99, 1979.
10. De Luca CJ: Control properties of motor units, *J Exp Biol* 115:125–136, 1985.
11. Dons B et al: The effect of weight-lifting exercise related to muscle fiber composition and muscle cross-sectional area in humans, *Eur J App Physiol* 40(2):95–106, 1979.
12. Duchateau J, Hainaut K: Isometric or dynamic training: differential effects on mechanical properties of a human muscle, *J App Physiol* 56(2):296–301, 1984.
13. Enoka RM: *Neuromechanical Basis of Kinesiology,* Champaign, IL, 1988, Human Kinetics Books.
14. Enoka RM, Fuglevand AJ: Neuromuscular basis of the maximum voluntary force capacity of muscle. In Grabiner MD (ed): *Current Perspectives in Biomechanics,* Champaign, IL, 1991, Human Kinetics Publishers.
15. Enoka RM, Stuart DG: Henneman's size principle: current issues, *Trends Neurosci* 7:226–228, 1984.
16. Ewing JL et al: Effects of velocity of isokinetic training on strength, power, and quadriceps muscle fiber characteristics, *Eur J App Physiol* 61:159–162, 1990.
17. Grimby L, Hannerz J: Firing rate and recruitment order of toe extensor motor units in different modes of voluntary contraction, *J Physiol* 264:865–879, 1977.
18. Häkkinen K, Komi PV: Electromyographic changes during strength training and detraining, *Med Sci Sports Exerc* 15(6):455–460, 1983.
19. Häkkinen K, Komi PV, Alén M: Effect of explosive type strength training on isometric force and relaxation time, electromyographic and muscle fibre characteristics of leg extensor muscles, *ACTA Physiol Scand* 125:587–600, 1985.
20. Häkkinen K et al: EMG, muscle fibre and force production characteristics during a 1-year training period in elite weight-lifters, *Eur J App Physiol* 56:419–427, 1987.

21. Hannerz J: Discharge properties of motor units in relation to recruitment order in voluntary contraction, *ACTA Physiol Scand* 91:374–384, 1974.

22. Ishida K, Moritani T, Itoh K: Changes in voluntary and electrically induced contractions during strength training and detraining, *Eur J App Physiol* 60:244–248, 1990.

23. Kandel ER, Schwartz JH: *Principles of Neural Science,* ed. 2, New York, 1985, Elsevier.

24. Kanehisa H, Miyashita M: Specificity of velocity in strength training, *Eur J App Physiol* 52:104–106, 1983.

25. Komi PV: Training of muscle strength and power: interaction of neuromotoric, hypertrophic, and mechanical factors, *Int J Sports Med* 7(suppl):10–15, 1986.

26. Komi PV, Viitasalo HT: Signal characteristics of EMG at different levels of muscle tension, *ACTA Physiol Scand* 96:267–276, 1976.

27. Komi PV et al: Effect of isometric strength training on mechanical, electrical, and metabolic aspects of muscle function, *Eur J App Physiol* 40:45–55, 1978.

28. Loeb GE: Hard lessons in motor control from the mammalian spinal cord, *Trends Neurosci* 10(3):108–113, 1987.

29. Milner-Brown HS, Stein RB: The relation between the surface electromyogram and muscular force, *J Physiol* 246:549–569, 1975.

30. Milner-Brown HS, Stein RB, Lee RG: Synchronization of human motor units: possible roles of exercise and supraspinal reflexes, *Electro Clin Neurophysiol* 38:245–254, 1975.

31. Moffroid MT, Whipple RH: Specificity of speed of exercise, *Physical Therapy* 50(12):1692–1700, 1970.

32. Moritani T, deVries HA: Neural factors versus hypertrophy in the time course of muscle strength gain, *Am J Phys Med* 58(3):115–129, 1979.

33. Moritani T, Muro M: Motor unit activity and surface electromyogram power spectrum during increasing force of contraction, *Eur J App Physiol* 56:260–265, 1987.

34. Person RS: Rhythmic activity of a group of human motoneurons during voluntary contraction of a muscle, *Electro Clin Neurophysiol* 36:585–595, 1974.

35. Person RS, Kudina LP: Discharge frequency and discharge pattern of human motor units during voluntary contraction of muscle, *Electro Clin Neurophysiol* 32:471–483, 1972.

36. Petersen SR et al: The influence of velocity-specific resistance training on the in vivo torque-velocity relationship and the cross-sectional area of quadriceps femoris, *J Ortho Sports Phys Ther* May:456–462, 1989.

37. Rasch PJ, Morehouse LE: Effect of static and dynamic exercises on muscular strength and hypertrophy, *J App Physiol* 11(1):29–34, 1957.

38. Schmidtbleicher D, Haralambie G: Changes in contractile properties of muscle after strength training in man, *Eur J App Physiol* 46:221–228, 1981.

39. Tax AAM et al: Differences in the activation of m. biceps brachii in the control of slow isotonic movements and isometric contractions, *Exp Brain Res* 76:55–63, 1989.

40. ter har Romeny BM, Denier van der Gon JJ, Gielen CCAM: Changes in recruitment order of motor units in the human biceps muscle, *Exp Neurol* 78:360–368, 1982.

41. Thorstensson A et al: Effect of strength training on EMG of human skeletal muscle, *ACTA Physiol Scand* 98:232–236, 1976.

CHAPTER 3

CARDIOPULMONARY CONDITIONS

Nino Marino
Peter Bruno

I. THE HEART AND ITS FUNCTION

As the central organ of the cardiovascular system, the heart acts as a continuously self-regulating pump. This pump's function is crucial to the supply of blood to every organ of the body. The vessels of the arterial system deliver oxygenated blood with other nutrients throughout the body. Clearing of blood depleted of its oxygen is mediated via the vessels of the venous system.

Of vital importance, especially in sports-related activity, is the heat transport or cooling function of the blood via the blood vessels to maintain a core body temperature within a precise and critical range. It is not far-fetched to consider the skin surface and mucosa of the body as "radiators." The athlete's body would likely fail during exercise as enzyme systems and other proteins were denatured or "cooked" by undissipated heat.

Finally, the cardiovascular system performs a vital messenger function as it carries important hormones in the blood that act as distant mediators of metabolic processes.

We traditionally have measured the parameters of the heart's pump function by, among others, terms such as *stroke volume, ejection fraction, cardiac output,* and *cardiac index*. The following is a short glossary of terminology.

- *Stroke volume* is a measure of the quantity of blood, in cubic centimeters, that is ejected from the ventricles of the heart with each contraction.
- *Ejection fraction* is a measure of that quantity of diastolic blood volume that is pumped from the ventricles during systole or contraction. This measure is expressed in as a percentage.
- *Cardiac output* is a measure, usually in liters per minute, of the volume of blood circulated by the heart.
- *Cardiac index* is a measure of the cardiac output divided by the subject's body surface area in square meters.
- *Myocardial oxygen consumption (MVO_2)* is the amount of oxygen consumed by the heart per contraction.

The foregoing are perhaps the most important and widely used measures of cardiac function.

THE HEART IN EXERCISE

The cardiovascular systems will adapt to increasing loads of activity by first displaying an anticipatory response, which will be initiated by the central nervous system. Higher cortical brain centers will stimulate a catecholamine surge before the actual activity begins. This surge of neural hormones (epinephrine and norepinephrine) acts on the heart. By causing the sinoatrial node to depolarize more rapidly, the impulse for heart muscle contraction will become more frequent. In the highly trained athlete, heart rate may go from a low of 30 to 35 beats per minute to more than 200 beats per minute via catecholamine mediation. This increase in heart rate (and contractile force of the heart) is mediated by the sympathetic nervous system, which signals for the pumping of catecholamines.[13]

Whereas sympathetic discharge is increased, there is an inhibition of parasympathetic discharge. The heart begins to free itself of parasympathetic restraints and prepares itself for higher performance.

PERIPHERAL VASCULAR RESPONSES

To understand the heart in exercise, we must view it as the central organ of an exquisitely adaptable vascular system. With the anticipation of exercise, higher cortical stimulation is accompanied by stimulus from other brain centers, such as the diencephalon and vasomotor areas of the medulla. The result of this stimulation is a constriction of resistance and capacitance (arteries and veins) vessels. This mechanism allows blood to flow "downhill" to the right atrium. As a result, the more active heart will be adequately supplied by sufficient venous return.

Although the previously mentioned mechanisms may predominate just before exercise begins, other factors come into play during exercise. Contraction of muscles and intensifying neural discharge will increase cardiac output.

Local vascular changes enhance delivery of oxygen and metabolic substrates to muscles. There are local vasodilator responses mediated by hypoxemia and, in some vessels, enabled by substances (such as nitric oxide) generated by the vascular endothelium.

Muscle contractions serve to "milk" veins to increase venous return to the right heart, further priming the heart.

The increasing sympathetic discharge that continues into the active phase of exercise serves to redistribute blood throughout the body. Vasoconstriction in the splanchnic organs (liver, spleen) and skin surface shunts blood volume to exercising muscles. It is in this manner that blood pressure increases and cardiac output can be made to match muscular demands. Local muscle vascular dilations facilitate increased blood delivery to the muscles involved in any particular athletic endeavor.

Whether there is a true anticipatory phase in a particular situation, as the exercise phase is undertaken, a steady state in cardiac output soon develops. There may be small variations and adjustments in preload, afterload, and mean arterial pressure. For a relatively fixed exercise task, a very efficient interplay of peripheral variables appears to adjust delivery of blood to the left ventricle. Stroke volume is not fixed but will vary to accommodate for changes in heart rate. With a slight increase in heart rate or stroke volume, metabolic needs of mild exercise can be met. As the exercise advances beyond moderate, increase in heart rate added to stroke volume increase will supply the fivefold or greater increase in cardiac output required.

Larger stroke volumes are observed in subjects performing supine exercise. In erect exercise, stroke volume increases that measure more than double the resting volumes can be observed.

Several neurogenic adjustment mechanisms that may alter cardiac output not only originate from central neurologic impulses but also from sympathetic afferents from working muscle. These impulses will result in increases in heart rate, contractility, and peripheral vascular tone (Table 3-1).

Volume Status in Exercise

In the early phase of exercise, there is an alteration in intravascular volume that allows for flow of plasma from capillaries into the interstices of muscles involved. Lymphatic drainage generally returns plasma back to the intravascular space, and intravascular fluid loss remains at 10% to 45% early on.

It is almost intuitive that as the period of vigorous athletic activity increases, the steady state becomes less "steady." Heart rate tends to increase to compensate for any further drop in intravascular volume and central venous pressure. Stroke volume and arterial pressure continue to fall gradually. The body continues, with heart-rate increase, to try to maintain a constant cardiac output.

Temperature Regulation

As mentioned previously, vasoconstriction in vessels of the skin during exercise serves to shunt blood to working muscles. With prolonged intense activity and generation of heat, the body begins to be less able to dispose of this heat. Thermoregulatory centers in the brain respond by dilating the skin vessels. The "radiator" function of the skin performs well but at a certain cost. Blood volume shunted to skin vessels diminishes mean circulatory pressure and central venous pressure.[12] The heart's stroke

Table 3-1. Summary of integrated chemical, neural, and hormonal adjustments before and during exercise

Condition	Activator	Response
Preexercise "anticipatory" response	Activation of motor cortex and higher areas of brain causes increase in sympathetic outflow and reciprocal inhibition of parasympathetic activity.	Acceleration of heart rate; increased myocardial contractility; vasodilation in skeletal and heart muscle (cholinergic fibers); vasoconstriction in other areas, especially skin, gut, spleen, liver, and kidneys (adrenergic fibers); increase in arterial blood pressure.
Exercise	Continued sympathetic cholinergic outflow; alterations in local metabolic conditions resulting from hypoxia, $\downarrow$ pH, $\uparrow$ PCO_2, $\uparrow$ ADP, $\uparrow$ Mg^{2+}, $\uparrow$ Ca^{3+}, and $\uparrow$ temperature.	Further dilation of muscle vasculature.
	Continued sympathetic adrenergic outflow in conjunction with epinephrine and norepinephrine from the adrenal medullae.	Concomitant constriction of vasculature in inactive tissues to maintain adequate perfusion pressure throughout arterial system. Venous vessels stiffen to reduce their capacity. This venoconstriction facilitates venous return and maintains the central blood volume.

volume diminishes, and heart rate increases. An unchanging cardiac output under these circumstances supplies skin vessels at the expense of blood flow to working muscles. It is this mechanism that helps to explain the time course of the drift phase and eventual fatigue.

TRAINING AND THE HEART

Endurance training appears to make the cardiovascular system more efficient. After prolonged (several months) endurance activity, the athlete's heart becomes slow at rest and during exercise. This bradycardia may become diagnostic and include benign forms of heart block. Athletes who endurance train the leg muscles enjoy a greater bradycardic response than those who do upper body training. There may be a change in autonomic balance emanating from conditioned musculature. After long-term endurance training, intravascular blood volume is higher.

With an increase in oxygen extraction at the muscle level, cardiac output may not need to be so high to maintain a certain level of performance. The acclimatization response also will see that metabolic heat is dissipated efficiently (Table 3-2).

With the improvement of oxygen extraction at the cellular level of muscle fibers, exercise of up to 50% of maximal oxygen consumption (VO_2 max) does not induce a rise in heart rate. It is speculated that increased vagal resulting from training explains these observations. If exercise becomes more intense in the aerobically conditioned athlete, sympathetic discharge is relatively reduced.

In the trained athlete, stroke volume is increased. This increase probably occurs as a secondary function of bradycardia (longer filling time). It does not seem that there are primary myocardial charges that increase stroke volume. Stroke volume is a secondary or dependent vari-

able. Whereas ejection fraction may remain constant, maximal cardiac output in the trained athlete will reflect an increase in end-diastolic volume. It is likely that the Frank-Starling mechanism may be operative in maximal exercise. This mechanism is operative as preload (venous return) increases with high-intensity activity.

Diastolic properties of left ventricular function become more important in athletes as they age. We are becoming more aware of concepts such as active and passive filling characteristics of the ventricles. Abnormal diastolic properties of the left ventricle can cause the heart to fail during increasing activity. In the aging heart, it is often the diastolic filling properties that will be altered. An understanding of these alterations is helping us better understand the inexorable decline in cardiac performance observed in aging athletes.

CARDIOVASCULAR SCREENING OF THE ATHLETE

Perhaps because the athlete is considered to be the one who carries the standard of which we all would like to become, his or her sudden unexpected death is a heavy blow to us. Although less dramatic, his or her long-term health and the effect that participation in certain sports could have on the athlete should also be our concern. At the outset, it is imperative that the highest level of importance be rendered to the good of the athlete. As a principal decision maker regarding participation screening, it is vital that pressures that might be brought by team organizations, scholastic or otherwise, be resisted if they place the athlete at risk.[7]

Although preexercise cardiovascular screening for sedentary men aged 40 or older has been a general rule, the presentation of acute myocardial infarction, especially in men aged 35 or younger, prompts us to advise taking a detailed cardiovascular history to include suggestive risk factors, such as family and smoking history. In this age group, a careful cardiac examination to search for abnormal murmurs and heart sounds should be followed by an electrocardiogram (ECG) and screening stress test.

Should the results of cardiovascular examination, ECG, or stress test prove to be equivocal or abnormal, one should refer the patient to a cardiologist for additional evaluation or exercise prescription. The task for the cardiologist is not totally clear. In some series, most highly trained young athletes have audible murmurs. Furthermore, many of our testing modalities may be too sensitive.

In the young athlete, the cardiovascular abnormalities that threaten health are overwhelmingly congenital, however, many times more middle-aged athletes die each year while exercising because of acquired coronary heart disease. Nevertheless, although in numbers, exercise-related death in the young is rare, we are compelled to do all that we can to identify those at great risk. The task is difficult because we are not certain of the prevalence of certain congenital cardiac abnormalities in the general population. We do not have reliable statistics regarding mortality rates for participating athletes who carry congenital cardiovascular abnormalities.

The revised eligibility recommendations for competitive athletes with cardiovascular abnormalities set forth

Table 3-2. Physiologic adjustments during heat acclimatization

Acclimatization response	Effect
Improved cutaneous blood flow	Transports metabolic heat from deep tissues to the body's shell
Effective distribution of cardiac output	Appropriate circulation to skin and muscles to meet demands of metabolism and thermoregulation; greater stability in blood pressure during exercise
Lowered threshold for start of sweating	Evaporative cooling begins early in exercise
More effective distribution of sweat over skin surface	Optimum use of effective surface for evaporative cooling
Increased sweat output	Maximizes evaporative cooling
Lowered salt concentration of sweat	Dilute sweat preserves electrolytes in extracellular fluid

From McArdle WD, Katch FI, Katch VL: *Exercise physiology energy, nutrition, and human performance,* Philadelphia, 1981, Lea and Febiger. Reprinted by permission of the publisher.

at the 26th Bethesda Conference held January 6, 1994, are an indispensable guide to screening the competitive athlete. We frequently consider its recommendation when evaluating athletes who may have cardiac abnormalities.

Congenital Cardiac Abnormalities

In screening for the presence of significant cardiac abnormalities, care must be taken to establish whether the subject has ever experienced cardiac symptoms. Although not yet carrying a cardiac diagnosis, he or she may have experienced syncope or chest pain that could represent the first warning of grave events to follow. Careful questioning about sudden death and cardiac disease in the subject's kin is vital.

We briefly will review the most important cardiac abnormalities to consider in a preexercise screening.

Hypertrophic Cardiomyopathy

With the growth of echocardiography, we have become increasingly aware of this congenital heart muscle disease that Maron confirmed to be a major cause of sudden cardiac death in the young athlete.[9] With echocardiography, we are able to identify those subjects with this disordered heart muscle morphology, although the obstructive nature of this disease had been described during cardiac catherizations before the widespread use of echocardiography.

The primary screening of hypertrophic cardiomyopathy (HCM) can be difficult because the subject might never have complained of suggestive symptoms. Such symptoms could include unexplained chest pain, dizziness, palpitations, frank syncope, or, more frequently, exertional dyspnea. It is probable that he or she might never have undergone more than a cursory heart examination. If such an examination had been conducted, the subject might either not have had an audible murmur or had a murmur dismissed as "functional." It is common for HCM to produce a murmur of varying intensity from examination to examination. During screening, a changing murmur should raise the suspicion of HCM.

The gradient developing within the left ventricle in HCM is dynamic and has to do with acceleration of blood through an ever-narrowing left ventricular outflow tract. Certain maneuvers can change the outflow gradient and alter its resultant murmur. By having the subject perform a Valsalva maneuver (straining against a closed glottis or blowing against the thumb placed in the mouth), the systolic outflow murmur's intensity will increase.

The increase in systolic murmur loudness results from the reduction of preload on the left ventricle, making its internal diameter smaller, which accelerates the blood being ejected, drawing the mitral valve leaflets into the path of the blood by a Venturi effect (Fig. 3-1).

Extensive study of HCM also has elucidated its important diastolic abnormalities. In many subjects, these diastolic abnormalities appear to predominate in symptom generation. Inadequate and slowed diastolic filling is the most important abnormal mechanism to obtain, especially when the subject has tachycardia (Fig. 3-2).

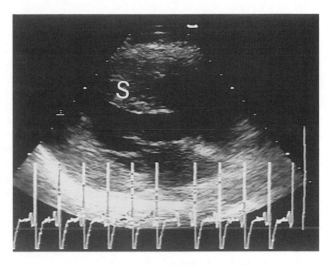

Fig. 3-1. Long axis view of a heart with hypertrophic obstructive cardiomyopathy. Note the markedly thickened interventricular septum (S).

These diastolic abnormalities may result from the characteristic disordered morphology of myofibrils found on myocardial biopsy specimen. Called myofibrillar disarray, it is considered histologically characteristic of HCM. Of note, although evidence for a left ventricular outflow gradient may be absent in as many as half of subjects with HCM, diastolic abnormalities are common to all sufferers of HCM. It has been postulated that these

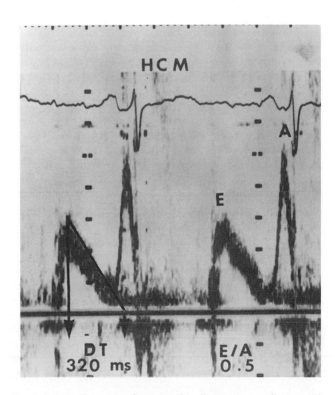

Fig. 3-2. Doppler tracing hypertrophic obstructive cardiomyopathy below mitral valve in diastole reveals abnormal relaxation in a patient with hypertrophic obstructive cardiomyopathy. Note the prolonged deceleration time (DT). From Oh JK, Seward JB, Tajik JA: *The echo manual,* Boston, 1994, Little Brown and Co. Reproduced with permission.

diastolic abnormalities may further result from a disorder of calcium metabolism in the myocardial cells of the left ventricle and sometimes the right ventricle. Small coronary vessel and conduction abnormalities may contribute to symptom generation in HCM.

DNA testing is increasingly being used with some success in screening of subjects suspected of having HCM. Unfortunately, we are learning that HCMs are a whole spectrum of diseases with multiple genetic determinants.

There are those who believe that certain other types of testing, such as electrophysiologic testing, may be able to stratify those with HCM according to risk. We someday may be able to screen and prescribe with greater confidence. The more widely followed approach prohibits participation in most competitive sports for those who carry the diagnosis of HCM.

Coronary Artery Disease

A second relatively important cause of sudden cardiac death in young athletes is coronary artery disease. In one study by Corrado et al 23% of deaths in young athletes appeared to result from coronary artery disease. Most appeared to have lesions of the proximal left anterior descending coronary artery. We should be suspicious of coronary artery disease in subjects aged 10 to 29 years. In younger patients, Kawasaki's disease, an acquired childhood febrile disorder, may leave coronary lesions in as many as 25% of subjects.

Congenital anomalies of the coronary arteries can cause sudden death in young subjects. Diagnosis of an aberrant coronary artery should be suspected in the subject who complains of anginal pain on exertion or exercise-induced syncope. Patients who present with such symptoms should undergo echocardiographic evaluation of their coronary ostia, thallium or echo stress testing, and coronary angiography, if necessary.

Complaints of chest pain related to position, respiration, or palpation are common in the young athlete and rarely suggest coronary artery disease. They often can be managed with explanation and reassurance. Conversely, exertion-related chest pain, sometimes accompanied by near-syncope or syncope, must be given careful scrutiny.

Complex Congenital Disorders

When considering sudden death from the time of birth, congenital valvular cardiac abnormalities play a large role. The young athlete arriving for screening will have been diagnosed with many of the severe complex malformations that would limit his or her activity. Also because of the subject's symptoms, the diagnosis is less likely to be missed.

When chest pain or syncope are the subject's complaints, there often will be no gross and obvious congenital cardiac abnormality detected, and the possibility of abnormal coronary arteries must be entertained. About 50% of young sufferers of sudden cardiac death will have reported previous prodromal symptoms.

Marfan Syndrome

Marfan syndrome, a congenital disease with the aorta its most important target organ, has been implicated in the sudden cardiac death of some star athletes. Recently,

there has been more awareness of this disorder, especially because it appears to present in tall, slender athletes. There have been high-profile sudden deaths of volleyball players and basketball players who seemed apparently well until their deaths.

Marfan syndrome is believed to be a fibrillin disorder that weakens the walls of the major vessels and may lead to aortic rupture. Some affected subjects may have very long spidery fingers and lax joints. There apparently are many grades of the clinical expression of this disease. Some subjects might have aortas so dilated that on reaching a certain diameter, prophylactic replacement of the aortic root must be undertaken. This course might be recommended after close regular follow-up evaluation, even if the young subject is asymptomatic (Fig. 3-3).

Competitive sports for those with Marfan syndrome are believed to increase the shear stress on the ascending aorta resulting from the augmented hemodynamic shear force that results from increased cardiac contractility during exercise.

Myocarditis

Myocarditis, or inflammatory disease of the heart muscle, is a potential cause of sudden death in young athletes and in older athletes.

Whereas myocarditis might be implicated in infant deaths, severe pump impairment and arrhythmia generation sometimes strike adult athletes with this disorder. The patient may or may not be aware of a recent bout of gastroenteritis or "flu" symptoms. The disease may present with recent dyspnea on exertion. The athlete might complain only of unexplained palpitation or lightheadedness. These latter symptoms might represent potentially dangerous ventricular or atrial arrhythmia. On examination, the findings could be minimal, but a pericardial rub suggesting coexistent pericarditis or a displaced apex heart beat should prompt the prohibition of exertion. An echocardiogram would reveal reduced ejec-

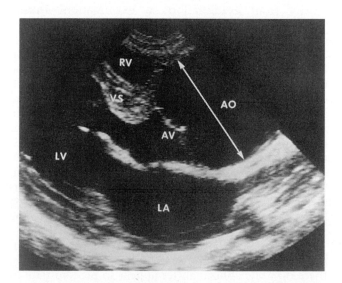

Fig. 3-3. Two dimensional long axis view of a typically dilated aortic root (AO) in a patient with Marfan syndrome. From Oh JK, Seward JB, Tajik JA: *The echo manual,* Boston, 1994, Little Brown and Co. Reproduced with permission.

tion fraction and perhaps a pericardial effusion. The most important viral agent responsible for myocarditis is *Coxsackie B* virus.

Dilated Cardiomyopathy

Dilated cardiomyopathy may be the final result of myocarditis, although there are some cardiomyopathies that may be familial. The diagnosis is relatively straightforward with echocardiography and careful history, although the etiology may be unclear. Systolic left ventricular function may be severely impaired. With exertion, this patient might experience an arrhythmia death.

Right Ventricular Dysplasia

In some sudden death series, particularly in one representing sudden death in northern Italy, right ventricular dysplasia, a congenital cardiomyopathy, predominates as an etiology.[4] On echocardiography, this patient, who may only have a right bundle branch block pattern on ECG, will have a thinned right ventricular wall. The patient may have syncope and death on exertion. This subject would require extensive electrophysiologic testing, perhaps combined with repeated stress testing to stratify his or her sudden death risk.

Commotio Cordis

Commotio cordis is the event after which a young athlete will fall to the ground unconscious after a blow to the precordium. Maron, in a recent study, described the disturbing scenario. A young athlete, perhaps playing sandlot baseball, will sustain a blow to the precordium and collapse immediately or briefly thereafter. Most no-table is how little force will appear to have been delivered, but the subject will collapse and die. The subject appears remarkably resistant to resuscitation attempts. It does not appear that the integrity of the chest wall or mediastinal structures are compromised. Instead, it is postulated that a force is transmitted to the heart during its electrically vulnerable period, which apparently triggers a lethal ventricular arrhythmia.[8] Work is ongoing in attempting to protect young athletes from these tragedies by redesigning chest padding and the missiles that the athlete might encounter during sporting events.

Mitral Valve Prolapse

Mitral valve prolapse is a rare cause of sudden death in young athletes. Nevertheless, there are some series in sudden death in young adults that implicate this etiology. This malformation of the mitral valve forces the leaflet farther into the left atrium in systole and is more often present in women. It may be symptomatic.[7] It may generate atrial or, more importantly, ventricular arrhythmias that could lead to sudden death.[3] Careful history may reveal a family history of this disease. Physical examination may reveal a midsystolic click or a late systolic blowing murmur. Sometimes mild or severe mitral regurgitation will be present. Echocardiography is perhaps the most sensitive test for the establishment of the diagnosis (Fig. 3-4). In the subject who wishes to exercise vigorously, stress testing and Holter monitoring is in order. Abstention from stimulants, such as caffeine and tobacco, is recommended. Some patients will become more symptomatic, requiring the use of beta-blocker medications. Good hydration of these patients is an important rule to

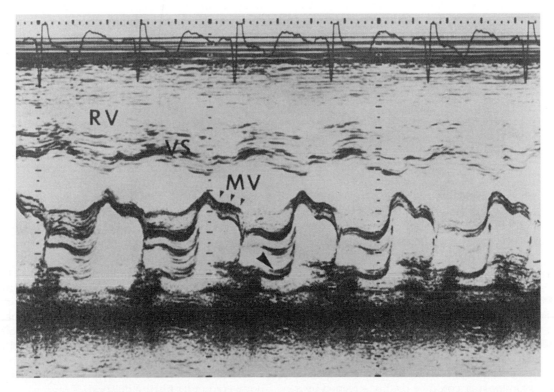

Fig. 3-4. Note the thickened appearing mitral valve (MV) prolapsing posterior mitral leaflet (large arrow) in this subject with mitral valve prolapse (MVP). From Oh JK, Seward JB, Tajik JA: *The echo manual,* Boston, 1994, Little Brown and Co. Reproduced with permission.

follow. Perhaps lengthening of the mitral apparatus relative to the left ventricular dimension may worsen mitral valve prolapse. Hydration, increasing intravascular volume and preload, may tighten up on this apparatus and reduce ventricular irritability and any mitral regurgitation.

Other Cardiac Anomalies

Careful history taking and physical examination will screen many of the remaining major anomalies. As with mitral prolapse, congenital aortic valvular disease has not been incriminated as among the important causes of sudden death in the athlete. Congenital aortic valvular disease in the relatively asymptomatic patient will most often be detected by careful auscultation. Although congenital (or acquired) aortic stenosis may be mimicked by coarctation of the aorta, an aortic abnormality will be the rule-out. The subject should be scheduled for an echocardiogram to clarify the issue. Significant aortic regurgitation also may produce a loud systolic murmur and a diastolic "blow." The important issue is that the athlete be screened and scheduled for additional testing to more clearly identify the problem.

The same is true for most other congenital or acquired cardiac abnormalities. Although the examiner may have difficulty deciding whether the systolic murmur one hears is aortic stenosis or pulmonic stenosis, he or she will know that the issue deserves additional investigation. An echocardiogram, ECG, and cardiology consultation will be needed before clearing the subject for competitive athletic activity. In congenital aortic stenosis, peak instantaneous Doppler gradients are of value, whereas in acquired aortic stenosis, mean gradients are measured.[5]

After a careful history is taken and a careful cardiac examination is performed (at rest and after exercise), the need for noninvasive testing may arise if the diagnosis is in doubt. The basic tests should include an ECG, an echocardiogram, and a stress test. Additionally, ambulatory rhythm monitoring (Holter monitoring), chest radiograph, and in rare cases, coronary angiography or arrhythmia testing in an electrophysiology laboratory may be required.

Although the absolute number of sudden cardiac deaths in young athletes is few, one can only imagine the impact general screening with echocardiography would have on this number. Most epidemiologists and public health authorities agree that general echocardiographic screening of athletes would be a huge expenditure. The hope is that the cost of these studies will come down, and a more general application of cardiac sonography in the screening of athletes could be the positive result.

DIAGNOSTIC TESTING MODALITIES

The Electrocardiogram

The resting ECG, although not part of the standard screening examination for the athlete, can be a vital tool. In those athletes who were victims of sudden death, review of any ECGs in their history would have pointed to the need for additional examinations.[9] Most patients with hyperthropic cardiomyopathy could be readily screened by a standard 12-lead ECG. As mass ECG testing would not be cost-effective, reserving these traces for any subject with

dizziness, syncope, or chest pain on exertion could reduce sudden athletic death by as much as 50%.

Typically, the ECG of the patient with hypertrophic cardiomyopathy would show high voltage resulting from characteristic wall thickening. Often, there also are abnormal q waves and t waves. The abnormal q waves and t waves are sometimes referred to as "pseudo infarct" patterns. Not uncommonly, the ECG might vary considerably.

Other important abnormalities, including those of rhythm disorders, might be detected by the 12-lead ECG. In the athlete complaining of rapid heart action, irregular heart beat, dizziness, or shortness of breath, an ECG could be diagnostic. Ventricular premature beats can signal more serious sustained ventricular arrhythmias. A short PR interval could warn of Wolff-Parkinson White syndrome, which sometimes can cause life-threatening atrial arrhythmias.

Atrioventricular block, from generally benign first degree atrioventricular block and Type-1 second degree (Wenkeback) atrioventricular block to more important second degree and complete heart block and congenital long QT interval, can be revealed by ECG techniques.

To further investigate ventricular and atrial arrhythmias and their daily frequencies, 24-hour ambulatory ECG monitoring is useful. The newest models of these devices are very light and can be worn during vigorous athletic activity. We are now able to monitor the athlete with arrhythmias while he or she is performing most sports at high intensity. In the event that the athlete suffers from arrhythmias that require medical therapy, ambulatory monitoring will enable us to monitor the effectiveness of the antiarrhythmic therapy as he or she performs exercise at various intensities to measure effectiveness of arrhythmia suppression.

Cardiac Stress Testing

Cardiac stress testing is used frequently to screen patients in populations in which there is a high incidence of coronary disease, particularly in men aged more than 35 years. Its reliability is greatest in this group when stress ECG is used. Greater sensitivity is afforded by the use of echocardiography and nuclear isotope techniques that attempt to add information about left ventricular wall motion to each test. The subject's tendency to develop arrhythmias with increasing workloads is addressed by an ECG-graded stress test.

The standard ECG stress test can be performed by using any one of several well-known protocols (Bruce, Naughton) or custom protocols that address the particular needs of a testing population. Tests could be modified to most closely reproduce the loads the athlete would encounter when engaging in his or her sport. Information about the subject's fitness or aerobic capacity can be obtained by calculating the subject's double product. This value can be obtained by multiplying the peak systolic blood pressure times peak heart rate.

There are treadmill or bicycle stress tests and upper body ergometer testing methods.

In preparation for the test, the subject is asked to fast. Before testing, ECG electrodes are attached to the chest.

The subject is requested to exercise to exhaustion. Blood pressure and ECG are monitored periodically throughout the test. The test is stopped only if the subject requests to stop or shows dangerous arrhythmias or ECG changes. An inappropriate drop in blood pressure, heart rate, pallor, or diaphoresis may also prompt cessation of the test.

When echocardiography or radionuclide studies are part of the test, the images are reviewed to render more information about myocardial perfusion and dynamics.

There are treadmill-based tests and bicycle-ergometer tests. Both techniques have their proponents. Treadmill testing has the advantage of more easily achieving higher peak heart rates, although echocardiographic image acquisition is delayed momentarily. We have not found this to be a problem. Bicycle stress-testing has the advantage of image acquisition without delay, but the subject must be coached (and familiar with cycling) to best use this technique and achieve the desired end point.

The use of Doppler wave techniques during echo–stress testing can add useful information and is an interesting investigational tool that helps better elucidate mechanics during exercise.

Echocardiography

The use of ultra-high frequency sound waves to render an ultrasound picture of cardiac structures has become an indispensable tool in the evaluation and screening of the athlete's heart. Without echocardiography, we would still have to rely on invasive or nuclear techniques to screen and measure the heart and major vessels. Echocardiography enjoys the combined unique advantages of sensitivity, technique, safety, repeatability, and portability. A major and ever-growing part of what we know about cardiac morphology and function in the healthy and at-risk athlete is because of echocardiography and Doppler echocardiography.

In the diagnosis of hypertrophic cardiomyopathy, Marfan syndrome, right ventricular dysplasia, mitral valve prolapse, congenital abnormalities of the heart valves and great vessels, myocarditis, and pericarditis, echocardiography is an essential diagnostic tool.

We also are able to evaluate wall thickness, systolic thickening, diastolic properties, and changes in these parameters over time and how these vary with type and intensity of sport in the training athlete.

Hemodynamics are evaluated by Doppler techniques that project a beam of ultra-high frequency sound waves into flowing blood. Erythrocytes act as Doppler beam reflectors that inform us of the direction and speed of the blood flow being interrogated. With these methods, we can readily determine whether there is a dynamic intraventricular or left ventricular outflow tract obstruction in the subject being screened. Doppler echocardiography also is useful in noninvasively determining cardiac output in varying loading conditions during exercise. With this testing modality we can detect and evaluate intracardiac shunts and stenosis and regurgitation of any of the cardiac valves.

The following figures represent Doppler studies revealing a typical dynamic obstructive left ventricular outflow tract obstruction that worsens with provocation by Valsalva maneuver and by the inhalation of amyl ni-

trate, which dramatically decreases afterload (Fig. 3-5).

Despite the powerful noninvasive techniques we now can use readily, sometimes more invasive techniques are the tests of last resort to be used in evaluating cardiac abnormalities in the athlete, from the "semiinvasive" modality called transesophageal echocardiography (TEE) to the clearly invasive cardiac catheterization and electrophysiologic studies.

With TEE, complex congenital abnormalities, aberrant coronary arteries, and cardiac and aortic trauma are evaluated. In catheterization tests, coronary arteries and assessing conduction velocities in the heart clarify causes of supraventricular arrhythmias and heart block. Ventricular stimulation techniques attempt to induce potentially lethal sustained ventricular arrhythmias in a controlled setting. These tests appear to be useful in stratifying athletes with ventricular arrhythmias as high or low risk for life-threatening cardiac events.

GENERAL EXERCISE CLASSIFICATION

We generally have categorized exercise into the large general groups of static and dynamic. As Mitchell has described,[10] static exercise includes athletic activity that involves a large mass of muscle with little movement through space of bones and joints. Dynamic exercise produces movement of joints and changing muscle lengths, often performed rhythmically.

Many studies have elucidated the hemodynamic changes that occur during each type of exercise. Dynamic exercise increases cardiac output and oxygen consumption while not greatly increasing systolic and mean arterial blood pressure. Total peripheral resistance is reduced. Static exercise increases systolic, diastolic, and mean arter-

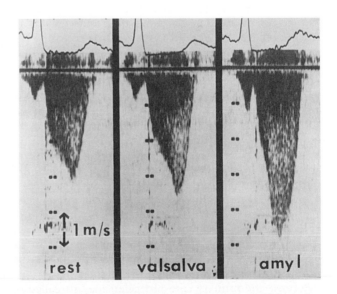

Fig. 3-5. Dynamic left ventricular outflow tract (LVOT) gradients recorded from the cardiac apex with continuous wave Doppler. During the Valsalva maneuver and after inhalation of amyl nitrate, outflow velocities increase, suggesting dynamic increase in obstruction under different loading conditions. From Oh JK, Seward JB, Tajik JA: *The echo manual,* Boston, 1994, Little Brown and Co. Reproduced with permission.

ial pressure while heart rate and cardiac output remain unchanged. Oxygen consumption is only increased mildly. Clinically, jogging would be considered dynamic, whereas isometric weight exercises would be considered static because static exercise place a pressure load on the heart; the walls of the heart thicken, whereas the chamber dimension does not significantly increase. Echocardiography assessments of these hearts are characteristic.

As dynamic exercise generates a volume load on the heart, the ventricular chamber will enlarge without dramatic wall thickening or hypertrophy. Nature's correlates of these circumstances yield a concentrically hypertrophied left ventricular wall in pressure load lesions. An obvious example would be the left ventricular hypertrophy of severe aortic stenosis. Where the volume to be ejected by the heart increases (as in mitral regurgitation), the left ventricular chamber becomes enlarged with proportionately little wall thickening. As opposed to the pressure loaded heart that has concentric hypertrophy, the volume load heart with eccentric hypertrophy is associated with a high maximal oxygen uptake during exercise. If we consider the determinants of myocardial oxygen consumption, we can understand how exercise can increase it. Heart rate, myocardial wall tension, and contractility are these determinants. The product of these three determinants yields maximal oxygen consumption in exercise.

Certain cardiac abnormalities cannot safely sustain the load that certain sport-related activities can place on the heart. Certain sports, such as cycling, share a high dynamic and static character. Other sports may involve a mostly static sports load on the heart. All the high static sports should be contraindicated for the subject with heart abnormalities intolerant of static loads.

In subjects with some degree of aortic stenosis, for example, dynamic exercise would be contraindicated. Such exercise depends on an increase in heart rate to maintain cardiac output. An increase in heart rate increases the gradient across the stenotic valve, thus unacceptably increasing myocardial oxygen demand and decreasing perfusion of the brain and other vital organs.

In subjects with hypertrophic cardiomyopathy, competitive high intensity athletics generally are to be prohibited. As there is a very large gray zone in the disease, especially where the left ventricular thicknesses may not be dramatically increased, a very exhaustive history (including family history), physical examination, and noninvasive (and perhaps even invasive) work-up is required. Presently, we do not have a fool-proof method of stratification of risk in these patients.

Athletes with Marfan syndrome often present the dual problems of aortic regurgitation, which requires prescription of exercise according to severity, and dilated aorta. The potential for aortic dissection is real. Static exercise and any exercise that would increase myocardial contractility may pose increased risk to the athlete.

Because the primary care physician may be called on to generally screen athletes before sport participation, an understanding of the principles governing cardiac clearance is essential. Final patient-by-patient recommendations should only be undertaken after an in-depth history, physical examination, and noninvasive evaluation in consultation with a cardiologist.

CARDIAC BENEFITS OF EXERCISE

We are well aware that regular exercise benefits all levels of fitness; there also is evidence to suggest regular exercise may help reduce coronary death.

Regular aerobic exercise has been labeled cardioprotective. Bassler once postulated that marathon runners who completed a full marathon were granted a certain immunity to coronary death,[1] but this claim has been disputed. Nevertheless, regular vigorous exercise appears to raise the favorable component of serum cholesterol, called HDL-C.[6] Perhaps, through increased insulin sensitivity in tissues, lipase activity and HDL-C levels increase.

More recently, direct rheologic effects of accelerated blood flow in coronary arteries have been studied. There is an enhanced efficiency of the natural arterial dilating system mediated by nitric oxide that results from vigorous exercise. Finally, the development of rich collateral arterial coronary networks seem to be the result of graded regular exercise when performed by patients with known symptomatic coronary artery disease.

Exercise in the athlete, be he or she an amateur, scholastic, or professional, is beneficial to the cardiovascular system. It increases fitness and quality of life and perhaps promotes cardioprotective mechanisms.[11]

II. THE LUNGS AND THEIR FUNCTION

As the heart is the pump of the vascular system, the respiratory system is responsible for the delivery of oxygen contained in the air to the blood and the removal of waste products like carbon dioxide back to the air. Any medical condition that alters this delivery will either increase or decrease the ability of exercising muscles and the athlete to perform. Changes in the oxygen and carbon dioxide content of the air and changes in the intraerythrocytic concentration of 2,3 biphosphoglyceric acid (2,3-BPG) will cause shifts in the oxygen dissociation curve.

The respiratory system includes the lungs, the central nervous system, the chest wall, and pulmonary circulation.

RESPIRATORY SYMPTOMS

Dyspnea

Dyspnea is defined as an abnormally uncomfortable awareness of breathing. Normally, our pattern of breathing is controlled by mechanisms that can vary ventilation to meet the demands of physical exertion. In addition, emotional states, such as anxiety and fear, can cause a change in normal ventilatory patterns. When evaluating the degree of dyspnea in a patient, one must take into consideration factors such as the overall level of fitness of the subject and the individual's perception of how bad the shortness of breath is.

Dyspnea may be related directly to the amount of physical exertion or may be sudden and related to specific underlying conditions, such as pulmonary embolism, spontaneous pneumothorax, or anxiety. In any athlete with dyspnea, it is important to look thoroughly for the cause.

TYPES OF DYSPNEA. *Orthopnea* is defined as dyspnea on assuming the supine posture.

Paroxysmal nocturnal dyspnea is defined as attacks of dyspnea that usually occur at night and awaken the patient from sleep. It also is known as *cardiac asthma*.

Tripopnea describes dyspnea only in the left or right lateral decubitus position, which usually occurs in patients with congestive heart failure.

Platypnea describes dyspnea that only occurs in the upright position, specifically in situations where the abdominal viscera has no diaphragmatic support because of herniation when the individual stands. Platypnea would be managed with an abdominal binder or surgical repair.

The actual mechanism of dyspnea is unknown, and the differential diagnosis of dyspnea is included in box below.

CAUSES OF DYSPNEA

Obstructive disease of airways
    Extrathoracic airway obstruction
        Aspiration of food or a foreign body (gum, dental prosthesis)
        Angioedema of the glottis or acute allergic reaction
        Fibrotic stenosis of trachea
        Acute respiratory infections (intermittent)

    Obstruction of intrathoracic airways
        Asthma
        Chronic bronchitis
        Bronchiectasis
        Chronic obstructive pulmonary disease

Diffuse parenchymal lung diseases
    Pneumonia
    Sarcoidosis
    Pneumoconiosis
    Carcinoma

Pulmonary vascular occlusive diseases
    Pulmonary embolism

Diseases of the chest wall
    Kyphoscoliosis
    Pectus excavatum
    Spondylitis

Heart disease
    Congestive heart failure
    Mitral stenosis
    Cardiogenic pulmonary edema

Anxiety neurosis

Noncardiogenic pulmonary edema
    Liver disease
    Nephrotic syndrome
    Protein-losing enteropathy
    Narcotic overdose
    Exposure to high altitude
    Neurogenic

Anemia

Obesity

Hypoxia

Arterial hypoxia is a fall in the oxygen content in the arterial blood, noted as a fall in the partial pressure of oxygen or the $PaCO_2$.

Cyanosis

Cyanosis is a dark bluish or purplish coloration of the skin and mucous membrane resulting from deficient oxygenation of the blood in the lungs or from an abnormally great reduction of the blood in its passage through the capillaries. It appears when the reduced hemoglobin in the minute blood vessels is 5 mg or more per 100 mL. A false cyanosis can be caused by the presence of an abnormal pigment such as methemoglobin (carbon monoxide poisoning). It usually is most marked in the lips, nail beds, ears, and malar eminences.

When hypoxia occurs as a result of a respiratory problem, the $PaCO_2$ level usually rises and displaces the oxygen dissociation curve to the right, which allows the percentage saturation of the hemoglobin in the arterial blood at a given level of alveolar oxygen tension (PaO_2) to decline. Thus, arterial hypoxia and cyanosis are likely to be more marked in proportion to the degree of depression of PaO_2 when such depression results from pulmonary disease.

Clubbing

Clubbing is the broadening and thickening of the ends of the fingers. Although in some patients, the cause may be unknown, it may be inherited or seen with a variety of diseases. The mechanism of clubbing is unclear, but it appears to be secondary to humoral substance, which caused dilatation of the vessels of the fingertip. As part of the physical examination, the presence of clubbing should elicit a differential diagnosis. See box below.

Clubbing in patients with primary and metastatic lung cancer, mesothelioma, bronchiectasis, and hepatic cirrhosis may be associated with hypertrophic osteoarthropathy. Hypertrophic osteoarthropathy is the subperiosteal formation of new bone in the distal diaphyses of the long bones of the extremities, which causes pain and symmetric arthritis-like changes in the shoulders, knees, ankles, wrist, and elbows. It may be confirmed by radiography.

CAUSES OF CLUBBING

Primary lung carcinoma

Metastatic lung carcinoma

Bronchiectasis

Lung abscess

Cystic fibrosis

Mesothelioma

Regional enteritis

Ulcerative colitis

Cirrhosis

CAUSES OF COUGH

Acute
   Upper respiratory infections
   Asthma
   Bronchitis
   Bronchogenic carcinoma
   Foreign body inhalation
   Gastroesophageal reflux
   Left ventricular failure

Chronic
   Post-nasal drip
   Asthma
   Chronic bronchitis
   Gastroesophageal reflux
   Postinfective cough
   Psychogenic
   Carcinoma
      Interstitial lung disease
      Benign tumors of the lung
      Drugs (*e.g.,* ACE inhibitors)

Cough

Coughing is a form of violent exhalation by which irritant particles in the airways can be expelled. Stimulation of the cough reflexes results in the glottis being kept closed until a high expiratory pressure has built up, which suddenly is released. The causes are listed in box above.

Chest Pain

Chest pain or tightness is a common sign of many diseases and is important in the diagnosis of pulmonary-related disorders. See box below.

VENTILATORY FUNCTION

Ventilation is the process of exchange of air in the lungs with atmospheric air, which has higher oxygen and lower carbon dioxide contents.

COMMON CAUSES OF CHEST PAIN

Asthma

Exercise-induced asthma

Infection

Chest wall injuries

Referred pain from the thoracic spine

Cardiac ischemia

Carcinoma

Interstitial lung disease

Herpes zoster (shingles)

Measurement of ventilatory function includes total lung capacity (TLC), which is the volume of gas contained within the lungs after a maximal expiration, and residual volume (RV), which is the volume of gas remaining within the lungs at the end of a maximal expiration.

Vital capacity (VC) is the volume of gas that is exhaled from the lungs when going from the TLC to the RV.

Common clinical measurements of airflow include

- *FEV1* is the volume of gas exhaled during the first second of expiration (forced expiratory volume in 1 second).
- FVC is the total volume exhaled, the forced vital capacity.
- MMFR is the maximal midexpiratory flow rate or the FEF 25% to 75% forced expiratory flow between 25% and 75% of the VC. This is the average expiratory flow rate during the middle 50% of the VC (Fig. 3-6).

By evaluating these values in a pulmonary laboratory, one can classify the type of disorder (Fig. 3-7).

CIRCULATORY FUNCTION

Circulatory function depends on cardiac output and pulmonary vascular resistance. The peripheral vascular resistance (PVR) typically is obtained in an intensive care unit using a flow-directed pulmonary arterial catheter (Swan-Ganz). The normal value for PVR is approximately 50 to 150 dyn.s/cm^5.

A healthy individual at rest inspires 12 to 16 times per minute, each breath having a TV of approximately 500 mL. A portion of each breath (about 30%) never reaches the alveoli; this portion is known as the *dead space.*

The most commonly used measures of gas exchange are the partial pressures of O_2 and CO_2 in the arterial blood (PaO_2 and $PaCO_2$).

The alveolar–arterial O_2 difference ($PAO_2–PaO_2$), or the A–a gradient, is a useful calculation. The alveolar

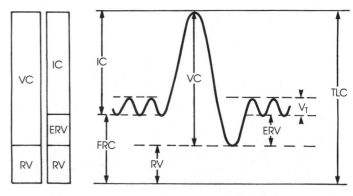

Fig. 3-6. Lung volumes, shown by block diagrams (left) and by a spirographic tracing (right). TLC = total lung capacity; VC = vital capacity; RV = residual volume; IC = inspiratory capacity; ERV = expiratory reserve volume; FRC = functional residual capacity; V_T = tidal volume. (From Weinberger SE: *Principles of pulmonary medicine, 2d ed.* Philadelphia, 1992, WB Saunders.)

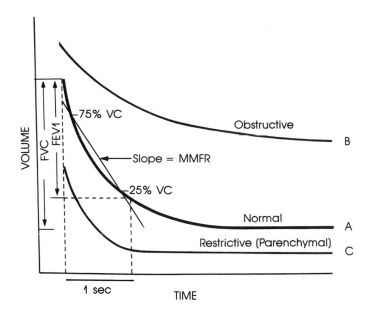

Fig. 3-7. Spirographic tracings of forced expiration, comparing a normal tracing (**A**) and tracings in obstructive (**B**) and parenchymal restrictive (**C**) disease. Calculations of FVC, FEV$_1$, and FEF$_{25-75\%}$ are shown only for the normal tracing. Because there is no absolute starting volume with spirometry, the curves are positioned artificially to show the relative starting lung volumes in the different positions. (From Weinberger SE, Drazen JM: Disturbances of respiratory function, In Isselbacher KJ, et al, eds: *Harrison's principles of internal medicine, 13th edition,* New York, 1994, figure 214-2, p. 1152, McGraw-Hill.)

and, hence, arterial PO$_2$ can be expected to change depending on the level of alveolar ventilation, reflected by the arterial PCO$_2$.

Pulse oximetry is a recent practical development in respiratory care and allows continuous monitoring of the patient's state of oxygenation. It is more practical than arterial puncture, which is required to measure the PaCO$_2$. Using a probe clipped to a patient's finger, it measures the absorption of wavelengths of light by hemoglobin in arterial blood. Because of differential absorption of the two wavelengths of light by oxygenated and nonoxygenated hemoglobin, the percentage of hemoglobin that is saturated with oxygen can be displayed instantaneously.

Radiologic testing and other diagnostic procedures have become more state-of-the-art and include many modalities. See box in second column. In all patients, a simple history and physical examination is important to make a diagnosis. A simple posteroanterior chest radiograph may suffice as an inexpensive diagnostic procedure. The examiner should always review the films him- or herself because the examiner has the best knowledge of the clinical state of his or her patient. Portable films are a necessary evil in some situations but never as reliable in quality.

Computed tomography (CT) has added amazing clarity to studies, and magnetic resonance imaging (MRI) is superior to differentiating pulmonary vessels *versus* lymph nodes. However, the added cost of these proce-

RADIOLOGIC AND DIAGNOSTIC PROCEDURES AVAILABLE

Pulmonary imaging
    Chest radiographs
    Portable chest radiographs
    Computed tomography
    Magnetic resonance imaging
    Ultrasound
    Ventilation/perfusion (V/Q) lung scan
    Interventional (computed tomography-guided
      biopsy)
Diagnostic procedures
    Skin tests (ppd, candida, RAST, etc.)
    Bronchoscopy/biopsy

dures must be considered. Lung scans are important in the diagnosis of pulmonary embolisms.

CLINICAL DISEASE STATES

There are three groups of individuals who experience asthma-like symptoms after exercise.

- Athletes with chronic asthma, 90% of whom will experience symptoms after exercise.
- Athletes with allergic rhinitis or atopic dermatitis who have a positive exercise challenge.
- Athletes who do not have underlying allergies or asthma and only experience symptoms of asthma after exercise.

Asthma

Asthma is an obstructive disease of airways that is characterized by increased responsiveness of the tracheobronchial tree resulting from a variety of stimuli. The airways narrow by contraction of their smooth muscle, by a swelling of the mucous membrane, and by edema of the bronchial wall and an increase in the production of mucous. Recurrent attacks of difficult breathing, particularly on exhalation caused by an increased resistance to airflow through the respiratory bronchioles, are typical of the disease. Status asthmaticus is the persistence of severe airway obstruction for days or weeks.

Asthma may be induced by exercise. Sports vary in their tendency to induce asthma, with running having the highest tendency, cycling a moderate tendency, and gymnastics and swimming a low tendency. Paradoxically, many sufferers gain relief from their bronchospasm by regular exercise, and exercise is not seen as negative in the management of asthma. Many drugs help to control asthma, but team physicians must be aware that some are on the International Olympic Committee list of banned substances.

The National Institute of Allergy and Infectious Disease estimates that 41 million Americans have asthma and allergies. Asthma is said to be found in 4% to 5% of the general population in the United States. Half of the cases occur in patients before age 10 years, and another one third in those before age 40 years. In children, there is a 2:1 male preponderance, which equalizes by age 30 years.

Allergy is a state of altered reactivity in the host that results from interaction between antigen and antibody. An antigen is an agent that stimulates the production of an antibody. An allergen is defined as an antigen that has been shown to initiate an allergic response. The antibody classically associated with allergy is the IgE immunoglobulin. After inhalation of an allergen, it penetrates the respiratory epithelium and combines with pairs of IgE molecules attached to underlying mast cells, thus signaling release of mediators that initiate an inflammatory response. Individuals who readily make IgE antibody are prone to allergic reactions of the respiratory tract.

Allergic asthma often is associated with a family history of allergic diseases, such as rhinitis, urticaria, and eczema. These individuals will have positive skin reactions to intradermal injections of allergens and a positive response to the inhalation of the antigen.

Idiosyncratic asthma refers to those individuals without a history of allergy, negative skin testing results, and normal levels of IgE.

Environmental and occupational factors may be potent bronchial irritants, such as ozone and the oxides of sulfur and nitrogen. Metal salts, wood and vegetable dusts, pharmaceutical chemicals and plastics, biologic enzymes, and animal and insect dusts can cause problems. The house dust mite (*Dermatophagoides pteronyssinus*) or fungal spores (*e.g., Aspergillus fumigatus*) can cause bronchial hyperactivity. Fumes from paint and household cleaners may precipitate an acute attack of asthma, as may some perfumes. A drop in temperature at night can trigger asthma and may be prevented by heating the bedroom at night.

The most common stimulus for an asthmatic attack is a respiratory infection. Exercise and emotional stress also can be stimuli.

The symptoms of dyspnea, cough, and wheezing are the hallmarks of asthma. One must be careful to differentiate asthma (see boxes on cough and dyspnea).

Every new patient with asthma should be examined. See box on p. 31.

The diagnosis is made by demonstrating reversible airway obstruction, which is defined as a 15% or more increase in FEV1 after two puffs of a beta-adrenergic agonist. Once the diagnosis is confirmed, the course of the illness and the effectiveness of therapy can be followed by measuring the peak expiratory flow rates (PEFR) or the FEV1.

Therapy should be aimed at elimination of the cause of the attack.

DRUG TREATMENT. There are five basic categories.

1) Beta-adrenergic agonists/adrenergic stimulants
2) Methylxanthines
3) Glucocorticoids
4) Mast cell stabilizing agents
5) Anticholinergics

Adrenergic stimulants include epinephrine and isoproterenol, which are not beta-2 selective, and have considerable side effects (palpitations and tremulousness). They are effective only as an inhalation or parentally. The usual dose is 0.3 cc of a 1:1000 solution administered subcutaneously.

The most commonly used inhalers are metaproterenol (Alupent®—Boehringer Ingelheim Pharmaceuticals, Ridgefield, CT), terbutaline (Brethaire®—Geigy Pharmaceuticals, Summit, NJ), fenoterol, albuterol (Proventil®—Schering Corporation, Kenilworth, NJ), biolterol (Tornalate®—Dura Pharmaceuticals, San Diego, CA), salbutamol (Ventolin®—Allen & Hanburys, Research Triangle Park, NC), salmeterol (Serevent®—Allen & Hanburys, Research Triangle Park, NC), and pirbuterol (Maxair™—3M Pharmaceuticals, St. Paul, MN). Isoetharine (Bronkosol®—Sanofi Winthrop Pharmaceuticals, New York, NY) is used less often. With the exception of metaproternol, these inhalers are highly selective for the respiratory tract and virtually devoid of significant cardiac effects except in high doses. The major side effect is jitteriness because of the stimulation of the beta receptors on skeletal muscles. They also may cause headaches and insomnia.

Inhalation is the preferred route as fewer side effects occur. The dose is up to two puffs every 4 hours while awake. Oral forms also are available, however, the International Olympic Committee has approved only *inhaled* albuterol, terbutaline, metaproterenol, and bitolterol. There is some debate whether these drugs improve performance in athletes without bronchospasm.

Methylxanthines (theophyllines) are medium-potency bronchodilators and are best used in maintenance therapy. Their dose has to be reduced in elderly patients. The most common side effects are nervousness, nausea, vomiting, anorexia, and headache. Because of a need for blood level monitoring, they have been less popular recently.

Glucocorticoids are not bronchodilators and have most benefit in patients with acute illness with severe airway obstruction that is not resolving. The usual dose is 6 mg/kg/day of hydrocortisone, and higher doses do not improve patients' symptoms.

Mast cell stabilizing agents, cromolyn sodium (Intal) and nedocromil sodium (Tilade), are not brochodilators. They inhibit degranulation of mast cells, preventing the release of the chemical mediators of anaphylaxis. They are most useful in atopic patients. A therapeutic trial of two puffs daily for 4 to 6 weeks frequently is necessary. Nedocromil may cause an unpleasant bitter taste about 10 to 15 minutes after inhalation.

Anticholinergics, such as atropine sulfate, can cause bronchodilation, but their side effects limit their usefulness. Inhaled anticholinergics, such as ipratropium bromide (Atrovent), are somewhat useful but not as much as they are in the management of chronic obstructive pulmonary disease.

Any athlete who is prescribed a new medication should be asked to report any deterioration in his or her asthma. Beta-adrenergic blocking agents, either oral or in eye drop form, aspirin, and other nonsteroidal anti-

ASTHMA MEDICAL HISTORY CHECKLIST

Evaluate the following areas with every new patient with asthma.

1. Current symptoms
   - ❑ Cough, wheeze, dyspnea, chest tightness, sputum production, exercise-related symptoms
2. Patterns of symptoms
   - ❑ Perennial, seasonal, or perennial with seasonal exacerbation
   - ❑ Continuous or episodic
   - ❑ Onset, duration and frequency of symptoms
   - ❑ Diurnal variation (with special reference to nocturnal symptoms)
   - ❑ Relation to exercise
3. Precipitating or aggravating factors (trigger factors)
   - ❑ Viral respiratory infections
   - ❑ Exposure to known allergens, *e.g.,* dust mite, pollens, animal dander, molds
   - ❑ Exposure to chemicals or other occupational sensitizers
   - ❑ Exposure to irritants, *e.g.,* cigarette smoke, perfume
   - ❑ Drugs, *e.g.,* aspirin and beta-blockers
   - ❑ Foods
   - ❑ Food additives—colorings, metabisulphite, monosodium glutamate
   - ❑ Changes in weather, exposure to cool air
   - ❑ Exercise
4. Development of disease
   - ❑ Age of onset, age at diagnosis
   - ❑ Progress of disease with time (better or worse)
   - ❑ Previous treatments and response
   - ❑ Frequency of symptoms
   - ❑ Frequency of exacerbations
   - ❑ History of accident and emergency room visits and admissions
   - ❑ History of life-threatening attacks and intensive care unit admissions
   - ❑ Limitation of physical activity
5. Present management
   - ❑ Current medication
   - ❑ Response
   - ❑ Current action plan
6. Profile of a typical exacerbation
   - ❑ Trigger
   - ❑ Usual time course, especially the amount of time between the first signs or symptoms and sudden deterioration
   - ❑ Usual management
   - ❑ Usual outcome
7. Home environment
   - ❑ Smoking
   - ❑ Othe factors including clinically relevant allergens—dust mite, pollens, animal danders, molds, birds

ASTHMA MEDICAL HISTORY CHECKLIST—cont'd

8. Impact of the disease
   - ❑ Time off school or work
   - ❑ History of life-threatening asthma
   - ❑ Emergency room visits and admissions
   - ❑ Limitation of physical activity
   - ❑ Effect on work, schooling, or physical activity
   - ❑ Effect on growth and development of children
   - ❑ Impact on the family when either a child or an adult family member is affected
9. Assessment of the patient's knowledge and self-assessment ability
10. Related atopic disorders
    - ❑ Family history of asthma, eczema, allergic rhinitis
    - ❑ Personal history of eczema or allergic rhinitis
11. General health, other medical conditions, and other prescribed medications

Enquire specifically about
   - ❑ Medications known to aggravate asthma, *e.g.,* beta-blockers for hypertension or glaucoma, aspirin, and nonsteroidal anti-inflammatory drugs
   - ❑ Sinusitis, nasal polyps

inflammatory drugs may cause or worsen asthma and should be avoided or used more cautiously. Nonproprietary preparations, such as Royal Jelly, are contraindicated in athletes with asthma.

There is evidence that microaspiration of stomach acid, or reflux of stomach acid over an inflamed lower esophagus, can lead to bronchospasm in patients with asthma. Asthma control may be better in these athletes if the reflux is managed.

Athletes with asthma should not smoke, and friends and relatives should be asked to avoid smoking around them.

The need for influenza vaccine in adults should be assessed. Influenza vaccine is not indicated routinely for children with asthma.

EMERGENT THERAPY. Aerosolized beta-2 agonists can be given every 20 minutes by a hand-held nebulizer for three doses in an emergency situation. This then can be followed by use of up to every 2 hours until the attack has stabilized. Aminophylline can be added to the regimen after the first hour to speed resolution. Salmeterol (Serevent®) takes 30 minutes to work, and it should not be used in emergencies.

In general, there is a correlation with the severity of the episode and the speed of resolution.

The mortality of asthma is small, less than 5000 deaths per year, but it is rising, especially in inner cities. The number of children having asthma 7 to 10 years after diagnosis is 26% to 78%. Arterial blood gases are essential in severe asthma. An increase in respiratory rate results in a decrease in PCO_2. An increase of the PCO_2 above 40 mm Hg may constitute a medical emergency, and intubation may be necessary. Important indications for hospital admission of patients with asthma include cyanosis, exhaustion, difficulty speaking, and pulsus paradoxus more than 20 mm Hg. Pulsus paradoxus is an exaggeration of the normal variation in the pulse volume with respiration, becoming weaker with inspiration and stronger with expiration.

Pulmonary function testing is an important part of diagnosis, but it should be performed when the patient is not in the midst of an acute attack.

Chest radiography usually will show hyperaeration, but it should be done to rule out concurrent infection or pneumothorax. Skin prick tests and radioallergosorbent tests (RAST) may be helpful in confirming the patient's atopic status and in establishing certain allergies. **They have no usefulness in testing for food allergies.**

Drugs may be implicated in the production of asthma, especially beta-blocking agents and prostaglandin inhibitors, such as aspirin.

Exercise-Induced Bronchospasm

Exercise-induced bronchospasm (EIB) is a condition in which vigorous physical activity triggers acute airway narrowing in people with heightened airway reactivity. The pathogenesis of EIB is associated closely with fluxes in heat and water that develop within the tracheobronchial tree during the conditioning (warming and humidification) of large volumes of air. It is more likely to occur in cold, dry environments and in the presence of environmental pollution. Twelve percent to 15% of the general population are affected by EIB. Seventy percent to 80% of patients with asthma have it. It occurs at any age, although 40% of children will have it at some time. It is distributed equally between male patients and female patients.

Vigorous exercise induces an initial bronchospasm, reaching a maximum in 5 to 10 minutes. Pulmonary function returns to normal in 20 to 60 minutes, which usually is followed by a refractory period lasting several hours (30 minutes to 120 minutes). Bronchospasm will not recur during this period, and an athlete may take advantage of this in timing his or her play. Warm-up exercises (either 20 minutes of **submaximal** exercise or 7×30-second sprints 30 minutes before exercise) are effective in diminishing EIB.

During the acute attack, the athlete may present with dyspnea, chest tightness, cough, and fatigue more than expected for the type of exercise performed. Recovery may be slow. If the testing is equivocal, an exercise challenge test using methacholine may be done. Methacholine is an inhaled bronchoconstrictor.

CRITERIA FOR DIAGNOSIS. A history should be taken for the types and levels of exercise that produce the problem, the timing, and the nature of the symptoms. Laboratory criteria for diagnosis and for severity are found in Tables 3-3 and 3-4. The severity of the disease is influenced by the same factors that affect asthma: the type, intensity, and duration of the exercise; the en-

Table 3-3. Criterion for diagnosis

Test	Criterion
Forced expiratory volume in one second (FEV1)	> 15% fall from baseline
Forced expiratory flow (FEF)	> 35% fall from baseline
Peak expiratory flow rate (PEFR)	> 10% fall from baseline
Residual volume (RV)/total lung capacity (TLC)	Increased volume reflects air trapping

vironmental conditions; the level of fitness of the athlete; the intercurrent infections; and time since the athlete's last bronchospastic episode.

EXERCISE TESTING FOR EXERCISE-INDUCED BRONCHOSPASM. Assessment by exercise testing is an integral part of pulmonary testing in the athlete. When performing the calculations, it is important to use a reputable laboratory so the results may be reproducible and easily comparable. When establishing a baseline, a 10% change in some results is enough to make a diagnosis, so that reproducibility is paramount.

The athlete should be told to sustain vigorous exercise for at least 5 minutes continuously, and the heart rate should exceed 70% of his or her maximum rate. Treadmills and cycle ergometers have had standard exercise programs developed for testing. It is important to note that for EIB, treadmill running is more asthmagenic than cycling.

Inexpensively, peak flow meters can be used to assess pulmonary function. Standardized readings should be taken immediately before and after exercise and at 1-, 3-, 5-, 10-, and 15-minute intervals after exercise. Spirometry is more sensitive but more expensive. In more sophisticated laboratories, histamine or methacholine challenge can be performed. Also, drugs used for therapy can be assessed running these tests with or without the various bronchodilators.

THERAPY. Patients with EIB will benefit from good conditioning, which will, however, reduce the severity of EIB but **not** prevent it.

Exercising with submaximal exercise will induce EIB. Waiting 30 minutes, one can restart exercising during the refractory period. About 50% of people who get EIB will have no more attacks for 1 to 2 hours after the first attack. These warm-up times are important for the athlete with EIB, as is the cool down afterward. Patients should avoid hyperventilation, try to use slow nasal

Table 3-4. Severity of exercise-induced bronchospasm

Category	Criterion
Mild	15–20% fall in FEV1
Moderate	20–30% fall in FEV1
Severe	> 30% fall in FEV1

breathing when possible, and wear a scarf or mask in the winter to warm the air and keep in the humidity. The cold, dry air is a precipitant of EIB. Exercising in a warm, more humidified environment will help minimize symptoms. Also trying to avoid exercise during times of high pollen counts is helpful. If one has the luxury of picking a sport, swimming and water sports are among the least asthmagenic. Baseball and volleyball are relatively easy for patients with EIB. Running is one of the hardest for these individuals, but long-distance running is better than sprinting.

Drug therapy remains the mainstay of management. Most physicians would prescribe an aerosolized selective beta-2 agonist, such as salbutamol or albuterol, one to two puffs, 5 to 20 minutes before exercise. This usually provides effective prophylaxis against the development of EIB for 2 to 3 hours. Alternatives include an inhaled cromoglycate (Intal) or nedocromil sodium (Tilade) two to four inhalations a few minutes before exercise. These drugs are used in athletes who do not tolerate the side effects of the inhaled beta-2 agonists, in those who appear to experience late-phase responses to exercise, and in those whose EIB is not prevented by beta-2 agonist therapy. Some athletes will need two to four inhalations of bronchodilators plus the same dose of cromoglycate (Intal) or nedocromil sodium (Tilade). Ipratropium bromide (Atrovent), an anticholinergic agent, may be beneficial, but for most athletes, it is less effective than the other classes of inhalers.

As in patients with asthma, beta blockers and sedatives are contraindicated, and their use can be fatal. Long-acting bronchodilators, such as Serevent, should be taken 30 minutes before exercise, preferably 2 hours before. Athletes should be told to keep their bronchodilator handy while exercising. If they have an attack, they should take two to four inhalations. If the attack is severe, the dose should be repeated 5 to 10 minutes later. Medical help should be sought if the attack does not go away.

Inhaled steroids do not prevent EIB if taken before exercise. If an inhaled steroid is taken regularly, the EIB will be less severe. Also, less bronchodilator medication or mast cell stabilizing agents will be needed before exercising. Oral forms of bronchodilators used to manage asthma may not prevent EIB.

If these management strategies are not successful, consider

- Poor drug delivery—check technique;
- Combining beta-2 agonist with four inhalations of cromoglycate sodium (Intal) or nedocromil sodium (Tilade);
- Poor cardiopulmonary fitness—some patients will need a graduated exercise program to develop fitness;
- Poor asthma control—check peak expiratory flow rates at home over a 2-week period;
- Check for another cause of breathlessness on exertion.

If symptoms still are occurring during or after exercise, the athlete should cease activity, rest, and use a short-acting beta-2 agonist.

Sinus-Related Symptoms

Sinusitis is a common disorder in athletes. In its acute state, it is easily recognized. Allergic rhinitis occurs in about 15% to 20% of the general population. Viral infections are common, but about 50% of these infections result from *Hemophilus influenzae* and *Streptococcus pneumoniae*. Other bacteria, such as *Branhamella catarrhalis,* and mixed oral anaerobes can cause this problem.

Chronic sinusitis may be a more subtle cause of respiratory difficulty in the athlete. Symptoms may present as facial pain, headache, toothache, post-nasal drip, cough, rhinorrhea, nasal obstruction, fever, and epistaxis.

Diagnosis is made on history and physical examination and supplemented by radiographs of the sinuses, looking for opacification or fluid levels. CT scan of the sinus also is a good, albeit more expensive, way to make the diagnosis.

Cultures of the nasal sinus often will just show normal flora and are not that helpful in diagnosis or management.

Management is aimed at hydration of the athlete, adequate humidification of the air, and appropriate antibiotic therapy. Decongestants are of some value. The use of intranasal steroids, such as fluticasone propionate (Flonase—Glaxo Pharmaceuticals, Research Triangle Park, NC), budesonide (Rhinocort—Astra Pharmaceutical Products, Westboro, MA), and flunisolide (Nasarel—Roche Laboratories, Nutley, NJ), is widely advocated in the acute situation, but there is a latent period of about 24 hours before these are effective.

The presence of polyps or anatomic deformity may be a reason for medical failure, and surgery may be required in these patients.

Exercise-Induced Anaphylaxis

Exercise-induced anaphylaxis is characterized by sensation of warmth, pruritis, cutaneous erythema, angioedema, urticaria (giant, more than 1 cm), upper respiratory obstruction, and occasionally vascular collapse. Risk factors include previous atopic history, family atopic history, food ingestion (shellfish, celery, nuts, alcohol), weather conditions (heat, high humidity), and drug ingestion (aspirin, nonsteroidal anti-inflammatory drugs).

Management includes decreasing the intensity of exercise, avoiding exercising on warm, humid days, and stopping exercise at the earliest sign of itching. Also, avoiding meals 4 hours before exercise will help.

Drug therapy includes antihistamines, cromglycate and epinephrine. Pretreatment does not prevent the onset of exercised-induced anaphylaxis.

Cholinergic Urticaria

Cholinergic urticaria is an exaggerated cholinergic response to body warming. The athlete will develop urticarial papules after exposure to heat and humidity and exercise. Generally, the papules appear first on the wrist or upper thorax and spread to the limbs. Antihistamines are used in management.

Exercise-Induced Angioedema

Exercise-induced angioedema is a nonitchy swelling occurring in the deep dermis and subcutaneous tissue. It tends to involve the face and oral region. Attacks may be life-threatening if the airway is involved. Prevention may be achieved with modification of exercise programs or with the use of antihistamines (diphenhydramine). In addition, selective H2-receptor blockers, such as cimetidine (Tagamet®—SmithKline Beecham, Philadelphia, PA), ranitidine (Zantac—Glaxo Pharmaceuticals), famotidine (Pepcid®—Merck & Co., West Point, PA), lansoprazole (Prevacid®—TAP Pharmaceuticals, Deerfield, IL), Prilosec®—Astra Merck, Wayne, PA, and nizatidine (Axid®—Eli Lilly and Company, Indianapolis, IN), have been used in the management of this condition.

Chronic Obstructive Pulmonary Disease

It has been shown repeatedly that exercise programs, although not accompanied by measurable improvement in lung function, result in increased exercise tolerance and an improved sense of well-being. Walking is an excellent exercise for these individuals. Arm exercises are poorly tolerated. If there is any evidence of malnutrition, improvement will yield dividends. The use of bronchodilators will be helpful for those who have some evidence of reversible bronchospasm.

Pulmonary Embolism

Pulmonary embolism is a leading cause of morbidity and mortality. Any athlete with dyspnea or chest pain and with a history of recent trauma or surgery to the lower extremities or history of deep vein thrombophlebitis should be suspect. Female athletes receiving estrogen therapy or birth control pills have a higher incidence of phlebitis.

Sleep Apnea

Sleep apnea is intermittent obstruction of airflow during sleep. It is no more common in athletes, but its diagnosis should be entertained when an overweight recreational athlete who snores is having trouble with alertness during the day.

BIBLIOGRAPHY

Barnes PJ: Drug therapy: inhaled glucocorticoids for asthma, *N Engl J Med* 332(13):868–875, 1995.

Mahler DA, Horowitz MB: Perception of breathlessness during exercise in patients with respiratory disease, *MSSE* 26(9):1078–1081, 1994.

McFadden ER, Gilbert IA: Current concepts: exercise-induced asthma: *N Engl J Med* 330(19):1362–1367, 1994.

Leff AR, ed: *Cardiopulmonary exercise testing,* Orlando, 1986, Grune and Stratton.

Cantu RC, Micheli LJ, eds: *ACSM's guidelines for the team physician,* Philadelphia, 1991, Lea and Febiger

Cishek MB, Moser KM, Amsterdam EA: Chest pain: working up nonemergent conditions, *J Respir Dis* 17(7):560–575, 1996.

Cecil textbook of medicine, 20th ed, Bennett JC, Plum F, eds. Philadelphia, 1996, WB Saunders.

Harrison's principles of internal medicine, 13th ed, Isselbacher KJ, Braunwald E, Wilson JD, Martin JB, Fauci AS, Kasper DL, eds. New York, 1994, McGraw-Hill.

Spector SL: Update on exercise-induced asthma, *Ann Aller* 71(6):571–577, 1993.

Brukner P, Khan K: *Clinical Sports Medicine,* Sydney, 1993, McGraw-Hill Book Company.

The Bantam medical dictionary, New York, 1990, Bantam Books.

Sports medicine for the primary care physician, Boca Raton, 1994, RCRC Press.

Oxford textbook of sports medicine, Harries M, Williams C, et al, eds. New York, 1994, Oxford University Press.

Stedman's medical dictionary, 21st ed. Baltimore, 1966, Williams & Wilkins.

Rupp N: Diagnosis and management of exercise-induced asthma, *Phy Sports Med* 24(1):77–87, 1996.

McFadden ER: Exercise-induced airway obstruction, *Clin Chest Med* 16(4):671–682, 1995.

REFERENCES

1. Bassler TJ: Better life expectancy and marathon running, *Am J Cardiol* 45:1292–1297, 1980.
2. Cheitlin MD: Mitral valve prolapse: key references, *Circulation* 59:610–612, 1979.
3. Chester E, King RA, Edwards E: The myxomatous mitral valve and sudden death, *Circulation* 67:632–639, 1983.
4. Corrado D, Thiene G, Nava A, Rossi L, Pennelli N: Sudden death in young competitive athletes: clinicopathologic correlations in 22 cases, *Am J Med* 89:588–596, 1990.
5. Graham TP Jr, Bricker TJ, James FW, Strong WB: 26th Bethesda conference: recommendations for determining eligibility in athletes with cardiovascular abnormalities, *J Am Coll Cardiol* 24:867–873, 1994.
6. Hartung GH, Squires WG, Gotto AM: Effects of exercise training on plasma high density lipoprotein cholesterol coronary disease patients, *Am Heart J* 101(2):181–184, 1981.
7. Hutter AM Jr: Cardiovascular abnormalities in the athlete: role of the physician. Keynote address 26th Bethesda Conference: recommendations for determining eligibility in athletes with cardiovascular abnormalities, *J Am Coll Cardiol* 24:851–852, 1994.
8. Maron BJ, Poliac LC, Kaplan JA, Mueller FO: Blunt impact to the chest leading to sudden cardiac arrest during sports activities, *N Engl J Med* 333(6):337, 1995.
9. Maron BJ, Roberts WC: Sudden death in young athletes, *Circulation* 62(2):218–229, 1980.
10. Mitchell JH, Blomqvist CG, Haskill WL, et al: Classification of sports. 16th Bethesda Conference. Cardiovascular abnormalities in the athlete: recommendations regarding eligibility for competition, *J Am Coll Cardiol* 6:1198–1199, 1985.
11. Paffenberger RS, Laughlin ME, Gina AS, et al: Work activity of long-shoreman as related to death from coronary heart disease and stroke, *N Engl J Med* 282:1109–1114, 1970.
12. Rowell LB: Human cardiovascular adjustments to exercise and thermal stress, *Physiol Rev* 54:75–159, 1974.
13. Rushmer RF, Smith O, Franklin D: Mechanisms of cardiac control in exercise. *Circ Res* 7:602–627, 1962.

CHAPTER 4

HEAD TRAUMA

Matthew E. Fink

EPIDEMIOLOGY OF SPORTS-RELATED HEAD INJURIES

Sports-related head injuries, except those incurred during boxing or combat sports, are accidental, and great efforts are being made to reduce their frequency. Unlike the more common musculoskeletal injuries associated with athletic activities, head injuries may first appear trivial; but there may be a progression of disability or the start of a lifelong process of neurologic impairment, which, if not recognized early with the appropriate interventions, can result in serious disability in later life.

The magnitude of the problem can be best appreciated from statistics compiled by the National Football Head and Neck Injury Registry.[19] It is estimated that there are 250,000 concussions in this country each year in football alone.[7] In the years between 1971 and 1984, there was a documented yearly average of eight deaths due to head injuries. At the high school level, about 20% of football players sustain a concussion during a single season, and some suffer two or more. In football, the risk of sustaining a concussion is four times greater for the player who has a history of concussion than for a player who has never sustained a previous concussion.[8] In Great Britain, a recent survey of 544 rugby players found that 56% had suffered at least one head injury associated with posttraumatic amnesia; this lasted more than an hour in 58 players, of whom only 38 had been admitted to the hospital for evaluation and treatment.[15] Repeated concussions, best documented in professional boxers, can cause long-term impairments in cognitive functions (dementia pugilistica) and have been associated with pathological changes in the brain on imaging studies.[9,11,20] Recent epidemiologic studies have also suggested that head injury with concussion is an independent and additive risk factor for the development of Alzheimer's disease in later life.[14] For all of the above reasons, it is crucial that a standardized program be instituted for the prevention and treatment of all head injuries during sports activities to prevent the long-term consequences.

In the United States the sports associated with the highest incidence of head injury are football, horseback riding, and bicycling, especially in children. In Glasgow, Scotland, a survey revealed that golf (club injuries), horseback riding, and rugby were the most common causes of head injury, reflecting the relative frequency of different sports in different countries.[13] The use of hard-shell helmets significantly reduces the risk of head injury during sports activities, and major efforts are underway to encourage their universal use by both children and adults.[3,10,16]

CLASSIFICATION AND PATHOLOGY OF HEAD INJURIES

Primary Brain Damage

Concussion, the most common brain injury during sports, refers to a syndrome of brief loss of consciousness (LOC) with a variable period of post-traumatic amnesia (PTA) and confusion. Some injuries do not have a documented period of unconsciousness, but there is a clear period of PTA; these episodes should also be defined as concussion. It is likely that the period of LOC was too brief to be recognized. Although there has been controversy regarding the underlying neuropathology of concussion, animal studies and recent neuroimaging studies in humans confirm that there are pathological lesions associated with concussion, specifically axonal swelling in subcortical white matter.[12,17]

The hallmarks of concussion are a period of post-traumatic confusion and amnesia for recent events. The severity of the concussion has been graded according to the duration of LOC and PTA, according the scheme of Cantu.[7]

Grade 1 (mild) No LOC, PTA less than 30 min
Grade 2 (moderate) LOC less than 5 min or PTA more than 30 min
Grade 3 (severe) LOC for 5 min or PTA for 24 hours or more

The above classification is important in determining when athletes may return to play after acute injury.

Cerebral contusions, or bruising of the surface of the brain, can occur as a result of a direct blow to the skull. Contusions may be focal underneath a skull fracture after direct impact to the head, or multifocal due to the whole brain being suddenly slammed against the interior of the skull and rigid dural membranes. Multifocal contusions generally occur during a rapid deceleration injury, such as occurs when the athlete falls to the ground and strikes the head against a hard surface. The most common locations are the anterior tips of the frontal and temporal lobes and the occipital poles. Although these lesions may not result immediately in loss of consciousness or focal neurologic signs, they can cause significant impairments in cognitive functions and personality and create a risk for posttraumatic epilepsy. Brain contusions in eloquent areas may cause focal deficits or aphasia. Brain imaging studies will reveal the extent of these lesions immediately.[4]

Diffuse axonal injury is caused by a combination of deceleration and rotational forces that cause shearing of large areas of white matter from the overlying cerebral cortex. This results in immediate coma and has a poor prognosis for recovery. This serious injury may occur in the absence of any external injuries or skull fractures, and initial brain imaging studies may appear normal.[4]

Secondary Brain Damage

Contusions and diffuse axonal injuries may secondarily cause brain edema, increased intracranial pressure, and subarachnoid, intracerebral, or subdural hematomas. A skull fracture across the path of meningeal arteries may cause an acute epidural hematoma. About half of all patients who develop coma from epidural and subdural hematomas are initially brought to the hospital awake and talking but deteriorate 6 to 24 hours later. Close observation, neuroimaging studies, and emergency neurosurgical consultation is required for any athlete who shows a decline in alertness after a lucid period.

Posttraumatic epilepsy may occur in patients with cerebral contusions with or without an underlying skull fracture. Overall, the incidence is about 5% in patients with these lesions. If a seizure occurs within the first week following injury, there is a high risk of recurrent seizures, and antiepileptic medication is usually required on a long-term basis.

The "Second Impact Syndrome" is the development of malignant brain edema after a second concussion occurs before the injured athlete has fully recovered from the first.[18] This syndrome is most common in young children but also occurs in teenagers and young adults.[5] The mechanism is thought to be persistence of vasomotor paralysis in the brain from the first concussion, resulting in severe vasogenic edema after the second insult. This potentially fatal disorder is a major reason for enforcing a period of rest and abstinence from play until the athlete has fully recovered from the effects of a concussion.

The "postconcussive syndrome" refers to a constellation of symptoms that may persist for weeks or months after a concussion—loss of intellectual capacity, poor recent memory, personality changes, headaches, dizziness, lack of concentration, and fatigue. In the past, many of these symptoms were thought to be psychologically based. However, it is now accepted that these symptoms represent the subacute and chronic effects of brain injury and reflect the underlying neuropathology of concussion.

EVALUATION AND TREATMENT ON THE FIELD

Following head injury, there may be a scalp wound with extensive bleeding. Hemorrhage should be controlled with pressure and players immediately removed from the field because of the risk of HIV transmission. Using sterile gloves, the wound should be explored to determine if there is a fracture. A depressed skull fracture may cause underlying brain contusion without loss of consciousness, but could result in a delayed epidural or subdural hematoma. An athlete with a scalp laceration, even without LOC, should be immediately moved to a hospital for neuroimaging studies and observation.

If the athlete is unconscious on the field, the cervical spine should be immobilized, and before any movement, the athlete should be examined for chest and abdominal injuries and limb fractures. The injured player should be placed in a semiprone position to protect the airway, and neurologic assessment on the field should consist of the Glasgow Coma scale (see Table 4-1), pupil size and responses to light, examination of the ears and nose for

Table 4-1. Glasgow coma scale

	Score 3–15
Eye Opening	
Spontaneous	4
To voice	3
To pain	2
None	1
Best Verbal Response	
Oriented	5
Confused	4
Inappropriate	3
Incomprehensible	2
None	1
Best Motor Response	
Obeys command	6
Localizes pain	5
Withdraws from pain	4
Flexes to pain	3
Extends to pain	2
None	1

HEAD INJURY CARD

This patient has received an injury to the head. A careful examination has been made, and no sign of any serious complication has been found.

It is expected that recovery will be rapid, but in such cases it is not possible to be quite certain.

If you notice any change of behavior, vomiting, dizziness, headache, double vision, or excessive drowsiness, please telephone the hospital at once.

No alcohol. No analgesics. No driving.

From McLatchie G: Brit Med J *308:1620–1624, 1994.*

blood, cerebrospinal fluid, and hemotympanum, and tests for perception of pain, tendon reflexes, and plantar responses. Search for an associated spinal injury should be paramount in the mind of the examiner. After examination, the injured athlete should be rapidly transported to the nearest trauma hospital.

Fortunately, most players have a brief LOC and are awake by the time a physician arrives on the field. The mental status examination should consist of tests for orientation (time, place, person, situation), concentration (digits forward and backward, the months of year in reverse), and memory (names of teams in prior games, President, Governor, Mayor, recent newsworthy events, 3 words at 0 and 5 minutes, details of current contest). Neurologic tests should include symmetry and light reactivity of pupils, coordination tests with finger-nose-finger and heel-shin tests, heel to toe standing with eyes open and closed, and standing on one foot. Challenge tests may include a 40-yard sprint, 5 push-ups, 5 sit-ups, and 5 deep knee bends. If the above activities cause headaches, dizziness, nausea, unsteadiness, photophobia, blurred or double vision, emotional lability, or mental status changes, the athlete should be transferred immediately to a hospital for brain imaging studies and observation. If there are no other abnormalities on the examination other than posttraumatic amnesia, the player should undergo brain imaging studies to look for a fracture or contusion. If these studies are normal, the athlete may return home for observation by family members for any change in neurological condition, as instructed by the medical staff. It is useful to provide instructions on a Head Injury Card similar to the one described in the box above.

RECOMMENDATIONS FOR RETURN TO ATHLETIC ACTIVITIES

The decision to allow an athlete to return to play is based on empiric guidelines rather than scientifically based knowledge. The guidelines are designed to ensure that the athlete has fully recovered from his head injury before allowing return to play, recognizing that there is a cumulative effect from recurrent brain injuries. According to the criteria developed by Cantu, guidelines are as follows:[1,6,7]

Grade 1 Concussion (Mild)

First Concussion—May return to play if asymptomatic for 1 week

Second Concussion—Return to play in 2 weeks if asymptomatic at that time for 1 full week

Third Concussion—Terminate season; may return to play next season if asymptomatic

Grade 2 Concussion (Moderate)

First Concussion—Return to play if asymptomatic for 1 week

Second Concussion—Minimum of 1 month of no play; may then return if asymptomatic for 1 week; Consider terminating season

Third Concussion—Terminate season; may return next season if asymptomatic

Grade 3 Concussion (Severe)

First Concussion—Minimum of 1 month of no play; may then return if asymptomatic for 1 week

Second Concussion—Terminate season; may return next season if asymptomatic

Third Concussion—Terminate season; consider permanent retirement from contact sports

PREVENTION OF HEAD INJURIES

In 1904, President Theodore Roosevelt urged the formation of the National Collegiate Athletic Association after 19 athletes were killed or paralyzed from football injuries.[2] Since then, prevention of head injuries in sports has been a high priority, although this may be impossible in boxing and other combat sports. Contact sports such as football, rugby, and basketball have a significant risk that can be reduced with the use of headgear, and this has already been well established in motorcycle and autoracing accidents. In children under the age of 16, accidental injuries are the leading cause of death, and head injuries from skateboarding, bicycling, horseback riding, rollerblading, and rock-climbing are a major cause of death and disability. Most states in the U.S. now require children to wear helmets while riding bicycles; similar helmets should be worn for other activities where there is a risk for head injury.[3,10,16] Golf club injuries among children under age 16 are common and point to the need for stronger rules of play on golf courses to ensure that spectators stand clear of players.

Boxing represents a special situation, since the goal of professional boxing is to cause a concussion (i.e., a knock-out). Professional boxers enter the ring voluntarily knowing the risks. But we certainly have an obligation to protect amateur athletes, and we should ensure that headgear is always used in amateur competition to prevent head injuries. In addition, professional boxers should have their total number of fights limited if they have sustained repeated knock-outs or dazed states. In other combat sports, the use of padded and spring flooring may protect against serious injuries during falls.

REFERENCES

1. Akau CK, Press JM, Gooch JL: Sports Medicine. 4. Spine and head injuries, *Arch Phys Med Rehabil* 74:S443-446, 1993.
2. Albright JP, McCauley E, Martin RK, et al: Head and neck injuries in college football: an eight-year analysis, *Amer J Sports Medicine* 13:147-152, 1985.
3. Ashbaugh SJ, Macknin ML, Medendorp SV: The Ohio Bicycle Injury Study, *Clin Pediatrics* 34:256-260, 1995.
4. Becker DP, Gudeman SK: *Textbook of Head Injury*, Philadelphia, 1989, WB Saunders.
5. Bruce DA, et al: Diffuse cerebral swelling following head injuries in children: the syndrome of "malignant brain edema," *J Neurosurg* 54:170-178, 1981.
6. Cantu RC: Guidelines for return to contact sports after cerebral concussion, *Physician and Sports Medicine* 14:75-83, 1986.
7. Cantu RC: When to return to contact sports after a cerebral concussion, *Sports Med Digest* 10:1-2, 1988.
8. Gerberich SG, et al: Concussion incidences and severity in secondary school varsity players, *Amer J Public Health* 73:1370-1375, 1983.
9. Gronwall D, Wrighttson P: Cumulative effects of concussions. *Lancet* 2:995-997, 1975.
10. Hamilton MG, Tranmer BI: Nervous system injuries in horseback-riding injuries, *J Trauma* 34:227-232, 1993.
11. Jordan BD, Zimmerman RD: Computed tomography and magnetic resonance imaging comparisons in boxers, *J Amer Med Assoc* 263:1670-1674, 1990.
12. Levin HS, et al: Magnetic resonance imaging and computerized tomography in relation to the neurobehavioral sequelae of mild and moderate head injuries, *J Neurosurg* 66:707-713, 1987.
13. Lindsay KW, McLatchie GR, Jennett B: Serious head injury in sport, *Brit Med J* 281:789-791, 1980.
14. Mayeux R, et al: Genetic susceptibility and head injury as risk factors for Alzheimer's disease among community-dwelling elderly persons and their first-degree relatives, *Ann Neurol* 33:494-501, 1993.
15. McLatchie G, Jennett B: ABC of Sports Medicine. Head injury in sport, *Brit Med J* 308:1620-1624, 1994.
16. Nelson DE, Bixby-Hammett D: Equestrian injuries in children and young adults, *Amer J Dis Child* 146:611-614, 1992.
17. Ommaya AK, Gennarelli TA: Cerebral concussion and traumatic unconsciousness. Correlation of experimental and clinical observations on blunt head injuries, *Brain* 97:633-654, 1974.
18. Saunders RL, Harbaugh RE: The second impact in catastrophic contact sports head trauma, *J Amer Med Assoc* 252:538-539, 1984.
19. Torg JS, et al: The national football head and neck injury registry. 14-year report on cervical quadriplegia, 1971 through 1984, *J Amer Med Assoc* 254:3439-3443, 1985.
20. Unterharnscheidt F: About boxing: Review of historical and medical aspects, *Texas Reports Biol Med* 28:421-495, 1970.

CHAPTER 5

GASTROINTESTINAL SYSTEM

Seth A. Cohen
Jerome H. Siegel

Gastrointestinal problems are common among athletes, especially in those persons who participate in endurance events such as long-distance running. Although much remains to be understood concerning the effects of exercise in the gastrointestinal tract, a large amount of new information has come to light in the past 15 years. The most common gastrointestinal complaints reported by athletes include diarrhea, fecal urgency, abdominal pain, bloating, nausea, vomiting, heartburn, chest pain, and occult or overt gastrointestinal hemorrhage. In this chapter we will review the pathophysiology, clinical presentation, and treatment for the various problems affecting the gastrointestinal tract of athletes.

GENERAL OVERVIEW

Gastrointestinal symptoms are common among athletes, but the problems vary widely according to the specific sport, level of exertion, degree of anxiety, and possibly gender of the athlete. Most studies reporting these problems are in general agreement in terms of the spectrum of gastrointestinal symptomatology. Studies have concentrated on endurance athletes—long-distance runners and triathletes, but specific recreation or competitive team sports such as football and tennis have not been studied. All studies report that the incidence of gastrointestinal symptoms is proportional to the level of exertion, while some studies have found more than 80% of endurance athletes experience "often" or "occasional" gastrointestinal symptoms. This high incidence of gastrointestinal symptomatology is remarkable even though it reflects some selection bias. Lower GI symptoms—watery bowel movements, fecal urgency or incontinence, cramps or GI bleeding—are more commonly reported than upper GI symptoms—nausea, vomiting, belching, heartburn—which are perceived as more intermittent and milder.

Most studies of endurance athletes have focused on men; less information is available concerning women.

Women, however, appear to experience more frequent GI problems (40% to 70%) than men, and this is exacerbated during menses. More information on female athletes is needed. Younger runners (age less than 35) and less experienced runners experience a high incidence of GI symptoms compared to those reported by older and more experienced runners. Anxiety concerning performance is a well recognized factor in provoking or exacerbating GI symptoms among athletes.

Most athletes note a "training effect" upon gastrointestinal symptoms; that is, the symptoms occur more commonly during the initial training period and diminish as the athletes "get into shape." However, exercise exceeding an athlete's usual threshold provokes GI symptoms again. Paradoxically, there are reports that preexisting functional GI complaints (such as the irritable bowel syndrome) improve in athletes after they have been in training.

TRAUMA

Contact sports can lead to traumatic injury of the abdominal organs. The most serious injuries include laceration or rupture of the spleen, laceration of the liver, and contusion or disruption of the pancreas. Typically, affected individuals will develop signs and symptoms of an acute abdomen possibly with vascular collapse. Persons with these injuries require immediate referral for resuscitation and surgical evaluation. Further discussion will not be included here.

GASTROESOPHAGEAL REFLUX

Belching, regurgitation, heartburn, chest pain, or acid reflux are common, occurring intermittently in about 10% of the general population. Symptoms of reflux are provoked by vigorous exercise. Of long-distance runners, 20% to 25% experience symptoms. Belching and regurgitation are more common than heartburn. Although the mechanism for belching and regurgitation is not known, it is probably related to aerophagia, large volumes of liquids or food contained in the stomach, gastric agitation, and, possibly, increased intragastric pressures generated during exertion. Esophageal spasm is another possible cause for chest pain and is often misinterpreted as heartburn. Abnormal relaxation of the lower esophageal sphincter does not occur with exercise to explain reflux symptoms. Athletes are more likely to develop reflux symptoms if they eat just before exertion. Some athletes, however, experience heartburn if they eat after exercise, especially if they imbibe foods that either relax the lower esophageal sphincter or are acidic (e.g., alcohol, citrus drinks). Heartburn is also reported among anxious competitive players of team sports either before or during games.

Treatment of reflux symptoms is empiric and is based on clinical judgment. Young people who only complain of intermittent symptoms can be treated empirically without undergoing investigation. If upon closer questioning patients report frequent or persistent symptoms or other abnormalities such as weight loss or dysphagia, they should be evaluated with endoscopy. Older patients with new or persistent symptoms should be referred for evaluation to exclude significant esophagitis or neoplasia. In middle-aged men and women who are at risk for coronary artery disease, the complaint of exertional chest pain should always prompt a consideration of angina. Acid perfusion of the esophagus can lead to chest pain *and* myocardial ischemia. Most patients, as well as physicians, cannot accurately distinguish between esophageal pain and angina. Exclusion of coronary disease should take priority in patients at risk.

Patients should be counseled not to eat for several hours prior to exercise. They should also be cautioned

Table 5-1. Medicines available for peptic ulcer disease (PUD) and gastroesophageal reflux disease (GERD)

H-2 Blockers	Cimetidine (Tagamet) 400 mg BID or 800 mg qhs
	Famotidine (Pepcid) 20 mg BID or 40 mg qhs
	Nazitidine (Axid) 150 mg BID or 300 mg qhs
	Raniditine (Zantac) 150 mg BID or 300 mg qhs
Antacids	Calcium carbonate
	Magnesium hydroxide
	Aluminum carbonate
	Aluminum hydroxide and alginic acid
Proton pump inhibitor	Omeprazole (Prilosec) 20 mg qd
	Lansoprazole (Prevacid) 30 mg qd
Cytoprotective agents	Misoprostol (Cytotec) 100 or 200 mcg QID
	Sucralfate (Carafate) 1 gm QID

not to "gulp" down fluids when drinking, as this action increases aerophagia. Simple symptoms of heartburn are readily treated with antacids. An alginate-based antacid, such as Gaviscon (SmithKline Beecham), is preferred by many authorities. Care must be taken with magnesium-containing antacids, as they can precipitate or exacerbate diarrhea. On the other hand, while calcium-based antacids are a good source of this essential element, they may lead to constipation. Patients with more severe symptoms can take an antisecretory agent such as a histamine type 2 receptor antagonist (H-2 blocker) before exercising, but this approach should not be necessary for most athletes. The optimal treatment for peptic esophagitis and refractory symptoms of reflux is omeprazole, a member of a new class of medications (see Table 5-1).

NAUSEA, CRAMPING, VOMITING

Symptoms of nausea, cramping, and vomiting commonly occur in athletes who are not "in shape," exceed their exertional capacity, or have eaten too soon before exertion. Of endurance runners, 5% to 10% vomit and wretch after finishing a "hard" run. Gastric emptying is retarded during severe exertion, but, clinically, this phenomenon is not relevant to most athletes. Symptoms are inversely related to aerobic training capacity and may be exacerbated by dehydration as the result of prolonged exercise in hot weather. Treatment consists of rest and oral rehydration. Rarely, patients with severe dehydration will require parenteral hydration.

ABDOMINAL PAIN

A "stitch," located in a person's side, is frequent among athletes. It is characterized as a sharp, subcostal pain which may occur on either side and is exacerbated by breathing and relieved by rest. The frequency and severity of a stitch diminishes with aerobic training endurance. Although the cause of a "stitch" is unknown, speculative causes include ischemia, a trapped gas bubble in the intestine, or spasms of the diaphragm. Clinical diagnosis is evident and no treatment is required. Other types of abdominal pain that do not meet the criteria for a stitch should be evaluated systematically as one would in a nonathlete. There are rare reports of cecal volvulus, ischemic bowel, incarcerated or strangulated hernia, colon cancer, or Crohn's disease presenting as abdominal pain during exercise. Evaluation of abdominal pain in the athlete is the same as in other patients: What is the nature of the pain? What are the associated symptoms? Over what period of time does the pain present? etc.

IRRITABLE BOWEL SYNDROME

The irritable bowel syndrome (IBS) is common among the general population. It is characterized by altered bowel habits with abdominal pain or bloating in the absence of organic disease. IBS generally affects younger people and women more than men. The pathophysiology remains unknown, but possible explanations include disordered intestinal and colonic motility, increased sensitivity to colonic distension, exaggerated gastrocolic reflexes, carbohydrate intolerance, psychoneurotic disorders, and stress. The physiologic abnormalities and symptoms of IBS are believed to be common, however, only a minority of people seek medical evaluation. Those patients who do seek medical help have significantly more psychoneurotic disorders. There appears to be an association between functional abdominal pain and a history of physical and sexual abuse, but this remains debatable. Some studies have noted a higher frequency of IBS among athletes, but exercise ameliorates the symptoms. IBS is a clinical diagnosis of exclusion. Treatment options include dietary restrictions (e.g., lactose products and high residue foods), fiber supplementation, antispasmodic agents, and medical and psychological counseling.

PSYCHOGENIC ABDOMINAL PAIN

Psychogenic abdominal pain is seen among young, anxious athletes. Although it is a diagnosis of exclusion, it does have certain characteristics. It can be a sharp, epigastric pain without radiation or associated with symptoms of nausea, vomiting, fever, or altered bowel habits. It has no relationship to food intake or other physiologic stimuli but may be associated with stress and anger. On examination the abdomen is flat, soft, with normal bowel sounds, and no guarding or peritoneal irritation. Generally, the history is chronic and repetitive. Acute presentation of epigastric pain in a young person could represent, among other causes, gastroenteritis, esophagitis, appendicitis, peptic ulcer disease, pancreatitis, or bowel obstruction, but these are unusual. The patient's history, associated symptoms, physical examination, and laboratory results along with observation will identify those people with organic disease. The most important aspect of treatment is recognition of the nonorganic cause of the pain to avoid unnecessary and costly testing.

DIARRHEA

Watery bowel movements, cramps, fecal urgency, and incontinence are the most common and troubling gastrointestinal symptoms among athletes who exercise strenuously. As many as 50% to 60% of marathon runners experience one or more of these symptoms. The urge to defecate is the most common reason for endurance runners to interrupt a race. Interestingly, in a survey of triathalon athletes, lower gastrointestinal symptoms were significantly reduced during the swimming and cycling portions of the event compared to during running. This observation highlights the fact that running specifically triggers colonic symptoms.

Although there is no proof that running increases intestinal transit, it is widely believed that running increases the frequency of bowel movements. The jarring of repetitive footfalls during running may stimulate mass movements in the colon or alter the absorption of fluids and electrolytes. Alternative hypotheses include the release of various prokinetic gastrointestinal hormones or inflammatory mediators such as prostaglandins. Runners note that the frequency and intensity of lower gastrointestinal symptoms are proportional to the level of exertion, their aerobic training capacity, and their level of anxiety. Symptoms are significantly more common in women than men and among younger runners when compared to older runners.

Athletes who experience diarrhea and/or fecal urgency associated with running, and not at other times, do not require a work-up. Most runners have adopted their own approach to handling exercise-induced diarrhea. The majority of runners abstain from eating 3 to 6 hours before running. Many consciously evacuate their bowel before running. Others always know where they can find a toilet on their usual running route. Individual runners may take fiber supplements to "bulk up" the stool to prevent a watery bowel movement, while others take an antimotility agent, such as Loperamide, or a nonsteroidal anti-inflammatory agent. The goal of treatment for exercise-induced diarrhea is to control symptoms so as not to interrupt the person's performance.

A patient with an alteration of bowel habits independent of exercise should be evaluated as any other patient: What is the pattern of bowel movements? A colitis pattern (urgency, tenesmus, bloody) or a small bowel pattern (less frequent, large volume, watery)? Is the onset of the problem acute or chronic? Are blood or fecal leukocytes present in the stool? Are there any risk factors for infectious causes of diarrhea? After obtaining a complete history and physical examination the work-up of diarrhea includes a stool sample for fecal leukocytes and occult blood, a complete blood count and an erythrocyte sedimentation rate (ESR). If fecal leukocytes are present, this finding suggests colitis, which can be infectious or idiopathic. Stool cultures will diagnose bacterial etiologies. Pseudomembranous colitis should always be considered in any patient who has taken antibiotics in the past several months; a stool specimen for *Clostridium difficile* toxin is the best test to establish the diagnosis. *Giardia lamblia*, the only parasitic infestation commonly seen in practice, produces large volume liquid stools and weight loss and can be diagnosed on examination for ova and parasites. An elevated ESR will help identify patients who have inflammatory bowel disease. A flexible sigmoidoscopy is important in diagnosing colitis, and, often, the combination of the endoscopic findings and the mucosal biopsies can be diagnostic of Crohn's disease, ulcerative colitis, or pseudomembranous colitis. Treatment consists of supportive care and specific treatment for the illness (see Table 5-2).

TRAVELER'S DIARRHEA

Athletes who travel to foreign countries to compete are always at risk for contracting "traveler's diarrhea." This syndrome occurs predominantly as a result of exposure to the different strains of toxigenic *Escherichia coli* present in foreign areas. The best measures are preventative, encouraging travelers to avoid tap water, ice cubes, and fresh vegetables. It is best to drink bottled water or carbonated beverages and eat only thoroughly cooked or peeled foods.

Table 5-2. Etiologies and treatment of diarrhea

Etiology	Diagnosis	Treatment
Toxigenic *E. coli*	Clinical dx, exclusion	Bismuth subsalicylate, loperamide, fluids
*Salmonella, Shigella, Yersinia, Campylobacter**	Stool culture	Ciprofloxacin 500 mg BID or erythromycin 500 mg BID × 5 days
Pseudomembranous colitis, *Clostridium difficile*	Stool for toxin sigmoidoscopy	Metronidazole 250 mg QID or vancomycin 125 mg QID × 10 days
Irritable bowel syndrome	Clinical dx, exclusion	Fiber supplements, antispasmodics, antidiarrheals
Runner's diarrhea	Clinical dx	See text
Inflammatory bowel disease	Sigmoidoscopy	Sulfasalazine
	Barium radiography, exclusion	Mesalamine Glucocorticoids

Clinical dx = clinical diagnosis, exclusion = diagnosis of exclusion
Yersinia is not sensitive to erythromycin

Bismuth subsalicylate (Pepto-Bismol, Proctor & Gamble) taken 4 times a day has been shown to be effective in preventing travelers diarrhea, but such a regimen is impractical. The administration of prophylactic antibiotics to protect against diarrhea (e.g., ciprofloxacin or trimethoprim-sulphamethoxazole) is effective, but the benefit does not justify the incidence of side effects, and it is not cost effective. A better strategy is to counsel the travelers in preventive measures and have them carry an antidiarrheal agent and antibiotics should symptoms arise. At the onset of the first liquid bowel movement, the patient should be instructed to take loperamide 4 mg once and ciprofloxacin 500 mg by mouth twice a day for several days. Loperamide 2 mg can be taken as needed several times a day. If the patient has persistent fever or blood is present in the stool, he should seek medical consultation.

LACTOSE INTOLERANCE

Lactose (mild sugar) is a disaccharide and requires enzymatic hydrolysis by lactase before it can be absorbed in the small intestine. Inherited lactose intolerance results when lactase is deficient, leading to carbohydrate malabsorption and osmotic diarrhea. Lactase deficiency occurs in 50% to 80% of African-Americans and Asians and 5% to 15% of Caucasians. Typically, affected persons develop bloating, abdominal pain, and foul-smelling watery diarrhea shortly after ingesting milk products. Similar symptoms can be provoked in all people by the ingestion of nonabsorbable disaccharides like sorbitol or mannitol, which may be found in medicinal elixirs and "sugar-free" products. Lactase deficient individuals should either abstain from lactose or use lactase supplements to enzymatically split the lactose into absorbable components.

GASTROINTESTINAL BLEEDING

Gastrointestinal bleeding is uncommon among athletes with the exception of long distance runners. Up to 20% of marathon runners have occult blood in their stool after competition when tested by the guaiac reagent. More sensitive assays for hemoglobin have shown that almost all long distance runners experience occult GI blood loss. A much smaller percentage of patients will experience overt gastrointestinal bleeding either as hematochezia (bright red blood per rectum) or melena (black tarry stool). It is not clear why runners experience gastrointestinal bleeding while other athletes do not. Two major theories are proposed. The first is related to intestinal ischemia. During marked exercise, splanchnic blood flow decreases 60% to 80%, and this may provoke a low-flow ischemia to vulnerable areas of the bowel, especially if patients become dehydrated and hypovolemic. The second theory suggests that bleeding is related to the trauma of repetitive footfalls and consequent jarring during running. This explanation is similar to that of runners' hematuria, which probably results from trauma to the bladder. Most episodes of bleeding are self-limited. There are, however, well-reported cases of ischemic colitis associated with running involving significant bleeding and, at times, colonic infarction requiring surgical resection. There is one case report of fatal hemorrhagic gastritis of unknown etiology that occurred in a marathon runner.

Evaluation and Treatment

All gastrointestinal bleeding should be interpreted in the complete clinical setting. Clinical decision making always begins with a good history and physical examination. Any athlete may suffer from organic gastrointestinal disease such as peptic ulcer, inflammatory bowel disease, or colonic neoplasm. As with any patient with gastrointestinal symptoms if orthostatic hypotension, signs of peritoneal irritation, melena, or significant or persistent bleeding are present, the patient should be urgently referred for evaluation. The amount of blood loss, hemodynamic parameters, physical examination, and laboratory assessment dictate whether the patient should be admitted to the hospital or treated as an out-patient. Young, fit patients without any remarkable history and who experience minimal blood loss related to strenuous exercise, particularly endurance events, probably can be observed without evaluation. Young patients with gross hematochezia are best evaluated by preforming a flexible sigmoidoscopy. Almost all cases of hematochezia are benign and self-limited. Ischemic colitis is unusual and is usually self-limited. Occult blood loss needs to be interpreted on the basis of the person's age and risk factors for colon cancer. Patients under age 40 with no family history of colon cancer probably do not require colonic evaluation. Older people or those with a family history of colon cancer should be evaluated by either performing total colonoscopy or by a barium enema and a flexible sigmoidoscopy. Guidelines now recommend that if a patient has had a normal colonoscopy without any colon polyps, he does not need another examination for 5 years.

Athletes with iron-deficiency anemia should have serial fecal occult blood testing after light exercise and independent of exercise; if occult blood loss is present, evaluation is indicated. Bloody diarrhea with urgency, tenesmus, fever, and lower abdominal pain suggests colitis that is either infectious, idiopathic, or ischemic. These patients should be referred for evaluation and treatment.

Bleeding from the stomach or duodenum leads to melena, the by-product of bacterial degradation of hemoglobin as it passes through the intestine. Melena indicates a significant amount of upper GI bleeding, and the affected person should be referred urgently for resuscitation and evaluation, i.e., endoscopy.

EATING DISORDERS

Anorexia nervosa and bulimia are prevalent and a serious problem among adolescent women. It is estimated that 5% to 20% of female college students suffer from eating disorders, and it has been suggested that participation in competitive athletics may contribute to their development. Anorexia nervosa is characterized by a severely distorted body-image with pathologic fear of food and weight gain. Psychologic disturbances which often accompany anorexia include a feeling of inadequacy, lack of control, perfectionism, interpersonal distrust, and maturity fears. Bulimia is characterized by episodes of uncontrolled binge eating, followed by vomiting. Affected women often have a pathologic fear of not being able to voluntarily control their eating, control their weight, have low self-esteem, and experience episodes of depression. Both disorders can seriously impair a person's health, resulting in malnutrition, growth retardation, electrolyte abnormalities, and even death at times.

Anorexia and bulimia are most prevalent among well-educated young women who are achievement oriented. Thus, it is found frequently among high school and college female athletes. One study analyzed the tendency toward eating disorders in three groups of college women: (1) non-athletes; (2) athletes in sports which do not emphasize thinness (swimming, track and field, and volleyball); and (3) athletes in sports that do emphasize thinness (ballet, cheerleading, gymnastics). The study found an exceptional preoccupation with weight or tendency towards eating disorders in 6% of non-athletes,

10% of all athletes, and 20% of athletes in sports which emphasize thinness. Anorexia athletica is characterized by symptoms of early anorexia nervosa prevalent among young female athletes. The relationship between competitive athletes and eating disorders may not be causal, however, because specific sports may attract women who already have eating disorders.

Many athletes occasionally use vomiting as a form of weight reduction, like a wrestler who has to "make weight." This is not classified as bulimia because these people do not have a morbid fear of becoming obese, nor do they experience uncontrolled binging. Persistent vomiting, however, even when not part of bulimia, can be harmful, leading to electrolyte abnormalities, myopathies, muscular weakness and esophageal laceration, bleeding (Mallory-Weiss syndrome), or perforation. Laxatives and enemas are abused also by some individuals as a form of weight control. Such activity is also associated with electrolyte imbalance such as hypokalemia and contraction alkalosis, which can lead to weakness, postural hypotension, and syncope.

It is imperative that coaches and physicians who care for young athletes, particularly women, be aware of the prevalence and severity of eating disorders. These disorders are easiest to treat when detected early before they become serious. Furthermore, coaches can supply the ultimate motivation for these young people by not making inclusion on the team dependent on specific behavior or minimum weight. Conversely, misguided coaches who place competitive performance above the health and well-being of their athletes place additional stresses on these women, exacerbating the eating disorders and leading to serious consequences.

NSAID-RELATED GASTROINTESTINAL PROBLEMS

Nonsteroidal antiinflammatory drug (NSAID) use is common in the United States, mostly among people with arthritis, but also among athletes. This class of medication provides moderate analgesia and good antiinflammatory action appropriate for treating bruises, strains and sprains. NSAIDs inhibit the production of prostaglandins that are mediators of inflammation and pain. There are more than 20 varieties of nonaspirin containing NSAIDs, several of which are now available over the counter. Acutely, aspirin and NSAIDs induce superficial gastric erosions (NSAID gastropathy or erosive gastritis) in most people, which are typically located in the antrum of the stomach. These erosions are not clinically significant and cause neither symptoms nor gastrointestinal bleeding. The gastric mucosa adapts, and the lesions heal spontaneously. When people take NSAIDs on a continuous basis for more than 4 to 5 days, up to 50% of users begin to experience symptoms of abdominal pain, dyspepsia, heartburn, and nausea. The presence of symptoms does not correlate well with significant mucosal abnormalities such as ulcers, and, conversely, patients with ulcers can be asymptomatic. While short term NSAID use can lead to superficial gastric erosions, chronic NSAID users (greater than 4 weeks) are at risk for developing significant peptic ulcers and their complications. Young, healthy patients who take NSAIDs intermittently only have a slightly increased risk of ulcer disease.

Evaluation and treatment of NSAID-associated symptoms includes identifying the indication for NSAID use and the other risk factors for peptic ulcer disease. Established risk factors for ulcer disease and their complications include prior history of ulcers, age greater than 60, cigarette smoking, female gender, chronic pulmonary or liver disease, and probably *Helicobacter pylori* gastritis. For patients with self-limited inflammatory conditions, discontinuing the NSAID is the most effective treatment for relieving symptoms and healing mucosal disease. In patients taking NSAIDs simply for analgesia, acetaminophen or mild narcotics can be substituted. For people who have a chronic need for NSAIDs (e.g., osteoarthritis), treatment options include: changing to an alternative agent (because symptoms can be idiosyncratic to a specific agent), reducing the agent to the lowest effective dose, administering NSAIDs with meals, or treating the person with antiulcer medication (see Table 5-1). Misoprostol and omeprazole are most promising for the treatment of NSAID-associated ulcers when ongoing NSAID use is obligatory. A minimal amount of data is available concerning the treatment of symptomatic NSAID gastropathy, but antacid use as needed is the most cost effective method. Symptomatic older patients and those at high risk for ulcers or with persistent symptoms require endoscopic evaluation. Other people at low risk for ulcer disease with NSAID-associated symptoms should discontinue NSAID use and do not require further evaluation.

Rarely, chronic NSAID use can lead to small bowel ulceration, chronic GI blood loss, and stricture formation. There are also reports of colonic ulceration and colitis induced by NSAIDs, but, again, these entities are uncommon.

ELEVATED LIVER CHEMISTRIES

Mild elevations of liver chemistries are commonly detected incidentally during routine examination with the use of multi-channel analyzers and automated chemistry profiles. The most common pattern is the isolated elevations of alanine aminotransferase (ALT or SGPT) and aspartate aminotransferase (AST or SGOT) in an asymptomatic person. The history should focus on any prior liver disease, episodes of hepatitis, prior abnormal blood tests, rejection as a blood donor, hemolytic disorders, blood transfusion, intravenous substance use, alcohol intake, and medication use, including NSAIDs, anabolic steroids, and acetaminophen. Physical examination should look for icterus, stigmata of chronic liver disease, and hepatosplenomegaly. The most common etiologies for mild elevations of the AST and ALT are obesity, alcohol use, and NSAID use. Suspected medications should be discontinued and blood chemistries should be repeated in 3 to 4 weeks. Abnormal liver chemistries due to fatty liver require no treatment.

Serologies to exclude hepatitis C, and less commonly, hepatitis A and B, may be appropriate in people with an unremarkable history and physical examination. Chronic hepatitis C tends to be an indolent disease, but it is increasingly being diagnosed with the new serologic tests available. The mode of acquisition of hepatitis C is unknown in 80% to 90% of patients, but a significant number of affected patients will progress to chronic liver disease and cirrhosis. Patients with symptoms, progressing abnormalities, or chronic hepatitis should be referred for evaluation.

Anabolic steroids, which are used by some athletes for muscle growth and strength, can cause a reversible cholestasis similar to that caused by estrogens. Chronic anabolic steroid use is associated with peliosis hepatis (blood lakes in the liver), hepatic adenoma, and malignant neoplasms. The use of these agents is to be discouraged, and they are banned in many competitive sports.

HELICOBACTER PYLORI

Helicobacter pylori infection of the stomach was first described in 1983 in association with chronic active antral gastritis. *H. pylori* is now recognized as the most important treatable risk factor for peptic ulcer disease, present in 90% and 60% of duodenal and gastric ulcers respectively. Infection with *H. pylori* is common and increases with age to about a 50% prevalence in the United States among people 60 years old or older. The vast majority of these patients, however, are asymptomatic and do not have ulcers. For patients with ulcer disease and *H. pylori*, treatment to eradicate this infection is recommended to reduce ulcer recurrence (see Table 5-3). Treatment of *H. pylori* has no proven benefit in patients with "nonulcer dyspepsia" and, at this time, is not recommended.

Table 5-3. Treatment regimes for *Helicobacter pylori*

Tetracycline	500 mg QID or amoxicillin 500 mg QID
or	
Clarithromycin	500 mg TID
Metronidazole	250 mg TID
and	
Bismuth subsalicylate	2 tabs QID for 14 days
Amoxicillin	500 mg QID or clarithromycin 500 mg TID
and	
Omeprazole	40 mg qd for 14 days
Amoxicillin	1 gm BID
or	
Metronidazole	500 mg BID
Clarithromycin	500 mg BID
Omeprazole	20 mg BID for 7 days

BIBLIOGRAPHY

Borgen JS, Corbin CB: Eating disorders among female athletes, *Physician Sports Med*, 15:89–95, 1987.

Fries JF, Williams CA, Block DA, et al: Non-steroidal anti-inflammatory drug-associated gastropathy: incidence and risk factor models, *Am J Med* 91:213–222, 1991.

Halvorsen FA, Ritland S: Gastrointestinal problems related to endurance event training, *Sports Med* 14:157–163, 1992.

Kam LW, Pease WE, Thompson PD: Exercise-related mesenteric infarction, *Am J Gastroenterol* 89:1899–1900, 1994.

McCabe ME, Peura DA, Kadakia SC, et al: Gastrointestinal blood loss associated with running a marathon, *Dig Dis Sci* 31:1229–1232, 1986.

Mellow MH, Simpson AG, Watt L, et al: Esophageal acid perfusion in coronary artery disease: induction of myocardial ischemia, *Gastroenterology* 85:306–312, 1983.

Moses FM: The effect of exercise on the gastrointestinal tract, *Sports Med* 9:159–172, 1990.

Moses FM, Berer TG, Peura DA: Running-associated proximal hemorrhagic colitis, *Ann Int Med* 108:385–386, 1988.

Riddoch C, Trinick T: Gastrointestinal disturbances in marathon runners, *BJ Sports Med* 22:71–74, 1988.

Smith NJ: Excessive weight loss and food aversion in athletes simulating anorexia nervosa, *Pediatrics* 66:139–142, 1980.

Sullivan SN: Exercise-associated symptoms in triathletes, *Physician Sports Med* 15:105–108, 1987.

Worobetz LJ, Gerrard DF: Gastrointestinal symptoms during exercise in Enduro athletes: prevalence and speculations on the aetiology, *NZ Med J* 98:644–646, 1985.

CHAPTER 6

GENITOURINARY INJURIES

Stuart H. Popowitz
Harris N. Nagler

Participation in team sports and individual exercise, for health and recreation, has assumed increasing importance in our society. Aerobics, running, swimming, bicycling, racquet sports, and "pick-up" ball games can all produce significant physiologic stresses on the body, forcing one to go from rest to intense physical exercise. In addition to these physiologic stresses and their effects, exercise may result in pathologic stress from falls, collisions with individuals or objects, and otherwise abnormal motions. The genitourinary tract is one of the many organ systems susceptible to the effect of these extremes. This chapter will review the potential impact of these physiologic and pathologic processes on the kidneys, bladder, and reproductive organs.

SPORTS-RELATED HEMATURIA

The most visible sign of injury to the genitourinary system of athletes is hematuria, either gross or microscopic. Gross hematuria in runners, the first reported exercise-induced urinary abnormality, was noted in 1793 by Italian physician Bernaedini Ramazziani.[22] Later, Collier in 1907 and Barach in 1910 reported similar findings in athletes following both rowing and long-distance running.[7,29] Hematuria subsequently has been reported in a wide variety of sporting activities.

Hematuria in athletes has been well documented in contact as well as noncontact sports. Alyea and Parish[4] published an in-depth review of urinary findings in a wide variety of sporting activities. They found that 60% to 80% of all athletes had red blood cells, albumin, and casts in their urine samples after exercise. There was no significant difference in the incidence of hematuria in athletes involved in contact as compared to noncontact sports; however, contact sport participants were more likely to have *gross* hematuria. Thus, it appears gross hematuria is caused by direct trauma. This concept was supported by Boone et al. in a study of urine samples from football players. The incidence of hematuria paralleled the players' participation in games and was more prevalent immediately following game day. Of the 37 players who participated in this study, 60% had hematuria, 16% of which was gross.[14] All hematuria resolved with bedrest. A similar study by Fletcher reported the results of urine samples obtained from 15 hockey players immediately after a game, and then 24, 48, and 72 hours thereafter. All players had some degree of hematuria that resolved within 72 hours.[30] Amelar and Solomon studied 103 boxers who gave urine samples before and after their fights. Microhematuria was noted in 73% of the boxers after the bout. The only significant factor associated with hematuria was the length of the fight. Surprisingly, the location and number of blows to the flank had no predictive value. In fights that lasted less than six rounds, 65% of the fighters had hematuria compared to 89% of the fighters in bouts lasting beyond six rounds. Gross hematuria was only found in boxers whose fights lasted longer than six rounds.[51]

In noncontact sports, the presence of hematuria is directly correlated with the duration and intensity of the activity. This relationship was originally documented by Kachadorian, who exercised male subjects on a treadmill. As the treadmill speed increased, so did the number of episodes of microscopic hematuria.[41] There have also been numerous reports on the effect of long distance running on both microscopic and gross hematuria.[6,13] Fassett et al. reported that 69% of athletes completing runs of 9 and 14 km had hematuria.[29] Siegel studied 50 physicians with no preexisting medical or renal disease who ran the Boston Marathon. Of these doctors, 18% developed hematuria immediately after the race.[60]

There are several potential mechanisms by which sports-related hematuria may occur. Aside from the usual mechanisms of trauma, there are complex pathophysiologic effects on renal function from exercise that cause sports hematuria (Fig. 6-1). The kidney at rest receives approximately 20% of the cardiac output or close to

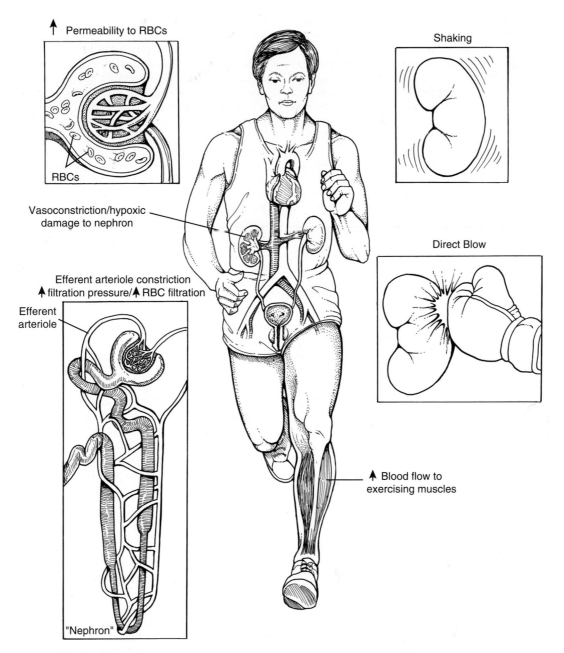

Fig. 6-1. Mechanisms of sports hematuria in the kidney. (Modified from Abarbanel J et al: J Urol 143:887, 1990.)

1200 ml/min. Renal plasma flow is approximately 700 ml/min. Thus, the blood flow to the kidney exceeds that to other metabolically active organs, such as the brain, liver, and heart, by three- to fivefold. Nonetheless, renal blood flow does not adjust to satisfy altered metabolic needs. When the body is stressed, the skeletal muscles, heart, and lungs require increased blood flow. As a result, there is a concomitant decrease in kidney and splanchnic blood flow, with the renal plasma flow decreasing to approximately 200 ml/min.[42] The decrease observed is proportional to the intensity of the exercise. Poortman demonstrated that moderate exercise resulted in a 30% reduction in plasma flow; heavy exercise resulted in a 75% reduction.[57] This decreased flow causes hypoxic damage to the nephrons, resulting in an increased per-

meability of the glomerulus, thereby allowing blood cells to pass through into the urine.[42]

A second pathophysiologic mechanism by which exercise may result in hematuria is renal vasoconstriction. Vasoconstriction resulting from exercise is more prominent in the efferent arteriole vasculature. This results in an increased filtration pressure, thereby producing stasis within the glomerular capillaries, which allows red blood cells to escape into the urine.[21] These physiologic hypotheses help to explain why 80% of swimmers, noncontact athletes, had hematuria compared to 55% of the football players in Alyea and Parish's study. Despite football's traumatic nature, the amount of exercise and *physiologic* stress involved in swimming is more profound.

Not all exercise-associated hematuria, however, is an

innocuous pathophysiologic response. The differential diagnosis of exercise-associated hematuria is identical to that of nonexercise-associated hematuria (see box below). The physician must also be aware of two entities that present with red colored urine yet fail to demonstrate red blood cells on urinalysis. The first is *march hemoglobinuria*. This occurs 1 to 3 hours after exercise in an upright position. Marching on hard surfaces results in mechanical trauma to the red blood cells in the feet. Hemolysis results, releasing hemoglobin which then binds to haptoglobin. The excess unbound hemoglobin is cleared into the urine, giving the urine a reddish appearance.[16,56]

Exercise myoglobinuria is the second entity causing red colored urine without the presence of red blood cells. Exercise myoglobinuria appears 24 to 48 hours after the event and is the result of muscle fiber breakdown that releases myoglobin into the plasma. Myoglobin is readily cleared into the urine, resulting in the red discoloration.[25]

The important complications of sports hematuria that demand medical attention include anemia and renal failure. Anemia has been noted in athletes who are involved in daily exercise.[17] Renal dysfunction may result from prolonged strenuous exercise in the heat. The resultant dehydration will further decrease the renal blood flow which is already diminished in response to the exercise. This lowers the perfusion pressure below the critical threshold of the kidney, producing renal ischemia. Additionally, exercise results in muscle injury causing rhabdomyolysis and myoglobinuria, either of which can cause renal dysfunction by obstructing the renal tubules. Hemoglobinuria from intravascular hemolysis (see march hemoglobinuria) may also contribute to renal dysfunction by causing tubular necrosis.[36] Adequate fluid replacement to maintain urine output is critical to prevent acute renal failure.

Management of "physiologic" sports hematuria begins with recognition of this condition and reassuring the anxious athlete of the benign nature of this process. In the acute setting, dehydration should be corrected. The initial consultation should consist of a proper history and physical, a urinalysis, and a urine culture. The urinalysis should be repeated 48 to 72 hours after the insult. A normal urinalysis will essentially exclude significant renal and urologic disease. If the hematuria fails to resolve, further investigation is warranted. Sports hematuria should never be assumed to be the cause of hematuria in an athlete, rather it is a diagnosis of exclusion. Radiologic evaluation and cystoscopy are reserved for persistent hematuria. Additional investigation for intrinsic renal causes is indicated if the patient continues to exhibit hematuria or a change in renal function.

No clear guidelines exist for the resumption of activity after an episode of gross hematuria. Some authors advocate bedrest until the hematuria has completely resolved. Most authors recommend that the athlete should not exercise until the gross hematuria has resolved; activity may resume if only microscopic hematuria persists. If all athletes adhered to the dictum that bedrest was required until hematuria resolved completely, numerous athletes, including possibly the entire starting lineup of your local football, lacrosse, or swim team would be sidelined. It appears that as long as gross hematuria becomes microscopic hematuria within 24 to 72 hours, activity may be resumed without adverse sequelae.[1]

RENAL INJURIES

The growing participation in sports has resulted in the increased frequency and diagnosis of sports related injuries. Abdominal and genitourologic trauma literature report that 5% to 10% of all trauma is related to sporting activities.[9,10,18,28,44,48,54,58] Sport-related injuries to the genitouri-

CAUSES OF HEMATURIA

Kidney
Acute renal failure

Cystic disease

Glomerulonephritis

Hemorrhagic Disorders: Hemophilia

Hydronephrosis

Infectious Diseases: Tuberculosis

Ischemia

Neoplasm

Pyelonephritis

Renal calculus

Renal infarct

Trauma

Vascular diseases

Ureter
Neoplasm

Strictures

Trauma

Ureteral calculus

Bladder
Bladder calculus

Cystitis

Neoplasm

Trauma

Prostate
Benign prostatic hypertrophy

Neoplasm

Prostatitis

Urethra
Foreign body

Neoplasm

Stricture

Trauma

Urethral calculus

Urethritis: Sexually transmitted disease

nary system may be the result of blunt or penetrating forces to the chest, abdomen, pelvis, perineum, or external genitalia. Genitourinary injury should be suspected when gross anatomical pathology is apparent. The severity of the hematuria, however, has not proven to be indicative of the severity of the injury. In the absence of visible signs or symptoms, the recognition and subsequent treatment requires a fundamental knowledge of the mechanism of injury, the anatomy and pathophysiology of the organs involved, and the appropriate diagnostic tests and treatment.

The kidney and its vasculature are well protected in the retroperitoneum surrounded by the abdominal wall, abdominal viscera, ribs, and back musculature (Fig. 6-2). A significant blow to the abdomen or flank is normally necessary to cause visible injury. Organs adjacent to the kidney may also be injured when trauma is sufficient to injure the kidney. The left kidney, proximal ureter, and adrenal gland are surrounded by Gerota's fascia. Adjacent structures include the spleen, diaphragm, tail of the pancreas, posterolateral chest wall, lower three ribs, and descending colon. The right kidney, proximal ureter, and adrenal gland within Gerota's fascia are displaced approximately 1 to 2 cm below the left kidney by the liver and are in close proximity to the duodenum.

The kidney is the most common urologic organ injured from both blunt and penetrating trauma, and in certain sports, such as skiing, may be the most commonly injured thoracoabdominal organ.[58] The exact incidence of renal trauma due to sports injuries has not been well defined. The trauma literature for children and adults report an incidence of renal injuries due to sports of between 10% to 33%. A review of all urologic trauma in the Pacific Northwest by Krieger et al. found 184 urologic injuries, of which 154 injuries included the kidney. Of these renal injuries, 20% were directly sports related.[44] Bergqvist reported on all abdominal trauma over a 30-year period in Sweden and found that 29% of the injuries involved the kidney.[10] Renal trauma in children is related to sports activities in 10% to 25% of the cases.[18,38,48,54] Virtually every sporting activity has been associated with renal trauma and its consequences.[9,10,14,18,28,33,40,43,48,58,63]

Renal injuries are classified as minor or major based upon the severity of damage to the parenchyma, collecting system, and vasculature. Minor injuries include contusions, perirenal hematomas, and parenchymal lacerations confined to the cortex (Fig. 6-3). They are most commonly associated with direct blunt flank trauma or a contrecoup injury whereby the kidneys are thrown forward as the athlete encounters rapid deceleration forces. The kidneys are quite mobile within Gerota's fascia, and a direct blow to the flank or abdomen can cause parenchymal lacerations or contusions by compression of the kidney against the surrounding musculature or vertebral bodies.[23] The result of these contusions or lacerations is local extravasation of blood beneath the renal capsule. These injuries are not usually serious and complete recovery is expected. Infection of the hematoma is a rare late complication.

Major injuries, which are rarely seen in sporting events, include deep parenchymal disruption with extension into the collecting system, a vascular injury, or a shattered kidney (Fig. 6-4). These injuries are usually caused by associated fractures of the lower ribs or transverse processes. A severe laceration may extend into the collecting system or cause the renal capsule to rupture with subsequent development of a perirenal hematoma. The most violent injuries cause either avulsion or thrombosis of the renal artery and/or vein. Because the kidney is quite mobile, deceleration injuries result in the stretching of the renal vessels, producing a tear in the renal vein or intimal tears in the artery with subsequent spasm and thrombosis.[26] Injuries of this magnitude usually require exploration and an attempt to salvage the kidney, depending on the status of the patient and the associated injuries.

It is important to realize that abnormal organs are more susceptible to injury. Thus renal cancer, ureteropelvic junction obstructions, renal cysts, horseshoe kidneys, and duplex or ectopic kidneys will usually require less trauma to cause significant injury.[50] The incidence of renal abnormalities in children is reported to range between 1% and 23%,[49] making children more likely to experience renal injury after apparently minor trauma. Furthermore, as discussed by Kuzmarov, children have less perirenal fat, weaker abdominal musculature, and proportionately larger kidneys relative to abdominal size of an adult. Therefore, children deserve special attention, as they are more prone to renal injury after blunt trauma than adults. The child may also still have fetal lobulations that are more susceptible to parenchymal laceration.[46] This point was highlighted by Sparnon and Ford's article on bicycle handlebar injuries. In this report no child showed signs or symptoms immediately following the trauma. Subsequently, five children presented with severe renal lacerations requiring three nephrectomies.[63]

Evaluation begins with a history, detailed physical exam, and appropriate laboratory studies. Because the kidneys are so well protected by the ribs and surrounding musculature, the magnitude of force required to injure the kidney will also result in injuries to other organs. Associated injuries are observed in 60% to 80% of patients with blunt renal injuries and 90% of penetrating injuries.[26] Fractures of the extremities, injuries to the head, and lacerations of the liver and spleen are the most common concurrent injuries.

The most common presenting sign in renal injury is gross or microscopic hematuria. A minor renal injury may present without hematuria if the collecting system is not involved. However, it cannot be emphasized enough that the absence of hematuria does not exclude the possibility of a severe renal injury. A major injury such as an avulsed ureter or a lacerated or thrombosed renal vessel may also present without gross or microscopic hematuria. Dixon and McAninch reported that 19% to 36% of renal pedicle injuries have normal urinalyses.[26] The diagnosis of renal injury thus requires a high index of suspicion. Therefore, even without significant signs or symptoms, any injury to the lower chest, abdomen, or flank warrants attention to the genitourinary tract.

The signs or symptoms which may be associated

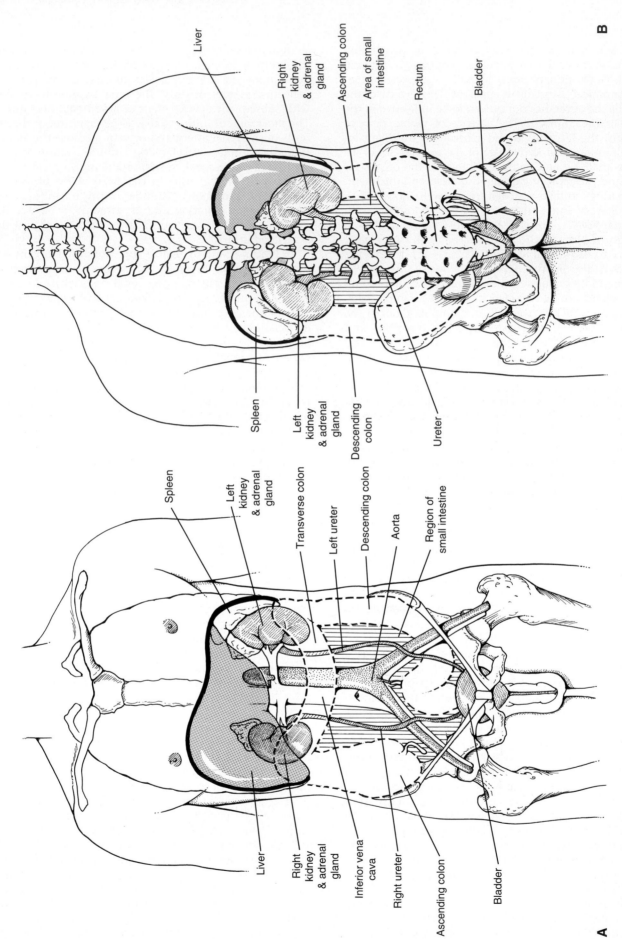

Fig. 6-2. Anatomic relationships of the kidneys and ureters. **A**, Anterior anatomic positions of frequently injured organs. **B**, Posterior anatomic positions of frequently injured organs.

Liver

Right kidney & adrenal gland

Ascending colon

Area of small intestine

Rectum

Bladder

Spleen

Left kidney & adrenal gland

Descending colon

Ureter

Spleen

Left kidney & adrenal gland

Transverse colon

Left ureter

Descending colon

Aorta

Region of small intestine

Liver

Right kidney & adrenal gland

Inferior vena cava

Right ureter

Ascending colon

Bladder

B

A

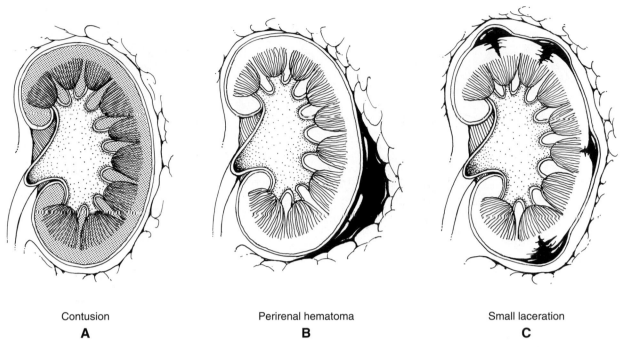

Contusion	Perirenal hematoma	Small laceration
A	**B**	**C**

Fig. 6-3. Classification of minor renal injuries. **A**, Contusion; **B**, perirenal hematoma; **C**, small parenchymal laceration less than 1 cm in length that does not extend into the collecting system.

with renal injury include a palpable mass, muscle tenderness or spasm, rib fractures, flank pain, or colic. Severe injuries may have similar findings; however, these patients are often in clinical shock and become surgical emergencies.

The initial diagnostic study in a stable patient should be an excretory urography with tomograms. An abdominal film may show loss of renal contour or psoas shadow, a fractured rib or transverse process, bowel displacement, or elevation of the hemidiaphragm. Intra-

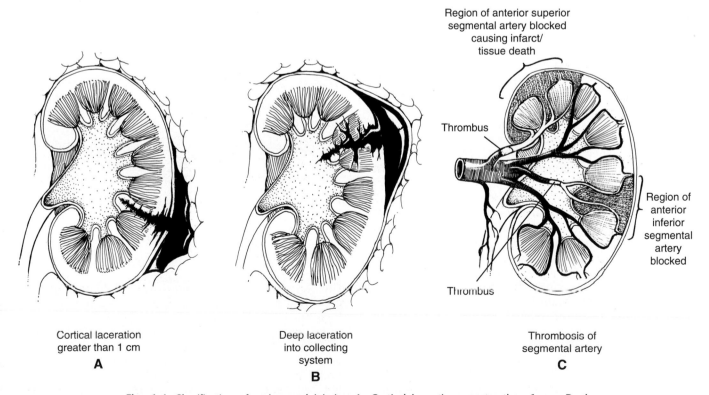

Cortical laceration greater than 1 cm	Deep laceration into collecting system	Thrombosis of segmental artery
A	**B**	**C**

Fig. 6-4. Classification of major renal injuries. **A**, Cortical lacerations greater than 1 cm; **B**, deep parenchymal lacerations extending into the collecting system; **C**, thrombosis of a segmental renal artery.
Continued.

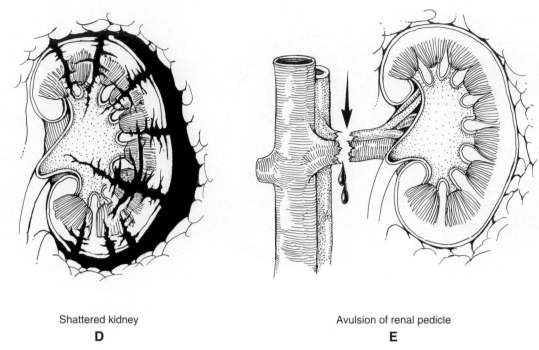

Shattered kidney

D

Avulsion of renal pedicle

E

Fig. 6-4, cont'd. D, Multiple lacerations (i.e., a shattered kidney); **E**, renal pedicle avulsion.

venous pyelography (IVP) will detect most major renal injuries, including diminution or nonvisualization of a portion of or the entire renal unit, pelvicalyceal displacement, cortical mass defects, or extravasation of contrast, but may not provide adequate staging information when expectant treatment is planned for high risk patients. In fact as many as 33% to 60% of IVPs may not be adequate to exclude a major renal injury.[26] In these cases a CT scan of the abdomen and pelvis is warranted. Because patients with urologic trauma frequently have associated injuries, a CT scan may be the first test of choice. The CT scan is more accurate in differentiating between minor and major renal injury (Figs. 6-5, 6-6). Renal nuclear scans are of limited value but may be used in patients with contrast allergies when there is concern about renal perfusion. Angiography is utilized only when there is evidence of a vascular injury severe enough to require surgical intervention in an otherwise stable patient.

The majority of sports-related trauma to the kidneys results in minor injuries such as contusions and small lacerations, which can be treated conservatively with bedrest and supportive therapy. The athlete with a parenchymal laceration should abstain from contact sports for 6 weeks with a repeat IVP at 3 months. Of patients with blunt trauma and minor injuries, 97% can be managed in this manner.[26] Surgical intervention is rarely required for sports-related trauma and is reserved for a major laceration, fracture, vasculature, or pedicle injury. All patients with severe renal trauma should be followed at 3-month intervals with a urinalysis and an IVP for at least 1 year. Athletes with severe renal trauma should not return to contact sports for 6 to 12 months, if at all.[22]

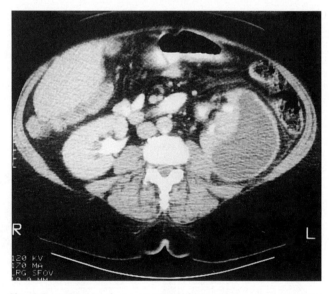

Fig. 6-5. A CT scan demonstrating a large subcapsular hematoma.

URETERAL INJURIES

Ureteral injuries secondary to external trauma are exceedingly rare, accounting for less than 1% of all urologic trauma.[24] The right ureter lies behind the duodenum proximally and the mesentery, terminal ileum, and appendix distally. The right colic, ileocolic, and gonadal vessels cross the ureter anteriorly. The left ureter lies behind the sigmoid colon, and the gonadal, left colic, and sigmoid colon vessels. The ureter, with its narrow caliber and retroperitoneal location, is sur-

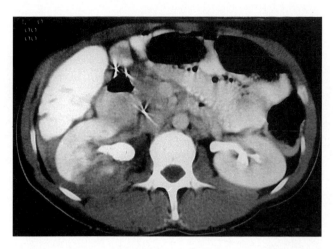

Fig. 6-6. A 20-year-old male with right flank pain while playing football. The CT scan demonstrates a fracture of the posterior medial parenchyma of the kidney.

rounded by fat and muscle and is well protected from injury (Fig. 6-2).

Ureteral trauma is most often the result of penetrating injury, rarely occurring from blunt trauma. Due to associated abdominal injuries and mechanism of the injury, diagnosing a ureteral injury is usually not an immediate concern. Signs and symptoms of ureteral injury are not specific but instead are common to abdominal, renal, and bladder injuries. An IVP is the study of choice for documenting ureteral injuries, followed by retrograde pyelography if the IVP is indeterminate. Abdominal exploration is often required due to the associated injuries. When ureteral injuries are diagnosed, the ureter is primarily reconstructed over a nephroureteral stent. However, the operative decision is based upon the findings and the mechanism of injury. A nephrectomy is rarely necessary.

BLADDER INJURIES

The incidence of bladder injury, as in ureteral injury, is also extremely uncommon in sports. The bladder is a pelvic organ behind the pubic symphysis. In children the bladder assumes an abdominal position and thus is more susceptible to injury. The bladder is protected anteriorly and laterally by the pubic arch, supported inferiorly by the pelvic diaphragm and superiorly by the peritoneum and intraperitoneal structures. The superior surface of the bladder is in close contact with the uterus and ileum in the female and with the ileum and portions of the colon in the male. The base of the bladder is separated from the rectum by the uterus and vagina in the female and by the seminal vesicles, vas deferens, and ureter in the male (Fig. 6-7A, B).

There is approximately a 5% to 10% incidence of bladder injury in the trauma literature.[9,10,18,40,44,66] Bladder rupture is rarely an isolated injury, and associated injuries are found in 94% to 97% of the cases.[66] Blunt trauma accounts for up to 80% of all bladder injuries with the remainder due to penetrating injuries. Al-

though up to 80% of patients with blunt injuries to the bladder will have an associated pelvic fracture, only 10% to 16% of patients with pelvic fractures will have an associated bladder injury.[27,66]

Bladder injuries are classified as contusions, extraperitoneal ruptures, intraperitoneal ruptures, or a combination of both extra- and intraperitoneal ruptures. Extraperitoneal rupture is twice as common as intraperitoneal rupture, with both occurring in 12% of cases. Contusions of the bladder are diagnosed after the exclusion of more severe injuries in patients with hematuria and account for 45% of bladder injuries.[15]

The mechanism of bladder injury differs between adults and children. In the child, the bladder is an abdominal organ; in the adult the bladder is a pelvic organ. Therefore, bladder injuries in children are usually intraperitoneal. Abdominal pain in a child after trauma may indicate a bladder injury.

Bladder rupture from blunt trauma occurs by three mechanisms. Intraperitoneal rupture may occur secondary to the hydraulic forces resulting from compression of a full bladder. The bladder thus ruptures at its weakest point—the dome. A direct blow to a full bladder may cause a bladder wall contusion and result in urinary extravasation into the extraperitoneal perivesical space or into the peritoneum. Pelvic fractures may result in the formation of bony spicules which lacerate the bladder and lead to extraperitoneal urinary extravasation. Additionally, shear forces may cause the ligaments attached to the bladder to forcefully disengage and lacerate the bladder.[66]

The diagnosis of bladder injuries may be delayed due to the associated major trauma. An inability to void is frequently observed. The first indication of a bladder rupture may be a nonpalpable bladder with absence of urine output after placement of a Foley catheter. Intraperitoneal urine will irritate the peritoneum, causing tenderness, muscle guarding, and abdominal rigidity. There may be ecchymosis of the lower abdomen, pubic region, or perineum. Gross or microscopic hematuria is present in 82% to 97% of the cases. Of patients with gross hematuria, 50% have significant bladder injuries compared with 2% with microscopic hematuria.[66]

A cystogram with a postdrainage film is the diagnostic test of choice in patients suspected of having bladder injuries. If a pelvic fracture is diagnosed on the basis of clinical findings or x-ray findings, a retrograde urethrogram should be performed to rule out urethral pathology prior to the insertion of a urethral catheter. After placement of the Foley catheter, the initial plain abdominal x-ray may show free air. A properly performed cystogram with instillation of up to 400 cc of contrast by gravity filling can achieve close to 100% diagnostic accuracy. The bladder should be completely filled, thus stretching the bladder and dislodging blood clots that may have sealed off a bladder tear. A postdrainage film is essential and by itself will result in the diagnosis of small extraperitoneal ruptures in 13% of the cases (Fig. 6-8).[66] Intraperitoneal rupture will be demonstrated by contrast around loops of

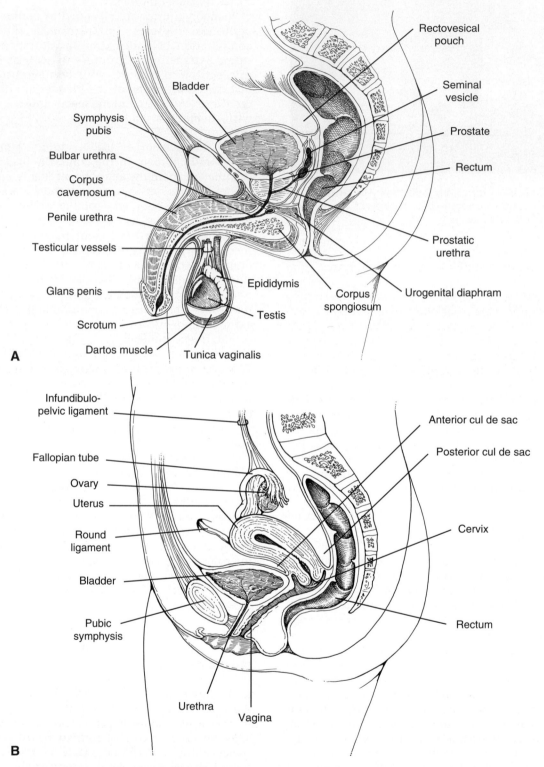

Fig. 6-7. A, Anatomic relations of the male bladder, prostate, penis, urethra, and scrotum. **B,** Anatomic relations of the female bladder, urethra, uterus, ovaries, and vagina.

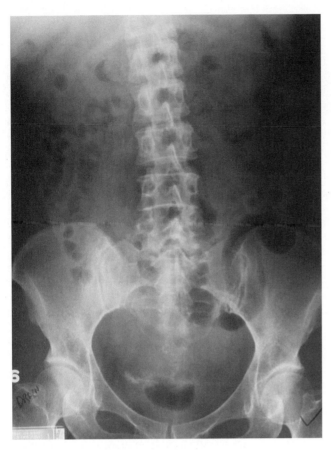

Fig. 6-8. A post urinary drainage film documenting a small extraperitoneal bladder rupture.

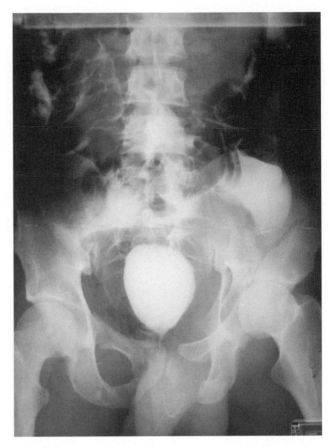

Fig. 6-9. Intraperitoneal bladder rupture with contrast extravasating throughout the peritoneum. Of note is the pubic rami fracture.

bowel within the peritoneal cavity. Contrast may also be visualized streaming along the "gutters" of the posterior peritoneum along the psoas muscles (Fig. 6-9). A CT scan, usually performed to aid in the diagnosis of the associated injuries, may demonstrate both intraperitoneal and extraperitoneal extravasation. Extraperitoneal ruptures are seen as "flamelike" or "star burst" areas of contrast extravasation. Another common finding is the "tear drop" or "spindle shape" bladder due to the compression of the bladder by a large pelvic hematoma (Fig. 6-10). Cystography is rarely warranted in patients with blunt trauma without gross hematuria, as the incidence of a significant bladder injury is less than 2% with microscopic hematuria.

The most common sports related bladder injury is the bladder contusion. Cystography is usually normal or may demonstrate clots in the bladder. Generally, no treatment is required, although a urethral catheter may be placed if the patient experiences difficulty in voiding. Bladder contusions were first described by Blacklock, who noted characteristic cystoscopic findings in long distance runners with hematuria, in whom no upper tract pathology was noted. Within 48 hours of the injury, bladder contusions appeared on specific areas of the dome and base of the bladder and the bladder neck. These observations suggest that the contusions are the result of the posterior bladder wall striking the base of the empty bladder. Running with even a small amount

of urine to absorb the trauma can prevent this type of benign hematuria.[12]

Extraperitoneal bladder ruptures should be treated with drainage by a urethral catheter for 10 to 14 days. Intraperitoneal rupture, however, requires surgical exploration, repair of the laceration, and catheter drainage. If the patient is to undergo surgical exploration for associated injuries, an extraperitoneal laceration may then be concurrently repaired.[66]

URETHRAL INJURIES

Urethral injuries are more common in sports than one would expect. These injuries are the result of straddle injuries to the perineum and are commonly seen in gymnastics, bicycling,[32,47,83] horseback riding,[31] and winter sports accidents.[39,40,67] A urethral injury may present with blood at the urethral meatus or hematuria.

The male is far more likely than the female to sustain a urethral injury. The male urethra is divided into anterior and posterior portions (Fig. 6-7,A). The anterior urethra is distal to the urogenital diaphragm, which surrounds the external sphincter. The anterior urethra includes the bulbar and pendulous or penile urethra. In spite of its mobility, the anterior urethra, which is contained within the corpus spongiosum, is most commonly injured by blunt trauma. In straddle type injuries,

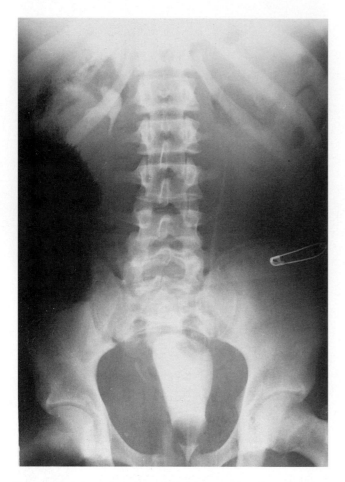

Fig. 6-10. A tear drop-shaped bladder resulting from the compression of a large extraperitoneal hematoma.

the bulbar urethra is crushed against the undersurface of the pubic rami. Reports of even minor trauma to the urethra such as occurs from hard banana type bicycle seats can cause urethral pathology.[32,47,53] Hematuria is the common presenting sign to these injuries. Anterior urethral injuries can usually be avoided with proper use of genital supporters and protectors.

The posterior portion of the urethra is above the urogenital diaphragm and includes the membranous and prostatic urethra. The membranous urethra is muscular and comprises both smooth muscle and skeletal muscle that form the external sphincter. The proximal prostatic urethra enters the bladder neck that constitutes the internal sphincter. Rupture of the posterior urethra is usually associated with pelvic fractures. Significant shearing forces are required to tear the prostate and prostatic urethra from the fixed membranous urethra. These will not only avulse the urethra but may damage the erectile neurovascular bundles alongside the prostate, causing hemorrhage and potential impotence. Whenever a pelvic fracture is present, a urethral injury should thus be suspected. An inability to void, blood at the meatus, a distended bladder out of the pelvis, and a high riding prostate gland on rectal exam are all indications of a posterior urethral injury.

The fascial planes of the perineum, penis, and scro-

tum help limit and delineate the boundaries of blood and urine extravasation that are associated with lower genitourinary tract injuries (Fig. 6-11, A). The corporal bodies of the penis are surrounded by Buck's fascia. Colles' fascia is attached to the triangular ligament and fascia lata of the thigh and is continuous with Scarpa's fascia of the abdominal wall. Buck's fascia will limit urinary/blood extravasation associated with an injury to the anterior urethra to the penile shaft. The result is a swollen ecchymotic distorted phallus. Because of the strong fascial planes of the urogenital membrane, an injury limited by Buck's fascia is not usually associated with extravasation of blood and urine into the scrotum or perineum. If an injury to the urethra is severe enough to violate Buck's fascia, blood and urine may reach the perineum, scrotum, and abdominal wall, being limited only by Colles' fascia (Fig. 6-11, B).

In a posterior urethral injury, blood and urine will be contained within the extraperitoneal or retroperitoneal space due to the strong fascial planes. With posterior urethral injuries, there should be no perineal ecchymosis unless there is disruption of the fascial planes. However, extravasation above the level of the membranous urethra may track along the spermatic cord into the scrotum, causing a swollen ecchymotic scrotum without disruption of normal fascial planes (Fig. 6-11, C).

A retrograde urethrogram is the most important diagnostic study to establish the presence of a partial or complete disruption of the urethra. Partial tears in the anterior urethra can be adequately managed with urethral catheter drainage, however, complete urethral disruptions will require placement of a suprapubic catheter and a formal repair at a later date. Most authors favor delayed repair of posterior urethral injuries to allow for the resorption of the associated pelvic hematoma. With resorption, the distance between the two portions of the urethra is shortened.[2] Recently, there has been a renewed enthusiasm for primary repair of posterior urethral injuries. The long term complications of the injury and the repair include impotence, urethral stricture, incontinence, diverticula, and fistulas.[49]

In the female, most injuries to the urethra involve lacerations from prolonged labor, instrumentation, or pelvic trauma. These injuries often go unrecognized, with the only presenting signs and symptoms being an inability to void or labial or vulvar edema. A successful urethral catheter placement does not rule out pathology. A cystoscopy is necessary for definitive diagnosis because a retrograde urethrogram may not be diagnostic. There have also been reports of urethral injuries in women with genital injuries during water sporting activities.[38,45,51,55] Urethral catheter drainage is usually sufficient treatment.[34]

GENITAL INJURIES

Injuries to the male genitalia are the most common genitourinary injuries in sports trauma with an incidence of 10% to 15%.[3,19,40] With an increasing participation of females in sports, there will certainly be more case reports of female genital injuries. Genital injuries are the most anxiety provoking of all genitourologic trauma for many

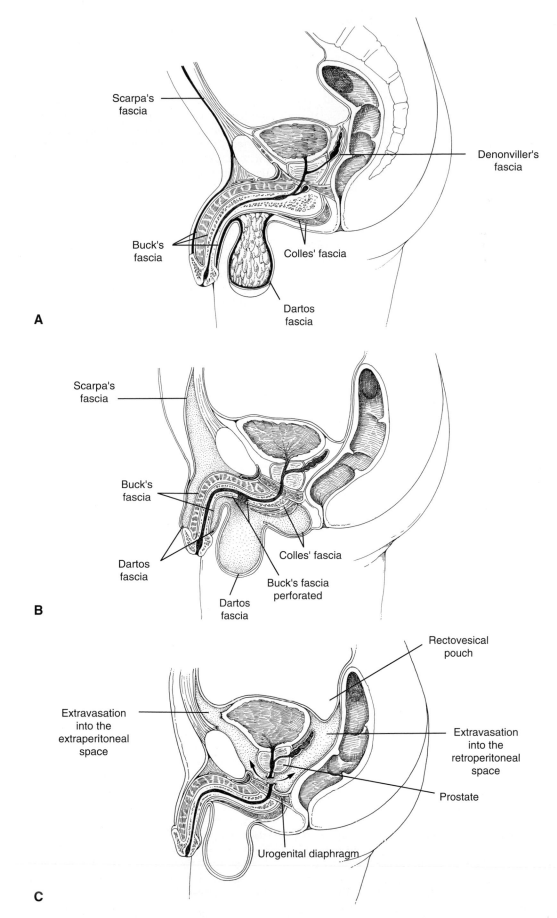

Fig. 6-11. A, The fascial planes of the male perineum, penis, and scrotum. **B,** An anterior urethral injury through Buck's fascia will allow extravasation of blood and urine into the perineum, scrotum, and anterior abdominal wall being limited by Colles' fascia. **C,** A posterior urethral injury will be contained within the extraperitoneal and retroperitoneal space as long as there are intact fascial planes. The scrotum may be swollen if the extravasation extends along the spermatic cord into the scrotum.

reasons. As most injuries occur in children, teenagers, and young adults where sexual identity is most important, the physician must be prepared to deal with not only the injury but the emotional concerns of the individual.

The testicle lies within the scrotal sac consisting of skin, dartos muscle, and external and internal spermatic fascia and is suspended by the spermatic cord that contains the testicular vessels (Fig. 6-7, A). The tunica albuginea is a tough, resilient capsule that encompasses the entire testicle. The scrotal sac is also surrounded by the tunica vaginalis, which was once continuous with the peritoneal cavity and surrounds the testicle, except posteriorly, where the epididymis attaches to the testicle.

Due to their mobility, the testes are not generally injured unless trapped against a fixed structure, as may occur in a straddle injury. In this circumstance the testicle is caught between a forceful object and the pubic bone or ischial rami. This is less common in the infant and young child due to the small size of the testicles. The right testicle is more often injured than the left, perhaps due to the higher position of the right testicle within the scrotum.[49]

Scrotal and testicular trauma have been widely reported in active team sports such as football, rugby, soccer, and baseball. Individual sports have also resulted in severe genital injuries. Children have sustained severe scrotal injuries on the handlebars of a BMX bicycle while jumping over obstacles. Severe scrotal skin avulsion with exposure of the testicles may be repaired with split thickness skin grafts.[64]

Testicular rupture may occur after forceful blunt trauma or penetrating trauma. The severe scrotal pain and swelling may make a physical examination very difficult to perform. Ruptured blood vessels may cause either ecchymosis in the overlying scrotal skin or a hematocele or hematoma within the tunica vaginalis. This renders palpation of the testicle very difficult.[59] Severe scrotal trauma may produce hematoceles, traumatic hydroceles, dislocation, contusion, and/or testicular rupture. Testicular torsion has also been attributed to testicular trauma with approximately a 10% incidence.[49] One must also be aware that testicular tumors may present with scrotal pain after minor trauma. Therefore, patients with scrotal injuries should be carefully followed until the swelling and hematoma have subsided to be certain that there are no underlying testicular abnormalities.

Ultrasound examination, a relatively quick, noninvasive test, is extremely helpful in differentiating between contusion, hematoma, and testicular rupture. If testicular torsion is suspected, a duplex ultrasound or radionuclide scan will provide a definitive answer in up to 95% of the cases.

Not all scrotal and testicular trauma is quite so dramatic. Adno reported on marathon runners who presented with perineal pain due to "jogger's testicles."[2] Vuong et al. observed perineal nodular indurations in cyclists that were referred to as "accessory" or third testicles. These developed from chronic microtrauma to the perineum and histologically consisted of pseudocysts with central areas of necrosis.[68] Mandell et al. discussed the "highball syndrome" seen in a lacrosse player and other athletes. The resulting testicular trauma occurred because of perineal trauma causing a forceful cremasteric contraction that drew the testicle into the inguinal region. The athlete subsequently complained of inguinal pain that resulted from the testicle pushing against the external ring. The treatment was orchiopexy.[50]

Treatment of testicular injuries is individualized according to the history, physical, and diagnostic tests. Testicular dislocation that results from a severe blow to the scrotum displaces the testicle to the inguinal, perineal, penile, pubic, or crural regions. This can usually be treated by manual reduction and rarely requires exploration and orchiopexy.[50] A contusion of the testicle will tamponade within the hydrocele sac and can be followed, with return to physical activity as the signs and symptoms abate.

In all cases of hematoceles and ecchymosis of the scrotum after trauma, a ruptured testicle should be suspected and scrotal exploration is warranted.[59] A hematocele or contusion of the testicle presents minimal risk to the patient. Blood clots and necrotic or nonviable tissue should be removed and the remaining tunica albuginea closed over the defect. Ruptured testicles can be salvaged by exploration when accomplished within 3 days of injury. Morbidity and duration of bedrest are decreased with early exploration.[35] These athletes should not return to athletic participation until completely recuperated from surgery. Any injury to the testicle should be taken seriously, as it has recently been reported that there is an unexpected increased incidence of infertility in men who sustained testicular trauma in adolescence.[52]

The penile shaft is composed of two cavernosa corpus and a corporus spongiosum that surrounds the urethra. The three corporal bodies are surrounded by Buck's fascia, a dense fibrous layer of tissue. Each corpora cavernosum is separately attached to the pubic arch. This attachment along with the suspensory and fundiform ligaments provide fixation and stability to the erect penis. The corporus spongiosum surrounds the urethra and expands at its distal end to form the glans penis.

Most penile injuries are not sport related. The most common injuries are zipper injuries and fractures of the erect penis during a sexual act. There have, however, been various individual reports of sports-related penile trauma. Penile insensitivity and impotence have both been reported as a result of bicycling on a standard narrow hard leather seat. Both vascular and neural compression have been implicated in these cases.[37,62] Perineal trauma associated with impotence was reported in a young basketball player, who while descending after dunking a basketball, slammed his perineum into an opponent's knee. Work-up revealed a total occlusion of his deep and dorsal penile arteries from either an intimal tear or disruption of the vessels.[65] Weakening of the corporal bodies secondary to the trauma of horseback riding has also been implicated as a cause of impotence.[11] Finally, two soccer players in one report presented to the physician with partial skin thickness burns of the penis, scrotum, and inner thigh as a result of the soda lime used to mark the lines on the playing field.[8]

Trauma to the penis may affect one or all of the corporal bodies. The physical examination may show a subcutaneous hematoma. Penile deviation and swelling may be prominent and occasionally result in voiding difficulties. Urethral injuries coexist in approximately 20% of patients with penile trauma.[34] The physical findings are determined by the fascial compartments. With an intact Buck's fascia, ecchymosis will be limited to the penis, while violation of the fascial plane may allow extravasation of the hematoma into the perineum or abdomen, as seen with urethral injuries (Figs. 6-11 A, B). Cavernosography usually identifies the site of extravasation and the fracture. A retrograde urethrogram is performed if a urethral injury is suspected. The treatment is individualized. A skin injury can be primarily repaired. If the corpora and urethra have been injured, then a primary surgical repair is warranted.

Female external or internal genital injuries are rare occurrences in conjunction with athletics and are associated with straddle type injuries seen in horseback riding, bicycling, and gymnastics. These injuries include labial contusions or lacerations, clitoral tears, vaginal and cervical lacerations, and urethral injuries. A variety of genital tract injuries have also been reported in association with water sports, particularly waterskiing and jetskiing. These include injury to the cervix, vaginal lacerations, perineal lacerations, salpingitis, tubo-ovarian abscess, and incomplete abortion.[45,51,55] In one case report, Haefner et al. describes a vaginal laceration requiring pudendal artery ligation when a jet skier fell behind the jet ski and the full force of the jet nozzle was directed into the vagina.[38]

As these patients are usually quite anxious and in a state of shock due to the tremendous bleeding associated with this injury, a sufficient initial assessment is usually very difficult. The patient may be present urinary retention requiring placement of a suprapubic catheter. Contusions or minor lacerations to the external genitalia can usually be controlled by manual compression. Deeper lacerations involving the vagina or cervix will require exploration and repair under general anesthesia. On exploration the surgeon must be aware of the possibility of both rectal and urethral injuries. Urethral injuries can usually be treated with catheter drainage. Long-term complications include vesicovaginal fistulas and urethral strictures.

THE ATHLETE WITH A SOLITARY PAIRED ORGAN

Having reviewed the genitourinary system with regard to sports trauma, one is left with the question of whether the athlete with a solitary testicle or kidney should be allowed to participate in contact sports. All too often physicians are approached by athletes, their parents, and coaches asking for recommendations and advice on this subject. Whether the absence of the testicle or kidney is the result of a congenital malformation or due to a previous injury, there is always the possibility of injury to the remaining organ.

Historically, physicians have recommended that the individual with the absence of one of the paired organs avoids participation in contact sports. However, current epidemiologic studies of sports injuries, clinical experience, and changing attitudes toward sports have prompted most physicians to avoid this attitude and instead to provide informed counseling to prospective athletes and their parents regarding risks, equipment for protection, and sports alternatives.[61]

However, even today, a consensus at all levels of athletic participation is still lacking. In order to gain some insight into the attitudes of college team physicians and athletic directors, Mandell et al. conducted a survey of 40 major universities across the country. This study found varied philosophical and individualized opinions. First there was a broad interpretation of what was a contact or collision sport. Only five universities had unrestricted athletic participation, while seven opposed any participation. Some schools required waivers to be signed by the athlete and the parents. Almost 80% of the respondents stated they would advise directing the athlete with a single paired organ into an alternative noncontact sport. The authors concluded from the study that the single organ athlete can compete, even at the college level, as long as the athlete and parents are correctly counseled as to the dangers of possible loss of the organ in question and the appropriate protective measures.[50]

When a child with a solitary organ wishes to compete in athletics today several considerations must be addressed. The child and parents should first be counseled in the pros and cons of contact sports and if possible should attempt to direct the child into a noncontact sport. If they still wish to participate in contact sports, proper counseling regarding the use of protective equipment as well as close supervision is warranted.

As discussed above, abnormal kidneys are more likely to suffer injury from otherwise innocuous trauma. Therefore, it is imperative that the normalcy of the solitary paired organ be assessed prior to participation in a contact sport. Although the possibility of loss of the organ in question is low, this complication and its consequences should be discussed with the parents, child, and coach. Those athletes with a solitary kidney or testicle and an anatomical variant, such as ureteropelvic junction abnormality, ectopic location, or a functional abnormality should not be allowed to participate in contact sports due to the increased susceptibility to injury.[50]

The overall incidence of genitourologic trauma in sporting events is low. In general terms, the prevention of serious urologic injuries, as with any injuries, include proper athletic physical conditioning, use of protective equipment, and reliable supervision. Successful management requires prompt assessment, diagnosis, and treatment.

REFERENCES

1. Abarbanel J, et al: Sports hematuria, *J Urol* 143:887–890, 1990.
2. Adno J: "Jogger's testicles" in marathon runners, *S Afr Med J* 65:1036, 1984.
3. Altarac S, et al: Testicular trauma sustained during football, *Acta Med Croatica* 47:141–143, 1993.
4. Alyea EP, Parish HH Jr: Renal response to exercise: urinary findings, *JAMA* 167:807, 1958.
5. Amelar RD, Solomon C: Acute renal trauma in boxers, *J Urol* 72:145–148, 1954.
6. Anonymous: The hematuria of a long distance runner, *Br Med J* 2:159, 1979.
7. Barach J: Physiological and pathological effects of severe exertion (marathon race) on circulatory and renal systems, *Arch Intern Med* 5:382, 1910.
8. Benmeir P, et al: Chemical burn due to contact with soda lime on the playground: a potential hazard for football players, *Burns* 19:358–359, 1993.
9. Bergqvist D, et al: Abdominal injuries in children: an analysis of 348 cases, *Injury* 16:217–220, 1985.
10. Bergqvist D, et al: Abdominal trauma during thirty years: analysis of a large case series, *Injury* 13:93–99, 1981.

11. Bissada NK: Penile joint, (letter) *South Med J* 85:1266–1267, 1992.

12. Blacklock NJ: Bladder trauma in the long-distance runner: "10,000 metres hematuria," *Br J Urol* 49:129–132, 1977.

13. Boileau M, et al: Stress hematuria: athletic pseudonephritis in marathoners, *Urology* 15:471–474, 1980.

14. Boone AW, Haltiwanger E, Chambers RL: Football hematuria, *JAMA* 158:1516, 1955.

15. Brosman SA, Fay R: Diagnosis and management of bladder trauma, *J Trauma* 13:687–694, 1973.

16. Buckle RM: Exertional (march) haemoglobinuria. Reduction of haemolytic episodes by use of sorbo-rubber insoles in shoes, *Lancet* 1:1136, 1965.

17. Carlson DL, Mawdsley RH: Sports anemia: a review of the literature, *Am J Sports Med* 14:109–112, 1986.

18. Cass AS: Blunt renal trauma in children, *J Trauma* 23:123–127, 1983.

19. Cass AS: Testicular trauma, *J Urol* 129:299–300, 1983.

20. Cass AS: Urethral injury in the multiple-injured patient, *J Trauma* 24:901–906, 1984.

21. Castenfors J: Renal function during prolonged exercise, *Ann N Y Acad Sci* 301:151–159, 1977.

22. Cianflocco AJ: Renal complications of exercise, *Clin Sports Med* 11:437–451, 1992.

23. Coady C, Stanish WD: Emergencies in sports: The young athlete, *Clin Sports Med* 7:625–640, 1988.

24. Corriere JN Jr: Ureteral injuries. In Gillenwater JY, ed: *Adult and Pediatric Urology* St Louis, 1991 Mosby–Year Book, 491–497, 1991.

25. Demos MA, Gitin EL, Kagen LJ: Exercise myoglobinemia and acute exertional rhabdomyolysis, *Arch Intern Med* 134:669–673, 1974.

26. Dixon AM, McAninch JW: Traumatic renal injuries, Part 1: Patient assessment and management, *AUA Update Series* 11:274–279, 1991.

27. Dretler SP, Schiff SF: Urologic emergencies. In Earle Wilkins Jr, ed: *Emergency Yearbook*, 674–700, 1989.

28. Emanuel B, Weiss H, Gollin P: Renal trauma in children, *J Trauma* 17:275–278, 1977.

29. Fassett RG, et al: Urinary red-cell morphology during exercise, *Br Med J* 285:1455–1457, 1982.

30. Fletcher DJ: Athletic pseudonephritis. Lertter to the editor, *Lancet* 1:910–911, 1977.

31. Flynn M: Disruption of symphysis pubis while horse riding: a report of two cases, *Injury* 4:357–359, 1973.

32. Frey JJ: Banana-seat hematuria (letter), *New Engl J Med* 287:938, 1972.

33. Fujita S, et al: Perirenal hematoma following judo training, *NY State J Med* 88:33–34, 1988.

34. Gill IS, McRoberts JW: New Directions in the Management of GU Trauma, *Mediguide to Urology* 5:1–8, 1992.

35. Goldman MS: Repair of shattered solitary testicle, *Urology* 24:229–231, 1984.

36. Goldzer RC, Siegel AJ: Renal abnormalities during exercise. In Straus R, ed: *Sports Medicine*, Philadelphia, 1984, WB Saunders.

37. Goodson JD: Pudendal neuritis from biking (letter), *New Engl J Med* 304:365, 1981.

38. Haefner HK, Anderson F, Johnson MP: Vaginal laceration following a jet ski incident, *Obstet Gynecol* 78:986–988, 1991.

39. Hildreth TA, Cass AS, Khan AU: Winter sports-related urologic trauma, *J Urol* 121:62–67, 1979.

40. Jakse G, Madersbacher H: Winter sports injuries in the urogenital tract, *Urologe A* 16:315–319, 1977.

41. Kachadorian WA, Johnson RE: Athletic pseudonephritis in relation to rate of exercise, *Lancet* 1:472, 1970.

42. Kachadorian WA, Johnson RE: Renal response to various rates of exercise, *J Appl Physiol* 28:748–752, 1970.

43. Kleinman AH: Hematuria in boxers, *JAMA* 168:1633–1640, 1958.

44. Krieger JN, et al: Urological trauma in the Pacific Northwest: etiology, distribution, management and outcome, *J Urol* 132:70–73, 1984.

45. Kuntz WD: Water-ski spill and partial avulsion of the uterine cervix, *New Engl J Med* 309:990, 1983.

46. Kuzmarov IW, Morehouse DD, Gobson S: Blunt renal trauma in the pediatric population: a retrospective study, *J Urol* 126:648–649, 1981.

47. LeRoy JB: Banana-seat hematuria (letter), *New Engl J Med* 287:311, 1972.

48. Linke CA, et al: Renal trauma in children, *NY State J Med* 72:2414–2420, 1972.

49. Livine PM, Gonzales ET: Genitourinary trauma in children, *Urol Clin North Am* 12:53–65, 1985.

50. Mandell J, et al: Sports related genitourinary injuries in children, *Clin Sports Med* 1:483–493, 1982.

51. Morton DC: Gynaecological complications of water-skiing, *Med J Aust* 1:1256–1257, 1970.

52. Nolten WE, et al: Association of elevated estradiol with remote testicular trauma in young infertile men, *Fetil Steril* 62:143–149, 1994.

53. O'Brien KP: Sports urology: the vicious cycle (letter), *New Engl J Med* 304:1367–1368, 1981.

54. Persky L, Forsythe WE: Renal trauma in childhood, *JAMA* 132:709, 1962.

55. Pfanner D: Salpingitis and water-skiing, *Med J Aust* 1:320, 1964.

56. Pollard TD, Weiss IW: Acute tubular necrosis in a patient with march hemoglobinuria, *N Engl J Med* 283:803–804, 1970.

57. Poortman JR: Exercise and renal function, *Sports Med* 1:125–153, 1984.

58. Scharplatz D, Thurleman K, Enderlin F: Thoracoabdominal trauma in ski accidents, *Injury* 10:86–91, 1978.

59. Schuster G: Traumatic rupture of the testicle and a review of the literature, *J Urol* 127:1194–1196, 1982.

60. Siegel AJ, et al: Exercise related hematuria. Findings in a group of marathon runners, *JAMA* 241:391–392, 1979.

61. Smith NJ: Participation of athletes with one testicle (letter), *Am J Dis Child* 140:89–90, 1986.

62. Solomon S, Cappa KG: Impotence and bicycling: A seldom reported connection, *Postgrad Med* 81:99–102, 1987.

63. Sparnon AL, Ford WDA: Bicycle handlebar injuries in children, *J Pediatr Surg* 21:118–119, 1986.

64. Sparnon T, Moretti K, Sach RP: BMX handlebar: A threat to manhood? *Med J Aust* 2:587–588, 1982.

65. St Louis EL, et al: Basketball-related impotence (letter), *New Engl J Med* 308:595–596, 1983.

66. Thomas CL, McAninch JW: Bladder Trauma, *AUA Update Series* 8:242–246, 1989.

67. Towers RJ: Complete transection of urethra: a urogenital ski injury, *Rocky Mount Med J* 74:81–82, 1977.

68. Vuong PN, Camuzard P, Schoonaert M: Perineal nodular indurations ("Accessory testicles") in cyclists, *Acta Cytol* 32:86–90, 1988.

CHAPTER 7

PREPARTICIPATION EVALUATION

Andrew M. Tucker
John A. Bergfeld

The preparticipation physical examination for athletes is frequently looked upon with some contempt by participant and health care provider alike. The health care provider often is taking time from a busy schedule to face large numbers of athletes, sometimes in a less than ideal setting. The athlete, too, dreads the endless lines, medical scrutiny, and potentially embarrassing situations. Many of us remember this, perhaps accepting it as a right of passage or form of 'hazing' mandatory to pursuing dreams of athletic glory.

Despite possible personal biases, the preparticipation evaluation deserves the best effort from those caring for our athletic population. Much has been written about the screening encounter, and while some areas may be continuing sources of confusion and controversy, our present knowledge should allow us to conduct an examination that is effective and efficient. This chapter will review the many considerations for evaluation of our athletes and their preparation for athletic competition.

OVERVIEW OF THE PREPARTICIPATION PHYSICAL EXAMINATION (PPE)

Philosophy

There are differing philosophies that govern the approach to the PPE. One school of thought suggests that the PPE should be broad in scope, based on data that indicates approximately 80% of adolescents report the PPE serves as their annual health evaluation.[13,24] Many less privileged adolescents, as may live in the inner city of many metropolitan areas, often do not have a source of regular health care.[27] Thus, expanding the examination would be important to provide for the opportunity for early detection of medical disorders in these young people.

An opposing philosophy has emphasized that the primary goal of the PPE is to identify conditions that only impact on safe participation; thus the scope of the exam can be limited. Proponents point out that it is inappropriate for the screening examination to be expanded to serve as the adolescent's primary care visit, and expanding the examination potentially serves to decrease its efficiency and effectiveness.[11] While the authors favor the latter school of thought, we also would emphasize that different settings will dictate the scope of the PPE. Collegiate and professional teams have the resources to perform in-depth evaluations of potential team members. Also, in these situations, the team physician is becoming the primary care physician for the athlete. Thus an expanded examination is appropriate. At the high school or community level, the larger number of athletes and limited resources often require a PPE that is efficient and focused on the issues of safe participation.

Outcomes

To gain a different perspective on the PPE, a number of studies allow evaluation of outcomes of PPE screening.[13,14,16,24,29,30] Although differing methodologies make direct comparison between these studies somewhat difficult, the available data can give important information (see Table 7-1).

The studies underscore the low rates of disqualification for the PPE. This would be expected as the population being screened is young and generally very healthy, and therefore the incidence of potential disqualifying conditions is quite low. In addition, some conditions being screened for (e.g., hypertrophic cardiomyopathy) can be both asymptomatic and undetectable on routine physical examination. Thus false negative examinations will occur.[32]

Also contributing to these low rates of referral and disqualification would be an element of under reporting in this population. From adolescent to professional, athletes intent on playing their sport of choice may withhold information if they perceive they could be

Table 7-1. Outcomes of recent preparticipation evaluations

Study	Method	Number	Temporary disqualification requiring evaluation	Eventual disqualification	No disqualification but "MD attention advised"
Risser et al., 1982	Station/individual	763	16	2	213
Tennant, 1981	Station	271	32	N/A	217
Goldberg et al., 1980	Station	701	104*	9	N/A
Linder et al., 1981	Station	1268	64	2	N/A
Thompson et al., 1982	Station	2670	31	N/A†	257‡
Hough and McKeag, 1982	N/A	989	10%	1.1%	N/A

*Includes 40 with proteinuria. None had positive work-up.
†One found to have hypertrophic cardiomyopathy; one found to have severe mitral stenosis.
‡Includes 2 or greater proteinuria on dipstick urinalysis.
From Matzen RN, Lang RS: *Clinical Preventive Medicine,* 1993, Mosby–Year Book.

jeopardizing their own clearance to play. Likewise, some athletes may unknowingly omit or withhold information because they might think it is irrelevant or unimportant.[32]

It is helpful to note that the outcome of the PPE can depend significantly on the examiners themselves. The type of specialists involved and their knowledge of sports medicine may affect the findings and rates of referrals.[32] Examining physicians tend to be more sensitive to parts of the examination that are related to their particular interest or expertise.[16] In another study, the authors pointed out the high incidence of musculoskeletal findings was attributable to the large number of orthopedists involved.[30]

The cost effectiveness of preparticipation screening has been questioned. With low rates of disqualification and referral, it is not surprising that the PPE would not stand up to rigid cost-benefit analyses. One study performed a cost-benefit analysis of screening examinations for two groups of high school students in Houston and demonstrated a cost of $4537.00 for each disqualification.[24] The authors of the study made recommendations that could increase the cost effectiveness of the screening examination: (1) having subspecialty consultation available at the examinations, thus minimizing the expensive referrals; (2) by using a station examination method, large groups of athletes can be screened in a relatively short period of time; (3) require physical examinations at only entry levels of competition (junior high, high school, college) with encounters scheduled in the intervening years to screen for new problems; and (4) avoiding unnecessary tests (e.g., urine, hemoglobin) that have been shown to be cost ineffective screening methods.[24] Although the PPE may not stand up to cost-benefit analyses, the authors feel the real emphasis on outcomes of PPEs should be ensuring the safe participation of as many as possible as opposed to the restriction of activity of few.

State Requirements

A review of state guidelines for scholastic PPEs indicates significant variability and inconsistency among requirements governing these evaluations.[8] Thirty-five of 45

states that responded to a questionnaire indicated their requirement was for annual examinations. Six states actually had no requirement regarding the frequency of examination. Nine states had no official medical history and physical examination form. Of 36 states with forms, 9 did not include any medical history questions. Of those with medical history questions, the number of questions ranged from 1 to 200. A few of the states required specific laboratory testing, such as urinalysis, TB testing, and hemoglobin. Three states provided examiners with a list of AMA recommended contraindications for participation or recommendation for further evaluation. Although most states authorized only physicians to perform the PPE, some states allowed nurse practitioners or physician assistants, and three states did not specify who was authorized. Many are urging that current knowledge and understanding of the PPE needs to be applied to encourage more uniform standards across the country for this important evaluation.[32]

GOALS OF THE PPE

Defining the goals of the examination helps to define the appropriate content of the encounter. Most agree that the primary goal of the examination "should be the detection of athletes who would be at medical risk if they engage in competition."[1a] This includes the detection of those rare underlying conditions which may increase the risk of sudden death (e.g., hypertrophic cardiomyopathy) as well as medical conditions which might manifest or be worsened with participation (e.g., exercise-induced asthma or trauma-induced headaches). Relatively few athletes are disqualified on the basis of an underlying medical condition. Knowledge or awareness of a condition that might be worsened or manifested with participation is important for the athlete and the medical staff, as preventive measures can be instituted that hopefully will decrease the likelihood of morbidity from a given condition.

Another important goal is the uncovering of physical deficiencies that may put a participant at increased risk for injury.[23] These deficiencies may include incompletely rehabilitated injuries, developmental, or congenital problems of the musculoskeletal system. Data has shown that identification of physical deficiencies or residual injury and subsequent rehabilitation of these deficiencies, can decrease the risk of further injury.[1]

Another important goal is the fulfillment of state and local legal and insurance requirements.[17] As noted above, requirements may vary considerably from state to state. A physician should be knowledgeable of the state and local requirements where he practices.

The authors emphasize that these three goals must be met when planning and executing the PPE. Besides this "bare minimum," other worthwhile goals exist and depend on many variables and circumstances.

There are many secondary objectives proposed by several sources. One is the determination of the general health of the athlete.[23] Although many would agree that the PPE is not meant to replace the athlete's regular health maintenance examination, the fact remains that for many young athletes, the PPE remains the only contact with the health care system. Thus, attention to general health maintenance issues would be an important added benefit.[23]

As a related goal, the PPE may offer an opportunity for a health care provider to counsel the young athlete on various health related questions.[19] This goal may be difficult to meet in certain examination set-ups (e.g., station type). Counsel regarding such important topics as drug and alcohol use, tobacco use, nutrition, seat belt use, breast and testicular self-examination, and birth control are all worthy topics for discussion.

One controversial potential goal of the PPE is the evaluation of level of maturity of the younger athlete as it relates to recommendations for safe participation.[4,7,17] The open epiphyseal plates in a skeletally immature athlete represent potential sites of injury.[20] Exposing the skeletally immature athlete to collision sports against more mature counterparts may be an important risk factor for injury.[19] In addition, the immature athlete is usually at a competitive disadvantage in regards to speed, strength, and power, and thus may be more likely to fail in his or her efforts to make the team. This potentially negative psychologic trauma may have lasting effects. Thoughtful counselling with the participant and parents may help avoid this situation. Therefore, proponents would favor separating athletes for competition by maturity rather than age, especially as it relates to contact and collision sports.[23]

Opponents of this philosophy argue that the assessment is embarrassing for athletes and that there has been no definite data linking greater physical or psychological damage occurring when less mature athletes compete against more mature counterparts.[23] Male Tanner staging is easily accomplished during the genital examination, however, assessing breast bud size or pubic hair distribution in young females is more difficult and embarrassing. One alternative is self-rating of pubic hair and breast stage and has been shown to correlate well with that of an examining physician.[6,15] It is the authors' opinion that "maturity mismatching" in contact and collision sports is worthy of thoughtful counselling but should not be the basis for exclusion of participation until further data can prove this is warranted.

Another potential goal is the assessment of fitness so that performance and participation can be maximized.[2,4,13] Evaluation of parameters such as flexibility, strength, and body composition can be the basis for appropriate training modifications. Exercise physiologists, athletic trainers, and physical therapists are often utilized to help carry out these determinations. This is often accomplished during collegiate and professional PPEs where there is a heightened "vested interest" in the performance of the athletes. Assessment of body composition and determination of appropriate weight is important, especially in sports where weight loss techniques are frequently abused (e.g., wrestling, gymnastics).[32]

And finally, the PPE can serve as the entry of an athlete into a local health care or sports medicine system.[19] The establishment of a relationship with a trusted physician can be an important resource for the athlete regarding health-related issues.

To summarize, the basic goals of the PPE must be accomplished with every evaluation. Circumstances at higher levels of competition may dictate the pursuit of additional goals that enhance and maximize the evaluation process.

METHODOLOGY OF THE PPE

Methods

The evaluation has been conducted in three basic types of setting; office based, multiple station mass screening, and "the line-up" examination. Examination in the primary care physician's office offers many advantages. It usually is the most comfortable and private setting, which encourages patient rapport. The discussion of private and sensitive issues is more likely in this setting.[19] The availability of medical records enables the physician to follow up old injuries or previously treated medical conditions, thus promoting continuity of care.[16] The private office evaluation obviates the organizational challenges presented by scheduling mass screening examinations in a given location.[16]

The disadvantages of office-based examinations include decreased efficiency and cost-effectiveness and increased cost to the athlete.[19] Also, as physician's knowledge and interest in sports medicine varies greatly, the examinations may lack consistency in findings and recommendations.[19]

The station examination is commonly utilized to perform large numbers of screening examinations. The organization varies but usually involves a physician or physicians in conjunction with support personnel that may include nurses, trainers, therapists, coaches, or parents. An example of the typical station set-up is indicated in Fig. 7-1. Additional stations may be involved if other parameters are measured, such as body composition, flexibility, muscle strength, or other fitness parameters.

There are a number of advantages to this type of examination.[16] It is a standardized examination that offsets the physician variability that may be problematic in office examinations. Station examinations can be administered to large numbers of athletes over shorter periods of

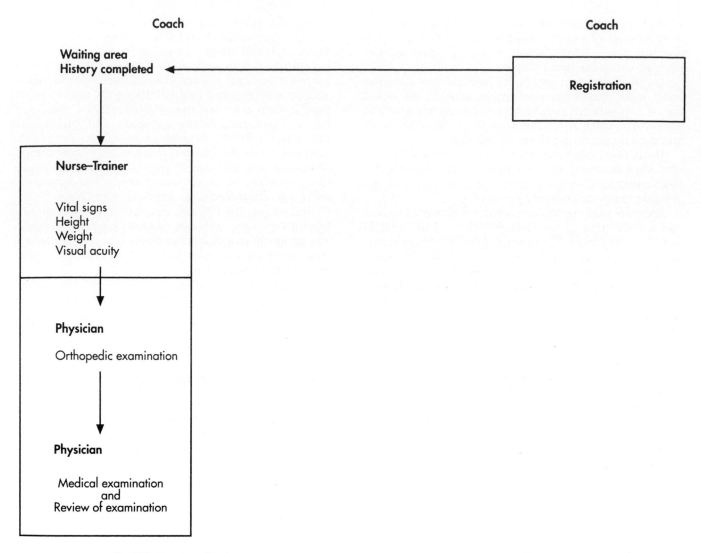

Fig. 7-1. An example of a station examination (from McKeag DB: Preparticipation screening of the potential athlete, *Clin Sp Med* 8(3):373, 1989).

time, and thus are more efficient than office examinations. Often specialty consultation can be made available, thus potentially minimizing referral. The mass station examination often is administered by physicians who have a genuine interest in sports medicine and thus may bring more knowledge that is pertinent to the examinations. Other potential benefits include fostering of cooperation among health professionals, the involvement of the coaching staff with the care of the athletes, and the development of a data base for research purposes.[16]

A potential disadvantage of this type of evaluation is a relative lack of privacy, which lessens the opportunity to discuss personal issues. Adequate planning would enable at least one private station to be available where this type of exchange could occur, thus combining the best of both the private and station examinations.[17] Table 7-2 summarizes the potential advantages and disadvantages of the office based and station screening PPE.

The line-up examination was commonly utilized in the past, and indeed offered a very efficient method of

evaluation. However, this type of exam has drawbacks. Invariably the patient has to endure lack of privacy. The physician's examination accuracy is also potentially compromised in this difficult setting. Many sports medicine authorities have condemned this type of examination.[32]

Frequency of Examination

The PPE is often required on an annual basis. The survey of state examination requirements indicated over three-fourths of the states required annual evaluations for sports participation.[9] Some schools engage in screening evaluations before each new sports season. The American Academy of Pediatrics recommends a complete evaluation every two years with an interim history prior to any new sports season.[7]

Many authorities now recommend a screening physical examination at the beginning of a new level of competition (e.g., junior high, high school, college) with intercurrent interviews at the start of each new sports season to screen for new problems or evaluation of rehabilitation of old injuries.[17,19,23]

Table 7-2. Potential advantages and disadvantages of office-based and station screening PPEs

Office-based PPE	Station screening PPE
Advantages	**Advantages**
Physician-patient familiarity	Specialized personnel
Continuity of care	Efficient and cost effective
Opportunity for counseling	Good communication with school athletic staff
	Opportunity for performance testing
Disadvantages	
Many athletes do not have a primary care physician	**Disadvantages**
Limited time for appointments	Noisy, hurried environment
Varying knowledge of and interest in sports medicine problems	Lack of privacy
	Difficulty following up on medical problems and concerns
Greater cost	
Lack of communication with school athletic staff	Lack of communication with parents

From American Academy of Family Physicians, American Academy of Pediatrics, American Medical Society for Sports Medicine, American Orthopaedic Society for Sports Medicine, American Osteopathic Academy for Sports Medicine: *Preparticipation Physical Evaluation Monograph,* 1992.

While the authors feel these recent recommendations are very appropriate in most settings, situations in which continuity of care is not optimal lend themselves best to a screening process which is performed annually.[23]

Timing of Examination

The timing of PPE must allow sufficient time for adequate rehabilitation and treatment of injuries or further investigations of new findings. However, the evaluation should not take place so far in advance of a season or school year that the development of new problems may become a significant factor. Four to six weeks before a season seems to satisfy both considerations.[17,19,23] For scholastic athletes, this timetable would place the PPE in the middle of summer vacation and thus be logistically not optimal. Therefore, the end of a school year may be the best time to perform the evaluations for the following sports season. In this case, a brief intercurrent history when an athlete reports for the fall sports season would be ideal for updating any problems.[23]

HISTORY

The medical history is the cornerstone of diagnosis and its role in the PPE is no less important. Many authors have emphasized the need for an effective screening history.[8,13,17,19,25] The effectiveness of the history as a screening tool has been borne out by studies. In one survey the history was positive in seven of nine students restricted from activities and in 74% of the students requiring further evaluation.[13] The history is generally regarded as the most sensitive and specific part of the screening evaluation.

Adherence to the specific goals of the PPE allows effective history taking with relatively few questions. The number of history questions will vary depending upon the depth of the evaluation. A setting where the team physician is becoming the primary care physician of an athlete will necessitate more in-depth history taking, and a survey of all organ systems is appropriate. However, it should be noted that an effective PPE can be accomplished with relatively few history questions; some authors recommend a history form with fewer than a dozen questions.[4,7,8,25,30]

The history that is focused primarily on the issues pertaining to safe participation will be directed toward the cardiovascular, neurologic, and musculoskeletal systems as well as adequately covering questions of general health.[8] There is no single correct history form. An example of the form used in PPE by the Cleveland Clinic Foundation is given in Fig. 7-2. In addition to covering the necessary areas, the forms should be brief, easy to read, and understandable by the athletes/parents, and allow adequate space for elaboration of positive findings.

A primary focus of the PPE is directed toward detection of cardiac abnormalities that may place the athlete at increased risk for participation. The common causes of sudden cardiac death in patients under 35 years of age are listed in the box on p. 67. While coronary artery disease is the most common cause of death in those older than 35, structural abnormalities (e.g., hypertrophic cardiomyopathy) are the most common causes of sudden cardiac death in the younger population.[28]

Although sudden death may be the initial presentation of such cardiac problems, premonitory symptoms can, at times, identify the at-risk individual. The examiner should specifically ask the prospective participant about a history of syncope/near-syncope with exercise, which may be associated with hypertrophic cardiomyopathy, conduction abnormalities, or valvular problems.[23] A sensation of palpitation or skipped beats may indicate conduction problems (e.g., Wolff-Parkinson-White syndrome). It is also helpful to ask about a history of heart murmur or hypertension. It is important to inquire about a family history of atraumatic sudden death under the age of 50. Conditions such as hypertrophic cardiomyopathy, Marfan's syndrome, and prolonged QT syndrome may have a significant genetic component.[23]

Chest pain with exercise and easy fatigability are two complaints that are felt by some to be rather nonspecific in young athletes.[27] The examiner must carefully sort out the history in every case to determine if these symptoms are of legitimate concern. Chest pain that is described as substernal pain or pressure associated with exercise that improves with rest should alert the examiner for the possibility of an anomalous coronary artery or premature atherosclerosis.[23] A complaint of easy fatigability that does represent an abnormal response to exercise in comparison to peers may be an important clue to underlying valvular abnormalities or lung pathology.[23]

Asthma and specifically exercise induced bronchospasm are common in the athletic population. The physician should inquire about wheezing, tightness of the chest, or postexercise coughing, all of which may be important clues to an underlying asthmatic condition.

Date of Exam_____ /_____ /_____

School Official _____

Exam Doctor _____

Cleveland Clinic Foundation

PREPARTICIPATION
SPORTS EXAM

A   B   C

Contact: Coach ☐

School Nurse ☐

Family Doctor ☐

Family Dentist ☐

THIS IS NOT A SUBSTITUTE FOR A REGULAR PHYSICAL EXAM PERFORMED BY YOUR FAMILY DOCTOR

Name_____   Grade _____ Age _____ Birthdate _____ /_____ /_____

School _____   Sport _____   Sex _____

Parents _____   Address _____   Phone _____

Family Doctor _____   Address _____   Phone _____

HISTORY: Answer **No** or **Yes** with details and dates. Use reverse side if necessary.

I.   Have you ever sustained **an injury** which prevented you from playing sports for **more than one day and** have you had any injuries **such as** (circle):   skull fracture - **brain surgery concussion** - knocked out, **neck pain**/injury - arm/finger **numbness**, **back pain**/injury - leg/toe numbness, heatstroke/fainting - exhaustion, broken bone - **fracture**, joint **dislocation** - out of place, **deep bruise** - muscle pull, ligament **sprains**, tender kneecap/shin, **trick knee** - catching/locking,

_____

_____

II. Do you have a history of **and/or** take medicine (specify) for any medical problems **such as** (circle): **asthma** - allergy - wheezing - short of breath, heart **murmur**/palpitation - rheumatic fever - **high blood high blood pressure**, diabetes - high/low **sugar**, fainting - **seizure**, yellow jaundice - **hepatitis**, severe influenza/cold - **mononucleosis** - weakness, **anemia** - bruise easily - bleeding - sickle cell, loss of eyesight, hearing, testicle, kidney, etc., **hernia** - rupture - bulging, skin disease - boils - **rash**, or other?

_____

_____

III. Are you allergic to any medicine such as (circle) penicillin, iodine, novocaine or other?

_____

IV. Any family history of medically unexplained or cardiac caused sudden death under age 50?

_____

V.   L.M.P. _____

BP____/____ P_____ Ht_____ Wt_____ Gross Vision: R_____ L_____, Pupils R_____ L_____ LAB: UA_____

EXAM:

1. Upper Extr: AC jts _____   4. Heart:_____
           Symm _____   5. Lungs: _____
           ROM _____   6. Skin: _____
2. Spine: Neck _____   7. Abdo: Spleen _____
           Fwd Bend_____   Liver _____
           Curve_____   8. GU: Hernia _____
3. Lower Extr: Gait _____   Testicles _____
           1-Hop_____   9. Dental _____
           Duck _____   10. Other _____
           Symm _____   _____
           ROM _____   _____

IMPRESSION:

☐ Satisfactory Exam

☐ Recommend further evaluation/rehabilitation regarding: _____

     Contact your: School Nurse — Coach — Family Doctor — Family Dentist
_____

CLEARANCE:

A — Cleared for: Collision — Contact — Noncontact sports

B — Cleared for: Collision — Contact — Noncontact sports after completing eval/rehab

C — NOT cleared for: Collision — Contact — Noncontact sports due to: _____

_____

2285570 Rev. 9/90

Fig. 7-2. Cleveland Clinic Sports Exam form.

COMMON CAUSES OF SUDDEN DEATH IN YOUNG ATHLETES

Hypertrophic obstructive cardiomyopathy

Idiopathic concentric left ventricular hypertrophy

Atherosclerosis

Aberrant origin of the left coronary artery

Hypoplastic coronary arteries

Ruptured aorta

From Strong WB, Steed D: Cardiovascular evaluation of the young athlete, *Pediatr Clin North Am* 29(6):1325, 1982.

A careful review of the neurologic system is important. Inquiries should be made regarding a previous history of concussion. Each occurrence, along with the time missed and any specific testing or hospitalization, should be reviewed. A history of severe concussion resulting in loss of consciousness for several minutes or more, or history of repeated concussion requires special attention to the neurologic examination and possible consultation before clearance for a contact or collision sport. A history of surgery on the skull/brain necessitates a deferred clearance decision to a neurosurgeon.[23] Resources are suggested that review clearance issues for these problems.[5]

A history of temporary paresis or paralysis may be caused by a number of conditions, including cervical spinal stenosis, congenital fusion, cervical instability, or cervical disc protrusion.[23] Any history of bilateral or four limb paresis, paralysis, or paresthesias necessitates a careful physical evaluation and further cervical spine radiographic evaluation. Consultation with a spine surgeon with experience in dealing with athletes is recommended to sort out the participation issues.[31]

Brachial plexus stretch injuries, commonly called "stingers" or "burners," are frequently seen in collision sports such as football and wrestling. This common injury is characterized by unilateral arm weakness and paresthesias that usually resolve in seconds to minutes. Rarely, symptoms are persistent for weeks or months. A history of brachial plexus injuries does not preclude participation but should spark further investigation regarding playing techniques, proper fit of equipment, recommendations for equipment changes, and a cervical spine rehabilitation program. Again, a careful history will differentiate the common brachial plexus injury from the more serious conditions reviewed above.

Information should be sought regarding history of prior heat-related illness. Research indicates that those who have suffered from heat-related illness have an increased likelihood of experiencing a recurrence.[8] An individual with such a history deserves close monitoring during practices and competitions held during conditions of high heat and humidity.

A menstrual history is important for the female athlete, including the history of onset of menses, the most recent menstrual period, and the regularity of cycles.[23]

Menstrual irregularities are common in female athletes involved in a variety of sports, most notably dancing, gymnastics, and the aerobic sports such as cross country running. Menstrual irregularities are sometimes linked to poor nutritional status and can be associated with an increased risk of stress fractures in the female athlete.

The musculoskeletal history is an obvious point of emphasis. In one study, musculoskeletal findings represented two thirds of all identified risk factors.[30] In another study, the results of the health history form indicated the most frequent positive response was a history of previous injury (about 27%).[16] Inquiry should be made regarding past sprains or strains, dislocations, fractures, or other injuries of bones and joints. Another approach to this topic includes a history of use of braces, splints, or other appliances, which may point the examiner's attention toward a problem that the athlete may omit.

A brief survey of previous medical problems, hospitalizations, and surgeries may uncover other medical problems that the athlete may omit. It is also important to record a history of allergies to medications or insect stings and tetanus status.

The athlete should have an opportunity to indicate a desire to discuss any health related issues. Athletes of all ages, like their nonathletic counterparts, are confronted with important decisions regarding alcohol and drug use, smokeless tobacco, and issues of sexuality. As previously noted, the encounter in a private physician's office is ideally suited to accomplish this counseling, however, important issues can be identified during mass screening examinations with appropriate follow up arranged.[32]

Ideally, the history form should be completed by the athlete in advance of the PPE. For a minor, the athlete's parents/guardians should also review and sign the form. At the time of the evaluation, it is helpful to have the history form reviewed with a health care provider prior to the examination so that any clarification or elaboration may take place prior to the physical examination.

The importance of the history in the overall evaluation process cannot be overemphasized. A history directed toward those few items that are most pertinent to safe participation by a scholastic athlete can be accomplished with relatively few questions. The response to those questions will go a long way in determining the fitness of an individual for participation.

PHYSICAL EXAMINATION

The content of the physical examination is governed by the same principles that directed the history. Examination should be relatively brief and should focus on the areas which are most pertinent to safe participation, namely the cardiopulmonary and musculoskeletal systems. However, the examiner must be prepared to pursue other areas of the examination should the athlete's medical history indicate. Also, the physical examination should be performed with the examiner's awareness of the intended sport of participation. This allows the examiner to pay particular attention to parts of the examination that are most relevant to a given sport.[19]

The examination should begin with accurate measurements of height, weight, visual acuity, and blood pressure. For pediatric athletes, standard tables can be used to evaluate height and weight. Significant variations from the norms may warrant further investigation. The examiner should be aware of the possibility of anabolic steroid use in an extremely well muscled athlete who has made rapid weight gains in a short period of time. Judgments must be made carefully, as adolescent bodies are capable of rapid changes. Significantly underweight athletes may arouse concern for eating disorders. Special awareness is needed for those involved in sports where weight control is especially important (e.g., wrestling, gymnastics).[32]

Visual acuity may be screened using the standard Snellen chart. Visual problems are often noted in screening examinations and are a frequent cause of referral. Eye protection is available for those with significant visual impairment, but thorough discussion of the risk of contact and collision sports is essential.

Blood pressure determinations are done with particular attention to the appropriate size cuff. If the blood pressure is elevated, repeat measurements are indicated. The Preparticipation Physical Examination monograph developed in 1992 lists an easy rule to remember regarding blood pressure: further evaluation is required prior to clearance if blood pressure is greater than 125/75 for athletes under 10 or greater than 135/85 for athletes older than 10.[23]

The head and neck examination is often included, although personal experience indicates that significant findings that affect participation are unusual. However, swimmers and divers are a special group of athletes that deserve careful examination of the ears. In addition, checking pupil equality in athletes is important. In the case of head injury, it is extremely beneficial to have prior documentation of physiologic anisocoria.

The cardiopulmonary examination deserves special emphasis and care. The detection of a subtle abnormality on examination may be the only clue to an underlying cardiac abnormality that may place the individual at increased risk to participation.

Peripheral pulses should be palpated to screen for coarctation of the aorta. Auscultation of the heart can be performed with the athlete in the seated and supine positions, utilizing the various maneuvers that can help differentiate functional murmurs from pathologic murmurs.[23] Innocent murmurs are common in young athletes, but any murmur that is questionable to an examiner should be evaluated. The question of when to obtain further testing frequently arises. The authors feel that further testing, such as electrocardiogram, chest x-ray, echocardiogram and/or stress echocardiogram, is indicated when there is a worrisome history (see above) and/or a questionable finding on physical examination. If a physician is not comfortable with this type of problem, then cardiac consultation should be obtained. The issue of mass screening for cardiac abnormalities is discussed in a later section.

Rhythm disturbances may be detected on physical examination and deserve further electrocardiographic evaluation. Rhythm variations may be supraventricular or ventricular in origin. Further complicating the clinician's investigation is the finding that highly trained athletes commonly have rhythm variations of both supraventricular and ventricular origin. In general, ventricular ectopic beats that disappear with exercise usually indicate a benign origin.[23]

A number of electrocardiographic variations are found in a higher percentage of the athlete population, including bradycardia, first-degree heart block, Wenckebach type of second-degree heart block, junctional rhythm, and ST-T wave abnormalities.[26]

Lungs are auscultated for pathologic sounds. If exercise-induced bronchospasm is suspected by history, the athlete may be exercised in an effort to bring out audible wheezing.

Abdominal examination is accomplished to rule out areas of tenderness, mass, or organomegaly. Infectious mononucleosis is a common cause of splenomegaly in the adolescent population and requires deferred clearance for participation until resolution in most contact/collision and strenuous aerobic sports.

The male genitourinary examination may detect an undescended testicle or testicular mass. Those with testicular absence should be counseled regarding risks in contact or collision sports. Inguinal hernia may require further consultation to assess the risk of possible complication with this condition. Inguinal hernia does not necessarily preclude competition, and clearance is decided on an individual basis.[23]

The genitourinary examination also allows assessment of Tanner staging in the male. The pros and cons of this were described in a previous section.

The pelvic examination in the female athlete, although not a basic part of the PPE, may be indicated if the medical history dictates. Although clearance for participation does not usually need to be delayed, the athlete should be encouraged to follow up with her personal physician for further evaluation if menstrual abnormalities exist.

The skin examination is important for those involved in contact or collision sports. A number of dermatologic infections require deferred clearance, including herpes, impetigo, louse, or scabies infestation.

A screening musculoskeletal examination can be accomplished efficiently. There are numerous examples of this examination, with one example outlined in Table 7-3. The emphasis of the screening musculoskeletal examination is to document full range of motion and symmetrical strength about the major joints. Special attention and further evaluation also should be paid to those areas that (1) have been previously injured, and (2) are of particular importance for the sport to be played.

It is controversial whether normal physical examination findings, such as ligamentous laxity or joint tightness, predispose to injury. One study indicated that excessive joint flexibility and ligamentous laxity was related to an increased risk of injury.[18] Others have indicated that the rapid growth of puberty may cause excessive joint tightness in adolescents and may be a predictor of injury.[23] However, other investigators have been unable to correlate examination findings with predictors for injuries among athletes.[12,21]

Table 7-3. Example of a screening musculoskeletal examination

Athletic activity (instructions)	Observations
1. Stand facing examiner	AC joints; general habitus
2. Look at ceiling, floor, over both shoulders, touch ears to shoulder	Cervical spine motion
3. Shrug shoulders (examiner resists)	Trapezius strength
4. Abduct shoulders 90° (examiner resists at 90°)	Deltoid strength
5. Full external rotation of arms	Shoulder motion
6. Flex and extend elbows	Elbow motion
7. Arms at sides, elbows at 90° flexed; pronate and supinate wrists	Elbow and wrist motion
8. Spread fingers; make fist	Hand and finger motion and deformities
9. Tighten (contract) quadriceps; relax quadriceps	Symmetry and knee effusion, ankle effusion
10. "Duck walk" four steps (away from examiner)	Hip, knee, and ankle motion
11. Back to examiner	Shoulder symmetry; scoliosis
12. Knees straight, touch toes	Scoliosis, hip motion, hamstring tightness
13. Raise up on toes, heels	Calf symmetry, leg strength

From McKeag DB: Preparticipation screening of the potential athlete, *Clin Sport Med* 8(3):373, 1989.

As noted previously, assessment of various parameters of fitness may be a goal of the PPE. These items are commonly evaluated during the PPE of collegiate and professional athletes. Variables such as body composition, aerobic fitness, flexibility, and strength may aid coaches and trainers in the modification of an athlete's training program to optimize performance. These evaluations may be impractical for office-based examinations but may be accomplished with the involvement of athletic trainers, physical therapists, or exercise physiologists in a station approach.

LABORATORY TESTS AND PROCEDURES

There has been controversy regarding the helpfulness of laboratory tests as part of the PPE. Tests commonly employed include CBC, blood chemistry tests, serum ferritin, lipid profiles, and urinalysis.

Urinalysis has often been utilized as part of the screening PPE. Complicating the utility of this test is the fact that proteinuria is commonly seen during childhood and adolescence. One study of junior high and high school preparticipation evaluations showed proteinuria was seen in 62% of all urinalyses, 17% when trace protein was excluded.[22] In another study, 40 of the 701 students had a positive dipstick test for urine protein. None of the 40 had a significant urologic abnormality after

further consultation.[13] In addition, strenuous physical activity can result in transient proteinuria and may give false positive tests for the urinalysis performed during a screening examination. Urine dipstick testing for blood can also be very misleading due to contamination of specimens in female athletes during their menstrual periods. Because of the lack of proof of the effectiveness of the routine urinalysis as a screening tool, many authorities are recommending that this not be part of screening PPE.[4,7,17,19] The authors agree with this policy.

Hemoglobin and hematocrit determination have also been included in the PPE but are also acknowledged to be of questionable benefit. Without a positive history, hemoglobin testing is not likely to detect an anemia that would adversely affect performance.[19] Many team physicians perform hemoglobin and ferritin testing in their higher risk athletes, especially at the collegiate level where iron deficiency is not uncommon in female athletes. In these athletes, poor iron intake combined with menstrual blood losses and increased iron requirements place the individual at risk for iron deficiency anemia and impaired performance.

The utility of other tests for routine screening, such as sickle cell test, blood chemistries, and lipid profiles, is also unproven. These tests are also not recommended for screening purposes.[23] Again, when the team physician becomes the primary care physician, such as seen at the collegiate and professional levels, the physician may choose to perform these screening lab tests, especially when the athlete is joining a particular team. This approach may be no different than a primary care physician dealing with a healthy young adult who is a new patient in their own private practice.

Some authors have proposed more extensive cardiovascular screening, utilizing such tests as chest x-ray, ECG, and echocardiography to screen for abnormalities that may cause sudden death.[23] Others have pointed out that mass screening with these types of tests is unnecessary and costly except in cases where the history and physical exam warrant such testing.[33] It has been estimated that 200,000 athletes would have to be screened to detect 1000 athletes who are at risk for sudden cardiac disease, and one person would actually die from that cardiac disorder.[9] The authors agree that mass screening with these type of tests is not indicated and should be reserved to only those instances where careful history and physical examination uncover a finding that requires further testing.

CLEARANCE

At the conclusion of the PPE, the examiner must make a decision regarding an individual's participation. A decision regarding participation must be made with (1) consideration of any abnormality found on initial history, physical examination, or further work-up, and (2) the requirements of the proposed activity.

The Preparticipation Physical Evaluation joint statement published in 1992 offers five questions the examiner should keep in mind when determining clearance: (1) Does the problem place the athlete at increased risk for injury? (2) Is any other participant at increased risk because of the problem? (3) Can the athlete safely participate with treatment (medication, rehabilitation, bracing, or padding)? (4) Can limited participation be allowed while treatment is being initiated? (5) If clearance is denied only for certain activities, in what activities can the athlete safely participate?[23] These questions provide an excellent foundation for the decision making process of the physician.

An excellent resource for decisions regarding clearance for participation is the American Academy of Pediatrics policy statement for Participation in Competitive Sports.[3] The policy statement takes into consideration that different sports impose varying demands on a participant. The sports are divided into five different categories based on the demands of each activity and is seen in Table 7-4. The conditions of the various organ systems and the panel's recommendations for participation are summarized in Table 7-5. It is worth reemphasizing that a given condition may be a contraindication to participation in certain types of sports but may not be so in other sports. For example, atlanto-axial instability is a clear contraindication to collision sports such as football, but is not a contraindication to various noncontact sports.

It should be reemphasized that these recommendations are to be considered as guidelines and individual circumstances may supersede published recommendations.

At the end of the PPE, a physician should have an option whether to clear or defer clearance for participation. This should be indicated on the PPE form. Various authors have proposed different classification schemes, and an example of one such scheme is indicated on the PPE form used by the Cleveland Clinic Foundation. In summary, an examiner has a choice of three categories of clearance:

a. complete clearance for participation in a designated sports classification (collision/contact/noncontact).
b. clearance pending notification of a responsible person (e.g., coach, family doctor, parent/guardian). This represents a scenario when special treatment or equipment is required but activity is not limited.
c. clearance deferred until further evaluation, treatment, or rehabilitation is accomplished (e.g., evaluation of a questionable heart murmur).

When working with young athletes such as seen at the junior high or high school levels, copies of the PPE should be made available for the school, parents/guardians, the examining physician, and the athlete's primary care physician. It should be emphasized that any abnormal findings must be clearly communicated by the examining physician.

SUMMARY

Available information should allow standardization of the PPE of young athletes, whether the encounter takes place in a private office setting or as part of mass screening examinations. Many authorities now advocate a complete screening examination only for new levels of competition, with annual or seasonal limited encounters to update information. The authors feel this is an appropriate schedule for the PPE, with exceptions as indicated in the text.

The encounter can be accomplished in an efficient manner that focuses on those items that pertain to safe sports participation. The history, which can be covered in relatively few questions, is the most sensitive portion of the examination. The physical examination focuses on the cardiovascular and musculoskeletal systems with flexibility to expand the evaluation depending on the participant's history. The history and physical examination may be expanded in certain situations as discussed, such as would be seen at the collegiate and professional levels where the physician is going to assume primary care of an athlete. Laboratory testing is of questionable benefit as a screening tool but may be appropriate in certain situations.

Determining clearance may be a difficult challenge for a physician. Guidelines exist to assist clinicians in making appropriate decisions, and consultations should be sought out whenever questions exist. The authors hope that the end result of a carefully planned and executed preparticipation evaluation will be safe and enjoyable sports participation for countless young athletes.

Table 7-4. Classification of sports by contact

Contact/ collision	Limited contact	Noncontact
Basketball	Baseball	Archery
Boxing*	Bicycling	Badminton
Diving	Cheerleading	Body building
Field hockey	Canoeing/kayaking	Bowling
Football	(white water)	Canoeing/kayaking
Flag	Fencing	(flat water)
Tackle	Field	Crew/rowing
Ice hockey	High jump	Curling
Lacrosse	Pole vault	Dancing
Martial arts	Floor hockey	Field
Rodeo	Gymnastics	Discus
Rugby	Handball	Javelin
Ski jumping	Horseback riding	Shot put
Soccer	Racquetball	Golf
Team handball	Skating	Orienteering
Water polo	Ice	Power lifting
Wrestling	Inline	Race walking
	Roller	Riflery
	Skiing	Rope jumping
	Cross-country	Running
	Downhill	Sailing
	Water	Scuba diving
	Softball	Strength training
	Squash	Swimming
	Ultimate Frisbee	Table tennis
	Volleyball	Tennis
	Windsurfing/surfing	Track
		Weight lifting

*Participation not recommended. From American Academy of Pediatrics: Medical conditions affecting sports participation, *Pediatrics* 94(5):491, 1994.

Table 7-5. Medical conditions and sports participation
This table is designed to be understood by medical and nonmedical personnel. In the "Explanation" section below, "needs evaluation" means that a physician with appropriate knowledge and experience should assess the safety of a given sport for an athlete with the listed medical condition. Unless otherwise noted, this is because of the variability of the severity of the disease or of the risk of injury among the specific sports in Table 7-4, or both.

Condition	May participate?
Atlantoaxial instability (instability of the joint between cervical vertebrae 1 and 2)	Qualified Yes
Explanation: Athlete needs evaluation to assess risk of spinal cord injury during sports participation.	
Bleeding disorder	Qualified Yes
Explanation: Athlete needs evaluation.	
Cardiovascular diseases	
Carditis (inflammation of the heart)	No
Explanation: Carditis may result in sudden death with exertion.	
Hypertension (high blood pressure)	Qualified Yes
Explanation: Those with significant essential (unexplained) hypertension should avoid weight and power lifting, body building, and strength training. Those with secondary hypertension (hypertension caused by a previously identified disease), or severe essential hypertension, need evaluation.	
Congenital heart disease (structural heart defects present at birth)	Qualified Yes
Explanation: Those with mild forms may participate fully; those with moderate or severe forms, or who have undergone surgery, need evaluation.	
Dysrhythmia (irregular heart rhythm)	Qualified Yes
Explanation: Athlete needs evaluation because some types require therapy or make certain sports dangerous, or both.	
Mitral valve prolapse (abnormal heart valve)	Qualified Yes
Explanation: Those with symptoms (chest pain, symptoms of possible dysrhythmia) or evidence of mitral regurgitation (leaking) on physical examination need evaluation. All others may participate fully.	
Heart murmur	Qualified Yes
Explanation: If the murmur is innocent (does not indicate heart disease), full participation is permitted. Otherwise the athlete needs evaluation (see congenital heart disease and mitral valve prolapse above).	
Cerebral palsy	Qualified Yes
Explanation: Athlete needs evaluation.	
Diabetes mellitus	Yes
Explanation: All sports can be played with proper attention to diet, hydration, and insulin therapy. Particular attention is needed for activities that last 30 minutes or more.	
Diarrhea	Qualified No
Explanation: Unless disease is mild, no participation is permitted, because diarrhea may increase the risk of dehydration and heat illness. See "Fever" below.	
Eating disorders	Qualified Yes
Anorexia nervosa	
Bulimia nervosa	
Explanation: These patients need both medical and psychiatric assessment before participation.	
Eyes	Qualified Yes
Functionally one-eyed athlete	
Loss of an eye	
Detached retina	
Previous eye surgery or serious eye injury	
Explanation: A functionally one-eyed athlete has a best corrected visual acuity of < 20/40 in the worse eye. These athletes would suffer significant disability if the better eye was seriously injured as would those with loss of an eye. Some athletes who have previously undergone eye surgery or had a serious eye injury may have an increased risk of injury because of weakened eye tissue. Availability of eye guards approved by the American Society for Testing Materials (ASTM) and other protective equipment may allow participation in most sports, but this must be judged on an individual basis.	
Fever	No
Explanation: Fever can increase cardiopulmonary effort, reduce maximum exercise capacity, make heat illness more likely, and increase orthostatic hypotension during exercise. Fever may rarely accompany myocarditis or other infections that may make exercise dangerous.	
Heat illness, history of	Qualified Yes
Explanation: Because of the increased likelihood of recurrence, the athlete needs individual assessment to determine the presence of predisposing conditions and to arrange a prevention strategy.	
HIV infection	Yes
Explanation: Because of the apparent minimal risk to others, all sports may be played that the state of health allows. In all athletes, skin lesions should be properly covered, and athletic personnel should use universal precautions when handling blood or body fluids with visible blood.	

Continued.

Table 7-5. Medical conditions and sports participation—cont'd

Condition	May participate?
Kidney: absence of one	Qualified Yes
Explanation: Athlete needs individual assessment for contact/collision and limited contact sports.	
Liver: enlarged	Qualified Yes
Explanation: If the liver is acutely enlarged, participation should be avoided because of risk of rupture. If the liver is chronically enlarged, individual assessment is needed before collision/contact or limited contact sports are played.	
Malignancy	Qualified Yes
Explanation: Athlete needs individual assessment.	
Musculoskeletal disorders	Qualified Yes
Explanation: Athlete needs individual assessment.	
Neurologic	Qualified Yes
History of serious head or spine trauma, severe or repeated concussions, or craniotomy.	
Explanation: Athlete needs individual assessment for collison/contact or limited contact sports, and also for noncontact sports if there are deficits in judgment or cognition. Recent research supports a conservative approach to management of concussion.	
Convulsive disorder, well controlled	Yes
Explanation: Risk of convulsion during participation is minimal.	
Convulsive disorder, poorly controlled	Qualified Yes
Explanation: Athlete needs individual assessment for collision/contact or limited contact sports. Avoid the following noncontact sports: archery, riflery, swimming, weight or power lifting, strength training, or sports involving heights. In these sports, occurrence of a convulsion may be a risk to self or others.	
Obesity	Qualified Yes
Explanation: Because of the risk of heat illness, obese persons need careful acclimatization and hydration.	
Organ transplant recipient	Qualified Yes
Explanation: Athlete needs individual assessment.	
Ovary: absence of one	Yes
Explanation: Risk of severe injury to the remaining ovary is minimal.	
Respiratory	Qualified Yes
Pulmonary compromise including cystic fibrosis	
Explanation: Athlete needs individual assessment, but generally all sports may be played if oxygenation remains satisfactory during a graded exercise test. Patients with cystic fibrosis need acclimatization and good hydration to reduce the risk of heat illness.	
Asthma	Yes
Explanation: With proper medication and education, only athletes with the most severe asthma will have to modify their participation.	
Acute upper respiratory infection	Qualified Yes
Explanation: Upper respiratory obstruction may affect pulmonary function. Athlete needs individual assessment for all but mild disease. See "Fever" above.	
Sickle cell disease	Qualified Yes
Explanation: Athlete needs individual assessment. In general, if status of the illness permits, all but high exertion, collision/contact sports may be played. Overheating, dehydration, and chilling must be avoided.	
Sickle cell trait	Yes
Explanation: It is unlikely that individuals with sickle cell trait (AS) have an increased risk of sudden death or other medical problems during athletic participation except under the most extreme conditions of heat, humidity, and possibly increased altitude. These individuals, like all athletes, should be carefully conditioned, acclimatized, and hydrated to reduce any possible risk.	
Skin boils, herpes simplex, impetigo, scabies, molluscum contagiosum	Qualified Yes
Explanation: While the patient is contagious, participation in gymnastics with mats, martial arts, wrestling, or other collision/contact or limited contact sports is not allowed. Herpes simplex virus probably is not transmitted via mats.	
Spleen, enlarged	Qualified Yes
Explanation: Patients with acutely enlarged spleens should avoid all sports because of risk of rupture. Those with chronically enlarged spleens need individual assessment before playing collision/contact or limited contact sports.	
Testicle absent or undescended	Yes
Explanation: Certain sports may require a protective cup.	

From American Academy of Pediatrics: Medical conditions affecting sports participation, *Pediatrics* 94(5):492–493, 1994.

REFERENCES

1. Abbott HG, Kress JB: Preconditioning in the prevention of knee injuries, *Arch Phys Med Rehabil* 50:326–333, 1969.
1a. Goldberg B, et al: Pre-participation sports assessment - an objective evaluation, *Pediatrics* 66(5):736–745, 1980.
2. Allman FL, McKeag DB: Prevention and emergency care of sports injuries, *Fam Prac Recert* 5(4):141–163, 1983.
3. American Academy of Pediatrics Policy Statement, Recommendations for participation in competitive sports, *Pediatrics* 81(5):737–739, 1988.
4. Blum RW: Preparticipation evaluation of the adolescent athlete, *Postgrad Med* 78(2):52–69, 1985.
5. Cantu RC: Guidelines for return to contact sports after a cerebral concussion, *Phys Sportsmed* 14(10): 75–83, 1986.
6. Duke PM, Litt IF, Gross IT: Adolescents' self-assessment of sexual maturation, *Pediatr* 66(6):918–20, 1980.
7. Dyment PG: Another look at the sports preparticipation examination of the adolescent athlete, *J of Adolescent Health Care* 7:130S–132S, 1986.
8. Epstein SE, Maron RJ: Sudden death and the competitive athlete: Perspectives on preparticipation screening studies, *J Am Coll Cardiol* 7:220–230, 1986.
9. Feinstein RA, Soileau EJ, Daniel WA: A national survey of preparticipation physical examination requirements, *Phys and Sportsmed* 16(5):51–59, 1988.
10. Fields KB, Delaney M: Focusing the preparticipation sports examination, *J of Fam Prac* 30(3):304–312, 1990.
11. Garrick JG, Smith NJ: Pre-participation sports assessment, *Pediatrics* 66(5):803–806, November 1980.
12. Godshall RW: The predictability of athletic injuries: an eight year study, *J of Sp Med* 3(1), 50–54, 1975.
13. Goldberg B, et al: Pre-participation sports assessment—an objective evaluation, *Pediatrics* 66(5):736–745, November 1980.
14. Hough DO, McKeag DM: Preparticipation examination results from Michigan State University (unpublished data), 1982.
15. Kreipe RE, Gewanter HL: Physical maturity screening for preparticipation in sports, *Pediatr* 75(6):1076–1080, 1985.
16. Linder CW, et al: Preparticipation health screening of young athletes, *Amer J Sp Med* 9(3):187–193, 1981.
17. Lombardo JA: Pre-participation physical evaluation, *Primary Care* 11(1):3–21, 1984.
18. Lysens R, Steverlynck A, van der Auweele Y: The predictability of sports injuries, *Sports Med* 1:6–10, 1984.
19. McKeag DB: Preparticipation screening of the potential athlete, *Clin Sp Med* 8(3):373–397, 1989.
20. Micheli LJ: Overuse injuries in children's sports: the growth factor, *Orth Clin North Am* 14:337–360, 1983.
21. Nicholas JA: Risk factors, sports medicine and the orthopedic system: an overview, *J of Sp Med* 3(5), 243–259, 1975.
22. Peggs JF, Reinhardt RW, O'Brien JM: Proteinuria in adolescent sports physical examinations, *J Fam Practice* 22(1):80–81, 1986.
23. A joint publication. American Academy of Family Physicians, American Academy of Pediatrics, American Medical Society for Sports Medicine, American Orthopaedic Society for Sports Medicine, American Osteopathic Academy of Sports Medicine, Preparticipation Physical Evaluation, 1992.
24. Risser WL, et al: A cost-benefit analysis of preparticipation sports examinations of adolescent athletes, *J School Health* 55(7):270–273, 1985.
25. Runyan DL: The pre-participation examination of the young athlete, *Clin Pediatr* 22(10):674–679, 1983.
26. Salem DN, Isner JM: Cardiac screening for athletes, *Orth Clin North Am* 11(4):687–695, 1980.
27. Strong WB: Preparticipation physical examination: it should be required, *Arch Pediatric Adolesc Med* 148(1):99–100, 1994.
28. Strong WB, Steed D: Cardiovascular evaluation of the young athlete, *Pediatr Clin of North Amer* 29(6):1325–1339, 1982.
29. Tennant FS, Sorenson K, Day CM: Benefits of preparticipation sports examination, *J of Fam Prac* 13(2):287–288, 1981.
30. Thompson TR, Andrish JT, Bergfeld JA: A prospective study of preparticipation sports examinations of 2670 young athletes: method and results, *Clev Clin Q* 49(4):225–232, 1982.
31. Torg JS, Glasgow SG: Criteria for return to contact activities following cervical spine injury, *Clin J Sports Med*, 1:12–26, 1991.
32. Tucker AM: Examination of school athletes and their preparation for competition. In Matzen RN, Lang RS, eds: *Clinical Preventive Medicine*, St. Louis, 1993, Mosby–Year Book.
33. VanCamp SP: Sudden death in athletes. In Grana WA, Lombardo JA, eds: Advances in sports medicine and fitness, Chicago, 1988, Mosby–Year Book.

CHAPTER 8

ON-FIELD EMERGENCIES

Richard A. Marder

The tragic occurrence of a young, healthy athlete collapsing on the court from an unsuspected cardiac arrhythmia is a vivid reminder of the paramount importance of having a medical team poised to deliver effective emergency treatment. Of added significance is that, in many instances, the initial treatment may positively or negatively impact the final outcome. Although more likely in contact sports such as football, every team physician must be prepared to deal with a catastrophic occurrence.[24,32]

"Sudden death," head and neck injuries with and without cardiopulmonary arrest, heatstroke, blunt chest and abdominal trauma, open fractures, and limb threatening dislocations are among the many potential serious injuries the medical staff must be able to handle. Although an up-to-date knowledge of emergency treatment, proper and functioning resuscitative equipment, and ancillary emergency services are vital components, the key to successful management of most on-field emergencies remains a well-organized, preinjury plan developed and executed by the medical staff under the leadership of the team physician(s).

PRINCIPLES

Prior to the start of the season, the team physician(s) and trainer(s) identify potential emergencies for their sport and establish or review treatment protocols. This will include identifying any athletes on the team at particular risk, developing responses to specific on-field emergencies that are coordinated with the chosen emergency medical service, selecting and learning to use needed resuscitative equipment, and arranging for potential hospital services.

Foremost is implementation of the capability to provide emergent care to the athlete in cardiopulmonary arrest. The ability to provide basic life support (BLS) procedures by two or more members of the medical staff is an absolute necessity; ideally, at least one member of the medical team will be certified in advanced life support techniques (ACLS).

Basic Life Support

The singular goal of this is to provide oxygen to the brain and heart until definitive medical treatment can restore normal cardiac and pulmonary functions. Cardiopulmonary resuscitation (CPR) consists of three components: airway, breathing, and circulation (the "ABCs") and can be performed without any equipment.[10]

Advanced Life Support

Advanced life support improves upon the organ perfusion accomplished during basic life support. This is achieved by securing adequate ventilation and maintaining cardiac output and blood pressure through correction of cardiac arrhythmias.[11] Essential components of therapy include early defibrillation of those athletes with ventricular tachycardia or fibrillation, tracheal intubation and ventilation with oxygen, intravenous fluid replacement, and appropriate resuscitative medications as indicated. The ability to defibrillate the heart in ventricular tachycardia or fibrillation within minutes of cardiac arrest greatly improves the odds of survival.[6,7] In advance of an emergency, the medical staff should divide and assume the component responsibilities of ACLS: leader of the resuscitation effort; airway, ventilation, and intubation; cardiac compression; cardiac monitoring/defibrillation; and intravenous access and administration.

EMERGENCY PERSONNEL, EQUIPMENT, AND TRANSPORTATION

Before the season the medical staff will decide what emergency equipment to maintain during games and practices and will need to contract with an ambulance or emergency medical service to provide on-field coverage along with transport of the seriously injured athlete to a hospital or medical center. If the selected hospital facility is not a Level I center, the medical team should make arrangements to have appropriate specialists readily available by call.[1] At each away game, the visiting team physician and trainer should meet with their counterparts from the home team in order to review standard emergency procedures including the level of training of emergency medical personnel, location and method of obtaining the assistance of such personnel during the game, and evacuation of the seriously injured player requiring hospital services.

Providers of emergency medical services differ markedly in their levels of training.[12,39] An Emergency Medical Technician-Ambulance (EMT-A) is trained in basic life support only and has skills in routine splinting, use of oxygen, and transport. More highly trained EMTs have experience in defibrillator use, tracheal airways, and central lines. Whenever possible, especially in high risk sports, emergency personnel trained in ACLS, such as an EMT-P (Paramedic), should be utilized. The medical staff, through a pre-arranged signal, must be able to immediately call the emergency medical services personnel on to the field or court. Familiarity of the medical staff with the abilities and equipment of the emergency services personnel, in conjunction with a preemergency plan for resuscitation and transport, can optimize treatment of the injured athlete.

Equipment for dealing with on-field injuries will vary by sport and medical staff preferences. Although no standards exist, by reviewing the potential injuries to each organ system, each medical staff can develop a checklist of useful equipment (see box below). This is in addition to the usual medications and equipment available for nonemergencies.[26] Experience and advances in therapy will result in season to season modifications. Depending on individual circumstances, the medical staff

may decide to maintain their own equipment for advanced life support (cardiac defibrillator, oropharyngeal and endotracheal airway tubes, intravenous set-ups, cardiac medications, etc.) or have these items provisioned by the emergency medical service. Certain equipment should be carried 'on-person' by one of the medical staff, including a pocketknife, scissors, penlight, and padded tongue blade. All other equipment must be immediately available on the sidelines.

INJURY PATTERNS

As observed from the sidelines, injuries that occur during sporting events can be categorized according to one of the following presentations. (1) athlete down from contact and not moving, (2) athlete down from contact and moving, (3) athlete down without contact, and (4) athlete injured but moving to the sidelines under his own power. Examination begins with an assessment of the level of consciousness, airway, breathing, and circulatory status. Subsequently, a secondary survey is performed to evaluate potential neurologic, chest, abdominal, and extremity injuries.

ATHLETE DOWN FROM CONTACT AND NOT MOVING

A sense of urgency is quickly detected as fellow players frantically motion to the sidelines for help. The previously designated medical staff who will provide the initial assess-

---

EMERGENCY MEDICAL EQUIPMENT AND MEDICATIONS CHECKLIST

For resuscitation

airway	oro- and nasopharyngeal airways, endotracheal tubes, laryngoscope, 14-gauge catheter for cricothyrotomy Other: bolt cutters in sports with obstructing face mask
breathing	supplemental oxygen, mask with oxygen inlet, bag-valve mask, epinephrine kit, albuterol inhalers, aminophylline
circulation	cardiac monitor/defibrillator, intravenous catheters, tubing, and solutions (crystalloid), cardiac drugs (epinephrine, atropine, lidocaine, etc.) Other: PASG if hospital transit time excessive

For transport

spineboard, rigid cervical collar, sandbags, ambulance bed or stretcher, blankets

Diagnostic equipment

stethoscope, sphygmomanometer, penlight, combination oto-opthalmascope, thermometer, reflex hammer

For fracture care

splints (air, plaster, prefabricated), Thomas (per Dorland's) or Hare femoral traction splints, knee immobilizers, cast padding, finger splints, ace and bias bandages, slings, clavicle loops, shoulder immobilizers, crutches, and cervical collars (rigid and soft).

Other

Minor surgical and suture sets, scalpels, eye patches, fluroscein, irrigation sets, alcohol, betadine, lidocaine, ethyl chloride spray, tongue blades, adhesive tape, sterile gloves, needles, syringes, sponge pads, drapes, bandages, etc.

ment runs to the player without delay. This may be the team trainer(s) alone or with the team physician depending on preference. A number of possibilities must be considered: concussion and other cerebral trauma, fracture-dislocations of the spine, blunt chest trauma, as well as the fact that the athlete, as a consequence of injury, is in frank cardiopulmonary arrest. The medical team must be prepared to initiate resuscitation on the field. On reaching the player, the injury plan goes into action.

Assessment

Without moving the player, the designated medical staff member kneels, lightly touches the player with a hand, and inquires, "are you okay" or "where are you hurt." Even in a prone position, it is usually possible to deter-

mine if there is spontaneous breathing by either observing chest expansion or feeling air movement during exhalation. Three possible scenarios exist: the player is (a) unconscious and not breathing, (b) unconscious but breathing, or (c) conscious and breathing.

PLAYER UNCONSCIOUS AND NOT BREATHING. Upon determining this, the on-field examiner raises his or her hand in a prearranged signal to the other sidelines medical staff who will start onto the field with the emergency medical equipment. If one of the medical staff is not ACLS trained, signal the emergency medical crew to come onto the field. Using the universal algorithm for adult emergency cardiac care, CPR is started (Fig. 8-1). At this point, the predetermined leader for CPR assumes control. The player must be positioned

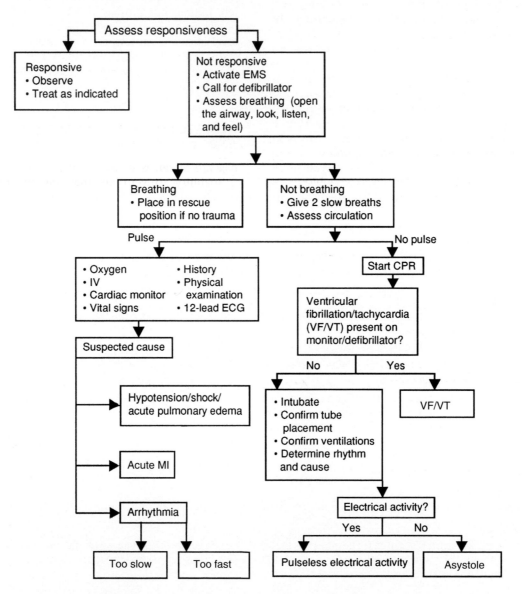

Fig. 8-1. Universal algorithm for adult emergency cardiac care (ECC). (From Emergency Cardiac Care Committee and Subcommittees, American Heart Association: Guidelines for cardiopulmonary resuscitation and emergency cardiac care, III: Adult advanced cardiac life support, *JAMA* 268:2199–2241, 1992; with permission.)

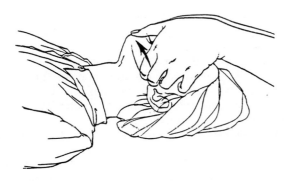

Fig. 8-2. Jaw-thrust maneuver for opening airway in player with suspected cervical spine injury. (From American Heart Association: Basic Life Support for Healthcare Providers, Dallas, 1994, American Heart Association; with permission.)

supine using techniques to protect the cervical spine, which must be presumed injured. While a physician or trainer applies gentle longitudinal traction to the head to maintain the head and neck in line with the body, at least three other staff members, positioned at the shoulders, hips, and legs, log-roll the athlete into the supine position onto a rigid, long spine board.[36] If there is no spontaneous breathing, CPR must be initiated. If not already present, the emergency medical services personnel should be notified by signal to assist on the field.

Airway and Breathing. A face mask may block access to the airway. Without removing the helmet, a window in the face mask can be cut using a bolt cutter, or when present, the helmet anchoring plastic loops can be detached by a knife. If it is deemed necessary to remove the helmet, the neck and head should be stabilized by a

rescuer inserting his hands under the helmet from below. If so, placement of a rigid cervical collar with adjunctive immobilization using towel rolls, sandbags, and/or forehead taping to the spine board is performed at this time. A rigid collar, by itself, is unable to control motion of the occipital-cervical junction or the upper two cervical segments.

The most common cause of airway obstruction in the unconscious patient is the tongue. Opening the airway using the jaw-thrust maneuver protects the cervical spine. This method (Fig. 8-2) relies on forward displacement of the mandibular angles by the resuscitator with minimal backward tilt of the head.[27] Using the chin-lift, head-tilt method, however, may improve the effectiveness of opening the airway and should be used if needed to ensure adequate ventilation (Fig. 8-3).[9] If present, remove the mouth guard and clear vomitus or foreign material from the airway using the index finger to sweep in a hooking fashion along the base of the tongue. An oral (oropharyngeal) airway can be inserted.

Ventilation is started with two initial breaths, followed by a rate of 10 to 12 breaths/min, using either mouth to mouth, mouth to sealed mask, or a bag-valve to mask device.[10,11] It appears that the risk of HIV or HBV cross-infection is minimal with mouth to mouth breathing.[28] In vitro studies have shown that mouth to mask ventilation may deliver greater tidal volumes as compared to bag-valve to mask devices.[19] Nevertheless, bag-valve devices are commonly employed.

Inability to ventilate may be due to an aspirated tooth, blood, or chewing gum, as well as laryngeal edema or fracture. Laryngeal fracture is suggested by subcutaneous emphysema of the anterior neck. If laryngeal fracture is suspected and the player is not breathing, careful orotracheal intubation or emergency tra-

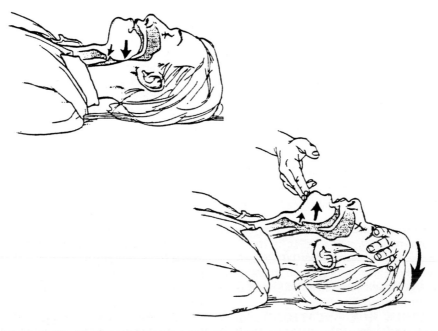

Fig. 8-3. Head-tilt, chin-lift method of opening airway. (From American Heart Association: *Basic Life Support for Healthcare Providers.* Dallas, 1994, American Heart Association; with permission.)

cheostomy is necessary.[17,33] To relieve intraluminal obstruction, perform up to five manual upper abdominal thrusts (Heimlich maneuver).[18] If this is unsuccessful, laryngoscopy can be used to remove the object or cricothyrotomy done to perform bypass ventilation.[21]

Circulation. After the airway is opened and two initial breaths have been given, determine whether or not cardiac arrest has occurred by noting the presence or absence of the carotid pulse. If the athlete is pulseless, cardiac compression is started using sternal compression at a rate of 80 to 100 compressions/min with a compression to ventilation ratio of 5:1.[10,11]

Cardiac monitoring is the next priority. Attachment of the cardiac/monitor defibrillator unit allows rhythm monitoring through "quick-look" paddles. Rhythm recognition is an essential component of ACLS training. Inability of the rescuer to analyze cardiac rhythms does not, however, preclude defibrillation. Automatic external defibrillators (AEDs) detect ventricular tachycardia and fibrillation, discharging automatically. The success of AEDs compares favorably with trained personnel using manual defibrillators.[5]

Prior to defibrillation, manual cervical stabilization must be replaced, if not already done, by a hard cervical collar supplemented by additional immobilization. Once ventricular tachycardia or fibrillation has been detected, defibrillation is carried out using up to three sequentially stacked shocks of increasing energy (Fig. 8-4). Early defibrillation takes precedence over endotracheal intubation and intravenous therapy due to the responsiveness of ventricular tachycardia and fibrillation to early shocking.[11]

The presence of electrical activity without a pulse (electromechanical disassociation) is most often due to hypovolemia. Other causes include tension pneumothorax and cardiac tamponade. Relieving hypoxemia and hypovolemia may reverse this condition. Therefore, endotracheal intubation and rapid intravenous fluid replacement are indicated. If spontaneous circulation does not return following these measures, epinephrine 1 mg is administered intravenously and repeated every 3 to 5 minutes.[11] Atropine is used for bradycardia.

If ventricular tachycardia or fibrillation persists or recurs after initial attempts at defibrillation, endotracheal intubation and intravenous access are necessary.[11] Epinephrine is administered and defibrillation repeated with an energy of 360 J. Intravenous bolus followed by drip infusion of an antiarrythmic drug (lidocaine and/or bretylium) is indicated for persistent ventricular tachycardia or fibrillation in conjunction with repeated defibrillation attempts following drug administration (Fig. 8-4).

Following cardioversion, the athlete may be responsive and breathing spontaneously. The athlete is transported to the hospital, receiving supplemental oxygen and intravenous fluids. A lidocaine or bretylium infusion is continued or started when the cause of cardiac arrest is ventricular tachycardia or fibrillation.

PLAYER UNCONSCIOUS BUT BREATHING. Assume the player has sustained a severe head and/or neck injury. If in the prone position, the player is log-rolled to the supine position for further evaluation, while manually maintaining the head and neck "in line" to the body using gentle, longitudinal traction.

Airway and Breathing. Secure an open airway with the neck neutral; if present, remove the mouthguard. The jaw-thrust maneuver can be used for improved airway patency. Be alert to the potential for respiratory arrest, depression, or aspiration.

Circulation. The adequacy of circulation (systolic blood pressure) is first estimated by the ability to palpate the radial (80 mm Hg or >), femoral (70 mm Hg or >), and carotid (60 mm Hg or >) pulses. Note the pulse rate and quality. An absent or thready radial pulse, extremity coolness, or delayed capillary refill (> 2 seconds) suggests hypovolemic shock. Measure the blood pressure using a sphygmomanometer. The combination of elevated blood pressure and bradycardia suggests increasing intracranial pressure, whereas spinal shock accompanying cervical fracture-dislocation is more likely to produce a decrease in both pulse and blood pressure owing to loss of sympathetic tone.[8]

Neurologic. The exam is directed at determining the level of consciousness and the presence of any focal neurologic deficits. Continue to monitor breathing and circulation. Do not reduce the head neck to align with the long axis of the body, but manually maintain their position relative to the body. Rotary dislocation of C_1-C_2 and unilateral facet dislocations may produce asymmetric positioning of the neck. Note any unusual flexion (decorticate) or extension (decerebrate) posturing of the extremities. Determine the best eye, verbal, and motor responses according to the Glasgow Coma Scale (Table 8-1).[29] Coma is defined as absence of any eye opening, motor, and sensory responses (Glasgow score of 3). Measure pupillary diameters and response to light. Differences in diameter greater than 1 mm and asymmetry of reactivity to light are abnormal.[38] Lateralized extremity motor weakness is difficult to detect in the unresponsive patient. Subtle differences in extremity response to stimuli may be the only finding. A palpable depressed skull fracture or signs of a basilar skull fracture (orbital ecchymosis, mastoid ecchymosis, or cerebrospinal fluid leaking from the ear or nose) may be evident.

The presence of abnormal posturing, lateralized weakness, pupillary asymmetry, vomiting, prolonged unconsciousness, bradycardia, and elevated blood pressure are symptoms and signs of increasing intracranial pressure and portend imminent cerebral herniation. If any of these are noted or subsequently develop, immediately transport the athlete, with the head and neck securely immobilized, to an alerted neurosurgical team for evaluation and treatment. Adjunct measures to combat rising intracranial pressure may be performed en route so as not to delay transport. These include endotracheal intubation for hyperventilation to reduce pCO_2 to between 25 to 30 mm and intravenous Mannitol (50 to 100 g).[20] If the player regains consciousness while being attended, proceed with the screening neurologic examination. Inquire about the presence of neck pain or headache as well as numbness, tingling, or weakness of the extremities. Perform a mental status

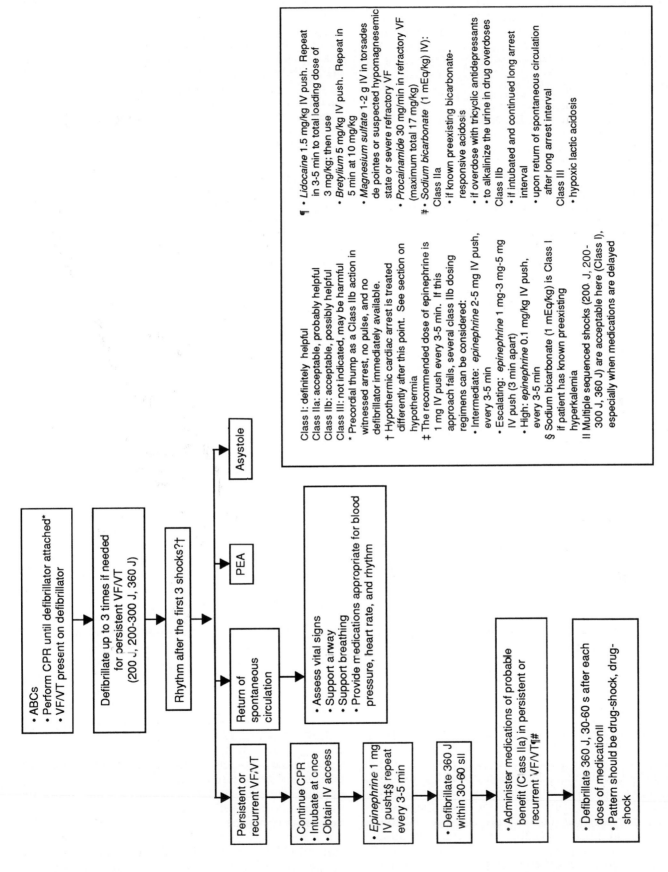

Fig. 8-4. Algorithm for ventricular fibrillation and pulseless ventricular tachycardia (VF/VT). (From Emergency Cardiac Care Committee and Subcommittees, American Heart Association: Guidelines for cardiopulmonary resuscitation and emergency cardiac care, III: Adult advanced cardiac life support. *JAMA* 268:2199–2241, 1992; with permission.)

Table 8-1. Glasgow coma scale

Eye opening	Spontaneous	4
	To voice	3
	To pain	2
	None	1
Motor response	Obeys commands	6
	Purposeful movement	5
	Withdraws to pain	4
	Flexion posturing	3
	Extension posturing	2
	None	1
Verbal response	Oriented	5
	Confused	4
	Inappropriate words	3
	Incomprehensible sounds	2
	None	1
Possible score		3–15

check to determine orientation and if there is amnesia, either post-traumatic or retrograde. Test extraocular movement. Palpate the cervical spine for any tenderness or hematoma, and step-off of the lower cervical and upper thoracic spinous processes. Prolonged unconsciousness (> 3 to 5 min), retrograde amnesia, focal neurologic deficit, abnormal cervical finding, complaints of neck pain, numbness, tingling, and/or extremity weakness are indications for immediate hospital transfer, while maintaining spinal immobilization.

If the cervical exam and screening neurologic are negative, the player is allowed to perform active range of motion of the neck. If no pain or limitation of cervical motion is noted, the player, with assistance, can walk off the field. After suffering a concussion, the player may experience headache, confusion, blurred vision, amnesia, and unsteadiness. The player who has sustained only a mild concussion may usually return to the same game after resolution of all symptoms and signs.[20,36,37] However, cognizant of the significant number of sports fatalities from cerebral trauma and the difficulty of performing close and frequent observation along the sidelines, the team physician may prefer to have a player hospitalized for evaluation and further observation.

PLAYER CONSCIOUS AND BREATHING BUT NOT MOVING. Injury may range from a player having his "wind knocked out" from a blow to the upper abdomen causing temporary paralysis of the diaphragm, to a fracture-dislocation of the cervical spine, with quadriplegia and potential respiratory arrest. The trainer and/or physician, as they arrive, should kneel by the player, touching him to provide reassurance. Even if the player complains of abdominal pain, for example, proceed with the standard protocol ("ABCs") for evaluating the injured player. Manually immobilize the head and neck whether the player is supine or prone while the assessment is started. Determine the player's level of consciousness and then assess the airway and breathing status.

Airway and Breathing. Without moving the player, the trainer and/or team physician observe respira-

tory rate and pattern. If dyspnea, stridor, wheezing, or a respiratory rate above 30 breaths/min are noted, ventilatory support is needed. Before proceeding, the player needs to be log-rolled to the supine position onto the spine board, protecting the cervical spine as described earlier. If the player is helmeted, the face mask will need to be cut away to provide airway access. Remove the mouthguard. If respirations are abnormal, check the chest for asymmetrical chest wall motion, palpate for crepitus and tenderness over the sternum and ribs, and auscultate the chest, listening for diminished breath sounds. Stridor, hoarseness, and/or subcutaneous emphysema of the anterior neck should alert the examiner to the possibility of laryngeal fracture.

If a flail chest (paradoxical wall motion due to multiple rib fractures) is noted, initial management consists of direct pressure manually or with a sandbag over the flail segment, which can improve the efficiency of ventilation. Intubation and mechanical ventilation may be necessary. If a tension pneumothorax develops (progressive respiratory distress, tracheal shift, and shock with distended neck veins), immediate decompression of the affected lung by inserting a 14-gauge needle in the second intercostal space in line with the midclavicle is necessary. Simple pneumothorax although causing tachypnea and pain usually does not require on-field decompression.

Control of the airway is a dilemma in the player with suspected laryngeal fracture. While milder injury may be able to be managed without the need for airway intervention, the risk of complete airway loss is possible. While careful orotracheal intubation has been used to ventilate successfully in some cases, emergency tracheostomy is recommended for severe laryngotracheal separation.[17,33]

Circulation. Palpate the radial pulse, noting its quality and rate. Use a sphygmomanometer to follow blood pressure. If shock is present, start treatment as described previously while continuing with the neurologic examination. Compression may be needed to control external hemorrhage.

Neurologic. Ask the player whether he has any head, neck, or back pain. Determine whether he has active movement of each extremity and note if sensation is present or absent. If neck or back pain is present or the player has abnormal or lost sensation, weakness or loss of active extremity motion, great caution must be exercised by the medical team to prevent further injury to the injured spine. While maintaining manual control of the head and neck, palpate for any cervical tenderness, soft tissue swelling, or deformity.

Once there is symptomatic or physical evidence of a cervical injury, immobilization in preparation for transport should be performed before proceeding with additional examination of the player. Securing the player to the spine board together with continued manual traction maintaining the neck in neutral may prevent additional cervical trauma. Although respiratory failure occurs quickly in cervical lesions above C_4 due to paralysis of the diaphragm, even in lower level injury, airway and breathing need to be monitored due to the potential for respiratory insufficiency. Without unduly delaying transport, an adequate peripheral neurologic examination is done to establish a baseline. The player who is less than fully responsive must be checked with a comprehensive cranial examination as discussed previously.

A stretcher or ambulance bed should be used for transport. A neurosurgical and orthopedic spine team should be on alert at the receiving hospital. One of the team physicians should accompany the injured player.

In the fully responsive player with a negative screening examination, active cervical spine motion can be assessed. Again, any limitation of motion or pain requires continued protected immobilization and transport for further evaluation. In this case, if no limitation of motion or pain is experienced during active motion, the player can walk off the field without immobilization and undergo more detailed examination on the sidelines.

Secondary Survey. If present, the abdominal or extremity injury is now addressed by the examiners.

ATHLETE DOWN FROM CONTACT AND MOVING

The player writhing on the field or court after a collision is likely to have sustained a musculoskeletal, chest, or abdominal injury. The athlete may be clutching the injured area, or deformity of an extremity may be readily apparent.

Assessment
The trainer kneels and establishes verbal contact with the player. The level of responsiveness is quickly established.

Airway, Breathing, and Circulation
Remove the mouthguard, if present. Observe the player's breathing rate and pattern; check the adequacy of circulation by palpating the peripheral pulse. If respiratory or circulatory distress is present, initiate CPR as described previously. If vital signs are stable, proceed to the neurologic and secondary survey.

Neurologic
Start by reviewing the level of responsiveness of the athlete. Inquire as to head or neck pain, presence of any numbness, tingling, or weakness of the extremities. Palpate the neck. If no neurologic abnormalities are present, proceed to the area of complaint.

ATHLETE DOWN ON THE FIELD WITHOUT CONTACT

A number of potentially life threatening conditions present in this manner, including "sudden death," anaphylaxis from an insect bite or drug reaction, seizure, heatstroke, as well as nonemergent, noncontact musculoskeletal injuries of the lower extremity (e.g., ACL tear, ankle sprain).

Assessment
As in the preceding examples, the trainer approaches the player, kneels, and without moving him, determines responsiveness to the question, "are you okay" or "where are you hurt?" If the player is not breathing, the trainer signals the sideliness for help from the other medical staff. In this situation, where the athlete has been seen to collapse without contact, the likelihood of cervical injury is minimal. Therefore, the player can quickly be turned supine to secure a patent airway and prepare for resuscitation.

Airway and Breathing
If the patient is experiencing "sudden death," he may be semi-conscious and agonal respirations may be noted. Using the chin-lift, head tilt method, open the airway. Remove the mouthguard and any foreign matter. Give two initial breaths and begin ventilation.

Circulation
Without a palpable carotid pulse, sternal compressions are initiated as described previously. The rapidity with which the cardiac monitor/defibrillator is attached in the player presenting in this manner cannot be overemphasized. As Maron et al. have reported, hypertrophic cardiac myopathy is the most common condition associated with "sudden death" in the athlete.[22] A potential sequence of arrhythmia occurrence is ventricular tachycardia, progressing to ventricular fibrillation, and finally asystole if untreated.[16] Defibrillation is performed as described previously (Fig. 8-5).

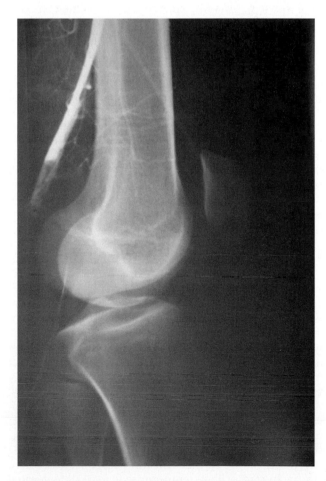

Fig. 8-5. Arteriogram demonstrating in situ thrombosis of popliteal artery following knee dislocation.

ATHLETE INJURED BUT MOVING OFF THE FIELD UNDER HIS OWN POWER

Most of these injuries are nonemergent, consisting of a variety of musculoskeletal conditions such as shoulder and finger dislocations, ankle and knee injuries, and acute muscle strains. However, a number of potentially serious injuries, including transient quadriparesis,[31] acute brachial plexus traction injuries,[3] pneumothorax, or aspiration of a foreign body may also present in this fashion.

OTHER SPECIFIC EMERGENCIES

Anaphylaxis

Antibody (IgE) mediated systemic reactions can result from exposure of a sensitized individual to pollens, insect stings, or drugs. Shock due to decreased peripheral resistance, and pulmonary distress due to bronchospasm and/or laryngeal edema, may develop quickly. Local erythema and edema from a bite or sting and generalized urticaria and pruritis may be present. There may be no known history or previous episodes.

MANAGEMENT. The first line of treatment is epinephrine, oxygen, and fluid replacement.[34] Epinephrine in a dose of 3 to 5 cc (1:1000 dilution) is administered subcutaneously and repeated as necessary. Pre-filled syringe kits (e.g., Ana-Kit, EpiPen) facilitate emergent use. If shock is severe and the player markedly dyspneic, epinephrine can be used intravenously (3 to 5 ml of a 1:10,000 dilution) or delivered through an endotracheal tube.[8,34]

The airway must be ensured. Laryngeal stridor dictates immediate need for ventilation by intubation or cricothyrotomy. Wheezing and dyspnea from bronchospasm not responsive to initial epinephrine and supplemental oxygen is managed with a beta-agonist inhaler (albuterol), followed by intravenous aminophylline (250 to 500 mg over 20 to 40 minutes) if necessary.[8,34]

Rapid fluid resuscitation using crystalloid is started and the patient is transported to the hospital for observation and further treatment as necessary.

Heat Illness

A number of heat-related disorders can affect the athlete, the most serious of which is heatstroke.[25] Heatstroke results from a derangement of the normal sweating response that maintains the core body temperature. If fluid lost from sweating is not replaced, the hypovolemia that develops may result in cerebral mediated cessation of sweating to preserve circulatory volume. This in turn causes a rapid rise in internal body temperature.

Clinically, heatstroke can present with lightheadedness, nausea, confusion, uncoordination, or most dramatically, loss of consciousness with collapse. Characteristic are the findings of hot and dry skin, indicating shut-down of the normal sweating response associated with tachycardia. Body temperature is markedly elevated and, due to unreliability of oral temperature readings, is best followed with rectal temperatures.

MANAGEMENT. If the player is not breathing, CPR is started. Further treatment is directed at immediate lowering of body temperature to prevent permanent damage to the brain, kidneys, and liver. Rapid cooling with ice packs, immersion in cold water, and rapid intravenous fluid replacement should be started immediately with transport to the hospital for further treatment.

Abdominal Injury

Intraabdominal injuries may occur in contact sports. A direct blow to the abdomen or flank can cause injury to the abdominal wall itself (e.g., rectus abdominis contusion) or to an underlying organ, usually the spleen, liver, and kidney. Abdominal wall injuries are associated with localized pain and tenderness, especially with active muscle contraction, but may be difficult to differentiate from intraabdominal injury in certain cases. Characteristically, intraabdominal injuries exhibit diffuse abdominal pain and tenderness, signs of peritoneal irritation, and shock from bleeding.

If the abdominal injury consists of solid organ bleeding, and especially with retroperitoneal (kidney) injury, early clinical findings may be minimal, and diagnosis may depend upon a high index of suspicion.[14] When assessed on the field immediately after injury, pain and abdominal tenderness may be the only significant clinical findings in the patient with a serious abdominal injury. Bleeding, either intracapsular of the organ involved or even intra-peritoneal, may not initially result in signs of peritoneal (pain with body motion, referred and rebound tenderness, guarding, loss of bowel sounds) or diaphragmatic (referred shoulder pain) irritation. Additionally, blood loss of 15% or less total volume may produce only slight tachycardia (Class I shock),[4] which may be difficult to determine in the acutely injured athlete. Renal injury may go undetected until gross hematuria is subsequently noted by the player after the game.

MANAGEMENT. Obviously, nothing should be given orally to the player with a suspected intraabdominal injury. If shock is developing (tachycardia and hypotension) or if there are abdominal symptoms and signs such as nausea, vomiting, referred shoulder pain, guarding, rebound tenderness, or diminished bowel sounds, then start resuscitation and prepare for immediate transport to the hospital. With no neck complaints, turn the head and neck to the side in case of vomiting to prevent aspiration. Keep the airway clear as necessary. Record the pulse rate and quality and determine the blood pressure with a sphygmomanometer. Without delaying transport, insert a 16-gauge catheter and start intravenous therapy with a crystalloid fluid challenge, maintaining the systolic blood pressure above 90 mm Hg. Cover the player with warm blankets, elevate the lower extremities, and transport. For shock not responding to rapid infusion of 2 to 3 L of intravenous crystalloid solution, a pressurized antishock garment (PASG) may be used to stabilize the player en route to the hospital, although its use remains controversial.[23]

If the player has localized abdominal pain in the absence of other symptoms and signs, the medical staff must decide whether to monitor the player on the sidelines or in the hospital setting. The importance of serial examinations and immediate transport because of a change in status cannot be overstated.

Knee Dislocation

Dislocation of the tibiofemoral joint is infrequent but is associated with a high incidence of vascular injury that can lead to amputation above the knee if circulation cannot be restored.[15] Disruption of the popliteal artery is most likely with posterior dislocations (tibia displaced posteriorly), whereas intimal injury with in situ thrombosis is noted more often with anterior dislocation due to stretching of the artery (Fig. 8-5). A key reminder is that vascular injury can occur in the dislocated knee with spontaneous reduction, potentially lulling the examiner into a false sense of security. Whereas an unreduced dislocation will readily be apparent (Fig. 8-6), a probable dislocation (dislocation with spontaneous reduction) requires careful examination. Probable dislocation should be suspected when one of the following is noted: greater than 30° of genu recurvatum (knee hyperextension), more than 1 cm of anterior-posterior tibial excursion on knee laxity exam (indicating probable anterior and posterior cruciate ligament rupture), and rapid hemarthrosis or soft tissue swelling.[35]

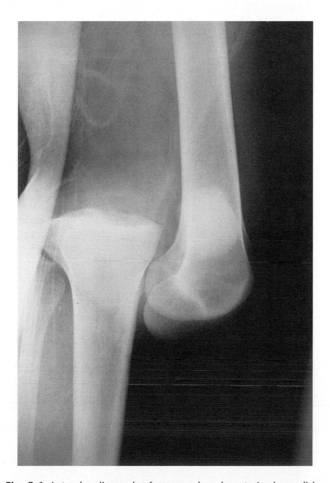

Fig. 8-6. Lateral radiograph of an unreduced posterior knee dislocation.

MANAGEMENT. Attention is first directed at determining adequacy of distal circulation and noting any impairment of distal motor and sensory function due to associated peroneal nerve injury. Check the dorsum of the first webspace to detect subtle peroneal nerve injury. If gross deformity is present and pedal pulses are absent, reduction should be attempted on the field. Longitudinal traction is usually sufficient to effect reduction of both anterior and posterior dislocations. For anterior dislocations, longitudinal traction may be combined with gentle lifting of the femur anteriorly. Hyperextension of the knee should be avoided to prevent further injury to the popliteal structures. Infrequently, a posterior dislocation may be irreducible.

After reduction, the knee may be stable in 5° to 10° of flexion with an immobilizer or posterior splint. If not, maintain longitudinal traction during transport. Repeat the distal neurovascular examination. The return of pedal pulses does not eliminate the need for immediate transport of the player to the hospital for vascular study with arteriography. Limited ligamentous surgery can be performed at the time of vascular repair, if needed, or delayed safely until 7 to 10 days, at which time delayed primary ligamentous repairs and/or reconstructions can be performed with the expectation of improved extremity perfusion and diminished soft tissue swelling.[13]

Extremity Fractures

After routine assessment of the overall physical condition of the athlete ("ABCs"), the first priority is to determine the status of distal pulses and peripheral neurologic function. Adjacent joint injury may be present, especially in fractures of the tibia and femur.[30] Bleeding from long bone fractures can be significant, leading to shock, especially in the already dehydrated athlete. Pelvic and femoral shaft fractures can result in blood loss of 2 L or more. Bleeding from fractures of the elbow, forearm, thigh, and leg rarely can lead to acute compartment syndromes.

MANAGEMENT. If pulses are absent and marked deformity exists, longitudinal traction is applied to improve alignment of the distal extremity without necessarily attempting to reduce the fracture. Otherwise, the fractured extremity is not manipulated but splinted in its position. A diligent examination of the skin about the fracture site is necessary to recognize the potential open fracture. In open fractures, no attempt is made to replace exposed bone within the soft tissue envelope. Open fracture-dislocations and open dislocations of the ankle, subtalar, knee, and elbow joints, however, are best treated by early reduction.[2] Instead, the open wound is covered using sterile gauze soaked with povidone-iodine solution secured with a gently compressive, sterile gauze bandage roll. The fracture should be splinted, with the joints immediately above and below immobilized as well. Most fractures can be splinted with an inflatable air splint or plaster, if preferred. Femoral shaft fractures are best immobilized with a commercial traction splint (Fig. 8-7) to maximize stability en route to the hospital. Observe the player for any signs of shock. Use blankets to warm the

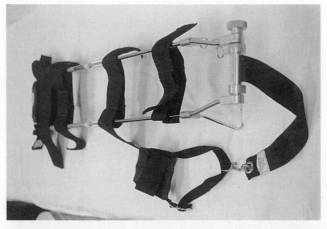

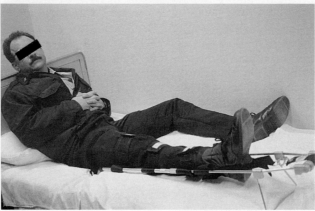

Fig. 8-7. Commercial traction splint for immobilization of femur fractures showing traction applied to the foot through the ankle hitch counterbalanced by padded ring at the ischial tuberosity of the pelvis.

player, and if indicated, insert a peripheral, large bore intravenous catheter for crystalloid infusion during transport.

SUMMARY

On-field emergencies do occur, and the fundamental key to organized and hopefully successful management is advance preparation. The medical staff should develop and rehearse preinjury plans for dealing with potential life threatening injuries. This foresight will help to ensure that functioning resuscitative equipment, the knowledge to perform life-saving CPR and other therapeutic interventions, and the ability to safely transport the injured athlete to a prepared hospital setting will be in place and operative before an actual emergency occurs.

REFERENCES

1. American College of Surgeons: *Resources for the optimal care of the injured patient.* Chicago, 1990, American College of Surgeons.
2. Chapman MW: Open fractures. In Chapman MW, ed: *Operative Orthopaedics,* ed 2, Philadelphia, 1993, JB Lippincott.
3. Clancy WG, Brand RL, Bergfeld JA: Upper trunk brachial plexus injuries in contact sports, *Am J Sports Med* 5:209–216, 1977.
4. Committee on Trauma, American College of Surgeons: *Advanced Trauma Life Support Course,* Chicago, 1985, American College of Surgeons.
5. Cummins RO, et al: Automatic external defibrillators used by emergency medical technicians: a controlled clinical trial, *JAMA* 257:1605–1610, 1987.
6. Cummins RO, et al: Improving survival from sudden cardiac arrest: the 'chain of survival' concept. A statement for health professionals from the Advanced Cardiac Life Support Subcommittee and the Emergency Cardiac Care Committee, American Heart Associaton. *Circulation* 83:1833–1847, 1991.
7. Cummins RO: From concept to standard-of-care? Review of the clinical experience with automated external defibrillators, *Ann Emerg Med* 18:1269–1275, 1989.
8. Eisenberg PR, Schuller D: Shock. In Stine RJ, Chudnofsky CR, eds: *A practical approach to Emergency Medicine,* ed 2, Boston, 1994, Little, Brown.
9. Elam JO, et al: Head-tilt method of oral resuscitation, *JAMA* 172:812–815, 1960.
10. Emergency Cardiac Care Committee and Subcommittees, American Heart Association: Guidelines for cardiopulmonary resuscitation and emergency cardiac care, II: Adult basic life support, *JAMA* 268:2184–2198, 1992.
11. Emergency Cardiac Care Committee and Subcommittees, American Heart Association: Guidelines for cardiopulmonary resuscitation and emergency cardiac care, III: Adult advanced cardiac life support, *JAMA* 268:2199–2241, 1992.
12. Emergency Medical Services System Act of 1973. Laws of

the 93rd Congress. Public Law 93-154, Washington, DC, 1973.

13. Ertl JP, Marder RA: Traumatic knee dislocations. In Chapman MW, ed: *Operative Orthopaedics*, ed 2, Philadelphia, 1993, JB Lippincott.

14. Freeman MB, Anderson CB: Abdominal emergencies. In Stine RJ, Chudnofsky CR, eds: A practical approach to Emergency Medicine, ed 2, Boston, 1994, Little, Brown.

15. Green NE, Allen BL: Vascular injuries associated with dislocation of the knee. *J Bone Joint Surg* 59A:236–239, 1977.

16. Greene HL: Sudden arrhythmic cardiac death: mechanisms, resuscitation, and classification, *Am J Cardiol* 65:4B–12B, 1990.

17. Gussack GS, Jurkovich GJ: Treatment Dilemmas in Laryngotracheal Trauma, *J Trauma* 28:1439–1444, 1988.

18. Heimlich HJ: The Heimlich maneuver to prevent food choking, *JAMA* 234:398–401, 1975.

19. Hess D, Baran C: Ventilatory volumes using mouth-to-mouth, mouth-to-mask, and bag-valve-mask devices, *Am J Emerg Med* 3:292–296, 1985.

20. Lehman LB, Ravich SJ: Closed head injuries in athletes, *Clin Sports Med* 9:247–261, 1990.

21. Mace SE: Cricothyrotomy, *J Emerg Med* 6:309–319, 1988.

22. Maron BJ, Epstein SE, Roberts WC: Causes of sudden death in competitive athletes, *J Am Coll Cardiol* 7:204–214, 1986.

23. Mattox KL, et al: Prospective MAST study in 911 patients, *J Trauma* 29:1104–1112, 1989.

24. Mueller FO, Blyth CS: Fatalities from head and cervical spine injuries in tackle football, *Clin Sports Med* 6:185–196, 1987.

25. Murphy RJ: Heat illness in the athlete, *Am J Sports Med* 12:258–261, 1984.

26. Ray RL, Feld FX: The team physician's medical bag, *Clin Sports Med* 8:139–146, 1989.

27. Safar P: Cardiopulmonary Cerebral Resuscitation, Philadelphia, 1981, WB Saunders.

28. Sande MA: Transmission of AIDS: the case against casual contagion, *N Engl J Med* 314:380–382, 1986.

29. Teasdale G, Jennett B: Assessment of coma and impaired consciousness: A practical scale, *Lancet* 2:81–83, 1974.

30. Templeman DC, Marder RA: Injuries of the knee associated with fractures of the tibial shaft. Detection by examination under anesthesia: A prospective study, *J Bone Joint Surg* 71A:1392–1395.

31. Torg JS, et al: Neuropraxia of the cervical spinal cord with transient quadriplegia, *J Bone Joint Surg* 68A:1354–1370, 1986.

32. Torg JS, et al: The National Football Head and Neck Injury Registry: 14-year report on cervical quadriplegia, 1971 through 1984, *JAMA* 254:3439–3433, 1985.

33. Trone TH, Schaefer SD, Carder HM: Blunt and penetrating laryngeal trauma: A 13 year review, *Otolaryngol Head Neck Surg* 88:257–261, 1980.

34. Valentine MD: Anaphylaxis and stinging insect hypersensitivity, *JAMA* 268:2830–2833, 1992.

35. Varnell RN, et al: Arterial injury complicating knee disruption, *Am Surg* 55:699, 1989.

36. Vesgo JJ, Lehman RC: Field evaluation and management of head and neck injuries, *Clin Sports Med* 6:1–15, 1987.

37. Wilberger JE, Maroon JC: Head injuries in athletes, *Clin Sports Med* 8:1–9, 1989.

38. Wilberger JE: Emergency care and initial evaluation. In Cooper PR, ed: *Head Injury*, Baltimore, 1993, Williams & Wilkins.

39. Williams KA: Emergency medical services system. In Stine RJ, Chudnofsky CR, eds: *A Practical Approach to Emergency Medicine*, ed 2, Boston, 1994, Little, Brown.

CHAPTER 9

WOMEN IN SPORTS

Letha Y. Griffin

Does opportunity bring enlightenment or does enlightenment bring opportunity? Both statements characterize women's athletics in the 1970s. In 1972, Title IX of the Educational Amendments was passed,[10] which mandated that in physical education and athletics in public schools women were to have equal opportunities to those of men. Because of this governmental action, increased sport participation was made available to women at both the high school and collegiate level. As the number of women participating in sports increased, research was funded to learn how to maximize benefits of athletic programs for women. Myths regarding training and performance limitations were for the first time scientifically scrutinized, and many were proven to be false.[8,19,53,72] The value of conditioning and rehabilitation, and of sport itself, was realized and soon women of all ages were being encouraged to participate in sports, not only for the advantage of competitive play, but for recreation and fitness.

Much of what is known regarding sport parameters, including data on preparticipation evaluations, conditioning and rehabilitation techniques, nutritional demands, psychologic support, and the prevalence of and approach to the diagnosis and treatment of injuries, has been gathered from experiences with male athletes. A great deal of this knowledge is applicable to female athletes. For example, in order to improve their upper body skills, women, like men, must participate in upper body conditioning programs,[78] and training aerobically improves VO_2max in both sexes.[89] However, the unique anatomic and physiologic characteristics of the female give her an identity of her own as an athlete, and understanding these characteristics and their effect on sport performance is important not only to those involved in the training, conditioning, and coaching of women athletes, but also to those involved in caring for their medical needs. Highlights of these differences and their effects on sport performance and injury will form the basis of this chapter.

INFLUENCE OF ANATOMIC AND PHYSIOLOGIC CHARACTERISTICS OF WOMEN ATHLETES ON SPORT PERFORMANCE

Although there are wide variations, the average adult female is shorter and weighs less than her male counterpart. She has shorter limbs and smaller articular surfaces, resulting in less power for striking, kicking, and throwing.[4,76] Women have narrower shoulders and a smaller thorax than men, but a larger abdomen and pelvis.[37,41,76] The length of their legs per total body height is less than men's, resulting in women having a lower center of gravity and hence better balance than men.[4,37] For example, most men would have a difficult time balancing on a 4½-inch beam and yet women gymnasts do this with ease.

Females have less muscle mass per total body weight than equally trained and conditioned males.[41,82] Because of this, males can run faster, jump higher, and lift greater weight than equally trained and conditioned females. Female athletes, because they have a greater percent of body fat per body weight, are more buoyant and better insulated than their male counterparts.[41,82,86,87] They, therefore, have an advantage in water sports, particularly those done in cold water. It is not surprising then that many English Channel swim records have been set by women.[57] Moreover, women have most of their subcutaneous fat in their hips and lower body regions, whereas men carry their subcutaneous fat in their abdomen and upper body.[82] This distribution of body fat also contributes to the lower center of gravity in the female.

Greater breast development in the female requires modification of sporting gear to include wide strap, maximally supportive bras of soft, sweat absorbent material.[32,38,90] Although at one time there was concern that contact sports and jumping activities would harm the female uterus and ovaries, we now know that as with other pelvic organs, the uterus and ovaries are well suspended and protected in the pelvis. Uterine prolapse will not occur unless the abdominal floor is weakened by pathologic processes.[53]

Because of their smaller body size, women have a

smaller heart size and heart volume, resulting in a smaller stroke volume and thus an increased heart rate for a given submaximal cardiac output (cardiac output = stroke volume × heart rate).[41,54,82] Because woman's stroke volume is less, even with an increased heart rate, her cardiac output is approximately 30% lower than an equally trained man's.[82] Her systolic blood pressure is also lower than a man's.[41,82] Because men have approximately 6% more red blood cells and 10% to 15% more hemoglobin per 100 cc of blood than women, their blood has a greater oxygen carrying capacity.[5,22]

Adult men, because of their larger chest size, have a greater vital capacity than women.[4] Vital capacity (VC) is the maximal volume of air that can be moved through the lungs from a maximal inspiration to a maximal expiration.[54] A man's residual volume (RV), the volume of air that remains in the lungs following maximal expiration, is also greater. Because VC and RV are less in women, total lung capacity (TLC) is also smaller. In fact, an adult woman's breathing capacity is approximately 10% less than her age-matched male partner's.[82]

Furthermore, at the same submaximal respiratory minute volume (tidal volume × respiratory rate) women have a smaller tidal volume but a faster respiratory rate than men.[82] Oxygen pulse, which is a measure of the efficiency of the heart and respiratory systems, that is, the quantity of oxygen used by the body per heart beat, is approximately three times higher in adult males.[4] All these differences in physiologic parameters combine together to give men a greater maximum oxygen uptake (VO_2max).[54,82] VO_2max is accepted as the best single measure of cardiovascular fitness or aerobic ability. It measures the lungs' ability to extract oxygen from the air and deliver it to the blood, the blood's ability to circulate that oxygen to muscle tissue, and the muscle's ability to effectively use oxygen in energy pathways. Prior to puberty, VO_2max is about the same for both sexes, and although both sexes reach their peak VO_2max by the late teenage years, the VO_2max of the post-pubertal male is greater than that of the female. In fact, expressed per total body weight, men's VO_2max is on the average 28% greater than women's.[82] Even if you express VO_2max relative to fat-free weight rather than total body weight, the differences between the sexes is still considerable. A man's VO_2max per fat-free weight is, on the average, 15% to 25% greater than that of a woman's.[4,82]

At one time, it was felt that women exercising in warm weather were at an increased risk for hyperthermia because, unlike males, they could not effectively decrease core body temperature by sweating. Research has since shown this not to be true. Both men and women can increase the amount and rate they sweat by conditioning in warm weather.[28,39,61,83]

Women physiologically mature earlier than men. Even in infancy, girls have more advanced skeletal ossification than boys. The adolescent growth spurt, which precedes sexual maturation, occurs in girls at about 11 years of age; the adolescent growth spurt in boys does not begin until approximately 1 to 3 years later.[74,82] Bone growth in girls ceases at about age 20, but in boys growth continues until the early 20s. Tables 9-1 and 9-2 summarize these anatomic and physiologic differences.

Menstrual Dysfunction in Athletes

Another factor unique to the female athlete is monthly hormonal cycling that begins at puberty. Athletes fre-

Table 9-1. Men and women athletes: Impact on performance of anatomic differences*

	Anatomic differences		
System	Women	Men	Impact
Height	64.5"	68.5"	
Weight	56.8 kg	70.0 kg	
Limb length	Shorter	Longer	Men can achieve a greater force for hitting or kicking.
Articular surface	Smaller	Larger	May provide men with greater joint stability; men have greater surface area to dissipate impact force.
Body shape	Narrow shoulders Wider hips Legs 51.2% of height More fat in lower body	Wider shoulders Narrower hips Legs 52% of height More fat in upper body	Women have lower center of gravity and therefore greater balance ability; women have an increased valgus angle at the knee that increases knee injuries; women and men have different running gaits.
% Muscle/TBW*	~36%	~44.8%	Men have greater strength and greater speed.
% Fat/TBW**	~22%–26%	~13%–16%	Women are more buoyant and better insulated; they may be able to convert to fatty acid metabolism more rapidly.
Age at skeletal maturation	17–19 yrs	21–22 yrs	Women develop adult body shape/form sooner than men.

* Comparisons are made for "average" post pubertal male and female
** Varies somewhat with age, sport, and level of conditioning

Table 9-2. Men and women athletes: Impact on performance of physiologic differences*

	Physiologic differences		
System	Women	Men	Impact
Cardiovascular			
Heart size	Smaller	Larger	Women's stroke volume is less, necessitating an increased heart rate for a given submaximal cardiac output; cardiac output in women is ~30% less than in men; women may be less at risk of developing hypertension.
Heart volume	Smaller	Larger	
Systolic blood pressure	Lower	Higher	
Hemopoietic			
Hemoglobin		10%–15% > per 100 cc blood	Men's blood has a greater oxygen carrying capacity.
Pulmonary			
Chest size	Smaller	Larger	Total lung capacity in men is greater than in women.
Lung size	Smaller	Larger	
Vital capacity (VC)	Smaller	Larger	
Residual volume (RV)	Smaller	Larger	
Efficiency of cardiorespiratory system			
Oxygen pulse	Lower	Higher	Higher oxygen pulse provides men an advantage in aerobic activity.
Level of aerobic fitness (reflects performance of cardiorespiratory and muscular systems)			
VO_2max	Lower	Higher	Men have greater aerobic ability.
Metabolism (BMR)	~6%–10% lower (when related to body surface area)	~6%–10% higher (when related to body surface area)	Women need fewer calories to sustain same activity level as men.
Thermoregulation	Female = Male	Female = Male	Both sexes can adequately sweat in hot weather to decrease core body temperature.

* Comparisons are made for "average" post pubertal male and female

quently have alterations in their monthly cycling. For example, puberty is often delayed by several years in women athletes, especially those who rigorously control their diet to achieve a "lean look"[11,12,79] and those who begin intense training at a very early age.[30] It has been proposed that the delay in puberty is secondary to an alteration of hypothalamic function caused by (1) the athlete's lack of body fat and the restriction of dietary fat resulting in a decreased concentration of circulating estrogen[31,73] and/or progesterone,[40] (2) the physical or psychological stresses of intense training,[27,33] (3) yet undefined genetic factors that are shared by those who are good athletes,[47] or (4) other influencing factors (see box). More research is needed in this area. The mean age for menarche in the U.S. is 12.8 years. Studies have reported the mean age of menarche in dancers to be 15.4 years[81]; in national level runners to be 14.1 years[27]; and in collegiate track and field athletes to be 13.6 years.[48] A delay in the onset of menses beyond the age of 16 is called primary amenorrhea.

Athletes may also experience oligomenorrhea or secondary amenorrhea. Risk factors for developing oligomenorrhea or secondary amenorrhea include low body weight, rapid weight loss, marked increase in the amount or intensity of training, genetic factors, and late menarche (see box on p. 89 at top of left column). Oligomenorrhea is infrequent menses, that is three to six menstrual cycles per year or cycles at intervals of greater than 38 days.[43] Secondary amenorrhea is the cessation of monthly menstrual cycles for at least 3 consecutive months after regular cycling has been established.[43,60] Although menstrual

THEORIES CONCERNING THE DELAY IN PUBERTY IN ATHLETES

- Athlete's lack of body fat and the restriction of dietary fat, resulting in a decreased concentration of circulating estrogen and/or progesterone
- Physical or psychologic stresses of intense training
- Undefined genetic factors that are shared by those who are good athletes
- Other influencing factors

RISK FACTORS ASSOCIATED WITH DEVELOPING OLIGOMENORRHEA OR SECONDARY AMENORRHEA

- Low body weight
- Rapid weight loss
- Marked increase in the amount or intensity of training
- Genetic factors
- Late menarche

dysfunction is not uncommon in women athletes, one should not assume the cessation of normal periods to be secondary to athletic participation until other potential causes have been excluded through a thorough history and physical examination including appropriate laboratory studies, which typically include tests for thyroid, pituitary, and ovarian function.[69]

Ovulatory oligomenorrhea is associated with chronic unopposed estrogen, resulting in infrequent, heavy bleeding at unpredictable times. If an athlete with amenorrhea responds to a 5-day course of medroxyprogesterone acetate by experiencing withdrawal bleeding, she is producing adequate estrogen.[70] If no withdrawal bleeding occurs, however, then the athlete has hypoestrogenic amenorrhea. It is felt that athletes with hypoestrogenic amenorrhea are at risk of developing osteoporosis, or at least low bone mass, when compared to eumenorrheic athletes performing the same sport.[20,23,45,62]

Eating disorders are frequently present in those athletes with menstrual dysfunction.[17,23] This association of amenorrhea, eating disorders, and osteoporosis has been termed the "Female Athletic Triad" (see box below). The athlete's menstrual history should be a routine part of the preparticipation examination. If menstrual irregularities are discovered, one should inquire about the athlete's eating habits.

Puberty is a time of tremendous physiologic change in both sexes. It is a time of growth when both weight and height are added. In male athletes, most of the weight gain is muscle mass. In women, both muscle and fat are increased during puberty.[15,52] Many women feel such weight gains adversely affect their performance and may resort to disorder eating, the extremes of which are anorexia and bulimia, to change their body image.[12] The incidence of eating disorders has been reported to be as

high as 60% in female athletes and is most common in young athletes 15 to 26 years of age.[21,85] When eating disorders are discovered, psychologic counseling should be considered because abnormal eating patterns have a significant effect on the general health of the female athlete, especially her bone health.[13,25,51,77]

Nutritional Concerns

Counseling on nutrition is important in all female athletes. Because females have a lower metabolic rate than males, they need to structure their diets to include all basic nutritional requirements in fewer calories than those traditionally recommended for male athletes. Moreover, most women need 1000 to 1200 mg of calcium/day in their diets; 1500 mg/day is recommended for post menopausal and adolescent women.[42] As much as possible, women should obtain their calcium needs by eating calcium-rich foods such as low fat cheese, milk, or yogurt. However, if they cannot obtain their daily requirement from natural foodstuffs, calcium supplements taken as carbonate or citrate is advisable.[7] Because women lose blood through monthly menstrual cycling, their dietary iron needs are greater than men's.[46,66] Women need to eat iron-rich foods like raisins, dates, apricots, broccoli, spinach, iron-fortified cereals, and lean red meat, which includes the dark meat of chicken and turkey.[46] Cooking in an iron skillet also helps to increase the iron in the diet.[18] Vitamin C (found in fresh fruits and vegetables), if eaten with iron-rich foods, will enhance iron absorption.[18]

CONDITIONING

Conditioning is an important part of both men's and women's sport programs. Conditioning not only maximizes performance, but also aids in preventing injuries. Conditioning programs should include strength and flexibility exercises for all muscle groups in the upper and lower extremities and trunk as well as techniques for proprioceptive skill development.

At one time, some women feared that weight training would result in bulky, undesirable muscles and unfavorably alter their looks. However, it has been proved that women can increase their strength by 44% without any increase in muscle bulk.[88] Muscle bulk is a genetically determined, hormonally controlled trait. Men can, with strength training, "bulk up" more than women because of their greater testosterone levels. Strength training can only maximize one's genetic potential.

Overuse injuries have been reported to be more common in females than in males. One reason advanced to explain this increase is that women have traditionally participated in greater numbers than men in sports where training extends throughout the year (such as skating, dancing, gymnastics, and running) rather than in sports where training typically is seasonal (i.e., football in the fall, basketball in the winter, and baseball in the spring and summer). It is thought that if one narrows the base of conditioning early in one's training, especially during the growth and development years, one

THE "FEMALE ATHLETIC TRIAD"

- Amenorrhea
- Eating disorders
- Osteoporosis

risks having a "faulty substructure," i.e., an unevenly balanced muscle base resulting in the occurrence of a high number of overuse injuries with intense sport participation. To try and prevent such injuries, in the single sport athlete, one should include in conditioning programs a variety of cross-training activities so that all muscle groups are equally developed, both in strength and flexibility.

INJURY RATES AND TYPES

Since the establishment of well structured conditioning programs for women, the number of minor injuries, especially overuse injuries, have decreased markedly, and now injury rates parallel very closely those seen in male athletes. In fact, injury types and rates seem to be more sport than sex specific (Tables 9-3, 9-4).[16,84] A few injuries, however, do appear to be somewhat more common in women than in men. These include stress fractures, patellofemoral tracking problems, anterior cruciate ligament injuries of the knee, and overuse injuries of the foot such as bunions, corns, and calluses.

Stress Fractures

The incidence of stress fractures has been reported to be 10 times greater in women athletes than in men athletes.[65] Initially, this increase was felt secondary to inadequate conditioning, but even after well structured conditioning programs became an integral part of women's sports programs, the incidence of stress fractures remained high. A potential cause for this increase is the decrease in bone mass that occurs with prolonged secondary hypoestrogenic amenorrhea.[13,59] Although studies have shown decreases in the bone mineral density of the vertebrae of women with hypoestrogenic amenorrhea, they have not shown loss of bone in the appendicular skeleton, the location of the majority of stress fractures.[14,20,34] On the other hand, a study done with runners reported that those using oral contraceptives for more than a year were less likely to develop

Table 9-3. Number and relative frequency (R) of men's and women's reportable injuries*

	1975–1977	
	No.	**R****
Women		
Basketball	383	19.5
Gymnastics	95	9.4
Softball	76	3.1
Men		
Basketball	566	15.9
Gymnastics	95	7.7
Baseball	133	2.9

* From Clark K, Buckley W: *Women's Injuries in Collegiate Sports,* **AJSM** 8(3):187–191, 1980.
** Cases/1000 athletic exposures.

Table 9-4. Injury rates for men and women athletes in comparable sports*

Sport		**Years sampled**	**Injury rate****
Softball	Women	4	3.39
Baseball	Men	5	2.08
Lacrosse	Women	4	3.46
	Men	5	3.93
Basketball	Women	2	4.18
	Men	2	4.14
Soccer	Women	4	5.07
	Men	4	4.52

* Adapted from NCAA Injury Surveillance Report, 1990–91.
** Injury rate/1000 athletic exposures.

stress fractures than those who did not use oral contraceptives.[6] The data lead one to believe that the amenorrheic athlete does have a decrease in bone mass of the appendicular skeleton, despite our inability to detect this loss with present day bone mineral density studies.

The evaluation and treatment of stress fractures in women athletes is similar to that in men, with the exception that in the female athlete with a stress fracture one should inquire about menstrual irregularities. Many now are recommending that athletes with menstrual irregularities be prescribed low dose birth control pills.[70] However, the estrogen level in such supplements is lower than that present if the athlete is cycling normally. Therefore, although such therapy may help to prevent bone loss, it is not the ultimate answer. More research is needed to better understand the multifactorial etiology and pathophysiology of the amenorrheic state so that effective treatment programs can be developed to restore normal menses in the athlete with menstrual dysfunction.

Knee: Patellofemoral Stress Syndrome

The patellofemoral stress syndrome, also called the lateral patella compression syndrome,[58] is the name given to the clinical syndrome of anterior knee pain thought to be caused by functional lateralization of the patella in the trochlear groove secondary to one or more of the following factors: an increased Q angle, a deficient VMO, and/or a tight lateral retinaculum (see box below).[58] The wider pelvis of the female (Fig. 9-1) results in a greater valgus angle of her knee when compared to a male's.[36] This produces an increased Q angle, making a woman

---

FACTORS CONTRIBUTING TO FUNCTIONAL LATERALIZATION OF THE PATELLA

- Increased Q angle
- Deficient VMO
- Tight lateral retinaculum

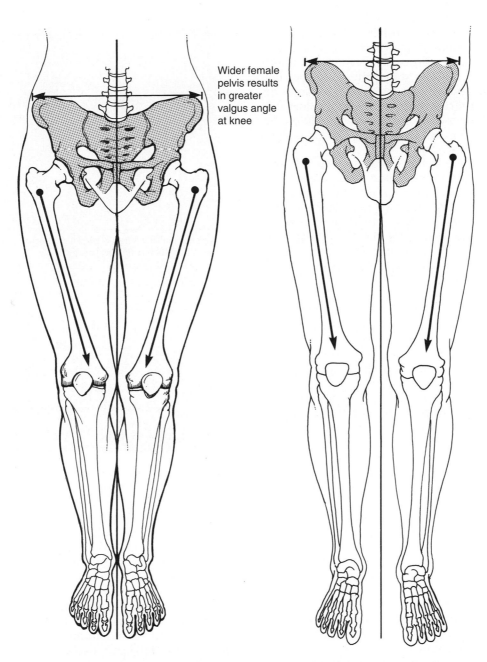

Wider female pelvis results in greater valgus angle at knee

Fig. 9-1. The wider female pelvis causes a greater valgus angle at the knee.

more at risk to develop patellofemoral stress or lateral patella compression syndrome. (The Q angle is the angle formed by the intersection of lines drawn from the anterosuperior iliac spine to midpatella and from midpatella to the anterior tibial tuberosity.) Because women have less muscle mass than men, their medial quadriceps, especially the vastus medialis obliquus muscle fibers, are frequently not well enough developed to effectively counterbalance this lateral angle. Femoral anteversion and foot pronation, if present, accentuate the functional lateralization of the patella.[3]

Athletes with patellofemoral stress typically complain of pain when running, especially down hills or when kicking or lunging, i.e., high quadriceps loading activities. Initially, the pain may be present only after activity,

but then develops during activity and eventually is present with normal activities of living like walking down stairs, squatting, or picking up an object off the floor.[26] The athlete may also experience give-way episodes. These episodes may mimic ligamentous or meniscal give-way symptoms. However, in the athlete with patellofemoral stress syndrome, the knee gives out with straight ahead, high quadriceps loading activities such as getting up from a squatted position or running down hills, rather than with twisting activities as is typically the case with ligamentous and meniscal give-way episodes.

The syndrome is commonly seen in women during the early teenage years (i.e., about or shortly after puberty at which time knee valgus increases with development of the woman's gynecoid pelvis).[63] Girls who participate primarily in running activities (i.e., soccer and cross country) seem to be particularly predisposed to develop it. During the running stride, the knee does not completely extend, and without terminal extension, the VMO does not maximally contract and hence does not become as well developed as the lateral muscle of the quadriceps groups (the vastus lateralis), which is contracting throughout extension.

Treatment for the patellofemoral stress or lateral patella compression syndrome centers about exercises to build VMO strength, in order to balance the pull of the quadriceps for better alignment of the patella in the femoral groove. These exercises should be combined with stretching exercises for the lateral retinaculum and the iliotibial band. Recommended exercises to strengthen the medial quadriceps include cross training with bicycling (done with the seat elevated), fast walking, with attention to extension of the back leg at push off, and terminal knee extension exercises performed with light weights.[35] When prescribing treatment for young girls (ages 12 to 18), who have limited time to work on an outside exercise program, creative ways to incorporate straight-leg raises and short-arc extension exercises into their prepractice warm-up is beneficial. For example, with soccer players, one can recommend they arrive at practice 10 to 15 minutes early and do three sets of 10 repetitions of short-arc extension exercises using their soccer ball as the "bump" under the affected knee. Strengthening exercises for the VMO should be combined with stretching exercises for the lateral patella stabilizers, i.e., the vastus lateralis and iliotibial band.

Climbing stadium stairs—a popular quadriceps strengthening exercise for boys—can increase patellofemoral symptoms in girls and should be avoided. Step classes can occasionally precipitate patellofemoral stress syndrome. Therefore, such classes should begin slowly, gradually increasing duration of participation and height of the step. Classes that incorporate numerous "repeat maneuvers" may be more difficult for those who tend to have patellofemoral stress syndrome than classes where the stepping sequence is more varied.

In women, as in men who pronate, arch supports may help in altering foot strike and hence improve patellar tracking. Similarly, braces that either lift the patella up, i.e., infrapatellar straps that fit under the knee below the patella at the level of the patella tendon (Fig. 9-2) or braces that dynamically try to "push" the patella more medially in the groove may be helpful (Fig. 9-3).[80] McConnell taping, a technique of knee taping developed by Australian physical therapist, Jenny McConnell, is another means to alter the glide, tilt, and rotation of the patella in the femoral groove.[56] This technique requires the athlete to be taped frequently. Therefore, it is helpful if the athlete or a member of her family learns the taping technique. Icing following activity or oral nonsteroidal anti-inflammatory medications may be prescribed for the acutely symptomatic athlete.

When treating athletes for patellofemoral stress syndrome, one needs to explain the frustrating nature of

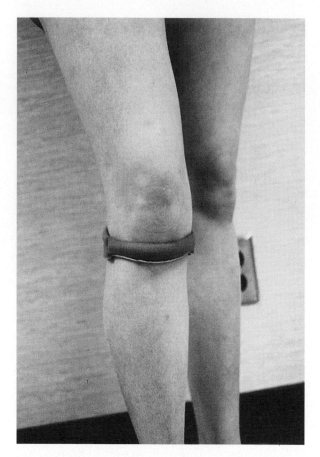

Fig. 9-2. Infrapatellar strap applies gentle pressure to infrapatellar area in attempt to favorably alter patella tracking.

this problem to the athlete, and when appropriate, to her family. It should be stressed that a muscle strengthening program to alter patellar tracking, combined with stretching of the lateral patella stabilizers, is the basis of the athlete's treatment program, and this exercise program may need to be diligently pursued for weeks or often months before positive effects are realized and pain subsides. Activity modification, knee braces, shoe orthotics, and, if the pain necessitates, anti-inflammatories and physical therapy modalities are helpful, but must be used in conjunction with an exercise program (see box in the left column on p. 93). Surgery is rarely necessary.

Knee: Ligament Injuries

Early injury data reported an equal number of ligamentous injuries in men and women athletes. It appeared to sports medicine specialists caring for women athletes, especially women involved in high risk sports such as soccer and basketball, however, that women were sustaining more anterior cruciate ligament (ACL) injuries than men. Indeed, on closer scrutiny of injury data statistics, such as the Injury Surveillance System Reports compiled by the National Collegiate Athletic Association (NCAA), it was discovered that although the total number of complete ligamentous tears was similar in men and women for soccer and basketball, the number of anterior cruciate ligament tears was greater in women participat-

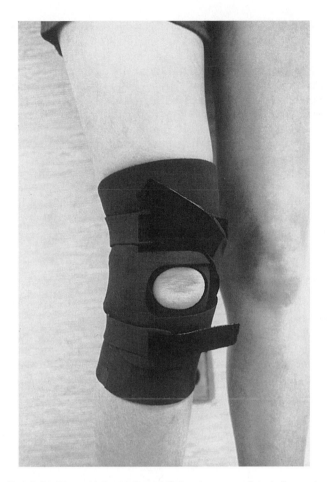

Fig. 9-3. "Dynamic" patella stabilizing brace used to help center the patella in the trochlear groove.

Table 9-5. Comparisons of the rate of complete ligament tears to the rate of anterior cruciate ligament injuries in men and women soccer players*

Sport		Incidence of complete ligament tears**	Incidence of ACL injuries
Soccer	Women	0.23	0.27
	Men	0.20	0.13

* Adapted from NCAA Injury Surveillance Report 1991–92.
** Injury rate/1000 athletic exposures.

been advanced to explain this increase in ACL injuries include: (1) Women have less muscle mass per total body weight and increased flexibility, resulting in less effective secondary restraints; (2) women's wider pelvis, lower center of gravity, and increased valgus angle of the knee may result in a different gait or jumping style than men, making them more injury prone; (3) women have smaller articular surfaces and thus less stability from their bony architecture; and (4) women have a narrower femoral notch, which may result in greater shear forces on the ACL during pivotal activities (see box below). To establish effective, preventative programs for this serious knee injury, a better understanding of these risk factors is needed.

When considering reconstructive surgery for anterior cruciate ligament injuries in women athletes, one has to carefully evaluate whether it is wise to use the patella tendon as a replacement graft. Women have been reported to have an increased incidence of patellofemoral problems, and patella graft harvesting may further increase patellofemoral symptoms.

Overuse Injuries of the Feet

The styles of dress shoes have been blamed for the increase in the number of overuse injuries of the feet in

ing in these sports (Table 9-5). Recent reports indicate that ACL injuries in women basketball players are four to six times less common in men basketball players.[48]

Since this increase in ACL injuries is even seen in highly competitive, well conditioned athletes, lack of adequate hamstring or gastrocnemius strength is not felt to be the only causative factor.[55] Other theories that have

TREATMENT OF PATELLOFEMORAL STRESS SYNDROME

- Muscle strengthening program for the vastus medialis obliquus of the quadriceps group
- Stretching of the lateral patella stabilizers
- Activity modification to avoid high patella load activities
- Knee bracing
- Shoe orthotics
- Anti-inflammatories
- Physical therapy modalities

THEORIES CONCERNING THE INCREASE IN THE NUMBER OF ACL INJURIES IN WOMEN

- Women have less muscle mass per total body weight and increased flexibility, resulting in less effective secondary restraints.
- Women's wider pelvis, lower center of gravity, and increased valgus angle of the knee may result in a different gait or jumping style than men, making them more injury prone.
- Women have smaller articular surfaces and thus less stability from their bony arhitecture.
- Women have a narrower femoral notch, which may result in greater shear forces on the ACL during pivotal activities.

women.[29,67] Bunions, corns, and calluses can result from pointed-toe, high-heeled shoes, particularly if the length of the shoe is shorter than that needed for the toes. Soft corns occur between the toes, and hard corns occur on the top of the toe or the sole of the foot. Both are formed by the skin in response to pressure and/or friction, i.e., the shoe rubbing or putting pressure over the toe's bony prominences or the shoe constricting lateral spread of the foot resulting in increased pressure over bony prominence between the toes.[50] When shoes are too short, they can force the toes to "cock up," causing the metatarsal head to be more prominent on the sole of the foot.[49] A callus can develop over this prominence. A callus can also develop over the PIP joint in this deformity, as this joint now is higher than the normal shoe toe box (Fig. 9-4).[1] Calluses on the bottom of the foot can be particularly worrisome in athletes, as friction over a callus can result in sufficient bleeding under the callus to form a hematoma. Such a hematoma can become infected if not properly treated by shaving the callus, evacuating the hematoma, and keeping the area clean and dry until it is healed.

Although the development of a bunion or the valgus drift of the great toe may be, in part, genetically determined, a pointed-toe, high-heeled shoe may aggravate this drift and also cause pressure over the medial flare of the first metatarsal head, producing thickening or enlargement of this bone. The thicker the medial flare of the MP joint, the more prominent the bunion deformity. Most shoes are not made to accommodate a thickened metatarsal head, and hence the injury cycle of overuse is established: greater rubbing and friction by the shoe over the medial metatarsal head results in greater bony hypertrophy, which makes the shoe fit even tighter and cause more rubbing.

In the athlete, treatment of these common foot problems should emphasize buying shoes to accommodate the foot and not trying surgically to make the foot fit the shoe. Low-heeled shoes of soft leather with a wide, high-toe box are recommended.

PSYCHOLOGIC CONCERNS

The psychologic ramifications of increased sport participation by women are many. For example, in the 1990s it is acceptable for a woman to be tall, aggressive, competitive, and a leader.[19] Being feminine does not preclude sweating and "pumping iron." Through sport participation, young women learn that winning comes only with

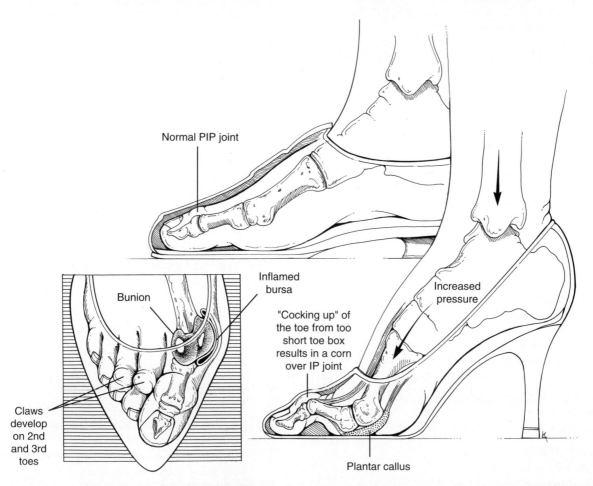

Normal PIP joint

Bunion

Inflamed bursa

Increased pressure

"Cocking up" of the toe from too short toe box results in a corn over IP joint

Claws develop on 2nd and 3rd toes

Plantar callus

Fig. 9-4. "Cocking up" of the toe from a toe box that is too short can result in a corn over the PIP joint due to increased pressure from the shoe on this area. The metatarsal head also becomes more planar flexed, resulting in the development of a plantar callus under it.

hard work and determination. Additionally, it is felt that women participating in team sports develop skills that will help them function more effectively in the workplace.[68]

Sport can enhance father-daughter relationships.[75] Fathers now can share sport experiences with their daughters as they have done for years with their sons. Not only can they be their daughters' greatest fan, but they can be their coaches and advisors. In fact, sport enjoyment can be a common family bond—a center focus for play, conversation, and socialization.

SUMMARY

Sport has added another dimension to the character of women. It is now not only acceptable for women to enhance their beauty, sharpen their artistic talents, and develop their intellectual skills, but it is also acceptable for them to maximize their physical abilities through sport participation.

REFERENCES

1. American Academy of Orthopaedic Surgeons: *Athletic Training and Sports Medicine,* Park Ridge, IL, 1991, American Academy of Orthopaedic Surgeons.
2. American College of Sports Medicine. *Conference on The Female Athlete Triad: Disordered Eating, Amenorrhea and Osteoporosis,* American College of Sports Medicine, June, 1992.
3. Arendt E: Orthopaedic issues for active and athletic women; In Agostini R, ed: *Clinics in Sports Medicine-The Athletic Woman,* Philadelphia, 1994, WB Saunders.
4. Arnheim D: *Modern Principles of Athletic Training,* ed 7, St. Louis, 1989, Mosby–Year Book.
5. Astrand P, Rodahl K: *Textbook of Work Physiology,* ed 2, New York, 1977, McGraw-Hill.
6. Barrow G, Saha S: Menstrual irregularity and stress fractures in collegiate female distance runners, *Am J Sports Med* 16(3):209–216, 1988.
7. Benardot D: *Sports Nutrition: A Guide for the Professional Working with Active People,* ed 2, 1993, The American Dietetics Association.
8. Benas D: Special considerations in women's rehabilitation programs, In Hunter LY, Funk FJ, eds: *Rehabilitation of The Injured Knee,* St. Louis, 1985, Mosby Year Book.
9. Brooks-Gunn J, Gargiulo J, Warren M: The menstrual cycle and athletic performance, In Puhl J, Brown C, eds: *The Menstrual Cycle and Physical Activity,* Champaign, IL, 1986, Human Kinetics.
10. Burke P: American women, 1800–1860: The effect of current sports legislation on women in Canada and the USA, Title IX, In Howell R, ed: *Her Story in Sport: A Historical Anthology of Women in Sports,* West Point, 1982, Leisure Press.
11. Calabrese L: Nutritional and medicine aspects of gymnastics, *Clinical Sports Medicine* 4:23–30, 1985.
12. Calabrese L, Kirkendall D, Floyd M, et al: Menstrual abnormalities, nutritional parameters and body composition in female classical ballet dancers, *Physician Sports Med* 11(2):86–98, 1983.
13. Caldwell F: Light boned and lean athletes: Does the penalty outweigh the reward? *Physician Sports Med* 12(9):139–149, 1984.
14. Cann C, Genant H, Ettinger B, et al: Spinal mineral loss in oophorectomized women, *JAMA* 244(18):2056–2059, 1980.
15. Clark M: Women and weight, *Physician and Sports Med,* 20(3):41–42, 1992.
16. Clark K, Kenneth S, Buckley W: Women's injuries in collegiate sports, *Am J Sports Med* 8(3):187–191, 1980.
17. Clark N, Nelson M, Evans W: Nutritional education for elite female runners, *Physician and Sports Med* 16(2):124–136, 1988.
18. Clark N: Supplements: What they are, what they aren't, *Sports Nutrition Guidebook,* Champaign, Illinois, 1990, Human Kinetics.
19. Comes the revolution, *Time* pp. 54–60, June 26, 1978.
20. Cook S, Harding A, Thomas K, et al: Trabecular bone density and menstrual function in women runners, *Am J Sports Med* 15(5):503–507, 1987.
21. DeMoss V: When thin is too thin, *Nautilus Magazine* 5(2):54–58, 1983.
22. DeVries H: *Physiology of Exercise for Physical Education and Athletics,* ed 3, Dubuque, IA, 1980, Wm C Brown.
23. Drinkwater B, Nilson K, Chesnut C, et al: Bone mineral content of amenorrhea and eumenorrheic athletes, *N Engl J Med* 311(5):277–280, 1984.
24. Drinkwater B, Bruemner B, Chesnut C: Menstrual history as a determinant of current bone density in young athletes, *JAMA* 263(4):545–548, 1990.
25. Drinkwater B, Nilson K, Ott S, et al: Bone mineral density after resumption of menses in amenorrhea athletes, *JAMA* 256(3):380–381, 1986.
26. Eilert R: Adolescent anterior knee pain, In Heikman J, ed: *AAOS Instructional Course Lectures,* 42:497–516, 1993.
27. Feicht C, Johnson T, Martin B, et al: Secondary amenorrhea in athletes, *Lancet* 2(8100):1145–6, 1978.
28. Ferstle J, Wells C: Asking the right questions, *Physician and Sports Med* 14(7):157–160, 1982.
29. Frey C, Thompson F, Smith J: American orthopaedic foot and ankle society: Woman's shoe survey, *Foot and Ankle* 14:78–81, 1993.
30. Frisch R: Delayed menarche and amenorrhea of college athletes in relation to age of onset of training, *JAMA* 246:1559–1563, 1982.
31. Frisch R: Fatness and Fertility: A Review, *Scientific America* 258(3):88–95, 1988.
32. Gehlsen G, Albohm M: Evaluation of sports bras, *Physician and Sports Med* 8(10):89–96, 1980.
33. Gendel E: Psychological factors and menstrual extraction, *Physician and Sports Med* 4(3):72–76, March 1976.
34. Gonzalez E: Premature bone loss found in some nonmenstruating sportswomen, *JAMA* 24(5):513–514, 1983.
35. Griffin L: Revolution of the knee extensor mechanism. In Fox J, Del Pizzo W, eds: *The Patella Femoral Joint,* New York, 1993, McGraw Hill.
36. Hale RW: Women and sports: Keeping up with female athletes' needs, *Contemporary OB/GYN,* 13:85–95, 1979.
37. Hale RW: Factors important to women engaged in vigorous physical activity, In Strauss R, ed: *Sports Medicine,* Philadelphia, 1984, WB Saunders.
38. Haycock C, Gillette G: Susceptibility of women athletes to injury: Myths versus reality, *JAMA* 236:163–165, 1976.
39. Haymes E: Physiological response of female athletes to heat stress: A review, *Physician and Sports Med* 12(3):45–59, 1984.
40. Kaiserauer S, Snyder A, Sleeper M, et al: Nutritional, physiological and menstrual status of distance runners, *Med Sci Sports Exerc* 21(2):120–125, 1989.
41. Klafs C, Lyon J: *The Female Athlete,* ed 2, St. Louis, 1978, Mosby-Year Book.
42. Kleiner S: Bone up on your diet, *Physician and Sports Med* 21(5):27–28, 1993.
43. Lebrun C: Effects of the menstrual cycle and birth control pill on athletic performance, In Agostini R, Titus S, eds:

Medica and orthopaedic issues of active and athletic women, St. Louis, 1994, Mosby-Year Book.

44. Lesmes G, Fox E, Stevens C, et al: Metabolic responses of females to high intensity interval training of different frequencies, *Med Sci Sports Exerc* 10(4):229–232, 1978.

45. Lloyd T, Triantafyllou S, Baker E, et al: Women athletes with menstrual irregularity have increased musculoskeletal injuries, *Med Sci Sport* 18(4):374–379, 1986.

46. Loosli AR: Reversing sports related iron and zinc deficiencies, *Physician and Sports Med* 21(6):70–78, 1993.

47. Malina R: Menarche in athletes: A synthesis and hypothesis, *Annals of Hum Biology* 10:1–24, 1983.

48. Malina R: Age at menarche in athletes and nonathletes, *Med Sci Sport* 5(1):11–13, 1973.

49. Mann R, Conghlen M: *Surgery of the Foot and Ankle,* ed 6, Philadelphia, 1993, Mosby-Year Book.

50. Mann R, Conghlen M: *Surgery of the Foot and Ankle,* ed 6, Philadelphia, 1993, Mosby-Year Book.

51. Mansfield M, Emans S: Anorexia nervosa, athletes and amenorrhea, *Rad Clinics N America* 36(3):533–549, 1989.

52. Marino D, King J: Nutritional concerns during adolescence, *Rad Clinics N America* 1980, 27:125–139.

53. Marshall JL: Myths about women and sports, In Marshal JL, ed: *The Sports Doctor's Fitness Book For Women,* New York, 1981, Delacorte Press.

54. Marshall JL: The physiological differences between women and men, In Marshal JL, ed: *The Sports Doctor's Fitness Book for Women,* New York, 1981, Delacorte Press.

55. McCallum J: Out of joint, *Sports Illustrated* 13:44–53, 1995.

56. McConnell J: The management of chondromalacia patellae: A long term solution, *Aust J Physiother* 2:215–223, 1986.

57. McWhirter N: Guinness book of women's sports records, New York, 1979, Sterling Publishing.

58. Merchant A: The lateral patella compression syndrome, In Fox J, Del Pizzo W, eds: *The Patella Femoral Joint,* New York, 1993, McGraw Hill.

59. Myburgh K, Hutchins J, Fataar A, et al: Low bone density is an etiology factor for stress fractures in athletes, *Ann Int Med* 113(10):754–759, 1990.

60. Nattive A, et al: The female athlete triad: The interrelatedness of disordered eating, amenorrhea and osteoporosis, *Clin Sport Med* 13(2):405–418, 1994.

61. Nunnaley S: Physiological response of women to thermal stress: A review, *Med Sci Sports Exerc* 10(4):250–255, 1978.

62. Otis C, Lynch L: How to keep your bones healthy, *Physician and Sports Med* 22(1):71–72, 1994.

63. Paglinano J: Injury prevention. In *The Complete Woman Runner,* Mountain View, CA, 1978, World Publications.

64. Pate R, Maguire M, Wyk J: Dietary iron supplementation in women athletes, *Physician and Sports Med* 7(9):81–86, 1979.

65. Protzman R, Griffis C: Stress fractures in men and women undergoing military training, *JBJS* 59-A(6):825–826, 1977.

66. Risser W, Risser J: Iron deficiency in adolescents and young adults, *Physician and Sports Med* 18(12):87–107, 1990.

67. Rudicel S: The shod foot and its implication for American women, *J Southern Ortho Assoc* 3(4):268–272, 1994.

68. Schwimmer L: Women executives: What holds so many back? *US News and World Report* 63–64, 1982.

69. Shangold M: Evaluating menstrual irregularity in athletes, *Physician and Sports Med* 10(2):21–24, 1982.

70. Shangold M, Mirkin G: Menstruation, In Shangold M, ed: *Women and Exercise: Physiology and Sports Medicine,* Philadelphia, 1988, FA Davis.

71. Sherman M, Baugher H: Introduction, In Marshal JL, ed: *The Sports Doctor's Fitness Book for Women,* New York, 1981, Delacorte Press.

72. Shlerman G: Conditioning the athlete, In Haycock C, ed: *Sports Medicine for the Athletic Female,* Oradell, NJ, 1980, Medical Economics.

73. Snow R, Barbieri R, Frisch R: Estrogen 2-hydroxylase oxidation and menstrual function among elite oarswomen, *J Clin Endocrinol Metab* 1989:69(2):369–376.

74. Tanner J: *Growth At Adolescence,* ed 2, 1962, Oxford Blackwell Scientific Publications.

75. Harris D, Sabo D, Schafer S, ed: *The Wilson Report: Moms, Dads, Daughters, and Sports,* New York, 1988, Women's Sports Foundation Conference: Proceedings.

76. Thomas C: Factors important to women participants in vigorous athletics, In Strauss R, ed: *Sports Medicine and Physiology,* Philadelphia, 1979, WB Saunders.

77. Thornton J: How can you tell when an athlete is too thin, *Physician Sports Med* 18(12):124–133, 1990.

78. Tomasi L, Peterson J, Pettit G, et al: Women's responses to army training, *Physician and Sports Med* 5(6):32–37, 1977.

79. Vandenbroucke J, Van Laar A, Valkenburg H: Synergy between thinness and intensive sports activity delaying menarche, *Br Med J* 284:1907–1908, 1982.

80. Walsh WM: The knee: patella femoral joint, In DeLee J, Drez D, eds: *Orthopaedic Sports Medicine, Principles and Practice vol 2,* Philadelphia, 1994, WB Saunders.

81. Warren M: The effects of exercise on pubertal progression and reproductive function in girls, *J Clin Endocrinol Metab* 51(5):1150–1157, 1980.

82. Wells CL: *Women, Sport & Performance,* ed 2 Champaign, IL, 1991, Human Kinetics.

83. Wells CL: Response of physically active and acclimatized men and women to exercise in a desert environment, *Med Sci Sports Exerc* 12(1):9–13, 1980.

84. Whiteside P: Men's and women's injuries in comparable sports, *Physician and Sports Med* 8(3):130–140, 1980.

85. Wichmann S, Martin D: Eating disorders in athletes, *Physician and Sports Med* 21(5):126–135, 1993.

86. Wilmore J, Brown C: Physiological profile of women distance runners, *Med Sci Sports Exerc* 6(3):178–181, 1974.

87. Wilmore J, Brown D: Body physique and composition of the female distance runner, In Milvy P, ed: *The Marathon: Physiological, Medical, Epidemiological and Psychological Studies,* New York, 1977, New York Academy of Sciences.

88. Wilmore J: Alteration in strength, body composition and anthropometric measure consequent to a 10-week training program, *Med Sci Sport* 6(2):133–138, 1974.

89. Wilson H: Rehabilitation of the injured athlete. In Haycock C, ed: *Sports Medicine for the Athletic Female,* Oradell, NJ, 1980, Medical Economics.

90. Women marathoners describe bra needs: Results of an informal survey, *Physician and Sports Med* 5(2):12–13, 1977.

COMMON
SPORTS INJURIES

CHAPTER 10

WOUND HEALING

Susan Craig Scott

GENERAL CONSIDERATIONS

Primary wound healing is the goal of management in all wounds; scar tissue composed of collagen is the material that the body uses to repair wounds. In optimal circumstances, the body is able to heal a wound in the predictable orderly sequence of events commonly known as *wound healing.*

Certain local and systemic factors can influence wound healing. To the extent that physicians are able to control these factors, a durable healed wound will result.

Initial wound assessment begins with an accurate history and a careful physical examination. If the patient is able, he or she must be carefully questioned regarding the time and the mechanism of injury. The physician makes every effort to elicit factors that might influence the decision regarding how and whether to proceed with wound closure, e.g., severe contamination from a human bite or crush from a garbage compactor. With this accomplished, the physician taking the patient's history addresses questions of systemic factors—clotting abnormalities, diabetes, immune compromise—that will influence how the wound and the patient will be treated.

Attention is then turned to the wound itself, which is examined for bleeding, contamination, and foreign bodies. Control of bleeding by local pressure is indicated. Local contamination must be eliminated before a wound can be closed. A careful inspection for shards of glass or pieces of dirt or gravel is done, and any other obvious contaminants are removed; this inspection is followed by vigorous irrigation.

Bleeding vessels ordinarily stop bleeding spontaneously as vasospasm and the formation of a platelet plug herald the beginning of the clotting cascade. Under certain circumstances, bleeding can be difficult to control. If a vessel is only partially transected and cannot contract adequately to allow the cessation of bleeding or if, alternatively, a vessel is rigid with atherosclerotic plaque and is unable to contract sufficiently, persistent bleeding may be a problem. In both instances, although control is of the essence, clamps must never be blindly

stabbed into a wound in an attempt to halt bleeding. This will injure tissue unnecessarily and add to the burden of debris that must be cleared for healing to progress. Pressure should be maintained until adequate help—sufficient personnel, adequate anesthesia, and proper equipment—is available. When these conditions are met, the vessel responsible for bleeding can be precisely clamped and irrigated or repaired as necessary. After bleeding is controlled, the wound is examined. Wound margins are inspected, and any crushed components are evaluated for viability; crushed tissue, beveled edges, and missing tissue present specific problems (Fig. 10-1). As the physician gains experience in wound management, he or she does not hesitate to débride severely crushed tissue, which will invariably be a source of contamination and a nidus for infection. The beveled wound requires attention to detail to coapt accurately. (Fig. 10-2) Missing tissue requires a decision to allow for healing by 2° intention or to proceed with coverage (Fig. 10-3). The coverage decision is best made in conjunction with a plastic surgeon.

WOUND HEALING PHASES

Early experience with gains of tensile strength in wound healing led to the description of the three classical phases of wound healing; the first phase is initiated immediately after the wounding occurs.[7] The three phases overlap in time, with the last phase resolving up to 18 months after injury. The initial *inflammatory phase* is predominant in the first 48 hours; the function of the inflammatory phase is the cleaning of the wound in preparation for wound repair. The initial vasoconstriction yields to vasodilatation and increased vessel permeability; histamine is thought to be responsible for these events. Large numbers of neutrophils, monocytes, and fibroblasts enter the area of the wound in preparation for the *proliferative* or second phase of tissue repair, which begins the second or third day after injury.

When extensive contamination is present, however, the inflammatory phase will persist until control of con-

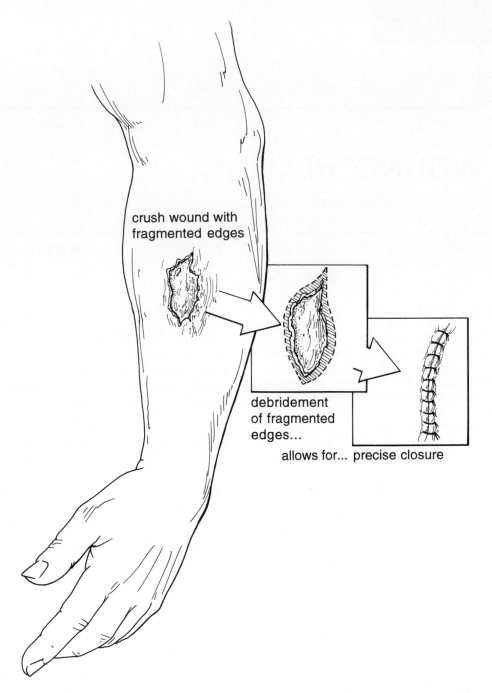

crush wound with
fragmented edges

debridement
of fragmented
edges...

allows for... precise closure

Fig. 10-1. Crushed or damaged wound edges may be judiciously débrided to provide clear edges for suturing.

tamination is gained in the area. Until local contaminants in the form of damaged tissue, bacteria, or foreign material are removed, the inflammatory phase remains active. In this situation, unless and until vigorous and accurate mechanical débridement of the wound takes place, proper and complete wound repair may never occur. Bacterial colonization and proliferation, aided by impaired circulation, may overwhelm the body's reparative processes by feeding on necrotic tissue and by outflanking in their own clever way our attempts to eliminate them.

In this early phase of wound repair, there is simply no substitute for a clean wound and as much débridement as is necessary to achieve it. No amount of antibiotic, oral or intravenous, can substitute for adequate elimination of necrotic or contaminated debris in which bacteria can dwell.

The second phase of wound repair, the fibroblastic or proliferative phase, already begins by 48 hours after injury. If it progresses normally, this phase lays down the protein and fiber network on which the scaffolding of the collagen matrix of soft tissue repair is built. Initially, the strength of

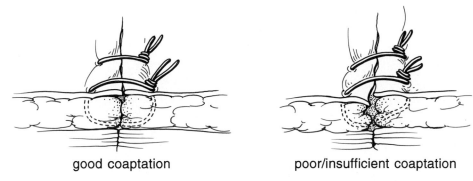

good coaptation   poor/insufficient coaptation

Fig. 10-2. Perfect edge-to-edge suturing is necessary for most satisfactory wound healing.

this collagen is virtually nonexistent, but as time passes, tropocollagen is converted to collagen fibrils, which gain strength as their numbers increase. As wound collagen accumulates after 3 weeks, the third or *remodeling phase* of wound healing begins when the collagen deposited as type III (embryonic collagen) is gradually replaced by type I collagen and the multiple crosslinks of this more stable and mature collagen forge a wound that can withstand mechanical stresses comparable with the strength of intact skin.[1,9] Although strength gains are greatest in these early weeks and the rate of gain then slows, the wound continues to gain strength for months after injury as it responds to the mechanical stresses.

FACTORS THAT AFFECT WOUND HEALING

Although most wounds heal normally and uneventfully, a reason must be sought when healing does not proceed as expected. A brief review of the factors that influence wound healing is in order.

Wound-Related Factors

LOCAL TISSUE OXYGENATION (PO$_2$). This is the single most important factor in wound healing. It is poor local PO$_2$ that ultimately accounts for healing problems in irradiated tissue or in a patient with diabetes mellitus, peripheral vascular disease, chronic infection, and pressure sores.[8]

Interestingly, the fibroblast, which lays down the collagen for wound healing, is oxygen-sensitive. Collagen synthesis requires a PO$_2$ (tissue partial pressure of oxygen) in the range of 90 to 95 mm Hg; in patients on a normal diet with adequate vitamin C, the availability of O$_2$ to the fibroblast is the rate-limiting cofactor for collagen production.

Adequate local PO$_2$ depends on several factors. There must be adequate inspired O$_2$, and hemoglobin must be adequate in level and normal in structure to allow the transfer of O$_2$ on demand by local tissue. From this, it is easy to infer the types of systemic illness that may predictably interfere with O$_2$ delivery to healing tissue and, by extrapolation, interfere with wound healing.

INFECTION. Local accumulations of bacteria can overwhelm the body's ability to fight infection. Certain virulent organisms, such as beta hemolytic streptococcus, can cause greater damage in smaller numbers than less virulent organisms. A bacterial inoculation of 10^5 mg per gram of tissue is necessary for infection with most organisms.[12]

Patient-Related Factors

DIABETES MELLITUS. Diabetes mellitus predisposes to poor healing of soft tissue because of impaired microcirculation, associated neuropathy, and predisposition to infection. Excellent control of blood glucose is especially helpful in delaying and decreasing these known complications of the disease and is essential when wound healing is critical in the postsurgical period.[11]

NUTRITIONAL STATUS. Nutritional status must be severely impaired, with a serum protein below 2 gm %, before any effect on wound healing is seen. Isolated nutritional deficiencies, such as the vitamin C deficiency that causes scurvy or severe elemental zinc deficiency, are well known and commonly accepted causes of deficient healing. Interestingly, vitamin E, commonly touted as an aid to healing, has no known beneficial healing properties, and given systemically in large doses, it can lower the collagen accumulation and decrease the tensile strength of a healing wound.

SMOKING. Smoking has been blamed as a culprit in wounds that fail to heal; its mechanism seems to be via the sympathetic nervous system, causing severe vasoconstriction that impairs the oxygenation of healing tissues. In addition, carbon monoxide present in inhaled smoke has a predictable effect on the oxygen–hemoglobin dissociation curve, shifting the curve to the left and at the same time forming carboxyhemoglobin. The effect can impair local PO$_2$ levels enough to cause skin necrosis.[3]

ANEMIA. There is no evidence that hematocrit levels that fall to even 50% of normal levels significantly decrease the tensile strength of the healing wound. The crucial importance of local tissue oxygenation for adequate healing would argue that a low hematocrit level will at least delay wound strength gain, but the evidence for this is controversial.[4]

Medication-Related Factors

Medications can significantly affect wound healing.

STEROID ADMINISTRATION. Steroid administration orally or by injection results in the arrest of the inflammatory phase of wound healing; wound macro-

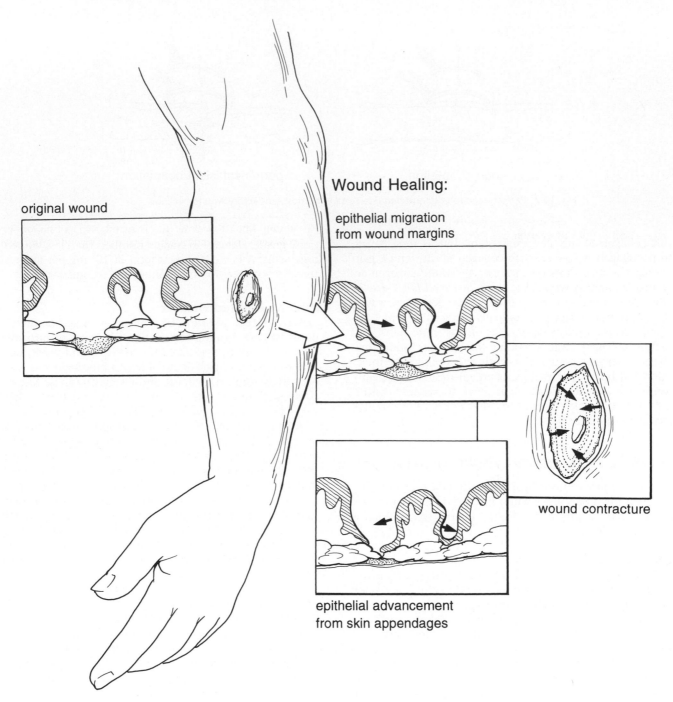

Wound Healing:

original wound

epithelial migration
from wound margins

epithelial advancement
from skin appendages

wound contracture

Fig. 10-3. Healing by secondary intention proceeds inward from the periphery and outward from the center.

phages, fibrogenesis, angiogenesis, and wound contraction are halted by the administration of steroids. Anabolic steroids and vitamin A can reverse this effect of steroids; although the exact dose of vitamin A is unknown, 25,000 IU per day orally or 200,000 IU of ointment applied topically is usually effective.[5,6] Vitamin A is an essential ingredient for normal wound healing; its absence impairs the macrophages' role in wound repair.

CHEMOTHERAPEUTIC AGENTS. Chemotherapeutic agents decrease the proliferation of fibroblasts in the healing wound; certain agents, such as actinomycin D and

bleomycin, are more detrimental than others to the gains of tensile strength in a healing wound. The question of wound healing arises when chemotherapy is planned in the postoperative period. Timing is important: in general, when chemotherapy treatment is begun 10 to 14 days after surgery, there is very little long-term effect on wound healing.[2]

GROWTH FACTORS. Growth factors, such as fibroblast growth factors and platelet growth factors, are proteins that appear to play an enormous role in cell synthesis and division; they also play a role in wound healing and are responsible for attracting collagen-synthesizing fibroblasts into the healing wound and stimulating their proliferative and division. Growth factors are being used experimentally and with great success to heal open wounds, burns, and skin graft donor sites.[10]

SUMMARY

Circumstances that support satisfactory wound healing are known; the physician's role is to minimize those conditions that negatively impact the healing process. Careful attention to detail in wound care, careful history taking, and an accurate current understanding of factors that might benefit the healing wound work to support this normal series of events.

REFERENCES

1. Chapman JA, Kellgren JH, Steven FS: Assembly of collagen fibrils, *Fed Proc* 25:1811, 1966.
2. Falcone RE, Nappi JF: Chemotherapy and wound healing, *Surg Clin North Am* 64:779, 1984.
3. Forrest CR, Pang CY, Lindsay WK: Dose and time effects of nicotine treatment on the capillary blood flow and viability of random pattern skin flaps in the rat, *Br J Plast Surg* 40:295, 1987.
4. Heughan C, Grislis G, Hunt TK: The effect of anemia on wound healing, *Ann Surg* 179:163, 1974.
5. Hunt TK: Vitamin A and wound healing, *J Am Acad Dermatol* 15(4 Pt 2):817, 1986.
6. Hunt TK, et al: Effect of vitamin A on reversing the inhibitory effect of cortisone on healing of open wounds in animals and man, *Ann Surg* 170:633, 1969.
7. Hunt TK, et al, eds: *Soft and hard tissue repair: biological and clinical aspects,* ed. 1, New York, 1984, Praeger Publishers.
8. Jonsson K, et al: Tissue oxygenation, anemia, and perfusion in relation to wound healing in surgical patient, *Ann Surg* 214:605, 1991.
9. Madden JW, Peacock EF: Studies on the biology of collagen during wound healing. III. Dynamic metabolism of scar collagen and remodeling of dermal wounds, *Ann Surg* 174:511, 1974.
10. McGrath MH: Peptide growth factors and wound healing, *Clin Plast Surg* 17(3):421, 1990.
11. Morain WD, Colen LB: Wound healing in diabetes mellitus *Clin Plast Surg* 17(3):493, 1990.
12. Robson MC, Stenberg BD, Hegggers JP: Wound healing alterations caused by infection, *Clin Plast Surg* 17(3):485, 1990.

CHAPTER 11

DERMATOLOGIC CONDITIONS

Robert S. Scheinberg

Text and illustrations adapted with permission from Scheinberg RS: Exercise-Related Skin Infection: Managing Bacterial Disease. *Phys Sportsmed* 1994;22(6):47–58, and Scheinberg RS: Stopping Skin Assailants: Fungi, Yeast and Viruses. *Phys Sportsmed* 1994; 22(7):33–39.

The athlete may get any of the dermatologic conditions seen in the sedentary individual. However, trauma, perspiration, and prolonged exposure to sunlight, cold, water, and protective equipment make the athletic patient particularly vulnerable to a number of dermatoses and neoplasms.

SKIN PROBLEMS CAUSED BY TRAUMA

Blisters, Erosions, and Scrapes

Repeated shearing force against a relatively small area of skin will cause epidermal separation and fluid accumulation. If such a blister breaks, a sensitive eroded area is uncovered, which may become a portal to secondary infection. A sudden shearing force will result in a scrape.

The best management is prevention of blisters with properly fitted equipment and shoes. Petroleum jelly applied to the feet or areas of rubbing (i.e., thighs and nipples of runners) reduces the coefficient of friction and may prophylax against blisters and irritation. Incipient blisters can be covered with moleskin. Alternatively, tincture of benzoin or tannic acid soaks (use strong tea) can "toughen" the skin to prevent blister formation. If a blister forms and is intact, it should be drained with a sterile lancet or needle in several places and then dressed with antibiotic ointment and gauze several times a day. If the blister roof has been sheared off, peroxide or antiseptic scrub followed by antibiotic ointment and gauze will speed healing. Alternatively, several of the newer occlusive or semipermeable dressings (i.e., Duoderm®— ConvaTec, Princeton, NJ; OP Site; Vigilon; Second Skin, etc.) can be used right over lanced blisters and erosions and most impressively over painful scrapes (such as the infamous "strawberry" on the thighs and buttocks of base stealers and on Astroturf burns) with almost immediate pain relief and accelerated reepithelialization.

Subungual Hematoma, Cauliflower Ear, and Talon Noir

Subungual hematoma, cauliflower ear, and talon noir all result from bleeding into or under the skin. The painful subungual hematoma is best managed by draining the blood through a small hole made in the nail by repeatedly twisting a 11 blade until it breaks through the nail or by heating a paper clip until it is red hot and then melting a hole in the nail. Pain relief is instantaneous, and the squirting blood prevents burning the nail bed with the hot paper clip.

A cauliflower ear (Fig. 11-1) results from bleeding into the thin subcutaneous space between the skin and the ear cartilage. The resulting hematoma organizes into fibrous tissue, which may calcify. Incision and drainage of the hematoma and pressure dressings should prevent the disfiguring sequelae. Recently, swimmer's noseclips applied over collodion-soaked cotton has been advocated as a simple way to provide constant compression on the pinna postaspiration of the hematoma.

Talon noir (black heel) occurs from repeated rapid movement of the calcaneal area against an athletic shoe. It needs no treatment but can be irregular and black, beautifully mimicking a malignant melanoma. Management consists of making an accurate diagnosis by paring away the surface of the skin and finding the pigment removed (chronic subungual hematoma can also mimic a subungual melanoma). If diagnosis is in doubt, drill through the nail and hematest the black material. Melanin will be negative, whereas dried blood will be strongly positive.

Corns and Calluses

Corns and calluses consist of thickened stratum corneum. Calluses are nontender and show the dermatoglyphic skin markings on the surface. They result as an adaptation to repeated shearing forces on the skin surface not strong enough to cause blisters, erosions, or scrapes. They need not be treated except for cosmetic reasons, and there is no reason to change shoes because large calluses have formed. Corns are tender compactions of stratum corneum resulting from compression of skin or callous between two unyielding surfaces. Paring a tender area of thickened skin (most typically under a prominent metatarsal head) reveals a translucent yellowish "kernel," which can be further pared away to give

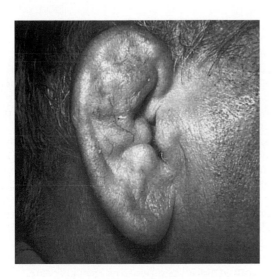

Fig. 11-1. Cauliflower ear.

pain relief. Repeated parings or the use of corn plasters (40% salicylic acid; Trans-vers-sal®—Tsumura Medical, Shakopee, MN; or Trans-Plantar®—Tsumura Medical) or keratolytics can make the area asymptomatic, but frequently new shoes or orthotics are needed to change the biomechanics of the area so the corns will not reform. Very painful and unresponsive corns may require surgery to realign foot bones. Collagen also can be injected as a cushion around a prominent metatarsal head, but the resulting pain relief usually only lasts for 4 to 12 months until the collagen is metabolized.

Fibrous Nodules
Fibrous nodules are firm bumps that feel as part of the skin but are elevated and are frequently some red or brown color and result from repeated blunt trauma causing dermal fibroblasts to produce more collagen. They are seen most frequently on the shins (usually termed *dermatofibromas*) and on the knuckles, dorsal feet, and sacral areas. Depending on the sport, they have been termed "surfer's nodules," "knuckle pads," "foot bumps," and "rower's bumps." No treatment is necessary, but the nodules sometimes persist long after the activity is stopped, making knowledge of a patient's past athletic activities helpful in arriving at the proper diagnosis.

Frostbite
As a response to cold, cutaneous blood vessels constrict and shunt blood away from the skin in an attempt to keep up the core temperature. Ice crystals form in the extracellular space, dehydrating the cells and resulting in irreversible injury. Wind accelerates heat loss from the skin as does direct contact with metal (such as a ski pole). If clothing is saturated with perspiration, it loses most of its insulating properties, so covered areas can experience severe cold injury.

The clinical signs of mild frostbite (also called frostnip) include a grayish white color to the skin and loss of sensation. Frostnip occurs most commonly on the nose, cheeks, hands, and feet. Once the diagnosis is made, the affected skin should be rewarmed rapidly as long as it is

certain that the area will not be exposed again to the cold. The rewarming can be done with tepid soaks or warm body parts applied to the frostnipped skin. The area will become warm and swollen and frequently severely painful requiring analgesia. Blisters may form in 12 to 24 hours, and throbbing and burning may persist for days to weeks. Ultimately healing is almost always complete with minimal scarring or functional impairment, however, deep frostbite is analogous to a third-degree burn with full-thickness loss of skin and possible damage to underlying muscle and bone, sometimes requiring amputation. Initial management is the same as for frostnip, but the area frequently remains anesthetic, indicating irreversible nerve damage, and the patient should be transported to the hospital immediately.

SKIN PROBLEMS CAUSED BY INFECTIOUS AGENTS

Heat and humidity are increased on the skin surface of athletes because exertion causes increased blood temperature, dilated cutaneous blood vessels, and copious sweating. The occlusion caused by uniforms, pads, and footwear worn for prolonged periods of time, direct contact with competitors, and cuts and abrasions on the skin surface create an almost ideal environment for bacterial proliferation and invasion of the skin. The most common cutaneous bacterial infections are those caused by *Staphylococcus aureus,* beta hemolytic *streptococcus,* and gram negative rods. These infections vary in clinical appearance and symptoms depending on the part of the skin infected, the extent of the infection, and whether the athlete irritates the area by continued sports participation.

The best management is preventive measures such as loose fitting clothing of "breathable" fabric changed frequently when saturated, dusting powder or antiinfective creams applied prophylactically before exercise, and blowdrying moist skin surfaces after exercise.

If an infection is suspected, it is best to make a precise diagnosis by means of wet mount, fungal and yeast, or bacterial culture. However, intertrigo, which is macerated and very malodorous, frequently consists of a mixed infection, and the best treatment is to dry the area with cool compresses, such as acetic acid (one-part vinegar to 10-parts water) or Burow's solution, followed by blowdrying the area until it is no longer "sticky" and applying antiseptic solutions, such as povidine.

Dermatophytic and other fungal conditions, such as athlete's foot, jock itch, and related infections, cause much discomfort, but they usually respond well to treatment and prevention. However, skin lesions caused by viruses, such as herpes simplex, herpes zoster, warts, and molluscum contagiosum, can be tougher to manage because they often require long-term therapy and activity restrictions.

Bacterial Infections
IMPETIGO AND ECTHYMA. Impetigo consists of honey-colored crusts with little surrounding redness. Symptoms may include itching or burning, and removal of crusts leaves a raw base with a tendency to weep. It may be caused by coagulase positive *S. aureus* alone or as a

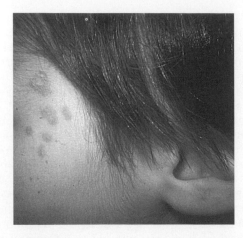

Fig. 11-2. This variation of impetigo appears as vesicles and bullae on this patient's cheek. (From Scheinberg R: Exercise-related skin infection; managing bacterial diseases, *Phys Sports Med* 1994.)

mixed infection including beta hemolytic *streptococcus*. One variant of impetigo (Fig. 11-2), produced by *S. aureus* phage type II, produces vesicles and bullae that may be centimeters in diameter and can be mistaken for poison oak or ivy, blistering insect bite reactions, herpes simplex or zoster, bullous drug eruptions, or blistering diseases such as pemphigus or pemphigoid.

Impetigo tends to favor body folds (Fig. 11-3) and areas subject to friction and occlusion, such as thighs and axillae. It also may complicate abrasions or areas of dermatitis, such as atopic dermatitis (the patient will have a history of asthma, hay fever, or eczema, and the crusts frequently will be on the face, popliteal, or antecubital fossae), contact dermatitis (especially from shoe materials and rubberized pads), and irritant dermatitis (such as hands chapped from frequent immersion or handling irritating substances as occurs when cleaning fish). Secondary impetiginization may complicate other infections such as herpes simplex. Fifteen percent to 20% of people carry coagulase positive *S. aureus* in their nares. Some will have a tiny fissure at the most anterior aspect of the nares, representing very localized impetigo. In im-

petigo, bacterial toxins cause a split near the cutaneous surface where the living epidermal cells are connected to the acellular stratum corneum.

Ecthyma is caused by the same organisms as impetigo, but it differs from impetigo in that the bacteria causes destruction of the entire epidermis and part of the superficial dermis, resulting in erosions or shallow ulcers surrounded by erythema (Fig. 11-4).

Diagnosis of impetigo and ecthyma is made by the clinical appearance, supplemented by a culture showing the causative organism, and its sensitivities whenever possible. Management with systemic antibiotics, such as dicloxacillin, cephalothin, and erythromycin, is preferable to topical therapy because the medication will be transported by the bloodstream to the whole cutaneous surface, making uninvolved skin resist the spread of infection. The organisms are highly contagious, and athletic competition quickly can make a mild infection widespread or transfer the bacteria to other competitors. Skin-to-skin contact must be avoided while crusts are present. Gentle cleansing with soap and water is valuable in removing the crusts. Uniforms, towels, etc. from infected individuals must be laundered in hot water to prevent inoculation back to the patient or to other individuals. Very localized impetigo or ecthyma may be managed with mupirocin (Bactroban®—SmithKline Beecham, Philadelphia, PA) ointment applied to the skin three times daily if the athlete is finished with competition or participating in a noncontact sport. Recurrent impetigo may mean a family member or competitor or the patient him- or herself is a carrier. Mupirocin in the nostrils three times daily for 1 week each month and regular use of antibacterial soap (Lever 2000, Dial, Safeguard, Irish Spring) may prevent future recurrences.

CELLULITIS. The term *cellulitis* refers to an infection in the deep dermis and subcutaneous tissues. It is very painful and tender and is primarily caused by beta hemolytic *streptococcus* and *S. aureus*, which are almost impossible to culture from the surface of the skin. Cellulitis is recognized as a somewhat ill-defined plaque of tender erythema of the trunk or extremities, usually appearing

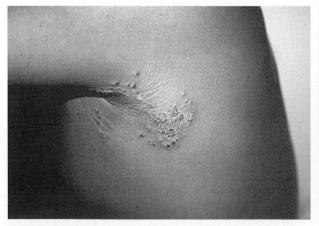

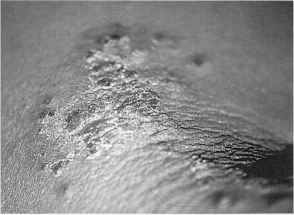

Fig. 11-3. Most commonly, impetigo consists of honey-colored crusts with little surrounding redness. (From Scheinberg R: Exercise-related skin infection; managing bacterial diseases, *Phys Sports Med* 1994.)

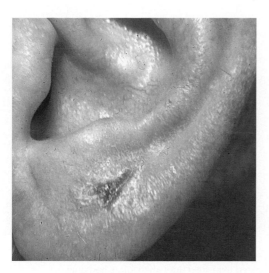

Fig. 11-4. The same organism that causes impetigo, *Staphylococcus aureus,* causes ecthyma, which appears as erosions or shallow ulcers on this patient's ear. (From Scheinberg R: Exercise-related skin infection; managing bacterial diseases, *Phys Sports Med* 1994.)

around a break in the skin from antecedent trauma or from bacteria entering a fissure caused by athletes' foot. The patient may have malaise and fever with intense pain and may have streaks along pathways of lymphatic drainage ("blood poisoning" or lympangitis). The athlete must be kept from competition to avoid systemic dissemination as additional trauma to an area of cellulitis can cause bacteremia. Hospitalization for intravenous antibiotics administration may be necessary as was with the case with Michael Jordan, who missed several games during the 1992–1993 season because of cellulitis around a foot corn. Milder cases of cellulitis can be managed with oral antibiotics, such as dicloxacillin or erythromycin, warm tapwater compresses for 15 minutes three times daily, elevation, and bedrest.

If the erythema is sharply defined and if the skin surface has a peau d'orange appearance, a *streptococcus* in-

fection of the upper dermis termed erysipelas is present. Management is the same as for cellulitis, but if erysipelas is in the periorbital area, ophthalmologic consultation should be obtained on an emergency basis because blindness can result from intense pressure on the globe or spread of the infection to the eye itself.

FOLLICULITIS, ACNEIFORM LESIONS, AND MILIARIA. The same forces of friction, heat, and humidity that can cause impetigo, ecthyma, and cellulitis will frequently cause occlusion of the skin's adnexal structures, and bacteria will proliferate behind the obstruction to cause folliculitis (hair follicle infection), acneiform lesions (pilosebaceous gland inflammation and infection frequently termed "acne mechanica" if rubbing and other mechanical factors are aggravating the condition), and miliaria (sweat gland and duct inflammation and infection).

Follicular papules and pustules are found most commonly on the scalp, chest, back, buttocks, and thighs (Fig. 11-5). If a pustule is surrounded by a small erythematous halo, it is caused most likely by coagulase-positive *S. aureus.* Dome-shaped follicular papules and pustules can be caused by *staphylococcus, streptococcus,* or gram negative organisms. Very extensive folliculitis may occur from shaving the legs of women and after total body shaving by men and women competitive swimmers, which is presumably because an infective focus is seeded to other follicles by the razor. Furuncles ("boils") are deep-seated inflammatory nodules resulting from rupture into the tissues of preexisting folliculitis.

Carbuncles occur when several furuncles merge in the subcutaneous tissue. Furuncles and carbuncles occur most commonly on the buttocks, neck, face, and axillae as complications of folliculitis subject to friction and repeated blunt trauma of athletic competition. Several weeks of systemic antibiotic therapy should be instituted, and in patients with severe cases, immobilization, incision and drainage, and hospitalization may be necessary.

Pseudomona organisms can produce a widespread folliculitis if there is a heavy innoculum of the organism while the patient is bathing in a hot tub that has inade-

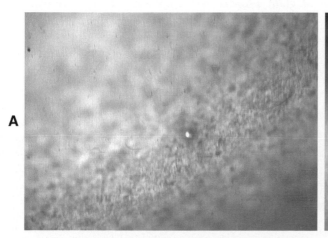
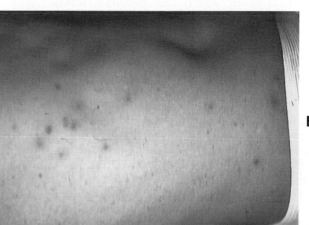

A　　　　　　　　　　　　　　　　　　　　**B**

Fig. 11-5. Folliculitis and pustular forms of acne and miliaria often are impossible to differentiate from one another. A pustule surrounded by a halo of erthema **(A)** that appears on this patient's trunk **(B)** is typical of staphyloccoccal folliculitis. (From Scheinberg R: Exercise-related skin infection; managing bacterial diseases, *Phys Sports Med* 1994.)

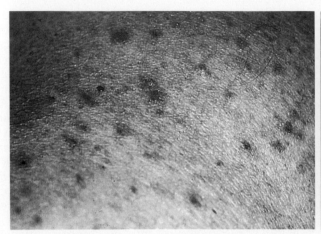 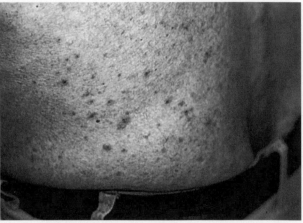

Fig. 11-6. Widespread folliculitis, as on this patient, can result from *Pseudomonas,* which thrive in underchlorinated hot tubs. (From Scheinberg R: Exercise-related skin infection; managing bacterial diseases, *Phys Sports Med* 1994.)

quate chlorination ("hot tub dermatitis" (Fig. 11-6)). Other gram negative organisms can cause folliculitis, especially if the patient has been receiving antibiotics with a primarily gram positive spectrum as treatment for acne. The pustular forms of acne and miliaria can be impossible to distinguish from folliculitis. If the patient with widespread presumed folliculitis has no systemic signs, such as malaise or fever, he or she should be treated empirically with a systemic antibiotic, such as erythromycin, tetracycline or minocycline, to cover for gram positive folliculitis and acne and miliaria pustulosa. In addition, the patient should be advised to begin measures to avoid maceration of the skin, such as the use of absorbent powders (Zeasorb, which contains cellulose so it does not cake like pure talcum powder and does not act as a nutrient medium, such as cornstarch, is preferred), changing clothing frequently, and decreasing sweating with aluminum chloride (Xerac™ AC—Person & Covey, Inc., Glendale, CA). Regular use of antiseptic soaps may also prevent recurrences (in addition to the soaps used to prevent impetigo, bar or liquid soap with benzoyl peroxide, which can penetrate follicles and sweat ducts, is recommended). Very localized folliculitis can be managed with the topical antibiotics developed for acne, such as erythromycin (Erycettes®—Ortho Pharmaceutical Corporation, Raritan, NJ; Emgel™—Glaxo Dermatology, Research Triangle Park, NC; TStat; etc.) and clindamycin (Cleocin T®—Upjohn Company, Kalamazoo, MI). Folliculitis is stubborn, and cultures and even skin biopsies are needed to establish the diagnosis and causative organism for appropriate antibiotic coverage. However, if the culture grows *Pseudomonas* organisms, topical therapy with acetic acid (1:10 vinegar solution) and meticulous drying along with avoiding underchlorinated hot tubs should clear the infection without having to resort to "big gun" systemic antibiotics.

Some patients with folliculitis, acne mechanica, and miliaria pustulosa will not have symptoms resolve until the competitive season ends and until the local factors that predispose the patient to the adnexal occlusive disease are finished.

OTHER BACTERIAL INFECTIONS. Corynebacteria, in addition to being the main pathologic organism implicated in acne, can cause two other common infections. Well-defined slightly scaling plaques in the inguinal folds and between the toes may result from *Corynebacterium minutissimae,* the causative organism of erythrasma. Diagnosis is confirmed by putting the patient under a Woods black light, which will cause the area to glow with a coral red fluorescence. The organism responds to topical erythromycin or clindamycin or systemic erythromycin. Well-demarcated 1- to 15-mm pits on the soles of patients with very sweaty, macerated, and malodorous feet are diagnostic of pitting keratolysis (Fig. 11-7) in which a corynebacterium lyses the very thick stratum corneum of the soles, giving a dramatic appearance. However, they may be treated with powders, vinegar soaks, and blowdrying the skin to make the environment inhospitable to the bacteria.

Erysipeloid looks like cellulitis but is somewhat more purple and typically occurs on the hands of people who fish and have been exposed to *Erysipelothrix rhusipathiae,* a gram positive rod commonly found on fish. It responds to penicillin and erythromycin. A more serious fish-borne infection is caused by *Vibrio vulnificus,* which can cause hemorrhagic bullae progressing to gangrenous-type lesions and sepsis if it enters the skin through a cut or abrasion. The organism is most prevalent in the Gulf coast and also may produce a severe gastroenteritis and severe skin infections after ingestion of rawfish and shellfish. Most susceptible are persons with poor liver function resulting from cirrhosis, in whom bacteria is not cleared from the bloodstream. Mortality in these individuals approaches 50%.

Rickettsial Disease
The major rickettsial disease to which an athletic patient has increased risk is Lyme borreliosis. In endemic areas, hikers, golfers, hunters, and ballplayers who retrieve balls in areas of heavy grass may be exposed to infected ticks. If the tick is not removed within 24 hours, the rickettsia can get into the patient's bloodstream causing Lyme dis-

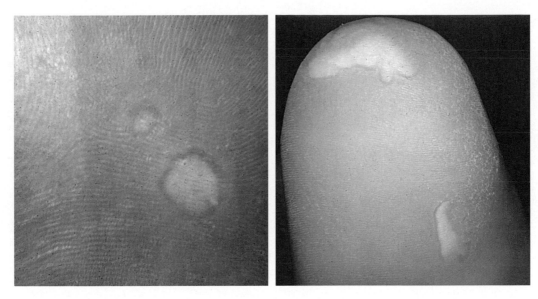

Fig. 11-7. Pitting kerotolysis appears on this patient's heel and sole. (From Scheinberg R: *Modern Med* 1993.)

ease. The majority of patients (but certainly not all) get a rash consisting of a ring of erythema, which may be mildly itchy, in the area of the tick bite. This ring may appear 3 to 12 days after the bite and may be associated with fever and malaise. Months to years later, peripheral and central neuropathies, arthritis, and cardiomyopathy may occur. Preferred management is a 21-day course of amoxicillin or doxycycline, although erythromycin and tetracycline also may be used. Most practitioners will treat persons bitten by ticks in endemic areas, but this treatment is controversial. All patients with the characteristic rash (erythema chronicum migrans) should be treated with antibiotics because the blood tests for Lyme disease are presently unreliable, and the causative organism has been cultured from cutaneous lesions repeatedly after negative results on blood tests.

Fungal and Yeast Infections

Dermatophytes and yeasts thrive in the same warm, moist environment that makes active patients susceptible to bacterial skin infections. Although fungus is the most common etiology of "athlete's feet" and "jock itch," it is essential to recognize that infections in intertrigenous areas may be caused by different organisms. Conversely, active, sweaty persons are particularly susceptible to extensive fungal infections in nonintertrigenous areas. Athlete's feet, when presenting dry and scaly and involving the toe webs and sole, is most commonly caused by dermatophyte fungus *(tinea pedis)* (Fig. 11-8). This diagnosis can be confirmed by collecting a scale with a scalpel blade and performing a potassium hydroxide microscopic examination or by culturing the scale in DTM (dermatophyte test medium), which turns red in the presence of dermatophytes. Blisters on the instep also may be caused by dermatophytes, which may be distinguished from contact dermatitis also by potassium hydroxide, and culture. The macerated toe web infection, also called athlete's feet, usually is a mixed infection caused by *Candida* or gram negative rods in addition to or replacing the original dermatophyte. Likewise, jock

itch, when forming pruritic, scaly rings involving the inguinal folds and sparing the scrotum and penis, is invariably dermatophytic, whereas a tender and itchy, bright red plaque with pustules peripheral to it ("satellites") that does involve the penis and scrotum most commonly is caused by *Candida albicans* (Fig. 11-9). Gram negative and gram positive bacteria also may cause a macerated inguinal intertrigo. As mentioned previously, erythrasma can form a dry, finely scaling infection in this area.

Management of athlete's feet and jock itch depends on recognizing the probable etiologic organisms and modifying the environment that is conducive to their growth. The dry dermatophyte infections can be cured with topical antifungal medication. Imidazoles such as clotrimazole (Lotrimin®—Schering Corporation, Kenilworth, NJ;

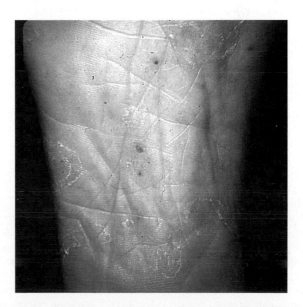

Fig. 11-8. Athlete's foot appears as scaling on the sole and blistering on the instep of a patient's foot. (From Scheinberg R: Fungal, yeast, and viral infections, *Phys Sports Med* 1994.)

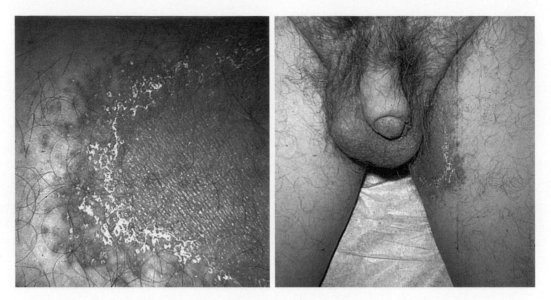

Fig. 11-9. Jock itch caused by *Candida albicans* appears as a bright red plaque with peripheral pustules. (From Scheinberg R: Fungal, yeast, and viral infections, *Phys Sports Med* 1994.)

Mycelex®—Miles Inc., Elkhart, IN), miconazole (Micatin), econazole (Spectazole®—Ortho Pharmaceutical Corporation), ketoconazole (Nizoral®—Janssen Pharmaceutica, Inc., Titusville, NJ), sulconazole (Exelderm®—Westwood-Squibb Pharmaceuticals, Inc., Buffalo, NY), and Oxistat® (Glaxo Dermatology), which have a spectrum including yeast and some bacteria are recommended. For recalcitrant scaling of the sole caused by fungus (sandal *t. pedis*), the new allylamines naftifine (Naftin®—Allergan Herbert, Irvine, CA) and terbinafine (Lamisil) are especially effective and may induce longer fungus-free periods than the imidazoles. Allylamines, however, are less effective against yeast, therefore, they are best not used if a fungal etiology has not been positively established. Florid inguinal *Candida* and bacterial intertrigo of groin and toe webs can be quickly cooled down with a regimen consisting of cool 1:10 vinegar soaks for 15 minutes three times daily followed each time by blowdrying or fanning the area until it is "bone dry" and the skin can be touched with a finger that will not stick to the surface when lifted. This can be followed by a moderate strength corticosteroid (two to three sample tubes of triamcinolone or flucinolone are recommended) and an imidazole cream or lotion. Within 2 to 3 days, the compresses and blowdrying usually can be stopped, and the imidazole can be used alone twice a day.

Active patients may require prolonged topical treatment because the area is continually subjected to the same forces that produced the infection initially. Topical management should be continued until the infection is clinically gone and then for an additional 2 weeks. Drying powders, such as Zeasorb, and measures to diminish sweating, such as Drysol™ (Person & Covey), XeracAc, and tannic acid soaks (made by adding two tea bags to a cup of boiling water, letting it steep, and then pouring it into a basin and adding enough water to cool the solution to a tolerable temperature) can prevent future infections. Changing socks, athletic shoes, bathing suits, and uniforms as soon as possible after athletic activity should be encouraged. If the patient has recurrent infections, daily imidazole cream on the feet and groin may prevent recurrences.

Patients with widespread fungus infections (*tinea corporus;* Fig. 11-10) should be treated with griseofulvin (Gris-PEG®—Albergan Herbert, Fulvicin®—Schering Corporation) in the newly recommended higher dosing schedules (i.e., 500 mg twice daily for a large man). Resistant cases may indicate fungal resistance or the patient's immunologic tolerance of the organism (this is especially true of atopics). Systemic ketoconazole (Nizoral®—Janssen Pharmaceutica, Inc.), fluconazole (Difulcan®—Roering, New York, NY), and itraconazole (Sporonox) have shown excellent results in many of these patients, but they may cause liver toxicity (especially ketoconazole). Systemic terbinafine at 200 mg once daily for 2 weeks will cure most *t. corporis* with minimal interaction with other medications and little chance of liver toxicity. Twelve-week courses of both oral itraconazole and

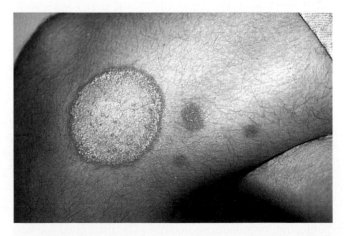

Fig. 11-10. *Tinea corporis* on a patient's leg demonstrates the typical ringworm pattern of this fungal infection. (From Scheinberg R: Fungal, yeast, and viral infections, *Phys Sports Med* 1994.)

terbinafine have higher cure rates for fungal infections of the toenails (onychomycosis) than a year of oral griseoful-vin. *Tinea versicolor* commonly affects active individuals because the causative yeast (pityrosporum) is lipophilic and a normal inhabitant of hair follicles and sebaceous glands, which colonize the skin when host factors of heat and moisture are increased. On unexposed skin, the colonies will be rust colored and asymptomatic or mildly pruritic. They are more dramatic during the summer months when the areas colonized do not tan or sunburn so they appear as well-defined white patches especially on the chest or back. Woods black-light examination shows yellow fluorescence, and potassium hydroxide examination has a characteristic appearance as spores and hyphae resemble "spaghetti and meatballs," whether the patches are white or rust-colored. Extensive cases of *t. versicolor* may involve the entire trunk and extremities. This same pityrosporum organism occasionally is responsible for patients with antibiotic-resistant folliculitis.

Management of pityrosporum can be topical or systemic. Selenium sulfide, 2.5% (prescription strength Selsun, Exel), applied to affected areas for 10 minutes each day for 1 week frequently will be curative (because the areas will remain white until the skin is tanned, a Woods black-light examination showing no yellow fluorescence or a negative potassium hydroxide examination may be needed to assure the physician and the patient that treatment was effective). Topical imidazoles also are effective in this infection, but treatment requires several weeks and is very expensive if large areas of skin are involved. Many clinicians favor systemic ketoconazole for extensive *t. versicolor*, and it frequently will be the only effective treatment for pityrosporum folliculitis. *T. versicolor* can be cured with a single dose of two tablets (400 mg) of ketoconazole taken with a carbonated beverage or cranberry juice to increase absorption. The drug is excreted in the sweat so patients are advised to work out for 1 hour or more after taking the two pills and to delay showering by additional hour. This treatment can be repeated in 1 week if Woods black-light or potassium hydroxide examination is still positive. If the patient has no history of liver disease, this minidose has not been associated with liver toxicity. Management of folliculitis may take several weeks of daily medication, and monitoring of liver function tests should be done. Alternatively, itraconazole at 100 mg bid for 2 weeks can be prescribed for resistant *t. versicolor* or pityrosporum folliculitis.

Viral Infections

Herpes simplex, herpes zoster, warts, and HIV may be transmitted during or precipitated by athletic participation. Routine hygienic measures, such as cleansing the skin after athletic competition and removing participants with open cuts on exposed skin from participation involving contact, may reduce or eliminate transmission of these pathogens. The full scope of HIV and athletics is beyond the scope of this chapter and will not be discussed further.

HERPES SIMPLEX AND ZOSTER. Because up to 80% of adolescents already have antibodies directed against herpes simplex, the main role of activity is reactivating the latent virus that resides in dorsal root nerve ganglia between attacks. The term "fever blister" has been used to indicate that increased body temperature can trigger an attack of herpes labialis. During many sports activities, body temperature may rise to 102°F or more. This thermal stress, combined with the stress of athletic competition and exposure to ultraviolet light, may precipitate frequent attacks of herpes in susceptible individuals (in labial and genital areas).

Management of recurrent herpes simplex is directed at reducing trigger factors whenever possible by cooling down the skin and taking nonsteroidal antiinflammatory drugs after competition and wearing sunscreens on a daily basis if attacks are precipitated by ultraviolet light. Acyclovir (Zovirax®—Burroughs Wellcome Co., Research Triangle Park, NC) tablets, 200 mg, taken five times a day for 5 days can shorten an episode if taken within 48 hours of the attack. Alternatives are famciclovir (Fanovir®—SmithKline Beecham) 125 mg bid for 5 days and valacyclovir (Valtrex®—Burroughs Wellcome Co.) 500 mg bid for 5 days. Ideally, antiviral therapy should be started at the first sign of tingling that presages such an attack. A prophylactic regimen of acyclovir, 400 mg, taken twice daily will prevent most herpes simplex and should be started the day before the active individual expects to be at risk. Topical acyclovir is of no use in these circumstances.

Those persons participating in contact sports must be kept away from other participants while they have an active herpetic lesion. The term *herpes Gladiatorum* was coined to describe epidemics of inoculation herpes occurring in wrestlers. Recent outbreaks have occurred in wrestling camps and on football and basketball teams.

Herpes zoster results from reactivation of the varicella (chickenpox) virus, and occasionally can be precipitated by local trauma in contact sports. Infected individuals should be kept from competition and treated with acyclovir, 800 mg, taken five times a day for 7 days, famciclovir, 800 mg q8h for 7 days, or valacyclovir, 1000 mg tid for 7 days. Because HIV also can precipitate herpes zoster in a young person, a test for HIV antibodies also is appropriate.

Herpes viruses typically produce clusters of painful blisters. Herpes simplex blisters are 1 to 3 mm in diameter and appear as localized clusters (Fig. 11-11). Herpes zoster blisters may be centimeters in diameter and follow a dermatome. If blisters are broken, shallow erosions may be present.

WARTS. Verrucae are caused by dozens of varieties of the human papilloma virus (HPV). They are recognized as papillomatous, flesh-colored, well-defined papules and nodules that occur predominantly on exposed skin parts (Fig. 11-12). Incubation is from several weeks to 5 years after exposure. Plantar warts will be round or oval and on close inspection interrupt the dermatoglyphic skin lines on the sole (Fig. 11-13). When the thick stratum corneum is pared, tiny bleeding puncta or black dots of dried blood are revealed, representing blood vessels projecting vertically toward the skin surface. In most young individuals, the body will mount an immunologic reaction against the virus within 6 months so any treatment, including no treatment, may be effective. However, a minority of persons will not mount an effective response to the virus, and almost any treatment will be ineffective. The people frequently are atopic, analogous to the sus-

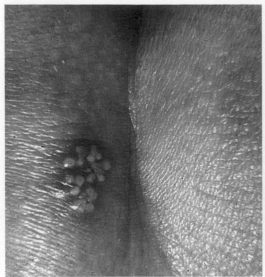
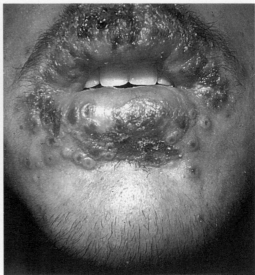

Fig. 11-11. Herpes simplex.

ceptible and hard-to-cure patients with impetigo and fungal and yeast infections.

The goal of therapy in an active individual is to minimize "down time" while maximizing the chance of cure. Treating a patient with one or two warts with liquid nitrogen cryocautery is recommended. A spray is directed at the wart for approximately 10 seconds or a cotton swab is applied to the wart with minimal pressure for the same time. Thicker warts might require a second spray or application during the same visit after they are allowed to thaw. Alternatively, the warts can be curetted or hyfrecated under local anesthesia. Care must be taken not to go too deeply in a misguided attempt to prevent recurrences because excessive morbidity and scarring can result. Most recurrences occur from subclinical infection by the HPV in the surrounding normal-appearing skin. For many competitive athletes who run a high risk of wound infection during their season, topical therapy with keratolytic liquids or pads (Compound W® (Whitehall Laboratories, Inc., New York, NY), DuoFilm, 40% salicylic acid plasters, Trans-versal, and Trans Plantar) is prescribed. These medications are all over-the-counter and are especially helpful in keeping painful plantar warts soft so they do not feel like a pebble in the shoe. Liquid nitrogen and surgical treatment of plantar warts should be avoided until the competitive season is over because postoperative pain can be disabling. CO_2 laser excision has the least chance of scarring and minimizes morbidity, but it can occasionally result in significant postoperative pain, and the excision site is an easy portal of entry for secondary bacterial infection if the patient is engaged in competitive sports before the 1- to 3-week healing period is finished. The author has been unimpressed with Bicloroacetic acid applications to plantar warts, but some practitioners use this therapy with success. Intralesional bleomycin by injection and scarification also is used by many dermatologists, but there is severe associated pain and risk of permanent nerve damage.

MOLLUSCUM CONTAGIOSUM. The molluscum virus belongs in the pox family and produces flesh-colored-to-yellow papules with a tiny punctum on the surface best visualized if the lesion is lightly frozen with liquid nitrogen. It represents a viral folliculitis and is easily spread by children at play, sexual activity, and athletic competition. It is primarily of cosmetic concern, although occasionally a molluscum will rupture from blunt trauma, resulting in a foreign body reaction that can mimic cellulitis and be disabling (Fig. 11-14).

Management is the same as with almost any destructive modality; they are easier to cure than warts because there is no subclinical extension of virus. Curettage, light hyfrecation, or topical 50% trichloroacetic acid applied only to the surface of the lesions is favored. Topical wart preparations sometimes can be effective, as can tretinoin (Retin-A®—Ortho Pharmaceutical Corporation), which is useful especially in uncooperative children. Athletes do not need to be kept from competition because they have warts or molluscum but the hygienic measures noted earlier should be emphasized, and affected areas whenever person-to-person contact is to be expected should be covered.

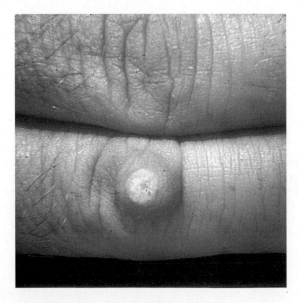

Fig. 11-12. Wart on right-hand index finger.

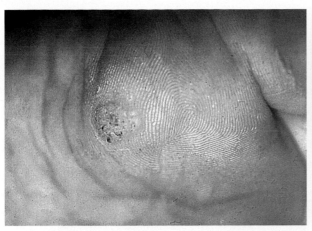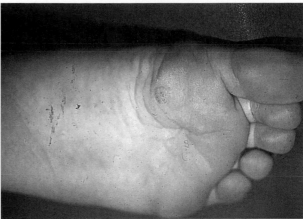

Fig. 11-13. Plantar wart.

Summary

A skin condition that is out of control can make participation uncomfortable or even unsafe. Physicians who know when to tell the patient to avoid participation are making sports safer not only for the patient, but for other competitors as well.

ALLERGIC AND IRRITANT CONTACT DERMATITIS

Contact dermatitis occurs when the eruption fits an area of exposure to a garment, liquid, medicament, or bandage. Most common causes are sweat (which can cause sweaty sock syndrome), rubber products in shoes, stretch garments and dressings, fragrances in medications and toiletries, topical antibiotics, herb and vitamin preparations, sunscreens, and plants such as poison oak.

Management consists of making the proper diagnosis and substituting less irritating substances wherever possible, and the use of cool compresses with topical and systemic corticosteroids for relief.

A unique reaction to an environmental agent is green discoloration of the hair of athletes with blond or gray hair who swim in chlorinated pools. This results from copper leached from pipes supplying the pool or from various pool-care products. If the pH of the pool is kept between 7.4 and 7.6, the copper will not attach to the hair. Hair already affected can be treated by application of hydrogen peroxide, 3%, for several hours.

PHOTODERMATITIS

A common rash in the athlete is the *phototoxic reaction.* The prototype is acute sunburn which can be prevented with sunscreens that are protective (i.e., Sun Protective Factor of 10 to 50) and substantive (i.e., resist wash-off by sweat and water). Some of the best are Sundown 15, 20, and 24; PreSun 15, 29, and 30 (this last one is nongreasy and waterproof); Eclipse 15; Solbar 15 and 50; Sea and Ski 15; Coppertone Supershade; and Bullfrog. PABA-sensitive patients can use Tiscreen, PAPBAFree, and PreSun 29. Patients who claim to be sensitive to all sunscreens can be protected by the so-called chemical-free sunscreens, which contain the physical-blocker titanium dioxide. Examples are chemical-free Neutragena and Tiscreen. Phototoxic reactions can be precipitated by medications, such as thiazide diuretics, sulfonamides (including TMP/SXT), griseofulvin, tetracycline, and Accutane®—E.C. Robbins Company, Inc., Richmond, VA. Doxycycline, commonly used to prevent "traveler's diarrhea," is a notorious photosensitizer, and patients using this on a trip to sunny Mexico or the Caribbean should be forewarned of this side effect. Phototoxic reactions are caused by the longer UVA ultraviolet light and are best protected by the above-mentioned chemical-free physical blockers and sunscreens containing parsol, such as UVA-guard.

Management of phototoxic reactions consists of cooling the skin, preferably in a tub of cool water. Ice compresses can be used on blistered areas, and nonsteroidal anti-inflammatory drugs are useful for pain relief. Although they have been used for years, systemic corticosteroids have been found no better than placebo in reducing pain and inflammation of sunburn. Topical anesthetics may result in sensitization, so the popular OTC benzocaine-containing products are not recommended. Nonsensitizing pramoxine (Pramasone®) is the preferred topical anesthetic.

The athlete who, while exercising, develops intensely

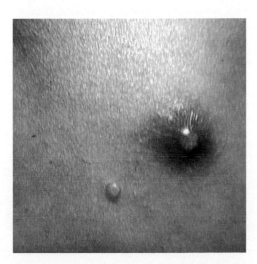

Fig. 11-14. Molluscum contagiosum papules appear on this patient's cheek. Cellulitis from trauma to the papule on the right induced a foreign-body reaction. (From Scheinberg R: *Modern Med* 1993.)

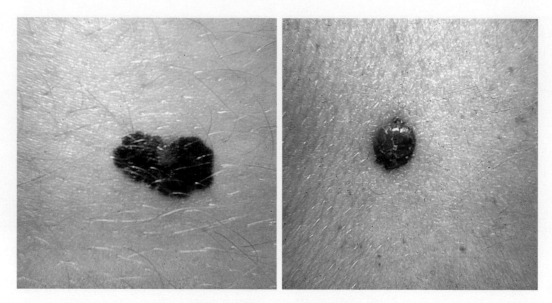

Fig. 11-15. Malignant melanoma.

itchy 1 to 2 mm papules surrounded by erythematous halos probably has cholinergic urticaria. This condition frequently begins during young adult life and interferes with exercise and any activities that raise body temperature. The etiology of this apparent hyperreactivity to acetylcholine in peripheral nerve endings is unknown, but it frequently responds to antihistamines, especially hydroxyzine. The recently released antihistamines, terfenadine (Seldane®—Marion Merrell Dow Inc., Kansas City, MO) and Hismanil, have no sedative effects, and although expensive, they may be helpful in managing cholinergic urticaria and seasonal rhinitis, urticaria, etc. in the athletic patient bothered by drowsiness from the more commonly used antihistamines. Exercise-induced anaphylaxis may result from food allergies and made more intense by the increased blood flow during exercise or from insect bites occurring during exercise. Dietary elimination of chocolate, nuts, dairy products, and preservatives before exercise may prevent this problem in some patients, although others may require constant availability of an epinephrine-containing anaphylaxis kit during exercise.

NEOPLASMS

Because chronic sun exposure frequently is a part of the life of an athlete, active patients should be warned about the risks of sun exposure and closely watched for skin cancers (15% of women professional golfers have skin cancers before aged 30 years). The usual skin cancers are represented, such as basal and squamous cell carcinomas, however, there has been an alarming increase in malignant melanomas (Fig. 11-15), and the skin of outdoor-loving patients should be examined once a year (especially fair-skinned patients) to catch melanomas in their earliest stage (before they have descended into the dermis) when they are virtually 100% curable by simple excision. The use of sunscreens (SPF 10 to 50) should be encouraged to prevent skin cancers and to prevent the aging of the skin caused by the sun. Patients with several large (greater than 7 mm) flat or slightly elevated ac-

quired nevi may have dysplastic nevus syndrome. This syndrome is relatively common but only recently recognized, and patients with this syndrome have a 20% to 100% chance of developing a melanoma during their lifetime (other whites have a 1.25% risk according to the latest figures). These patients should be examined every 3 months for their entire lives and should drastically reduce sun exposure to minimize this otherwise considerable risk.

If the increased risk of skin cancer does not impress athletic patients, the irony of having wrinkled, leathery, old-looking skin from the solar ultraviolet irradiation they were exposed to while keeping their cardiovascular and musculoskeletal systems in a "youthful" state should be stressed.

BIBLIOGRAPHY

Basler RS: Skin lesions related to sports activity, *Prim Care* 10(3):479–494, 1983.

Belongia EA, Goodman JL, Holland EJ, et al: An outbreak of herpes gladiatorum at a high school wrestling camp, *N Engl J Med* 325(13):906–910, 1991.

Conklin RJ: Common cutaneous disorders in athletes, *Sports Med* 9(2):100–119, 1990.

Dover JS: Sports-related dermatoses, *Curr Challenges Dermatol* Spring:1–9, 1992.

Fitzpatrick TB, Eisen AZ, Wolff K, et al (eds): *Dermatology in general medicine*, ed 4. New York, 1993, McGraw-Hill.

Levine N: Dermatologic aspects of sports medicine, *J Am Acad Dermatol* 3(4):415–424, 1980.

Magid DM, Schwartz B, Craft J, et al: Prevention of Lyme disease after tick bites: A cost effectiveness analysis, *N Engl J Med* 327(8):534–541, 1992.

Pro basketball power poll. *The Sporting News* 215(11):39, 1993.

Scheinberg RS: Exercise-related skin infection; managing bacterial disease, *Phys Sports Med* 22(6):47–58, 1994.

Scheinberg RS: Summer skin clinic: Recognizing and treating common derm problems in active adults, *Modern Med* 61(6):48–62, 1993.

Spruance SL, Hamill ML, Hoge WS, et al: Acyclovir prevents reactivation of herpes simplex labialis in skiers, *JAMA* 260(11):1597–1599, 1988.

CHAPTER 12

EYE INJURIES

Mary Mendelsohn
David Abramson

An eye injury can carry significant consequences for vision, disability, and future lifestyle. It is essential that health care professionals, trainers, and others involved in the care of athletes understand how to handle eye injuries. This chapter is organized in four sections. First, we review the anatomy of the eye. Second, we suggest a systematic method for examining the eye after injury. Third, we discuss how to diagnose and manage common ophthalmic injuries encountered in sports activities. Finally, we list useful contents of an emergency eye care kit.

ANATOMY REVIEW

Figures 12-1 and 12-2 show the basic anatomy of the eye. The labeled structures will be referred to throughout the chapter. The *cornea* is the clear covering in the front of the eye. The *sclera* is the visible white layer of the eye. The *limbus* is the junction of the cornea and the sclera. The sclera is covered by the *conjunctiva,* a thin transparent membrane with fine red blood vessels in it that can become thickened, reddened, and opaque from acute injury. The *iris* is the circular pigmented structure that gives the eye its color (blue, brown, hazel, etc.). The space between the iris and the cornea is called the *anterior chamber.* The anterior chamber is filled with a clear fluid called *aqueous humor.* The black *pupil* is simply a hole bounded by the iris. Behind the pupil and iris sits the *lens,* which is supported by fibers called "zonules." The zonules run radially from the lens to a structure called the *ciliary body,* which is attached to the inner eye wall. The ciliary body makes the aqueous humor and supports and focuses the lens. The ciliary body is continuous with the iris anteriorly and fuses with the retina and choroid posteriorly. Behind the lens is the large cavity of the eyeball that is filled with a clear gel called *vitreous humor.* The inner lining of the eye is the *retina,* a transparent neurosensory membrane with blood vessels running in it. The retina transforms light to neural impulses and sends that information to the brain via the *optic nerve.* The optic nerve transmits the visual informa-

tion to the brain. The *macula* is the area of the retina where the sharpest vision occurs. The optic nerve and the macula are posterior structures within the eye that can be identified with the direct ophthalmoscope (Fig. 12-3). Between the retina and the sclera is a middle layer of the eye wall called the *choroid.* The choroid is a blood vessel layer of the eye. Another common anatomic term is the "uvea"; it is a collective name for the three vascular structures of the eye: the iris, ciliary body, and choroid.

EXAMINATION OF THE EYE AFTER TRAUMA

Before attempting to examine an injured eye, protect it from further injury. While at the playing area, place a shield over the eye that rests on the brow and cheek; tape the shield in place. Do not use a patch or device that touches the eye or eyelids because this can worsen conditions such as ruptured globe or foreign body penetration. Do not put pressure on the eye; instruct the player not to rub the eye. If a specific eye shield is not available, taping a paper cup over the eye is an acceptable alternative. Remove the player to the examining area.

Once the eye is protected, take a history. The history will direct the examiner to the kind of injury sustained. Record the time, location, and mechanism of the injury. Was it a scraping, lacerating, chemical, or concussive injury? If concussive (sudden blunt trauma), was the object that hit the eye larger than the size of the orbit (basketball, baseball bat) or smaller than the orbit (elbow, squash ball)? Objects larger than the diameter of the orbital entrance have their forces absorbed by the bones of the orbit and are more likely to cause fracture of these bones. Objects smaller than the orbital entrance are more likely to cause injury to the globe itself.[11] What symptoms does the player have (decreased vision, double vision, photophobia, pain, tearing)? Symptoms can help direct the examiner to the part of the eye that was injured; symptoms are discussed more fully under each diagnosis in the next section. A complete history includ-

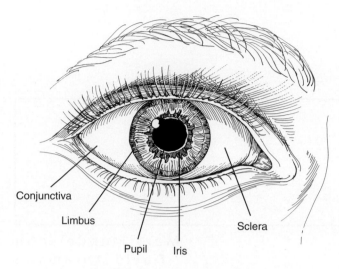

Fig. 12-1. Eye anatomy, front view.

Conjunctiva

Limbus

Pupil Iris

Sclera

ing allergies, medical illnesses, and other medication use is required before giving any antibiotic, eyedrop, or other medication.

Next, check the vision. Cover each eye and have the patient read an eyechart at 20 feet or a near card to the lowest line he or she can read. It is important to check vision before manipulating the eye in any way. If vision is being checked with a near card and the patient ordinarily uses reading glasses, a substitute pair of over-the-counter reading glasses of +2.50 diopters can be used to

assist near vision. If a patient's contact lenses or glasses were damaged or lost, the vision can be better approximated in each eye by having the patient read the chart while looking through a pinhole. (A small hole made in an index card will do if the diameter of the hole is approximately 1.2 mm.[1] This is about the size of a hole made with the end of a paper clip.)

Observe the lids and periorbita (area around the eye). If the lids are swollen shut, a lid speculum can be used to open them without putting pressure on the eye itself, but if this is necessary, it is better to refer to an ophthalmologist for further care. Note any lacerations, facial bone deformities, or irregular positioning of the eye. Test the extraocular movements: have the patient look in all directions of gaze (right, left, up, down, up and right, down and right, up and left, down and left). Note any limitations of movement; can it be explained by local swelling? Have the patient report any double vision seen in any direction. Palpate gently around the orbital rims, feeling for any discontinuity or excessive mobility of the facial bones. Brush a cotton swab on each cheek, testing for diminished sensation. Any findings such as limitation of eye movement, orbital rim discontinuity, or decreased sensation of the cheek can signal orbital fracture.

Check the pupil reactivity, an important indicator of damage to the iris or the optic nerve. Dim the room lights. Have the patient look into the distance (he should not look at the examiner or the light), and shine a bright light in one pupil while observing its reaction. It

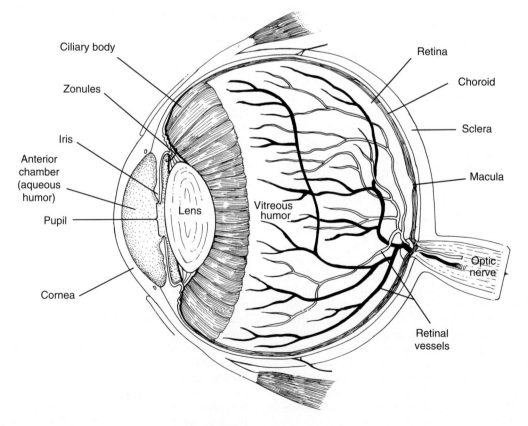

Ciliary body

Zonules

Iris

Anterior chamber (aqueous humor)

Pupil

Cornea

Lens

Vitreous humor

Retina

Choroid

Sclera

Macula

Optic nerve

Retinal vessels

Fig. 12-2. Eye anatomy, side view.

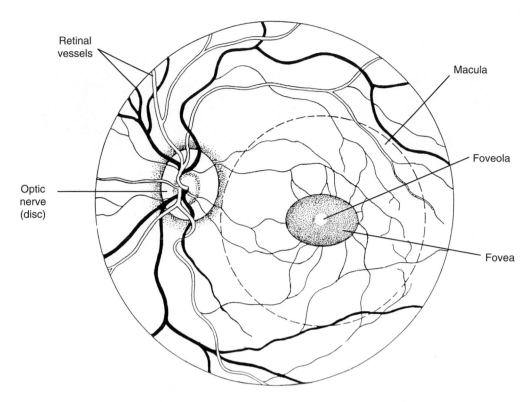

Fig. 12-3. Posterior structures of the eye: the macula, optic nerve, and retinal blood vessels.

should constrict briskly. Remove the light from the eyes. Next, shine the light on the second pupil. It should also constrict briskly to the same final size as the first pupil. A normal pupillary phenomenon called *hippus* may cause the pupil to slightly "bounce" (constrict and dilate) when light is held on it for an extended time, but its first reaction when a light is brought to it should be constriction. If one pupil is not responding, iris damage or optic nerve damage is likely. Subdural hematoma with herniation of the brain can also cause an ipsilateral, nonreactive, mid-dilated pupil.[4,7]

Next, do the "swinging flashlight" test, a good method of detecting optic nerve damage. Optic nerve damage diagnosed in this manner is called an *afferent pupillary defect.* The patient should look into the distance. Hold a bright light on the first eye, and watch as the pupil constricts. When it is fully constricted, quickly move the light to the other pupil—it should already be fully constricted and should not change much in size. Quickly return the light to the first pupil—it also should remain fully constricted. With normal eyes, light in one pupil will fully constrict both pupils simultaneously. (You may hold the light on a pupil for as long as you like, but the time spent crossing from one eye to the other should be minimal. You may swing the light to each eye several times to confirm your observations.) If one pupil dilates when the light is quickly returned to it, the eye has optic nerve damage. For example, if the right pupil constricts when the light is swung onto it but the left pupil dilates when the light is swung onto it, the left (dilating) eye has optic nerve damage. Swing the light back to the

right pupil, and it will constrict. Swing the light to the left pupil, and it will dilate. This dilation is an abnormal reaction, signaling optic nerve damage of the left eye. However, the constriction of the right eye when the light is swung to it is also abnormal, and it also signals optic nerve damage of the **left** eye. If the eyes were healthy each pupil would **already be constricted** when the light was swung to it from the other eye. Suppose the injured eye has blood obscuring the pupil or the pupil is nonreactive because of iris damage. Shine the light on the injured eye; the damaged eye's pupil is obscured or does not move. Quickly swing the light to the fellow eye; if the uninjured eye's pupil constricts when the light is swung to it, the injured eye has suffered optic nerve damage. Any patient with an afferent pupillary defect after trauma must be seen by an ophthalmologist immediately to identify the cause of the optic nerve damage.

Peripheral vision can be quickly checked by the *confrontation* technique to rule out a retinal detachment. Any patient who notes loss of peripheral vision or describes visual loss "like a curtain coming down" into his or her visual field should have a confrontation visual field test performed (Fig. 12-4). The examiner sits directly across from the patient. The patient covers his or her left eye while the right is tested. The examiner aligns his or her own left eye directly across from the patient's right eye about 3 feet away and closes his or her right eye. Each person stares into the other's eye throughout the entire test. The examiner holds his or her hand in a fist halfway between the two eyes but slightly off to the side, briefly raises a number of fingers, and then closes

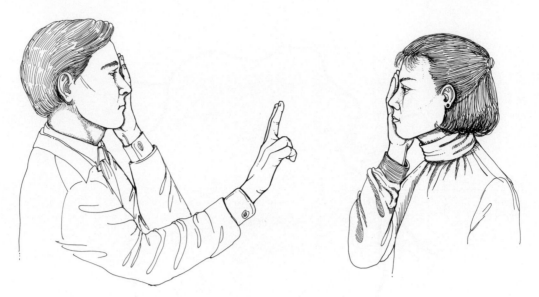

Fig. 12-4. A confrontational visual field test is done to detect losses of peripheral vision.

his or her fist again. The patient must respond by saying how many fingers were shown, which the examiner and patient see with their periperhal vision. The examiner should repeat the test showing different number of fingers while moving his or her hand around all clock hours and at different distances from the center of gaze to test the patient's peripheral vision against his or her own. To test the patient's reliability, the examiner should flash some fingers that are so far outside his or her own peripheral vision that he or she knows they cannot be seen. Test the uninjured eye for comparison.

The conjunctiva and sclera should be examined for hemorrhage, laceration, redness, and swelling. The cornea should be clear—any opacities may indicate ulcer or perforation. A drop of topical anesthetic—such as proparacaine, 0.5%—can be used to facilitate the examination if a ruptured globe has been ruled out. (A ruptured globe is an eye that has a perforating [full-thickness] tear through either the cornea or sclera into the uvea or humors of the inner eye. See the diagnosis section on how to diagnose and manage a ruptured globe. No drops should be used if a ruptured globe is present.) If a slit lamp is available, it can be used for a more magnified and detailed view; however, the procedure is the same whether a slit lamp or penlight examination is done. A fluorescein strip can be used to check for conjunctival abrasions, lacerations, corneal abrasions, or perforation. The fluorescein strip is moistened with water or anesthetic drop and touched briefly to the inside of the patient's lower lid to transfer some orange dye to the lid. The patient blinks to spread the dye evenly across the surface of the eye in a smooth green wash. (The orange dye turns yellow–green in water). If any geographic patches of dye stain brightly on the cornea because of pick-up of extra dye, the area is a corneal abrasion. Mucous threads and tear debris can also stain brightly, so the examiner should have the patient blink a few times. The items in the tear film will float about, but a corneal or conjunctival abrasion will remain stationary.

The fluorescein should remain an even green wash over the cornea. A blue-filtered light or Wood's lamp can be used to better visualize fluorescein stain because it causes the dye to fluoresce; any staining areas appear bright green. (Blue filters are available with many penlights, slit lamps, direct ophthalmoscopes, and muscle light attachments.) If there is a question of corneal perforation, the examiner should do the Seidel test. A dry fluorescein strip should be held up to the cornea just below the site in question. If there is a perforation, aqueous humor flowing from the perforation site will cause fluorescein to stream off the strip (Fig. 12-5). If a perforation is present, it must be surgically explored and repaired.

Make sure the iris and pupil are fully visible. If red or black blood is obscuring the view of any part of the iris, the patient has a hyphema, defined as blood in the anterior chamber. If the pupil is irregular or the sclera is obscured by pigmented material, a ruptured globe may be present. Iris tears or iridodialysis (iris disinsertion from its base at the ciliary body) can occur after blunt trauma and can cause irregular pupils.

The pressure in the eye should be checked, usually by Schiotz tonometer or applanation tonometry, if experienced personnel are present. (Any eye with a suspected rupture or possible perforation should not have pressure checked until examined by an ophthalmologist because pressure on the globe can worsen such situations.) Finger pressure can provide a rough guide to intraocular pressure if no other method is available. This is done by gently pressing on both sides of the globe at once through the patient's closed lids with the index fingers to get an idea of the pressure within the globe. The examiner can compare the firmness of the globe to the patient's uninjured eye and to his or her own to get an idea of normal pressure. An eye that is abnormally soft may indicate a ruptured globe—further examination should be deferred until seen by an ophthalmologist. An eye that is abnormally firm may have glaucoma or retrobulbar hemorrhage, blood collecting behind the eye—a potential oph-

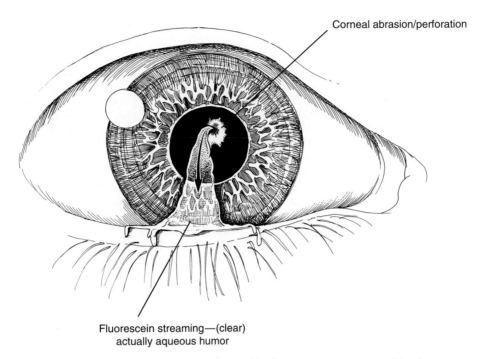

Corneal abrasion/perforation

Fluorescein streaming—(clear)
actually aqueous humor

Fig. 12-5. Seidel test: a corneal perforation detected by fluorescein streaming resulting from aqueous humor outflow.

thalmic emergency. Resistance to retropulsion can also be assessed to evaluate for retrobulbar hemorrhage: the eye should be pushed gently backward into the orbit by pressure on the globe through the closed lids. Healthy eyes can be retropulsed with a mild force; if the eye meets undue resistance, a retrobulbar bleed should be considered. This is especially significant if periocular tissue swelling is not sufficient to explain the degree of resistance.

If a direct ophthalmoscope is available, it can be used by experienced personnel to visualize the optic nerve, macula, and vitreous and to look for optic nerve edema. Optic nerve edema can indicate increased intracranial pressure (from subdural hematoma, usually bilateral) or severe hypotony (from ruptured globe). Retinal or vitreous hemorrhage, posterior retinal tears, or retinal detachment can also be seen. The direct ophthalmoscope can be easily used by following these simple steps. The examiner should set the displayed number to 0 (diopters) and stand facing the patient on the same side as the eye to be examined. The examiner should wear his or her glasses if applicable; the patient should remove his or her glasses. The examiner should ask the patient to look up slightly and to the side away from the examiner. For example, if the patient's right eye is being examined, the patient should look up slightly and to the left. (This brings the optic nerve directly in line with the examiner's view through the pupil.) The ophthalmoscope is held close to the examiner's eye and brought close to the patient's pupil. The patient should be instructed to keep his or her eyes open and still while maintaining gaze up and away, although his or her view will be largely blocked by the examiner's head. The examiner will see the red reflex of the pupil and should come closer, moving his or her

head and the scope as one unit and keeping a direct view through the scope, until he or she sees a linear, red retinal blood vessel. That vessel leads to the optic nerve by following any branching vessel back to its trunk. Vessels branch in a "Y" pattern; the optic nerve is at the base, or bottom, of all the Y's (see Fig. 12-3). The scope can be focused if necessary by slowly turning different plus (black or green) or minus (red) diopter values into the scope while looking at the vessels to get the clearest view. A nearsighted (myopic) patient will have the retina in clearest focus with minus diopters added to the scope; a farsighted patient may require plus diopters in the scope for a clear view. Before the examiner attempts to focus, he or she should be close to the patient and have a retinal vessel or optic nerve in view. Usually no more than 4 diopters need be dialed to achieve focus. Once the examiner has focused the optic nerve, he or she will see that it is generally a little larger than his or her field of view with the direct ophthalmoscope and will have to move his or her head slightly to assess all of its borders. The margins should be clear and sharp. To see the macula, the examiner turns the scope temporally toward the patient's ear and looks for the area where the blood vessels curve toward a darker area of retina and then stop, not reaching the center. This is the macula—the area of sharpest vision. The examiner should evaluate for blood or pallor and may have the macula brought directly to his or her view by telling the patient to look directly into the light of the scope. A limited examination of the posterior retina can be done by moving slowly around the periphery, looking for tears or blood. To fully evaluate the retina for tears or detachment, a dilated examination by an ophthalmologist is necessary. Naturally, if the symptoms cannot be explained after the initial examination or if any significant finding is encountered, an ophthalmologist should be consulted.

COMMON INJURIES—DIAGNOSIS AND TREATMENT

All medications have side effects and contraindications to usage in certain situations; eye medications are no exception. Anyone administering any of the medications recommended in this chapter must be familiar with their restrictions and must ascertain their safety for each patient on a case-by-case basis.

Conjunctiva, Cornea, and Sclera

The most common injuries to this region of the eye are abrasions and lacerations, subconjunctival hemorrhage, entrapped foreign bodies, and chemical injury.

LACERATIONS AND ABRASIONS. Lacerations and abrasions of the conjunctiva and cornea can be caused by any kind of scraping or wiping across the ocular surface. Lacerations and abrasions often cause symptoms of pain, tearing, a gritty sensation, or photophobia (sensitivity to light). If the central cornea is abraded, vision will be decreased. Signs include conjunctival hyperemia (redness) and conjunctival chemosis (swelling). If of long duration, lid swelling and a reactive ptosis (upper lid droop) may occur. Diagnosis is made by inspection, noting a defect in the conjunctival or corneal surface, and aided by a slit lamp if available. Fluorescein dye should be applied after initial inspection to better visualize any abrasions; they will stain brightly and be seen well with blue light (technique described previously).

Simple linear conjunctival lacerations usually heal well. The only treatment required is an antibiotic drop 3 to 4 times a day for 4 days to prevent infection. A broad-spectrum antibiotic ophthalmic drop—such as tobramycin, 0.3%, or sulfacetamide, 10%—can be used. If a geographic patch of conjunctiva has been removed, an antibiotic ophthalmic ointment (tobramycin or erythromycin ointment) and pressure patch can be applied (patching technique to be discussed). A patch worn for 24 hours is advised; then the area can be reexamined. Conjunctiva usually heals within 24 hours. If healed or the abrasion becomes smaller, the patient can use antibiotic drops as discussed previously for several more days. If the conjunctiva is in many shreds, surgical examination and débridement are warranted. The sclera below any conjunctival laceration must be carefully examined to rule out scleral laceration or penetrating injury. Any sign of laceration that involves the sclera requires a full dilated examination to rule out ruptured globe or underlying retinal injury. If the laceration worsens or becomes purulent, prompt referral to an ophthalmologist is necessary.

Corneal abrasions are superficial lacerations to the cornea that remove the epithelial layer of the cornea. On penlight examination the cornea may look normal, but with fluorescein staining the abraded area will stain bright green (also seen best with a blue light). Corneal abrasions can be managed with an antibiotic ointment (tobramycin, erythromycin) and a pressure patch worn for 24 hours. These abrasions are often painful because of the ciliary muscle spasm that often accompanies them. If the patient is very uncomfortable, a drop of cycloplegic can be given to relax the ciliary muscle. (Such drops, like homatropine, 5% [preferred for children; 2% for infants] or cyclopentolate, 1%, or 2% for adults, will dilate the pupil and blur the patient's vision of close objects for 24 hours or so.[2] The patient should be warned of this side effect. Atropine drops should not be used because their effects can last 1 to 2 weeks!) The examiner should apply the cycloplegic drop, the ointment directly over the cornea, and then the pressure patch as follows: fold an oval eye pad in half, and place over the closed eyelid. Put an unfolded eye pad over this, and place tape on the patient's forehead, across the pads, and onto his or her cheek. The patch should be taped tightly to prevent the eyelid from opening, but should not be uncomfortable for the patient. The next day, the patient should be examined by an ophthalmologist to ensure complete healing or repatching if necessary. Abrasions can become corneal ulcers if unhealed and will require much more intensive treatment. Any area of white or grey opacity in the normally clear cornea is a possible corneal ulcer and should be examined by an ophthalmologist. Corneal ulcers require intensive antibiotic management, possible scraping and culture, and may worsen if a patch is applied. They do not form in the acute injury period; it takes 1 to 2 days for an ulcer to form after injury.

The sclera is a tougher tissue and does not abrade. It can be lacerated, however, which is usually associated with an overlying conjunctival laceration and subconjunctival hemorrhage. A scleral laceration will appear as a discontinuity in the sclera. If the laceration penetrates the sclera, the underlying reddish-brown uvea may bulge through the wound. (The uvea is the vascular layer of the eye between the retina and sclera, comprising the choroid, ciliary body, and iris.) This bulge is a sign of a ruptured globe; a shield should be placed over the eye and further examination should be done by an ophthalmologist because surgical repair may be required. If there is a possibility of perforating scleral injury, but the sclera cannot be adequately visualized because of overlying subconjunctival hemorrhage, the eye needs to be explored surgically.

SUBCONJUNCTIVAL HEMORRHAGE. A subconjunctival hemorrhage can occur with any laceration or blunt injury, but also may result from Valsalva maneuvers during straining, weightlifting, constipation, or vomiting. It can also occur with aspirin use or spontaneously, unassociated with an injury. A subconjunctival hemorrhage is a collection of bright red blood under the conjunctiva but overlying the sclera, obscuring the white of the sclera (Fig. 12-6). The blood stops at the cornea and does **not** obscure the cornea, iris, or pupil. This bleeding is often startling, but is painless and not associated with other symptoms. Isolated hemorrhages do not require treatment and will resolve after a few weeks, changing color and clearing in the same manner as a bruise of the skin. The sclera below the hemorrhage should be carefully inspected to rule out laceration or perforation. If associated with other signs or symptoms

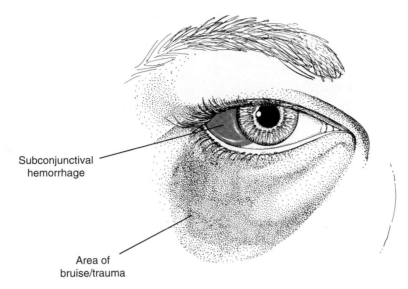

Subconjunctival hemorrhage

Area of bruise/trauma

Fig. 12-6. Subconjunctival hemorrhage: blood does not cross the limbus or obscure the iris.

such as decreased vision, pain, irregular pupils, or scleral irregularity, a dilated examination is needed to discover the cause.

FOREIGN BODIES. Foreign bodies are usually felt entering the eye. Before any topical anesthetic drop is applied, the patient should be asked to localize where he or she feels the foreign body to direct the examiner's search. Pain is the usual symptom of conjunctival or corneal foreign bodies. Conjunctival foreign bodies often show a localized hyperemia. The longer the time from injury, the more diffuse conjunctival irritation will be seen. A marked papillary reaction can be seen around many conjunctival foreign bodies (the conjunctiva shows many small elevated bumps, seen with a slit lamp for magnification). Corneal foreign bodies show a perilimbal (encircling the base of the cornea) or diffuse irritation. If lodged in the central cornea, a foreign body may be associated with decreased vision.

If a visible foreign body is located superficially in the conjunctiva, it can be removed with a fine forceps under direct visualization. A slit lamp or surgical loupes can be used to aid magnification. A drop of proparacaine and an antibiotic drop (such as tobramycin, 0.3%, or sulfacetamide, 10%) should be given before and after removal, and an antibiotic drop should be used 4 times daily for approximately 4 days while the conjunctiva heals. A small amount of conjunctival bleeding is expected and should stop momentarily or at most require local pressure with a cotton swab soaked in proparacaine (or phenylephrine, 2.5%, for hemostasis) for a few minutes.

Any foreign body in the cornea should be removed at a slit lamp by trained personnel. An antibiotic drop and anesthetic drop should be given before and after removal. If there are many scattered particles that are difficult to see, such as glass shards, the superficial pieces can be removed, but any that might be penetrating the eye should be left for an ophthalmologist to examine. If

there is a possibility of foreign bodies penetrating into the eye, orbit, or lids where they cannot be seen, radiographs or computed tomography (CT) scans can help localize them if they are of radioopaque material.

If there is a possibility of a ruptured globe, a shield should be placed over the eye and orbital rim. No drops, manipulation, or further examination should be done until seen by an ophthalmologist. Ruptured globes require surgical exploration and repair and will be discussed more fully.

The upper lid should be everted to remove any foreign particles that may have become trapped beneath it. (This should not be done if there is a risk of the eye having a perforating laceration because the maneuver puts increased pressure on the eye and may worsen a laceration.) The examiner should apply a drop of proparacaine and ask the patient to look down. The examiner should grasp the upper eyelashes, pull the upper lid toward him or herself and away from the patient's eye, and then push with a cotton swab or coin edge downward on the skin of the upper lid near the upper lid crease, while folding the lashes upward over the swab, and back toward the brow (Fig. 12-7). The examiner then checks the inner (tarsal) surface of the eyelid exposed in this way and removes or flushes away any particles; sweeping underneath the tarsus can be done with a cotton swab moistened with an anesthetic drop to ensure that no particles are trapped there. Care should be taken not to rub against the surface of the cornea during this procedure because the patient's natural reaction is to pull away from the swab and to roll his or her eyes upward. The patient should be instructed to look down during this maneuver.

After foreign body removal from the cornea, abrasions inevitably remain. If very small, they can be managed with antibiotic ointment (tobramycin or erythromycin) for 1 night—they should be examined the next day to ensure complete healing. The patient can then use an

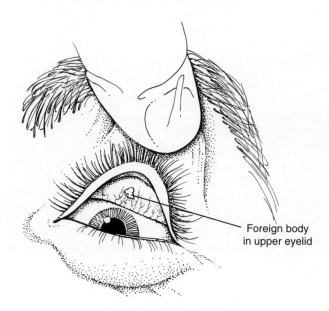

Foreign body
in upper eyelid

Fig. 12-7. Everted upper lid.

antibiotic drop (such as tobramycin or sulfacetamide) 4 times daily for 4 days. If the abrasion is larger, it should be pressure-patched as described previously.

Foreign bodies lodged in the sclera are penetrating injuries; these are most safely explored and removed by an ophthalmologist because of the possibility of ruptured globe.

CHEMICAL INJURIES. Chemical injuries occur when a toxic material, such as grass lime, enters the eye. The history is usually sufficient to diagnose the problem. The injury to most eyes will be painful and have varying degrees of photophobia and visual loss. The conjunctiva is usually red and may be chemotic. Even when the eye is white, the risk of damage from acidic or basic substances is high. In severe base burns, the eye is deceptively white because of extensive ischemic damage to the conjunctival and episcleral vessels. The cornea may be abraded, cloudy, or opaque. The eye should be flushed immediately with several liters of fluid. Rinses designed for the eye, sterile normal saline, or Ringer's lactate are preferred, but plain water should be used if it is the only fluid available. A drop of proparacaine in the eye as a topical anesthetic will allow the patient to open his or her eye during flushing, making it easier to get water past the lids, but flushing should begin immediately whether or not the drop is available. The eye should be flushed for 15 minutes with several liters of fluid. This is most easily done using a squeeze bottle, emergency eyewash sinks, or intravenous tubing connected to a bag of solution. The stream of water should not be sprayed directly onto the cornea if possible (to avoid abrasion), but rather rinsed on the sclera and allowed to flow over the cornea. The upper lid should be everted (technique as previously described), and the area beneath the lids should be flushed as well. Any foreign material should be removed. The pH of the tears (normally 7.0 to 7.7) can be tested several minutes after rinsing to ensure that no residual acidic or basic substances remain. Mild chemical injury that has only reddened the conjunctiva

can be managed with an antibiotic drop. A small corneal abrasion can be pressure-patched with antibiotic ointment and a cycloplegic drop as described previously. However, if symptoms, signs, or visual disturbances persist for more than a few hours, the patient should be referred to an ophthalmologist. Perilimbal blanching, large abrasions, or elevated intraocular pressure are ominous signs and require referral. Steroid drops are sometimes useful but should be used by an ophthalmologist because they can aggravate some situations, such as infections.[3]

Swimmers encounter frequent mild injuries to the cornea and conjunctiva from the hypotonicity, pH, chlorine, and chloramines of pool water. They develop conjunctivitis, corneal superficial punctate keratitis, microabrasions, and corneal edema, which have symptoms of eye irritation and halos seen around lights. No treatment is required if symptoms disappear several hours after cessation of swimming. Goggles greatly decrease the incidence of eye irritation.[6] If symptoms or signs persist, the patient should be examined for corneal abrasions and treated as outlined previously. If corneal opacities are noted, the patient should be referred to an ophthalmologist for possible corneal ulcer.

Anterior Segment (Anterior Chamber, Iris, Pupil, Lens)

Iritis (inflammation of the iris) is very common after concussive (blunt) trauma. The most prominent symptom is photophobia, with mildly decreased or normal vision, mild-to-moderate pain, and tearing. The eye is usually red, often more prominently around the limbus. Iritis is diagnosed at the slit lamp by observing cells and flare in the aqueous humor. The injured eye may have a lower intraocular pressure and poorly dilating pupil. It can be managed by steroid drops (prednisolone acetate, 1%, 4 times daily for 4 days can resolve a moderately traumatic iritis). Dosage is adjusted depending on severity. A cycloplegic drop (cyclopentolate, 1%, or homatropine, 5%) may be added for comfort and to prevent iris adhesions to the cornea or lens during the period of acute inflammation. Follow-up evaluation should ensure that the iritis is gone before the drops are no longer administered. Traumatic iritis should resolve within 1 week with drops; if additional treatment is required, the patient should be referred to an ophthalmologist.

Certain kinds of damage to iris structures and the ciliary body can be asymptomatic, with normal vision and general appearance. Examples are iridodialysis (a tear of the iris base from its attachment to the ciliary body) and angle recession (a tear through the muscle layers of the ciliary body). These injuries may not cause symptoms until months after the injury, when a late-onset glaucoma causes permanent visual loss. Patients with severe iridodialysis may appear to have an irregular pupil and have symptoms of iritis (Fig. 12-8). Even patients without symptoms are at risk for late-onset glaucoma. Any patient who had a concussive injury should have an eye examination done to evaluate these structures 1 to 2 weeks after injury.

A hyphema is a serious injury often associated with

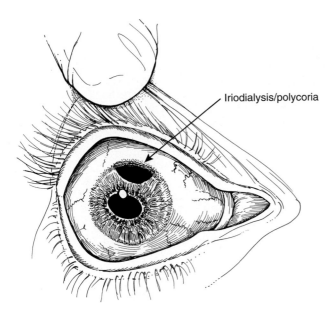

Fig. 12-8. Iridodialysis causing irregular pupil and "polycoria" (the appearance of multiple pupils).

blunt trauma to the globe. A hyphema is blood in the anterior chamber of the eye collecting behind the cornea and in front of the iris (Fig. 12-9). The blood partially obscures the view of the iris, sometimes the pupil, and layers by gravity. When the patient is sitting up, only the inferior part of the iris may be obscured. The patient may have no symptoms or may experience only the expected pain and photophobia from an associated iritis. Complete, or "eight ball," hyphemas fill the entire anterior chamber with blood so that behind the cornea the eye looks like a dark mass, with no iris or pupil seen. Vision is obviously decreased in such cases. Hyphemas are

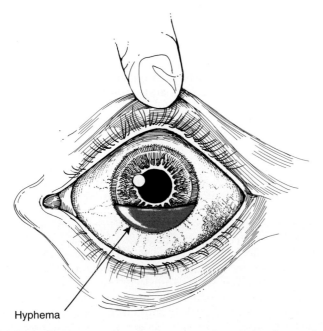

Hyphema

Fig. 12-9. Hyphema: blood layers in anterior chamber and obscures iris.

associated with a 10% incidence of rebleeding and risk of severe glaucoma. The patient must be referred immediately to an ophthalmologist and followed daily, usually with bedrest, until the blood clears. He or she may require hospitalization or surgery to clear the blood and control the intraocular pressure. While awaiting referral, the patient should be placed at bedrest with the head of the bed elevated 30° to allow the blood to settle into the inferior part of the eye; the patient should not be given aspirin, which can worsen bleeding. Vomiting can worsen bleeding; an antiemetic should be given if needed. If a ruptured globe can be ruled out, atropine, 1%, drops can be given every 6 hours. Elevated intraocular pressure can be controlled by topical beta blocker drops, oral carbonic anhydrase inhibitors (acetazolamide, methazolamide), and intravenous mannitol as needed.

Microhyphemas have erythrocytes floating in the anterior chamber but no layering of blood. This diagnosis can only be made with the slit lamp. Care must be taken to distinguish erythrocytes from the pigmented iris cells of iritis. When a microhyphema is present, the patient must also be put at bedrest and observed closely for rebleeding. A complete dilated examination is needed to evaluate for other trauma.

Blunt trauma can sublux (partially dislocate) or completely dislocate the lens of the eye. A symptom is decreased vision. Diagnosis is made by visualizing the lens' edge or eccentric center of the lens with a dilated examination or by observing the lens in the anterior chamber or in the vitreous (Fig. 12-10). Any patient with this problem should see an ophthalmologist. Lenses dislocated into the anterior chamber cause glaucoma and corneal decompensation and need to be removed. Lenses in the vitreous are often well tolerated, and surgery may not be necessary. Cataracts can form from trauma, especially after penetrating injuries when a foreign body enters the lens. Blunt trauma can also cause cataracts. If the lens capsule is intact, these findings can be observed. Rupture of the capsule may require removal to avoid the development of phacoanaphylactic inflammatory response to the lens proteins released inside the eye. Such reactions, which develop days to weeks after the injury, can be severe and can destroy the eye.

Posterior Segment (Optic Nerve, Retina, Vitreous)

Any patient with signs or symptoms of posterior segment trauma (as will be described) requires an immediate dilated examination to adequately evaluate the optic nerve, retina, vitreous, and choroid. In addition, any patient who has suffered concussive trauma but is asymptomatic should have a dilated examination in the next week to rule out asymptomatic injury.

Concussive trauma to the eye can cause retinal swelling called *commotio*, which is often asymptomatic. If the commotio involves the macula, the patient will have decreased vision. When commotio is present, the retina is whitened on examination. This condition is difficult to appreciate with the direct ophthalmoscope; it is more obvious with the indirect ophthalmoscope. Com-

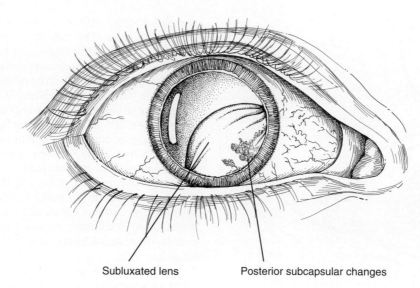

Subluxated lens   Posterior subcapsular changes

Fig. 12-10. Subluxed, or partially dislocated, lens. The lens' edge can be seen in the pupil.

motio usually resolves completely without treatment, but it can leave areas of retinal pigment changes with some visual loss. A dilated examination should be done for all patients who have commotio because of the possibility of retinal tears.

Retinal tears are important to diagnose because they may lead to detachment. Symptoms of new floating spots in front of the eyes or spontaneous flashing lights require examination by an ophthalmologist. Retinal tears appear as distinct retinal defects with the orange choroidal color showing through (Fig. 12-11). There may be pigment or retinal fragments floating in the vitreous above the tear. Retinal detachments and retinal tears are usually located more peripherally than can be

seen with the direct ophthalmoscope; a dilated examination with indirect ophthalmoscopy is necessary. Tears can also occur without signs or symptoms, so after concussive injury a dilated eye examination by an ophthalmologist should be done in the next week to rule out asymptomatic injury. Laser treatment, cryotherapy, or surgery may be required if tears are present.

Retinal detachment (Fig. 12-11) can occur without loss of central vision. The patient may notice, when covering one eye, that the other eye has lost part of its peripheral vision. This vision loss is often described as a "curtain coming down" into the patient's field of view. Such symptoms require an immediate dilated eye examination. A confrontation visual field test (as described previously) should be performed after concussive trauma, even for asymptomatic patients. If loss of vision is noticed, a dilated examination is required. Other signs of retinal detachment are pigment in the vitreous and the transparent membrane of the retina with the retinal blood vessels floating off the surface of the choroid. Retinal detachments require prompt surgical repair. They can progress if untreated and result in permanent visual loss.

Blood in the vitreous will obscure vision or give symptoms of floating spots or lines in front of the vision. Local clumps of heme or a diffuse red haze in the vitreous are seen, often obscuring the view of the optic nerve or macula. Although the blood will often clear without treatment, a dilated examination is needed to identify the source of the bleeding. Retinal tears or choroidal rupture (a tear in the choroid) are common causes of vitreous hemorrhage after trauma.

Optic nerve injury can occur from severe concussive trauma (more commonly seen after automobile collisions than after sports injuries). The vision will be decreased, and the patient will have an afferent pupillary defect. If results of the examination are otherwise normal, the afferent pupillary defect may be caused by compression of the optic nerve at the level of the optic canal.

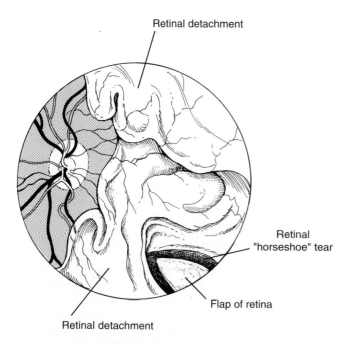

Retinal detachment

Retinal "horseshoe" tear

Flap of retina

Retinal detachment

Fig. 12-11. Retinal detachment.

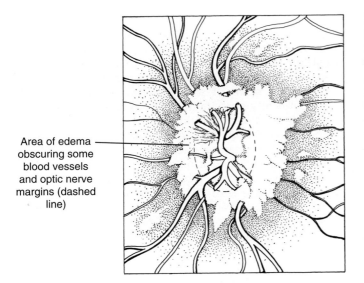

Area of edema obscuring some blood vessels and optic nerve margins (dashed line)

Fig. 12-12. Edema of the optic nerve. The optic nerve margins are blurred, and the blood vessels may by indistinct as they cross the optic nerve.

A new afferent pupillary defect should be considered an ophthalmic emergency; imaging studies (CT or magnetic resonance imaging [MRI] scan concentrating on the optic nerve from globe to chiasm and the brain) and an ophthalmologic examination should be obtained. Management may include consideration of high-dose steroid administration to decrease inflammation or surgery to relieve compression.[8,9]

Optic nerve edema, noted with a direct ophthalmoscope, may occur without symptoms or vision changes. Symptoms, when they occur, include central scotomas,

headache, and brief (seconds) periods of visual loss. The margins of the optic nerve appear blurred, either diffusely or focally, with partial obscuration of the blood vessels as they cross the optic nerve margin (Fig. 12-12). An ophthalmologic examination and imaging studies are required because optic nerve edema after trauma can signal increased intracranial pressure such as from subdural or epidural hematoma (usually affecting both optic nerves). Unilateral optic nerve edema may imply severe hypotony from a ruptured globe—this is usually obvious from other signs.[10]

Ruptured Globe

A ruptured globe is a perforation of the sclera or cornea. A direct blow with an object smaller than the size of the orbit (a squash ball or an elbow) is the most likely type of injury to cause ragged rupture of the globe. Other common causes of ruptured globe are lacerating injuries (darts, glass shards). The patient usually has poor vision but may not have much pain. The most obvious signs of a ruptured globe are disorganization of anterior structures. Without touching the eye, the sclera should be examined for signs of uvea (dark pigmented tissue) protruding through the sclera (Fig. 12-13). The weakest points of the sclera are near the insertion of the recti muscles, so ruptures most often occur at these sites (approximately 6 to 7 mm posterior, radially outward, from the limbus, at 12:00, 3:00, 6:00, and 9:00). There is often extensive subconjunctival hemorrhage. The pupil, instead of being round, may be misshapened or elongated as the iris is pulled toward the rupture site. There may be a hyphema that obscures the iris entirely or partially. An afferent defect is sometimes present. If there is a possibility of ruptured globe, the eye should not be manipulated in any way. Drops should not be used. An eye shield should be

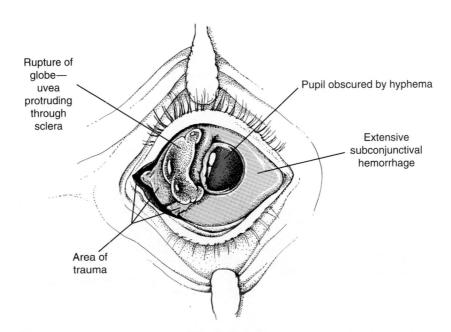

Rupture of globe— uvea protruding through sclera

Pupil obscured by hyphema

Extensive subconjunctival hemorrhage

Area of trauma

Fig. 12-13. Ruptured globe. Uvea is seen protruding through sclera from 7:00 to 9:00 just outside limbus. Also present are extensive subconjunctival hemorrhage and the pupil obscured by hyphema.

placed over the eye and the patient sent immediately to an ophthalmologist. Any pressure put on the eye from patches or examination may cause the rupture to enlarge and the contents of the eye to extrude. The patient should be kept at bedrest and receive no food or drink. Antiemetics should be administered if needed to avoid vomiting, which can worsen a rupture. Tetanus toxoid should be given if needed. Intraveneous antibiotics can be administered: for adults, cefazolin, 1 g intravenously every 8 hours plus gentamicin 2.0 mg/kg intravenous load, then cefazolin plus gentamicin, 1 mg/kg intravenously every 8 hours. For children, the dose is cefazolin 50 mg/kg/24 h intravenously in divided doses given every 6 or 8 hours, plus gentamicin, 2 mg/kg intravenously every 8 hours.[3] CT scan may be needed to rule out intraocular foreign body or to localize a rupture site.

Ruptured globes can occur posteriorly and be difficult to see. Findings associated with occult scleral rupture include severe vision loss (less than 20/400), hypotony (low intraocular pressure), extensive subconjunctival hemorrhage, hyphema, vitreous hemorrhage, afferent pupillary defect, abnormally deep or shallow anterior chamber, or unexplained loss of extraocular movement. If the eye looks intact but these findings suggest occult rupture, the patient should be referred to an ophthalmologist rather than risking a missed diagnosis. Imaging studies can sometimes be helpful in such cases. Ruptured globes require surgical repair.[5,12]

Orbital Bone Fractures

Blunt injury with an object larger than the orbital opening (basketball or baseball bat) has most of the force of the injury absorbed by the bones of the orbit, often sparing the globe. All the injuries mentioned in the previous section can be seen, but more commonly fractures of the orbital bones occur. Orbital floor fractures and medial wall fractures are the most common because the bones are thinnest at these locations. A greater force is needed to cause inferior orbital rim or lateral rim fractures. High impact forces are required for superior orbital rim fractures and tripod fractures (fractures of the zygoma at its three articulations: the arch, the lateral orbital rim, and the inferior orbital rim).

Symptoms of orbital fracture include local tenderness and binocular double vision (usually worse on upgaze for orbital floor fractures). It should be noted that binocular double vision (with both eyes open) in any field of gaze can be a sign of injury to an extraocular muscle or nerve or a result of soft-tissue swelling displacing the eye. Difficulty chewing or inability to open the mouth widely can indicate a tripod fracture because the coronoid process impinges on the mandible. Key physical findings that suggest a fracture include an irregularity or discontinuity in palpation along the orbital rims (there are normal notches along the inferior and superior rims—compare with the other orbit to detect asymmetry). Swelling and ecchymosis of the overlying eyelid are often present. Decreased sensation to the upper cheek below the injured eye often accompanies an orbital floor fracture, signaling injury to the inferior orbital nerve. Crepitus from emphysema of the lids or periorbital tissues occurs with floor or medial wall fractures, when the orbital wall fractures into a sinus and air from the sinus enters the periorbital tissues. (The patient may notice his or her lids swell after nose blowing. If so, he or she should avoid nose blowing.) An eye that appears enophthalmic (sunken in compared with the other eye) also suggests a floor or medial wall fracture. Limited vertical movement of the involved eye (an inability to look up or down) can mean that a floor fracture has trapped orbital tissue or extraocular muscle within it (Fig. 12-14). "Forced ductions" can be performed to test eye mobility. A topical anesthetic drop, such as proparacaine, should be given. The conjunctiva should be grasped near the cornea and the eye rotated in any direction. A normal eye is freely movable. If the eye is unable to be elevated with forceps and there is resistance against the pull of the forceps, there may be an orbital fracture. To diagnose any fracture with certainty requires radiographs and occasionally CT scans. Large fractures require surgical repair, but small fractures frequently do not. An ophthalmologist should be consulted to determine if surgery is necessary.

Other traumatic causes of binocular diplopia, such as damage to an extraocular muscle or nerve, are rare in sports injuries unless associated with obvious lacerations that require surgical exploration and repair. A binocular

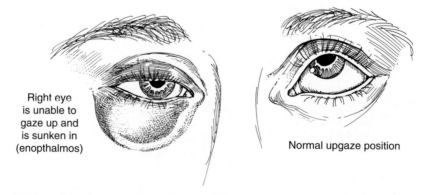

Right eye is unable to gaze up and is sunken in (enopthalmos)

Normal upgaze position

Fig. 12-14. Right orbital floor fracture. Patient is attempting to look up: note restricted upgaze and enophthalmos of right eye.

vertical diplopia can develop because of concussive trauma resulting from IVth nerve palsy; here, the double vision is worse (images appear farther apart) in gaze down and toward the nose of the affected side. The patient should be followed; if no resolution occurs when the soft-tissue swelling resolves, he or she should see an ophthalmologist.

Periorbital Injury

Bruising and swelling of the eyelids and tissues around the eye are common after blunt trauma. Localized pain is the usual symptom. Management consists of applying ice packs to the area as frequently as possible during the first 24 hours; after that, bruising will resolve with time. Swollen or lacerated lids should not prevent a thorough examination of the globe itself. The same blunt trauma may have caused a hyphema or other asymptomatic but potentially serious conditions. Obviously, no ice packs should be applied until a ruptured globe has been ruled out; the pressure from the pack can worsen a rupture.

Laceration of the skin around the eye is usually repaired with sutures after cleaning the wound with betadine in the same manner as other wounds. There are several areas of special concern to the eye. The lacrimal drainage system is one such area. If the laceration is between the corner of the eye and the nose, it may have cut the lacrimal apparatus (tear drainage system). Any incision in this area should be cleaned, covered with sterile gauze moistened with saline, and the patient referred for an immediate ophthalmic examination. If the laceration is through the eyelid margin, the repair must be done with a layered technique first closing the tarsus of the lid, then skin, to prevent lid notching when healed. The patient should be referred if the field surgeon is not familiar with lid-suturing techniques. Any patient with a laceration associated with poor eye movement (possibly involving an eye muscle), lid droop (damage to eyelid retractor muscles), or unusual anatomic position should be referred to an ophthalmologist. Tetanus prophylaxis should be given if needed for any laceration.

A retrobulbar hemorrhage is a collection of blood behind the eye and within the orbit. It is an ophthalmic emergency that can occur from any deep laceration around the eyelids. If the injury penetrates the orbital septum (the tissue barrier between the eyelids and the deep orbit), blood can collect behind the globe within the orbit where it cannot be seen. As the bleeding continues, the blood will push the globe forward, and the intraocular pressure will be severely elevated. This condition can cause permanent blindness within hours if not detected. The patient may not be aware of the condition, and any pain may be attributed to the laceration. The main symptoms are increasing pain and decreased vision, often rapidly worsening over several hours. Characteristic signs and symptoms of retrobulbar hemorrhage are pain, proptosis (forward protrusion of the eye), eyelid and subconjunctival hemorrhage, resistance to retropulsion, development of an afferent defect, and increased intraocular pressure. Any patient who has had a laceration around the eyelids should be instructed, after repair, to check the vision in each eye periodically and compare the appearance of the eyes during the first 24 hours; he or she should be sure nothing has worsened. The patient should report any increasing pain. Any surgical repair of a lid laceration should be taped with sterile adhesive strips and not covered by a patch that obscures the eye, so appearance and vision can be monitored. If a retrobulbar hemorrhage occurs, it is an emergency. A lateral canthotomy with inferior cantholysis should be done immediately by an ophthalmologist or trained emergency personnel. The canthotomy is done to allow the accumulated retrobulbar blood to exit and relieve the pressure on the eye. When performed promptly, permanent visual loss can be avoided. While waiting for the canthotomy, the intraocular pressure can be lowered by using topical beta blocker drops, carbonic anhydrase inhibitors, or intravenous mannitol as needed.

PREVENTION

The best method for managing eye injuries is to prevent their occurrence. Adequate eye protection is essential for any sport where injury is a risk; face and head protection are often needed as well. The standards set by the American Society for Testing and Materials (ASTM) are based on performance testing by committees (composed of physicians, manufacturers, and athletes) and are useful guidelines for minimum recommended protection. Any protective eyewear should have lenses made of polycarbonate, which is more impact resistant than other plastic or glass lenses. Such lenses are recommended for all racquet sports; none of the lensless eye protectors are adequate because balls traveling at high speeds can deform and mold into the opening sufficiently to strike the eye.[11]

CONTENTS OF AN EYE EXAMINATION KIT

Several useful items should be available to facilitate eye examination and management whether at fieldside or in the emergency room. The following list includes the contents of a basic eye examination kit, with more extensive equipment listed in brackets.

Emergency phone numbers (emergency room, ophthalmologist);
Near card for vision testing (usually read at 14 inches) [eye chart for vision testing, preferably read at a 20-foot distance];
Pinhole occluder for vision testing;
Pair of +2.50-diopter, over-the-counter reading glasses;
Penlight, with bright light [or halogen "muscle light" attachment of direct ophthalmoscope];
Blue filter for tip of penlight for reviewing fluorescein stain;
Sterile cotton swabs;
Topical anesthetic drop (i.e., proparacaine, 0.5%);
Antibiotic ophthalmic drop (i.e., tobramycin, gentamicin, sulfacetamide);
Antibiotic ophthalmic ointment (i.e., tobramycin, erythromycin, bacitracin);

Fluorescein strips;
Sterile large eye pads;
Paper tape;
Eye shields;
Eye fluid rinse bottle;
Sterile strips for closing lid skin wounds
[Direct ophthalmoscope, which may come with blue filter and bright light for fluorescein viewing, and slit lamp, useful for any examining area or emergency room].

REFERENCES

1. American Academy of Ophthalmology: *Basic and clinical science course, section 3—optics, refraction and contact lenses,* San Francisco, 1993, American Academy of Ophthalmology.
2. American Academy of Ophthalmology: *Basic and clinical science course, section 6—Pediatric ophthalmology and strabismus,* San Francisco, 1993, American Academy of Ophthalmology.
3. Friedberg M, Rapuano C: *Wills Eye Hospital: Office and emergency room diagnosis and treatment of eye disease,* Philadelphia, 1990, JB Lippincott.
4. Isselbacher K, ed: *Harrison's principles of internal medicine, Chapter 26,* New York, 1994, McGraw-Hill.
5. Kylstra JA, et al: Clinical predictors of scleral rupture after blunt ocular trauma. *Am J Ophthalmol* 115(4):530–535, 1993.
6. Pizzarello L, Haik B, eds: *Sports ophthalmology, Chapter 6,* Springfield, 1987, Charles C. Thomas.
7. Tasman W, ed: *Duane's clinical ophthalmology, vol 2, chapter 3,* Philadelphia, 1993, JB Lippincott.
8. Tasman W, ed: *Duane's clinical ophthalmology, vol 2, chapter 5,* Philadelphia, 1993, JB Lippincott.
9. Tasman W, ed: *Duane's clinical ophthalmology, vol 3, chapter 31,* Philadelphia, 1993, JB Lippincott.
10. Tasman W, ed: *Duane's clinical ophthalmology, vol 3, chapter 58,* Philadelphia, 1993, JB Lippincott.
11. Tasman W, ed: *Duane's clinical ophthalmology, vol 5, chapter 45,* Philadelphia, 1993, JB Lippincott.
12. Werner MS, et al: Predictors of occult scleral rupture. *Ophthalmology* 101:1941–1944, 1994.

CHAPTER 13

CRANIOFACIAL INJURIES

Alex M. Greenberg
Richard H. Haug

The craniomaxillofacial region is injured frequently by athletes engaged in various forms of sports-related activities. The role of the primary care provider involved in the treatment of athletes, whether as a generalist or specialist, should be to have a well-informed appreciation of the anatomy, pathophysiology, etiology, distribution, and classification of the craniomaxillofacial injuries that may be encountered. This way, preventive and management-oriented approaches to these many problems can be applied to the treatment of these patients. The broad scope of contemporary sports activities ranges from those with minimal interpersonal contact to high-energy contact, including high-velocity vehicular and high altitude-dependent activities,[3,9,29,33,38,49,50,65] thus many possibilities exist for variations in the form of trauma. It is important to begin with a definition of the craniomaxillofacial region and the types of classical injuries that can be sustained. The region is divided into hard- and soft-tissue structures that because of anatomic position, predilection to traumatic forces, and the presence or absence of protective garb will have specific types of injuries.

It is important to maintain a hierarchy of prioritization when evaluating these patients because certain head and neck organ systems will have greater immediate concern than others. Of paramount importance is the central nervous system (CNS), which in the head and neck region consists of the brain and cervical spine column. Injuries to the brain and spinal cord can range from mild concussion to severe paralysis and death. Certain sports activities have higher degrees of risk to the CNS than others, for example, boxing, automobile racing, boat racing, and other contact sports.[4,62] The primary sports care provider should be able to perform a basic neurologic examination to determine the integrity of the CNS, associated cranial nerves, and cervical spine structures. This also requires the ability to provide acute care services on the playing field to permit stabilization of the patient before hospitalization. Upon implementation of basic Advanced Trauma Life Support (ATLS) guidelines,[3] when neurologic integrity is determined, a more thorough history and physical examination of the patient may be performed.[3,38]

The most frequently injured organ system for athletes is the integumentary system.[9,29,33,50,65] External soft-tissue structures of the craniomaxillofacial region consist of the scalp, posterior neck, ears, face, and anterior neck. Internal soft tissues include the oral and oropharyngeal mucous membranes, ophthalmologic structures, nasal septum, and auditory canal. These sites are at risk for contusion, abrasion, hematoma formation, laceration, and avulsion. Numerous studies have attempted to categorize and classify the incidence of soft-tissue injuries encountered in sports activities.[33,46,62,65] In the craniomaxillofacial region, certain soft-tissue injuries may have functional and cosmetic implications because of the exposure of this anatomic site. Because many minor soft-tissue injuries are managed on an outpatient basis through on-site repair or private offices, it is difficult to obtain statistics for other than the more major types of injuries.[9,29,33,50,65] When injuries are classified according to certain parameters, it becomes possible to gain certain information regarding these injuries and whether they may result in any significant disability of a temporary or permanent nature.[4,21,57] The goal of this chapter is to provide information regarding the more commonly encountered American sports as opposed to the least frequent higher risk types of sports (i.e., bungee jumping, hang gliding, and sky diving). This way, common sport activities related to athletic competition that have a higher rate of injury because of interpersonal contact will be emphasized rather than injuries associated with high-risk individual sports that are machine-dependent activities.

Soft-tissue injuries will occur more frequently in some sports activities than others. For example, sports such as hockey and football will have a minimal incidence of scalp injuries because of the use of protective helmets.[6,52] Other sports such as soccer and basketball, which have a high degree of physical contact without the use of head and face protective equipment, will have higher numbers of scalp lacerations.[9,29,50] Facial and ear lacerations will occur more frequently in contact sports such as boxing, wrestling, and basketball.[9] Lacerations may be classified as simple, complex, or avulsive, and particular attention must be paid to the specific anatomic site. For example, a depressed skull fracture could be present with a scalp laceration. Ocular soft-tissue injuries may require further ophthalmologic evaluation before treatment. Soft-tissue injuries may mask underlying hard-tissue injuries.

Where indicated or suspected, radiography should supplement the physical examination to determine the presence of underlying skeletal injuries.[22] Plain radiography is useful for the facial skeleton, cervical spine, and dental structures.[22] Computed tomography (CT) and magnetic resonance imaging (MRI) scanning may be indicated in the presence of neurologic symptoms or where neurologic injuries are suspected, especially the brain and spinal cord.[22]

Injuries of the facial skeleton are generally studied as hospital populations.[9,29,33,50,65] The types of injuries are generally more severe with poor prognosis. Therefore, information concerning the distribution and etiology of facial injuries are generally within the context of the hospital emergency room or operating room. Sports injuries, on the other hand, are usually of a minor nature or may be managed at the athletic facility or in private offices. These injuries may include more significant facial lacerations or minor nasal, dentoalveolar, and mandibular fractures.[29] There have been few studies that have been directed toward the etiologies, distribution, and classification of maxillofacial sports injuries.[33,46,49,65] Perhaps the difficulty of engaging in such a study has to do with the large variety of sports activities that are available today at the amateur and professional levels. Sports activities and athletic competitions have become part of daily activities from the school aged to the elderly. Most studies have examined injuries severe enough to require treatment or cause disability, and yet there are variations that are seen between amateur and professional athletes that make these studies even more difficult. For example, Watson,[65] in studying four types of sports (endurance, contact, noncontact, and explosive) in Irish athletes, found that 6% of all injuries included head (5%) and dental (1%).[5,6] Therefore, it is more important for the primary care provider to be able to diagnose the various types of injuries that can occur in the craniomaxillofacial region and be able to either treat on a primary basis or be knowledgeable to make the appropriate referral to qualified specialists. Unlike orthopedics and sports medicine, there is no singular head and neck discipline that can claim specialty status in sports injuries. Rather, there are interested individuals who attend sporting events as team dentists, oral and maxillofacial surgeons, plastic surgeons, or otolaryngologists.

There are many studies that document the frequency of certain types of injuries in specific sports. In baseball, basketball, hockey, and football because of the high level of contact and the relative energies of impact, dental and craniomaxillofacial injuries are predictable.[6,9,46,52,62] Fortunately, these sports have evolved so that protective devices and regulations concerning their use have become more widespread and many of the injuries seen in the past occur less frequently.[6,52] For example, Torg et al[62] in the National Football Head and Neck Injury Registry reported a significant reduction in the incidence of quadriplegia between 1975 and 1984. This reduction reflected the change in the "spearing" rule of tackling in 1976, resulting in an immediate reduction in cervical spine injuries.

Of special interest are the pediatric populations between ages 5 and 14 years, in whom facial injuries in sports are frequent because of the learning stages of sports ability, the need for proving fearlessness to peers, and the ignorance of the consequences of taking greater risks.[49] Several recent studies have shown that 15% of pediatric facial fractures were sports-related, with 56% having associated soft-tissue injuries.[50] Polytrauma must always be considered as a cofactor, with head injuries comprising 42%.[50] Others have demonstrated that of those having facial fractures, children aged less than 12 years comprise less than 5% of all injuries, and children aged less than 6 years account for less than 1%.[54] Other authors claim a range of 1.5% to 8% of facial fractures in children aged less than 12 years, whereas children aged less than 1 year account for less than 1%.[29] Another study by the US Consumer Product Safety Commission in 1981 indicated a facial injury rate of 11% to 40% in children aged 5 to 14 years, depending on the type of sport.[46] Because of differences between the pediatric and adult facial morphology, there are differences in the fracture patterns. In infants and children, the cranium is large relative to the face. The cranial-to-facial ratio is 8:1 in infants and 2.5:1 in adults.[50] The accessory sinuses are poorly developed in children, and therefore high-energy injuries are less likely to be absorbed by the face than by the frontal bones. McGraw and Cole[42] observed age-related variations in a pediatric population, with a decrease in cranial fractures from 88% (in children aged less than 5 years) to 34% (children aged 12 to 16 years). Such studies may be skewed, based on the different hospital services that may treat these patients. For example, neurosurgeons may see more of the cranial injuries relative to craniomaxillofacial surgeons.[50]

With development, the paranasal sinuses become aerated and enlarged, and the mandible gains a more prominent position, allowing this structure to be more readily injured.[29,50,55] Maxillary and mandibular fractures will increase in occurrence with age. In the younger pediatric population, less developed sinuses, more flexible suture lines, and thicker adipose tissues result in fewer midfacial injuries.[29]

Because of soft-tissue edema, presence of lacerations, greater incidence of CNS involvement, poorly pneumatized sinuses, and presence of tooth buds (which can obscure fracture lines), CT axial and coronal scanning is the imaging method of choice in pediatric trauma patients.[29,50] The panoramic radiograph is still a highly cost-effective and accurate method for the determination of the presence of mandibular fractures, especially of the condylar region. Mandibular fractures are the most commonly reported fractures in the pediatric hospital population.[29,50,54]

EXAMINATION AND TREATMENT

It is important for the primary care provider involved in the management of acute sports-related craniomaxillofacial injuries to be able to diagnose, treat, or refer the patient to other specialists. To be able to perform these tasks, it is necessary to be cognizant of the types, distribution, and classification of these injuries and be able to perform accurate history taking and physical examination, which may include other diagnostic procedures and tests.

Soft-Tissue Injuries

Soft-tissue injuries may be described as clean or contaminated, and classified as contusions, abrasions, punctures, lacerations, and burns. Patients may present with combinations of the previously mentioned classifications and may have associated damage to vital structures and varying degrees of underlying skeletal involvement. In sports injuries of the face, most soft-tissue injuries can be considered to be contaminated because of the usual conditions under which they occur. If any athlete has a penetrating injury of the skin, tetanus immunization status must be determined, and appropriate tetanus coverage provided. Superficial burns, abrasions, and contusions should be gently washed and examined under good light. If particulate matter is embedded in the soft tissues, it should be meticulously debrided to avoid tattooing. Clean wounds may be dressed with antibiotic ointment preparations, such as Neosporin (Burroughs Wellcome, Research Triangle Park, NC), and light dressings may be applied where tissue protection is desired. Superficial lacerations should be cleansed with antimicrobial agents and then repaired primarily when possible with sutures or sterile strip dressings or a combination of the two. Deep lacerations may cause greater concern and often require more extensive diagnostic imaging or surgical intervention. Because traumatic forces can be so variable in sports, ranging from a boxing glove to a flying hockey puck, deep structures such as the CNS, eyes, tongue, ear, and base of skull should be carefully evaluated for damage. Penetrating wounds, especially of the scalp, ocular, and neck region, have particular anatomic concerns. Depressed skull fractures are easily masked by large scalp lacerations, and their radiographic examination should be carefully considered, rather than performed by blind digital or instrument techniques to avoid iatrogenic injuries. Radiologic examination, involving CT or MRI, may be necessary. Ocular injuries are seen frequently in sports-related trauma and must be carefully evaluated to determine the need for acute intervention.[47,63] Problems, such as hyphema, retinal tears, lens dislocation, penetrating globe injuries, optic nerve compression, orbital apex syndrome, superior orbital fissure syndrome, retrobulbar hematoma, and orbital floor and roof blowout fractures with adnexiae entrapment, should all be carefully considered. Neck soft-tissue considerations would include concern for the major vessels (carotid and jugular) and the laryngeal structures. Laryngeal injuries, although infrequent, can be devastating catastrophic problems if airway patency is compromised.

There can be many indications for intubation, cricothyrotomy, and tracheostomy depending on the circumstances, environment, and status of the patient. The unconscious athlete may require emergency airway treatment that is separate and distinct from laryngeal trauma. Basic life support considerations must always be considered in the initial assessment of these patients. Salivary gland injuries, although rare, should be considered when a laceration occurs in the midface where the parotid duct can be transected. The external ear is also of great concern, especially in athletes who engage in high-impact contact sports, such as boxing, wrestling, basketball, and football. Protective headgear should be worn by these athletes, but in certain situations it can be dislodged or not used (i.e., professional boxing). Hematoma and contusion of the external ear should be managed aggressively to avoid the "cauliflower ear," and lacerations are best treated immediately.[9]

Skeletal Injuries

Various sports committees have adopted specific guidelines for the prevention of dental and craniomaxillofacial injuries. Sports such as hockey and football have adopted full facial and cranial protective headgear.[6,52] Evolution of these protective devices has significantly reduced many types of head and neck injuries in these sports.[6,52,62]

Dentoalveolar Injuries

The craniomaxillofacial region (Fig. 13-1) can be divided into the cranium, facial bones, and dentition (primary and permanent). Injuries to these sites may be categorized according to the particular anatomy and various classification schemes. Dental injuries range from minor enamel fragments, complete coronal fractures, and even complete tooth avulsion.[4] For further discussion of dental injuries, see chapter 14. When the dental fracture involves the alveolar bone, whether in the maxilla or the mandible, these injuries are classified as *dentoalveolar* fractures and may include dental fractures and fractures of the supporting bone. Alveolar region fractures include more highly fragmented jaw fractures. These types of injuries are common in sports and are highly preventable with the use of mouthguards. The diagnosis of an alveolar fracture is made by physical and radiographic examination. Examination requires bimanual palpation and periapical dental or occlusal radiographs. More severe dentoalveolar fractures may involve laceration of the overlying mucosa, and displacement can occur with preservation of a lingual or buccal pedicle. Dentoalveolar fractures can be completely avulsed as well. Today, with open reduction and stabilization using techniques of microplate fixation, these fractures can be managed with retention of even completely avulsed segments. The classification of dentoalveolar fractures was discussed previously.

Facial Skeletal Fractures

Moving beyond dental and dentoalveolar fractures, the various facial bones of the craniomaxillofacial complex may be considered for their etiology, distribution, and classification of fractures. The craniomaxillofacial region may be defined anatomically as the cranium, which con-

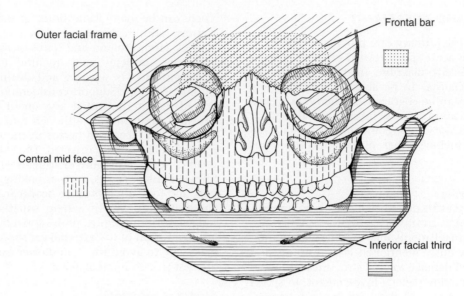

Fig. 13-1. Pancraniomaxillofacial skeletal regional landmarks. From Greenberg AM, ed: *Craniomaxillofacial fractures: Principles of internal fixation using the AO/ASIF technique*, New York, 1993, Springer-Verlag.

sists of the parietal, occipital, temporal, frontal, and sphenoid bones. The frontal, temporal, and sphenoid bones are most commonly associated with facial bone injuries. The facial skeleton is defined by the mandible, maxillae, palatine, zygomatic, nasal, ethmoid, and lacrimal bones.

Mandibular Fractures

The mandible is the most extensively studied facial bone, and there is a well-defined pattern of classically encountered fractures (Table 13-1).[1,2,5,13,21,24,25,28,31,44,53]

The particular fracture patterns seen are related to the particular biomechanics of the mandible and the insertions of the muscles of mastication (Fig. 13-2).[16] The frequency of occurrence at various mandibular fracture sites appears to be predominated by the body, followed by the angle, condyle, symphysis, ramus, and coronoid process (in that order).

Mandibular fractures may be classified as single, multiple, fragmented, or avulsive according to the Spiessl classification as modified by Haug and Greenberg (Fig. 13-3).[21,57] Localization of fractures is defined by the

Table 13-1. Mandible fracture locations

Study	Location (%)							Number of patients in study
	Symphysis	**Body**	**Angle**	**Ramus**	**Coronoid**	**Condyle**	**Alveolus**	
Rix et al. (1991)[53]	24	24	34	3	0	15	NI	80
Haug et al. (1990)[24]	20	30	27	2	0	21	NI	307
Abiose (1986)[1]	20	59	9	0	0	10	2	87
Bochlogyros (1985)[5]	7	42	24	3	0	23	1	853
Ellis et al. (1985)[13]	8	33	23	3	2	29	1	2137
Hill et al. (1984)[25]	4	14	12	0	0	15	25	214
Olson et al. (1982)[44]	22	16	25	2	1	29	3	580
James et al. (1981)[28]	14	27	31	6	3	19	NI	253
Khalil and Shaladi (1981)[31]	10	20	14	2	0	14	7	187
Adekeye (1980)[2]	26	48	15	1	0	11	NI	1106

From Greenberg AM: *Craniomaxillofacial fractures: Principles of internal fixation using the AO/ASIF technique*, Springer-Verlag, 1993.
NI—not investigated.

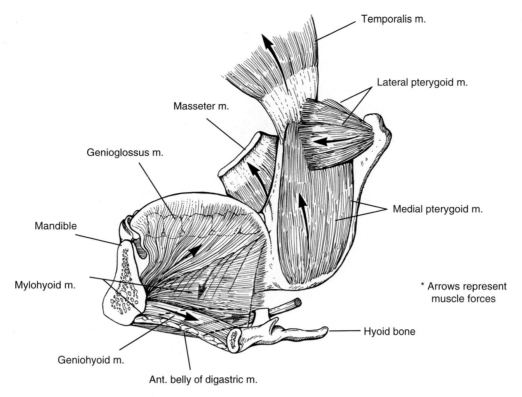

Temporalis m.

Lateral pterygoid m.

Masseter m.

Medial pterygoid m.

Genioglossus m.

Mandible

* Arrows represent
muscle forces

Mylohyoid m.

Hyoid bone

Geniohyoid m.

Ant. belly of digastric m.

Fig. 13-2. Diagram indicating muscles of mastication and their vectors of force during contraction. From Greenberg AM, ed: *Craniomaxillofacial fractures: Principles of internal fixation using the AO/ASIF technique*, New York, 1993, Springer-Verlag.

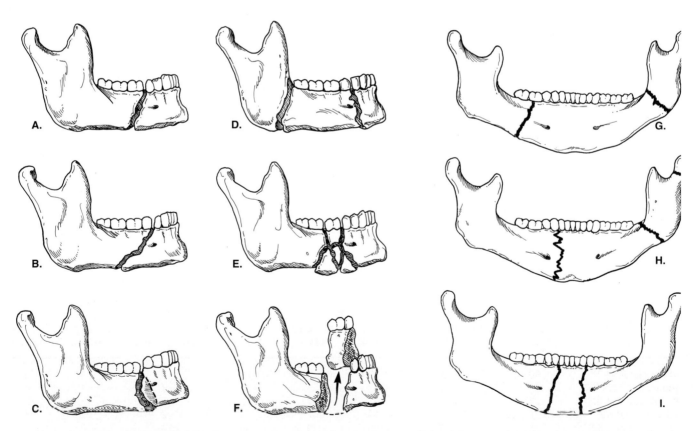

Fig. 13-3. Categories of mandibular fractures. From Greenberg AM, ed: *Craniomaxillofacial fractures: Principles of internal fixation using the AO/ASIF technique*, New York, 1993, Springer-Verlag, and Spiessl B: *Internal fixation of the mandible*, Berlin, 1989, Springer-Verlag; **A.** Single fracture (transverse fracture); **B.** Single fracture (oblique fracture); **C.** Single fracture (oblique-surface fracture); **D.** Unilateral (segmental fracture); **E.** Comminuted (fragmented) fracture; **F.** Fracture with bone defect; **G.** Multiple fracture (segmental fracture); **H.** Unilateral segmental fracture and contralateral single fracture; **I.** Bilateral segmental fracture.

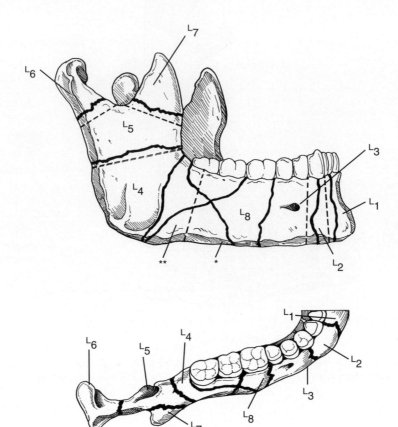

* Postcanine fracture. ** Angular fracture.

Fig. 13-4. Localization of mandibular fractures. L1, Precanine; L2, Canine; L3, Postcanine; L4, Angular; L5, Supraangular; L6, Processus articularis (condyle); L7, Processus muscularis (coronoid); and L8, Alveolar process. From Greenberg AM, ed: *Craniomaxillofacial fractures: Principles of internal fixation using the AO/ASIF technique*, New York, 1993, Springer-Verlag, and Spiessl B: *Internal fixation of the mandible*, Berlin, 1989, Springer-Verlag.

Table 13-2. Mandible fracture epidemiology

| | | | Cause (%) | | | | | |
Study	Male/ female	Most frequent age (yr)	MVA	Bicycle/ MCA	Assault	Occupational	Falls/ home	Sports
Rix et al. (1991)[53]	90	20–30	8	0	73	4	11	6
Haug et al. (1990)[24]	60	16–35	33	4	54	1	4	4
Bochlogyros (1985)[5]	77	20–29	41	17	19	7	13	3
Ellis et al. (1985)[13]	76	20–40	13	2	55	2	21	4
Olson et al. (1982)[44]	78	20–29	48	14	34	1	8	2

From Greenberg AM: Craniomaxillofacial Fractures: Principles of Internal Fixation Using the AO/ASIF Technique, Springer-Verlag, 1993. MVA—motor vehicle accidents; MCA—motorcycle accidents.

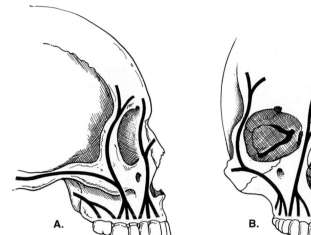
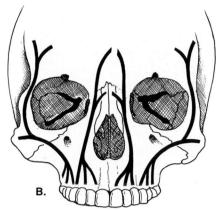
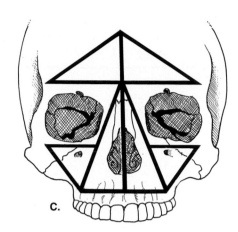

Fig. 13-5. Traditional concept of the distribution of masticatory forces throughout the face delineating the six facial buttresses. **A**, Lateral view. **B**, Anteroposterior view. Adapted from Sicher H, Tandler J: *Anatomie fur Zahnartze*. Wien, 1928, Verlag von Springer. **C**, Contemporary concept of facial trusses under tension during asymmetric mastication and facial muscle pull. From Greenberg AM, ed: *Craniomaxillofacial fractures: Principles of internal fixation using the AO/ASIF technique*, New York, 1993, Springer-Verlag.

anatomic site (Fig. 13-4).[57] There are a variety of causes for mandibular fractures (Table 13-2)[5,13,21,24,44,53] predominated by assaults and motor vehicle collisions, with sports as a smaller etiology (2% to 6%).[5,13,21,24,44,53]

Maxillary Fractures

Maxillary fractures were typically referred to in the context of LeFort's early anatomic studies.[35-37] This particular classification was useful in the era when management was done by closed reduction (jaw wiring). Current therapy is oriented toward aggressive anatomic open reduction with rigid internal fixation via miniplates and microplates.[20,51,60] Such surgical approaches have revealed to clinicians fracture patterns that differ from the classical LeFort classification system. The forces of function or impact are transmitted through the midfacial skeleton across the facial buttress system, which recently was well described by Manson and Gruss (Fig. 13-5).[17,18,40] The orientation and level of energy of impact will influence the type of fracture pattern that will develop. The LeFort system classifies Lefort I fractures at the level of the zygomaticomaxillary buttresses and inferior piriform rim with separation at the pterygoid plates.[35-37]

A LeFort II fracture is defined as fracture lines crossing through the zygomaticomaxillary buttress superiorly through the infraorbital rim and medially to the nasal bridge (naso-orbital-ethmoid complex).[35-37,55] A LeFort III fracture no longer simply involves the maxillary bones, but also the naso-orbital-ethmoid complex and zygomatic bones.[35-37,55] Such a fracture will in-

volve the bilateral frontozygomatic processes, nasofrontal suture, naso-orbital-ethmoid, sphenozygomatic, and zygomaticotemporal processes. LeFort I, II, and III fracture patterns are considered to be general terms to describe collections of bone fractures in close proximity, which at higher levels and as the result of higher energy have greater degrees of complexity and a higher predilection for complications from the injury and management methodologies. Previous studies have noted the distribution and frequency of such injuries (Table 13-3).[1,2,8,21,24,25,30,56,59]

There are four varieties of localized maxillary fractures, which range from high alveolar to the classical LeFort I and II types (Fig. 13-6).[21] We have separated our classification from the typical LeFort to an individual bone-based system because it facilitates diagnosis and subsequent management-oriented therapies and research methods.[21] Midfacial fractures are rarely equal bilaterally, with variations from one side to the other; for example, a higher level nasomaxillary fracture occurs on the side of impact *versus* a lower level piriform rim fracture on the opposite side, which results from the diminished transmission of forces. The greatest frequency of maxillary fractures results from assaults and motor vehicle collisions, with sports accounting for 5% to 8% of such fractures (Table 13-4).[21,24,30,59]

Zygoma Fractures

The zygoma is a separate bone of the facial region that becomes one of the interfaces between the skull base and the facial skeleton. Studies evaluating the inci-

Table 13-3. Maxillary fracture locations (LeFort classification)

Study	LeFort level (%)							Number of patients in study
	I	II	III	0/I	I/II	II/III	0/II	
Haug et al. (1990)[24]	38	28	17	9	2	6	0	53
Cook and Rowe (1990)[8]	32	47	21	NI	NI	NI	NI	95
Kahnberg and Göthberg (1987)[30]	29	35	13	23	—	—	—	266
Abiose (1986)[1]	47	24	24	NI	NI	NI	NI	17
Hill et al. (1984)[25]	35	61	3	NI	NI	NI	NI	31
Sofferman et al. (1983)[56]	14	33	10	0	0	43	0	21
Steidler et al. (1980)[59]	22	53	18	2	4	1	0	240
Adekeye (1980)[2]	6	34	6	20	4	0	21	212

From Greenberg AM: *Craniomaxillofacial fractures: Principles of internal fixation using the AO/ASIF technique,* Springer-Verlag, 1993.
NI—not investigated.

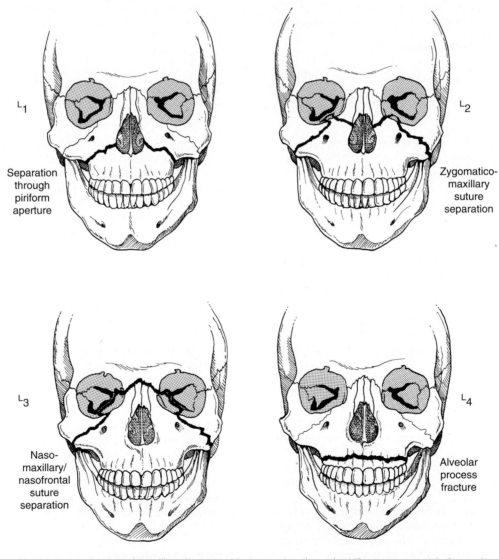

Fig. 13-6. Localization of maxillary fractures. L1, Separation through piriform aperture; L2, Separation through zygomaticomaxillary suture; L3, Separation through nasomaxillary and nasofrontal suture; and L4, Alveolar process. From Greenberg AM, ed: *Craniomaxillofacial fractures: Principles of internal fixation using the AO/ASIF technique,* New York, 1993, Springer-Verlag.

Table 13-4. Mandible fracture epidemiology

| Study | Male/female | Most frequent age (yr) | Cause (%) | | | | | |
			MVA	Bicycle/MCA	Assault	Occupational	Falls/home	Sports
Haug et al. (1990)[24]	83	26–30	66	8	13	4	2	8
Kahnberg and Göthberg (1987)[30]	NI	NI	35	11	27	27	—	—
Sofferman et al. (1983)[56]	71	25	76	NI	NI	NI	NI	NI
Steidler et al. (1980)[59]	83	20–29	69	8	9	4	1	5

From Greenberg AM (ed): Craniomaxillofacial Fractures: Principles of Internal Fixation Using the AO/ASIF Technique, Springer-Verlag, 1993.
MVA—motor vehicle accidents; MCA—motorcycle accidents; NI—not investigated.

dence of isolated zygomatic fractures are infrequently reported in the literature, which is a reflection of the lack (until more recently) of an appropriate classification system. The Knight and North classification was a management-oriented classification system based on the stability of fractures managed without fixation and the unstable fractures that would require fixation.[32] Haug and Greenberg have devised a system that is oriented toward the anatomic involvement of the bone and its suture articulations, which may be involved in fractures and become sites for internal fixation.[21] Zygomatic fractures are distributed based on the particular anatomic sites of involvement (Table 13-5),[12,14,24] whether they involve the arch, supra-arch, frontozygomatic, zygomaticomaxillary, zygomaticotemporal, or orbital floor regions (Fig. 13-7). Zygomatic fractures can be complicated by the involvement of the vital structures of the eye, and a thorough ophthalmologic examination is essential in their management, which requires consultation with an ophthalmologist (see box in second column). Visual acuity testing, extraocular muscle evaluation, pupillary reflexes, and globe position are the most important general ophthalmologic considerations after occurrence of these injuries. Zygomatic fractures most commonly result from assault, falls, and motor vehicle collisions, whereas 4% to 11% result from a sports injury (Table 13-6).[12,14,24]

OPHTHALMOLOGIC SEQUELAE OF COMPLEX INJURIES

Hyphema

Lens dislocation

Retinal detachment

Optic nerve compression

Vitreous hemorrhages

Superior orbital fissure syndrome

Orbital apex syndrome

Ophthalmoplegia

Carotid-cavernous fistula

Globe avulsion

Chemosis

Epiphora

Enophthalmus

Exophthalmus

Telecanthus

From Greenberg AM (ed): *Craniomaxillofacial fractures: Principles of internal fixation using the AO/ASIF technique*, Springer-Verlag, 1993.

Table 13-5. Zygoma fracture location

| Study | Location (%) | | | | | Number of patients in study |
	Nondisplaced	Arch	Body	Fragmented	Blow-out	
Haug et al. (1990)[24]	11	27	53	9	NI	98
Ellis et al. (1985)[12]	15	8	62	8	3	2067
Fisher-Brandies and Dielert (1984)[14]	8	9	80	2	NI	97

From Greenberg AM (ed): *Craniomaxillofacial fractures: Principles of internal fixation using the AO/ASIF technique*, Springer-Verlag, 1993.
NI—not investigated.

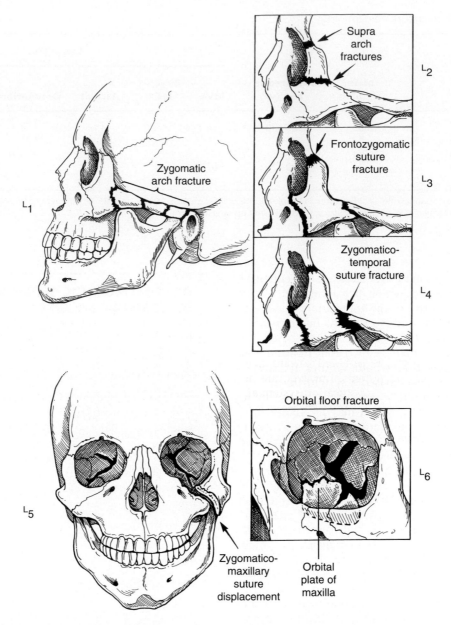

Fig. 13-7. Localization of zygoma fractures. L1, Arch; L2, Supra-arch; L3, Displacement at fronto-zygomatic suture; L4, Displacement at zygomaticomaxillary suture; L5, Displacement at zygomatico-temporal suture; and L6, Orbital floor. From Greenberg AM, ed: *Craniomaxillofacial fractures: Principles of internal fixation using the AO/ASIF technique*, New York, 1993, Springer-Verlag.

Table 13-6. Zygoma fracture epidemiology

| Study | Male/female | Most frequent age (yr) | Cause (%) | | | | | |
			MVA	MCA	Assault	Home/occupational	Falls	Sports
Haug et al. (1990)[24]	60	21–35	38	5	45	1	7	4
Ellis et al. (1985)[12]	80	20–40	11	1	45	3	22	11
Fisher-Brandies and Dielert (1984)[14]	86	16–20	NI	NI	NI	NI	NI	NI

From Greenberg AM (ed): *Craniomaxillofacial fractures: Principles of internal fixation using the AO/ASIF technique*, Springer-Verlag, 1993.
MVA—motor vehicle accidents; MCA—motorcycle accidents; NI—not investigated.

Table 13-7. Nasal fracture location

Study	Location (%)				Number of patients in study
	Entire nasal tip	**Nasal bone**	**Naso-orbital**	**Naso-orbital-ethmoid**	
Haug and Prather (1991)[23]	15	40	35	10	20
Williamson et al. (1981)[66]	NI	NI	54	46	13

From Greenberg AM (ed): *Craniomaxillofacial fractures: Principles of internal fixation using the AO/ASIF technique,* Springer-Verlag, 1993.
NI—not investigated.

Nasal and Nasoethmoid Fractures

Nasal and naso-orbital-ethmoid fractures are among the most frequently reported skeletal fractures because of their delicate bony structures and relative prominence in the face.[26,39] There are numerous classification systems for the nasal region that range from simple to complex,[15,19,43,61] with some systems oriented toward management approaches.[41] These systems, however, are not part of a uniform facial fracture classification system and are difficult to organize (Table 13-7).[23,66] Haug and Prather in a survey given in 1991 to 20 patients noted that the entire nasal bone had a higher frequency of fracture than the naso-orbital-ethmoid complex.[23] These fractures may be localized to the nasal tip; entire nasal bones; nasal bone and frontal process of the maxilla; nasal, ethmoid, frontal process of the maxilla; and nasal spine of the frontal bone (Fig. 13-8). The majority of these fractures result from assaults and motor vehicle collisions, whereas 0 to 27% result from sports injuries (Table 13-8).[7,23,66]

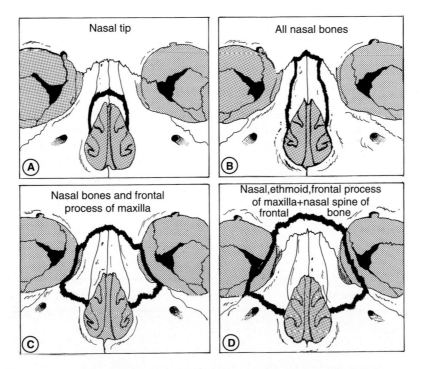

Fig. 13-8. Localization of nasal and naso-orbital-ethmoid fractures. **A,** Nasal tip; **B,** Entire nasal bones; **C,** Nasal bone and frontal process of maxilla; and **D,** Nasal, ethmoid, frontal process of maxilla, nasal spine of frontal bone. From Greenberg AM, ed: *Craniomaxillofacial fractures: Principles of internal fixation using the AO/ASIF technique,* New York, 1993, Springer-Verlag.

Table 13-8. Nasal fracture epidemiology

Study	Male/female	Most common age (yr)	Cause (%)				
			MVA/MCA	**Assault**	**Occupational**	**Falls/home**	**Sports**
Haug and Prather (1991)[23]	80	20–30	50	45	0	5	0
Clayton and Lesser (1986)[7]	73	23	27	46	0	0	27
Williamson et al. (1981)[66]	100	27	54	46	0	0	0

From Greenberg AM (ed): *Craniomaxillofacial fractures: Principles of internal fixation using the AO/ASIF technique,* Springer-Verlag, 1993.
MVA/MCA—motor vehicle accident/motorcycle accident.

Frontal Bone Fractures

Frontal bone fractures are less common compared with other fractures of the craniomaxillofacial skeleton because of their greater thickness and biomechanical advantages. Local anatomic considerations, such as the degree of pneumatization and nasofrontal duct configuration, may influence the tendency of certain individuals to be predisposed to fractures. Few studies have been reported, and all have evaluated small patient groups (Table 13-9).[11,27,45,58,64] Frontal bone fractures are classified according to the involvement of the supraorbital rim, anterior table, posterior table, or sinus floor (Fig. 13-9). Motor vehicle collisions, assault, and occupational causes are the most frequent reasons for frontal fractures, whereas 3% to 5% result from sports injuries (Table 13-10).[10,27,34,45,48,64]

Other cranial fractures and their incidence will be discussed elsewhere in this text. Various diagnostic algorithms can be developed to approach the treatment of patients who have craniomaxillofacial injuries. As with all trauma patients, the ATLS guidelines are an excellent resource that include primary and secondary assessments to determine patient stability and basic life support (see ATLS guidelines).[3] All patients must undergo a complete history and physical examination, with particular signs guiding the clinician to order more extensive tests and laboratory or radiologic investigational studies.

PHYSICAL EVALUATION

Primary providers who care for individuals who engage in sports and athletic competition must be well versed in disorders and injuries of the craniomaxillofacial region. Having reviewed the types of traumatically induced soft- and hard-tissue injuries common to the head and neck region, the practitioner must apply this knowledge in a systematic manner when caring for patients suspected of having sustained such injuries. As with all acute care, the ABCs of life support are always a place to start. The ATLS protocols for treatment of the trauma patient are also an excellent methodology, and the craniomaxillofacial aspects of the primary survey and the more detail-oriented examination of the secondary survey (American College of Surgeons) will be reviewed.[3] Given the wide range of sports played today, accidents may occur in a variety of unfavorable locations, such as swimming pools, fresh and salt water, and at high altitudes (alpine skiing, mountaineering, rock climbing, etc.). Ensuring that the patient's airway is intact is the examiner's first responsibility, and because the oral cavity and the dentition are often primary trauma sites, care must be taken to remove nonpermanent dentures, mouthguards, loosened bridges, avulsed teeth and to establish hemostasis if the tongue or oral mucosa is lacerated and profuse hemorrhage is present. If a cervical in-

Table 13-9. Frontal bone fracture locations

Study	Location (%)				Number of patients in study
	Supraorbital rim	**Anterior table**	**Anterior/posterior table**	**Floor**	
Onishi et al. (1989)[45]	77	61	19	12	42
Wallis and Donald (1988)[64]	NI	54	39	3	72
Stanley and Becker (1987)[58]	NI	44	56	64	50
Duval et al. (1987)[11]	NI	65	35	NI	112
Ioannides et al. (1984)[24]	48	43	13	NI	23

From Greenberg AM (ed): *Craniomaxillofacial fractures: Principles of internal fixation using the AO/ASIF technique,* Springer-Verlag, 1993.
NI—not investigated.

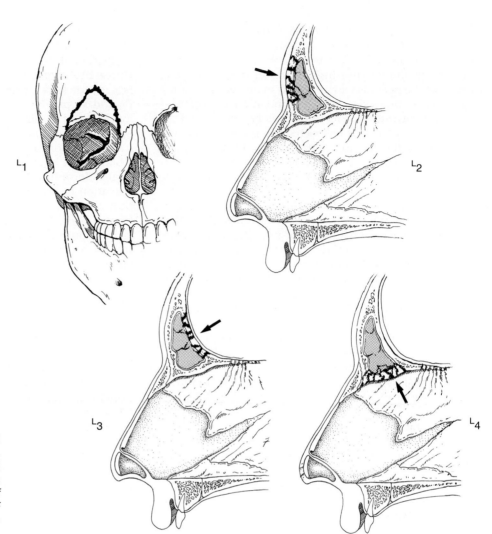

Fig. **13-9.** Localization of frontal fractures. L1, Supraorbital rim; L2, Anterior table; L3, Posterior table; and L4, Sinus floor. From Greenberg AM, ed: *Craniomaxillofacial fractures: Principles of internal fixation using the AO/ASIF technique*, New York, 1993, Springer-Verlag.

Table 13-10. Frontal bone fracture epidemiology

				Cause (%)			
Study	Male/ female (%)	Most frequent age (yr)	MVA/MCA	Suicide and Assault	Occupational	Falls/ home	Sports
Onishi et al. (1989)[45]	84	NI	84	0	5	5	5
Wallis and Donald (1988)[64]	85	32	71	17	7	0	6
Ioannides et al. (1984)[27]	83	33.5	70	4	17	9	0
Donald (1982)[10]	66	34.3	71	24	0	5	0
Peri et al. (1981)[48]	80	20–30	85	0	12	—	3
Larrabee et al. (1980)[34]	91	24	44	28	28	—	—

From Greenberg AM (ed): *Craniomaxillofacial fractures: Principles of internal fixation using the AO/ASIF technique,* Springer-Verlag, 1993.
MVA/MCA—motor vehicle accidents/motorcycle accidents; NI—not investigated.

jury is suspected, a cervical collar should be placed on patient until radiographs can establish the integrity of the spinal column. This limits the ability to position the head for opening or ensuring patency of the airway. Jaw thrust may be necessary as an initial maneuver until further measures are taken, such as intubation, cricothyrotomy, or tracheostomy. Breathing may be maintained or reestablished by manual or mechanical types of support, depending on the location of the patient (in the hospital or otherwise). A cursory neurologic examination should be performed, and control of any excessive hemorrhage should be obtained.

Clinical examination should begin with a thorough history of the trauma because details regarding the mechanism, magnitude and site of impact, and symptomatology will be important. If the patient is unconscious, it is important to ascertain the events from a witness. Past medical and surgical history, including pertinent medications and allergies, are required.

When cervical injuries are suspected, the head and neck examination should begin with the cervical collar in place on the patient. Radiographs may be taken first if a cervical injury is strongly suspected and should consist of a minimum of a lateral, posteroanterior (with all seven cervical vertebrae observed), and an open-mouth Water's view of the dens. If these initial radiographs are insufficient, a swimmer's view, CT, or MRI may be necessary to complete the radiologic examination. Once radiography has established skeletal integrity of the spinal column, the cervical collar may be removed to permit physical examination of the neck. The soft tissues of the neck should be observed for the presence of ecchymosis, edema, and lacerations, and manual palpation should proceed along the lateral vertebral processes first, followed by the posterior processes from caudad to cephalad to assess pain or tenderness and irregularities such as step defects or abnormal contours. Examination of the head should begin with the scalp, which should be inspected for lacerations, ecchymosis, edema, and Battle's signs around the ears, which may indicate a skull base fracture. Palpation of the cranium is performed, and care should be taken to elicit complaints of pain or tenderness, crepitus, or contour irregularities of bone, with special attention directed toward the presence of depressed skull fractures.

Neurologic Injuries

The neurologic examination should establish the patient's level of consciousness, orientation toward intellectual function, emotional stability, and cognition. Given the high incidence of brain injury in contact sports, this aspect of the examination should be thorough because initial signs of severe head trauma can be subtle. If the patient demonstrates progressive cerebral dysfunction, the possibility of evolving intracranial injury, hypoxia, or hypotension is indicated. Drug abuse must also be considered as an etiology of these symptoms. Cranial nerves need to be examined in a systematic manner because they may indicate the presence of injuries to the brain, cranium, eyes, ears, or facial skeleton. Cranial nerve I (olfaction) is not easily tested. Cranial nerve II should be evaluated for visual acuity, and

penlight testing for the light reflex, which when combined in an alternating manner between eyes, permits evaluation of the cranial nerve III consensual light reflex. Unreactive dilated pupils or a lack of the consensual reflex is indicative of severe CNS injury. Cranial nerve III, IV, and VI provide extraocular movement, which is easily evaluated by directional testing. Inability to move the eye in all directions may indicate extraocular muscle entrapment secondary to orbital fractures, severe edema, or a brain stem injury in the absence of gross structural orbital deformities. Cranial nerve V provides sensory innervation to the face, and the presence of altered sensation may indicate underlying facial bone fractures. Cranial nerve VII provides innervation to the muscles of facial expression, which when partially injured is reflective of a severed nerve trunk or its more peripheral branches, whereas complete loss of function indicates a skull base fracture or temporal bone involvement. Cranial nerve VIII is easily examined by hearing tests. Cranial nerve IX, X, and XII provide mobility and sensation to the soft palate, uvula, tongue, and pharynx. Altered taste sensation may indicate injury to the chorda tympani, which travels from the lingual branch of cranial nerve V to cranial nerve IX, and can indicate trauma to the glenoid fossa or temporomandibular joint (an occasional complaint of boxers). Cranial nerve XI will be intact if shoulder lifting is possible. Cerebellar function is established by testing for the ability to touch the nose with a forefinger with the eyes opened or closed, walking heel to toe in a straight line with eyes opened or closed. Additional general motor examination can include testing for reflexes and observing muscle tone and overall posture. Decerebrate or decorticate postures indicate serious brain injuries. The sensory system can be readily evaluated by pin testing, directional testing, and temperature sensitivity. Altered sensation posterior to the ears in the coronal plane is suggestive of cervical spine or skull base injuries. The presence of significant brain, spinal cord, cervical spine, or cranial injuries requires consultation with a neurosurgeon.

Soft Tissue Injuries (Integument and Oral Mucosa)

The skin of the scalp, neck, and face and oral and oropharyngeal mucosa should be examined thoroughly for the presence of lacerations, abrasions, contusions, edema, ecchymosis, emphysema, burns, or avulsive defects. Skin injuries may reflect more severe underlying skeletal or other vital structure problems. Deep lacerations need to be explored for the presence of debris, especially in the case of lip lacerations in which dental fragments may be embedded. Periapical dental radiographs are often helpful. Other deep vital soft-tissue structures must be considered, such as the major salivary gland ducts (submandibular duct under the tongue, parotid duct across the midface), which can be confirmed by dye studies (sialography). Hemorrhage from arterial sources often need to be ligated to achieve hemostasis and can often be significant, such as in scalp injuries and in deep neck and facial vessels. Underlying fractures of the cranium and facial bones can be a source of severe hemorrhage and often require reduction to achieve control of hemorrhage. Nerve injuries associated with lacerations often require repair, although because of their presence anterior to a line perpendicular to the Frankfort horizontal plane through the lateral canthus of the eye, they are often untreated because the nerve diameter is too small.

Ophthalmologic Injuries

Ophthalmologic injuries frequently result from sports trauma,[47,63] and they can consist of the full range of extraocular, intraocular, orbital bone, and neurologic problems—individually and in combination. These injuries may be as acute as penetrating globe injuries, globe avulsion, optic nerve compression or severence (with total blindness), retinal detachment, or orbital roof and floor blowout. Ocular injuries require immediate diagnosis and management in consultation with an ophthalmologist. Examination of the eye should begin with visual acuity because this is potentially the most important problem, followed by the neurologic examination of light and consensual reflexes. These signs will determine the extent of injuries to the optic nerve, orbital apex contents, and the superior orbital fissure contents. Fundoscopic examination will detect the presence of hemorrhages, lens dislocation, and retinal disorders. The external eye and the sclera, subconjunctiva, cornea, eyelids, and lacrimal apparatus need to be examined for lacerations, abrasions, penetration, ecchymosis, and emphysema. Certain sports have greater rates of eye injuries because of the high degree of contact, explosive nature, and use of accessory equipment, such as hockey pucks and sticks, and baseball bats and balls.

Mandible Fractures

Mandibular fractures need to be suspected in individuals with intraoral or extraoral ecchymosis, lacerations, edema, inferior facial asymmetry, lip and chin altered sensation, jaw hypomobility, altered dental occlusion, and other signs and symptoms (see box in second column). Patients may complain of the teeth not meeting correctly and the inability to bite appropriately. Clinical evaluation should begin with inspection of the skin, oral mucosa, dentition, alveolar bone, and dental prostheses, followed by bimanual palpation. It is necessary to first establish the status of the dentoalveolar region and the presence of fractured, luxated, avulsed, or displaced teeth and prostheses. The mandible should then be grasped with the thumbs along the incisal edges (cusps) of the teeth and the forefingers along the inferior border, moving around the dental arch to determine the presence of pain, tenderness (Fig. 13-10), or mobile segments. The finger positions are changed for the posterior mandibular body and ramus so that the forefingers grasp the mandibular body and ramus with the thumbs along the inferior border, looking for similar signs of pain, tenderness, or segment mobility. Palpate the preauricular region while asking the patient to open and close the jaw to search for the presence of pain, tenderness, or unusual protruding masses (indicative of condylar segment displacement). Otoscopic examination of the tympanic membrane is important to detect the presence of external auditory canal lacerations or hemotympanum,

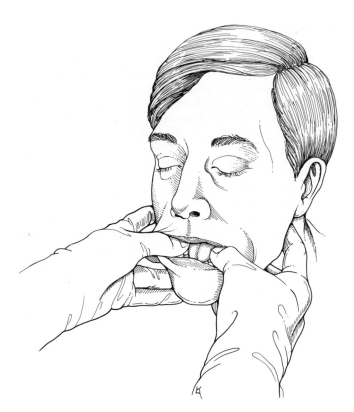

Fig. 13-10. Examination of a suspected mandibular fracture. Thumbs on occlusal surface edges and forefingers on inferior border of mandible. From Greenberg AM, ed: *Craniomaxillofacial fractures: Principles of internal fixation using the AO/ASIF technique*, New York, 1993, Springer-Verlag.

which are indicative of condylar fractures. When mandibular fractures are suspected, evaluation by radiographic examination should follow. The single-most important radiograph for mandibular evaluation is the panoramic radiograph.

SIGNS AND SYMPTOMS OF MANDIBULAR FRACTURES

Trismus

Edema

Laceration or abrasion

Ecchymosis

Malocclusion

Mental nerve paresthesia

Crepitus

Deviation upon opening

Asymmetry

Step defect along inferior border

From Greenberg AM (ed): *Craniomaxillofacial fractures: Principles of internal fixation using the AO/ASIF technique,* Springer-Verlag, 1993.

Maxillary Fractures

Similar to mandibular fractures, suspected maxillary fractures may be present in patients with intraoral or extraoral ecchymosis, lacerations, edema, midfacial retrusion, upper lip altered sensation, jaw hypomobility, altered dental occlusion, and other signs and symptoms (see box in second column). Patients may complain of the teeth not meeting correctly and the inability to bite appropriately. These patients often present with an "open bite" deformity and flattened midface. Clinical evaluation should begin with inspection of the skin, oral mucosa, dentition, and alveolar bone, dental prostheses, followed by bimanual palpation. It is necessary to establish the status of the dentoalveolar region and the presence of fractured, luxated, avulsed, or displaced teeth and prostheses. Because maxillary fractures occur at various levels of the midface, they may involve only the dental portion or more superiorly include the orbital, zygomatic, and nasal regions. Periorbital symptomatology includes ecchymosis, subconjunctival hemorrhage, and nasal hemorrhage, and if there is associated anterior cranial fossa involvement, there may be a dural tear with cerebrospinal rhinorrhea with its classical tramline appearance. Nasal involvement may be noted as a widened intercanthal distance or "traumatic telecanthus." Standard measurements are available for the

SIGNS AND SYMPTOMS OF MAXILLARY FRACTURES

Tenderness

Flattened face

Lengthened face

Periorbital ecchymosis

Air emphysema

Paresthesia of cheek or nose

Malocclusion

Crepitus

Edema

Ecchymosis of vestibule

Subconjunctival hemorrhage

Cerebrospinal fluid leak

Step defect at zygomatic or nasomaxillary buttress

From Greenberg AM (ed): *Craniomaxillofacial fractures: Principles of internal fixation using the AO/ASIF technique,* Springer-Verlag, 1993.

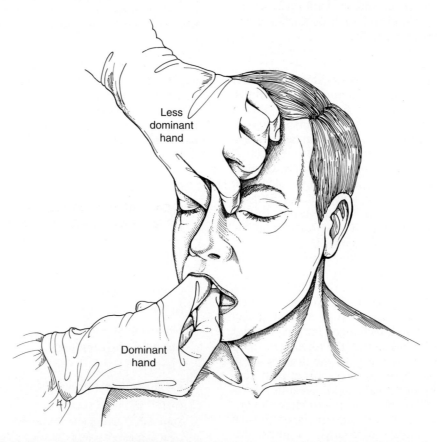

Fig. 13-11. Examination of a level II (LeFort II level) maxillary fracture. Thumb and forefinger of the dominant hand grasp the incisors and dentoalveolus, while the less dominant hand palpates the nasofrontal suture for movement. From Greenberg AM, ed: *Craniomaxillofacial fractures: Principles of internal fixation using the AO/ASIF technique,* New York, 1993, Springer-Verlag.

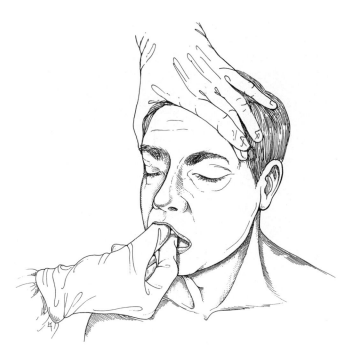

Fig. 13-12. Examination of a level III (LeFort III level) maxillary fracture. Thumb and forefinger of the dominant hand grasps the incisors and dentoalveolus, while the less dominant hand palpates the frontozygomatic suture for movement. From Greenberg AM, ed: *Craniomaxillofacial fractures: Principles of internal fixation using the AO/ASIF technique*, New York, 1993, Springer-Verlag.

intercanthal distance and may be useful for the diagnosis of nasoethmoid involvement (28.6—33.0 mm in women and 28.9–34.5 in men).[22] Commonly, the skin overlying the midface may have a crackling sensation on palpation, which is subcutaneous emphysema associated with the disrupted maxillary and paranasal sinuses. LeFort II (level

II) maxillary fractures will be clinically evident by grasping the maxillary incisors with the dominant hand and palapating the nasal bridge with the less dominant hand, and upon manipulation attempt to detect the presence of movement at the nasal bridge (Fig. 13-11). LeFort III (level III) maxillary fractures are detected by a similar maneuver: the less dominant hand will grasp the bilateral frontozygomatic sites to detect mobility upon manipulation (Fig. 13-12). If fractures are suspected, radiographic imaging of this region should be obtained and may range from plain radiographs to CT. In children, these fractures are less common, but because of the presence of tooth buds in the pediatric facial skeleton, CT scanning should be performed.[29,50]

Zygoma Fractures

Patients with zygomatic fractures will typically present with periorbital edema, ecchymosis, subconjunctival hemorrhage, malar flattening, difficulty with mandibular movement, and altered sensation of the posterior dental quadrant or overlying cutaneous region. Globe position may be altered with the presence of exophthalmus or enophthalmus, based on the degree of orbital floor or wall involvement and the disruption of the suspensory ligament. Other signs and symptoms (see the box in the left column on p. 146) must be fully determined, and radiography is especially helpful because of the extensive edema that may be present. Examination for zygomatic fractures should begin with palpation of the supraorbital region, moving from a lateral to medial direction and with care to observe for tenderness over the frontozygomatic region. The infraorbital rim should then be palpated, with simultaneous palpation of the contralateral side as a reference. Stepping may be noted over the infraorbital region because the zygomatic body is often medially and inferiorly displaced (Fig. 13-13). The zygomatic arch should be palpated to determine the presence of

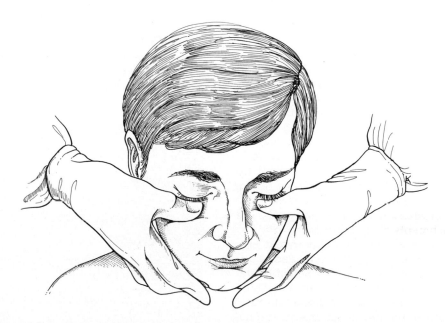

Fig. 13-13. Clinical examination of the infraorbital rims in a patient with a suspected zygoma fracture. From Greenberg AM, ed: *Craniomaxillofacial fractures: Principles of internal fixation using the AO/ASIF technique*, New York, 1993, Springer-Verlag.

SIGNS AND SYMPTOMS OF ZYGOMA FRACTURES

Periorbital ecchymosis

Lateral subconjunctival hemorrhage

Paresthesia of nose and cheek

Unequal pupil height

Downward slope of lateral canthus

Flattening of cheek contours

Trismus

Edema

Air emphysema

Diplopia

Exophthalmus/enophthalmus

Ecchymosis of buccal vestibule

Crepitus

Limited extraocular movements

Step defects at zygomaticomaxillary, frontozygomatic, or zygomaticotemporal sutures

From Greenberg AM (ed): *Craniomaxillofacial fractures: Principles of internal fixation using the AO/ASIF technique,* Springer-Verlag, 1993.

SIGNS AND SYMPTOMS OF NASOETHMOID FRACTURES

Periorbital ecchymosis

Medial subconjunctival hemorrhage

Bilateral epistaxis

Traumatic telecanthus

Nasal contour deformity

Cerebrospinal fluid leak

Crepitus

Diplopia

Tenderness

Edema

Laceration

From Greenberg AM (ed): *Craniomaxillofacial fractures: Principles of internal fixation using the AO/ASIF technique,* Springer-Verlag, 1993.

hematoma, or mucosal lacerations. If nasal fractures are suspected, imaging should be obtained, which may include plain radiographs (simple fractures) or CT scanning (complex fractures).

Supraorbital Rim and Frontal Sinus Fractures

Periorbital ecchymosis is the most frequently noted sign in supraorbital rim and frontal sinus fractures, followed by soft-tissue lacerations, and many other signs and symptoms (see box below). Soft-tissue edema may obscure the underlying frontal bone fracture. These injuries

of stepping or tenderness. Finally, intraoral examination is performed, which should include palpation of the zygomaticomaxillary buttress. Ophthalmologic examination should be thorough because there may be extraocular muscle entrapment with limitation of gaze, diplopia, enophthalmus, exophthalmus, and globe injury (see box on p. 137). Radiographic examination should consist of a minimum of a Waters' view and submentovertex with panoramic radiography, and CT axial and coronal examination are useful.

Nasoethmoid Fractures

Nasoethmoid fractures vary from simple nasal tip fractures to fracture dislocation of the nasoethmoid complex into the base of the skull. Simple nasal fractures may be limited to the nasal bridge and displacement of the nasal septum. There are many symptoms of nasoethmoid fractures that are seen in fractures of the maxilla and zygoma (see the box at the top of the second column). When nasal fractures involve more than the nasal tip and are complex naso-orbital-ethmoid fractures, severe problems, such as traumatic telecanthus, loss of nasal projection, and cerebrospinal rhinorrhea may result. The medial canthal attachments may be disrupted with loss of the medial canthal angle. Examination should proceed with inspection for edema, ecchymosis, and lacerations of the overlying skin and associated periorbital region. Palpation of the nasal bridge can determine whether the nasal bones are intact or displaced. Nasal speculum examination of the intranasal mucosa can determine the presence of septal displacement, septal

SIGNS AND SYMPTOMS OF SUPRAORBITAL RIM AND FRONTAL SINUS FRACTURES

Periorbital ecchymosis

Subconjunctival hemorrhage

Laceration

Flatness of forehead

Edema

Tenderness

Crepitus

Exposed bony fragments

Cerebrospinal fluid leak

Exophthalmus

Paresthesia of forehead

Step defect of supraorbital rim

From Greenberg AM (ed): *Craniomaxillofacial fractures: Principles of internal fixation using the AO/ASIF technique,* Springer-Verlag, 1993.

range from simple to severe, from minor nondisplaced supraorbital rim or outer table fractures to displaced inner table fractures with dural tears, brain injury, and cerebrospinal rhinorrhea. Other clinical complaints may include altered sensation of the brow and forehead, visual complaints, and headache. Examination of the patient should proceed from inspection to palpation, with the detection of crepitus suggestive of soft-tissue emphysema. If a deep laceration is present, bone fragments and foreign bodies may be palpable or directly visualized by exploration. If a frontal fracture is suspected, imaging is necessary and should include plain radiographs at a minimum, with CT scanning obtained if a penetrating injury or neurologic damage is suspected. Surgical exploration is often necessary to determine whether the posterior table is involved and the nasofrontal ducts are patent.

REFERENCES

1. Abiose PO: Maxillofacial skeleton injuries in the western states of Nigeria, *Br J Oral Maxillofac Surg* 24:31–39, 1986.
2. Adekeye EO: The pattern of fractures of the facial skeleton in Kaduna, Nigeria, *Oral Surg Oral Med Oral Pathol* 49:491–495, 1980.
3. American College of Surgeons: Initial assessment and management. In: *Advanced trauma life support course for physicians*, Chicago, 1989, American College of Surgeons.
4. Andreaseon JO: *Traumatic injuries of the teeth*, Philadelphia, 1981, WB Saunders.
5. Bochlogyros PN: A retrospective study of 1,521 mandibular fractures, *J Oral Maxillofac Surg* 43:597–599, 1985.
6. Castaldi CR: Prevention of craniofacial injuries in ice hockey, *Dent Clin North Am* 35:647–656, 1991.
7. Clayton MI, Lesser THS: The role of radiography in the management of nasal fractures, *J Laryngol Otol* 100:797–801, 1986.
8. Cook HE, Rowe M: A retrospective study of 356 midfacial fractures occurring in 225 patients, *J Oral Maxillofac Surg* 48:574–578, 1990.
9. Crow RW: Diagnosis and management of sports-related injuries to the face, in sports dentistry, *Dental Clin North Am* 35:719–732, 1991.
10. Donald PJ: Frontal sinus ablation by cranialization, *Arch Otolaryngol* 108:142–146, 1982.
11. Duval AJ, Porto DP, Lyons D, et al: Frontal sinus fractures, *Arch Otolaryngol Head Neck Surg* 113:933–935, 1987.
12. Ellis E, El Attar, Moos KF: An analysis of 2067 cases of zygomatico-orbital fracture, *J Oral Maxillofac Surg* 43:417–428, 1985.
13. Ellis E, Moos KF, El-Attar A: Ten years of mandibular fractures: an analysis of 2,137 cases, *Oral Surg Oral Med Oral Pathol* 59:120–129, 1985.
14. Fisher-Brandies E, Dielert E: Treatment of isolated lateral midface fractures. *J Maxillofac Surg* 12:103–106, 1984.
15. Giles HD, Kilner TP: The treatment of the broken nose, *Lancet* i:147–149, 1929.
16. Greenberg AM: Basics of AO/ASIF principles and stable internal fixation of mandibular fractures. In Greenberg AM, ed: *Craniomaxillofacial fractures: principles of internal fixation using the AO/ASIF technique*, New York, 1993, Springer Verlag.
17. Gruss JS, Babak PJ, Egbert MA: Craniofacial fractures, an algorithim to optimize results, *Clin Plast Surg* 19:195–206, 1992.
18. Gruss JS, Mackinnon SE: Complex maxillary fractures: role of buttress reconstruction and immediate bone grafts, *Plast Reconstr Surg* 85:9–22, 1986.
19. Harrison DH: Nasal injuries: their pathogenesis and treatment, *Br J Plast Surg* 32:57–64, 1979.
20. Haug RH: Basics of stable internal fixation of maxillary fractures. In Greenberg AM, ed: *Craniomaxillofacial fractures: principles of internal fixation using the AO/ASIF technique*, New York, 1993, Springer Verlag.
21. Haug RH, Greenberg AM: Etiology, distribution, and classification of fractures. In Greenberg AM, ed: *Craniomaxillofacial fractures: principles of internal fixation using the AO/ASIF technique*, New York, 1993, Springer-Verlag.
22. Haug RH, Likavec MJ: Evaluation of the craniomaxillofacial trauma patient. In Greenberg AM, ed: *Craniomaxillofacial fractures: principles of internal fixation using the AO/ASIF technique*, New York, 1993, Springer-Verlag.
23. Haugh RH, Prather JL: The closed reduction of nasal fractures: an evaluation of two techniques, *J Oral Maxillofac Surg* 49.1288–1292, 1991.
24. Haug RH, Prather J, Inderesano AT: An epidemiologic survey of facial fractures and concomittant injuries, *J Oral Maxillofac Surg* 48:926–932, 1990.
25. Hill CM, Crosher RF, Carroll MJ, et al: Facial fractures—the results of a prospective four year study, *J Oral Maxillofac Surg* 12:267–270, 1984.
26. Illum P, Kristenson C, Jorgenson K, et al: The role of fixation in the treatment of nasal fractures, *Clin Otolaryngol* 8:191–195, 1983.
27. Ioannides C, Freihofer HPM, Bruaset I: Trauma of the upper third of the face, *J Maxillofac Surg* 12:255–261, 1984.
28. James RB, Frederickson C, Kent JN: Prospective study of mandible fractures, *J Oral Surgery* 39:275–281, 1981.
29. Kaban CLB: Diagnosis and treatment of fractures of the facial bones in children 1943–1993, *J Oral Maxillofac Surg* 51:722–729, 1993.
30. Kahnberg KE, Gothberg KAT: LeFort fractures: a study of frequency, etiology, and treatment, *Int J Oral Maxillofac Surg* 16:154–159, 1987.
31. Khalil AF, Shaladi OA: Fractures of the facial bones in the eastern region of Libya, *Br J Oral Surg* 19:300–304, 1981.
32. Knight JS, North JF: The classification of malar fractures: an analysis of displacement as a guide to treatment, *Br J Plast Surg* 13:325–339, 1961.
33. Landry GL: Sports injuries in childhood, *Pediatric Annals* 165–168, 1992.
34. Larrabee WF, Travis LW, Tabb HG: Frontal sinus fractures their suppurative complications and surgical management, *Laryngoscope* 90:1810–1813, 1980.
35. LeFort R: Etude experimentale sur les fractures de la machoire superieure, *Rev Chir* 23:208–227, 1901.
36. LeFort R: Etude experimentale sur les fractures de la machoire superieure, *Rev Chir* 23:360–379, 1901.
37. LeFort R: Etude experimentale sur les fractures de la machoire superieure, *Rev Chir* 23:479–507, 1901.
38. Lephart SM, Fu FH: Emergency treatment of athletic injuries, *Dent Clin North Am* 35:707–717, 1991.
39. Lundun K, Ridell A, Sandberg N, et al: One thousand maxillofacial and related fractures at the ENT clinic in Gothberg, *Acta Otolaryngol* 75:359–361, 1973.
40. Manson PN, Hoopes JE, Su CT: Structural pillars of the facial skeleton: an approach to the management of LeFort fractures, *Plast Reconstr Surg* 66:54–61, 1980.
41. Markowitz BL, Manson PN, Sargent L, et al: Management of the medial canthal tendon in nasoethmoid orbital fractures: the importance of the central fragment in classification and treatment, *Plast Reconstr Surg* 87:843–853, 1991.
42. McGraw BL, Cole RR: Pediatric maxillofacial trauma, age related variations in injury, *Arch Otolaryngol Head Neck Surg* 116:41, 1990.

43. Murray JA, Maran AGD, Butsuttil A, et al: A pathological classification of nasal fractures, *Injury* 17:338–344, 1986.

44. Olson RA, Fonseca RJ, Zeitler DL, et al: Fractures of the mandible: review of 580 cases, *J Oral Maxillofac Surg* 40:23–28, 1982.

45. Onishi K, Nakajima T, Yoshimura Y: Treatment and therapeutic devices in the management of frontal sinus fractures, *J Craniomaxillofac Surg* 17:58–63, 1989.

46. *Overview of sports related injuries to persons 5–14 years of age.* Washington, 1981, US Consumer Product Safety Commission.

47. Pashby TJ: Eye injuries in hockey, In Vinger PF, ed: *Ocular sports injuries (International Opthalmology Clinics)* Boston, Little, Brown, 1981.

48. Peri G, Chabannes S, Menes R, et al: Fractures of the frontal sinus, *J Maxillofac Surg* 9:73–80, 1981.

49. Pinkham JR, Kohn DW: Epidemiology and prediction of sports-related traumatic injuries, *Dent Clin North Am* 35:609–625, 1991.

50. Posnick JC, Wells M, Pron GE: Pediatric facial fractures: evolving patterns of treatment, *J Oral Maxillofac Surg* 51:836–844, 1993.

51. Prein J, Hammer B: Stable internal fixation of midfacial fractures, *Facial Plast Surg* 5:221–230, 1988.

52. Ranalli DN: Prevention of craniofacial injuries in football, *Dent Clin North Am* 35:627–643, 1991.

53. Rix L, Stevenson ARL, Punnia-Moorthy: An analysis of 80 cases of mandibular fracture treated with miniplate osteosynthesis, *Int J Oral Maxillofac Surg* 20:337–341, 1991.

54. Rowe NL: Fractures of the facial skeleton in children, *J Oral Surg* 26:505, 1968.

55. Rowe NL, Williams JL: *Maxillofacial injuries,* Edinborough, 1985, Churchill Livingstone.

56. Sofferman RA, Danielson PA, Quatela V, et al: Retrospective analysis of surgically treated LeFort fractures, *Arch Otolaryngol* 109:446–448, 1983.

57. Spiessl B: *Internal fixation of the mandible: a manual of AO/ASIF Principles,* New York, 1989, Springer Verlag.

58. Stanley RB, Becker TS: Injuries of the nasofrontal orifices in frontal sinus fractures, *Laryngoscope* 97:728–731, 1987.

59. Steidler NE, Cook RM, Reade PC: Incidence and management of major middle third facial fractures at the Royal Melbourne Hospital, *Int J Oral Surg* 9:92–98, 1980.

60. Stoll P, Schilli W: Primary reconstruction with AO miniplates after severe craniomaxillofacial trauma, *J Craniomaxillofac Surg* 16:18–21, 1988.

61. Stranc MF, Robertson GA: A classification of injuries of the nasal skeleton, *Ann Plast Surg* 32:57–64, 1979.

62. Torg JS, Vesgo JJ, Sennett B, Das M: The national football head and neck injury registry: 14 year report on cervical quadriplegia, 1971–1984, *JAMA* 254:3439–3443, 1985.

63. Vinger PF: The incidence of eye injuries in sports. In Vinger PF, ed: *Ocular sports injuries (International Opthalmology Clinics),* Boston, 1981, Little, Brown.

64. Wallis A, Donald PJ: Frontal sinus fracture: a review of 72 cases, *Laryngoscope* 98:593–598, 1988.

65. Watson AWS: Incidence and nature of sports injuries in Ireland: Analysis of four types of sport, *Am J Sports Med* 21:137–143, 1993.

66. Williamson LK, Miller RH, Sessions RB: The treatment of nasofrontal ethmoidal complex fractures, *Otolaryngol Head Neck Surg* 89:587–593, 1981.

CHAPTER 14

DENTAL INJURIES

Michael D. Kurtz
Joe H. Camp
J.O. Andreasen

Preseason dental and oral screening should be the first step in the prevention of sports-related dental injuries.[63] The more information available before an injury occurs, the better from a management and medicolegal standpoint.[69] Experienced trainers, team physicians, and dentists know that logistically this may not always be convenient nor possible, especially in the case of visiting team players. Even if the information is incomplete, the more information gathered in advance the better. This information may include medical and dental histories, clinical examination and dental charting, radiographic survey, and customary photos and models.

Much of this information, especially radiographs, will serve as a baseline for comparison should an injury occur. Radiographs can also help identify problems that have the potential to remove the athlete from competition during the season. Such problems include impacted wisdom teeth, periapical radiolucencies, and teeth with deep decay. Panorex radiographs may be considered efficacious because they require less time to take than a full mouth series, do not subject the athlete to gagging, and show more of the maxillary and mandibular jaw bones.

Study models are good records. They can be used to fabricate a valuable piece of protective equipment—a custom mouthguard. Use of custom-made mouthguards has proven to reduce the number and severity of sports-related dental and orofacial traumatic injuries and cerebral concussions.

Sports participants are at risk for unique and distinct kinds of injuries. In turn, different diagnostic and treatment needs may be necessary.[68] For example, avid use of smokeless tobacco among baseball players would suggest greater significance for an oral cancer examination.

The exact mechanisms of injury to teeth are mostly unknown and not investigated. Direct trauma from a high-velocity object, such as a baseball that takes a bad hop and strikes the maxillary incisors, is likely to cause a fracture (Fig. 14-1). Alternatively, good lip coverage will diffuse the force of the blow, lower the velocity of the ground ball, and distribute the energy of impact over a wider area, causing greater surrounding hard- and soft-tissue damage, e.g., an avulsion. In other words, low-velocity trauma causes greatest damage to the hard and soft tissues that surround the teeth, whereas high-velocity trauma is more likely to fracture the teeth.[8,9,34]

Another mechanism, indirect trauma, occurs when the mandible whiplashes into collision with the maxilla. This trauma can occur from a blow to the chin, such as an uppercut in boxing, a football tackle, or a hockey stick. The concussion is capable of shattering posterior teeth (Fig. 14-2).[9,34]

Any traumatic dental injury has the potential to challenge pulp vitality even if not apparent initially. Electrical and thermal pulp tests on freshly traumatized teeth are unreliable, and their results should not be weighed heavily. Pain, palpation, percussion, and radiography are more indicative. Patients should be recalled to monitor pulp vitality at 1, 3, and 6 months after trauma. Thereafter, it is recommended pulp vitality be evaluated at 6-month intervals for several years.[27] A similar recall regimen may be instituted for teeth that have been displaced and are at risk of developing external root resorption or ankylosis.

The classification of dental sports injuries varies from author to author. The application of general standards for traumatic injuries to teeth is helpful especially when compiling or comparing statistics. Four basic categories of traumatic injuries to the oral cavity will be discussed: teeth, periodontal tissues, supporting bone, and gingival and oral mucosa.[9]

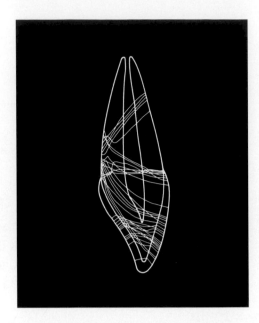

Fig. 14-1. Facio-lingual directions of 33 fracture lines caused by frontal impacts. (From Andreasen J: *Traumatic injuries of the teeth,* ed 2, Philadelphia, 1981, WB Saunders Co.)

TEETH

Crown Fractures

Crown fractures are most likely to result from high-velocity trauma. Pulpal vitality has a better chance of being maintained compared with low-velocity trauma, which is customarily associated with displacement injuries. Crown fractures occur more frequently in permanent teeth, whereas primary teeth are more likely to be displaced. Severe overjet will predispose a maxillary incisor to fracture, especially if there is lack of lip coverage (Fig. 14-3). Early interceptive orthodontics helps reduce this risk.[56]

CROWN FRACTURES INVOLVING ENAMEL. Enamel infraction is a crack in the enamel without loss of tooth substance. The crack usually runs parallel to the direction of the enamel prisms. The resulting craze line extends to the dentin-enamel junction and may lead to subsequent chipping of the tooth.

Enamel fracture is a loss of tooth substance confined to the enamel only. The attending dentist may need to round off sharp edges or consider acid-etch bonding of composite to prevent further injury to soft tissues or for aesthetics (Fig. 14-4).

CROWN FRACTURES INVOLVING ENAMEL AND DENTIN. Fractures involving dentin and exposing dentinal tubules often result in thermal sensitivity. The reduction of this sensitivity, usually taking 6 to 8 weeks, correlates to the formation of reparative dentin.[80] Restoration of the tooth can usually be accomplished by acid-etch composite bonding with adequate pulpal protection (Fig. 14-5).

CROWN FRACTURES INVOLVING ENAMEL, DENTIN, AND PULP. This is a complicated crown fracture exposing the pulp to bacterial infection and directly challenging tooth vitality. If left untreated, the fracture will usually lead to either a proliferative (pulpal hyperplasia) (Fig. 14-6) or destructive response (pulpal necrosis) (Fig. 14-7). Bacterial infection will necessitate pulpectomy and root canal therapy.[23] This may require a more significant restorative procedure, such as a post and crown. Whenever maintenance of vitality is important, the exposed pulp should be isolated and covered as soon as possible to prevent microorganisms from establishing an infection. Studies have demonstrated that injured pulpal tissues in germ-free animals usually heal, irrespective of the severity of the pulp exposure.[47,66] When possible, these procedures should be performed under rubber dam isolation. According to the Centers for Disease Control and Prevention in Atlanta, Georgia, dental rubber dam isolation also helps limit the transmission of all blood-borne pathogens, including HIV and HBV, by minimizing spatter of blood and blood-contaminated saliva.[83]

When immature teeth are injured, it is essential that pulpal vitality be maintained to allow completion of root development. This will permit better canal obturation should vitality be compromised and pulpectomy become necessary in the future. Afterward, a permanent restoration could be placed. One of the following two procedures should be selected as appropriate: (1) Pulp capping is used for small traumatic exposures free of inflammation and treated within hours of injury. A hard-setting calcium hydroxide material (e.g., Life—Kerr Corporation, Orange, CA; Dycal—Dentsply International Inc., L. D. Caulk Division, Milford, DE) is used to dress the exposure before placement of a temporary restoration. (2) Pulpotomy—using a sterile diamond bur[31] at high speed with copious cooling water, sufficient inflamed tissue, usually 2 to 3 mm, is removed to expose healthy uninflamed tissue. Damp cotton pellets are used to achieve hemostasis. Life or Dycal is then applied or $Ca(OH)_2$ United States Pharmacopia (USP) powder mixed with saline is carried to the pulp, and a hard-setting base can be placed over it. Signs of successful pulp capping and pulpotomy are (Fig. 14-8 on p. 154)[27] absence of pain, negative percussion, normal thermal sensitivity, negative palpation, and absence of radiographic periapical pathosis; radiographic dentin bridging; and radiographic evidence of continued root development. Possible complications include canal calcification, internal resorption, and pulp necrosis.

Crown–Root Fractures

There are two categories of crown–root fractures: (1) uncomplicated—involving enamel, dentin, and cementum only. Missing tooth structure can be restored by bonding, 3/4 crown, or full crown as appropriate (Fig. 14-9 on p. 154). (2) Complicated—involving enamel, dentin, cementum, and pulp (Fig. 14-10 on p. 155), usually requiring prompt root canal therapy (RCT) so that a post and crown may be fabricated (see Fig. 14-2).

Pulpal considerations are essentially the same as for crown fractures. After fragment removal, the remaining portion of the tooth can be surgically exposed, pro-*Text continued on p. 155.*

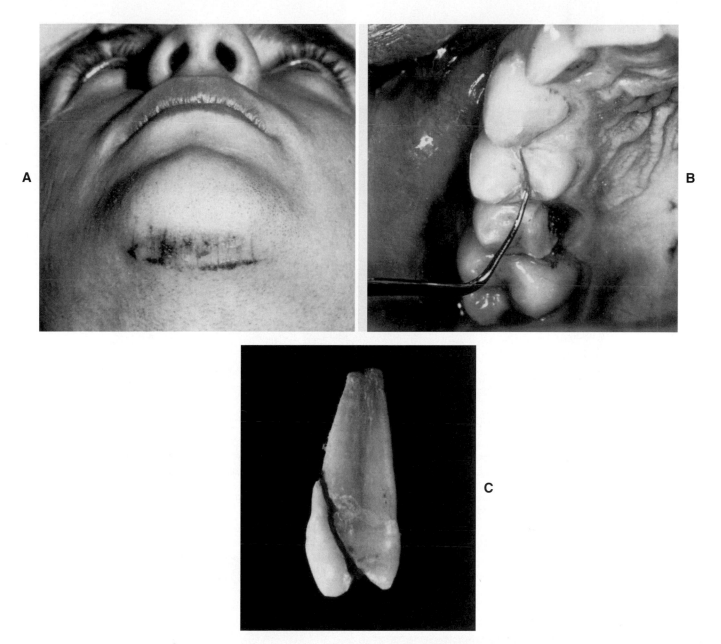

Fig. 14-2. Complicated crown–root fractures of posterior teeth. **A,** Trauma to the chin. **B,** Complicated crown–root fractures of both right first and second premolars. **C,** Lateral view of extracted first premolar. (From Andreasen J, Andreasen F: *Textbook and color atlas of traumatic injuries to the teeth,* ed 3, Mosby–Year Book, 1994.)

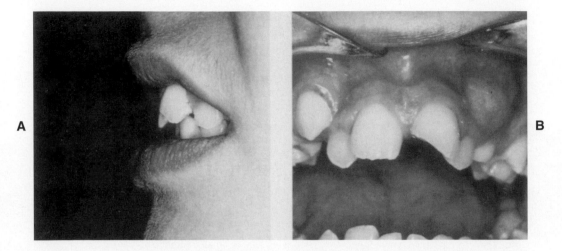

Fig. 14-3. Predisposition to crown fracture. **A,** Protruding central incisors with incomplete lip coverage. **B,** Crown fracture of a left central incisor. (From Andreasen J, Andreasen F: *Textbook and color atlas of traumatic injuries to the teeth,* ed 3, Mosby–Year Book, 1994.)

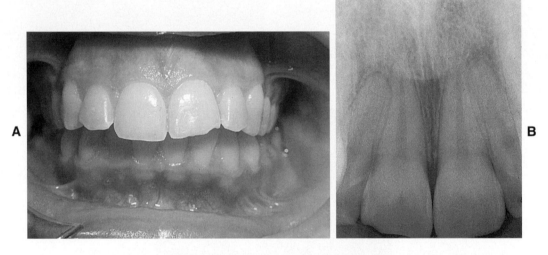

Fig. 14-4. Enamel fracture of the maxillary left central incisor involving the distoincisal angle. **A,** Photograph and **B,** radiograph of fracture.

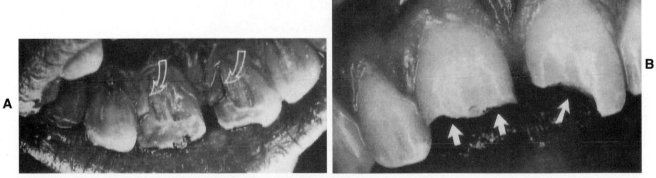

Fig. 14-5. Crown fractures involving enamel and dentin. **A,** Mirror view of palatal "chisel" type fractures. **B,** Direct facial view of incisal edge and mesio-incisal angle fractures. (From Bakland, Leif: Traumatic injuries in Ingle J, Taintor J: *Endodontics,* ed 3, Philadelphia, 1985, Lea & Febiger.)

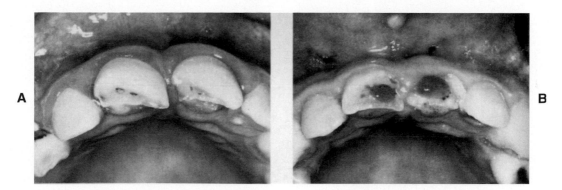

Fig. 14-6. Complicated crown fractures of central incisors. **A,** Small traumatic pulp exposures. **B,** Pulp proliferation in complicated crown fractures left untreated for 21 days. (From Andreasen J, Andreasen F: *Textbook and color atlas of traumatic injuries to the teeth,* ed 3, Mosby, 1994.)

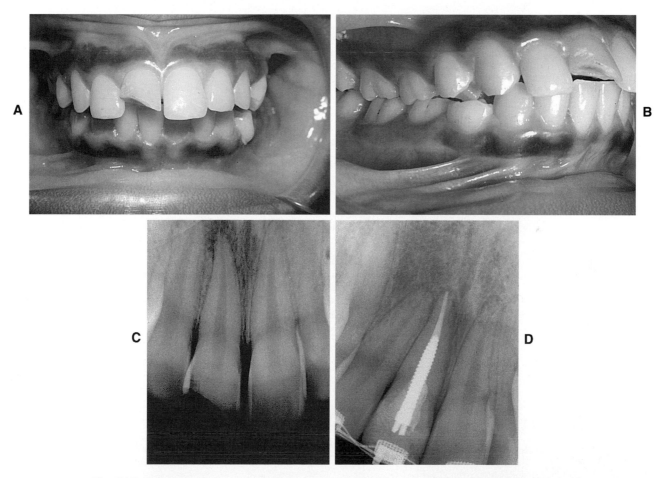

Fig. 14-7. Pulp necrosis in an untreated anterior tooth with a crown fracture involving enamel, dentin, and pulp. **A,** Fractured maxillary right central incisor. **B,** Untreated pulp exposure that has developed a necrotic response. Note staining where dentinal tubules have aspirated blood. **C,** Periapical radiolucency. **D,** Radiograph showing resolution of periapical pathology five years after root canal therapy. Note Dentatus screw post (distributed by Dentatus—Dentatus USA, New York, NY) and concurrent orthodontic treatment.

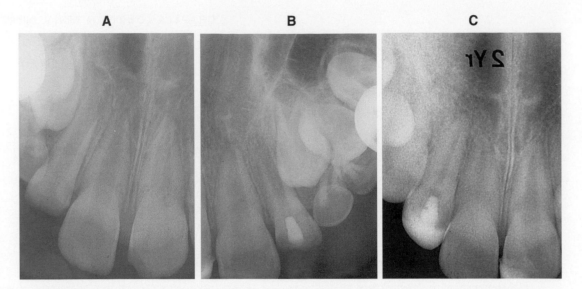

Fig. 14-8. Radiographs of continued root development following a pulpotomy. **A,** Maxillary lateral incisor with incomplete root development and a pulp exposure. **B,** Effects of calcium hydroxide following a pulpotomy. **C,** Two-year follow-up: root formation is completed and the pulp remains vital. Note the dentinal bridge just superior to the calcium hydroxide.

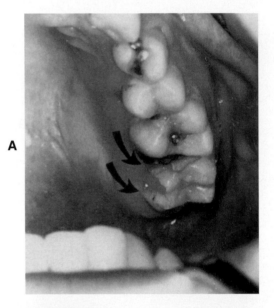

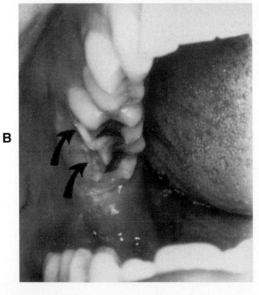

Fig. 14-9. Uncomplicated crown–root fractures (not exposing the pulp) resulting from a blow to the chin. The fractures of the lingual cusps in the maxillary arch correspond to the fractures of the buccal cusps in the mandibular arch. **A,** Maxillary arch. **B,** Mandibular arch. (From Andreasen J, Andreasen F: *Textbook and color atlas of traumatic injuries to the teeth,* ed 3, Mosby, 1994.)

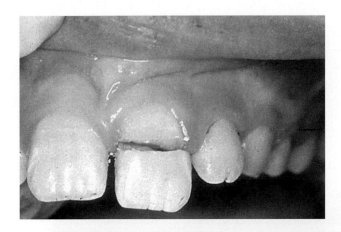

Fig. 14-10. Complicated crown–root fracture of an anterior tooth. *Courtesy of the Academy for Sports Dentistry.*

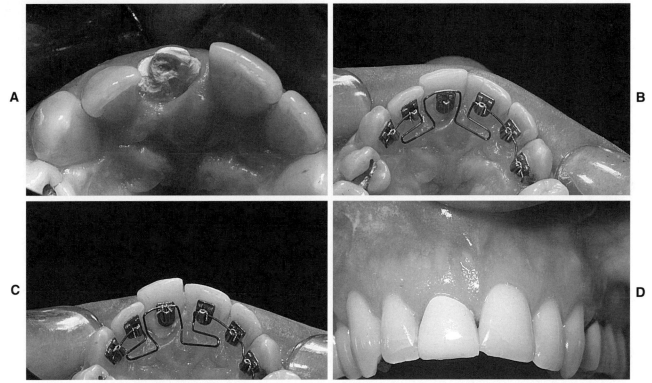

Fig. 14-11. Multidisciplinary extrusion of a complicated crown–root fracture involving an anterior tooth using lingual braces and periodontal surgery. **A,** Traumatically fractured maxillary right central incisor. **B,** Provisional restoration following cementation and placement of an orthodontic appliance. **C,** Activation of orthodontic appliance. **D,** Alterations of gingival margins immediately following eruption. *Continued.*

vided that the fracture site is less than 2 mm below the level of the alveolar bone. Otherwise, orthodontic or surgical extrusion to about 2 mm coronal to the alveolar crest must be considered. This extrusion will expose enough tooth structure to rebuild the tooth prosthetically if there is sufficient root length (Fig. 14-11). If the coronal fragment comprises more than one third of the clinical root length, the tooth is indicated for removal.[9] Extraction is also indicated for vertical fractures when the fracture line follows the long axis of the tooth.

Root Fractures

Root fractures involve dentin, cementum, and pulp and account for only 7% or fewer of injuries to permanent teeth.[5] Surprisingly, most teeth with radicular fractures remain vital, and only 20% to 40% become nonvital.[89] The patient's main complaint is sensitivity to biting pressure. Mobility of the tooth may be indicative of root fracture. Percussion accomplished with a mouth-mirror handle will assist in confirming the diagnosis. Fracture location can be determined by gentle digital palpation over the facial aspect of the suspected root fracture. This examination is done while holding and delicately rocking the crown of the suspect tooth between the thumb and forefinger of the clinician's other hand. Prompt reduction and fixation with a rigid acid-etched splint will promote healing by calcific callus formation internally (on the root canal wall) and externally (on the root surface) (Fig. 14-12). Experience has shown the farther coro-

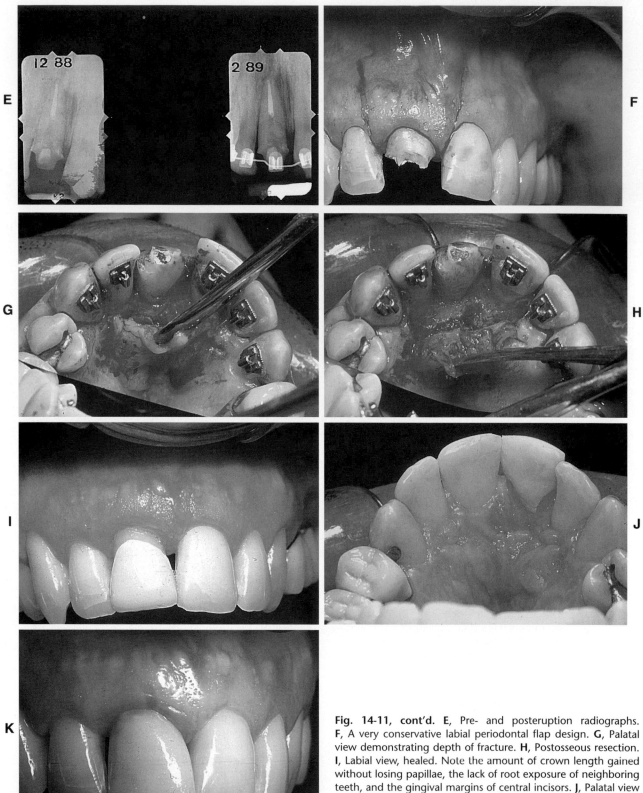

Fig. 14-11, cont'd. E, Pre- and posteruption radiographs. **F,** A very conservative labial periodontal flap design. **G,** Palatal view demonstrating depth of fracture. **H,** Postosseous resection. **I,** Labial view, healed. Note the amount of crown length gained without losing papillae, the lack of root exposure of neighboring teeth, and the gingival margins of central incisors. **J,** Palatal view showing amount of crown length gained. **K,** Final result. Restorative dentistry by Dr. Daniel Budasoff, NY, NY. (All photographs courtesy of Frank Celenza Jr., DDS, New York, NY.)

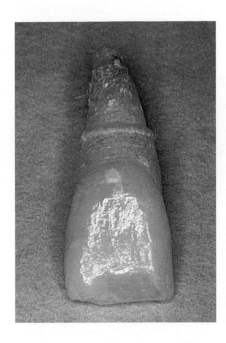

Fig. 14-12. Extracted tooth with a previous root fracture healed with a calcific callus. (From Fountain SB, Camp JH: *Pathways of the pulp*, ed 6, St. Louis, 1994, Mosby–Year Book.)

nally a radicular fracture is located, the longer a splint should be left in place. This period can vary from 3 to 6 months. A far coronal fracture may need to be left in place for 1 year or exchanged for a permanent-type splint, such as a Maryland bridge. If reduction is insufficient, edema has caused some separation, or if fixation is deficient, which allows too much mobility, then fibrous connective tissue healing similar to periodontal ligament may result. If these conditions are somewhat exaggerated, new alveolar bone may actually form between the fracture segments. Where there is severe dislocation, there will be nonunion (Fig. 14-13). Usually, the apical segment will remain vital, and the incisal segment will undergo necrosis with granulation tissue formation between the two segments. RCT can be confined to the incisal (coronal) segment. Filling the canal with Ca(OH)$_2$ initially and later with gutta percha is accomplished if there is evidence of resorption. This is also true if the root is sufficiently immature and wide open so as to interfere with the creation of a positive stop to prevent overfilling and extrusion of gutta percha or cement sealer.

PERIODONTAL TISSUES

Nondisplacement Injuries

Nondisplacement injuries are characterized by edema, bleeding, and trauma to periodontal ligament (PDL) fibers. These PDL fibers can be damaged by tearing, stretching, or compression. Clinically, there is sensitivity to percussion and palpation. Relief of the occlusion by selective grinding of the opposing teeth and a soft diet for several weeks are generally recommended. Radiographic follow-up evaluation for 1 year is advisable to rule out the need for endodontic therapy.

CONCUSSION. Concussion is an injury to the PDL with no visible loosening or displacement of the tooth from its alveolus. The chief complaint is tenderness to touch or biting pressure (Fig. 14-14).

SUBLUXATION. Subluxation is characterized by discernable loosening of the tooth in the horizontal direction without demonstrable clinical or radiographic displacement. It may be sufficient to cause bleeding in the periodontal ligament, with hemorrhage visible in the gingival crevice (see Fig. 14-14). If several teeth are involved and if there is significant mobility, short-term splinting may be used.

Displacement Injuries

Displacement injuries most likely occur as the result of low-velocity trauma.[8] Moderate overjet of the maxillary incisors with good lip coverage would predispose them to displacement rather than fracture. Early orthodontics might help to intercept this problem. Patients with displacement injuries may complain of discomfort, swelling, discoloration of the crown of the tooth, mobility, or a change in their occlusion. Primary teeth are more apt to be displaced than permanent teeth. About 50% of permanent teeth with displacement injuries will require RCT.[75] Pulpal necrosis, root resorption, pulp calcification and obliteration, and loss of alveolar crestal bone height are the major complications of displacement injuries. Ca(OH)$_2$ can be used to fill the root canal of teeth exhibiting root resorption. This will help arrest the process before future filling with gutta percha.[25] Ca(OH)$_2$ should be retained between 6 to 12 months for intruded teeth and about 12 months for avulsed teeth, depending on whether resorption is ongoing. Ca(OH)$_2$ powder is mixed with a liquid and delivered as a paste. Anesthetic carpule solution or physiologic saline can be used as a carrier solvent. Premixed pastes are available from commercial vendors. Some examples are Tempcanal (Pulpdent Corp., Watertown, MA), Hypo-Cal (Ellman International, Hewlett, NY), and Calasept (distributed by J. S. Dental Manufacturing Inc., Ridgefield, CT). Because it is absorbable, the paste should be removed and refreshed every 3 to 6 months as needed and cannot be used as a permanent root canal filler.[17] Displacement injuries may need splinting to limit mobility and promote healing. Splints that cause gingival inflammation or subject teeth or alveolar bone to active pressures or tensions will cause PDL inflammation, external root resorption, or ankylosis. Oral

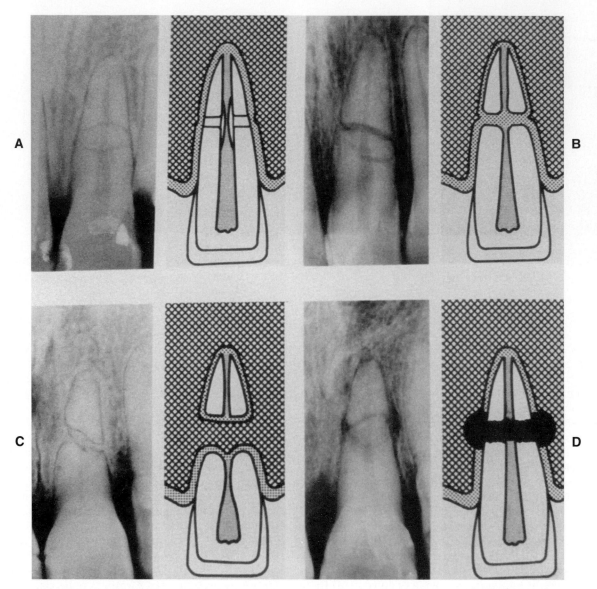

Fig. 14-13. Radiographs and diagrams illustrating various modalities of healing after root fracture. **A,** Calcified tissue. **B,** Interposition of connective tissue. **C,** Interposition of bone and connective tissue. **D,** Interposition of granulation tissue. (From Andreasen J: *Traumatic injuries of the teeth*, ed 2, Philadelphia, 1981, WB Saunders Co.)

surgical wire ligatures and arch bars should not be used in managing traumatized teeth (Fig. 14-15).[27] An arch wire between 0.015″ and 0.030″, about the size of paperclips, can be shaped to be bonded passively using acid-etch resin. According to Andreasen[2] prolonged rigid splinting of displaced teeth for more than 7 to 10 days may lead to external root resorption and ankylosis. Splinting time for displaced teeth can range between 2 to 3 weeks, depending on the severity of the injury and the patient's healing abilities (e.g., diabetes).

EXTRUSION. Extrusion is a partial avulsion of the tooth out of the alveolar socket. It is accompanied by radiographic evidence of increased width of the PDL space (Fig. 14-16).

LATERAL DISPLACEMENT. Lateral displacement is a sideways dislocation of the tooth accompanied by

comminution or fracture of the alveolar socket. Usually the coronal portion of the tooth is driven palatally or lingually, and the apical portion is driven in a facial direction. To free an apically locked tooth from a fenestration through buccal plate, coronally directed finger pressure over the apex of the root may be helpful (Fig. 14-17).[8]

INTRUSION. Intrusion is a displacement of the tooth in the direction of the alveolar bone caused by axially directed forces accompanied by comminution or fracture of the alveolar socket. The highest incidence of pulpal necrosis in teeth with displacement injuries occurs with intrusions. About 96% of intruded permanent teeth will undergo pulpal necrosis.[7] In mature teeth, after 7 to 10 days to allow some PDL healing, pulpectomy and Ca(OH)$_2$ therapy are necessary to decrease the likeli-

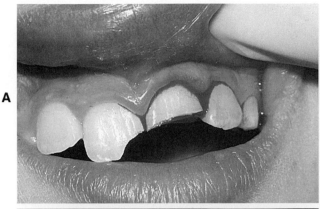

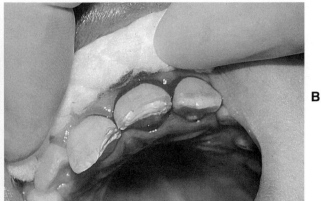

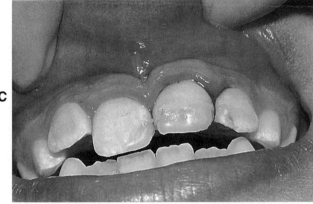

Fig. 14-14. Concussion and subluxation with accompanying crown fractures. **A,** The maxillary incisor fractured at the angle has suffered a concussion and is very sensitive to touch but exhibits neither mobility nor displacement. The horizontally fractured incisor has been subluxated, is bleeding from the periodontal ligament, and has a concomitant pulp exposure. **B,** Fracture after Dycal has been applied over the pulp exposure and the exposed dentin. **C,** Acid-etch composite has been placed to retain the Dycal dressing. No attempt is made at this phase to restore esthetics because of danger of further injury from manipulation of the teeth. Esthetics is addressed after periodontal healing.

hood of accompanying root resorption.[8,24] An intruded tooth with incomplete root formation will sometimes spontaneously reerupt. Mature teeth are best treated by prompt orthodontic extrusion back into position (Fig. 14-18 on p. 162). This extrusion will help reduce the complications of loss of alveolar crestal bone height and external root resorption or ankylosis. Severe intrusions may require surgical repositioning and splinting. Any intruded tooth that extends into the nasal cavity must also be surgically repositioned.

AVULSION. Avulsion is the complete displacement of the tooth from its socket. The maxillary central incisors are the most frequently avulsed teeth (Fig. 14-19 on p. 162). The sooner an avulsed tooth is replanted, the better its chances of survival.[35] Andreasen and Hjorting-Hansen's study[10] in 1966 showed that 90% of teeth replanted in less than 30 minutes will not demonstrate discernible external root resorption. Immature teeth with incomplete root formation have the greatest potential to revitalize and survive. In a sports setting, immediate replantation might be accomplished by the team trainer, physician, or dentist. Maintenance of periodontal ligament integrity is critical, therefore, no attempt to scrub, chemically clean, or sterilize the tooth should be made. The tooth should be handled by its crown rather than by its root. If there is some delay, clotted blood in the alveolar socket may prevent a tooth from being completely seated when replanted. No attempt to curette the socket or force the

tooth into position should be made because this could induce root resorption. Instead, the clot may be dislodged by gentle rinsing with saline or aspiration without damaging the socket. If an avulsed tooth cannot be replanted to its original position without force, it is probably safer to move it into correct position after healing using orthodontics. Avoid wrapping the tooth in tissue paper or gauze, which will encourage desiccation. Debris can be flushed with a transport media (i.e., Hank's Balanced Salt Solution), normal saline, or cold water according to availability in an emergency. Cotton pliers or a wet sponge can be used to gently remove persistent debris. Immediate systemic antibiotic therapy helps prevent infection of the pulp and PDL to promote healing. Precautions against *Clostridia tetani* as outlined in the section on lacerations should be considered within 48 hours.

In situations where replantation is delayed more than 30 minutes, the type of storage media and the method of handling become important issues. A tooth allowed to air dry will lead to PDL necrosis with replacement resorption (ankylosis) or inflammatory resorption (external root resorption). In ankylosis, the body attempts to repair the resorption by laying down new alveolar bone in direct apposition to the tooth. The PDL space is obliterated and becomes absent radiographically.[11] This clinically immobilizes the tooth. External (inflammatory) root resorption is the body's attempt to eliminate infected calcified tissue, bacteria,

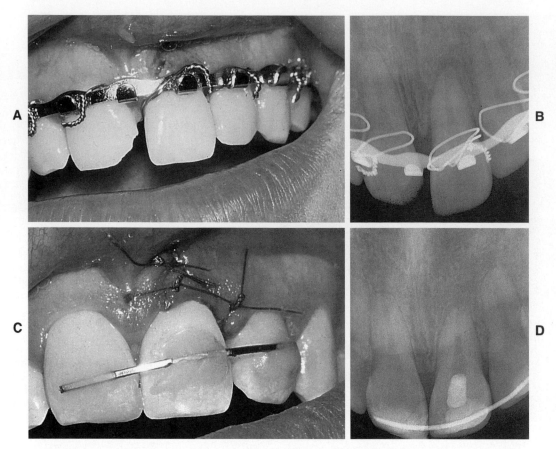

Fig. 14-15. An improperly treated avulsed central incisor. **A,** The maxillary left central incisor was avulsed and replanted, and an arch bar splint was placed. The replanted tooth has extruded either because of the force of the ligature wire on the root or because the tooth was not properly repositioned. The arch bar and wires are a gingival irritant. Note that the maxillary left central incisor has a crown fracture and that no sutures were placed in the torn gingival tissues. **B,** Corresponding radiograph showing the improper position of the replanted incisor. Note the degree of displacement of the tooth from its socket. **C,** The maxillary left central incisor following proper reposition and resplinting several hours following the mistreatment. The fractured left incisor has been restored with a Dycal base and composite restoration. The gingival tissues have been sutured. **D,** Corresponding radiograph showing the tooth back in its socket.

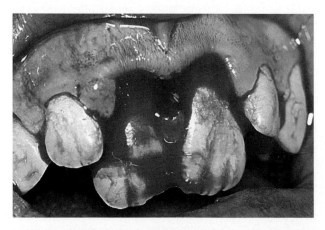

Fig. 14-16. Extrusion of the maxillary left central incisor. The tooth has partially left its alveolus and there is bleeding from the gingival sulcus. (From Kruger E, Schilli W: *Oral and maxillofacial traumatology,* Chicago, 1982, Quintessence Publishing Co., Inc.)

and their toxic lytic byproducts. It is characterized histologically by granulation tissue in the PDL adjacent to large areas of root resorption. External root resorption can be prevented by pulpectomy before a bacterial infection is established.[2,3,6] Infection prevention is also a good reason to initiate immediate antibiotic therapy after replantation.[37]

Revascularization is a possibility in replanted immature teeth with open apices. Conversely, untreated avulsed teeth with mature roots always develop pulpal necrosis and external root resorption. For this reason, RCT using $Ca(OH)_2$ to fill should routinely be done to replanted teeth with complete root development 1 to 2 weeks after replantation as a preventive measure. This time period corresponds with the time when the splint needs to be removed. Pulpectomy and RCT are not initiated in immature teeth unless signs of pulpal necrosis are observed. These teeth must be monitored closely for signs of degeneration. Replanted

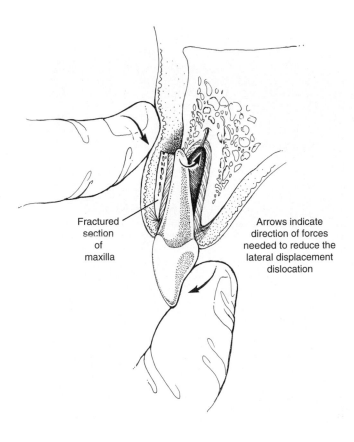

Fractured section of maxilla

Arrows indicate direction of forces needed to reduce the lateral displacement dislocation

Fig. 14-17. Repositioning a lateral displacement. (From Andreasen J, Andreasen F: *Textbook and color atlas of traumatic injuries to the teeth,* ed 3, Mosby–Year Book, 1994.)

immature teeth that lose their vitality have a poor prognosis.

Sterile solutions of Hank's Balanced Salt Solution or Viaspan, which have compatible physiologic osmolalities, qualify as superior storage media.[84] For avulsed teeth, Hank's Balanced Salt Solution is an older media that has been used to maintain mammalian cells in tissue culture. Viaspan, a newer media, has been used for organ-transplant storage. A packaged commercial product similar to Hank's Balanced Salt Solution called Save-A-Tooth (3M Health Care, St. Paul, MN) should be available in any training room, emergency field kit, gym, or sports complex.[27,51] It includes a built-in basket to allow the solution to reach all aspects of the PDL, and it cushions the tooth to prevent accidental crushing of the PDL (Fig. 14-20). This is important because crushing damage is a key source of resorption. With Save-A-Tooth, clinical success of 91% is reported.[27,51,52] Milk,[13] saliva for intraoral or extraoral transport, normal saline,[4] and polyethylene wrap[2] have been used with some success. Cold milk is a better storage medium than saliva because it has fewer bacteria and a more compatible physiologic osmolality.[13,57]

Replanted teeth undergo gradual ankylosis but are capable of functioning many years.

SUPPORTING BONE

Comminution of the Alveolar Socket
This is a shattering into a number of small fragments and crushing of the alveolus resulting from compressive trauma, such as that found with intrusions and lateral displacements.

Fracture of the Alveolar Socket Wall
This is a fracture limited to the facial or lingual (palatal) wall of the alveolar socket. These fractures are most often associated with lateral displacements.

Fracture of the Alveolar Process
When two or more neighboring teeth are able to be moved jointly as a block, a clinical diagnosis of fracture of the alveolar bone can be made (Fig. 14-21). This injury is common in ice hockey where sticks, frozen pucks, and fists abound. A fracture of the alveolar process may involve the alveolar socket.

Fracture of the Jaw
The patient should be examined clinically and appropriate radiographs ordered.[42] If a patient complains of having difficulty putting his or her teeth together, a fracture of the jaw should be ruled out. Conversely, some fractures do not exhibit occlusal disharmony.

FRACTURE OF THE MANDIBLE. Airway management is the most important aspect of emergent treatment with mandibular fractures. Fast-traveling frozen hockey pucks routinely deliver sufficient force to fracture a mandible (Fig. 14-22).

A mandible may be evaluated for fracture by having the patient open his or her mouth gently. Slight bilateral pressure is applied at the angles of the mandible. If there is a fracture, the patient will usually point to the area of discomfort.[42] As with a fracture of the alveolar process, a fracture of the mandible may or may not involve the alveolar socket.

It is believed that athletes may be predisposed to certain kinds of injuries based on existing anatomic conditions. For instance, impacted wisdom teeth may predispose the athlete to fracture of the mandible at the angle. Systemic or dental conditions yielding localized weakness, like mandibular cysts or semierupted mandibular wisdom teeth with accompanying pericoronitis, can also be contributory. Periodontal bony defects may also be related to the location of a fracture line.[53]

According to Haug and Greenberg,[32] mandibular fractures are the most frequently, completely, and consistently investigated facial fractures. The rank order of occurrence by anatomic location in the general population may be deduced from the total of studies cited and extrapolated to sports injuries (Table 14-1 and Fig. 14-23 on p. 164).

FRACTURE OF THE MAXILLA. This is an uncommon sports injury. To evaluate a fracture of the maxilla, hold the bridge of the nose with one hand while the other hand grasps the anterior maxilla and palate. If there is mobility of the maxilla without movement of the bridge of the nose, a horizontal fracture of the maxilla or a Le Fort I injury is suspected. If mobility is felt at

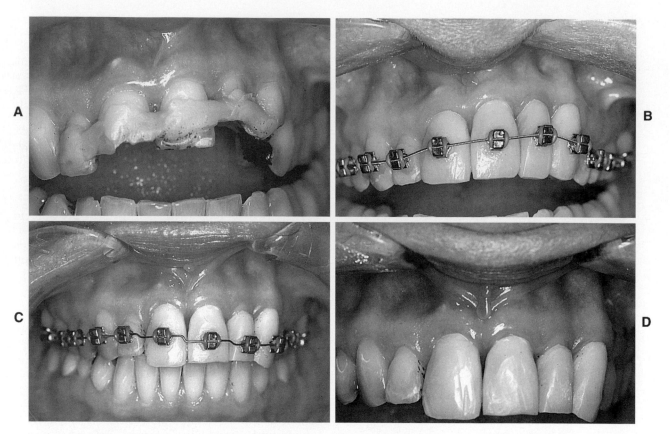

Fig. 14-18. Intrusive displacement of maxillary anteriors. **A,** Four maxillary teeth (#8 to #11) that have been traumatically intruded and splinted in a hospital emergency room. **B,** Later provisional restorations were placed and an orthodontic appliance activated to erupt the teeth back towards normal position. **C,** Posteruption. Note favorable alteration to free gingival margin architecture. **D,** Removal of orthodontic appliance. Provisional restorations will be removed and permanent restorations will be fabricated. (Courtesy Frank Celenza Jr., DDS, New York, NY.)

the bridge of the nose, a Le Fort II or Le Fort III fracture is possible.[42] Panoramic and Waters' view radiographs are useful in evaluating Le Fort fractures. Fractures of the maxillary sinus walls are best seen on Waters', Caldwell, or lateral plate views of the face.[67]

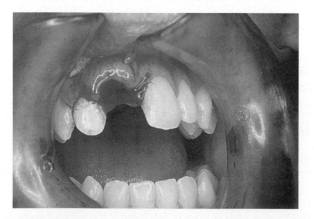

Fig. 14-19. Avulsed maxillary right central incisor. (Courtesy of Ray R. Padilla, DDS, West Covina, California.)

GINGIVAL & ORAL MUCOSA

Lacerations

A laceration is a tearing wound usually produced by a sharp object. These wounds must be explored for foreign matter and débrided before suturing (Fig. 14-24). Radiographic examination of a laceration will help locate radioopaque foreign objects, such as tooth fragments and orthodontic brackets. Careful inspection and cleansing of the wound are required to rule out contamination with nonradioopaque materials, such as glass, plastic, and wood. The need for antibiotic coverage and precautions against tetanus should be considered. Penicillin, amoxicillin, or erthyromycin seem to have the appropriate spectra and work well on nonallergic individuals for intraoral infections.

IRREGULAR LACERATIONS. Irregular lacerations can occur anywhere intraorally, including gingiva, oral mucosa, lips, tongue, palate, and pharynx. A through and through laceration of the lip with blunt trauma (e.g., a punch) is probably the most common maxillofacial injury and should be routinely examined for tooth fragments. Approximation of the vermillion border is crucial when suturing.[42]

The tongue is very vascular and its location strategic.

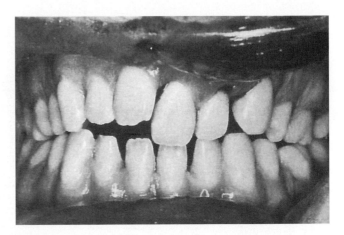

Fig. 14-21. Fracture of the alveolar process involving the maxillary left central and lateral incisors. (From Kruger E, Schilli W: *Oral and maxillofacial traumatology,* Chicago, 1982, Quintessence Publishing Co., Inc.)

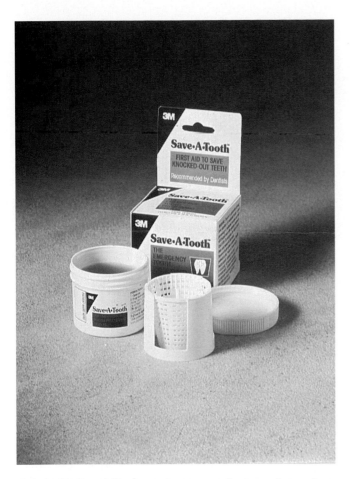

Fig. 14-20. Save-A-Tooth emergency tooth preserving system. (Courtesy of 3M Health Care, St. Paul, MN.)

Direct pressure may be necessary to control profuse bleeding and keep the airway patent. Injuries to the tongue can cause posttraumatic swelling leading to dysphagia, dysmasesis, drooling, dysgeusia, and dysphonia.

REGULAR LACERATIONS. Incisions and punctures are special kinds of lacerations containing geometric symmetry. Incisions are prevalent in hockey in which ice skate blades can cut lips and tongues (Fig. 14-25). These types of wounds may bleed profusely and can be a challenge to suture and achieve good approximation of the borders of the tissue.

Punctures are potentially dangerous. Commonly,

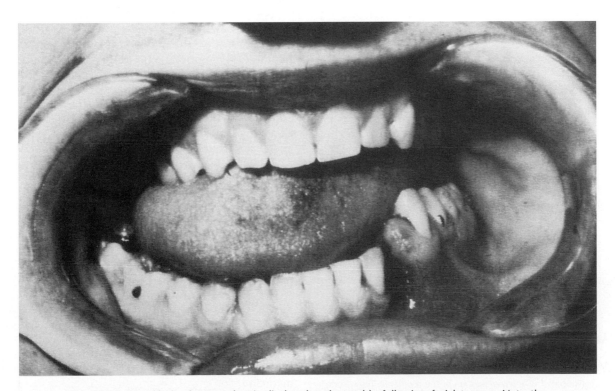

Fig. 14-22. Mandibular fracture that is displaced and unstable following facial trauma. Note the change in the occlusion. (From Ranalli: *Dent Clin North Am* 35(4):711, 1991.)

Table 14-1. Occurrence of mandibular fractures

Rank order of occurence	Anatomic location of mandibular fracture
1	Corpus (body)
2	Angle
3	Condylar process
4	Symphysis
5	Ramus
6	Coronoid process

baseball cleats have been known to cause puncture wounds when a player attempts to steal a base by sliding. *C. tetani* is an anaerobic spore-forming gram-positive bacillus found in soil and feces. It causes the infectious disease tetanus characterized by intermittent tonic spasms of voluntary muscles. Trismus of the masseter muscles accounts for the name "lockjaw." Its pathogenicity stems from the effects of its neurotoxin, *tetanospasmin*, produced by the introduction and germination of spores in host tissue. Toxin is released upon cell lysis. In clean wounds where the blood supply is good and O_2 tension is high, germination of the spores rarely occurs. This emphasizes the importance of prompt, thorough débridement. Generally, whenever a previously immunized patient sustains a wound, a booster of toxoid should be injected to produce protective antibodies within a couple of weeks. Patients who have not previ-

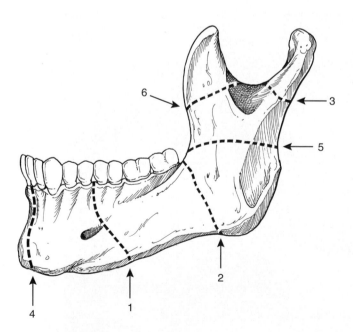

Fig. 14-23. Fractures of the mandible by rank order of occurrence. (Adapted from Spiessl B: *Internal fixation of the mandible,* New York, 1989, Springer-Verlag Co. Reproduced with permission.)

ously been immunized should receive human tetanus immune globulin (250 U) because the antibody response to an initial dose is too slow to be useful. Full-blown tetanus has a mortality rate of 50%, and should be managed by an infectious disease physician.

Contusions

A contusion is a bruise usually produced by blunt trauma that causes subgingival or submucosal hemorrhage with accompanying swelling, pain, and discoloration; i.e., hematoma. The majority of hematomas will resorb with no treatment. On rare occasions, a hematoma may become encapsulated. Proteolytic enzymes like papain given systemically are ineffective.[77] As liquefaction proceeds, aspiration with a large-bore needle (at least 18-gauge) is helpful.

Abrasions

An abrasion is an excoriation of the superficial epithelial layer of gingiva or mucosa resulting from shearing trauma e.g., a rubbing or scraping. This friction wound generally leaves a raw bleeding surface. Management usually consists of appropriate antibiotic coverage.

MOUTH PROTECTOR CONSIDERATIONS

Objectives

Protection from hard- and soft-tissue injuries, jaw fractures, and temporomandibular joint (TMJ) and miniscular injuries are obvious goals of mouth protection. More than half of all facial sports injuries involve either fractures of the alveolar process or luxation of teeth.[58] What are some of the other objectives that the ideal mouth protector needs to offer?

Retention, protection, and durability have been used as yardsticks to measure the efficacy of mouthguards. As an indication of the protection mouthguards provide, hardness, penetration, rebound, and dynamic resilience have been studied.[20,30] Mouthguards are exposed to high compressive stresses when in use. As an indication of durability, the tensile strength, tear strength, elongation, and moduli of elasticity have also been measured.[20,30] Generally, thickness of material correlates with impact energy absorption.[64]

Epidemiologic evidence exists suggesting that wearing a mouthguard will prevent dental and oral injuries.[40,55] This applies to contact and noncontact sports.[39] In 1973, the National Collegiate Athletic Association (NCAA) football rules committee adopted the mouth-protector rule. The following year, professional football followed suit by embracing a similar requirement.[14] In 1990, the NCAA mandated the use of brightly colored mouthguards to promote their use and facilitate the ability of officials to observe player compliance. More than half of officials surveyed believed this rule had resulted in more frequent use by athletes and a decrease in dental injuries.[73,74] Other than fluoridation, mouthguards rank as one of the most important contributions that dentistry has made to preventive medicine.

Basketball is supposed to be a noncontact sport de-

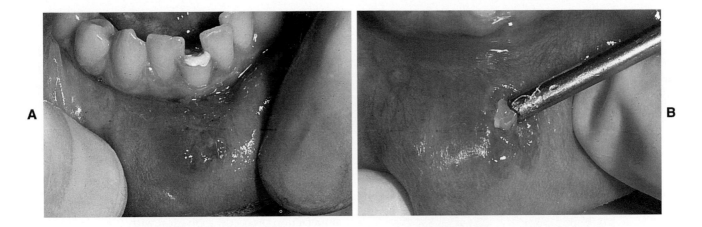

Fig. 14-24. Foreign object in the lip. **A,** The patient was seen in the emergency room after an injury. The lip was sutured and a dressing placed on the fractured mandibular incisor. The sutures were removed the following day because of patient complaints. **B,** A fractured tooth segment was found in the lower lip. (Courtesy of Dr. Dan Kolzet, Durham, NC.)

spite the flying elbows asserting possession after a rebound. Basketball, lacrosse, and wrestling are sports with a very high incidence of dental injuries.[55] This can be inferred from the nature of these sports and because most players are inattentive regarding mouthguard use. One can speculate this occurs because they are not regarded as contact sports or because there are no regulations requiring use of mouthguards.[18,55] Mandatory mouth protection in basketball may be necessary.[59]

A mouthguard needs to be comfortable for an athlete and minimize sore spots and gagging. It should have almost no effect on breathing.[44] The more oxygen an athlete is able to deliver to muscle tissue, the less lactic acid build-up and the less fatigue. The mouthguard should interfere little with speech and be time- and cost-effective to fabricate. The device needs to be able to negotiate orthodontic brackets, missing or erupting teeth, and tori. When not in use, a mouthguard should be soaked in mouthwash to keep it odor-free and tasting fresh. It should be rinsed in cold water before and after each insertion.

Cervical Injuries

Dr. John Stenger's classic 5-year clinical study on Notre Dame football players began in 1958 and was published in 1964 (Fig. 14-26).[82] Dr. Stenger, the initiator of the concept of physiologic dentistry, based much of his work on that of James B. Costen, MD, a Washington University otolaryngologist.[22] By means of before and after cephalometric radiographic tracings, Stenger demonstrated differences in the position of the mandibular condyle, the hyoid bone, and the cervical vertebrae (C2–C4) when the teeth were in centric occlusion *versus* when the bite was opened by a custom-made mouthguard to the vertical dimension of the freeway space (Fig. 14-27).

In the spring of 1963, with the encouragement of then trainer Gene Paszkiet, a decision was made to equip the entire Notre Dame football team with a new model ethylene vinyl acetate (EVA) mouthguard. As expected, the number of injuries to the teeth and jaws declined. There was also an impressive reduction in cerebral con-

Fig. 14-25. Incision inferior to vermillion border of left lower lip caused by an accident involving a skate blade during an ice hockey game. (Courtesy of Ray R. Padilla, DDS, West Covina, California.)

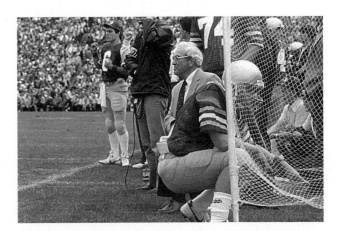

Fig. 14-26. Dr. John Stenger kneels at the sidelines watching his Notre Dame boys, mouthguards inserted, power their way to victory. (Courtesy of John Stenger, DDS, South Bend, IN.)

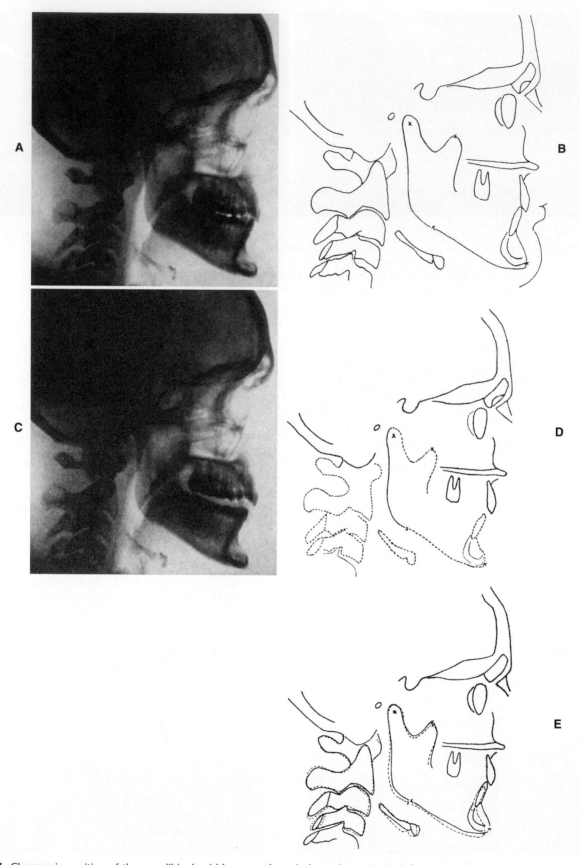

Fig. 14-27. Changes in position of the mandible, hyoid bone, and cervical vertebrae. **A,** Cephalometric radiograph with teeth in occlusion. **B,** Solid line tracing of A. **C,** Cephalometric radiograph showing mouthguard inserted. This film was taken 30 seconds after first film while the patient's position remained unchanged in the headholder. **D,** Dashed line tracing of C. **E,** Composite tracing of B (solid line) and D (dashed line). (From Stenger J et al: *JADA* 69:274–275, 1964.)

cussions. A serendipitous correlation between wearing the mouthguards and a decrease in neck injuries was an important finding.[81,82] "A reduction in the number of neck injuries was an unexpected result of wearing the mouthguards. Neck injuries had increased since the use of the face bar had become mandatory. During the 1962 season at Notre Dame, six or seven players had chronic neck problems, and four of them wore cervical collars. Cervical traction was routine therapy for these players. An automatic traction device was ordered by the athletic department and delivered during the summer to replace the manual one in use. Fortunately, because of the mouthguards worn by the players prone to neck injuries, the new machine, ordered in anticipation of more injuries, has never been unpacked. Furthermore, not a single Notre Dame player who faithfully wore his mouthguard during the 1963 season found it necessary to wear a cervical collar."[82]

Cerebral Concussions

In a 1967 study, Hickey et al[41] of the University of Kentucky used a cadaver to measure changes in intracranial pressure and bone deformation. The mandible was struck from below by a device designed to deliver a uniform repeatable force. Changes in intracranial pressure were measured by a tubing inserted through a hole drilled in the cranium and secured by acrylic resin. Changes in intracranial pressure were ascertained first without a mouth protector inserted, second with a natural rubber mouthguard in place, and lastly using a vacuum-formed mouth protector (Fig. 14-28). The results clearly demonstrated that mouthguards reduce intracranial shock wave propagation. Further, intracranial pressure differences between natural rubber and vacuum-formed vinyl mouth protectors were not significant.[41] Caution should be exercised concerning proprietary claims of mouthguard superiority regarding degree of shock absorbency.

Performance Enhancement

In 1977, a controversial article by Dr. Stenger[81] triggered an avalanche of clinical and experimental studies. He proposed that a lack of posterior bite support and malocclusion were factors that limited athletic performance. The first published study to test this hypothesis appeared in 1978.[79] Its author, Stephen D. Smith, DMD, Director of the TMJ Clinic at the Philadelphia College of Osteopathic Medicine, obtained permission from head coach, Dick Vermeil, to study 25 Philadelphia Eagles football players.

Using wax bites to reposition the mandible, Smith used a kinesiologic muscle challenge known as the Isometric deltoid press to determine the *ideal* three-dimensional occlusal position at which to construct a Mandibular Orthopedic Repositioning Appliance (MORA), which would mimic mouthguard design. A MORA similarly repositions the mandible anteriorly, increases the vertical dimension, and changes the head posture relationship.[28] Smith believed he demonstrated a positive correlation between the posture of the jaw and the ability of the arm musculature to give strong contraction. His critics denounced his applied kinesiologic methods, calling them unscientific, and dubbed his results statistically insignificant.

Since Smith's initial report, there have been numerous studies that have produced apparently conflicting results. An excellent review and critique of the salient studies has been presented by Forgione et al.[26] They charged "one commentator,[45] a reviewer,[21] and three authors of original studies[33,76,88] with having made emphatic general statements critical of the original results and later studies supporting Stenger's proposed

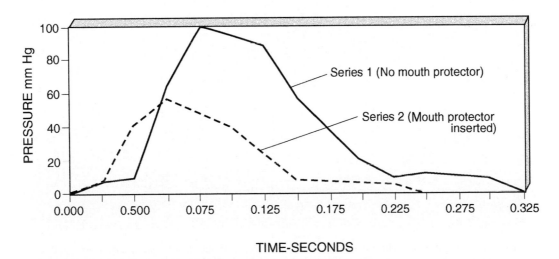

INTRACRANIAL PRESSUE

Fig. 14-28. Intracranial pressure changes Series 1. Without Mouth Protector Series 2. With Mouth Protector inserted. Notice the significant decrease in both shock wave amplitude and period. (Adapted from Hickey J et al: *JADA*, 74:735–740, 1967.)

relationship despite the following: (1) Most of these experiments used subjects with no apparent malocclusions or lack of posterior support[12,15,38,62,65,86,88] and others, mixed occlusions.[16,76,78,79,87] (2) Most researchers[1,12,15,16,33,38,60,62,65,76,85–87] set bite appliances by techniques other than kinesiologic guidance, a functional technique, assuming or implying that all MORAs are equivalent. (3) Researchers used data showing no increase in isokinetic tests of strength to criticize studies of isometric strength[1,15,16,33,38,65,76,85] while commenting on strength unqualifiedly. (4) Some researchers used either questionable statistics, experimental design or both.[15,16,38,76] (5) Some authors[16,21,33,76] and a commentator[45] have invoked placebo as a criticism of evidence that supports Stenger's proposal even though the placebo effect has not been demonstrated in any of the studies that have employed a placebo control condition. The belief that the placebo effect is omnipresent has even fostered an explanation for its lack of appearance."[60]

For the most part, criticism of performance enhancement has been aimed at study designs, controls, period (long-term *vs.* short-term), double blindness, and the placebo effect.[50]

There is almost universal agreement that designing one indisputable study is not an easy task. It would be very difficult to satisfy all investigators, scientists, and clinicians. At one point, Joseph J. Marbach, DDS, former Director of the world's first TMJ Clinic[54] at Columbia University's School of Dental and Oral Surgery stated, "There is no way that true double-blind studies can be done to measure any changes that occur as a result of repositioning because the researcher will know if he is testing a functional occlusal splint and the patient will know that the splint is in and something is supposed to change as a result."[61]

So, if you cannot prove something scientifically, how do you know it works? It is the opinion of this author that the kinesiologically adjusted mouthguards made by selected clinicians do work. Brainchild of Dr. Richard Kaufman of Oceanside, New York,[48] the Mouthpiece of Champions is a kinesiologically adjusted mouthguard that has gained tremendous patient acceptance. At this point, they are prized and sought after repeatedly by many prominent professional athletes who have had long experience with a variety of other mouthguards.

Mouth Protector Construction

EXTERNAL MOUTH PROTECTORS. Youth ice hockey is the rage in Canada. An external mouthguard has been designed into the helmet strap. It is reminiscent of a miniature baseball catcher's mask for the oral cavity (Fig. 14-29). Recently, Dr. Arthur Wood of Toronto received the Canada Medal for promoting its use as a cost-effective way to decrease dental injuries among Canadian youth.[19]

INTERNAL MOUTH PROTECTORS. The maxillary central incisors are the most frequently traumatized teeth, and consequently, a mouthguard will usually be constructed for the maxillary arch. However, in cases of mandibular prognathism, it may be desirable to reverse this or construct a bimaxillary appliance.

Stock mouthguards are inexpensive, can be purchased over-the-counter, and are ready for immediate use. They are often ill-fitting and may interfere with breathing and speech because they must be held in position by keeping the teeth together. However, they are convenient to have

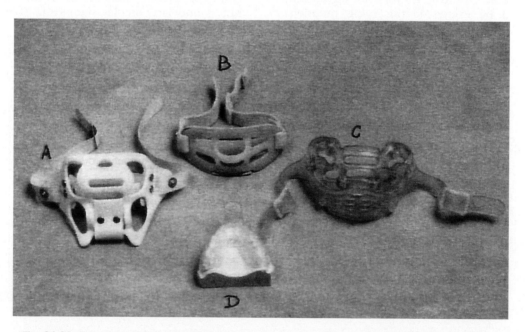

Fig. 14-29. Types of mouthguards: **A, B,** and **C,** are external mouthguards widely used from 1970 to 1980 in Sweden (A), Canada (B), and the United States (C). **D,** Custom-made mouthguard formed on a model of the player's maxillary teeth. (From Castaldi C et al: *The sports mouthguard: Its use and misuse in ice hockey, safety in ice hockey,* Vol 2, ASTM STP 1212, Philadelphia, American Society for Testing and Materials.)

available in case of loss or damage to an athlete's custom mouthguard during an event.

Mouth-formed mouthguards are a compromise between stock and custom-made. They are adapted by the direct method intraorally. One variety comes with a shell, often of ethylene vinyl chloride, that is lined with soft, chemically setting ethyl methacrylate. Another variety, commonly referred to as "boil and bite," is made of a thermoplastic material, usually EVA copolymer. It is softened by boiling water and adapted intraorally while warm by literally biting into the material.

Custom-made mouthguards are fabricated indirectly on a stone model of the athlete's dentition. This is made from a dental impression, usually alginate. Custom mouthguards are the most expensive but are superior in virtually every aspect. Smart athletes make a point to have spares in case of loss or damage. The majority of custom mouthguards are fashioned by first heating a 0.150"-thick sheet of EVA held in a frame on a vacuum-forming machine until it exhibits a specific amount of droop or sag (Fig. 14-30). The sheet is then vacuum-formed over a stone model that has either been previously soaked in water or coated with separator (Fig. 14-31). The material is allowed to cool, separated from the model, chilled with cold or ice water, trimmed and polished (Fig. 14-32). If a strap is needed to attach the mouthguard to a football facemask, before finishing, the EVA can be heated with a torch or flameless heat gun to spot weld an EVA strap. Also, an identification label can be placed anywhere. To accomplish this, the location for the label is selected, the mouthguard chilled, and channeled with a heatless stone. The label is placed inside the trough, and just enough EVA copolymer is added to cover the label. Applying heat will melt and seal the EVA. Finger pressure using a moistened cloth can be applied to smooth the area over the label. Gentle flaming can be used to establish a glossy finish.

Heated EVA can be formed in other ways. One method uses positive pressure rather than a vacuum to adapt the same EVA sheet material. Great Lakes Ortho-

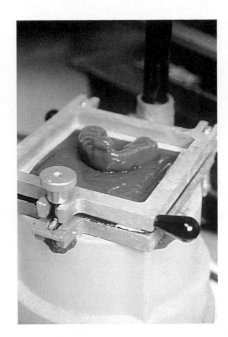

Fig. 14-31. Frame holding EVA material has been lowered and vacuumed over model on vacuum platform. (Courtesy of Ray R. Padilla, West Covina, California.)

dontics of Tonawanda, New York, imports one such machine, the Biostar, manufactured in Germany by Scheu Dental (Fig. 14-33). This machine is capable of producing admirable adaptation. If desired, positive pressure and the use of a jig allow a one-piece strap attachment to be incorporated into the mouthguard simultaneously.

Another technique used to fabricate superior custom mouthguards involves heat flasking. These are bimaxillary guards resembling orthodontic positioners. They are used in situations where it is important to maintain a precise jaw relationship indexed by a dentist. The flasking procedure is roughly the same whether the material is (nonsheet) EVA or vulcanized natural rubber (Fig. 14-34).

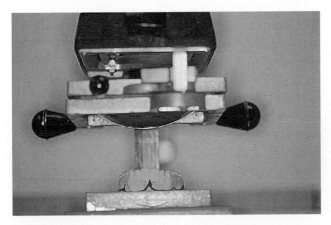

Fig. 14-30. Ethylene vinyl acetate heated and beginning to droop while soaked model sits ready on vacuum platform. (Courtesy of Ray R. Padilla, West Covina, California.)

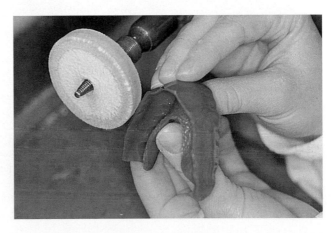

Fig. 14-32. Mouthguard being trimmed and polished after separation from model. (Courtesy of Ray R. Padilla, West Covina, California.)

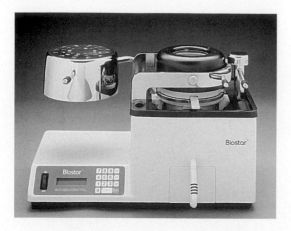

Fig. 14-33. Biostar Positive Pressure Machine. The Biostar is capable of fabricating many orthodontic appliances. (Courtesy of Great Lakes Orthodontics, Tonawanda, NY.)

Boxing and martial arts mouthguards need to provide an extra degree of protection to both dental arches, especially against TMJ injuries and cerebral concussions. Some believe that the posterior vertical dimension should be increased beyond rest to yield a larger mandibular condylar separation from the glenoid fossa.[43] These mouthguards need to be made of a firmer material to resist bite-through and change in "power bite" position that heavy clenching might produce.

Boxing and martial arts mouthguards need to be engineered with provisos for maximum oxygen exchange. Maintaining an adequate airway in the event of nasal obstruction from a blow is an important consideration.[43] One way to accomplish this is by eliminating the flange on the lower portion of the mouthguard, which uncovers the mandibular incisors and creates space for breathing. Barring allergy, its elasticity, resistance to deformation during clenching, and historic use since the beginning of the century give natural rubber a certain appeal to some professional boxers.

Presently, EVA copolymer has become the material of choice. When manufactured, the physical properties of a polymer can be varied by such additives as antioxidants and stabilizers, fillers, plasticizers, lubricants, coloring, and flavoring agents.[20] The thermoplastic abilities of EVA make it an attractive material with which to work. Commercial glue gun material is EVA to which a tackisizer has been added. Some orthodontic laboratories use a commercial glue gun to help maxillary and mandibular EVA mouthguards stick together to form a bimaxillary guard like those used in boxing and martial arts. The firmness of EVA can be controlled by adjusting the amount of plastisizer incorporated into the polymer. Allesee Orthodontic Appliances of Sturtevant, Wiscon-

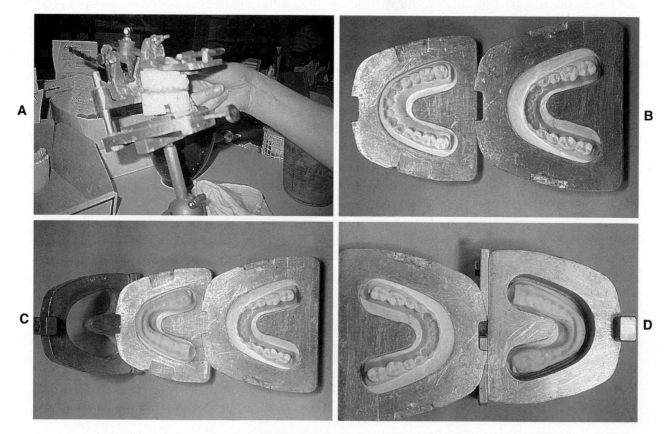

Fig. 14-34. Heat flasked mouthguard fabrication. **A,** Models mounted in three-dimensional articulator similar to Galletti. **B,** Individual models mounted into flask. **C,** Cavity unit prepared for mounting (note mouthguard material). **D,** Cavity unit mounted into flask.

Continued.

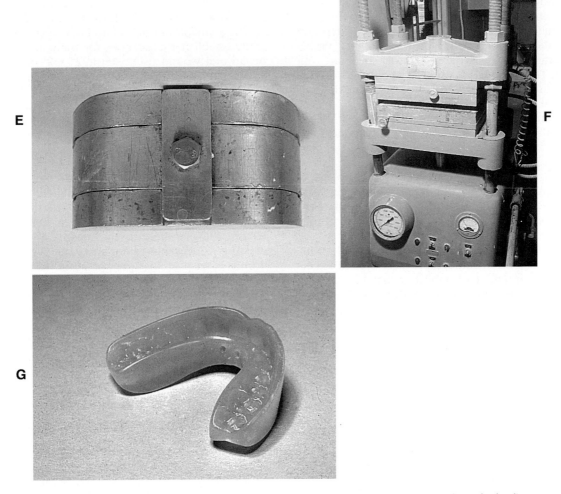

Fig. 14-34, cont'd. E, Mouthguard material inserted into closed flask. **F,** Flask inserted into hydraulic press. **G,** Bimaxillary mouthguard after finishing and polishing. (Courtesy of Allesee Orthodontic Appliances, Sturtevant, WI.)

sin, has a selection of colored, flavored, and scented EVAs. They report that by allowing athletes to personalize their appliances, there is a noticeable improvement in athlete compliance.

Recently, the use of another material has been described by Dr. Dennis N. Ranalli of the University of Pittsburgh.[71,72] Originally formulated by L.D. Caulk of Milford, Delaware, this material, known as Lite Line, was meant for soft-denture relines. According to Dr. Ranalli, one advantage this photopolymerized urethane diacrylate offers is better bonding than EVA.[36,71]

DENTAL SPORTS TRAUMA READINESS

Dental Injury Assessment

Dental injuries are seldom life-threatening and should be triaged only after more serious medical injuries. Naturally, a team physician, dentist, or trainer must first consider "ABC" injuries (airway, breathing, or circulatory), neurologic signs and symptoms, and the overall well being of the athlete. A history furnishes important infor-

mation regarding the nature and severity of an injury.[70] Where and what kind of dental or oral injury has been incurred should be determined. This would include how, when, and where did the injury occur? Was the injury witnessed? Can the athlete put his or her teeth together normally? Is there sensitivity to hot, cold, or biting pressure? When did the athlete receive a tetanus shot? Are antibiotics necessary?

If there is bleeding, an attempt to discover its source can be made in the field. A sterile 4" x 4" gauze sponge can be used to wipe away the blood. With repeated blotting and careful observation, the general source of bleeding may be identified.[18] Soft-tissue injuries are usually conspicuous. If the source of bleeding is apparently a tooth, digital palpation from a gloved hand can be used to explore and compare mobility, pain, and numbness, and detect sharp edges. Any fracture that involves more than just enamel will render the tooth sensitive to orally inhaled air. This is particularly noticeable in winter sports like ice hockey and football.[18]

The TMJ should be examined for capsular or miniscular injuries. Limitations on jaw movement and discomfort should be explored. Deviations when opening and closing, tenderness, or swelling of the affected joint should be noted. Crepitus and abnormalities of the head of the condyle can be detected by palpating externally with the index fingers over the area of the TMJ. Pinkie fingers inserted into the external auditory meati are also a good test. The patient is instructed to open, close, and go into excursions. Fractured mandibular condyles can sometimes be detected in this fashion.

TMJ traumatic injuries can be managed with cold compresses the first 24 hours, soft diet, nonsteroidal antiinflammatory medications and aspirin. Trismus, ankylosis, fracture, or dislocation of the condyle must also be considered.[34] Later, vigorous physical therapy to maintain the normal range of mandibular motion and prevent ankylosis is recommended.[49] For more information, refer to the excellent textbooks written by Dr. Harold Gelb.[29]

After clinical examination, all areas of possible traumatic injuries should be radiographed for immediate diagnostic purposes and to establish a baseline against which to compare at follow-up appointments.[17]

Dental and Oral First Aid
The contents of a dental field emergency kit will vary depending on the idiosyncrasies of the attending coach, trainer, dentist or physician, the particular sport, and the availability and sophistication of a nearby treatment facility. Contents should be planned in advance, and those items with limited shelf lives should be replaced at regular intervals to sustain trauma readiness. For example, Save-A-Tooth has a shelf life of about 2 years.

The principles of dental and oral first aid follow generally established guidelines for trauma. Direct pressure on an oral wound using sterile 2" x 2" or 4" x 4" gauze sponges is useful to achieve hemostasis and prevent the development of a hematoma. Elevation of the head is helpful. Rinsing, spitting, nose blowing, or sucking through a straw creating a negative intraoral pressure can sometimes exacerbate bleeding. If the episode continues, a decision may have to be made concerning the athlete's continued competition. Cold packs help reduce swelling, pain, and subsequent ecchymosis. Immobilization of loose or broken teeth can sometimes be achieved by gentle biting with or without a mouthguard in place. A Barton bandage is a circumferential head dressing that secures the mandible to the maxilla (Fig. 14-35). This dressing reduces movement and eases pain and suffering during transport of the patient with a suspected mandibular fracture. Medications for pain and prevention of infection may need to be prescribed in some patients.

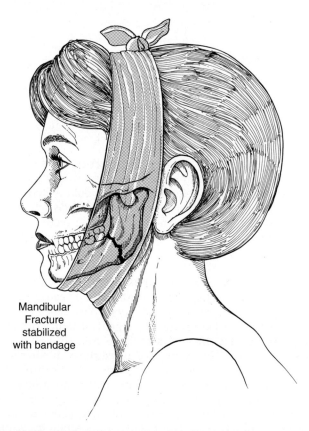

Mandibular
Fracture
stabilized
with bandage

Fig. 14-35. Barton bandage supporting the mandible for athlete transport. Illustration by Kibiuk.

REFERENCES
1. Allen M, et al: Occlusal splints (MORA) vs. placebos show no difference in strength in symptomatic subjects. Double blind cross-over study, *Can J Appl Sport Sci* 9(3):148–152, 1984.
2. Andersson L: Dentoalveolar ankylosis and associated root resorption in replanted teeth: experimental and clinical studies in monkeys and man, *Swed Dent J Supp* 56:1, 1988.
3. Andersson L, et al: Progression of root resorption following replantation of human teeth after extended extra-oral storage, *Endo Dental Traumatol* 5:38, 1989.
4. Andreasen J: Effect of extra-alveolar period and storage media upon periodontal and pulpal healing after replantation of mature permanent incisors in monkeys, *Int J Oral Surg* 10:43, 1981.
5. Andreasen J: Etiology and pathogenesis of traumatic dental injuries: a clinical study of 1298 cases, *Scand J Dent Res* 78:329, 1970.
6. Andreasen J: External root resorption: its implication in dental traumatology, paedodontics, periodontics, orthodontics and endodontics, *Int Endo J* 18:109, 1985.
7. Andreasen J: Luxation of permanent teeth due to trauma: a clinical and radiographic follow-up study of 184 injured teeth, *Scand J Dent Res* 78:273, 1970.
8. Andreasen J: *Traumatic injuries of the teeth*, ed 2, Philadelphia, 1981, WB Saunders.
9. Andreasen J, Andreasen F: *Textbook and color atlas of traumatic injuries to the teeth*, ed. 3, St. Louis, 1994, Mosby.
10. Andreasen J, Hjorting-Hansen E: Replantation of teeth, I. Radiographic and clinical study of 110 human teeth replanted after accidental loss, *Acta Odontol Scand* 24:263, 1966.
11. Andreasen J, Hjorting-Hansen E: Replantation of teeth. II. Histological study 22 replanted anterior teeth in humans, *Acta Odontol Scand* 24:287, 1966.
12. Bates R, Atkinson W: The effects of maxillary MORA's on strength and muscle efficiency tests, *J Craniomandib Pract* 1(4):37–42, 1983.
13. Blomlof L, et al: Storage of experimentally avulsed teeth in milk prior to replantation, *J Dent Res* 62:912, 1983.

14. Brotman I, Rothschild H: Report of a breakthrough in preventive dental care for a national football league team, *JADA* 88:553, 1974.

15. Burkett L, Bernstein A: Strength testing after jaw repositioning with a mandibular orthopedic appliance, *Physician Sports Med* 10(2):101–107, 1982.

16. Burkett L, Bernstein A: The effect of mandibular position on strength, reaction time and movement time on a randomly selected population, *NY State Dent J* 49(5):281–285, 1983.

17. Camp J: Diagnosis and management of sports-related injuries to the teeth, *Dent Clin North Am* 35(4):733–756, 1991.

18. Castaldi C: First aid for sports-related dental injuries, *Physician Sports Med* 15(9):81–89, 1987.

19. Castaldi C: The sports mouthguard: its use and misuse in ice hockey, safety in ice hockey vol 3, Philadelphia, 1993, ASTM STP.

20. Chaconas S, et al: A comparison of athletic mouthguard materials, *Am J Sports Med* 13(3):193–197, 1985.

21. Chiodo G, Rosenstein D: Mandibular athletic repositioning appliance and athletic performance, *JODA* Winter:31–33, 1986.

22. Costen J: Neuralgias and ear symptoms involved in general diagnosis due to mandibular joint pathology, *J Kansas Med Soc* 315–321, 1935.

23. Cvek M: A clinical report on partial pulpotomy and capping with calcium hydroxide in permanent incisors with complicated crown fractures, *J Endo* 4:232, 1978.

24. Cvek M: Endodontic treatment of traumatized teeth. In Andreasen J: *Traumatic injuries of the teeth*, ed 2, Philadelphia, 1981, WB Saunders.

25. Cvek M, et al: Treatment of non-vital permanent incisors with calcium hydroxide, *Odontol Rev* 25:43, 1974.

26. Forgione A: Strength and bite, Part I: An analytical review, *J Craniomandib Prac* 9(4):305–315, 1991.

27. Fountain SB, Camp JH: *Traumatic injuries in pathways of the pulp*, ed 6, St. Louis, 1994, CV Mosby Co.

28. Gelb H: A too-polite silence about shoddy science: dynamic strength testing and beyond, *J Craniomandib Prac* 10(1): 75–79, 1992.

29. Gelb H: *New concepts in craniomandibular and chronic pain management*, London, 1994, Mosby-Wolfe.

30. Going R, Loehman R, Chan M: Mouthguard materials: their physical and mechanical properties, *JADA* 89:132–138, 1974.

31. Granath L, Hagman G: Experimental pulpotomy in human bicuspids with reference to cutting technique, *Acta Odontol Scand*, 29:155, 1971.

32. Greenberg AM, Haug RH: *Etiology, distribution, and classification of fractures*, New York, 1993, Springer-Verlag.

33. Greenberg M, Cohen S, Springer P, et al: Mandibular position and upper body strength: a controlled clinical trial, *JADA* 103:576–579, 1981.

34. Greenberg M, Springer P: Diagnosis and management of oral injuries. In Torg J, ed: *Athletic injuries to the head, neck and face*, ed. 2, St Louis, 1991, Mosby-Year Book.

35. Grossman L, Ship I: Survival rate of replanted teeth, *Oral Surg* 29:899, 1970.

36. Guevara P, Ranalli P: Techniques for mouthguard fabrication, *Dent Clin North Am* 35:627–645, 1991.

37. Hammarstrom L, et al: Replantation of teeth & antibiotic treatment, *Endo Dental Traumatol* 2:51, 1986.

38. Hart D, et al: The effect of vertical dimension on muscular strength, *J Orthop Sports Phys Ther* 3(2):57–61, 1981.

39. Heintz W: Mouth protection for athletics today. In Godwin W, Long B, Cartwright C, eds: *The relationship of internal protection devices to athletic injuries and athletic performance*, Ann Arbor, 1982, University of Michigan.

40. Heintz W: Mouth protectors: a progress report, *JADA* 77:632, 1968.

41. Hickey J, et al: The relation of mouth protectors to cranial pressure and deformation, *JADA* 74:735–740, 1967.

42. Hildebrandt J: Dental and maxillofacial injuries, *Clin Sports Med* 1(3):449–468, 1982.

43. Hildebrandt JR, Garner-Nelson J: *Mouthguard protection for boxing*, US Olympic Committee, 1990.

44. Holland GJ, et al: Custom vs. commercial mouth guard use: effect on exercise metabolic-ventilatory response of trained distance runners, *NCSA J Applied Sports Sci Res* 3: 1989.

45. Jakush J: Divergent views: can dental therapy enhance athletic performance? *JADA* 104(3):292–298, 1982.

46. Jarvinen S: Incisal overjet and traumatic injuries to upper permanent incisors. A retrospective study. *Acta Odontal Scand* 36:359, 1978.

47. Kakehashi S, et al: The effects of surgical exposures of dental pulps in germ-free and conventional laboratory rats, *Oral Surg* 20:340, 1965.

48. Kaufman R, Kaufman A: An experimental study on the effects of the MORA on football players, *Basal Facts* 6(4): 119–126, 1984.

49. Keith D, Orden A: Orofacial athletic injuries and involvement of the temporomandibular joint, *J Mass Dental Soc* 43(4):11–15, 1994.

50. Kerr I, Lawrence: Mouth guards for the prevention of injuries in contact sports, *Sports Med* 415–427, 1986.

51. Krasner P: Treatment of tooth avulsion in the emergency department: appropriate storage and transport media, *Am J Emerg Med* 8:351, 1990.

52. Krasner P, Person P: Preserving avulsed teeth for replantation, *JADA* 123:80, 1992.

53. Krekeler G, Petsch K, Flesch-Gorlas M: Der Frakturverlauf in parodontalen Bereich, *Dtsch Zahnärztl Z* 38:355–357, 1983.

54. Kurtz M: Columbia University and those that made it the Mecca of dental education, *Bull Hist Dent* 26(2):86–103, 1978.

55. Lee-Knight C, et al: Dental injuries at the 1989 Canada Games: an epidemiological study, *JCDA* 58(10):810–815, 1992.

56. Lewis T: Incidence of fractured anterior teeth as related to their protrusion, *Angle Orthop* 29:128, 1959.

57. Lindskog S, et al: Mitosis and microorganisms in the periodontal membrane after storage in milk or saliva, *Scand J Dent Res* 91:465, 1983.

58. Linn E: Facial injuries sustained during sports and games, *J Max Fac Surg* 14:83–88, 1986.

59. Maestrello-deMoya M: Orofacial trauma and mouth-protector wear among high school varsity basketball players, *J Dent Child* 56(1):36–39, 1989.

60. McArdle W, et al: Temperomandibular joint repositioning and exercise performance: a double blind study, *Med Sci Sports Exerc* 16(3):228–233, 1984.

61. Moore M: Corrective mouth guards: performance aids or expensive placebos? *Phys Sports Med* 9(3):130, 1981.

62. Novich M, Schwartz R: The athletes mouthpiece, *Clin Proc Dent* 7(3):18–21, 1985.

63. Padilla R, Balikov S: Sports dentistry: coming of age in the '90s, *J CDA* 21:27–37, 1993.

64. Park J: Methods to improved mouthguards, First International Symposium on Biomaterials, Korea Research Institute of Chem Tech, Daedeog-Danji, Taejon, Korea, Aug 12–13, 1993: 1–18.

65. Parker M, et al: Muscle strength related to use of inter-occlusal splints, *Gen Dent* 32(2):105–109, 1984.

66. Paterson R, Watts A: Further studies on the exposed germ-free dental pulp, *Int Endo J* 20:112, 1987.

67. Pavlov H: Radiographic evaluation of the skull and facial bones, In Torg J: *Athletic injuries to the head, neck, and face*, ed 2, St. Louis, 1991, Mosby–Year Book.

68. Pinkham J, Kohn D: Epidemiology and prediction of sports-related traumatic injuries, *Dent Clin North Am* 35(4): 609–626, 1991.

69. Pollack B: Legal considerations in sports dentistry, *Dent Clin North Am* 35(4):809–829, 1991.

70. Powers M: Diagnosis and management of dentoalveolar inuries. In Fonseca R, Walker R: *Oral and maxillofacial trauma*, Philadelphia, 1991, WB Saunders.

71. Ranalli D, Guevara P: A new technique for the custom fabrication of mouthguards with photopolymerized urethane diacrylate, *Quintessence International* 23(4): 253–255, 1992.

72. Ranalli D, Guevara P: Protective mouthguards: a new technique for the custom fabrication of mouthguards with photopolymerized urethane diacrylate, *Penn Dent J* 62(1):22–24, 1995.

73. Ranalli D, Lancaster D: Attitudes of college football officials regarding NCAA mouthguard regulations and player compliance, *Public Health Dent* 53(2):96–100, 1993.

74. Ranalli D, Lancaster D: Comparative evaluation of college football officials' attitude toward NCAA mouthguard regulations and player compliance, *Pediatr Dent* 15(6):398–402, 1993.

75. Rock W, Grundy M: The effect of luxation and subluxation upon the prognosis of traumatized incisor teeth, *J Dent* 9:224, 1981.

76. Schubert M, et al: Changes in shoulder and leg strength in athletes wearing mandibular orthopedic repositioning appliances, *JADA* 108(3):334–337, 1984.

77. Schultz R: Facial injuries, ed 3, Chicago, 1988, Year Book Medical Publishers

78. Smith S: Adjusting mouthguards kinesiologically in professional football players, *NY State Dent J* 48(5):298–301, 1982.

79. Smith S: Muscular strength correlated to jaw posture and the TMJ, *NY State Dent J* 278–283, 1978.

80. Stanley H, et al: The rate of tertiary (reparative) dentin formation in the human tooth, *Oral Surg* 21:180, 1966.

81. Stenger J: Physiologic dentistry with Notre Dame athletes, *Basal Facts* 2(1):8–18, 1977.

82. Stenger J, et al: Mouthguards: protection against shock to head, neck and teeth, *JADA* 69:273–281, 1964.

83. Summers C: In personal communication to Department of Health and Human Services, Centers For Disease Control, Atlanta, GA, October 15, 1991.

84. Trope M, Friedman S: Periodontal healing of replanted dog teeth stored in Viaspan, milk, and Hanks Balanced Salt Solution, *Endo Dent Traumatol* 8:183, 1992.

85. Vegso J, et al: The effect of an orthopaedic intraoral mandibular appliance on upper body strength, *Med Sci Sports Exer* 13(2):115–116, 1981.

86. Verban E, et al: The effects of mandibular orthopedic repositioning appliance on shoulder strength, *J Craniomandib Pract* 2(3):232–237, 1984.

87. Williams M, Chaconas S, Bader P: The effect of mandibular position on appendage muscle strength, *J Prosthet Dent* 49(4):560–567, 1983.

88. Yates J, et al: Effect of a mandibular orthopedic repositioning appliance on muscular strength, *JADA* 108(2):331–333, 1984.

89. Zachrisson B, Jacobsen I: Long-term prognosis of 66 permanent anterior teeth with root fracture, *Scand J Dent Res* 83:345, 1975.

CHAPTER 15

OTORHINOLARYNGOLOGY

Gwen S. Korovin

When one thinks about sports medicine, the regions of the body encompassed by the field of otorhinolaryngology do not initially come to mind. However, many otorhinolaryngologic problems may result from a sports injury or may have a significant effect on the ability to perform various types of sports.

The head and neck area is a common site of injury in sports-related trauma. The injury may be isolated or may be associated with injuries to other parts of the body. The primary care physician or otorhinolaryngologist who cares for a patient who has sustained a sports-related injury must be aware of other associated injuries and must refer appropriately.

The head and neck area is the site of the body's breathing apparatus. Because breathing is a key aspect of achieving success in any sport, the otorhinolaryngologic region is of great importance. Any problem of the nose or throat that compromises breathing will subsequently compromise the athlete's ability.

This area of the body is also the site through which one hears. Any impairment of the ear or the hearing mechanism can have a detrimental effect on the athlete's performance. Hearing signals, whistles, or cues and communicating with teammates or colleagues is an important part of any sport.

The ability to create voice and sound is also housed within the head and neck region. The vocal mechanism is of great importance in communication between athletes. Voicing signals or cues to teammates may be a crucial part of the game. Any problem or injury that limits the ability to vocalize will therefore affect play in many types of sports.

GENERAL PRINCIPLES

Injuries

Sports injuries to the head and neck area have been a common problem for years. In managing these injuries, it is important to get the athlete back to playing the sport as soon as possible. Management should not be compromised, however, because of these pressures. Once treatment is given, the athlete must be informed of the risks of reinjury in this very vulnerable area of the body.

Fortunately, there has been a great decrease in the number and severity of these injuries, resulting from the wearing of face masks and guards, ear protectors, nose guards, and neck protection. Emphasis should be placed on the use of protective gear in all athletes, be they children or adults or professionals or amateurs.

Ear, Nose, and Throat Problems

The athlete being treated for a variety of medical problems in the head and neck area may be prescribed a variety of medications. These medications can have various side effects, leading to an alteration in the athlete's performance. The physician prescribing these medications must be aware of the demands of the various types of sports in which his or her patient may engage.

Infections of the upper respiratory system can lead to more widespread infections, locally and systemically. The physician managing a sports-related problem in another part of the body must be aware of this. This is especially important if a surgical procedure is being planned for the management of the injury. The body should be free of infection before elective surgery or treatment. If emergency or urgent care is necessary, proper coverage, including the use of antibiotics, may be needed.

EAR PROBLEMS

Trauma to the ear may occur at various sites. Fig. 15-1 shows the anatomy of the external, middle, and inner ear, any of which may be injured. The auricle, or the outer ear or pinna, is easily injured because of its prominent location on the head. An abrasion to this area must be cleansed well. Any foreign material in the wound must be removed. Antibiotic ointment may be useful to prevent local infection.

Lacerations of the auricle must be inspected carefully and repaired as soon as possible. If the injury only involves the skin, it must be carefully cleansed, and the skin can be reapproximated using 5-0 or 6-0 nylon. If the

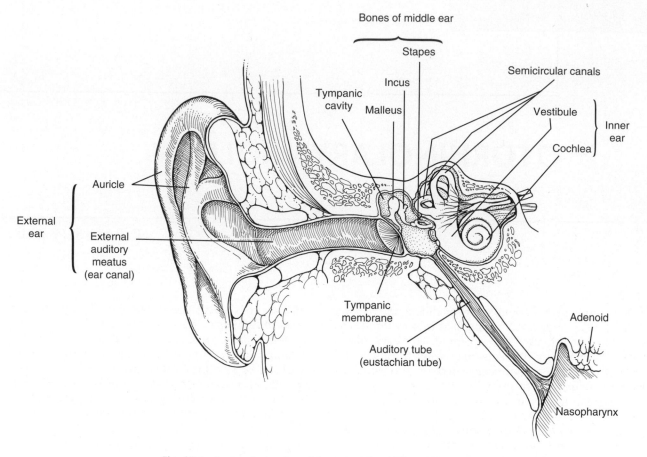

Fig. 15-1. Anatomic drawing of the external, middle, and inner ear.

injury also involves cartilage, the edges of the cartilage must be carefully approximated. This approximation should be done in a separate layer using 4-0 or 5-0 chromic. It is important to reapproximate the edges well for proper healing and good cosmetic results. If the laceration involves the external auditory canal, it may require packing to prevent stenosis.

Partial or total avulsion of the ear may also occur. If a partial avulsion is found, it can be reattached. The outcome is variable, depending on the extent of the avulsion and the available blood supply. Total avulsion, which is rare, most often results in an unfavorable outcome. The best chance for successful outcome may occur if the cartilage is buried in the postauricular region or superficial abdominal wall for use in a delayed reconstruction. Fig. 15-2 shows a healed partial avulsion that was not reattached.

Contusions of the auricle may also occur. If it is minor, the injury can be observed. If there is an area of ecchymosis, cold compresses and analgesia may be needed. If the injury is more severe, a hematoma may occur. More severe injury usually results from blunt trauma and results in sudden, painless swelling. It is a very common injury in wrestling. An auricular hematoma is seen in Fig. 15-3.

The bleeding only occurs on the anterior surface of the auricle where the skin is closely adherent to the perichondrium and cartilage.[13] Posteriorly, there is a cushion of subcutaneous fat, which acts as protection. The bleeding has been shown by Ohlsen et al[13] to occur between the perichondrium and the cartilage. If the hematoma is not drained, the blood is replaced by fibrous tissue. A cauliflower ear or perichondritis can result.

There are many different types of management published in the literature. The oldest type of management

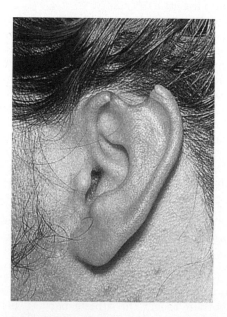

Fig. 15-2. Healed area of partial avulsion injury to the auricle without reattachment. (From Bull TR: *A color atlas of E.N.T. diagnosis*, ed 2, London, Mosby-Wolfe, 1987.)

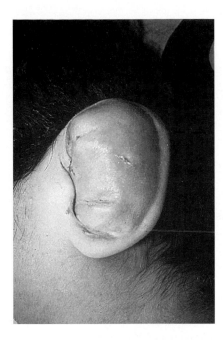

Fig. 15-3. An auricular hematoma involving the entire anterior auricle.

is that of performing needle aspiration of the hematoma. This procedure is demonstrated in Fig. 15-4. Incision and drainage are often needed, especially if there is a recurrence or the blood is clotted and fibrosed. Fig. 15-5 shows a hematoma that has been incised and drained. A bolster dressing of some type is usually needed. Various bolsters have been described, including cotton bolsters, dental rolls, and plaster molds. Occasionally a drain is left in place. Management of a cauliflower ear, which occurs rarely, requires excising and thinning of the deformed cartilage. An example of a cauliflower ear is seen in Fig. 15-6.

Perichondritis or chondritis may also occur, as seen in Fig. 15-7. The symptoms include pain, fever, and erythema and fluctuation of the affected part of the auricle. Management may include intravenous antibiotics. Chondritis can cause necrotic cartilage to develop, which must be débrided.

Thermal injury to the auricle may also occur. The pinna has a prominent exposed position on the head. It is vulnerable because of its poor insulation, its minimal subcutaneous tissue, and its tenuous distal blood supply. Frostbite can occur rapidly with wind and cold exposure during winter sports.

In its early stages, frostbite causes numbness of the pinna. Pallor and edema may occur with thawing, and vesicles and bullae may form. Cellular destruction and small vessel injury may cause necrosis and infection to occur in the more severe cases.

Management involves quick, but gentle rewarming. Analgesics may be needed. Blebs need sterile aspiration. If necrosis occurs, surgical débridement or antibiotic treatment may be necessary.

Sunburn may also cause significant problems. The superior portion of the pinna is exposed to direct sunlight and mild-to-severe burns may occur. Mild burns can be managed with cool compresses and emollients. More severe burns may result in erythema, pain, edema, and blistering. Infection can ensue. Management may include corticosteroids and possibly antibiotics.

In addition to trauma of the external ear, trauma may also have significant effects on the middle and inner ear. Blast injuries to the ear often occur during sports activities. Of 91 cases of blast injuries to the ear studied in Israel, 31 resulted from sports-related activities.[1] Sports accidents and ball games accounted for 13 of these cases, and swimming and water sport activities accounted for the other 18. The swimming accidents represent a special group because these injuries are often associated with water contamination of the ear. Problems that oc-

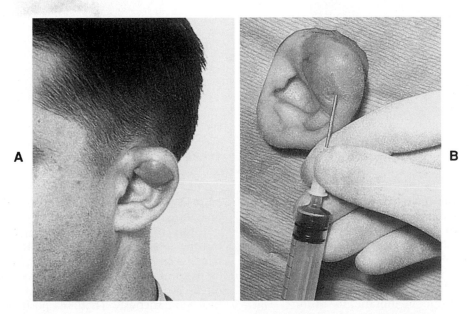

Fig. 15-4. A, Auricular hematoma of the upper auricle. **B,** Needle aspiration of the hematoma for drainage. (From Bull TR: *A color atlas of E.N.T. diagnosis,* ed 2, London, Mosby-Wolfe, 1987.)

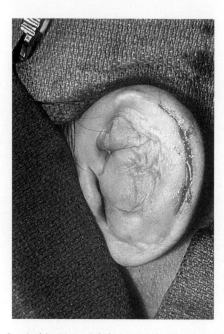

Fig. 15-5. Surgical incision and drainage of an auricular hematoma.

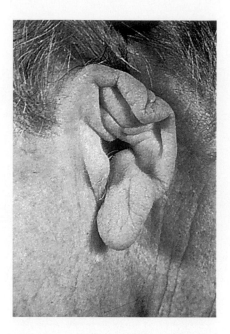

Fig. 15-6. Cauliflower ear after repeated septal hematomas that were untreated. (From Bull TR: *A color atlas of E.N.T. diagnosis*, ed 2, London, Mosby-Wolfe, 1987.)

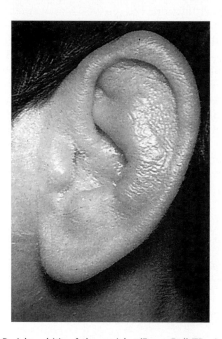

Fig. 15-7. Perichondritis of the auricle. (From Bull TR: *A color atlas of E.N.T. diagnosis*, ed 2, London, Mosby-Wolfe, 1987.)

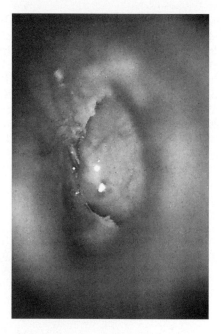

Fig. 15-8. Large tympanic membrane perforation with underlying middle ear cavity seen. (From Bull TR: *A color atlas of E.N.T. diagnosis*, ed 2, London, Mosby-Wolfe, 1987.)

curred in these 31 cases included hearing loss, earaches, tinnitus, vertigo, and purulent otorrhea.

The most common middle ear injury is perforation of the tympanic membrane which can result from penetrating injuries, blast injuries, or blunt trauma. A sudden blow that seals the external auditory meatus may cause a significant increase of ear pressure in the canal and cause the tympanic membrane to rupture. Fig. 15-8 shows a perforation of a tympanic membrane and

Fig. 15-9 shows a perforation with an associated hematoma.

Injury to the tympanic membrane may cause pain, hearing loss, bleeding, and possibly dizziness. An otoscopic examination is necessary, and audiogram should be performed. The ear must be kept dry. Antibiotics are often used prophylactically. Most traumatic perforations heal spontaneously. There is a positive correlation in the literature between the size of the tympanic membrane

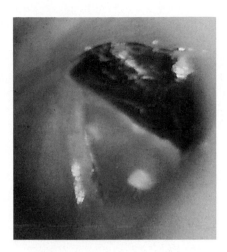

Fig. 15-9. Tympanic membrane perforation with associated hematoma. (From Bull TR: *A color atlas of E.N.T. diagnosis*, ed 2, London, Mosby-Wolfe, 1987.)

perforation and the recovery rate. If the perforation does not close, a tympanoplasty may be performed. This procedure would be desirable for either improving hearing or preventing infections in the nonhealing perforations.

Trauma may result in injury to the ossicular chain, causing a permanent conductive hearing loss. This hearing loss can occur in conjunction with a tympanic membrane perforation. An audiogram is needed for the evaluation. Middle ear exploration and repair may be necessary for this type of injury.

Trauma to the inner ear may be caused by blast or penetrating injuries. A labyrinth concussion may result from a severe blow to the head, causing either temporary or permanent dysfunction of either the cochlea or vestibular labyrinth or both. This concussion can result in sensorineural hearing loss or in mild-to-severe vertigo. Evaluation includes audiogram and possibly electronystagmogram (ENG). Management may include observation, antivertiginous medications, and avoidance of positions that induce the vertigo. Exercises designed specifically for the inner ear balance mechanism may be helpful in chronic cases.

Trauma may result in a perilymphatic fistula, which is a fistula between the middle and inner ears, resulting in a leakage of perilymphatic fluid. Symptoms may include the sudden onset of vertigo, nystagmus, or sensorineural hearing loss. Diagnosis is made by symptoms and an audiologic evaluation. Treatment is primarily observation and bedrest. The condition may require exploration of the middle ear and closure of the leak. Although some otologic surgeons do advocate immediate exploration, others believe this exploration may be of questionable long-term value.

Noise-induced trauma is another risk of certain sports activities. Rifle shooting is one example. The trauma may be temporary or permanent. Tinnitus can also occur. Management includes observation and subsequent ear protection to prevent further injury.

Severe blows to the head during sports activities can result in temporal bone fractures. This injury is often associated with other neurologic injuries. Fractures may re-

sult in conductive hearing loss caused by tympanic membrane perforation, hemotympanum or ossicular chain disruption, sensorineural hearing loss, facial nerve injuries, or cerebrospinal fluid otorrhea. Diagnosis is made by computed tomography scans and magnetic resonance imaging. Management depends on the extent of the injuries.

Infections in the ear may result from sports activities or impact ability to participate in the sport. External otitis or "swimmers ear" is an infection of the external ear canal. It may occur when there is local trauma to the skin of the external canal or the ear is in a hot and humid environment. Water can be a source of bacteria.

Symptoms of an otitis externa include mild-to-severe pain in the canal, which often seems to worsen when pulling on the auricle; itching; a feeling of fullness; hearing loss; and enlarged lymph nodes in the periauricular region. Examination of the ear reveals erythema and edema of the external ear canal with a varying amount of white, yellow, green, or black debris. The external canal may swell shut. The infection can be caused by different types of bacteria, including *Pseudomonas aeruginosa* and *Staphylococcus aureus*, and various types of fungi. Otitis externa with fungal debris is seen in Fig. 15-10. Management includes suctioning of debris and topical application of drops. Systemic antibiotics may be needed. A wick may be placed in the external canal if there is too much swelling and the drops cannot penetrate.

Otitis media, or middle ear infection, can also occur. Otitis media is an inflammation of the tympanic membrane and middle ear mucosa. Symptoms include pain, hearing loss, possible otorrhea, and possible vertigo. Examination may show erythema and bulging of the tympanic membrane. Purulent drainage may be seen in the external canal. Management includes antibiotics and analgesia.

Serous otitis media can also occur. Serous otitis media is a collection of fluid behind the tympanic membrane. It is seen with or after acute otitis media and it is often seen with barotuma.

Labyrinthitis may result from infection of the inner ear. It is usually caused by a virus, but rarely it is caused by a bacterial infection. The condition causes vertigo in most patients, and it is almost always self limited. Man-

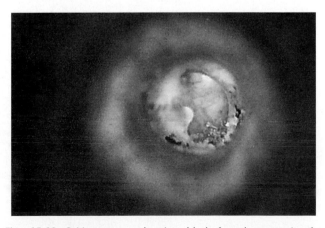

Fig. 15-10. Otitis externa showing black fungal spores in the external auditory canal. (From Bull TR: *A color atlas of E.N.T. diagnosis*, ed 2, London, Mosby-Wolfe, 1987.)

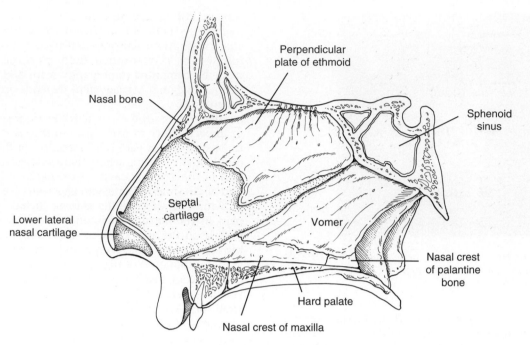

Fig. 15-11. Anatomy of the nose.

agement includes antivertiginous medications, such as meclizine and cyproheptadine, and supportive care.

NASAL PROBLEMS

Like the external ear, the nose occupies a prominent, vulnerable position on the head and is the site of some common sports-related problems. External trauma to the nose often results in epistaxis. If the nose is injured man-

ually or by an object such as a ball or puck, bleeding may occur. Figs. 15-11 and 15-12 illustrate nose anatomy and vascularity.

Most cases of bleeding cease spontaneously. Initial management is compression of the soft part of the nose for 5 to 10 minutes. Ice applied externally may be helpful for vasoconstriction. Topical vasoconstrictors, such as phenylephrine-containing nasal sprays, may be helpful. If bleeding occurs, the patient should lean forward to

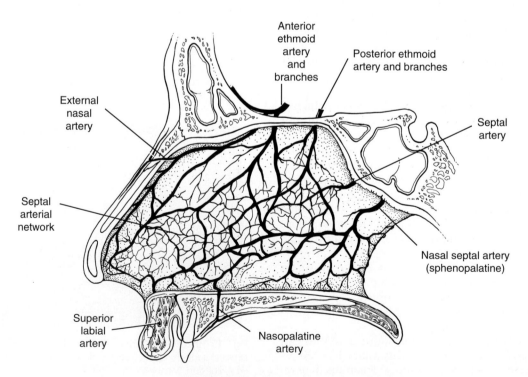

Fig. 15-12. Vascularity of the nose.

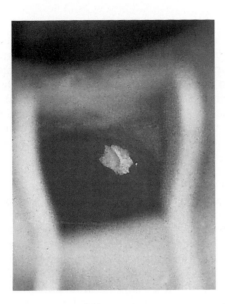

Fig. 15-13. Nasal septum viewed after application of silver nitrate to a bleeding spot. (From Bull TR: *A color atlas of E.N.T. diagnosis,* ed 2, London, Mosby-Wolfe, 1987.)

avoid swallowing the blood. Rarely, a roll of cotton placed under the upper lip may compress the labial artery and control bleeding.

If bleeding continues, the area must be examined to determine if the sight is anterior or posterior. A majority of nose bleeds occur on the anterior septum from a group of vessels known as Kiesselbach's plexus. Anatomic deformities of the anterior septum, including septal deviation and spurs, may predispose to this problem. Allergies or upper respiratory infections may also be contributory. Nasal cautery using silver nitrate or electrocautery may be necessary if the bleeding site is identified. Fig. 15-13 shows an area of the septum cauterized with silver nitrate.

If the bleeding site is either not controlled well with cautery, too posterior, or not identifiable, nasal packing may be necessary. Different types of packing include vaseline gauze strips, merocel packs, oxycel, and Gelfoam. Significant bleeding may require the use of a nasal catheter. Posterior bleeds will require a posterior pack and hospitalization. Rarely, surgical ligation of the bleeding vessels is necessary. An algorithm to help guide the management of epistaxis is seen in Fig. 15-14.

Fig. 15-14. Algorithm for the management of nose bleeds.

```
              Epistaxis [Nose Bleeds]
                       |
                       v
             Compression for 10 minutes
                       Ice
            Nasal Sprays [Vasoconstrictors]
                       |
                       v If continues to bleed

                   Locate site
              /                    \
             v                      v

   Anterior [90%]            Posterior [10%]
        |                           |
        v                           v
                             Place Packing
 Apply Cautery [Silver Nitrate]
               [Electrical]        May Use:
        |
        v If not effective         - Well placed vaseline gauze or
                                     merocel
 Place Packing [Unilateral]        - Posterior Pack
               [Bilateral]               Conventional
                                             [Rolled Gauze]
 May Use:                                Foley Type
                                   - Epistat
          - Vaseline Gauze                 |
          - Merocel Packs                  v
          - Oxycel                 Admit to Hospital
          - Gelfoam                   Monitoring
          - Nasal Catheters                O2
                                       Pack x3 days
          |    Remove in 2-3 days
          v                                |
 If bleeding persists:                     v
                                   If bleeding persists:
          Posterior Packs
          and/or Surgical               Surgical Management
          Management
                                   - Ligation of Anterior and/or
                                     Posterior Ethmoidal Arteries
                                   - Ligation of Int. Maxillary
                                     Artery
                                   - Others
```

Nasal fractures may occur in the context of sports activities either from manual trauma or being struck by an object. Diagnosis is made by the occurrence of epistaxis, observed external displacement of the nasal bones, localized bone tenderness, obstruction of the nasal airway, deformity, or swelling of the septum. Fig. 15-15 shows a fracture of the nasal bone.

Early treatment of the fracture is most important. Ice should be applied immediately. The epistaxis must be controlled. Simple reduction of the fracture can be performed in the first 1 to 2 hours. After several hours, increased swelling occurs. To then perform an adequate reduction, a wait of 3 to 5 days until the swelling subsides is necessary. A closed reduction is possible within 7 to 10 days of the injury. After this time, healing has occurred, and a wait of at least 1 month is needed to do an open reduction of the fracture. Nasal fractures in children should be reduced within 4 days. A displaced nasal fracture has the best chance of healing if a closed reduction is performed. The reduction may be done under a local anesthesia or a general anesthesia. Children usually require a general anesthetic. Once the bones are realigned, it may be necessary to place external tape, a splint, or packing. In the case of a comminuted or compound fracture, an open reduction may be necessary in the early stages after the injury. Open techniques in children should be conservative.

If the force of impact is greatest over the nasal bridge, injury to the mid-nasal bone may occur. There is no effective way to perform a closed reduction on this type of injury. Callous formation may occur, and this would require open reduction if so desired.

More extensive injury to the nasal region could cause fracture of the ethmoid bone or medial orbital wall. Injury to the roof of the ethmoid or cribriform plate could potentially cause a cerebrospinal fluid leak or anosmia. One case of pneumocephalus has been reported after a water jet injury to the nose resulting from a water skiing fall.[4] Injury could occur to the nasolacrimal apparatus, leading to persistent tearing of the eye, or to the medial canthal tendon, leading to pseudohypertelorism.

In addition to nasal fractures, injury to the nose could cause soft-tissue injuries. Contusions and abrasions require gentle cleansing. Bandaid or Steri Strip application may be needed, with possible application of antibiotic ointment. Ice compresses may be useful to minimize swelling.

Laceration and avulsion injuries may occur. These must be inspected for underlying nasal skeletal injury, and careful cleansing and suturing may be necessary.

A study performed in Oxford, England evaluating 50 consecutive children with nasal injuries revealed that 34% resulted from sports trauma.[6] Many of these injuries were abrasions or lacerations, however, 19 children did have skeletal injuries. Many of the fractures were of the greenstick variety and easily could have escaped diagnosis. In other fractures, there was little external deformity and a large disruption to the internal architecture. The study states the need for careful examination in children and adults when nasal injuries result from sports-related activities.

Another serious type of nasal injury is a septal hematoma, which may occur in conjunction with fractures or independently. In this injury, blood collects between the septal cartilage or bone and their mucosal covering. The hematoma deprives the cartilage of the blood supply.

Examination of the nose may reveal edema and ecchymoses of the septum with narrowing of the airway, and bulging into the nasal cavity may be seen. There is usually no bleeding externally. Nasal obstruction is noted. The presence of septal hematoma requires emergency treatment. Prompt drainage should be performed by either needle aspiration or by an open procedure. Placement of a drain may be necessary, and packing may be placed, dependent on the extent of the condition.

If the hematoma is not drained, a septal abscess may result, which can lead to necrosis of the septal cartilage and a subsequent saddle nose deformity.

Although septal hematomas are uncommon in children, they can cause devascularization of large segments of cartilage, on which the structural support and future nasal growth depend, when they do occur. Therefore, nasal injuries in children must be carefully examined to rule out this condition. Additionally, untreated septal abscess could lead to development of meningitis or cavernous sinus thrombosis.

Besides trauma, rhinitis is a very common nasal problem in sports and athletic events. Different types of nasal inflammation may be present and cause difficulties for the athlete. Rhinitis resulting from infection can cause nasal obstruction, nasal drainage, epistaxis, and headache. Allergic rhinitis may also cause these problems.

Vasomotor rhinitis could lead to persisting nasal drainage. Rhinitis medicamentosa causes nasal obstruction, dryness, and epistaxis. Nasal polyposis could lead to breathing problems and subsequent infection. Mucosal atrophy could also cause nasal obstruction and dry-

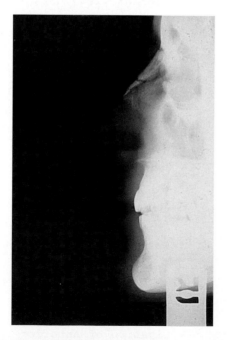

Fig. 15-15. Nasal fracture of the mid-nasal bone with minimal displacement.

ness. Endocrinologic abnormalities and hormonal and drug effects could significantly alter nasal physiology.

Changes in nasal anatomy and physiology caused by inflammation, infection, or other medical conditions could lead to difficulties in breathing, subsequently causing decreased oxygenation to the entire body. Decreased oxygenation will have a detrimental effect on the athlete's ability to perform.

In addition to the athlete's own anatomy and physiology, the environment in which he or she endeavors to perform the sport may have a significant effect on the nose. Cold air, polluted air, and extreme temperature or weather changes may affect the nasal airway. Sulfates, ozone, and particulate matter can also cause problems. Exposure to formaldehydes, glues, paints, cleaner, and vinyls such as in gymnasiums could have detrimental effects. The athlete could subsequently develop a variety of problems including rhinitis, sinusitis, nasal polyposis, eustachian tube dysfunction, and epistaxis.

Management of various forms of rhinitis may include the use of antihistamines, decongestants, cromolyn nasal sprays, steroid nasal sprays, and immunotherapy. Potential side effects of these must be considered when prescribing to the athlete.

A new concept in easing nasal congestion caused by structural problems or rhinitis is now used by many athletes. National Football League players have been shown wearing Breathe Right™ strips (CNS, Inc., Minneapolis, MN) across their noses. Breathe Right™ is a rigid drug-free strip that resembles an elongated butterfly-type bandage, and is illustrated in Fig. 15-16. It is said to pull open the nasal passages gently, increasing the flow of oxygen to the lungs. Breathe Right™ was approved for marketing by the Food and Drug Administration in 1993.[12] The company claims that Breathe Right™ reduces nasal airway resistance by up to 31%. Besides the National Football League players, many other athletes are using this latest trend to ease their congestion. With its continued use, more will be learned about the potential benefit of this product and applications to other types of nasal aids for the athlete.

THROAT AND LARYNX PROBLEMS

The throat is an area that is rarely involved in sports problems or injuries. An infection of the throat or tonsils, with its accompanying pain and fever, can be detrimental to an athlete's performance. Laryngitis can cause an inability to communicate with teammates or peers.

The larynx, however, is an area that has been associated with a variety of sports-related injuries. The thyroid cartilage, which serves as a shield to the larynx, can be injured with enough external force.

Blunt trauma to the larynx occurs most frequently in high-velocity sports, such as hockey, bicycling, and motorcycling. Direct trauma can actually crush the larynx and upper trachea, causing neck pain, odynophagia, and dyspnea. Even in a simpler laryngeal fracture, pain, tenderness, and swelling over the anterior neck can occur. Fig. 15-17 shows a tracheal cartilage fracture. In a simple fracture or a crush injury, hemoptysis and hoarseness or aphonia may occur. Examination of the neck may reveal ecchymosis or crepitus of the neck. There may be absence of the Adam's apple with injury of the thyroid cartilage or underlying structures.

Any injury to this area requires immediate examination. Initial evaluation must rule out airway obstruction. It may be necessary to intubate or perform a tracheostomy. Radiographs need to be taken to evaluate the extent of the injury. Plain films may give some useful information. Computed tomography scans will be needed for more detail. The throat and larynx must be visualized to look for mucosal tears, bleeding, and submucosal contusions or hematomas. There must be continued observation for development of airway obstruction of gradual onset.

Management of a nondisplaced fracture is observation. More severe injuries may require a thorough endoscopy. It may be necessary to do neck exploration and fix the laryngeal fragments.

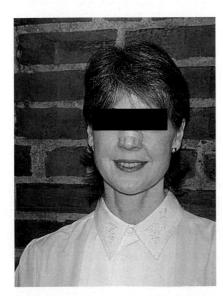

Fig. 15-16. Photograph of a Breathe Right™ strip placed across the nasal dorsum.

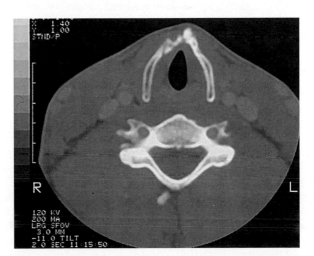

Fig. 15-17. Comminuted fracture of the tracheal cartilage. This patient also suffered a hemorrhage of his underlying vocal cord.

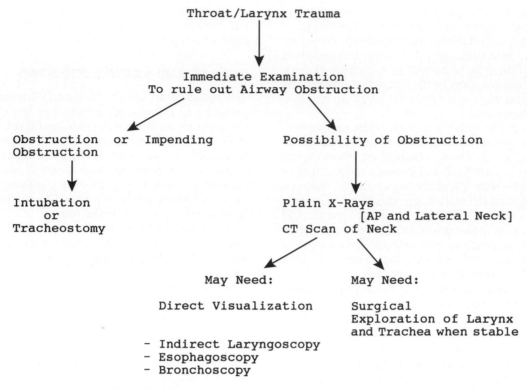

Fig. 15-18. Algorithm for the management of obstructed airway.

Penetrating trauma to the larynx falls under the category of "freak accidents" in sport events. The trauma may be accompanied by neck pain, dysphagia, dyspnea, crepitus, hemoptysis, or a change in the voice. Immediate management includes a careful check of the airway, clearing the airway of secretions, and performing lateral neck radiographs. Additional management may involve observation, endoscopy, or surgical exploration and subsequent repair, as in the management of blunt laryngeal trauma.

An algorithm for the management of airway obstruction from either blunt or penetrating trauma is seen in Fig. 15-18.

NECK INJURIES

Sports-related injuries to the neck range from superficial ones to those that are potentially life threatening. Minor abrasions or lacerations may result from blunt trauma, requiring simple local first-aid. A hematoma could occur, causing pain, swelling, and ecchymoses. Although most of these are self-limited, some may enlarge progressively. A persistent hemorrhage resulting from bleeding from a large vessel could cause continued difficulties, and intubation or tracheotomy may be needed to protect the airway. An angiogram may be necessary to determine the bleeding site, and hematoma may require drainage and vessel ligation. Potential complications include cranial nerve deficits and the formation of arteriovenous fistulas.

Penetrating trauma to the neck during sports injuries is very rare. Immediate evaluation of the airway is mandatory, and neurologic evaluation is important. If there is significant injury to the vasculature of the neck, excessive hemorrhage, absent pulses, and an expanding neck mass may be seen. Management includes pressure to the bleeding site, an angiogram, and probable surgical exploration. Although some experts believe that any penetrating injury of the neck that occurs deep to the platysma muscle mandates surgical exploration, others believe this procedure needs to be performed selectively.

SUMMARY

Otorhinolaryngology is an important area in the vast field of sports medicine. Problems of the ears, nose, throat, and neck can cause significant difficulties for the athlete. Trauma to these areas of the body can easily occur during any sports activities. Primary care physicians, otolaryngologists, orthopedists, and others who care for these athletes must work together to provide comprehensive medical care.

REFERENCES
1. Berger G, Finkelstein Y, Harell M: Nonexplosive blast injury of the ear. *Laryngol Otol* 108:395–398, 1994.
2. Carter RL: Prevention of springboard and platform diving injuries, *Clin Sports Med* 5(1):185–194, 1986.
3. Chandler JR: Avulsion of the larynx and pharynx as the result of a water ski rope injury, *Arch Otolaryng* 96:365–367, 1972.

4. David SK, Guarisco JL, Coulon JR: Pneumocephalus secondary to a high pressure water injury to the nose, *Arch Otolaryngol Head Neck Surgery* 116:1435–1436, 1990.

5. Dominguez RH: Water polo injuries, *Clin Sports Med* 5(1):169–183, 1986.

6. East CA, O'Donaghue G: Acute nasal trauma in children, *J Pediatr Surg* 22(4):308–310, 1987.

7. Fife D, Barancik JI: Northeastern Ohio trauma study III: incidence of fractures, *Ann Emerg Med* 14(3):244–248, 1985.

8. Griffin CS: Wrestler's ear: pathophysiology and treatment, *Ann Plast Surg* 28(2):131–139, 1992.

9. Handler SD, Wetmore R: Otolaryngologic injuries, *Clin Sports Med* 1(3):431–447, 1982.

10. Katz RM: Rhinitis in the athlete, *J Allergy Clin Immunol* 73 (5 pt 2):708–711, 1984.

11. Lucente FE, Defreitas J: Epistaxis. In Lucente FE, Sobol SM, eds: *Essential Otolaryngology*, New York, 1988, Raven Press.

12. Morrison J: Lateral radical chic. In *New York Times*, Styles section, p.43, Jan. 29, 1995.

13. Ohlsen L, Skoog T, Sohn S: Pathogenesis of cauliflower ear: an experimental study in rabbits, *Scand J Plast Reconstr Surg* 9:34–39, 1975.

14. Sarti EJ, Lucente FE: Ear trauma. In Lucente FE, Sobol SM, ed: *Essential Otolaryngology*, New York, 1988, Raven Press.

15. Starkhammar H, Olofsson J: Facial fractures: a review of 992 cases with special reference to incidence and aetiology, *Clin Otolaryngol* 7:405–409, 1982.

CHAPTER 16

THE CERVICAL SPINE, SPINAL CORD, AND BRACHIAL PLEXUS

Joseph S. Torg

This chapter will present clear, concise guidelines for the classification, evaluation, and management of athletic injuries that occur to the cervical spine, spinal cord, and brachial plexus.

Although all athletic injuries require careful attention, evaluation and management of these injuries require particular caution. The actual or potential involvement of the nervous system creates a potentially high-risk situation in which the margin for error is low. An accurate diagnosis is imperative because the clinical picture is not always representative of the potential seriousness of the problem. In general, athletic injuries to the cervical spine, spinal cord, and brachial plexus can be classified into two major groups: (1) catastrophic and potentially catastrophic, or those injuries in which permanent neurologic sequelae is a major factor; and (2) noncatastrophic, or those in which the major problem is the potential for chronic nonneurologic disability.

EMERGENCY MANAGEMENT

There are several principles that should be considered by those responsible for athletes who may sustain injuries to cervical spine and spinal cord.

(1) The team physician or trainer should be designated as the person responsible for supervising on-the-field management of a potentially serious injury. This person is the "captain" of the medical team.

(2) Planning must ensure the availability of all necessary emergency equipment at the site of potential injury. At a minimum, a spineboard, stretcher, and equipment necessary for the initiation and maintenance of cardiopulmonary resuscitation should be included.

(3) Planning must ensure the availability of a properly equipped ambulance and a hospital equipped and staffed to handle emergency neurologic problems.

(4) Planning must ensure immediate availability of a telephone for communicating with the hospital emergency room, ambulance, and other responsible individuals in case of an emergency.

Treating the spine-injured athlete is a process that should not be done hastily or haphazardly. Being prepared to handle this situation is the best way to prevent actions that could convert a repairable injury into a catastrophe. The necessary equipment should be readily accessible, in good operating condition, and all assisting personnel should be trained to use it properly. On-the-job training in an emergency situation is inefficient. Everyone should know what must be done beforehand, so that on a signal the "game plan" can be put into effect.

A means of transporting the athlete must be immediately available in a high-risk sport, such as football, and on-call in other sports. The medical facility must be alerted to the athlete's condition and estimated time of arrival so that adequate preparation can be made.

Having the proper equipment is essential! A spineboard is necessary and is the best means of supporting the body in a rigid position. It is essentially a full-body splint. By splinting the body, the risk of aggravating a spinal cord injury, which must always be suspected in the unconscious athlete, is reduced. In football, bolt cutters and a sharp knife or scalpel are also essential if it becomes necessary to remove the face mask. A telephone must be available to call for assistance and to notify the medical facility. Oxygen should be available and is usually carried by the ambulance and rescue squads, although it is rarely required in an athletic setting. Rigid cervical collars and other external immobilization devices can be helpful if properly used. Manual stabilization of the head and neck is recommended if other means are not available.

Properly trained personnel must know who is in charge. Everyone should know how to perform cardiopulmonary resuscitation and how to move and transport the athlete. Personnel should know where emergency equipment is located, how to use it, and the procedure for activating the emergency support system. Individuals should be assigned specific tasks beforehand so that duplication of effort is eliminated. Being well prepared helps to alleviate indecisiveness and second-guessing.

Prevention of further injury is the single most important objective. Any action that could possibly cause further injury should not be taken. The first step should be to immobilize the head and neck by supporting them in a stable position, and then, in the following order, check for breathing, pulse, and level of consciousness (Fig. 16-1).

If the victim is breathing, the mouthguard should be removed, if present, and the airway maintained. It is necessary to remove the face mask only if the respiratory situation is threatened or unstable or if the athlete re-mains unconscious for a prolonged period. The chin strap should be left on.

Once it is established that the athlete is breathing and has a pulse, neurologic status should be evaluated. The level of consciousness, response to pain, pupillary response, and unusual posturing, flaccidity, rigidity, or weakness should be noted.

At this point, the situation should be maintained until transportation is available. If the athlete is face down, change his or her position to face up by logrolling him or her onto a spineboard (Fig. 16-2). Gentle longitudinal traction should be exerted to support the head without attempting to correct alignment, and no attempt should be made to remove the helmet. There is controversy between emergency medicine physicians and technicians on one hand and team physicians and athletic trainers on the other. Existing emergency medical services guidelines mandate removal of protective headgear before transport of an individual suspected of having a cervical spine injury. These guidelines were implemented with full-face motorcycle helmets in mind to facilitate airway accessibility and application of cervical spine-immobilizing devices. Such a procedure contradicts the long-standing principle adhered to by team physicians and athletic trainers of leaving the helmet in place on the football player suspected of having a cervical spine injury until

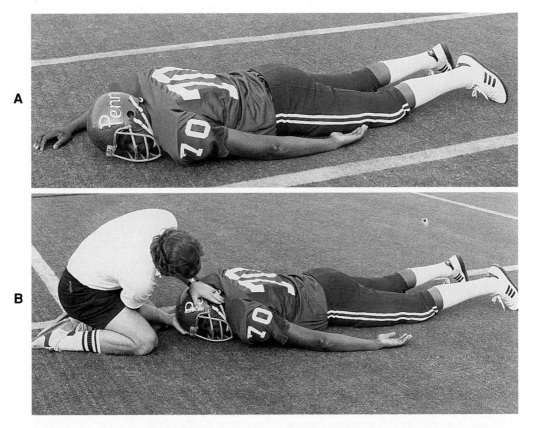

Fig. 16-1. A, Athlete with suspected cervical spine injury may or may not be unconscious. However, those who are unconscious should be treated as though they had a significant neck injury. **B,** Immediate manual immobilization of the head and neck unit. First, check for breathing. From Torg JS, ed: *Athletic injuries to the head, neck and face,* Philadelphia, 1991, Mosby–Year Book.

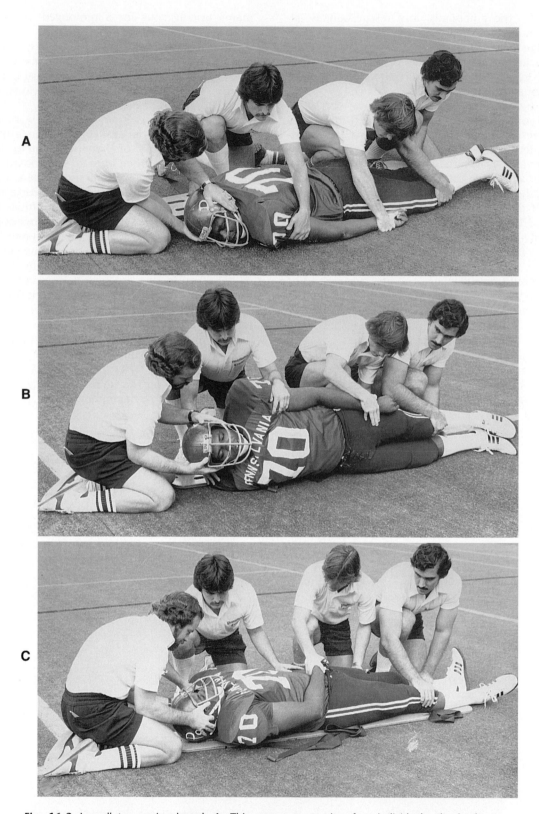

Fig. 16-2. Logroll to a spine board. **A,** This maneuver requires four individuals: the leader to immobilize the head and neck and to command the medical support team, and three individuals who are positioned at the shoulders, hips, and lower legs. **B,** The leader uses the crossed-arm technique to immobilize the head. This technique allows the leader's arms to "unwind" as the three assistants roll the athlete onto the spine board. **C,** The three assistants maintain body alignment during the roll. From Torg JS, ed: *Athletic injuries to the head, neck and face,* Philadelphia, 1991, Mosby–Year Book.

he or she is transported to a definitive medical facility. It must be emphasized that this particular problem is of more than academic interest. Specifically, there have been occasions where emergency medical technicians under the direction of the emergency room physicians unfamiliar with the nuances of the relationship between helmet, shoulder pads, and the injured cervical spine have precipitated in on-site turf battles by refusing to move the injured player before helmet removal. Such episodes represent more than an honest difference of opinion, and are clearly detrimental to the well-being of the injured player. It is the view of this author that removal of the football helmet and shoulder pads on-site exposes the potentially injured spine to unnecessary and awkward manipulation and disruption of the immobilizing capacity of the helmet and shoulder pads. Also, removal of the helmet subjects a potentially unstable spine to a hyperlordotic deformity. If there are no problems with respiration, the helmet of a football player suspected of having a cervical spine injury should remain on until he or she reaches a definitive medical facility.

If the athlete is not breathing or stops breathing, the airway must be established. If face down, he or she must be brought to a face-up position. The safest and easiest way to accomplish this is to logroll the athlete into a face-up position. In an ideal situation, the medical-support team has five members: the leader, who controls the head and gives the commands only; three members top roll; and one to help lift and carry when necessary. If time permits and the spineboard is on the scene, the athlete should be rolled directly onto it. However, breathing and circulation are more important at this point.

With all medical-support team members in position, the athlete is rolled toward the assistant—one at the shoulders, one at the hips, and one at the knees. They must maintain the body in line with the head and spine during the roll. The leader maintains immobilization of the head by applying slight traction and by using the crossed-arm technique. This technique allows the arms to unwind during the roll (see Fig. 16-2).

The face mask must be removed from the helmet before rescue breathing can be initiated. The type of mask that is attached to the helmet determines the method of removal. Bolt cutters are used with the older single- and double-bar masks. The newer masks that are attached with plastic loops should be removed by cutting the loops with a sharp knife or scalpel, and the entire mask should be removed so that it does not interfere with further rescue efforts.

Once the athlete has been moved to a face-up position, breathing and pulse should be evaluated quickly. If there is still no breathing or if breathing has stopped, the airway must be established. The jawthrust technique is the safest first approach to open the airway of a victim who has a suspected neck injury because in most cases, it can be accomplished by the rescuer grasping the angles of the victim's lower jaw and lifting with both hands, one on each side, displacing the mandible forward while tilting the head backward.

The rescuer's elbows should rest on the surface on which the victim is lying.

If the jaw thrust is not adequate, the head tilt–jaw lift should be substituted. Care must be exercised not to overextend the neck. The fingers of one hand are placed under the lower jaw on the bony part near the chin and lifted to bring the chin forward, which supports the jaw and helps to tilt the head back. The fingers must not compress the soft tissue under the chin, which might obstruct the airway. The other hand presses on the victim's forehead to tilt the head back.

The transportation team should be familiar with handling a victim with a cervical spine injury, and they should be receptive to taking orders from the team physician or trainer. It is extremely important not to lose control of the athlete's care; therefore, the team physician or trainer should be familiar with the transportation crew that is used. In an athletic situation, arrangements with an ambulance service should be made before the event.

Lifting and carrying the athlete requires five individuals: four to lift and the leader to maintain immobilization of the head. The leader initiates all actions with clear, loud, verbal commands (Fig. 16-3).

The same guidelines apply to the choice of a medical facility as to the choice of an ambulance; it should be equipped and staffed to handle an emergency head or neck injury. There should be a neurosurgeon and an orthopedic surgeon to meet the athlete on arrival. Radiographic facilities should be standing by.

Once the athlete is in a medical facility and permanent immobilization measures are instituted, the helmet is removed. The chin strap may be unfastened and discarded. The athlete's head is supported at the occiput by one person while the leader spreads the earflaps and pulls the helmet off in a straight line with the spine (Fig. 16-4).

Despite the advent of such high-tech imaging modalities as computed axial tomography and magnetic resonance imaging, the initial radiographic examination of a patient with suspected or actual cervical spine trauma remains routine. The preliminary study, while immobilization of the head, neck, and trunk are maintained, includes an anteroposterior and lateral examination of C1–C7. If a major fracture, subluxation, dislocation, or evidence of instability are not evident, the remainder of the routine examination, including open mouth and oblique views, should be obtained. Depending on the neurologic and comfort status of the patient, lateral flexion and extension views should be obtained at some point. Computed tomography and magnetic resonance imaging may provide more detailed information, although horizontally oriented fractures and subtle subluxation are best identified on the routine radiographs. The choice of imaging technique will depend on the results of routine examination, neurologic status of the patient, preference of the responsible physician, and availability of the imaging modalities.

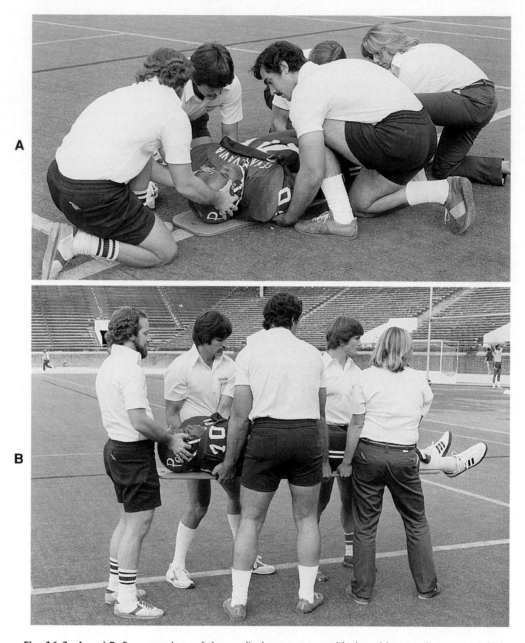

Fig. 16-3. A and **B,** Four members of the medical support team lift the athlete on the command of the leader. The leader maintains manual immobilization of the head. The spine board is not recommended as a stretcher. An additional stretcher should be used for transporting over long distances. From Torg JS, ed: *Athletic injuries to the head, neck and face,* Philadelphia, 1991, Mosby–Year Book.

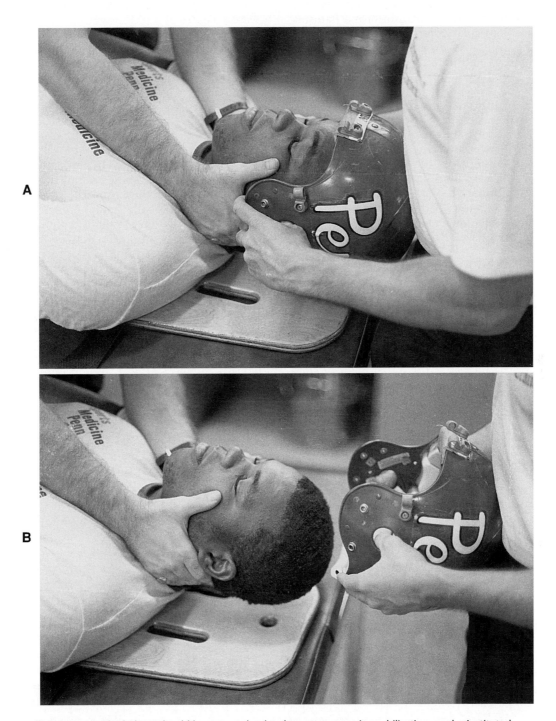

Fig. 16-4. A, The helmet should be removed only when permanent immobilization can be instituted. The helmet may be removed by detaching the chin strap, spreading the earflaps, and gently pulling the helmet off in a straight line with the cervical spine. **B,** The head must be supported under the occiput during and after removing the helmet. From Torg JS, ed: *Athletic injuries to the head, neck and face,* Philadelphia, 1991, Mosby–Year Book.

PREVENTION

Athletic injuries to the cervical spine resulting in injury to the spinal cord are infrequent but catastrophic events. Accurate descriptions of the mechanism or mechanisms responsible for a particular injury transcend academic interest. Before preventative measures can be developed and implemented, identification of the mechanisms involved in the production of the particular injury is necessary.

Injuries resulting in spinal cord injury have been associated with football, water sports, wrestling, rugby, trampolining, and ice hockey. The use of epidemiologic data, biomechanical evidence, and cinematographic analysis has: (1) defined and supported the involvement of axial load forces in cervical spine injuries, (2) demonstrated the success of appropriate football rule changes in the prevention of these injuries, and (3) emphasized the need for use of epidemiologic methods to prevent cervical spine and similar severe injuries in other high-risk athletic activities.

Data on cervical spine injuries resulting from participation in football have been compiled by a national registry since 1971.[11-13] Analysis of epidemiologic data and cinematographic documentation clearly demonstrate that the majority of cervical fractures and dislocations resulted from axial loading. On the basis of this observation, rule changes banning deliberate "spearing" and the use of the top of the helmet as the initial point of contact in making a tackle were implemented at the high school and college levels. Subsequently, a marked decrease in cervical spine injury rates has occurred. The occurrence of permanent cervical quadriplegia decreased from 34 instances in the 1976 season to one in the 1991 season (Fig. 16-5).

Identifying the cause and prevention of cervical quadriplegia resulting from football involves four areas: (1) the role of the helmet–face mask protective system; (2) the concept of the axial-loading mechanism of injury; (3) the effect of the 1976 rule changes banning spearing and the use of the top of the helmet as the initial point of contact in tackling; and (4) the necessity for continued research, education, and rules enforcement.

Classically, the role of hyperflexion had been emphasized in cervical spine trauma whether the injury resulted from a diving accident, trampolining, rugby, or American football. Epidemiologic and cinematographic analyses have established that most cases of cervical spine quadriplegia that occur in football resulted from axial loading. The protective capabilities provided by the modern football helmet resulted in the advent of playing techniques that have placed the cervical spine at risk of injury with associated catastrophic neurologic sequelae. Rather than an accidental event, techniques have been deliberately used that place the cervical spine at risk of catastrophic injury. Recent laboratory observations also indicate that athletically induced cervical spine trauma results from axial loading.

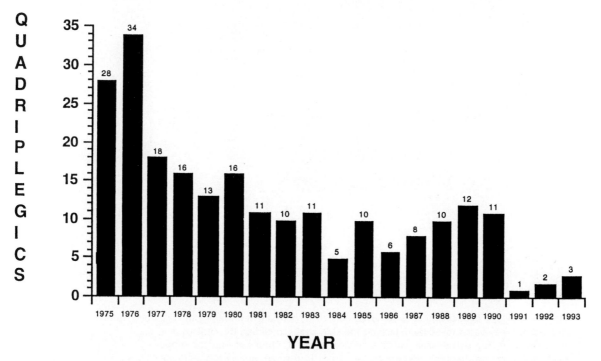

YEAR

The yearly incidence of permanent cervical quadriplegia for all levels of participation (1975 to 1993) decreased dramatically in 1977 following the initiation of rule changes prohibiting the use of head first tackling and blocking techniques.

Fig. 16-5. Yearly incidence of permanent cervical quadriplegia.

In the course of a collision activity, such as tackle football, most energy inputs to the cervical spine are effectively dissipated by the energy-absorbing capabilities of the cervical musculature through controlled lateral bending, flexion, and extension motion. However, the vertebrae, discs, and ligamentous structures can be injured when contact occurs on the top of the helmet with the head, neck, and trunk positioned in such a way that forces are transmitted along the longitudinal axis of the cervical spine.

With the neck in the anatomic position, the cervical spine is extended because of normal cervical lordosis. When the neck is flexed to 30°, the cervical spine straightens. In axial-loading injuries, the neck is slightly flexed, and normal cervical lordosis eliminated, thereby converting the spine into a straight segmented column. Assuming the head, neck, and trunk components to be in motion, rapid deceleration of the head occurs when it strikes another object, such as another player, trampoline bed, or lake bottom. This results in the cervical spine being compressed between the rapidly decelerated head and the force of the oncoming trunk. When the maximum vertical compression is reached, the straightened cervical spine fails in a flexion mode, and fracture, subluxation, or unilateral or bilateral facet dislocation can occur.

Refutation of the "freak accident" concept with the more logical principle of cause and effect has been most rewarding in dealing with problems of football-induced cervical quadriplegia. Definition of the axial-loading mechanism in which a football player, usually a defensive back, makes a tackle by striking an opponent with the top of the helmet had been key in this process (Fig. 16-6). Implementation of rules changes and coaching techniques eliminating the use of the head as a battering ram have resulted in a dramatic reduction in the incidence of quadriplegia since 1976 (see Fig. 16-5). The author believes that the majority, if not all, athletic injuries to the cervical spine also result from axial loading.

Tator et al[9] identified 38 acute spinal cord injuries resulting from diving accidents and observed that "In most cases, the cervical spine was fractured and the spinal cord crushed. The top of the head struck the bottom of the lake or pool." Scher,[6] reporting on vertex impact and cervical dislocation in rugby players, observed that "When the neck is slightly flexed, the spine is straight. If significant force is applied to the vertex when the spine is straight, the force is transmitted down the long axis of the spine. When the force exceeds the energy-absorbing capacity of the structures involved, cervical spine flexion and dislocation will result." Tator and Edmonds[8] have reported on the results of a national questionnaire survey done by the Canadian Committee on the Prevention of Spinal Injuries Due to Hockey, which recorded 28 injuries involving the spinal cord, 17 of which resulted in complete paralysis. They noted that in this series, axial loading was found to be the most common mechanism of cervical spine and spinal cord injury resulting from head impact into the boards, with the most frequent inciting event being a push or check from behind.

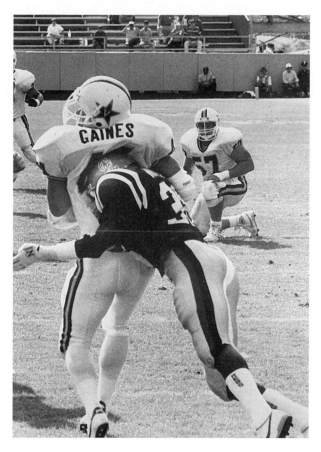

Fig. 16-6. With the advent of the polycarbonate helmet–face mask protective device, use of the top or crown of the helmet as the initial point of contact in blocking and tackling became prevalent. Contact is made; the head abruptly stops; the momentum of the body continues; and the cervical spine is literally crushed between the two. In this instance, the fracture–dislocation injured the spinal cord. The injured player collapses, having been rendered quadriplegic.

CLASSIFICATION

Catastrophic and Potentially Catastrophic Injuries

Catastrophic and potentially catastrophic injuries to the cervical spine and cord are as follows:

(1) cervical subluxation;
(2) unilateral and bilateral facet dislocation;
(3) unstable cervical fractures—axial-load teardrop fracture; and
(4) spear tackler's spine.

CERVICAL SUBLUXATION. Athletic injuries to the cervical spine resulting in either translatory or angulatory instability are uncommon. It is generally accepted that up to 2 mm of translatory displacement is normal. White and Panjobi[17] have defined clinical instability and established 3.5 mm translation and 11° of rotation as two factors to be used in determining indications for surgical stabilization. There are no data regarding the degree of risk presented by 2.0 to 3.5 mm of translation.

UNILATERAL AND BILATERAL FACET DISLO-CATION. Experience with unilateral and bilateral facet dislocations have been reported recently.[16] More favorable results of immediate reduction of unilateral and bilateral facet dislocations have been observed and deserve emphasis. Three cases of unilateral facet dislocation reduced within 3 hours of the injury and subsequently fused experienced significant neurologic recovery. Four other patients, two who were treated expectantly and eventually underwent an open reduction and laminectomy and two treated with closed reduction with skeletal traction have had no neurologic recovery. In four injuries of bilateral facet dislocation where reduction was achieved by either open or closed method, although there was no neurologic recovery, all four survived their injuries. However, three children whose dislocations were not successfully reduced all died. Prompt reduction of cervical dislocations to relieve cord deformation is recommended.

UNSTABLE CERVICAL FRACTURES—AXIAL-LOAD TEARDROP FRACTURE. The most frequently occurring cervical spine fracture associated with instability, cord compromise, and major neurologic sequelae is the three-part, two-playing axial-load teardrop fracture.[10] The fracture pattern, in addition to the anterior inferior vertebral body "teardrop" fracture, is associated with sagittal vertebral body and posterior neural element fractures (Fig. 16-7). In those sustaining this injury as a result of tackle football, 85% were rendered and remained quadriplegic.

SPEAR TACKLER'S SPINE. A subset of football players has been identified who demonstrated: (1) developmental narrowing (stenosis) of the cervical spinal canal, (2) persistence straightening or reversal of the normal cervical lordotic curve on erect lateral radiographs obtained in the neutral position, (3) concomitant preex-isting posttraumatic radiographic abnormalities of the cervical spine, and (4) documentation of having used spear-tackling technique.[15]

Of 15 patients evaluated because of complaints referable to the cervical spine or brachial plexus, four resulted in permanent neurologic deficit: (1) quadriplegia, two; (2) incomplete hemiplegic, one; and (3) residual long-track signs, one.

Although anecdotal, it is proposed that the permanent neurologic injury resulted from axial loading of a persistently straightened cervical spine from use of head impact playing techniques. It is recommended that individuals who possess the characteristics of spear tackler's spine be precluded from participation in collision activities that expose the cervical spine to axial energy inputs.

SPINAL CORD RESUSCITATION. Research obtained during the past 20 years have established the principles of brain resuscitation in the management of closed head injuries. It is recognized that regarding resulting morbidity, the same pathophysiologic and mechanistic phenomena occur in acute spinal cord trauma. Specifically, it is secondary spinal cord injury phenomena caused by hypoxia, edema, and aberration of cell membrane potential that are largely responsible for resulting neurologic deficits. The principles of spinal cord resuscitation are proposed as an attempt to reverse secondary changes that occur to obtain maximal neurologic recovery. These measures include:

(1) Management of any aberrations and neurovascular function with particular regard to maintaining blood pressure and spiratory function;
(2) Prompt initiation of measures to affect reduction of spinal deformity to relieve cord deformation;
(3) Prompt disabilization of the injured cervical segment;

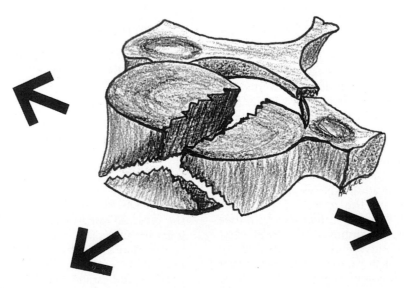

Fig. 16-7. Diagrammatic representation of the three part-two plane vertebral body compression fracture demonstrates the anteroinferior teardrop and the sagittal vertebral body fractures and associated fracture through the lamina. From Torg JS, ed: *Athletic injuries to the head, neck and face,* Philadelphia, 1991, Mosby–Year Book.

(4) Administration of corticosteroid intravenously in doses recommended by Bracken et al.[2] This measurement involves the administration within 8 hours of injury of methylprednisolone, 30 mg/kg, given as a bolus followed by an infusion of 5.4 mg/kg/hr for 23 hours. Patients who receive methylprednisolone within 8 hours of injury improved significantly after 6 months compared with those who received a placebo. It is believed that the steroid acts by suppressing the breakdown of the cell membrane by inhibiting lipid peroxidation and hydrolysis at the injury site. When lipid peroxidation is inhibited, the vascoreactive products of arachidonic acts metabolism reduce the blood flow at the site of injury; and

(5) Administration of cerebrogangliosides, such as Sygen, in an attempt to facilitate a neurologic recovery.

Noncatastrophic Injuries

Noncatastrophic injuries to the cervical spine, cord, and brachial plexus are those in which residual neurologic sequelae is not a problem. Rather, the major factor is whether nonneurologic disability will result, particularly if the individual returns to collision activities. Common injuries in this group are:

(1) Nerve root—brachial plexus injury;
(2) Cervical sprain and strains;
(3) Intervertebral disc injury;
(4) Cervical cord neurapraxia-transient quadriplegia; and
(5) Stable fractures.

NERVE ROOT AND BRACHIAL PLEXUS. Injury to the cervical spine, cervical discs, brachial plexus, and peripheral nerves can result in neurologic signs and symptoms involving the upper extremity. The most common are the cervical pinch–stretch neurapraxias of the nerve roots and brachial plexus. Often called "burners" or "stingers" by players and trainers, these injuries often go unreported and untreated. Injury to the cervical nerve roots and brachial plexus most frequently occurs in contact sports, particularly football, and rugby, wrestling, and soccer. In football, burners are usually diagnosed in defensive players and in offensive linemen. Clancy et al[3] reported that 49% of the football players at the University of Wisconsin had experienced at least one burner at some time during their playing career.

These injuries result from two distinct injury mechanisms: (1) traction to the brachial plexus, and (2) compression of the cervical nerve roots. Plexus traction neurapraxia occurs in younger athletes and results from ipsilateral shoulder depression and contralateral neck and head deviation. Cervical root injuries result from compression of the dorsal root ganglion in the intervertebral foramen and are the result of hyperextension and ipsilateral deviation of the cervical spine. They are often associated with degenerative changes and may be seen combined with developmental cervical stenosis.

Typically, burners occur after head and shoulder contact; the player often leaves the playing field complaining of pain and numbness and inability to move the involved upper extremity. Pain is usually experienced radiating from the base of the neck into the shoulder and down the arm, including the hand. Burning paresthesias and numbness may accompany the pain and also radiate into the arm and hand. Most often these symptoms are not dermatomal in distribution. Weakness may occur, and characteristically the deltoid, spinati, and biceps are affected; motor weakness is often not initially apparent and may not manifest until a few days after the injury. Repeated neurologic evaluation therefore is mandatory. Characteristically, the signs and symptoms are transient and resolve within minutes. In these athletes in whom pain and paresthesia abate, a normal neurologic examination is required, and, most importantly, a full pain-free range of cervical motion is needed before the athletes return to contact activity. Also, players must demonstrate normal strength on clinical examination before they return to participation. Those who have recurrent symptoms without weakness require careful follow-up evaluation; continued symptoms associated with weakness preclude further athletic participation.

Clancy et al[3] recommended classifying these injuries based on the staging system of Seddon. Neurapraxia, the mildest form of injury, represents a reversible aberration in axonal function. Focal demyelinization can occur, producing an electrophysiologic conduction block or conduction slowing. Complete recovery usually occurs immediately or within a maximum of 2 weeks. Axonotmesis is an injury in which the axon and myelin sheath are disrupted, but the epineurium remains intact. Wallerian degeneration occurs distal to the point of injury; functional recovery may occur, but it can be incomplete and unpredictable. The most severe injury, neurotmesis, is rarely seen in athletes and results in complete disruption of the nerve. Prognosis is poor, and generally the patient does not recover.

Brachial plexus injuries are more likely to occur in younger patients with less well-developed neck musculature. Usually, these are traction injuries resulting from lateral neck flexion away from the involved area and shoulder depression to the side of involvement. Neck pain can be present, but it is usually not a prominent feature. When present, cervical spine radiographs are indicated. Typically, pain and paresthesias involving the arm and shoulder are transient. On examination, a Spurling test result is negative. Weakness typically involves the deltoid, spinati, and biceps and might not be evident initially on clinical examination, and a follow-up evaluation becomes necessary.

Root lesions result from compression of the nerve root or dorsal root ganglion in the intervertebral foramen and are generally associated with radiologic evidence of cervical disc disease and developmental stenosis. In football players, these injuries usually occur when the player reaches the college or professional level. Hyperextension with ipsilateral neck flexion is the common mechanism of injury. Neck pain and a decreased cervical range of motion may be present, and Spurling's test is positive. Plain radiographs may be normal or demonstrate loss of normal cervical lordosis and degenerative disc changes. Magnetic resonance imaging is indicated in patients with a persistent neurologic deficit and prolonged or recurrent symptoms and will demonstrate either acute disc herniation or degenerative disc disease with asymmetric disc bulging. In the author's experience, patients often have developmental spinal stenosis, degenerative disc disease, and asymmetric disc bulging that results in root irritation with cervical hyperextension.

Initial management must be directed toward evaluation of the cervical spine, shoulder girdle affected upper extremity, and peripheral nervous system. The first obligation of the physician is to rule out serious cervical spine injury. A history of bilateral symptoms or symptoms including the lower extremities should alert the physician to the possibility of cord neurapraxia, cervical spine fracture, or ligamentous injury. In this instance, the spine should be immobilized until the possibility of severe injury is ruled out. If a player complains of neck pain, a complete cervical spine evaluation is mandatory, including radiographic examination.

In brachial plexus injuries, prevention is based on an aggressive neck and shoulder strengthening program. Neck rolls, or devices such as the cowboy collar, and high-profile shoulder pads also help prevent injuries by limiting the extent of lateral flexion and extension (Fig. 16-8).

Electrodiagnostic studies may be helpful but are not mandatory in the management of burners secondary to brachial plexus injury. Speer[7] demonstrated that although there was no correlation between initial physical findings and the results of electrodiagnostic testing, evidence of muscular weakness at 72 hours after the injury did correlate with a positive electromyogram. Bergfeld[1]

reported that electromyography findings continue to appear long after weakness has appeared resolved in clinical examinations, and therefore abnormal electromyography findings should *not* be used as a criterion for exclusion from athletic participation.

In individuals with cervical disc disease, the criteria for the return to sports activities is identical as for those with brachial plexus injuries. Neck and shoulder strengthening is the key to prevention. A neck roll or cowboy collar will help control recurrences by limiting extension. Athletes with large acute herniations or with large central disc components should refrain from participation in sports activities. Players with chronic symptoms and degenerative disc disease should be counseled as to the likelihood of recurrent symptoms with athletic participation. In those patients with subjective symptoms but who have normal strength, participation is not contraindicated if the player understands the possible implications of repetitive root trauma. In rare instances, discectomy and fusion may be considered if symptoms persist. A one-level fusion is not an absolute contraindication to athletic participation.

Conclusions

(1) The burner pain syndrome results from either of two distinct injury patterns: traction to the brachial plexus and compression of the cervical nerve roots;

(2) Brachial plexus injuries are typically traction neurapraxias occurring in younger athletes resulting from shoulder depression and lateral neck flexion away from the side of injury;

(3) Cervical root injuries typically occur in older players; they are hyperextension injuries, and they are associated with degenerative disc changes and often combined with developmental cervical stenosis;

(4) Criteria for return to athletics include the absence

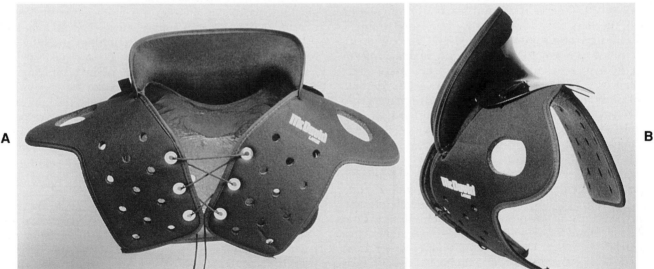

Fig. 16-8. Frontal (**A**) and lateral (**B**) views of the cowboy collar. This device, which is worn under the shoulder pads of an athlete, effectively limits the extremes of extension and lateral bending of the cervical spine.

of symptoms, normal strength, and painless, full range of motion of the cervical spine;

(5) Players who experience one or more burners should wear appropriate neck rolls or a cowboy collar to prevent extreme hyperextension and lateral bend of the cervical spine (see Figs. 16-8, 16-9); and

(6) A year-round neck and shoulder muscle strengthening program will aid in the prevention of the burner syndrome.

ACUTE CERVICAL SPRAIN SYNDROME. An acute cervical sprain is a collision injury frequently seen in contact sports. The patient complains of having "jammed" his or her neck with subsequent pain localized to the cervical area. Characteristically, the patient presents with limitation of cervical spine motion but without radiation of pain or paresthesia. Neurologic examination is negative, and radiographs are normal.

Stable cervical sprains and strains eventually resolve with or without treatment. Initially, the presence of a serious injury should be ruled out by thorough neurologic examination and determination of the range of cervical motion. Range of motion is evaluated by having the athlete: actively nod his or her head, touch his or her chin to his or her chest, extend his or her neck maximally, touch his or her chin to his or her left shoulder, touch his or her chin to his or her right shoulder, touch his or her left ear to his or her left shoulder, and touch his or her right ear to his or her right shoulder. If the patient is unwilling or unable to perform these maneuvers actively while standing erect, the evaluation should not proceed. The athlete with less than a full, pain-free range of cervical motion, persistent paresthesia, or weakness should be

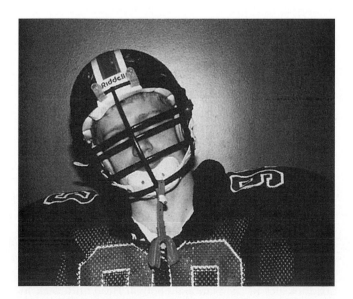

Fig. 16-9. The combined action of the football helmet, cowboy collar, and shoulder pads effectively limits the extremes of lateral bend of the neck. From Torg JS, ed: *Athletic injuries to the head, neck and face,* Philadelphia, 1991, Mosby–Year Book.

protected and excluded from activity. Subsequent evaluation should include appropriate radiographic studies, including flexion and extension views to demonstrate fractures or instability. If the patient has pain and muscle spasm of the cervical spine, hospitalization and head-halter traction may be indicated.

In general, management of athletes with "cervical sprains" should be tailored to the degree of severity. Immobilizing the neck in a soft collar and using analgesics and antiinflammatory agents until there is a full, spasm-free range of neck motion is appropriate. It should be emphasized that individuals with a history of collision injury, pain, and limited cervical motion should have routine cervical spine radiographs. Also, lateral flexion and extension radiographs are indicated after the acute symptoms subside. Marked limitation of cervical motion, persistent pain, or radicular symptoms or findings may require a magnetic resonance imaging scan to rule out intervertebral disc injury.

CERVICAL CORD NEURAPRAXIA-TRANSIENT QUADRIPLEGIA. The author has previously described the distinct clinical entity of the syndrome of neurapraxia of the cervical spinal cord with transient quadriplegia.[14] Sensory changes include burning pain, numbness, tingling, and loss of sensation, whereas motor changes range from weakness to complete paralysis involving upper and lower extremities. The episodes are transient, and complete sensory and motor recovery usually occurs in 10 to 15 minutes, although in some patients, gradual resolution may occur in 24 to 36 hours. Except for burning paresthesias, pain in the cervical area is not present at the time of injury, and there is complete return of motor function and full, pain-free motion of the cervical spine. This is a spinal cord phenomena, no root or plexus, as evident by its bilaterally.

Routine radiographs of the cervical spine are characteristically negative for fracture, subluxation, or dislocation. However, radiographic findings include developmental cervical spinal narrowing, either as an isolated finding or associated with congenital fusions; ligamentous instability; or intervertebral disc disease (Fig. 16-10). Pavlov et al[4] devised the ratio method for determining the sagittal spinal canal diameter (Fig. 16-11). The author compared the standard measurement of the canal with the anteroposterior width of the vertebral body at the midpoint of the corresponding vertebral body.

The ratio method of determining cervical spinal canal narrowing is independent of magnification factors caused by differences in target distance, object-to-film distance, or body type because the sagittal diameter of the spinal canal and that of the vertebral body are in the same anatomic plane and are similarly affected by magnification. There is normally a one-to-one relationship between the sagittal diameter of the spinal canal and that of the vertebral body, regardless of sex. A spinal canal-to-vertebral body ratio of less than 0.82 was recorded at one or more levels in all patients who experienced cervical cord neurapraxia.

The author's experience clearly indicates that those individuals who experience an episode of cervical cord neurapraxia manifested by sensory or motor symptoms

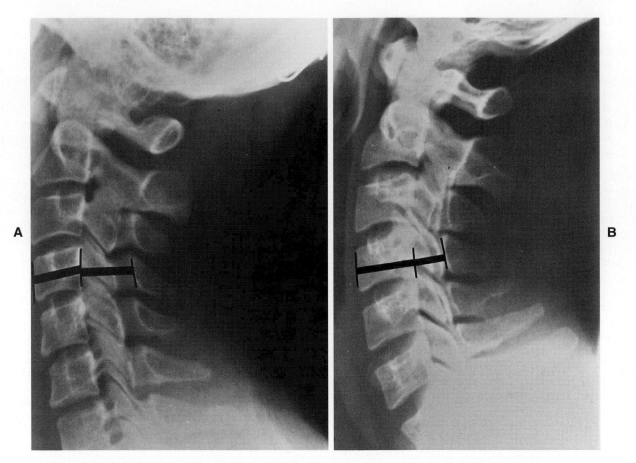

Fig. 16-10. Comparison between the ratio of the spinal canal to the vertebral body of a healthy control subject with that of a stenotic patient demonstrated on lateral view radiographs of the cervical spine. Pavlov's ratio is 1 : 1 (1.00) in the control subject (**A**) compared with 1 : 2 (0.50) in the stenotic patient (**B**). From Torg JS, Pavlov H, Genuario S, et al: *J Bone Joint Surg* 68-A:1370, 1987.

have, with very few exceptions, a spinal canal-to-vertebral body ratio of 0.80 or less at one or more levels. The sensitivity of the ratio, i.e., the probability of getting a positive result in a symptomatic individual, was 100% in the author's series.[14]

The author's initial report was based solely on radiographic findings—all of the patients were evaluated before magnetic resonance imaging was widely available. The importance of the radiographic ratio determination, in addition to standardizing the films that were taken by various techniques, was to explain the pathophysiologic basis for the occurrence of cord neurapraxia. Developmental narrowing of the spinal canal in the anteroposterior plane associated with extreme flexion or extension of the spine can result in a transient compression of the cord. Penning[5] described this effect as the "pincer mechanism." Specifically, with hyperextension of the cervical spine, the posteroinferior aspect of the superior vertebral body and the anterosuperior aspect of the lamina of the subjacent vertebra decrease; conversely, in flexion, the lamina of the superior vertebra and the posterosuperior aspect of the subjacent vertebral body approximate with a sudden decrease in the anteroposterior diameter of

the canal at that point, resulting in compression of the spinal cord (Fig. 16-12). In every instance of symptomatic developmental narrowing uncomplicated by instability or disc herniation, the neurologic manifestations are transient and completely reversible.

The low specificity of the ratio method in college and professional players results from anthropomorphic differences. Specifically, the cervical spines in these two groups are characterized by relatively larger vertebral bodies with subsequent lower ratios.

Permanent neurologic loss resulting from cervical spine injuries sustained in tackle football is a function of playing technique in which the cervical spine is axial loaded, resulting in unstable fractures or dislocations and irreversible neurologic compromise. The question of whether individuals who have experienced an episode of cord neurapraxia are predisposed to injury with permanent neurologic residua has been answered. None of the 117 known quadriplegics in the National Football Head and Neck Injuries Registry experienced previous episodes of cord neurapraxia, and none of the 110 patients in the transient cohort remained quadriplegic after an episode of cervical cord neurapraxia. Based on the random distribution of

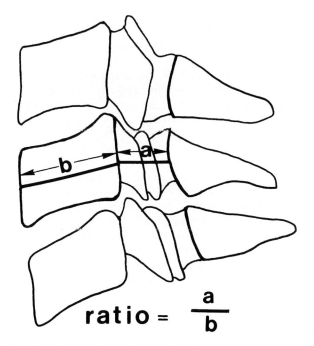

$$ratio = \frac{a}{b}$$

Fig. 16-11. The spinal canal-to-vertebral body ratio is the distance from the midpoint of the posterior aspect of the vertebral body to the nearest point on the corresponding spinolaminar line (**A**) divided by the anteroposterior width of the vertebral body (**B**). Pavlov's ratio is A/B. From Torg JS, Pavlov H, Genuario S, et al: *J Bone Joint Surg* 68-A:1354–1370, 1986.

ratio determinations and the lack of correlation between the occurrence of permanent quadriplegia and prodromal episodes of cord neurapraxia, it is clear that the occurrence of cord neurapraxia does not predispose an individual to an injury associated with permanent catastrophic neurologic sequelae. There was no correlation between occurrence of permanent quadriplegia and prodromal episodes

of cord neurapraxia in a tackle football population. Therefore, the author believes that the presence of uncomplicated developmental narrowing of the stable cervical spine is neither a harbinger of nor does it predispose for permanent neurologic injury.

Cervical cord neurapraxia is a transient totally reversible phenomenon that results from compressive deformation of the spinal cord. The syndrome is caused by developmental narrowing of the cervical canal either as an isolated entity or combined with degenerative changes, instability, or congenital abnormalities. Uncomplicated stenosis of the cervical canal in a patient with a stable spine does not predispose to permanent neurologic injury. The present data do not indicate that there is a correlation between developmental narrowing and permanent neurologic sequelae in a spine rendered unstable by football-induced trauma. Data also indicate that an episode of cervical cord neurapraxia is not a harbinger or indicator of susceptibility to permanent neurologic sequelae. However, the author has in the past recommended that continued participation in collision activities be restricted in those individuals who have had a documented episode of cervical cord neurapraxia associated with: (1) ligamentous instability, (2) intervertebral disc disease with cord compression, (3) significant degenerative changes, (4) magnetic resonance imaging evidence of cord defect or swelling, (5) symptoms of positive neurologic findings lasting more than 36 hours, and (6) more than one recurrence.

As stated previously, the author described cervical cord neurapraxia using radiographic measurements and identified narrowing of the anteroposterior diameter of the cervical canal as the etiologic factor. A more recent report classifies the various clinical manifestations, measures cord and canal diameters on magnetic resonance imaging with a newly developed computer technique, and delineates management guidelines.

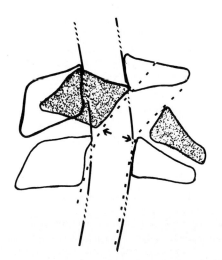
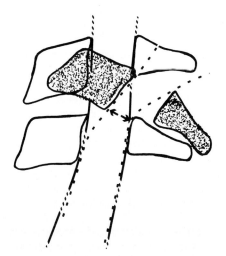

Fig. 16-12. The pincers mechanism, as described by Penning,[32] occurs when the distance between the posteroinferior margin of the superior vertebral body and the anterosuperior aspect of the spinolaminar line of the subjacent vertebra decreases with hyperextension, resulting in compression of the cord. With hyperflexion, the anterosuperior aspect of the spinolaminar line of the superior vertebra and the posterosuperior margin of the inferior vertebra would be the "pincers."

A retrospective review was performed of 110 cases of cervical cord neurapraxia seen in consultation by the author. Radiographs were measured as described previously, and a new technique with an MS-DOS-based system was developed to measure cord and canal diameters from the magnetic resonance imaging scans. All injuries were sports-related, and 86% occurred during football participation. Follow-up evaluation was available for 93 (85%) of the patients after an average of 22 months. Results of this study indicated that clinical manifestations (cervical cord neurapraxia type) were paralysis in 36%, weakness in 26%, and sensory changes alone in 38%. Duration of the symptoms (cervical cord neurapraxia grade) were: I—less than 15 minutes in 73%; II—more than 15 minutes but less than 24 hours in 16%; and III—more than 24 hours in 10%. The averages for the sagittal radiologic indices were: (1) Pavlov ratio, 0.69 (standard deviation [SD] = 0.11); (2) minimal magnetic resonance imaging canal diameter, 9.6 mm (SD = 1.8); (3) cord diameter, 8.1 mm (SD = 0.8); and (4) space available for the cord, 1.6 mm (SD = 1.4). There was no relationship between the various clinical manifestations and the radiologic indices. Overall, 65% of the patients returned to contact sports, with 56% of these patients having at least one recurrence of cervical cord neurapraxia. Patients with recurrence had smaller Pavlov ratios ($P < 0.05$), smaller absolute canal diameters ($P < 0.01$), and less space available for the cord ($P < 0.05$).

Based on this statistically significant data, it was concluded that: (1) individuals with uncomplicated cervical cord neurapraxia can be advised to return to play without greater risk of permanent neurologic injury, (2) the various clinical manifestations (cervical cord neurapraxia type and grade) are not related to the radiologic indices; and (3) there is a 56% recurrence rate that is correlated with the pathoanatomy, i.e., the smaller the canal, the greater the risk of recurrence.

INTERVERTEBRAL DISC INJURY. Acute cervical intervertebral disc herniation is exceedingly rare in high school, intercollegiate, and professional athletes. However, an acute central disc deforming the cord or the lateral disc associated with pain, limitation of full cervical motion, or neurologic symptoms are absolute contraindications to athletic participation.

A problem seen with an increasing frequency in older collegiate and professional players is degenerative disc changes associated with repetitive "microtrauma." Common radiographic findings include disc space narrowing, anterior bony ridging, and loss of normal cervical lordosis. If the individual is symptomatic and has associated loss of normal cervical motion, treatment consists of rest, including a cervical collar, heat, and analgesics until the individual is symptom-free and has full range of cervical motion.

To be noted is the association of chronic, recurrent cervical nerve root neurapraxia ("burner syndrome") resulting from cervical nerve root compression in the intervertebral foramina secondary to cervical disc disease. Whereas burners have been identified to result from brachial plexus stretch injury in high school and college football players presenting with symptoms, nerve root compression in the intervertebral foramina secondary to disc disease is a more common etiology in older collegiate and professional football players with chronic recurrent burners.

STABLE FRACTURES. An acute fracture of either the vertebral body or posterior elements with or without associated ligamentous laxity constitutes an absolute contraindication to participation.

The following healed, stable fractures in an asymptomatic patient who is neurologically normal and has a full range of cervical motion can be considered to present no contraindication to participation in contact activities: (1) stable compression fractures of the vertebral body without a sagittal component on anteroposterior radiographs and without involvement of either the ligamentous or posterior bony structures, (2) a healed stable endplate fracture without a sagittal component on anteroposterior radiographs or involvement of the posterior or bony ligamentous structure, and (3) healed spinous process "clay shoveler" fractures.

Relative contraindications apply to the following healed stable fractures in individuals who are asymptomatic, neurologically normal, and have a full pain-free range of cervical motion: (1) healed, stable displaced vertebral body compression fractures without a sagittal component on anteroposterior radiographs; the propensity for these fractures to settle with increased deformity must be considered and carefully followed, and (2) healed, stable fractures involving the elements of the posterior neural ring in individuals who are asymptomatic, neurologically normal, and have a full pain-free range of cervical motion. In evaluating radiographic and imaging studies to find the location and subsequent healing of posterior neural arch fractures, it is important to understand that, as pointed out by Steel (personal communication), a rigid ring cannot break in one location; thus, healing of paired fractures of the ring must be demonstrated.

An absolute contraindication to further participation in contact activities exists in the presence of the following fractures: (1) vertebral body fracture with a sagittal component, (2) fracture of the vertebral body with or without displacement with associated posterior arch fractures or ligamentous laxity, (3) comminuted fractures of the vertebral body with displacement into the spinal canal, and (4) any healed fracture of either the vertebral body or posterior components with associated pain, neurologic findings, and limitation of normal cervical motion.

REFERENCES

1. Bergfeld JA: Brachial plexus injury in sports: A five year follow-up, *Orthop Clin North Am* 23:743–744, 1988.
2. Bracken MB, Shepard MS, Collins WF, et al: A randomized, controlled trial of methylprednisolone or naloxone with treatment of acute spinal-cord injury, *N Engl J Med* 320:1405–1411, 1990.
3. Clancy WG, Brand RL, Bergfeld J: Upper trunk brachial plexus injuries in contact sports, *Am J Sports Med* 5:209–214, 1977.
4. Pavlov H, Torg JS, Robie B, Jahre C: Cervical spinal stenosis: Determination with vertebral body ratio method, *Radiology* 164:771–775, 1987.

5. Penning L: Some aspects of plain radiography of the cervical spine in chronic myelopathy, *Neurology* 12:513–519, 1962.

6. Scher AT: Vertex impact and cervical dislocation in rugby players, *South Afr Med J* 59:227–228, 1981.

7. Speer KP: The prolonged burner syndrome, *Am J Sports Med* 18:591–594, 1990.

8. Tator CH, Edmonds VE: National survey of spinal injuries in hockey players, *Can Med Assoc J* 130:875–880, 1984.

9. Tator CH, Edmonds VE, New ML: Diving: A frequent and potentially preventable cause of spinal cord injury, *Can Med Assoc J* 124:1323–1324, 1981.

10. Torg JS, Pavlov H, O'Neill MJ, Nichols CE, Sennett B: The axial load teardrop fracture: The isolated fracture and the three part-two plane fracture of the cervical spine . . . the clinical and roentgen analysis of 55 cervical spines, *Am J Sports Med* 19:355–364, 1991.

11. Torg JS, Vegso JJ, O'Neill J, Sennett B: The epidemiologic, pathologic, biomechanical and cinematographic analysis of football-induced cervical spine trauma, *Am J Sports Med* 18:50–57, 1990.

12. Torg JS, Vegso JJ, Sennett B: The national football head and neck injury registry: 14 year report on cervical quadriplegia, 1971 through 1985, *JAMA* 254:3439–3441, 1985.

13. Torg JS, Truex R, Quedenfeld TC: The national football head & neck injury registry: report and conclusions, *JAMA* 241:1477–1479, 1979.

14. Torg JS, Pavlov H, Genuario SE, Sennett B, Robie B, Jahre C: Neurapraxia of the cervical spinal cord with transient quadriplegia. *J Bone Joint Surg* 68A:1354–1370, 1986.

15. Torg JS, Sennett B, Pavlov H: Spear tackler's spine: an entity precluding participation in tackle football and collision activities that expose the cervical spine to axial energy inputs, *Am J Sports Med* 21:640–649, 1993.

16. Torg JS, Sennett B, Vegso JJ, et al: Axial loading injuries to the middle cervical spine segment, *Am J Sports Med* 19:6–20, 1991.

17. White AA, Johnson RM, Pajobi MM, et al: Biomechanical analysis of clinical stability in the cervical spine, *Clin Orthop* 109:85–93, 1975.

CHAPTER 17

THE THORACIC AND LUMBAR SPINE

Jeffrey E. Deckey
Mark Weidenbaum

Most injuries to the thoracic and lumbar spine that result from athletic activity are relatively minor and resolve without involvement of health care professionals. Limited data exist regarding the incidence of specific back injuries according to particular sports. Few studies have comprehensively documented spine injury rates in sports overall.[12] Because serious thoracic or lumbar spine injury occurs infrequently in sports, such injuries have received little attention within the field of sports medicine.

The goals of the sports physician should not only include diagnosis and management of sports-related injuries but should also emphasize screening of athletes for prevention of potential injury. Once diagnosis has been made and treatment has been initiated, the physician must evaluate the athlete to determine when and if he or she may return to sports participation. This decision is one of the most difficult tasks faced by the sports physician.

ANATOMY

Knowledge of pertinent spinal anatomy is central to understanding mechanisms of injury and principles of management.[9] The vertebral column involves a delicate balance between osseous and soft-tissue structures, with alternating bony vertebrae and fibrocartilaginous discs. The spine is divided into cervical (neck), thoracic (chest), lumbar (lower back), sacral, and coccygeal regions. The cervical spine is discussed elsewhere in this text.

Normally, there are 12 thoracic and five lumbar vertebrae and discs, and the sacral and coccygeal vertebrae fuse to form the sacrum and coccyx. The vertebrae increase in size as one descends caudally (toward the tail) to the sacrum. Vertebral connections with each other occur through the discs and through posterior articulations called facets. Despite great regional anatomic differences, the spine always functions to provide structural support, harmonious movement, and neural protection. Changes in one region may affect other regions and the spine as a whole.

Thoracic and Lumbar Vertebrae

The thoracic pedicles originate from the superior aspect of the vertebral body. Thoracic laminae are short, relatively thick, and overlap slightly. Thoracic spinous processes are long and are directed posteriorly and inferiorly. Thoracic facets generally face posteriorly and slightly outward, although orientation changes from frontal to sagittal with caudal progression. The inferior facet originates at the anterior part of the lamina and faces anteriorly and slightly inward. This facet configuration permits increased rotation in the thoracic spine. However, rotation is limited, in part, by the intact rib cage and sternum.

Thoracic vertebrae are unique because of their articulation with the ribs. The second through ninth ribs articulate with the corresponding superior and inferior vertebrae at the intervertebral disc. The head of the rib articulates with the superior costal facet of the adjacent vertebral body and the inferior costal facet of the vertebra above. The rib tubercle articulates with the corresponding transverse process costal facet. The first, tenth, eleventh, and twelfth ribs have complete facets for articulation with their respective vertebra. The eleventh and twelfth rib do not articulate with the transverse processes.

Viewed in the horizontal plane, lumbar vertebrae are kidney-shaped. Their pedicles are thick, originating from the superior posterolateral aspect of the vertebral body. They give rise to short broad laminae that meet to form wide horizontal spinous processes. Unlike the thoracic laminae, the lumbar laminae do not overlap, and there is a space between each lamina, which is spanned by the ligamentum flavum. The articular facets project vertically. The superior facet faces posteromedially and articulates with the inferior facet of the vertebrae above in a reciprocal fashion (Fig. 17-1). The sagittal alignment of the facets allows increased flexion and extension compared with the thoracic spine.

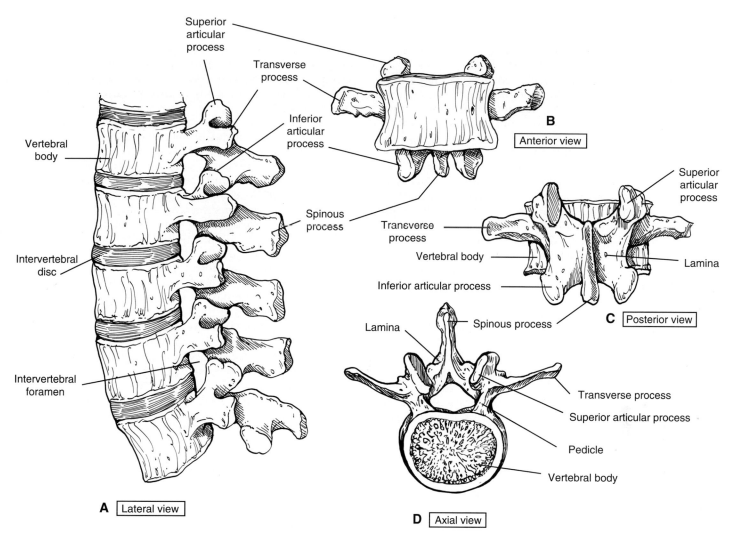

Fig. 17-1. Views of the lumbar spine. **A,** Lateral (sagittal plane). **B,** Anterior (frontal plane). **C,** Posterior (frontal plane). **D,** Horizontal (axial plane).

Intervertebral Disc

Interposed between the vertebral bodies are fibrocartilaginous intervertebral discs that become progressively larger and thicker as one descends the vertebral column, accounting for 20% to 30% of vertebral column height.[31] The discs connect the vertebrae, allow limited motion, and facilitate force distribution.

The disc includes an outer fibrocartilagenous ring, the annulus fibrosus, surrounding the inner gelatinous nucleus pulposus. The annulus fibrosus is composed of a series of concentric lamellae with alternating fiber orientations that function to contain the nucleus pulposus and to provide increased torsional strength. The nucleus pulposus assumes an eccentric position within the disc space as determined in part by the sagittal contour at each anatomic level of the spine. The outer portion of the annulus fibrosus attaches to the vertebrae above and below via Sharpey's fibers.[10] The inner portion of the annulus, the transition zone, blends with the nucleus pulposus. The annulus fibrosus and nucleus pulposus are contained above and below by cartilaginous vertebral endplates. Outer layers of the annulus fibrosus are vascularized, whereas the remainder of the disc receives its nutrition via diffusion through the endplates.

The annulus fibrosus contains approximately 60% to 70% water, and this figure remains relatively constant with age.[33] Collagen is the other major component of the annulus fibrosus, giving it tensile strength. Although the nucleus pulposus is approximately 80% water, much of its dry weight comes from proteoglycans. These proteoglycans are huge molecules with high concentrations of negative fixed charge, giving them a strong affinity for water (hydrophilic). Thus, water is pulled into the disc as a result of the electrochemical effect of the proteoglycans in the nucleus pulposus. Because external osmotic, hydrostatic, and mechanical forces tend to push water out of the disc, the proteoglycan hydrophilic effect is an essential part of the equilibrium necessary to maintain disc hydration. Water and proteoglycan content decrease with age and degeneration.

Ligaments

Numerous ligamentous structures support the thoracic and lumbar spine. The anterior longitudinal ligament (ALL) runs along the ventral surface of the vertebral bodies. The posterior longitudinal ligament (PLL) lies along the posterior aspect of the vertebral body within the spinal canal. Posteriorly, the ligamentum flavum (yellow ligament) at each level extends from the anterior surface of the proximal laminae to the lamina below. The facets are diarthrodial joints surrounded by capsules that provide stability, limit motion, and help to maintain the joint. The costovertebral joints are reinforced by ligamentous structures, including the radiate and the costotransverse ligaments. The supraspinous and interspinous ligaments connect the spinous processes posteriorly.

The ligamentous structures are more pronounced in the lumbar spine, which may result from the relative lack of bony stability present in the lumbar spine compared with the thoracic spine, which is reinforced by the rib cage. The ligamentum flavum, also thicker in the lumbar spine, serves as a barrier to the spinal canal between adjacent lumbar laminae (Fig. 17-2).

Muscles

The muscles of the spine are aligned longitudinally from the skull to the pelvis and provide support and motion to the axial skeleton. The musculature of the back may be divided into two layers: deep and superficial. The superficial muscles, which are associated with the shoulder girdle and upper limb, must not be overlooked when evaluating back injuries. The deep muscles of the spine consist of five major groups, including the splenius, the erector spinae, the transversospinalis, the interspinalis, and the intertransversarial.

The splenius consists of the splenius cervicis and splenius capitis and is located in the cervical spine.

The erector spinae is a massive group of muscles that occupy the vertebrocostal groove. It consists of the spinalis, longissimus, and the iliocostalis. It lies directly under the thoracic and lumbar fascia. It originates from the posterior aspect of the sacrum, iliac crest, and lumbar spinous processes. The muscle splits into three groups, consisting of the midline spinalis, the longissimus, and the iliocostalis. The erector spinae extends along the entire spine, however, it consists of short fasicles that span 6 to 8 segments.

The iliocostalis lumborum begins at the iliac crest and inserts on the angles of the lower six ribs. The next portion, the iliocostalis thoracis, originates from the upper border of the lower six ribs and attaches to the upper six ribs. Finally, the iliocostalis cervicis originates from the angles of the upper six ribs and inserts on the transverse processes of C4 to C6.

The longissimus consists of thoracic, cervical, and capital portions. The longissimus thoracis inserts onto

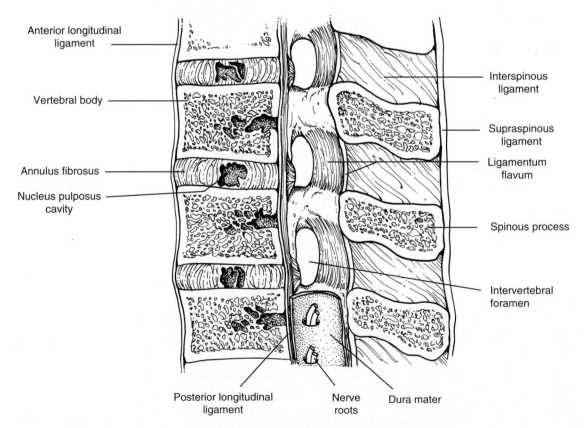

Anterior longitudinal ligament

Vertebral body

Annulus fibrosus

Nucleus pulposus cavity

Interspinous ligament

Supraspinous ligament

Ligamentum flavum

Spinous process

Intervertebral foramen

Posterior longitudinal ligament

Nerve roots

Dura mater

Fig. 17-2. Midline sagittal view illustrating important soft tissues in the lumbar spine.

the lower nine or ten ribs and their corresponding transverse processes. The longissimus cervicis originates from the upper four to six ribs and inserts onto the transverse processes of C2 through C6. The longissimus capitis bridges the articular processes of the lower four cervical vertebrae with the posterior margin of the mastoid process.

The spinalis muscle is the most medial and least defined of the erector spinae musculature. The spinalis capitis, cervicis, and thoracis originate and insert onto the spinous processes.

The erector spinae are actively involved in extension and lateral bending of the spine. The capitis portion of the longissimus muscle may also bend the neck laterally and rotate the head to the ipsilateral side. The erector spinae serves as an antagonist, controlling the extent and rate of flexion.

The next group of spinal musculature is the transversospinalis. This group lies deep to the erector spinae. The muscles originate on the transverse processes and insert onto the spinous processes four to six levels cephalad. They act as primary rotators of the spine and also participate in extension.

The final two groups of muscles, the interspinalis and intertransversarial, are less defined. In the lumbar and cervical regions, they consist of pairs of muscles running between the spinous and transverse spines. In the thorax, they exist as the levatores costarum, which originate from the transverse process and insert onto the rib below. They act to elevate the ribs during respiration.

The deep muscles of the thoracic and lumbar spine are enveloped by the thoracic and lumbar fascia. In the thorax, there is a thin, transparent layer covering the thoracic musculature that becomes thicker inferiorly as it enters the lumbar spine. This fascia attaches to the iliac crest and posterior sacrum.

Neural Structures

Neural structures include the spinal cord and nerve roots and all related entities. A detailed discussion of these is beyond the scope of this chapter, but a brief overview is presented here.

The spinal cord lies within the spinal canal, extending down from the cervical spine, through the thoracic spine, to the upper lumbar spine. The cord tapers to a terminal region called the *conus medullaris,* which usually lies at L1–L2. Below this level, the neural elements in the spinal canal continue as spinal nerve roots, collectively called the *cauda equina* (Fig. 17-3). The conus medullaris is anchored by the filum terminale, a tough structure that inserts into the top of the sacrum. The cord and the cauda equina are contained within a protective sac and are bathed in cerebrospinal fluid (CSF). The outer layer of this sac is the *dura mater.*

Each spinal nerve exits the spinal canal through an opening called the *intervertebral foramen.* The nerve courses out through the foramen, under the pedicle of the vertebra forming the roof of the foramen. The floor

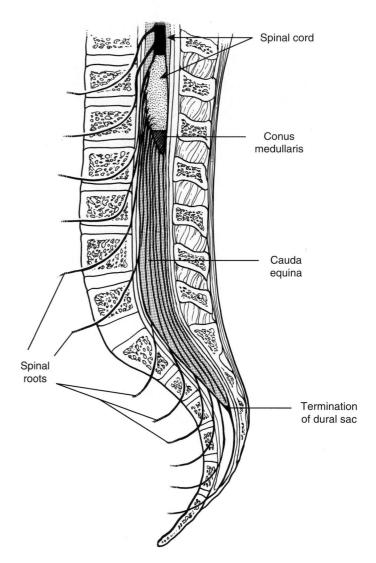

Spinal cord

Conus medullaris

Cauda equina

Spinal roots

Termination of dural sac

Fig. 17-3. Illustration of the spinal cord, conus medullaris, and cauda equina.

of the foramen is formed by the pedicle of the vertebra below.

The spinal nerves contain mixed fibers (motor, sensory, and visceral). They are composed of ventral and dorsal rootlets that unite and form the spinal nerve in the intervertebral foramen. The spinal nerve divides into a dorsal and ventral ramus as it exits the intervertebral foramen. The ventral rami supply a larger distribution, including the lumbosacral and coccygeal plexi. They also supply the intercostal nerves, which run in the groove along the inferior aspect of the rib.

The dorsal rami serve a limited distribution, consisting of the musculocutaneous innervation of the back. This area includes the spinous process to the angle of the rib in the thorax and to the lateral aspect of the paravertebral fascia in the lumbar spine. The dorsal rami enter the deep musculature of the back immediately after their exit from the intervertebral foramen. They divide into medial and lateral branches. In the lumbar region, the dorsal rami of L1, L2, and L3 provide cutaneous innervation via the superior cluneal nerves that exit over the posterior iliac crest. Branches of the dorsal rami may innervate the facet capsules and parts of the posterior annulus fibrosus. The dorsal rami of S1, S2, and S3 provide sensation via the middle cluneal nerves, and the dorsal rami of S4 and S5 provide sensation over the coccyx.

The L4, L5, S1, and S2 roots contribute to the sciatic nerve, a "cable-like" structure that includes the common peroneal and tibial nerves, which pass through the greater sciatic foramen, inferior to the piriformis muscle, lateral to the ischial tuberosity, and under the gluteus maximus muscle.

Vascular Supply

The blood supply to the thoracic and lumbar spine is predominantly from segmental arteries that originate directly from the aorta. These segmental arteries divide to form ventral and dorsal branches that supply the vertebral body. The dorsal branches provide the major blood supply to the dorsal musculature. A branch enters the intervertebral foramen and further divides, supplying blood to the nerve roots and spinal cord. The segmental arteries contain anastamosing branches that provide flow from segment to segment. There is significant variation in segmental arterial supply to the spinal cord.

The venous drainage parallels the arterial vasculature. An intervertebral plexus surrounds the spinal cord, which feeds into the segmental veins and drains directly into the vena cava.

BIOMECHANICS

As delineated previously, the spine includes bony and soft-tissue structures. The vertebral column must resist axial, torsional, and shear forces while allowing motion in the sagittal plane (flexion, extension), the frontal plane (left and right lateral bend), and the horizontal plane (axial rotation). This controlled motion is facilitated via the combined effects through the three-joint complex, *i.e.,* the disc and two facet joints at each level. Some motions, such as lateral bend, are coupled, which means they involve rotation in several planes, i.e., axial rotation and sagittal extension. Spinal biomechanics are extremely complex and are mentioned here primarily to alert the reader to review these matters in detail.

Although the spine is straight in the frontal plane, there are four curves in the sagittal plane. The cervical and lumbar regions are lordotic, whereas the thoracic and sacral regions are kyphotic. These balanced curves maintain the center of gravity over the pelvis and increase the load-carrying capacity of the spine. There is increased stress and susceptibility to injury at the junctions between the thoracolumbar and lumbosacral regions.

Forward flexion results in compression of the anterior disc and separation (distraction) of the facets. Active flexion is initiated by the musculature anterior to the vertebral column, such as the psoas and abdominal musculature. The posterior musculature and ligamentous structures primarily limit this motion. Active extension produces compression of the posterior vertebral disc and overlapping of the facet joints. It is initiated by the posterior musculature and is limited by the ALL and the posterior osseous structures. Flexion and extension are best accomplished in the lumbar region where the facets are oriented in a sagittal plane. The coronally oriented thoracic facets allow for maximum rotation, but the presence of the rib cage limits all motion and adds stability to these segments. Lateral bending combines flexion and rotation. Rotation is primarily limited by facet joint orientation and by disc thickness and integrity.

The disc must resist compressive, shear, and tensile forces. Axial forces are transmitted to the nucleus pulposus, which spans out radially against the annulus and creates a hoop stress.[26] The annulus is best suited to resist tensile and shear forces.

The soft tissue supports of the lumbar spine function like "guy wires." The abdominal muscles provide nearly 30% of lumbar support via hydrostatic column effects.[50] Accordingly, weakness in these structures results in abnormal increase in lordosis with higher stress on soft-tissue supports.

CLINICAL EVALUATION

The concepts outlined previously must be kept in mind when clinically evaluating athletes. With each patient, the examiner must attempt to correlate mechanism of injury with pertinent anatomy.

The history is perhaps the most important aspect of the clinical evaluation. The patient's chief complaint enables the clinician to remain focused while obtaining information concerning the timing, quality, and location of symptoms. If the patient is able to recall an exact cause of injury, it is extremely important to obtain a detailed description. For example, pain in the back after a direct blow from a football helmet is likely to be secondary to a contusion or posterior element injury. A description of the event may require the assistance of an observer present at the time of injury.

Questions related to the sequence of symptoms will also assist in establishing a diagnosis. First, it is important to clarify the time of onset of the patient's symptoms. Did the pain occur immediately after an injury or did it gradually occur hours later? These answers would help to differentiate between a break or contusion versus a muscular strain, which may not present in such an acute manner. Did the patient have pain before the injury? Is the pain constant, or is it intermittent? Is the pain associated with a certain activity? Does the pain occur at night? Pain that exists before the injury may be a chronic process possibly aggravated by the injury. Pain associated with upright activity may be a mechanical problem. Night pain should invoke concern about an infection or neoplasm. Pain radiating into the buttocks may result from spinal stenosis. Pain radiating into the groin should alert the clinician of possible hip abnormality.

Location of pain provides additional support for a specific diagnosis. Is the pain isolated to a certain site in the back? Is it midline, or does it include the paraspinal areas? What about the sciatic notch and the sacroiliac joints? Does the pain radiate into the buttocks or lower extremities? This information should be obtained carefully but without "leading" the patient.

It is fundamentally important to separate **back** pain from **leg** pain. Back pain may result from injury to one of the posterior structures. It may also result from irritation of the posterior primary ramus, the small branch coming posteriorly off the nerve root immediately after its exit from the foramen. This branch supplies the facet capsules, posterior annulus, and some of the local musculature.

In contrast, pain radiating to the leg, particularly below the knee, suggests irritation of the large ventral portion of the root exiting from the canal via the foramen and continuing distally into the leg. The term "sciatica" is often used to refer loosely to pain radiating down the leg for whatever reason, although it specifically refers to nerve root compression (most commonly L5 or S1) by a herniated nucleus pulposus. Pain radiating down the leg as a result of nerve root irritation is referred to as *radiculopathy*. Determining the dermatomal distribution of these symptoms within the leg is essential in identifying the specific nerve root involved.

The quality of pain and any associated symptoms are also very important components. Is the pain a dull ache, or is it a sharp, stabbing pain? Is there "electricity, tingling, or numbness" shooting down his or her leg? Is there any associated weakness? Does anything make the pain better or worse? Ask the patient to describe the condition in his or her own words. Does forward flexion relieve the symptoms (spinal stenosis)?

After obtaining the history of the present illness, one must carefully review the medical, surgical, family, and social history. When evaluating athletes with back complaints, it is important to realize that their symptoms may not be related to their athletic endeavors.

Having completed the history, the clinician should have formulated a working differential diagnosis, which will be further refined through physical examination of the spine by inspection, palpation, neurologic evaluation, and testing of range of motion. It is important to have the patient fully disrobe (down to underwear) before the examination. Inspection should begin with the patient standing in the upright position (if possible). Initially, one should observe the skin by looking for ecchymosis, swelling, old scars, cafe au lait spots (associated with neurofibromatosis), lipomata, and tufts of hair (associated with congenital defects).

Next, the alignment of the spine should be evaluated. Curvature of the spine can be best appreciated from behind with the patient leaning forward. Often, rotation of the vertebral column will accompany a scoliotic curve, resulting in a unilateral prominence of the rib cage known as a rib hump. Asymmetry of the shoulder or pelvis may also result from scoliosis, and a discrepancy in leg length may be another cause of pelvic tilt leading to back pain. Viewing the patient from the side will allow evaluation of the spine in the sagittal plane. One should look for changes in thoracic kyphosis or lumbar lordosis. Muscle spasm secondary to acute injury often leads to loss of lumbar lordosis.

The patient should be asked to perform several routine tasks, which will provide a quick assessment of his or her overall condition. For example, having the patient walk on his or her toes and heels provides information as to the general strength of the lower extremities. Having the patient walk (preferably without knowing he or she is being observed) may reveal a spinal radiculopathy with associated leg pain and weakness or Trendelenburg signs suggestive of hip abnormality. After inspection, the spine should be palpated in a systematic fashion to identify areas of tenderness. It is often helpful to begin palpating in a pain-free area. Touching the patient without causing pain will gain his or her confidence, reduce anxiety, and allow him or her to define more accurately areas of tenderness. The top of the iliac crests are a rough reference for L4–L5. Focal areas of tenderness, called *point tenderness,* usually represent acute trauma, such as a contusion, strain, musculoligamentous tear, or fracture.

The deep and superficial musculature of the back should be carefully palpated. The paraspinal muscles may demonstrate tenderness and rigidity, indicating spasm with loss of range of motion. The range of motion of the spine may be difficult to evaluate because, unlike the extremities, there is no matched control to serve as a reference. Furthermore, the segments act with the pelvis and hips to provide overall motion and may be difficult to isolate.

As noted previously, careful examination is essential to localize abnormalities involving the sacroiliac joints, iliac crests, and the greater sciatic notch. Often, conditions affecting these areas may present with complaints of "back pain" that is not really coming from the back. Because injury to these structures can also result in limited radiation of pain to the leg, it is particularly important to physically localize them.

Further distally in the pelvis lies the coccyx, which is injured frequently. Pain in the area of the coccyx is called *coccydynia* and is characterized by exquisite local tenderness. This pain may be better appreciated by palpating the anterior and posterior aspects of the coccyx during a rectal examination.

Physical examination should also include palpation of the costovertebral angles and the abdomen. Although kidney infections, stones, or contusions are not usually considered "sports injuries," these may present with back pain. Intraabdominal abnormalities, such as a dissecting aortic aneurysm, may also refer pain to the back. Although rare, this condition should be kept in mind, particularly when examining older athletes.

Flexion in the lower spine leads to the reversal of lumbar lordosis and rotation of the pelvis. Commonly with lower spine injuries, muscle spasm will prevent motion in the lumbar spine, and, thus, flexion will be performed solely through rotation of the pelvis while maintaining lumbar lordosis. Limitation of forward flexion may also result from hamstring tightness. Evaluation of extension should be performed in the standing position. Extension places stress on the posterior elements, including the pars interarticularis and facet joints, and it will decrease the opening of the intervertebral foramen. Symptoms secondary to abnormality in these regions may be exacerbated by this motion. A step off in the lower back may represent spondylolisthesis. Rotation and lateral bending can be best evaluated with the patient sitting on a chair securing the pelvis and lower extremities. Rotation and lateral bending should be symmetric. Lateral bending may compress the intervertebral foramen on the ipsilateral side, aggravating impingement of the spinal nerve in patients with radicular symptoms.

When there is a possibility of acute neurologic deficit with spinal cord injury, precaution must be taken regarding immobilization, oxygenation, and medical management. Protocols exist for this and must be strictly followed to minimize risk of neurologic deterioration. Neurologic status is determined by evaluation of the sensorium and the central nervous system and the cervical, thoracic, lumbar, and sacral spinal segments. Injury to the spinal cord may be classified as complete or incomplete. Early documentation of completeness of cord injury is essential because prognosis and management are vastly different for complete versus incomplete spinal cord injuries. Incomplete spinal cord injury refers to any situation where some but not all neurologic function is lost in the spinal cord or conus medullaris. Neurologic function remains normal proximal to the area of injury but is lost distally. Neurologic loss may be minimal as manifested by slight numbness or slight weakness in a limited area. Conversely, it may be near total, with apparent total loss of all sensory, motor, and reflex activity, including bowel and bladder function. In this setting, careful examination is crucial to identify **any** remaining function, no matter how limited. The integrity of sacral innervation is important to assess while conducting the neurologic examination. The S2, S3, S4, and S5 dermatomes provide sensation around the anus. Because the sacral plexus also supplies the intrinsic muscles of the foot and the sphincters of the bowel and the bladder, even a flicker of intrinsic foot function (toe motion) may indicate residual cord function and, therefore, incomplete cord injury. This condition is referred to as *sacral sparing*. With sudden and complete neurologic injury (paraplegia or quadriplegia), there is no hope for neurologic recovery. In contrast, if the injury is incomplete, there may be potential for some neurologic recovery, although the specific scope of return cannot be predicted. Numerous grading schemes (Frankel classification, Motor Index Score, etc.) have been developed to assess the scope of neurologic dysfunction. Of note, the Babinski reflex is a pathologic reflex, which, if present, indicates upper motor neuron injury.

The presence of spinal shock may confuse initial assessment of completeness of neurologic injury. Spinal shock refers to a physiologic state of paralysis, hypotonia, and areflexia after an acute spinal cord injury. This state may be reversible and often lasts 24 to 72 hours. The return of the bulbocavernosus reflex indicates the end of spinal shock. This reflex is evaluated by noting anal sphincter contraction in response to squeezing the glans penis in men or pulling gently on the Foley catheter in women. If the reflex is not present, the cord is in a state of spinal shock, indicating the possibility of future neurologic recovery.

Fortunately, spinal cord injury is very rare, particularly to the thoracic and lumbar regions. In part, this is because of the excellent protection and limited mobility of the thoracic region. In the more mobile lumbar region, there is no spinal cord because the conus terminates at L1–L2, with the cauda equina continuing distally. The conus is susceptible to injury, in part because of its location near the thoracolumbar junction, the area most often associated with vertebral fracture. Compression of the cauda equina may be caused by acute disc herniation, osseous fragments, hematoma, and a host of other entities. When this condition is acute, it is a surgical emergency known as *cauda equina syndrome*. This situation presents with bowel and bladder dysfunction (usually urinary retention), saddle anesthesia in the perineal area, and varying degrees of lower extremity weakness and loss of sensation. Failure to immediately decompress the involved neural elements results in permanent functional loss.

These acute neurologic conditions are rare, however. The neurologic examination should routinely focus on motor, sensory, and reflex evaluation of the thoracic and lumbar regions. Sensory testing should be conducted with attention to individual dermatomes. Motor testing should also be performed according to known segmental innervation patterns (see first box below).[19] Of note, manual strength testing by the examiner may fail to reveal relative weakness of an athlete's trunk or legs because an examiner's hands and arms may not be strong enough to overcome these muscle groups, even when partially weakened. Therefore, when possible, heel and toe walking and squatting and rising from full squat are important motor tests. Evaluation of deep tendon reflexes will also assist in identifying the level of neurologic involvement (see second box below).

LOWER EXTREMITY INNERVATION

Hip flexion: T12, L1, L2, L3

Knee extension: L2, L3, L4 femoral nerve

Hip adduction: L2, L3, L4 obturator nerve

Ankle dorsiflexion: L4 deep peroneal nerve

Toe dorsiflexion: L5 deep peroneal nerve

Ankle eversion: S1 superficial peroneal nerve

Ankle plantar flexion: S1 posterior tibial nerve

LOWER EXTREMITY DEEP TENDON REFLEXES

Patellar reflex: L4

Posterior tibialis reflex: L5 (difficult to elicit)

Achilles tendon reflex: S1

Multiple maneuvers have been described that place tension on the sciatic and femoral nerves to elicit radicular findings. Straight leg raising places tension on the sciatic nerve.[34] The test result is considered positive if radicular symptoms are reproduced when the straight leg is raised above 30° with the patient supine. Dorsiflexion of the ankle will place greater tension on the nerve and should exacerbate the patient's symptoms. The Lasègue test,[39] performed in the supine position, also places tension on the sciatic nerve. With the hip and knee initially flexed to 90°, the knee is slowly extended to elicit the radicular symptoms. Like the Valsalva maneuver, the Milgram test[18] is designed to increase the intrathecal pressure. In the supine position, the patient is asked to maintain both extended legs approximately three inches off the table for 30 seconds. If there is root impingement, the increase in intrathecal pressure will exacerbate radicular symptoms.

The Patrick (FABER) test is used to detect hip or sacroiliac abnormality. The patient lies supine on the examining table with the foot of the involved side placed on the opposite knee, which positions the hip in flexion, abduction, and external rotation, i.e., FABER. Downward force applied to the knee with the pelvis secure produces pressure on the sacroiliac joint. Pain radiating to the groin is suggestive of hip abnormality.

When injured on the field, the athlete should not be moved before examination. This precaution also applies to the athlete's equipment, which should not be removed until a targeted history and physical examination have been performed. Any suspicion of potential spinal injury should be managed with great caution, and the patient should be immobilized on a backboard. Complaints of numbness, tingling, or weakness in the legs, significant back pain after a high-velocity injury, or significant muscle spasm limiting movement should be managed with immobilization.[12] Off the field, the clinician has the luxury of being able to obtain a detailed history, perform an exhaustive examination, and request diagnostic testing.

On or off the field, the clinician should have a working differential diagnosis after completing the history and physical examination. When necessary, radiographic examinations should be performed to confirm this clinical diagnosis. Importantly, these tests should not be ordered in a "shotgun" manner, wherein the test is being ordered to make the diagnosis. Rather, each test requested should be designed to answer a specific question. Test results must be clinically correlated, so the entire picture makes sense. Some radiographic studies are particularly sensitive and may produce false-positive results, which have virtually no connection with the issue at hand. Clinical judgment is essential in directing management.

Plain radiographs are routinely used as the first step in the radiographic evaluation of the spine. They allow assessment of the alignment and integrity of the osseous structures within the vertebral column. Radiographs are commonly obtained in the anteroposterior, lateral, and oblique planes. Spinal curvature in the frontal plane (scoliosis) may be assessed on the anteroposterior view.

In addition, the status of the transverse processes may be determined. Widening of the interpedicular distance associated with loss of vertebral height may represent a burst fracture with possible involvement of the spinal canal. The lateral projection clearly demonstrates the vertebral bodies, intervertebral disc spaces, posterior structures, and the overall alignment of the spine in the sagittal plane. This view is especially helpful in evaluating compression fractures, dislocations, and degenerative changes within the spine. The oblique projection permits identification of defects within the pars interarticularis and evaluation of the intervertebral foramina. In this view, the pars is known as the "neck" of the "Scottie dog." Occasionally, lateral flexion and extension views are obtained to assess segmental instability demonstrated by increased angulation or translation of the vertebral bodies.

Computed tomography enables the clinician to evaluate the osseous and the soft tissues of the spine. Axial cuts permit assessment of the spinal canal for evidence of encroachment by herniated discs or retropulsed bony fragments from vertebral body fractures. Multiple sections in various planes may be performed, making this technique especially useful in evaluating fractures. Using computerized software, two- and three-dimensional views of the spine may be reconstructed, facilitating three-dimensional evaluation.

Magnetic resonance imaging (MRI) has become extremely popular in evaluating the soft tissues of the spine, including the intervertebral discs, neural structures, and musculoligamentous components. It is especially valuable in demonstrating degeneration and herniation of the intervertebral discs. The MRI is also able to evaluate surrounding soft tissues for evidence of trauma, including edema and hematoma formation, and intrinsic cord abnormalities such as syringomelia. Contrast material (gadolinium) that highlights vascularized areas can help to differentiate scar from disc.

Myelography, in conjunction with computed tomography, remains an excellent but invasive diagnostic technique for evaluating the contents of the spinal canal and exiting nerve roots. With the advent of MRI, the use of myelography has declined, but it remains a powerful diagnostic tool in certain settings, such as severe deformity and revision surgery. Nuclear imaging, such as the technetium bone scan, is an extremely sensitive modality that is invaluable for detection of increased osteoblastic activity throughout the skeleton. Such increase in activity may reveal occult stress fractures, healing fractures, response to infection or tumor, metabolic bone disease, and a host of other conditions. For example, a bone scan may assist in evaluating patients in whom there is a high suspicion of spondylolysis, even though plain radiographs appear normal. Similarly, a bone scan may be used to screen the skeleton for metastatic lesions and infection. Although the bone scan is extremely sensitive, it is not very specific. Other more specific nuclear imaging methods (SPECT, indium, and gallium scanning) are available.

There are many variations and degenerative changes in the healthy spine. Whenever possible, diagnostic tests should be reviewed with the radiologist, providing him or her with the pertinent history and physical findings. This will allow the correlation of the patient's history and physical findings with abnormal results on the diagnostic examination.

Back Pain and Injury in Sports

Rates of thoracic and lumbar injury vary greatly by sport. Keene[23] noted that "Surveillance and prevention of back injuries in athletes should be predicated upon studies that document the incidence and types of injuries that occur in each sport."

Participation in competitive tennis, volleyball, and cycling correlated significantly with increased back pain in children aged 8 to 16 years.[3] As noted by Hresko,[21] the most common mechanism of injury is through repetitive microtrauma, resulting in fatigue injuries. This applies to contact and noncontact sports, including gymnastics, ballet, figure skating, hockey, football, weightlifting, rowing, and diving.[22,24,27,35]

Because the growth plate is the weakest tensile link in the axial skeleton, physeal injuries may accompany disc injury in children. Annular protrusion produces traction on the ring apophysis and may avulse bony endplate fragments.[4] Traumatic vertebral ring apophyseal injury may be followed by disc prolapse and degeneration.[43]

Vertebral apophysitis resulting from microfractures may present with point tenderness or with vague pain. Management is rest followed by stretching and strengthening rehabilitation. Similarly, anterior ring apophyseal fracture caused by recurrent flexion results in wedging of thoracolumbar or lumbar vertebral bodies.[35] Management is semirigid bracing to unload anterior elements until symptoms abate.

A recent study on competitive wrestlers, gymnasts, and soccer and tennis players found unusually high frequencies and a significant relationship between back pain (50% to 85%) and radiologic abnormalities (36% to 55%).[44] Radiologic findings indicated direct traumatic changes and disturbed vertebral growth. These findings emphasize the vulnerability of the spine during the growth period and raise significant questions about when vigorous athletic training should begin, what loads are acceptable, and who takes responsibility to prevent and detect injury in the young athlete.

Most serious cases of spinal injury occur in high-velocity or contact sports. A 5-year review of 129 wrestlers identified only three back sprains, an incidence of only 2.3% for back injury.[37] In contrast, review of 70 female gymnasts revealed nine injuries to the thoracic and lumbar spine, including two spinal fractures, two spondylolyses, and five back strains.[38] Incidence of back injury was 12.8%, more than five times higher than that of the wrestlers. Only 50% of adolescent gymnasts sustaining herniated lumbar discs were able to return to their previous level after conservative therapy without experiencing further back pain.[30] Furthermore, interspinous osteoarthrosis and spondylolysis were more common among gymnasts.[18]

Keene[23] found a 7% incidence of back injuries sustained by 4700 varsity collegiate athletes over a 10-year period. Eighty-one percent of these injuries were to the lumbar spine. Notably, 80% of these injuries occurred during practice, and 14% occurred during preseason conditioning. Only 6% of these injuries occurred during competition. An acute injury occurred in 59% of cases, overuse in 12%, and aggravation of a preexisting condition in 29%. Football and gymnastics demonstrated the highest incidence of injury, 17% and 11%, respectively. Sixty percent of all back injuries were diagnosed as muscle strains, particularly common in football players.

Other studies have documented increased frequency of back injury in oarsmen, presumably because of the high physical demands of the sport.[20,40] Up to 82% of elite female rowers have significant low back pain.[19] Williams reported that 15% of all athletic injuries in England occur to the spine.[51] These injuries are most prevalent in automobile racing, horseback riding, parachuting, mountaineering, and weightlifting.

INJURIES

Soft-Tissue Injuries

The majority of injuries to the thoracic and lumbar spine are self-limiting and do not come to the attention of a clinician. Many of these injuries are contusions, musculotendinous strains, and ligamentous sprains. Contusions result from blunt trauma sustained by a direct blow. Often, the athlete is able to recollect an incident responsible for the injury. On physical examination, a contusion will present as a relatively discrete area of point tenderness with occasional overlying ecchymosis. Given a history of blunt trauma to the spine and point tenderness over the posterior elements on physical examination, the examiner should consider conventional radiographs to rule out the possibility of a fracture. A contusion may result in paraspinal muscle spasm that limits range of motion of the spine. Management of this injury includes an initial period of icing followed by stretching and strengthening of the supporting structures. The athlete should not be permitted to return to competition until normal range of motion and strength have been restored. If these criteria are not met, the spine's ability to withstand trauma may be limited, and the athlete will be susceptible to further injury.

Muscular or ligamentous injury affecting the spine may result from an acute event or from repetitive stress producing a chronic, insidious process. In the latter case, injury may be subtle, and the athlete may not be able to recall a particular incident. Further probing may expose need for altering the training regimen.

Acute musculoligamentous strains and sprains of the thoracic and, more commonly, lumbar and lumbosacral spine are the most common injuries to these regions. These injuries are characterized by nonradiating back pain whose etiology may be unclear. Common causes include change in level of activity, overuse activity, inadequate conditioning, poor posture, and improper lifting. Initially, a radiograph is not needed, particularly in young patients, but one should be taken if symptoms persist 2 to 3 weeks. Management consists of rest, icing for the first 72 hours, nonsteroidal anti-inflammatory drugs (NSAIDs), muscle relaxants, followed by physical modalities and controlled exercise with focus on strength and endurance, heat, transcutaneous electrical nerve stimulation, and education. Ninety percent of injuries resolve within 2 months.[47]

Chronic muscular or ligamentous injuries often present with vague symptoms of back discomfort. The origin of these symptoms is difficult to localize on examination. Movement placing stress on the injured structure may reproduce symptoms. As mentioned previously, an initial period of icing followed by stretching and strengthening is required. The chronicity of this condition must be reinforced to the patient. The athlete may need to stop or alter the training regimen possibly responsible for the injury. NSAIDs may be considered as adjuncts to rehabilitation.

Because the intervertebral disc is susceptible to herniation and degeneration, this area has an important potential for pathology. With age, there is a decrease in the proteoglycan content of the nucleus pulposus, leading to loss of hydration. The nucleus loses its ability to absorb stress and increases the demands placed on the annulus fibrosus and other supporting structures. Repetitive axial and torsional stresses applied to the disc lead to tears of the annulus and subsequent herniation of the nucleus pulposus.[14]

The majority of disc herniations occur in the lumbar spine. Symptoms of disc herniation may present acutely after a traumatic insult or may develop gradually without an inciting event, especially in the middle-aged or older athlete. Lumbar disc herniation is most common in the third and fourth decades, however it may occur at any age, including adolescence. The chief complaint is usually pain, often described as radiating from the back or buttock into the leg, which may be accompanied by numbness and weakness involving the lower extremity. It is important to obtain the exact distribution of the patient's symptoms. Complaints of bilateral leg pain or bowel and bladder symptoms should alert the clinician to the possibility of cauda equina compression syndrome. Pain is exacerbated with coughing or Valsalva maneuver because this increases intrathecal pressure and may increase contact between the irritated nerve root and its surrounding structures. Symptoms are often exacerbated in the sitting position, particularly with driving. Sitting reduces lumbar lordosis. As a result of the three-joint complex, this position unloads the facets but increases load on the disc, increases intradiscal pressure, and, therefore, symptoms, at the affected level.

On inspection, the patient may lean toward or away from the involved side, depending on the location of the herniation (Fig. 17-4). This leaning relieves pressure on the compressed nerve root by opening the intervertebral foramen. Midline tenderness in the lower back is common and often accompanied by paraspinal spasm. Radicular symptoms may be reproduced by performing femoral or sciatic nerve tension tests or by performing a

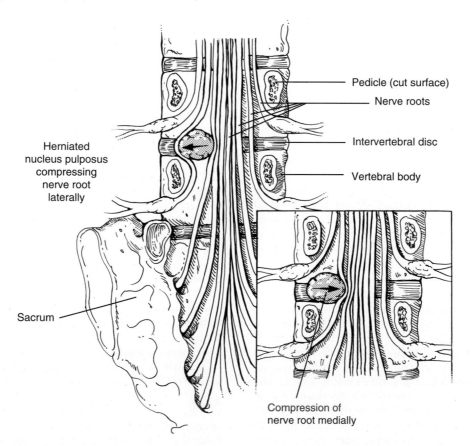

Pedicle (cut surface)
Nerve roots
Intervertebral disc
Vertebral body

Herniated nucleus pulposus compressing nerve root laterally

Sacrum

Compression of nerve root medially

Fig. 17-4. Herniated disc material impinging on adjacent nerve roots. Patients will involuntarily position themselves to minimize pressure on nerve roots.

Valsalva maneuver. The nerve tension tests must reproduce the patient's radicular symptoms to be considered significant. Straight leg testing in the sitting position (along with a host of other clinical examinations) may help differentiate real abnormality from malingering. A careful neurologic examination, noting a specific dermatomal sensory deficit, corresponding segmental motor weakness, and decreased deep tendon reflexes, may identify the compressed nerve root. If there is concern of cauda equina compression syndrome, evaluation of sacral innervation is imperative. This evaluation should include sensory testing around the anus and rectal tone evaluation.

Of note, adolescent athletes with disc herniations may present with back pain and hamstring tightness and minimal neurologic or radicular symptoms.

Plain radiographs may demonstrate indirect evidence of disc degeneration, such as decreased or irregular disc spaces. However, plain radiographs do not directly demonstrate disc herniations. MRI has become the initial procedure of choice for delineating disc abnormality although other techniques (computed tomography, myelography) are used as well.

In the absence of an acute neurologic deficit, the mainstays of management include rest, NSAIDs and antispasmodic medications, and physical therapy. Bedrest should be kept to less than 2 to 7 days, and controlled activity (therapy, rehabilitation) is initiated as soon as it is tolerable. If the pain is extreme, narcotics may be necessary. Many patients will markedly improve within 10 days, but conservative treatment should continue for 6 weeks before other measures are attempted. If leg pain persists beyond this period, a series of epidural steroid injections may be considered. Maximum benefit is usually within 2 weeks, with a maximum of three injections given per year. Responses vary greatly, with short-term improvement seen in roughly 40% of patients, but no significant long-term results have been demonstrated.[49] Rehabilitation must include stretching, strengthening, and modalities. Abdominal strengthening and lumbar extension exercises are beneficial. Therapy should be started early to prevent deconditioning. Return to athletic competition must be considered on an individual basis. Patients with significant pain relief, no neurologic sequelae, and normal range of motion may resume unrestricted activities. Education and lifestyle changes may be necessary to prevent recurrence.

Absolute surgical indications include cauda equina compression syndrome and progressive neurologic impairment. Patients without neurologic deficit who have not responded to conservative therapy may also be considered as elective candidates for surgical intervention if there is clear correlation between symptoms, physical findings, imaging, and electrodiagnostic (electromyography, somatosensory-evoked potential) testing. Successful return to vigorous athletic activity may be possible after surgery. More than 80% of athletes returned to sports after percutaneous or open discectomy, usually 8 weeks after surgery.[28] After surgical decompression, careful evaluation is necessary before return to athletics because functional impairment increases risk for further injury.

Degeneration of the intervertebral disc without herniation may be another source of low back pain. With disc degeneration, more stress is transferred to the ligamentous and osseous structures of the spine, which may lead to arthrosis of the facet joints and hypertrophy of the supporting ligaments.

The presentation of degenerative disc disease varies. Symptoms may consist of pain isolated to the back or pain radiating into the buttocks and lower extremities. These symptoms are usually aggravated with increased activity, especially forward flexion. On physical examination, findings may include midline tenderness and paraspinal muscle spasm, resulting in a limited range of motion. Disc degeneration is extremely common in the older population, regardless of symptoms. It is important to consider other possible etiologies responsible for the patient's complaints before making the diagnosis of degenerative disc disease. Management of a symptomatic degenerative disc includes NSAIDs, exercises, and modalities. Exercises should concentrate on strengthening abdominal and paraspinal musculature to relieve stress on the vertebral column.

Certain sports appear to contribute to an increased incidence of disc degeneration. In particular, a study on retired world-class gymnasts in their second and third decades of life demonstrated an increased incidence of disc degeneration on MRI that correlated with increased incidence of back pain (Fig. 17-5).[45] Signs of disc degeneration on MRI were present in 75% of gymnasts in the study. A similar study performed on younger participants (mean age, 12 years) demonstrated no signs of increased disc degeneration in the gymnasts.[46]

Although rare, thoracic disc herniations exist and are most common in the fourth decade of life.[1] The signs and symptoms of thoracic disc herniation vary widely and often may be subtle and associated with mild, but persistent, back pain. With a posterolateral herniation, impingement of a thoracic nerve root may lead to chest-wall pain that follows a dermatomal distribution. Often the neurologic symptoms are absent or subtle with mild changes in trunk sensation and lower extremity weakness. An athlete with a central herniation leading to direct impingement of the cord may demonstrate long track signs on examination, including Babinski's sign and clonus. The most important feature in establishing the diagnosis is a high degree of suspicion. The diagnosis is best confirmed by MRI or myelography. Management is usually conservative, including bedrest and NSAIDs followed by rehabilitation consisting of stretching and strengthening. Epidural injection with steroids may provide some relief if symptoms persist. Surgery is indicated if there is significant neurologic involvement. Anterior approaches are safest.

Sprains of the sacroiliac joint are another common source of back pain. This important joint within the pelvis is subject to large stresses and has strong restraining ligaments. Sudden and repetitive low-grade movements may result in injury. These injuries are often overlooked and are characterized by unilateral pain over the sacroiliac joint that may radiate to the buttock, leg, and groin. Symptoms may be exacerbated with standing and

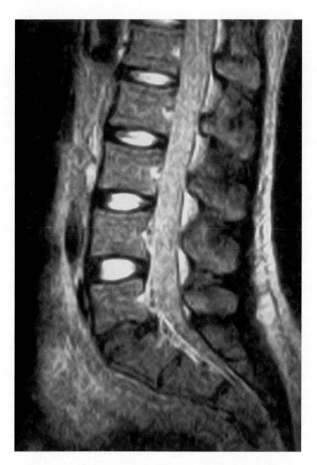

Fig. 17-5. Magnetic resonance imaging showing disc degeneration at L5–S1. Note loss of bright white signal at L5–S1 compared with other discs, suggestive of loss of water content and degeneration.

sitting as these impart shear and rotational forces across the joint. Stabilizing the pelvis by maintaining the opposite hip extended while flexing the hip on the affected side will usually reproduce the symptoms as will the FABER maneuver. Result of straight leg raising is normal, as is neurologic examination. Management consists of NSAIDs, sacroiliac mobilization and manipulation, modalities, heat, sacroiliac and trochanteric belts, stretches, and sacroiliac injections. Many patients are relieved to learn that their problem is "not their back" and will resume activity despite residual pain.

The facet syndrome is another painful condition, primarily of the lumbar spine, characterized by local back pain with paralumbar tenderness. Pain may be exacerbated with lumbar extension, whereas straight leg raising leads to hip, buttock, and back pain, but not leg pain. Management is limitation of activity, NSAIDs, modalities, and manipulation. Facet injections do not exceed placebo effects.

"Kissing spines," commonly found in female gymnasts, refers to interspinous bursitis wherein the interspinous ligament develops a pseudobursa and there is chronic inflammation and even osteophyte formation on the adjacent spinous processes.[18] Injections of local anesthetic and steroids have been described to manage this condition.

The piriformis syndrome is another pain syndrome wherein the sciatic nerve is irritated as it passes near the piriformis muscle. This often vague condition leads to deep pain along the posterior aspect of the hip that often radiates down into the leg. Unlike disc disease, there is no correlation of radicular pain with Valsalva maneuver. The condition occurs six times more frequently in women than men. It is suspected pain is triggered on active hip external rotation and with passive internal rotation of the hip. Management is with rest, NSAIDs, stretching, local injections, and, rarely, partial surgical release of the piriformis.

Osseous Conditions

FRACTURES. Fractures of the thoracic and lumbar spine occur infrequently in athletics and are usually associated with high-velocity or contact sports. The stability of the spinal column must be evaluated after each injury. Denis[11] described an anatomic classification of fractures according to a three-column system. The anterior column is composed of the ALL and the anterior two thirds of the vertebral body and annulus. The middle column consists of the PLL and the posterior third of the vertebral body and annulus. The posterior column includes the facets and spinous processes and the posterior ligamentous structures, including the ligamentum flavum, facet capsules, and interspinous and supraspinous ligaments. This classification has been modified to highlight the importance of bone soft-tissue components in each of the three columns.[13,48] Trauma to the vertebral column results from excessive application of compression, distraction, rotation, or shear forces. The resulting injuries include compression fractures, burst fractures, flexion–distraction fractures, and fracture dislocations. Instability is unusual with anterior column involvement only but becomes an issue with disruption of the middle column. Fractures of the anterior column followed by posterior ligamentous disruption may also lead to spinal instability.

Compression fractures are the most common type of fracture in the thoracic spine. In these injuries, flexion or axial loading lead to failure of the anterior cortex of the vertebral body. The amount of trauma necessary to produce this injury depends on the quality of the bone within the vertebral body. Skydiving has a high incidence of spine compression fractures as these injuries account for 17% of skeletal injuries in this sport.[32] Axial loading while seated, such as in falls in alpine or cross-country skiing, commonly leads to compression fractures.[21]

In healthy athletes, a great deal of energy is required to produce a compression fracture. In individuals with osteoporosis, the amount of force necessary for compression fracture may be trivial. This issue is of increasing concern as more older patients with decreased bone mass pursue sports.[17] If the fracture occurs in a young individual with minimal trauma, the possibility of an abnormal fracture should be investigated.

Compression fractures may be classified according to the amount of anterior compression. Most compression fractures do not have associated neurologic conditions and are relatively stable. Plain radiographs, especially the lateral view, will allow evaluation of the anterior and posterior cortices, and the amount of compression and angulation can be determined. Most fractures involve less than 25% loss of anterior body height (Fig. 17-6). As compression approaches 50%, there are concerns of instability caused by posterior ligamentous failure.[16]

Compression fractures are extremely painful, resulting in paraspinal muscle spasm and limited range of motion. On physical examination, the patient will exhibit diffuse tenderness surrounding the fractured vertebra. A thorough neurologic examination should be conducted. It is important to document any neurologic symptoms after the injury, even if transient. Any signs of neurologic involvement require further evaluation for possible spinal injury.

Initial management of compression fractures includes pain control and bedrest. Management of stable fractures involves bracing in a rigid hyperextension orthosis. Stabilization will provide pain relief and will also prevent progression of kyphosis during fracture healing. The length of bracing depends on the patient's bone quality and healing potential, although 8 to 12 weeks are usually needed. Progression of kyphosis must be monitored in patients with severe compression fractures or multiple compression fractures. After bracing and resolution of pain, the patient is started on a rehabilitation regimen including strengthening and stretching to regain range of motion. Fractures with more than 50% compression or 20° of angulation are potentially unstable and must be observed closely for progression. Surgical decompres-

sion and stabilization are indicated for instability and progressive neurologic involvement.

Burst fractures involving the posterior vertebral body cortex have serious implications. Disruption of the middle column leads to mechanical instability and the possibility of neurologic injury resulting from retropulsed fragments within the spinal canal. On the anteroposterior view, an increased distance between the pedicles may represent disruption of the posterior cortex, indicating a possible burst fracture. Computed tomography is most effective in demonstrating the fracture configuration and integrity of the spinal canal. Surgical decompression and stabilization are often necessary for burst fractures.

Flexion–distraction (seatbelt injuries) and fracture–dislocation injuries rarely occur in sports and are usually related to high-velocity activities, such as highdiving, automobile racing, and skydiving. These injuries have a high incidence of spinal cord trauma and usually require surgical decompression and stabilization. It is the responsibility of the clinician on the field to recognize the seriousness of the injury and to immobilize properly the patient before evacuation. Neurologic evaluation is crucial, and evidence of progression requires emergency decompression. Plain radiographs and computed tomography are standard for evaluating the osseous integrity of the vertebral column. MRI is extremely helpful in assessing trauma to the surrounding soft tissues, including the ligamentous structures, intervertebral disc, and spinal cord.

Transverse process fractures generally result from a direct blow. Frequently, the athlete is able to recall an incident responsible for the injury, and pain is localized to the fracture site. Overlying tissues may be contused. Diagnosis of a fracture is confirmed by plain radiographs. This fracture pattern is stable, and management is aimed at pain relief and followed by restoration of range of motion. When these goals are achieved, the patient may return to athletic participation. Cold therapy for the first 48 to 72 hours is followed by heat, rest and immobilization until the patient is nearly asymptomatic. Stretching and strengthening exercises can then begin. Protection with a flak jacket may be necessary if contact sports are resumed before complete resolution of symptoms.

Participation in noncontact sports may begin after an appropriate period of immobilization and rehabilitation from a spinal fracture. Involvement in contact sports must be considered on an individual basis. In a young athlete without surgical intervention, contact sports may be considered after proper discussion regarding potential risks involved.

SPONDYLOLYSIS AND SPONDYLOLISTHESIS. Athletes of all ages commonly complain of mild lumbar symptoms after strenuous workouts, but these symptoms generally resolve quickly without affecting the training schedule and requiring medical evaluation. In contrast, recurrent complaints of vague, but persistent, back pain, buttock ache, and hamstring tightness associated with activity should alert the clinician to an underlying spondylolysis or spondylolisthesis.[25]

Spondylolysis refers to a defect in the pars interarticularis (Fig. 17-7). The defect is believed to be a fatigue

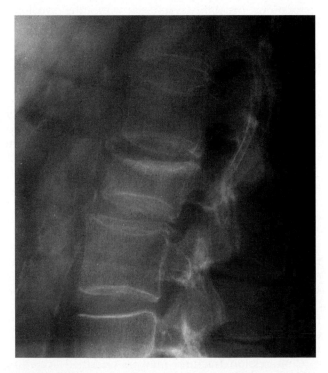

Fig. 17-6. Compression fracture at L2. Note mild loss of anterior vertebral body height.

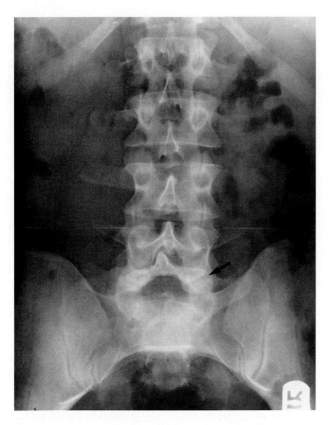

Fig. 17-7. Anteroposterior radiograph of spondylolysis with pars defect seen at L5 (arrow).

fracture secondary to repetitive stresses placed on the pars during hyperextension.[52] Repetitive stress on the pars from impingement by the inferior facet of the cephalad vertebra may result in microfractures, with continued stress leading to overt fracture. As a result, the disc bears excessive shear loads, and spondylolisthesis (slippage) may occur if excessive loading continues.[27] The incidence of spondylolysis in the general population is approximately 5%.[2] Studies demonstrate a hereditary predisposition, with Eskimo populations having an incidence as high as 50%.[42] Spondylolysis is believed to be the most common cause of back pain in children and adolescents, although many people with spondylolysis are asymptomatic. The presence of spondylolysis does not necessarily implicate it as the pain source. Clinical correlation is essential to establish a causal relationship.

Certain athletic activities including gymnastics, diving, wrestling, weightlifting, and football are associated with an increased incidence of spondylolysis.[15] Certain features of these sports, such as upright weightlifting, dismounts from gymnastics, three-point stance contact in football, hard tennis overhead serve, and competitive diving, result in repetitive axial loading with the spine in extension.[8,50] Often, a single event responsible for the symptoms cannot be recalled. The pain is often unilateral, nonradiating, increased with activity (especially on extension), and relieved with rest. Physical examination may reveal decreased lumbar motion and hamstring tightness, a slight list caused by spasm, and exacerbation

of pain with rotation and extension. Result of neurologic testing is normal, and result of straight leg raising is negative.

Diagnosis can be established radiographically using plain films, bone scanning, and single photon emission computer tomography imaging. Oblique radiographs may demonstrate the defect in the pars interarticularis, i.e., the "neck" of the "Scottie dog." During the first several weeks, radiographs may appear normal. A bone scan may help in establishing an early diagnosis. Diagnostic bone scanning can be used when plain films are negative for determining defect acuteness and to rule out other conditions.

Management of spondylolysis remains controversial and ranges from benign neglect to surgical stabilization.[6] Management may vary depending on when the diagnosis is first established. Early on, the lesion in the pars represents a stress reaction with an increased potential for healing. Radiographs may appear normal, but a bone scan will demonstrate increased activity within the pars. Some clinicians recommend limiting activity, wearing a soft corset, and beginning flexion exercises.[53] Many others achieve excellent results with cessation of all extension exercises and immobilization in a rigid polypropylene orthosis. In the acute setting, patients need 8 to 12 weeks of rest and corset wear, with a brace or cast if full relief does not occur within 2 to 3 weeks of initial rest. Casting or bracing in an antilordotic position has been recommended.[29] Eighty-eight percent of athletes with low back pain from spondylolysis became symptom-free and were able to return to full athletic participation after rigid bracing.[41] In contrast, Blanda[5] reported an 82% success rate using bracing with maintenance of lumbar lordosis for 3.5 months to approximate the fragments. He also emphasized the importance of abdominal exercises, hamstring stretching, and pelvic tilt once patients had become asymptomatic. Premature return to activity resulted in continued pain with activities of daily living. Early aggressive nonoperative management was essential to prevent long-term effects.

The patient must be fully asymptomatic before returning to activity. As a note of caution, some enthusiastic patients may not complete bracewear for the recommended period. Permanent avoidance of upright overhead weightlifting is prudent because fusion may be needed if symptoms become chronic. Education and reassurance are essential.

A visible pars defect on plain radiographs in conjunction with a normal bone scan most likely represents a chronic spondylolysis with limited healing potential. This defect should be managed conservatively with limitation of extension activities, lightweight corset for comfort, and abdominal muscle strengthening until symptoms resolve.

Surgical intervention is rarely necessary for spondylolysis, although symptoms persisting at least 6 months despite bracing may warrant surgical stabilization.

Spondylolisthesis is an anterior displacement of one vertebral body over another. The most common type in childhood is isthmic spondylolisthesis secondary to elongation or fracture of the pars interarticularis (Fig. 17-8).[52]

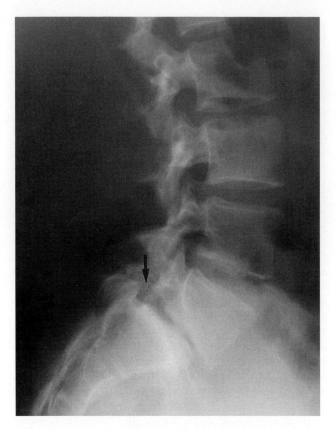

Fig. 17-8. Lateral radiograph of Grade I spondylolisthesis of L5 on S1, with clear pars interarticularis defect (arrow).

This type is believed to be a continuum of bilateral spondylolysis with loss of soft-tissue integrity leading to slippage, usually of L5 on S1. The severity of the slip is based on the amount of displacement compared with the width of the vertebral body below. Grades I to IV refer to slippage of 25%, 50%, 75%, or 100%. Grade V, where L5 is completely off, is called spondyloptosis.

The patient will usually present with low back pain. Occasionally, particularly with high-grade slips, patients will experience radicular symptoms, hamstring spasm, and symptoms of stenosis (Fig. 17-9). Physical examination may reveal flattening at the lumbosacral articulation because this is a kyphotic deformity of L5–S1. There may be compensatory lumbar hyperlordosis above the spondylolisthesis. A palpable step off may exist, along with a transverse abdominal crease, limited forward flexion, and trunk shortening. Results of neurologic examination and straight leg raising are generally negative, but subtle L5 radicular signs should be specifically pursued.

The anteroposterior radiograph may reveal the classic "Napoleon's hat" caused by superimposition of the body of L5 over the sacrum. Diagnosis is confirmed by lateral radiographs.

Grade I spondylolisthesis is managed similarly to spondylolysis. After resolution of symptoms, the patient is allowed to return to contact sports. Grade II lesions are also managed conservatively, but return to contact or hyperextension sports, such as gymnastics, is not recommended. Progression of low-grade slips is uncommon, but risk factors include young age at presentation, fe-

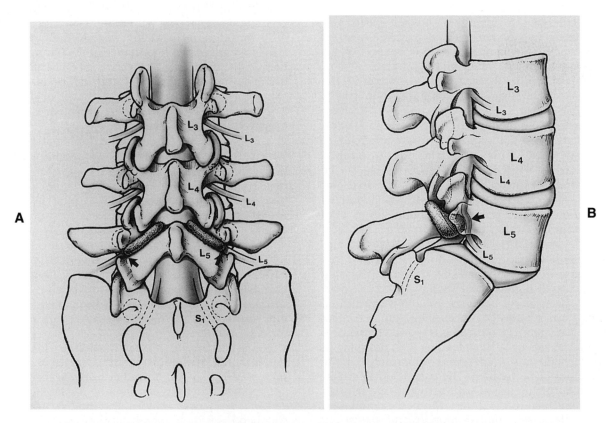

Fig. 17-9. Posterior (**A**) and lateral (**B**) views of spondylolisthesis, illustrating how a defect in the pars interarticularis may lead to L5 nerve root compression, resulting in back and leg pain.

male sex, domed-shaped sacrum, and high slip angle. Symptomatic patients with Grade I or II slips after 6 to 12 months of conservative treatment may be considered for fusion.

It is imperative that all children with high-grade slips be followed for possible progression regardless of symptoms. Grade III and IV lesions are likely to progress, and surgery is likely indicated.[5] Spondylolysis and spondylolisthesis are complex conditions, and their management is under constant review. The reader is encouraged to pursue this topic more fully in the literature.

DEFORMITY. Many children and adults wonder if their spinal deformity will affect sports participation. The majority of spinal deformities do not require bracing or surgery and have virtually no effect on the athlete (Fig. 17-10). When bracing is required, activity should be promoted to prevent deconditioning, stiffness, and weakness resulting from bracewear disuse. Clinical outcomes regarding scoliosis progression at cessation of management were similar when bracewear was liberalized to include 3 to 4 hours of aggressive sports participation each day compared with conventional 23-hour per day bracing.[36]

In the absence of structural defects, the major limitation related to spinal deformity results from chest wall deformity and reduction in vital capacity.[7] In the presence of a structural alteration (congenital scoliosis or kyphosis), contact sports should be avoided because structural effects may result in abnormal ranges of motion and decreased mechanical strength.

Deformity in the sagittal plane (kyphosis) may present as postural roundback. This flexible, smooth curvature is reducible with supine hyperextension and may be accompanied by pain. Reassurance and an exercise program to strengthen the posterior musculature are appropriate. Alternatively, kyphosis may present as Sheuerman's disease, a condition of unclear etiology characterized by short and sharp curvature that is stiffer, often accompanied by pain, and characterized by radiographic changes in the vertebral endplates and ring apophyses. Activity should be restricted, followed by a posterior strengthening program. Whether bracing is required, the patient should be instructed to avoid overhead weightlifting. If pain recurs, activity should be restricted again. Optimum bracing is with a Milwaukee brace. Surgery is indicated for stiff, progressive, large curves (Fig. 17-11).

Lumbar hyperlordosis (sway back) may present with lumbar pain and tight hamstrings. If the curve is flexible,

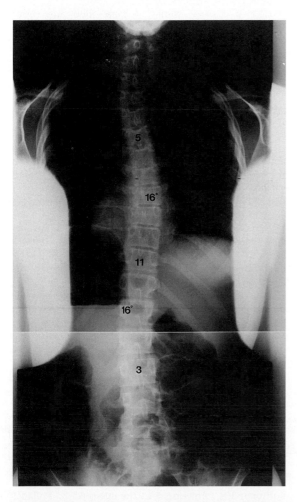

Fig. 17-10. Posteroanterior radiograph showing balanced 16° scoliotic curves in a skeletally mature 15-year-old girl 2 years past onset of menses. This minimal deformity does not require any management and does not affect athletic activity.

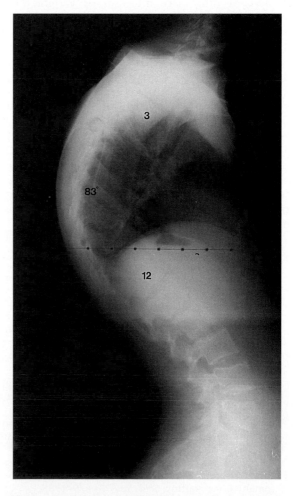

Fig. 17-11. Lateral radiograph showing severe kyphosis in 14-year-old boy. A deformity of this magnitude requires surgical correction.

antilordosis exercises and abdominal strengthening are adequate. Antilordosis bracing is necessary for more rigid curves.

There are no established guidelines for return to sports after fusion for spinal deformity. Care must be individualized, although, in general, patients undergoing short fusions may return to more vigorous activity than those undergoing longer fusions. A return 1 year after surgery with radiographically proven solid fusion and absence of symptoms is reasonable for short fusions. If long metal implants have been used, contact sports must be eliminated because of the risks of stress at the ends of the fusion. The specific long-term effects of fusion on adjacent discs are still unknown.

Patients with ankylosing spondylitis should attempt to maintain normal posture, and activity should be encouraged, along with judicious use of NSAIDs.

General Caution

Young athletes are at the age typical for the initial presentation of musculoskeletal tumors, such as osteoid osteoma and osteoblastoma, aneurysmal bone cysts, and osteogenic sarcoma. Disc space infection (discitis) is another possibility. Although these entities are rare, they must be kept in mind, particularly if symptoms persist.

In all patients, persistent fever is worrisome, possibly suggestive of disc space infection or vertebral osteomyelitis. Has there been recent surgery or an invasive procedure? Elevation of erythrocyte sedimentation rate and leukocytes, positive bone scanning, or disc space narrowing with endplate irregularity are suspicious. Weight loss, anorexia, or pain at rest raise concern for malignancy.

Finally, there are a host of conditions resulting in back pain that have nothing to do with the back. Pain referred to the back may originate from vascular, abdominal, and pelvic disorders, genitourinary and renal disorders, and others. Compulsive physical examination, including abdominal, rectal and pelvic examination when necessary and appropriate blood, urine, and radiographic testing, will minimize the chance of missing these potentially elusive disorders.

REFERENCES

1. Arce CA, Dohrmann GJ: Herniated thoracic discs, *Neurol Clin* 3:383, 1985.
2. Baker DR, McHollic W: Spondyloschisis and spondylolisthesis in children, *J Bone Joint Surg* [Am] 32:933, 1956.
3. Balague F, Nordin M, Skovron ML, Dutoit B, Yee A, Waldburger M: Non-specific LBP among schoolchildren: a field survey with analysis of some associated factors, *J Spinal Disord* 7:374–379, 1994.
4. Banks GM, Transfeldt EE: Biomechanics: clinical applications. In Weinstein S, ed: *The pediatric spine principles and practice*. New York, 1994, Raven Press.
5. Blanda J, Bethem D, Moats W, Lew M: Defects of pars interarticularis in athletes: a protocol for nonoperative treatment, *J Spinal Disord* 6:406–411, 1993.
6. Bradford DS, Iza J: Repair of the defect in spondylolysis or minimal degrees of spondylolisthesis by segmental wire fixation and bone grafting, *Spine* 10:673–679, 1985.
7. Chong KC, Letts RM, Cumming GR: Influence of spinal curvature on exercise capacity, *J Pediatr Orthop* 1:251–254, 1981.
8. Ciullo JV, Jackson DW: Pars interarticularis stress reaction, spondylolysis and spondylolisthesis in gymnasts, *Clin Sports Med* 4:95–110, 1985.
9. Clemente CD: *Anatomy—a regional atlas of the human body.* Philadelphia, 1975, Lea and Febiger.
10. Coventry MB: The intervertebral disc—its microscopic anatomy and pathology, *J Bone Joint Surg* [Am] 27:105–112, 1945.
11. Denis F: The three column spine and its significance in the classification of acute thoracic and lumbar spinal injuries, *Spine* 8:817–831, 1983.
12. Eismont FJ, Kitchel SH: *Orthopaedic sports medicine. Principles and practice.* vol 2. Philadelphia, 1994, WB Saunders.
13. Farcy JPC, Weidenbaum M: A preliminary review of the use of Cotrel-Dubousset instrumentation for spinal injuries, *Bull Hosp Jt Dis Orthop Inst* 48:44, 1988.
14. Farfan HF, et al: The effects of torsion on the lumbar intervertebral joints: the role of torsion in the production of disc degeneration, *J Bone Joint Surg* [Am] 52:468–497, 1970.
15. Flemming JE: Spondylolysis and spondylolisthesis in the athlete, *Spine: state of the art reviews* 4:339–345, 1990.
16. Floman Y, Farcy JP, Argenson C: *Thoracic and lumbar spine fractures.* New York, 1993, Raven Press.
17. Frymoyer JW, Pope MH, Kristiansen T: Skiing and spinal trauma, *Clin Sports Med* 1:309–318, 1982.
18. Hazlett J: Kissing spines, *J Bone Joint Surg* [Am] 46:1368–1369, 1964.
19. Hoppenfeld S: *Physical examination of the spine and extremities,* New York, 1976, Appleton-Century-Crofts.
20. Howell DW: Musculoskeletal profile and incidence of musculoskeletal injuries in lightweight women rowers, *Am J Sports Med* 12:278–282, 1984.
21. Hresko MT, Micheli LJ: Sports medicine and the lumbar spine, In Floman Y, ed: *Disorders of the lumbar spine.* Rockville, MD, 1990, Aspen.
22. Jackson DW, Wiltse LL, Circncoine RJ: Spondylolysis in the female gymnast, *Clin Orthop* 177:68–73, 1976.
23. Keene JS, et al: Back injuries in college athletes, *J Spinal Disord* 2:190–195, 1989.
24. Keene JS: Thoracic and lumbar fractures in winter sports, *Am J Sports Med* 216:39, 1987.
25. King H: Back pain in children. In Weinstein S, ed: *The pediatric spine—principles and practice.* New York, 1994, Raven Press.
26. Kulak RF, et al: Non-linear behavior of the human intervertebral disc under axial load, *J Biomech,* 9:377, 1976.
27. Letts M, Smallman T, Afanasie, Gouw G: Fracture of the pars interarticularis in adolescent athletes: A clinical-biomechanical analysis, *J Pediatr Orthop* 6:40–46, 1986.
28. Matsunaga S, Sakou T, Taketomi E, Iijiri K: Comparison of operative results of lumbar disc herniation in manual laborers and athletes, *Spine* 18:2222–2226, 1993.
29. Micheli LJ: Low back pain in the adolescent: differential diagnosis, *Am J Sports Med* 7:362–364, 1979.
30. Micheli LJ: Back injuries in gymnastics, *Clin Sports Med* 4:85–93, 1985.
31. Panjabi MM, White III AA: *Clinical biomechanics of the spine.* ed 2. Philadelphia, 1990, JB Lippincott.
32. Petras AF, Hoffman EP: Roentgenographic skeletal injury patterns in parachute jumping, *Am J Sports Med* 11:325–328, 1983.
33. Rothman RH, Simeone FA: *The spine* ed 3. Philadelphia, 1992, WB Saunders.
34. Schamm S, Taylor T: Tension signs in lumbar disc prolapse, *Clin Orthop* 75:195–204, 1971.

35. Semon RL, Spengler D: Significance of lumbar spondylolysis in college football players, *Spine* 16:172–174, 1981.

36. Shelokov AP, Herring JA: Spinal deformities and participation in sports, In Hochschuler SH, ed: *The spine in sports.* Philadelphia, 1990, Hanley & Belfus.

37. Snook GA: Injuries in women's gymnastics—a 5 year study, *Am J Sports Med* 7:242–244, 1979.

38. Snook GA: Injuries in intercollegiate wrestling—a 5 year study, *Am J Sports Med* 10:140–144, 1982.

39. Spangfert E: Lasegue's sign in patients with lumbar disc herniation, *Acta Orthop Scand* 42:459, 1971.

40. Stallard MC: Backache in oarsman, *Br J Sport Med* 14:105–108, 1980.

41. Steiner EM, Micheli LJ: The use of a modified Boston brace to treat symptomatic spondylolysis, *Orthop Trans* 7:20, 1983.

42. Stewart TD: The age incidence of neural arch defects in Alaskan natives considered from the standpoint of etiology, *J Bone Joint Surg* [Am] 35:937–950, 1953.

43. Sward L, Hellstrom M, Jacobsson B, Nyman R, Peterson L: Acute injury of the vertebral ring apophysis and intervertebral disc in adolescent gymnasts, *Spine* 15:144–148, 1990.

44. Sward L, Hellstrom M, Jacobsson B, Peterson L: Back pain and radiologic changes in the thoraco-lumbar spine of athletes, *Spine* 15:124–129, 1990.

45. Sward L, et al: Disc degeneration and associated abnormalities of the spine in elite gymnasts: a magnetic resonance imaging study, *Spine* 16:437–443, 1991.

46. Tertti M, et al: Disc degeneration in young gymnasts: a magnetic resonance imaging study, *Am J Sports Med* 18:206–208, 1990.

47. Triano JJ, Hyde TE: Nonsurgical treatment of sports-related spine injuries. In Hochschuler SH, ed: *The spine in sports.* Philadelphia, 1990, Hanley & Belfus.

48. Weidenbaum M, Farcy JPC: Surgical management of thoracic and lumbar burst fractures. In Bridwell KH, DeWald RL, eds: *The textbook of spinal surgery.* Philadelphia, 1991, JB Lippincott.

49. Wiesel SW, Boden SD: Diagnosis and management of cervical and lumbar disease. In Weinstein JN, Rydevik BL, Sonntag VKH, eds: *Essential of the spine.* New York, 1995, Raven Press.

50. Wilhite J, Huurman WW: Thoracic and lumbosacral spine. In Mellon MM, Walsh WM, Shelton GL, eds: *The team physicians handbook.* Philadelphia, 1990, Hanley & Belfus.

51. Williams JDA: Biomechanical factors in spinal injuries, *Br J Sports Med* 14:14, 1980.

52. Wiltse LL, Widell EH, Jackson DW: Fatigue fracture—the basic lesion in isthmic spondylolisthesis, *J Bone Joint Surg* [Am] 57:17–22, 1975.

53. Wiltse LL, Jackson DW: Treatment of spondylolisthesis and spondylolysis in children, *Clin Orthop* 117:92–100, 1976.

CHAPTER 18

THE SHOULDER

Ken Yamaguchi
Ira Wolfe
Louis U. Bigliani

Recent gains in the understanding and awareness of shoulder dysfunction have led to an increase of interest in sports-related shoulder injuries. The shoulder is now recognized as a primary and common source of functional disability in a large variety of sports, particularly those with repetitive overhead motions. Most athletes will experience some disabling shoulder pain requiring, at the minimum, a period of rest or inactivity.

In addition to overuse-acquired problems, traumatic injuries of the shoulder, such as seen with dislocations, fractures, or acromioclavicular separations, have been seen with increasing frequency with the involvement of larger, more physical athletes. Nontraumatic and traumatic injuries require early recognition and management to provide a better functional result and faster return to activities.

In this chapter, the authors will try to convey a systematic approach to the understanding, evaluation, and treatment of the athlete's shoulder. Relevant anatomy and biomechanics will be discussed to provide a basis for understanding. A discussion on shoulder evaluation in the initial, acute stages and in the recurrent or chronic stages and also on the office examination will follow. Evaluation and management will focus on unique problems associated with specific injuries, which will be divided into nontraumatic and traumatic types. Specifics of acute and conservative management and indications for surgical referral will be discussed.

ANATOMIC AND BIOMECHANICAL CONCERNS

Bony Anatomy

The shoulder is comprised of three bones: the clavicle, the scapula, and the proximal humerus. Each is uniquely shaped to articulate with each other and provide a foundation for stability while allowing the large degree of motion capable in the shoulder.

The clavicle, when viewed anteriorly, appears relatively straight but is actually an S-shaped bone that spans from the sternum medially to the acromial portion of the scapula laterally. It serves as a frame for muscle attachment, as a bony shield for underlying, major arteries and nerves, and as an osseous strut preventing the shoulder girdle from medial and inferior displacement.[15] This laterally directed strut is important to shoulder motion because it allows major muscular actions to be directed toward humeral or scapular motion rather than medial displacement.

Functionally, the clavicle can be divided into three parts: the medial third, which is important for neck strap muscle attachments and sternal articulation; the central third, which is more tubular and relatively muscle-free; and the distal third, which is important for the acromioclavicular articulation and scapular–clavicular stabilization.

The scapula is a complex, triangular-shaped bone that serves as a base for muscle attachment. Seventeen muscles attach to the scapula, allowing for mobility and stability for the otherwise inherently unstable shoulder joint. The scapulothoracic position is maintained with bony articulation to the axial skeleton through the clavicle and axioscapular muscles: trapezius, serratus anterior, rhomboid major, rhomboid minor, and the levator scapulae. The normal resting position is over the posterior–lateral aspect of the thorax between the second and seventh spinal segments. Because of its articulation with the rounded thorax, the scapula rests about 30° anterior to the coronal plane.

In addition to the axioscapular muscular attachments, the scapula serves as the origin for the all-important rotator cuff, which is formed by the confluence of the subscapularis, supraspinatus, infraspinatus, and teres minor muscles.

There are three important bony processes of the

scapula: the coracoid, acromion, and glenoid. The coracoid serves as an anterior point for muscular and ligamentous attachment between the axial and appendicular portions of the body. The coracobrachialis and short head of the biceps originate from the coracoid for distal, arm insertions, and the pectoralis minor inserts there from chest wall origins. Additionally, there are important ligamentous attachments to the clavicle, proximal humerus, and intrascapular to the acromial process.

The acromion is a flat, lateral expansion of the scapular spine that projects superiorly over the humeral head. The acromion forms from two or three ossification centers that fuse at around the age of 22 years. Unfused epiphysis can be mistaken for a fracture in the younger athletic population. In older individuals, a nonunion of one or more of the ossification centers, known as os acromiale, can also be mistaken for fractures. Os acromiale is seen approximately 1.6% of the time and is bilateral 60% of the time.[30,38]

The acromion serves with the scapular spine and distal clavicle as the point of origin for the deltoid. Additionally, it is important for the clavicular articulation and coracoacromial ligament attachment. The acromion together with the coracoacromial ligament forms the coracoacromial arch, the roof of the subacromial space through which the posterior rotator cuff, primarily supraspinatus, passes. Because pathology in this location has been implicated in the mechanical abutment and impingement of the supraspinatus tendon, the coracoacromial arch has been the source of much investigational study.[9,21,38,40] Bigliani and Morrison described a simple, clinically relevant way to classify acromial morphology. They found that acromions can be divided into three types: Type I, flat; Type II, curved; and Type III, hooked, with an anterior–inferior facing spur. Type III, hooked acromions were associated with a significantly higher incidence of rotator cuff tears.[9]

Articular Anatomy

As opposed to most other articulations in the body, the glenohumeral joint is inherently unstable. It is more of a plate and ball articulation as compared with the cup and ball configuration seen in the inherently stable hip joint. The glenoid socket is relatively shallow, with a surface area for articular contact that is disproportionately small, ranging from only 25% to 33% of the humeral head surface.[30,38,42,43] The lack of bony contribution to joint contact allows for a less constrained and more mobile joint. Stability, however, is inherently compromised and depends on static capsular restraints and dynamic muscular contribution from the rotator cuff.

The capsular restraints have been well characterized.[8,18,30,38,45] There are three ligamentous thickenings of the capsule, which are divided into superior, middle, and inferior bands. The inferior glenohumeral ligament is further divided into superior and posterior components and is commonly thought of as a sling on the inferior portion of the joint. This ligament is considered to be the most important capsular restraint to anterior and posterior glenohumeral subluxation. Glenohumeral dislocations usually occur in the upper elevations of arm position where these ligaments become taunt, acting as checkreins to dislocation at the extremes of motion. Laxity in the ligaments, either as part of an avulsion from the glenoid rim or acquired intrasubstance from repetitive micro or macro trauma, can cause clinically significant instability from several mechanisms: loss of checkrein function in sudden shifts of motion where muscular activity cannot compensate, loss of appropriate proprioceptive feedback for coordinated muscular contraction, and loss of checkrein function causing repeated stresses on surrounding musculature and overuse failure over time. All of these mechanisms are commonly seen in disorders of the athlete's shoulder.

The glenoid labrum is also considered important to glenohumeral stability by deepening the socket.[42,43] Up to 50% of the glenoid cavity depth is provided by the labrum. This increase in glenohumeral conformity provided by the labrum may also contribute to a "suction effect" of negative intraarticular pressure, further increasing stability.

The coracohumeral ligament is an additional checkrein to motion, primarily to external rotation and inferior translation. Technically extracapsular, the ligament spans from the anterior portion of the greater tuberosity to the coracoid. Significant contraction in this ligament and concomitant loss of external rotation is seen in frozen shoulder or adhesive capsulitis.

Muscular Anatomy

The proximal humerus is enveloped within a thick muscular sleeve responsible not only for gross movement of the extremity but also stabilization of the glenohumeral joint during motion. The muscles can be thought of in three groups: (1) primary glenohumeral muscles, which are the deltoid, subscapularis, supraspinatus, infraspinatus, teres minor, and teres major; (2) scapulothoracic musculature, which includes the trapezius, rhomboids, levator scapulas, serratus anterior, and pectoralis minor; and (3) multiple joint muscles, which include the pectoralis major, latissimus dorsi, biceps brachia, and triceps brachia. This review will focus primarily on the glenohumeral muscles.

The deltoid, which is the prime mover of the shoulder, can be functionally divided into three parts: anterior deltoid, responsible for flexion; middle deltoid, responsible for scapular plane abduction (elevation); and posterior deltoid, responsible for extension. Additionally, the anterior and posterior portions of the deltoid can work together for abduction. Among the three parts of the deltoid, loss of the anterior deltoid is most devastating because its function cannot be replaced.

The rotator cuff, which is comprised of the supraspinatus, infraspinatus, teres minor, and subscapularis, works in concert with the deltoid to provide arm elevation. The primary vector of muscle pull through the deltoid is vertical, which leads to superior translation of the humerus and impingement of interposed soft tissues, like the rotator cuff, if not properly controlled. The rotator cuff protects itself from this impingement by stabilizing the humeral head in the glenoid socket during arm elevation. In addition to humeral head stabilization, the posterior rotator cuff is important in external rotation and prevention of anterior subluxation of the humerus. The subscapularis is important for extremes of internal rotation and humeral head stabilization. The teres major also is an internal rotator of the humerus.

As muscular contraction of the rotator cuff is important for glenohumeral stability in the superior, anterior, and posterior directions, luxation in these directions could be a sign of cuff dysfunction or conversely lead to cuff disease.

Radiographic Anatomy

As with other parts of the body, during the radiographic evaluation of the shoulder there should be at least two views taken perpendicular to each other. Because of the relative difficulty in obtaining a good lateral view of the shoulder, this basic principle is often neglected, especially in the trauma setting where it is most important.

The standard trauma views for the shoulder are basic to all radiographic evaluations. They consist of a scapular plane anteroposterior, Y-scapulolateral, and axillary views. The scapular plane lateral view is taken at 45° from the anteroposterior plane of the thorax to account for scapular inclination. This allows for a true profile projection of the glenohumeral joint with superimposition of the anterior and posterior glenoid rims, minimizing overlap by the humeral head.

The Y-scapulolateral and axillary views provide right-angle projections to the anteroposterior view. The Y-scapulolateral view taken from posteromedial to anterolateral along the spine of the scapula is a true lateral view of the scapula. The "Y" is formed by the coracoid anteriorly, scapular spine posteriorly, and the scapular body inferiorly; the glenoid and humeral head is found at the center of the "Y." The axillary view is a true lateral view of the glenohumeral joint and is taken with some arm abduction and neutral rotation in a cranially directed fashion through the axilla. Because this view requires some abduction, it is often not done in the acute, trauma setting. It is important to note that only 30° to 40° of abduction is required, which is generally well tolerated. In the rare circumstance where a true axillary view cannot be obtained, a velpeau axillary view can suffice. The velpeau axillary view is taken from superior to inferior by having the patient lean backward over the film. Usually, the injured extremity can remain in its immobilizer.

In addition to the standard trauma series, several specialized views can be helpful depending on the clinical situation. The 10° cephalic tilt view highlights the acromioclavicular joint. The scapular outlet view is helpful for evaluating acromial morphology. Magnetic resonance imaging can give a highly accurate representation of the rotator cuff tendons and muscles.

Relevant Biomechanics

Glenohumeral motion is generally considered to have three degrees of freedom: flexion and extension, abduction and adduction, and rotation. This glenohumeral motion is amplified and augmented by a coordinated contribution of scapulothoracic motion. Without coordinated scapulothoracic motion, glenohumeral motion would be limited to about 80° to 90° from the mechanical abutment of the greater tuberosity against the acromion. Generally, glenohumeral motion is accompanied by scapulothoracic motion at a 2:1 ratio, although the exact relationship varies depending on the relative position during abduction.

Overhead throwing is considered to occur in five distinct phases.[13] These have been divided into: (1) wind-up, during which the rhythm and momentum for throwing is initiated, (2) cocking, where the shoulder is abducted and at extreme external rotation and the lower extremity is beginning rotation toward the target, (3) acceleration, where the arm begins horizontal adduction and internal rotation to accelerate the arm toward ball release (remember the hand is moving as fast as the ball at this point), (4) ball release, where the arm is forward to the body and elbow extension occurs to generate the last portion of velocity; and (5) follow-through, during which tremendous rotator cuff and biceps exertion strain is developed to decelerate the arm and stabilize the shoulder. Although described primarily for the baseball pitcher, all sports-related overhead activities are generally variations of this theme.[3,23,30,38]

EVALUATION OF THE PAINFUL SHOULDER

Acute Assessment and First Aid

When covering athletic events, acute assessment of a shoulder injury is sometimes necessary. The initial evaluation should be performed promptly, starting with a brief, directed history. Important considerations can be mechanism of injury, presence of any neurologic symptoms, and preexisting medical problems. After the history, a careful neurovascular assessment should be made of the upper extremity. This cannot be overemphasized. Whereas most injuries in the athletic setting can lead to some short-term disability or inconvenience, vascular compromise can lead to loss of the limb. The radial and ulnar arterial pulses should be palpated, and capillary refill, coloration, and warmth should be assessed. Careful documentation of the vascular status will not only ensure prompt recognition, but will also allow for serialized observations when subtle injuries are present.

Additionally, gross neurologic status should be determined. Neurologic injuries are not uncommon because of the proximity of the brachial plexus to the shoulder girdle. This is especially relevant to glenohumeral dislocations. Early recognition can lead to prompt reduction and decrease the severity of neurologic injury.

Once the neurovascular status is confirmed to be intact, an examination for more subacute problems can be performed. Any interfering athletic clothing or equipment should be removed to carefully observe the shoulder. Gross deformities, lacerations, swelling, or bruising should be appreciated. Palpation can pinpoint possible injuries. If the examination does not indicate obvious dislocation or fractures, active range of motion can be attempted. Any significant pain preventing range of motion should be an indication to stop and immobilize the extremity in a sling and swathe for transport of the athlete to an emergency facility where radiographs can be taken.

The acute management of a witnessed anterior dislocation of the shoulder is controversial. With appropriate experience and training, a physician can accurately diagnose a dislocation and perform a relatively atraumatic relocation in the acute setting before muscle spasm takes place. However, in rare circumstances where fracture accompanies dislocation, an inappropriate reduction maneuver can cause either displacement or propagation—a very serious complication.

Office Assessment

As with any other medical evaluation, obtaining an accurate history is essential in the overall clinical assessment of shoulder dysfunction.[4] It is important initially to determine whether the shoulder pain had a traumatic etiology. The nature of trauma will often clarify diagnosis. A thorough history and physical examination and appropriate diagnostic tests will allow the diagnosis of the majority of shoulder disorders. Conditions such as cervical radiculopathy, tumors, acromioclavicular joint disorders, and systemic rheumatologic diseases must be carefully considered.

HISTORY

A thorough history is essential to gather as much information as possible for evaluation. It is best obtained in a systematic fashion to avoid overlooking things that the patient may think unimportant but which may nevertheless be relevant to evaluating the shoulder problem (see box). Hand dominance, occupation, and athletic activities should be recorded to understand functional demands and future expectations. The dominant shoulder of a throwing athlete is a different challenge than the nondominant shoulder of a sedentary executive. In addition, certain activities may contribute to the pathology: the relationships between weightlifting and osteolysis of the distal clavicle,[12,39] and between repetitive minor injury (e.g., gymnastics or butterfly swimming) and shoulder instability[6] are well established.

A general medical history should be obtained, with special care to elicit any symptoms suggestive of a systemic or rheumatologic disorder. Conditions such as diabetes mellitus and metastatic cancer can cause a frozen shoulder. Furthermore, a family history may often be helpful, e.g., generalized ligamentous laxity in a patient with shoulder instability.

The precise nature of the patient's chief complaint, usually pain, weakness, stiffness, or instability, should be well understood. It is important to document the duration, provocation, severity, and timing of symptoms, especially pain. Rest pain and night pain are especially common in patients with shoulder pathology. Anatomic and mechanical conditions, such as impingement and glenohumeral arthritis, usually cause these symptoms, but infection and tumor must also be considered.

The mechanism of any injury and the nature of exacerbating activities should be documented. An accident or trauma may initiate a shoulder problem, but often there

HISTORY

Patient
  Hand dominance
  Occupation
  Athletics
    Sports
    Level of competition
    Relation to shoulder problem (e.g., weightlifting and osteolysis of the distal clavicle)
  Other medical disorders (e.g., diabetes, genetic disorders, cancer)
  Family history (e.g., arthritis, ligamentous laxity)

Shoulder disorder
  Chief complaint
    Pain
    Weakness
    Stiffness
    Instability
  Symptom pattern
    Duration
    Provocation
    Severity
    Location
  Injury
    Traumatic
    Atraumatic
    Repetitive microtrauma
    Preexisting condition
  Level of disability
    Athletics
    Occupation
    Daily tasks

Related symptoms
  Cervical pain
  Neurologic
    Cervical radiculopathy
    Brachial plexus
    Peripheral nerve
  Chest (e.g., cardiac, lung, herpes zoster)

is no history of injury. Frequently, a patient may have had shoulder symptoms before an injury that exacerbated them, as in a patient who suffers an acute extension of an impingement rotator cuff tear. The pattern of pain should be recorded. An episodic history of severe pain and inflammation may suggest calcium, whereas recurrent pain with the arm in abduction and external rotation after a hard injury in the same position may implicate anterior instability.

It is important to elicit complaints of other adjacent regions such as the neck, chest, heart, upper back, and arm. Cervical disease can be difficult to separate from intrinsic mechanical shoulder disorders, and the two frequently coexist. Nevertheless, neck pain is often referred to the posterior shoulder and trapezius and may be felt into the hand. Shoulder disorders more frequently hurt deep inside or down the front of the upper arm, and do not usually extend beyond the elbow. Furthermore, neck pain is often related to the position of the cervical spine and becomes more severe after driving or long periods of sitting.

Numbness or tingling in the hand may indicate cervical disease or peripheral nerve entrapment. However, shoulder instability, especially when a significant inferior component is present, can produce episodic brachial plexus stretch symptoms. Similarly, conditions that result in loss of shoulder suspension, such as acromioclavicular dislocation and trapezius palsy,[28] can cause brachial plexus traction.

EXAMINATION

Inspection
Muscle atrophy
Bone prominences
Deformity (e.g., biceps long-head rupture)
Generalized laxity (e.g., thumb, elbow)

Palpation
Sternoclavicular joint
Acromioclavicular joint
Rotator cuff and tuberosities (e.g., calcium deposits)
Glenohumeral joint line
Trapezius muscle spasm

Cervical spine
Rotation
Flexion–extension
Pain with motion

Range of motion
Elevation
    Active
    Passive
External rotation
Internal rotation

Strength
External rotation
"Lift-off" test (internal rotation)

Provocative tests
Subacromial impingement sign
Anterior apprehension
Posterior stress test
Horizontal adduction

Shoulder laxity
Sulcus
"Drawer"

PHYSICAL EXAMINATION

Physical examination is also performed in a systematic fashion (see box). The patient should be examined with both shoulders fully exposed: men disrobe above the waist, and women are given gowns that are tied under the shoulder in the axilla so that they are "strapless" (Fig. 18-1). Inspection is performed from the front and the rear. Careful note should be made of muscle atrophy and contour, bone prominences, and deformity. Atrophy of the spinati is best evaluated from behind (Fig. 18-2).

Standing behind the patient, palpation is performed, checking for areas of localized tenderness (Fig. 18-3). The acromioclavicular joint should always be carefully palpated because it is a frequently overlooked source of symptoms. Localized tenderness over the rotator cuff may result from calcific tendinitis and should be correlated with rotational radiographs of the humerus (Fig. 18-4). Anterior and posterior joint-line tenderness may be present with glenohumeral instability, and posterior joint-line tenderness is commonly noted in glenohumeral arthritis. The cervical spine should be gently rotated, flexed, and extended. If this maneuver reproduces the patient's "shoulder" pain, consideration should be given to a cervical etiology.

Range of motion is evaluated and recorded (Fig. 18-5). Elevation is measured in the scapular plane. Passive elevation is more accurately measured supine, because sub-

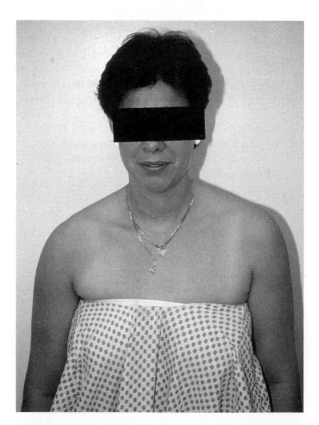

Fig. 18-1. The arms are not placed through the sleeves of the gown. Rather, the gown is tied under the arms to be "strapless." This allows full inspection throughout the examination.

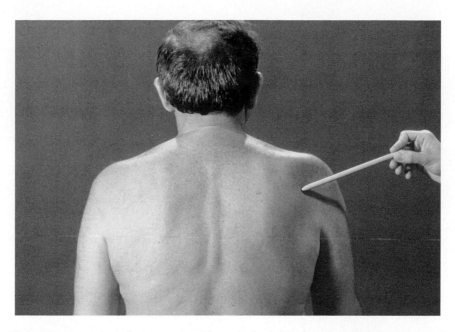

Fig. 18-2. Spinati atrophy is best appreciated from the back. The scapular spine becomes prominent relative to the adjacent hollowed-out supraspinatus and infraspinatus. This patient had spinati atrophy from a massive rotator cuff tear.

stitution through arching of the back is minimized. No effort is made to "isolate" glenohumeral motion; total elevation, consisting of glenohumeral and scapulothoracic motion, is more reproducibly measured and more functionally relevant. Active elevation is measured erect. External rotation, with the arm at the side, is measured supine to eliminate trunk rotation. Internal rotation is measured erect by the highest vertebral level to which the thumb may be brought up the patient's back.

Manual strength testing may be difficult because of pain, precluding quantitative assessment. External rota-

tion weakness can be present in long-standing rotator cuff tears, but may be secondary to pain, cervical radiculopathy, or suprascapular nerve palsy. It is best to test external rotation power with the elbow flexed and the arm at the side to avoid a contribution from the deltoid mus-

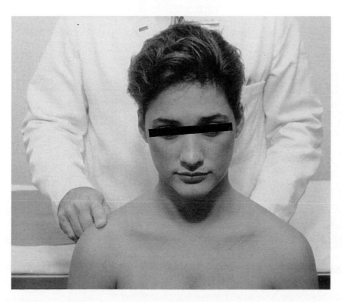

Fig. 18-3. Palpation is carefully performed to elicit any areas of localized tenderness. Here the acromioclavicular joint is being palpated.

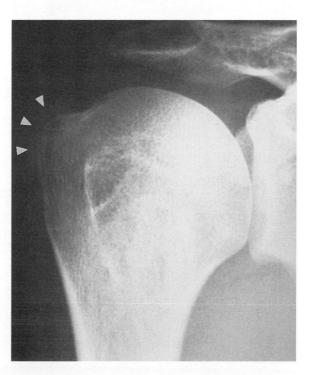

Fig. 18-4. This patient was referred because of shoulder pain unresponsive to arthroscopic labral débridement. Only one of three rotation views brought the calcium deposit (arrows) into view. A steroid injection completely relieved the symptoms, and the patient continues pain-free 1 year after the injection.

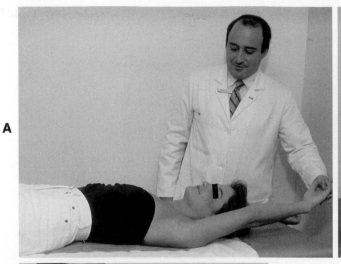

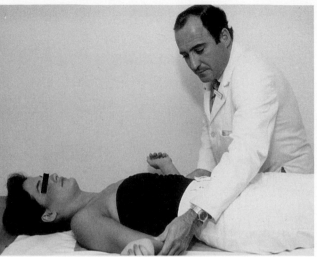

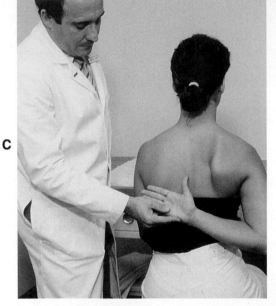

Fig. 18-5. A, Passive total elevation is measured supine in the scapular plane and is a combination of glenohumeral and scapulothoracic motion. **B,** Passive external rotation is measured supine, which minimizes trunk rotation. **C,** Passive internal rotation is measured by the highest vertebral level to which the thumb may be brought up the patient's back. This technique may be invalidated if there is a significant restriction of elbow motion.

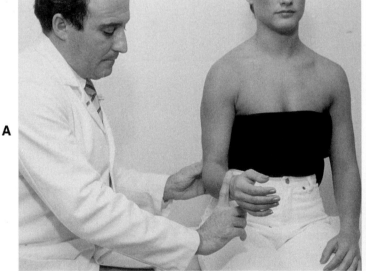

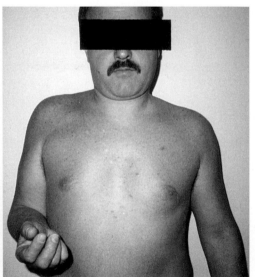

Fig. 18-6. A, External rotation strength is evaluated with the arms at the side. Weakness may be mimicked by pain and in some cases may be more reliably measured after a subacromial injection of local anesthetic.[7] **B,** Patients with massive rotator cuff tears may have severe weakness of external rotation. This patient had 11 passive external rotation supine, but in the standing position, his arm "drops off" to internal rotation despite his efforts to actively externally rotate.

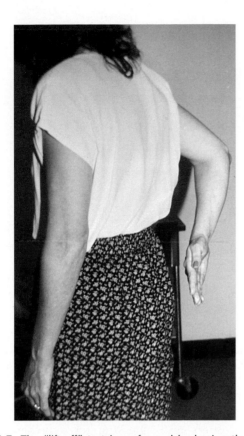

Fig. 18-7. The "lift-off" test is performed by having the patient lift his or her hand from the resting position on the lumbar region of the back. Alternatively, the examiner may place the patient's arm in internal rotation with the hand elevated above the back and buttocks and ask the patient to maintain this position. A patient with subscapularis pathology will be unable to perform this maneuver.

cle (Fig. 18-6). Recently, the role of rupture or incompetence of the subscapularis muscle has been described.[16] Because weakness or loss of the subscapularis can be masked by the other internal rotators, it is best to test for this in isolation. Gerber and Krushnell[16] have noted that to fully internally rotate the extended arm, an intact and functioning subscapularis is required. A "lift off" test is positive (and loose subscapularis function demonstrated) when there is a lag between passive and active internal rotation: the patient cannot lift the hand posteriorly off the lumbar region of the back (Fig. 18-7). A careful neurologic assessment is mandatory when there is significant weakness of the muscle groups, and electromyography may be indicated.

Specific "provocative" tests are also helpful. The subacromial impingement sign will elicit pain in patients with subacromial impingement syndrome (Fig. 18-8). The examiner stabilizes the scapula with one hand and brings the arm up into forced elevation with the other. A positive test elicits pain as the greater tuberosity is forced against the coracoacromial arch. It is important to realize that a frozen shoulder will invalidate this test because there will be restricted motion in all directions, not just elevation, with pain at the extremes. The subacromial injection test is positive when a subacromial injection of local anesthetic eliminates pain from the impingement sign. Pain from the acromioclavicular joint is usually increased with horizontal adduction of the arm across the chest and internal rotation of the arm up the back, but this sign is not specific for the acromioclavicular joint. A local anesthetic injection into the acromioclavicular joint can be of diagnostic value. Because of the frequent overlap of acromioclavicular arthritis and impingement syndrome, especially in older patients, a "differential" injection test is often helpful. The most symptomatic element is generally injected first.

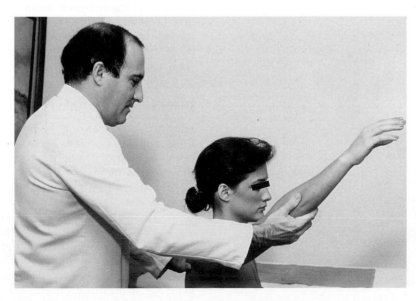

Fig. 18-8. The impingement sign is elicited by stabilizing the scapula with one hand and bringing the arm up into forced elevation with the other. This will elicit pain in a patient with subacromial impingement syndrome.

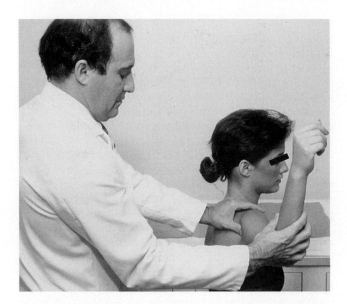

Fig. 18-9. The anterior apprehension maneuver is performed by bringing the arm up into a position of extension, abduction, and external rotation and by placing forward pressure on the proximal humerus. A patient with instability will generally be apprehensive and guard against this position for fear of shifting or dislocating anteriorly. A patient with subluxations may only have pain.

The anterior apprehension sign is the classic provocative test for anterior instability. The arm is brought up into a position of extension, abduction, and external rotation, and forward pressure is placed on the proximal humerus (Fig. 18-9). Patients with instability will generally guard against this position because of fear of shifting or dislocating anteriorly. Patients with subluxations may only have pain. Posterior instability is tested with the

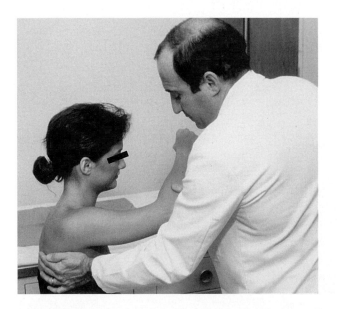

Fig. 18-10. The posterior stress test[1] is performed with the arm in 90° forward flexion and internal rotation while applying posterior pressure to the elbow with the scapula stabilized.

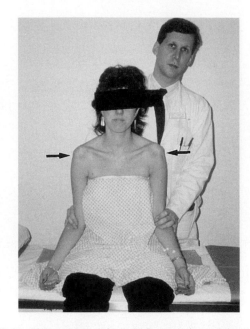

Fig. 18-11. This patient with multidirectional instability has bilateral sulcus signs (arrows) elicited by placing downward traction on the arms. A sulcus is formed between the acromion and the inferiorly translating humerus.

"posterior stress test" checking for apprehension or, more commonly, pain with the arm in 90° forward flexion and internal rotation while applying posterior pressure to the elbow (Fig. 18-10).[10,34] The scapula must be stabilized. Posterior inferior instability is checked by elevating the arm to 120°. Inferior laxity is assessed by pulling downward on the arm to create a sulcus sign (Fig. 18-11), which is a separation of the superior humerus from the acromion.

Generalized ligamentous laxity (Fig. 18-12) may be present in patients with multidirectional instability, but may be absent in those with acquired shoulder laxity after repetitive microtrauma (e.g., butterfly swimming). Both shoulders should be assessed for anteroposterior translation, a shoulder "drawer" sign (Fig. 18-13).

DIAGNOSTIC MODALITIES

Routine blood tests may be obtained to check for conditions such as systemic rheumatologic disorders, infections, and tumors, which may cause shoulder symptoms (box on p. 230).

All patients should have routine radiographs taken to assist in the diagnosis of tumors, fractures, or dislocations. This should include anteroposterior views of the scapular plane in neutral, internal, and external rotations, a lateral view in the scapular plane, and an axillary view. Rotational views are of value in detecting calcium deposits. The internal rotation anteroposterior view will generally demonstrate a Hill-Sachs defect, which is an impression fracture caused during anterior dislocations (see Fig. 18-11). The external rotation anteroposterior view shows the greater tuberosity in profile, and patients

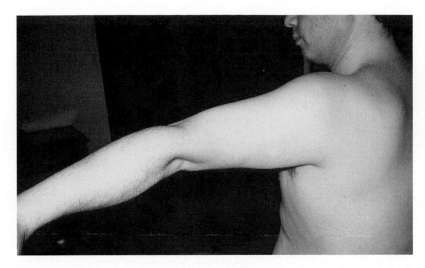

Fig. 18-12. Another common finding with generalized laxity is the ability to hyperextend the elbow.

with impingement may have sclerosis, cysts, or excrescences of the greater tuberosity. Spurs and sclerosis of the anterior acromion may be apparent on anteroposterior views, but acromial morphology may be best appreciated on a lateral view, especially if taken with slight caudal tilt. Such an "outlet view" can also be helpful in assessing the technical success of arthroscopic acromioplasty.

The axillary view will demonstrate posterior dislocations, which may be missed on anteroposterior views, and glenoid reactive changes or fractures associated with instability.

The acromioclavicular joints are frequently overpenetrated on standard views, and acromioclavicular films with "soft-tissue technique," anteroposterior and cephalic tilt anteroposterior views, may pick up subtle arthritis, fractures, or osteolysis.

Additional views are occasionally necessary and include special views to demonstrate the Hills-Sachs defect, such as the Stryker notch view (Fig. 18-14), modified axillary views that do not require removing an acutely injured arm from the sling, weighted acromioclavicular views to check for an acromioclavicular separation, and other views. Cervical spine radiographs are often obtained because of associated neck pain, especially in older patients.

Conventional arthrograms are highly accurate in detecting full-thickness tears of the rotator cuff and may detect some deep-surface partial thickness tears.[14] Ultrasonography has been reported to be an inexpensive,

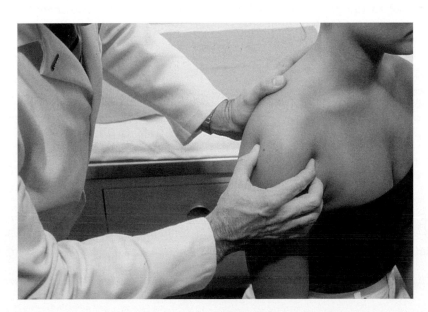

Fig. 18-13. Anteroposterior laxity may be assessed by stabilizing the scapula and by attempting to translate the humerus forward and backward in the glenoid, a shoulder "drawer sign."

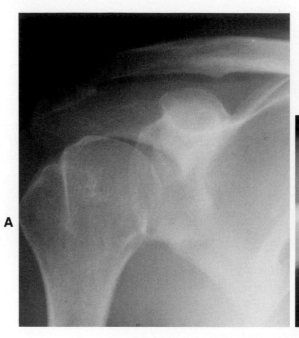
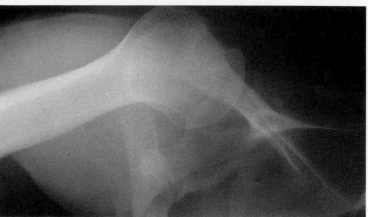

Fig. 18-14. The posterolateral humeral head impression fracture (Hill-Sachs defect[10]) associated with recurrent anterior dislocations is usually well demonstrated on the internal rotation anteroposterior view. Occasionally, other views are helpful in assessing its extent. **A,** Internal rotation anteroposterior view. **B,** Stryker notch view.

noninvasive imaging modality for the rotator cuff that can detect partial tears. However, reliability has varied with investigators and criteria for cuff pathology. Magnetic resonance imaging scans have become increasingly reliable in detecting rotator cuff tears but may overread minor degrees of cuff damage (Fig. 18-15).[19]

Electromyograms and nerve conduction studies are useful in distinguishing peripheral nerve injuries and entrapments, brachial plexus disorders, and cervical radiculopathies. Somatosensory-evoked potential testing may also be useful, especially when the predominant symptoms are sensory. Cybex testing can document func-tional deficits and serve as a baseline for the evaluation of rehabilitation protocols.

SPECIFIC NONTRAUMATIC INJURIES

Rotator Cuff Disorders

SPORTS COMMONLY INVOLVED. Rotator cuff disease is seen in participants of virtually all sports but should be especially suspected in athletes involved in sports with repetitive overhead motions. These include baseball, football (quarterbacks), swimming, tennis (racket sports), volleyball, field events (javelin), gymnastics, and weightlifting.

DIAGNOSTIC MODALITIES

Routine blood studies
CBC, ESR, SMAC, latex fixation

Others as indicated

Radiographs, routine
Anteroposterior in internal rotation, external rotation, neutral

"Outlet" view

Axillary

Radiographs, special
Anteroposterior and cephalic tilt anteroposterior views with "soft-tissue technique" to demonstrate C joint

Special views (e.g., Stryker, Hermodssen) to demonstrate Mil-Sachs defect

Modified axillary views (e.g., "velpeau axillary")

Cervical spine

Special diagnostic modalities
Arthro–computed tomography scan
    Labral pathology
    Glenoid bone changes

Three-dimensional computed tomography reconstruction

Arthrogram

Ultrasonography

Magnetic resonance imaging

Arthro–MRI

Electrodiagnostic studies (e.g., EMG, SSEP)

Isokinetic muscle testing

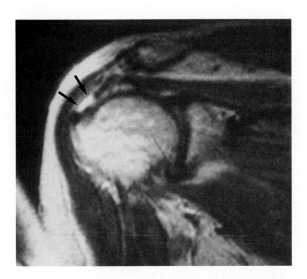

Fig. 18-15. T2-weighted magnetic resonance imaging shows a bright signal (arrows) consistent with fluid in a supraspinatus tear. This was confirmed at surgery.

BACKGROUND. Subacromial bursitis and rotator cuff tendinitis and tears are common disorders in the shoulder and can result in pain, weakness, and diminished athletic performance.[5,11,20,22,23,25–27,29,31,32,36–38,46] The central role the rotator cuff has in shoulder function almost precludes its involvement in most painful disorders. Commonly referred to as *impingement syndrome*, rotator cuff-associated pain can be primary bursitis, tendinitis from overuse, impingement from mechanical abutment, or secondary from glenohumeral instability. Whatever the primary etiology, there is a progression of pathology that describes the stages of impingement syndrome. In Stage I, seen in those aged less than 24 years, there is edema and hemorrhage of the tendon, which are generally considered reversible. In Stage II, seen in those aged 25 to 40 years, there is tendinitis and fibrosis, which can become chronic. In Stage III, seen in those aged more than 40 years, there is full-thickness rotator cuff tearing, requiring operative repair. This age-related characterization of rotator cuff disease is accelerated in athletes involved in sports with repetitive overhead motions, who not only increase the forces on the cuff tendons, but also the repetitions of aggravating motions.

PATHOMECHANICS. Many factors have been implicated in rotator cuff pathology, including extrinsic tendon injury resulting from compression from an abnormal coracoacromial arch, internal abutment against the glenoid rim, tendon and bursal swelling in a confined space, tensile overload from glenohumeral instability, and intrinsic tendon injury from tendinitis.[2,9,23,29,30,31,38]

Whether a primary factor or a secondary effect, subacromial impingement is thought to be an ongoing cause of tendon injury by the time surgical intervention is considered. The supraspinatus insertion on the greater tuberosity must repeatedly pass under the coracoacromial arch when the arm is used for vigorous overhead activity. As described in the anatomy section, the rotator cuff passes between the coracoacromial arch above and humeral head below. Comprised of the anterior acromion and coracoacromial ligament, any abnormality of the coracoacromial arch, such as an acromial spur, osteophyte formation, or ligament thickening, can encroach on the cuff below. Conversely, alterations in rotator cuff function from stress overload or tendinitis seen with instability can decrease humeral head stabilization, leading to superior migration and secondary impingement. Bigliani et al have demonstrated a relationship between acromial morphology and rotator cuff tears in cadavers, and contact studies on the subacromial space at the Columbia-Presbyterian Orthopaedic Research Laboratory have found that contact was centered on the supraspinatus insertion where cuff tears generally initiate, supporting an impingement etiology to rotator cuff disease.

Recently, an internal impingement mechanism has also been implicated in select patients with glenohumeral instability who are involved in overhead sports.[23] In this proposed mechanism, anterior translation of the humeral head with abduction and external rotation (seen during cocking for throwing) can cause abutment of the articular surface of the rotator cuff against the posterior–superior glenoid rim.

Calcific bursitis is a variety of rotator cuff disease unrelated to impingement. Acute pain is thought to be caused by the intermittent release of calcium from the tendon, irritating the bursa. Calcific bursitis usually responds well to steroid injection.

SPECIFICS OF HISTORY AND EXAMINATION. The majority of rotator cuff disorders can be diagnosed after a history, a physical examination, and appropriate imaging studies. These patients usually present with pain of insidious onset exacerbated with overhead activities. The pain is usually in the anterior deltoid, but it can be referred anywhere on the deltoid and down to mid-arm. The pain is often felt at night and can awaken patients from sleep.

On examination, the typical pain can be reproduced with forward flexion in internal rotation (impingement sign). This pain is often reduced with a subacromial injection of lidocaine (impingement test). Three specific manual muscle tests are performed to assess the possibility of a tear. To examine possible anterior, subscapularis involvement, the "lift-off" test as described by Gerber[16] is very reliable. Posterior tear involvement is tested by determining strength with thumb-down abduction at 70° in the scapular plane and by testing external rotation strength at the side. Weakness with thumb-down elevation is more specific for supraspinatus involvement, whereas loss of external rotation strength at side is more indicative of infraspinatus and teres minor extention. Profound and complete posterior cuff involvement is seen in patients who are unable to maintain their arms in external rotation (drop-arm sign).

In the young athlete, the examination should also focus on possible instability as the primary etiology for rotator cuff disease. In contrast to primary impingement, pain is often posterior deltoid in location, and the patient will sometimes complain of a "dead arm" with overhead activities. Apprehension and relocation tests and sulcus and range of motion examinations should be performed. These impingement signs and tests will also be positive from the secondary bursitis.

Routine radiographs, including supraspinatus outlet films, should be taken on initial visit. Additional studies, such as magnetic resonance imaging, should generally be reserved until conservative therapy has failed and until operative intervention is being considered. One exception would be for the high-performance athlete, who requires immediate rotator cuff evaluation for prognosticating return to sports.

CONSERVATIVE MANAGEMENT. Generally, initial management is rest and antiinflammatory medication to overcome the acute inflammation. When the pain persists, a subacromial injection of lidocaine and steroid preparation is often helpful to break the inflammation. However, there are no long-term benefits from the either the oral or injected antiinflammatory medication without a directed physical therapy regimen. Physical therapy first focuses on stretching exercises to regain complete range of motion and then on strengthening of the rotator cuff with external rotation. Care should be taken not to overstretch the shoulder.

INDICATIONS FOR ORTHOPEDIC REFERRAL. Patients should be considered for orthopedic referral when conservative treatment has failed to provide any meaningful improvement or if the care provider is uncomfortable with conservative measures, such as subacromial injections.

OPERATIVE MANAGEMENT. Operative management involves decompression of the subacromial arch by coracoacromial ligament excision and anterior–inferior resection of acromial bone (Fig. 18-16). Specific operative management is predicated on the presence or absence of a significant rotator cuff tear. When a rotator cuff tear is absent or small, surgery is performed arthroscopically. If a significant tear is present, formal open repair is preferred.

Glenohumeral Instability

SPORTS COMMONLY INVOLVED. Glenohumeral instability is seen in athletes involved in high-energy sports where dislocations are more common and in those with repetitive overhead motions where microtrauma is prevalent. These sports include football, basketball, baseball, hockey, swimming, tennis (racket sports), volleyball, field events (javelin), gymnastics, and weightlifting.

BACKGROUND. Multidirectional or unidirectional instability of the shoulder is more common than previously realized.[2,17,18,25,30,32,33,38,41,45] These patients have symptomatic glenohumeral instability in one or more than one direction: anterior, inferior, and posterior. There is a common misconception that multidirectional instability is limited to young sedentary patients with generalized ligamentous laxity who often present with bilateral symptoms and signs as opposed to unidirectional patients, who are thought to have a unilateral traumatic etiology. Multidirectional instability is classically thought of as acquired in an atraumatic fashion. Although there is a group of such patients, shoulders with multidirectional instability are often in athletic patients, many of whom have had significant injuries.[6] Repetitive microtrauma, seen for example in butterfly swimming or gymnastics, can also lead to multidirectional instability by selectively "stretching out" shoulders compared with other joints, which may not be lax on examination.

In the authors' experience, patients with shoulder instability do not always easily fall into distinct categories (unidirectional *vs.* multidirectional) (Fig. 18-17). This is especially true of athletes, often lax to begin with, who subject their shoulders to repetitive microtrauma on a daily basis but may also suffer a superimposed injury. The authors have found athletes with anterior instability to constitute a spectrum from unidirectional anterior instability to frank multidirectional instability with pronounced inferior capsular laxity rather than fall into simple discrete groups.

PATHOMECHANICS. The primary pathology in shoulders with acquired instability (without a specific traumatic event) is capsular laxity and redundancy, with

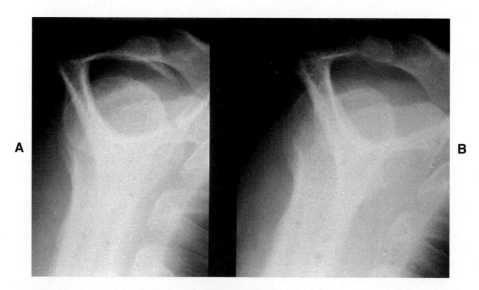

Fig. 18-16. A, Preoperative outlet view (left) demonstrates a large anterior acromial spur extending into the coracoacromial ligament. The spur was removed arthroscopically as confirmed by a postoperative view (right). **B,** This patient had a prominent, curved anterior acromion (left), which was converted to a flat acromion (right) arthroscopically.

The Spectrum of Instability

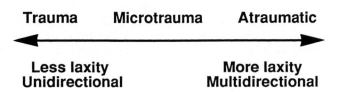

Fig. 18-17. Spectrum of instability.

instability possible in anterior, inferior, or posterior directions. In addition to capsular laxity, avulsion of the capsular ligaments from the anterior glenoid rim may occur, destabilizing the joint.

SPECIFICS OF HISTORY AND EXAMINATION. Patients with acquired instability may present in a variety of ways. A previous dislocation may have occurred without significant injury and spontaneously reduced or self-reduced. An extremely hypermobile shoulder can become symptomatic without unusual trauma and possibly from the activities of daily living. A common presentation appears to be an individual with a relatively loose shoulder who stresses it repetitively or incorrectly in athletic activities or work-related events. Symptoms can be complex, vague, and difficult to sort, but certain complaints may suggest the directions of instability involved. Inferior instability may present with the patient's description of pain associated with carrying heavy suitcases or shopping bags. Occasionally, these symptoms are accompanied by traction paresthesias. Pain associated with weight training (bench press), pushing open heavy or revolving doors, or use of the arm in a forward flexed and internally rotated position usually suggests a component of posterior instability.

The physical examination may demonstrate evidence of generalized ligamentous laxity, such as hyperextension at the elbows, the ability to approximate the thumbs to the forearms, hyperextension of the metacarpophalangeal joints, or patellofemoral subluxation. In some of these patients, hypermobile acromioclavicular and sternoclavicular joints can be sources of symptoms. It is important, therefore, to examine these joints for tenderness, inferior humeral subluxation with stress on the arm in neutral (sulcus sign) (see Fig. 18-8), or abduction, which suggests inferior laxity. Additionally, close inspection of the scapulothoracic articulation should be performed because concomitant scapulothoracic instability may occasionally be present. There may be multiple positive findings using the following maneuvers: anterior and posterior load and shift tests, anterior and posterior apprehension tests, relocation test, and the push–pull test. The aim is to produce humeral translations either anteriorly, posteriorly, or inferiorly (relative to the glenoid), and to document that these translations are reliably accompanied by the patient's report of the usual pain and discomfort.

It can be difficult to determine the primary direction of instability on physical examination. Determining

whether the shoulder is moving from a dislocated to a reduced position or from a reduced to a dislocated position can be challenging. Maintaining the fingers of one hand on the coracoid anteriorly and on the posterolateral acromion can aid in this determination. For this reason, multiple physical examinations are helpful in assessing these patients.

It is important that symptoms be reproduced with such maneuvers because laxity is not an indication for surgical stabilization procedures. Asymptomatic shoulders may show substantial translation on clinical testing. In addition, joint laxity may be remarkable enough to distract the examiner from the primary source of pain, such as a painful acromioclavicular joint or a cervical radiculopathy. Conversely, laxity may be hard to demonstrate even in a shoulder with multidirectional instability if pain, muscle spasm, and guarding prevent subluxation. It is helpful to examine the contralateral, asymptomatic shoulder for laxity. If it is extremely loose, it may be a clue to the multidirectional nature of the affected side.

Plain radiographs are generally normal but should be evaluated for the presence of humeral head defects or glenoid lesions, such as osseous Bankart fragments, reactive bone, or wear. An arthro CT scan is the diagnostic image procedure of choice because capsular and labral lesions can be detected. Magnetic resonance imaging is less satisfactory in demonstrating the redundant capsule because of the lack of joint distension or labral lesions. Stress radiographs can demonstrate laxity, especially inferior subluxation, but are not generally needed.

CONSERVATIVE MANAGEMENT. Once the diagnosis of instability has been established, a prolonged course of rehabilitation is instituted with emphasis on strengthening the deltoid and rotator cuff muscles with the arm below the shoulder. The scapulothoracic stabilizing muscles are strengthened as well. Patients with multidirectional instability may occasionally develop a secondary impingement syndrome. At times, a subacromial injection of a steroid preparation will provide relief sufficient for the patient to resume his or her exercise regimen.

During the rehabilitation program, motivation should be carefully assessed to ensure the patient is mature enough to cooperate in the rehabilitation effort required after surgery and to screen out those manipulating their disease for secondary gain.

Patients with acquired instability may have developed the ability to dislocate the shoulder at will or on command. This is especially true if certain positions will reliably result in a dislocation (e.g., the humeral head falls out posteriorly whenever the arm is raised in the forward plane in internal rotation). Such "positional dislocators" may demonstrate this for the examiner, if requested, but otherwise patients should do their best to avoid such positions. Although "positional dislocators" can demonstrate instability on command, they do not necessarily have accompanying psychiatric disorders and are amenable to surgical correction.

These patients must be differentiated, however, from true voluntary dislocators who have underlying psychiatric problems and who use asymmetric muscle pull to dislocate their shoulder, or even to hold it out, for a great dramatic effect. To complicate matters, there is a small group of patients who have developed a habitual initiation of improper muscle firing patterns, which also produce dislocations by asymmetric muscle pull. These patients can be unaware of this pattern and may be without psychiatric disturbance. Nevertheless, both groups of "muscular dislocators" are poor candidates for stabilization procedures. Those with psychiatric disturbances need counseling and, with respect to the shoulder, skillful neglect. The group with habitually improper muscle use may be treated successfully with muscle retraining and biofeedback.

INDICATIONS FOR ORTHOPEDIC REFERRAL. Any patient sustaining a traumatic dislocation should be immediately referred for orthopedic consultation. A patient may have a subtle fracture or be a candidate for early operative intervention. Additionally, a patient with episodes of multiple, recurrent dislocations should be referred because conservative treatment is unlikely to help. If the patient has prolonged symptoms of subluxation or pain, without dislocation, and has not responded to conservative management, including an exercise regimen, surgery may be indicated, and the patient should be referred.

OPERATIVE MANAGEMENT. Operative management involves imbrication or "tightening" of the redundant inferior joint capsule coupled with repair of any capsular–labral avulsion from the anterior glenoid rim (Fig. 18-18). Presently, a relatively higher rate of failures associated with arthroscopic repairs have narrowed indications for this approach. The preferred surgery is an open approach to restore anatomy by correcting existing pathology, most commonly either capsular laxity or labral avulsion.

Adhesive Capsulitis

SPORTS COMMONLY INVOLVED. Adhesive capsulitis is rare in active healthy people involved in athletics. It is not generally associated with any particular sport, but it can be seen in older athletes or in those with diabetes in whom concomitant tendinitis can lead to periods of immobility and subsequent stiffness.

BACKGROUND. Adhesive capsulitis, also known as frozen shoulder, is a primary shoulder disorder of unknown etiology characterized by progressive pain and restriction of glenohumeral motion. The condition can occur after any injury or inflammation around the shoulder joint that requires a period of immobilization. Other associated factors include diabetes, trauma, breast surgery, and hypothyroidism.[30,38] Because missed dislocations, osteoarthritis, and impingement can lead to a loss of range of motion, frozen shoulder is a diagnosis of exclusion, and other factors should be carefully ruled out.

PATHOMECHANICS. Frozen shoulder is characterized by chronic inflammation and fibrosis of the glenohumeral capsule, leading to marked restriction of joint volume and later adhesions from articulating surfaces to the capsule. The inflammatory process also extends to the subacromial bursa and coracohumeral ligament. The disease has been characterized clinically to involve three stages: I—early diffuse pain with range of motion largely intact, II—adhesive stage where there is progressive loss of range of motion, and III—gradual resolution of motion.

SPECIFICS OF HISTORY AND EXAMINATION. A patient with adhesive capsulitis initially has diffuse pain often indistinguishable from impingement. The pain is accompanied by a reduction in passive and active range of motion. The loss of motion is generally global but always involves a reduction in external rotation. Classically, a patient with frozen shoulder has pain at

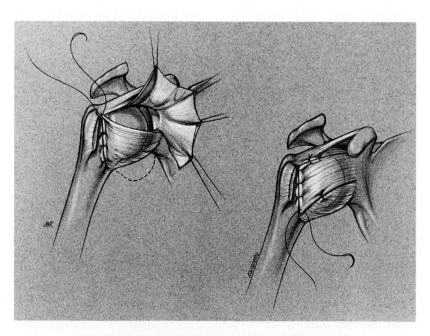

Fig. 18-18. Schematic of anterior–inferior capsular shift.

the end of the range of motion. He or she can be comfortable within the restricted range of motion but have pain—often severe—when inadvertently extending past his or her range. Because painful splinting can cause a loss of motion, selective lidocaine injections are often helpful.

CONSERVATIVE MANAGEMENT. Nonoperative management with physical therapy emphasizing stretching for the range of motion is successful in the majority of patients. The physical therapy is augmented with symptomatic support, such as nonsteroidal and injected steroid medication. Improvement can be slow, with recovery taking up to 1 year.

INDICATIONS FOR ORTHOPEDIC REFERRAL. Because many conditions, some severe, can cause loss of motion, referral should probably be made early to confirm the diagnosis of adhesive capsulitis. The advent of scalene block catheters and relatively less-invasive arthroscopic procedures has provided for more aggressive management of refractory cases.[35]

Distal Clavicle Osteolysis

SPORTS COMMONLY INVOLVED. Distal clavicle osteolysis is classically seen in the power weightlifter but can also be found in athletes prone to blunt trauma on the point of the shoulder. Those sports include hockey, football, rugby, wrestling, skiing, skating, and bicycling.

BACKGROUND. This condition, characterized by pain and osteolysis of the distal clavicle, is seen in athletes who undergo repetitive stress on the acromioclavicular joint or have had an acute injury, such as acromioclavicular separation.[12,39] It is most commonly associated with power weightlifters, especially after bench pressing and military, overhead pressing.

PATHOMECHANICS. The pathomechanics of osteolysis are poorly understood. Characteristic radiographic changes include osteoporosis, osteolysis, or osteophyte formation of the distal clavicle without acromial changes. Usually, the condition is unilateral and self-limiting with respect to symptoms. Bony reconstitution is uncommon.

SPECIFICS OF HISTORY AND EXAMINATION. A patient will present with a dull ache centered over the acromioclavicular joint. Often, there is an accompanying trapezius spasm. Pain is also exacerbated by flexion and cross-body adduction. Clavicular view radiographs with a 35° cephalic tilt are helpful in making the diagnosis.

CONSERVATIVE MANAGEMENT. Successful conservative management includes rest and activity modification. Activity modification in the weightlifter includes adjustment to a lower amount of weight and increased repetitions or substitution of exercises. If rest does not help, acromioclavicular joint injections of steroid can be helpful.

INDICATIONS FOR ORTHOPEDIC REFERRAL. Orthopedic referral can be sought after a trial of conservative therapy has failed to bring significant improvement.

OPERATIVE MANAGEMENT. Operative management consists of distal clavicle excision of 4 to 5 mm from an arthroscopic approach if the joint is stable.[7] If the acromioclavicular joint is unstable, an open excision with transfer of the coracoacromial ligament may be indicated.

SPECIFIC TRAUMATIC INJURIES: BONY

Bony injuries or fractures of the shoulder can be difficult clinical entities that would require an extensive discussion beyond the scope of this section.[1,3] This section is necessarily abbreviated and tailored to athletic concerns. Because of the complex nature of shoulder fractures, these injuries should be referred for at least an initial orthopedic evaluation.

Proximal Humerus Fractures

SPORTS COMMONLY INVOLVED. Proximal humerus fractures are generally rare in the athletic population but can occur in any high-energy contact sports such as football, hockey, rugby, skiing, and wrestling. In the skeletally immature population, growth-plate stress fractures can occur in baseball pitchers from repetitive overhead throwing. Additionally, proximal humerus fractures should be suspected in the context of glenohumeral dislocations, especially in patients aged more than 40 years.

BACKGROUND. Proximal humerus fractures are generally rare in the young athletic population with good bone stock. However, in high-energy contact sports or in those with repetitive overhead motions, fractures occur. Mechanism of injury usually involves a fall on the outstretched hand, causing an axial load to be transferred to the humeral head. In younger, skeletally immature athletes, surgical neck stress fractures can occur through the growth plate. Less commonly, a fracture can occur secondary to a direct blow to the lateral shoulder. Two of the most common patterns involve a physial fracture of the surgical neck and greater tuberosity fracture-associated dislocations. The surgical neck physis of the proximal humerus does not fuse until one is in his or her early 20s, and a younger athlete can fracture this relatively weak area. Known as a "little league shoulder," these stress fractures heal quickly with rest if recognized early.

PATHOMECHANICS. Fractures of the proximal humerus occur in predictable patterns based on old physial scars. These injuries can include some combination of fractures involving the lesser tuberosity, greater tuberosity, anatomic neck, and surgical neck. As stated previously, in the athletic population, surgical neck and greater tuberosity fractures predominate. The surgical neck fracture can tolerate a relatively large degree of angulation and displacement and is usually managed nonoperatively. The greater tuberosity fracture, in contrast, will not tolerate much displacement and is often surgically reduced and repaired in the younger population. Because the rotator cuff is attached to the greater tuberosity, any significant displacement implies a tear, which is another reason for surgery.

SPECIFICS OF HISTORY AND EXAMINATION. The patient should relate a history of significant trauma or dislocation of the shoulder. The trauma is usually accompanied by immediate pain that diffuses around the upper arm and is exacerbated by any movement. On examination, there often is ecchymosis and swelling around the shoulder. As stated previously, careful neurovascular examination should be performed because of the significant incidence of associated injuries.

Antecedent trauma may not be present in a younger child with physial stress fractures. Adolescents with "little league shoulder" can have a history of repetitive overhead throwing and associated nondisplaced physial fractures.

CONSERVATIVE MANAGEMENT. If any suspicion of fracture, the extremity should be immobilized in a sling and swathe, and the patient should be sent for appropriate radiographic analysis.

OPERATIVE MANAGEMENT. Operative management of proximal humerus fractures can take numerous forms. Management usually involves reduction of the displaced fracture fragments in an anatomic fashion followed by fixation using heavy, nonabsorbable sutures or wire that incorporate the rotator cuff for strength. Alternatively, percutaneous pin fixation can be used in select surgical neck fractures. More severe fractures require more extensive fixation methods or even prosthetic replacement.

Clavicle Fractures

SPORTS COMMONLY INVOLVED. Clavicle fractures are the most common bony injuries seen about the shoulder. They are most commonly seen in high-energy, contact sports, most notably football and hockey or in bicycling and skiing resulting from falls.

BACKGROUND. The most common mechanism for fracture of the clavicle is a fall or blow to the point of the shoulder. A less-prevalent mechanism is a fall on the outstretched arm or direct blow with an object, as can occur in hockey or lacrosse. The fractures predominate in the shaft (80%), followed by distal (15%), and medial (5%).[30,38] Associated neurovascular injuries are rare despite their close anatomic proximity, and most fractures heal uneventfully within 8 weeks.

PATHOMECHANICS. Because the primary function of the clavicle is to strut the shoulder girdle away from the thorax, fractures result in inferior and anterior displacement. Gravity or the weight of the arm is the major deforming factor.

Fractures of the clavicle are different clinical entities depending on location relative to ligamentous insertions. Distal clavicle fractures occur in the lateral third of the shaft where the coracoclavicular ligaments originate. These fractures usually involve a tear or bony avulsion of the coracoclavicular ligaments and functionally simulate acromioclavicular joint separations (see section on acromioclavicular separations). Because the small distal fragment displaces inferiorly and anteriorly away from the proximal shaft, these fractures have a high incidence of painful nonunions when not surgically stabilized. In contrast, fractures of the mid-shaft reduce relatively well and a majority of the time heal with conservative management. Medial third fractures are rare and do not displace very much. These fractures heal very well with just symptomatic management. It is important to remember that the medial growth plate of the clavicle fuses as late as age 22 years. Therefore, a fracture before this age is often through the epiphysis and is commonly a slate II-type of epiphysis fracture. These injuries are managed conservatively.

SPECIFICS OF HISTORY AND EXAMINATION. Displaced clavicle fractures are very apparent on inspection secondary to the subcutaneous location. Nondisplaced fractures can be more difficult to detect because of the lack of deformity, however, palpable pain and swelling are readily examined. Associated problems, such as skin compromise or neurovascular injury, should be carefully evaluated because they can easily be missed, leading to serious complications.

Although standard anteroposterior radiographs are commonly sufficient, cephalic tilt clavicle views show the fracture more clearly.

CONSERVATIVE MANAGEMENT. Conservative management of mid-shaft fractures can be accomplished with a figure of eight strap or simple sling or both. The figure of eight strap must be fitted properly with a snug fit, which can be uncomfortable. Because the arm sling has been shown to be equally effective, it is generally preferred. When using the sling, it is important to adequately support the weight of the arm to counteract the anterior and inferior displacement.

OPERATIVE MANAGEMENT. Operative management of acute clavicle fractures historically has been reserved for distal third fractures. These fractures are generally managed with operative reduction and fixation with circlage wires or sutures and screws. Additional fixation is secured to the coracoid process, depending on the relative integrity of the ligaments.

Acromial, Glenoid, and Scapular Body Fractures

SPORTS COMMONLY INVOLVED. Acromial and scapular body fractures are rare but can be seen in athletes who participate in high-energy contact sports, such as football, skiing, or bicycling. Glenoid fractures are relatively more common and in the athletic population are seen in the context of glenohumeral dislocations.

BACKGROUND. Acromial fractures can result from either a direct blow or fall on the point of the shoulder. More typically, this will result in either an acromioclavicular separation or clavicle fracture. Because these fractures are rare, the clinician should not mistake an unfused growth plate for fracture. Previously discussed in the anatomy section, fusion of the growth plates takes place around the age of 22 years. In older individuals, an os acromiale, which is a nonunion of the growth plate, may also be present. Os acromiale occurs approximately 1.6% of the time and is bilateral 60% of the time.[30,38] The growth plates occur in a characteristic location at the junction between the anterior and middle third of the acromion. Fractures, in contrast, generally occur near the scapular spine base.

Scapular fractures represent high-energy injuries to the posterior thorax and are usually undisplaced in the context of athletics. These fractures are stable and heal well because of the abundant surrounding musculature. An athlete sustaining this fracture should have a careful work-up for associated blunt thorax injuries, such as pneumothorax.

PATHOMECHANICS. Acromial fractures must be watched carefully. Because the lateral deltoid originates here, these fractures tend to angulate inferiorly, closing down the coracoacromial arch. A small reduction of the subacromial space is poorly tolerated, and these fractures often require operative fixation.

Scapular fractures, as stated previously, usually heal well because of the abundant investing musculature. However, secondary problems such as adhesions or fibrosis of the subscapular bursa can occur, causing pain and alteration of scapulothoracic mechanics.

In the athletic population, glenoid fractures occur usually in the context of glenohumeral dislocations. These fractures are seen on the anterior–inferior glenoid rim and, when significant in size, can severely affect glenohumeral stability. Also referred as bony Bankart fractures, these fractures represent a combination axial load and bony avulsion injury from pull of the inferior glenohumeral ligaments.

SPECIFICS OF HISTORY AND EXAMINATION. A patient with an acromial fracture will have sustained injury directly to the point of the shoulder. Pain will be palpable directly on the acromial base with associated ecchymosis. This contrasts with os acromiale or growth plate injuries, which show less evidence of trauma and have more anterior acromial pain. Specific radiographic studies that should be taken include the West Point and axillary views.

Scapular fractures are diagnosed with true anteroposterior radiographs of the shoulder. They are often seen as incidental findings on athletes who have sustained significant thorax trauma. In the context of athletics, these fractures are usually nondisplaced and difficult to detect. Palpable tenderness on the scapula should direct clinical suspicion on radiographic interpretation. The clinical examination should include evaluation for associated injuries such as rib fractures, pneumothorax, kidney contusions, and aortic dissections.

Glenoid fractures seen in athletics most commonly are associated with anterior, traumatic dislocations; it is very rare to see more complex fractures. Careful evaluation of standard anteroposterior and axillary radiographs will often show the displaced fragment of glenoid rim displaced in an anterior and inferior direction. When necessary, special views, such as the West Point or computed tomography scan images, help visualize the presence and extent of these fractures.

CONSERVATIVE MANAGEMENT. All the previously discussed fractures should be acutely immobilized with a sling and swathe for further evaluation. If nonoperative management is elected, the sling is continued. For acromial fractures, 4 to 6 weeks of arm support is required with careful follow-up evaluation for any displacement. For nondisplaced scapular fractures, motion is encouraged as soon as tolerated to prevent scapulothoracic adhesions. Larger glenoid fractures associated with instability are usually managed oppressively.

OPERATIVE MANAGEMENT. Displaced or angulated acromial fractures are managed with operative reduction and fixation using parallel screws or figure of eight wires. A patient with a scapular body fracture rarely undergoes surgery and only if the fracture involves significant glenoid displacement. Anterior rim glenoid fractures are managed usually with operative reduction and fixation with screws. Rarely, small or severely comminuted fragments are excised and a coracoid transfer performed. These procedures are achieved through a standard instability repair approach, using some elements of capsular repair.

SPECIFIC TRAUMATIC INJURIES: SOFT TISSUE

Rotator Cuff Tear

SPORTS COMMONLY INVOLVED. Traumatic tears of the rotator cuff are rare in younger athletes. In older athletes who have been involved for many years in repetitive overhead sports like baseball, tennis, swimming, or football (quarterback), these partial tears usually represent acute extensions of chronic tendinitis or partial tears. In younger athletes, traumatic tears may occur when playing in football or wrestling.

BACKGROUND. Traumatic rotator cuff tears are seen with violent internal rotation of the arm against resistance or in falls on the outstretched arm. Rarely, they are seen when trying to throw heavy objects. Because the rotator cuff tends to be thick and robust, these traumatic avulsion injuries are rare in the younger, athletic population.

PATHOMECHANICS. Because the rotator cuff functions in external rotation and stabilization of the humeral head, violent rotation or luxation can cause avulsion. These acute injuries are different clinical entities from chronic, attrition rotator cuff disease. The tendons tend to be comprised of healthy, well-vascularized tissue with muscle atrophy or scaring. When repaired in a timely fashion, a patient tends to have excellent functional recovery. For an older athlete with acute extension of a chronic process, the same principles outlined previously for nontraumatic rotator cuff disease still apply.

SPECIFICS OF HISTORY AND EXAMINATION. The patient will generally complain of sudden, intense pain after one of the previously mentioned injury mechanisms. Pain is accompanied by significant weakness in shoulder motion. When an acute tear is suspected, early imaging with magnetic resonance imaging is appropriate to confirm the diagnosis. Other specifics of history and examination are outlined previously for nontraumatic rotator cuff disease.

CONSERVATIVE MANAGEMENT. Initial conservative management is usually a sling for symptomatic relief. However, once a diagnosis of acute, full-thickness tear is confirmed, early operative repair provides the best chance for functional recovery. Partial tears can be managed with early symptomatic management followed by a directed physical therapy program.

INDICATIONS FOR ORTHOPEDIC REFERRAL. Acute tears diagnosed by magnetic resonance imaging should be referred early for surgery. A patient with partial-thickness tears can be referred after failure to progress with conservative treatment.

OPERATIVE MANAGEMENT. Because acute tears tend to be mobile without chronic scaring, they often can be repaired in an arthroscopically assisted fashion through small incisions. Larger chronic tears require open repair.

Glenohumeral Dislocation

SPORTS COMMONLY INVOLVED. Initial, traumatic dislocations are seen in participants of high-energy impact sports or result from significant falls. These sports include football, rugby, hockey, wrestling, boxing, skiing, skating, or bicycling.

BACKGROUND. Dislocations in the athlete are almost always anterior, involving an abducted and externally rotated arm position. This dislocation type can occur when bracing for a fall or when the arm is violently caught by another player. Uncommonly, a direct blow to the shoulder can cause a dislocation.

In the young athletic population, these dislocations tend to recur. Recurrence rates vary from 50% to 90% after initial, traumatic dislocation, with higher rates associated with athletes who participate in sports with repetitive overhead motion and younger individuals.[18,30,38,44]

PATHOMECHANICS. Anterior glenohumeral dislocations always involve some element of anterior–inferior capsular attenuation.[8,24] Additionally, frequently there is an avulsion of the anterior–inferior glenoid labrum with attached anteroinferior glenohumeral ligament. In the younger population, this acute capsular damage does not incite a vigorous inflammatory response with subsequent scarring and joint retraction. Rather, the capsule remains lax and can no longer serve as an adequate checkrein to extremes of motion. Recently, an alteration in capsular, proprioceptive feedback has been suggested as a mechanism for recurrent instability. In this model, the attenuated capsule cannot relay adequate proprioceptive feedback to initiate contraction of protective, surrounding musculature.

SPECIFICS OF HISTORY AND EXAMINATION. Diagnosis of an acutely dislocated shoulder is usually obvious by examination and history. The athlete will usually relate a history of significant trauma involving some external rotation and abduction of the shoulder. Rarely, insignificant trauma can cause a first-time dislocation. The dislocated shoulder will show deformity with a subacromial sulcus and palpable fullness anterior and inferior from the humeral head. The arm is generally held in some external rotation and abduction. A careful neurovascular examination should be performed, especially for axillary nerve injury.

On radiographs, anteroposterior and axillary views should be inspected carefully for any fractures. This inspection is especially important on prereduction radiographs because a missed, nondisplaced fracture can be propagated or displaced by an inappropriate reduction maneuver.

CONSERVATIVE MANAGEMENT. Once anatomic reduction is achieved, nonoperative management is preferred. The arm is immobilized in a sling. Although the exact length of time is controversial, 4 to 6 weeks of wearing the sling is generally accepted. After 4 to 6 weeks, a directed physical therapy program that stresses rotation-strengthening internally is prescribed. However, strengthening exercises should begin as soon as the patient is comfortable. These exercises should strengthen the internal and external rotation, deltoid, and scapular muscles so there is a balanced approach.

INDICATIONS FOR ORTHOPEDIC REFERRAL. Because of the possibility of subtle fractures, acute traumatic dislocation should generally be referred for initial evaluation.

OPERATIVE MANAGEMENT. Operative management for an acute dislocation is rare, but it may be indicated in the dominant arm in throwing athletes and in individuals who will return to repetitive, stressful, overhead activity.

Acromioclavicular Separations

SPORTS COMMONLY INVOLVED. Acromioclavicular separations are relatively common injuries seen in participants of contact sports, especially hockey, and in victims of significant falls. Those sports include hockey, football, rugby, wrestling, skiing, skating, and bicycling.

BACKGROUND. These injuries generally result from a blow or a fall directly on the shoulder. The separations are graded as follows: Grade I—pain and swelling at the acromioclavicular joint without radiographic subluxation, Grade II—subluxation without complete dislocation, and Grade III—complete dislocation of the joint.[38] Grade I and II injuries heal well with conservative, symptomatic management. Management of Grade III injuries is somewhat controversial. Although most of these injuries heal without significant functional limitations, conservative management will result in a persistently dislocated joint that may be at higher risk for painful arthrosis. Most physicians prefer nonoperative management, however in the high-performance, athlete engaging in overhead motion there may be a role for acute stabilization. Other commonly accepted indications for operative fixation include herniation of the distal clavicle through the trapezius and locking of the clavicle posterior to the acromion.

PATHOMECHANICS. The distal clavicle is stabilized to the acromion primarily through three ligaments: the superior acromioclavicular joint capsule and ligament and two coracoclavicular ligaments. Under normal, physiologic loads, the superior acromioclavicular ligament is most important for stabilizing the joint-form luxation. With higher loads, the coracoclavicular ligament becomes more important for stabilizing against superior displacement, and the superior acromioclavicular ligament remains the primary restraint against anterior–superior–posterior displacement.

With Grade I injuries, there is only a sprain of the acromioclavicular ligaments and no tear. In Grade II separations, there is a tear of the acromioclavicular ligaments, leaving the coracoclavicular ligaments as the primary restraint. In Grade III separations, the acromioclavicular and coracoclavicular ligaments are torn, destroying the remaining ligamentous restraints.

SPECIFICS OF HISTORY AND EXAMINATION. Patients with acromioclavicular separations relate a history of fall or force directly on the shoulder. With Grade I separations, there is tenderness and edema at the joint. Grade II and III separations will also show deformity from a more prominent distal clavicle. These separations should be checked for reducibility. If a partial reduction cannot be obtained, herniation through the trapezius should be suspected.

Distal clavicle anteroposterior radiographs with the arm in the dependent position should be obtained. Bilateral views help make the diagnosis when subtle luxation is present. Because the clavicle displaces posterior and anterior views, an axillary radiograph is also necessary.

CONSERVATIVE MANAGEMENT. Nonoperative management consists of a snug-arm sling to support the weight of the arm. Special slings are available to hold the distal clavicle in the reduced position, but they are ineffective and have problems of skin breakdown at the top of the acromioclavicular joint.

INDICATIONS FOR SURGICAL REFERRAL. Surgical fixation of a separated acromioclavicular joint is achieved by open reduction and stabilization of the distal clavicle with sutures secured to the coracoid. The coracoacromial ligament is then transferred from the acromion to the distal clavicle to reconstruct the torn coracoclavicular ligaments.

Peripheral Nerve Injuries

SPORTS COMMONLY INVOLVED. Peripheral nerve injuries to the suprascapular, axillary, long thoracic, and spinal accessory nerves are rare. Suprascapular nerve injury is seen in athletes who participate in activities with repetitive overhead motion, especially baseball pitchers and volleyball players. Other nerve injuries are seen in those who participate in contact sports where there is blunt trauma to the shoulder girdle.

BACKGROUND. All of these peripheral nerve injuries are uncommon but should always be considered in the differential diagnosis for atrophy, diffuse tenderness, and weakness about the shoulder.[28] These injuries can occur from seemingly insignificant injury, but more often are associated with significant injuries or overuse episodes.

Suprascapular nerve deficits can occur as isolated nerve compression syndromes from entrapment at the suprascapular or spinoglenoid notch or from ganglia. These syndromes often occur with insidious onset. Conversely, they can result from a blow to the shoulder or from repetitive overhead and cross-body motions. Conservative management of rest and nonsteroidal medication is often helpful. Surgical management of exploration and decompression, if necessary, has a good prognosis if significant muscle atrophy has not occurred.

Axillary nerve injuries are the most common and are often associated with dislocations or fractures of the proximal humerus. Rarely, a direct blow to the lateral shoulder can result in axillary nerve injury. These injuries are almost always neurapraxias, and there is a good prognosis for recovery with conservative management.

Long thoracic and spinal accessory nerve injuries associated with blunt trauma, in contrast to axillary and suprascapular injuries, have a more guarded prognosis. Nerve explorations and decompressions are usually not successful, and prolonged observation is generally used. Conservative management involves strengthening of the periscapular, adjunctive musculature. Long thoracic nerve palsies can be idiopathic, usually in throwers, and have a good prognosis for recovery. A 1-year observation period is recommended for the long thoracic nerve, and a 3-month period is recommended for the spinal accessory nerve.

PATHOANATOMY. The suprascapular nerve is formed from C5 and C6 spinal roots and branches from the upper trunk of the brachial plexus. The nerve enters the superior border of the scapula through the scapular notch, which is bridged by a thick, transverse ligament. The nerve gives off branches to the supraspinatus and courses around the scapular spine laterally to enter the infraspinatus fossa where it terminates into a number of muscular branches. In 50% of patients, the nerve passes the spinoglenoid ligament—an aponeurotic band separating the spinati. Compression of the nerve usually occurs at the notch or spinoglenoid ligament.[38]

The axillary nerve is responsible for innervation of the important deltoid muscle, teres minor, and overlying skin. The nerve also forms from C5 and C6, but it branches distally from the posterior cord. It courses anterior to the subscapularis muscle until it travels posterior directly under the glenohumeral joint to give off a circumflex branch, which innervates the deltoid. The close proximity of the nerve to the anterior–inferior glenohumeral joint results in susceptibility to concomitant injury with dislocations and fractures.

The long thoracic nerve originates directly from the confluence of the C5, C6, and C7 spinal roots, after which it courses down the anterolateral chest wall to innervate the serratus anterior muscle. Injury to this nerve can occur with blunt chest wall trauma or through several poorly understood mechanisms, including viral illness, prolonged recumbency, or overhead throwing.

The spinal accessory nerve is a cranial nerve that enters the neck from the jugular foramen to descend through the posterior triangle to innervate the trapezius muscle. Injuries can result from traction from a blow to the point of the shoulder or from direct blows.

SPECIFICS OF HISTORY AND EXAMINATION. Each of the previously discussed nerve injuries are characterized by specific muscle atrophy or dysfunction and diffuse pain. Thus, suprascapular nerve injuries result in weakness to external rotation; axillary nerve injuries result in weakness to elevation; long thoracic nerve injuries result in scapular winging seen best when pushing forward against a wall; and spinal accessory nerve injuries result in weakness to elevation and shoulder shrug. When suspected, electromyographic studies, in conjunction with a clinical examination, will confirm the diagnosis.

CONSERVATIVE MANAGEMENT. Nonoperative management consists of supportive, symptomatic care during observation. Range of motion and strengthening of adjacent, overlapping musculature is used. Serial electromyography can be helpful for following recovery or determining prognosis.

INDICATIONS FOR ORTHOPEDIC REFERRAL. Confirmed nerve injuries or documented muscle dysfunction, especially in the presence of significant atrophy, indicate orthopedic referral.

OPERATIVE MANAGEMENT. Operative management of peripheral nerve injuries to the suprascapular and axillary nerve are directed toward exploration, neurolysis, repair, or grafting as good muscle transfers are unavailable. In contrast, there are good muscle transfers for reconstituting serratus anterior and trapezius palsies, and they are generally preferred.

REFERENCES

1. Anderson T: Difficult sports-related shoulder fractures, *Clin Sports Med* 9:31–37, 1990.
2. Andrews JR, Kupferman SP, Dillman CJ: Labral tears in throwing and racquet sports, *Clin Sports Med* 10:901–911, 1991.
3. Bigliani LU: Fractures about the shoulder. In Rockwood CR Jr, Green DP, eds: *Fractures in adults*, ed 2, vol 1, Philadelphia, 1984, JB Lippincott.
4. Bigliani LU, Flatow EL: History, physical examination, and diagnostic modalities. In J.B. McGinty, et al, eds: Operative arthroscopy, New York, 1991, Raven Press.
5. Bigliani LU, Kimmel J, McCann PD, Wolfe I: Repair of rotator cuff tears in tennis players, *Am J Sports Med* 20:112–117, 1992.
6. Bigliani LU, Kurzweil PR, Schwartzbach CC, Wolfe IN, Flatow EL: Inferior capsular shift procedure for anterior-inferior shoulder instability in athletes, *Am J Sports Med* 22:578–584, 1994.
7. Bigliani LU, Nicholson GP, Flatow EL: Arthroscopic resection of the distal clavicle, *Orthop Clin North Am* 24:133–141, 1993
8. Bigliani LU, Pollock RG, Soslowsky LJ, Flatow EL, Pawluk RJ, Mow VC: Tensile properties of the inferior glenohumeral ligament, *J Orthop Res* 10:187–197, 1992.
9. Bigliani LU, Ticker JB, Flatow EL, Soslowsky LJ, Mow VC: The relationship of acromial architecture to rotator cuff disease, *Clin Sports Med* 10:823–838, 1991.
10. Bloom MH, Obata WG: Diagnosis of posterior dislocation of the shoulder with use of velpeau axillary and angle-up roentgenographic views, *J Bone Joint Surg* 49A:943–949, 1967.
11. Burnham RS, May L, Nelson E, Steadward R, Reid DC: Shoulder pain in wheelchair athletes. The role of muscle imbalance, *Am J Sports Med* 21:238–242, 1993.
12. Cahill BR: Osteolysis of the distal part of the clavicle in male athletes, *J Bone Joint Surg* 64A:1053–1058, 1982.
13. Dillman CJ, Fleisig GS, Andrews JR: Biomechanics of pitching with emphasis upon shoulder kinematics, *J Orthop Sports Phys Ther* 18:402–408, 1993.
14. Flannigan B, Kursunoglu-Brahme S, Snyder S, Karzel R, Del Pizzo W, Resnick D: NM arthrography of the shoulder: comparison with conventional NM imaging, *AJR Am J Radiol* 155:829–832, 1990.
15. Flatow EL: The biomechanics of the acromioclavicular, sternoclavicular, and scapulothoracic joints, *Instr Course Lect* 42:237–245, 1993
16. Gerber C, Krushnell RJ: Isolated ruptures of the tendon of the subscapularis muscle, *Orthop Trans* 14:261, 1990.
17. Gross ML, Brenner SL, Esformes I, Sonzogni JJ: Anterior shoulder instability in weight lifters, *Am J Sports Med* 21:599–603, 1993.
18. Higgs GB, Weinstein D, Flatow EL: Evaluation and treatment of acute anterior glenohumeral dislocations, *Sports Med Arthroscopy Rev* 1:190–201, 1993.
19. Iannotti JP, Zlatkin MB, Esterhai JL, Kressel HY, Dalinka MK, Spindler KP: Magnetic resonance imaging of the shoulder. Sensitivity, specificity, and predictive value, *J Bone Joint Surg* 73A:7–29, 1991.
20. Ireland ML, Andrews JR: Shoulder and elbow injuries in the young athlete, *Clin Sports Med* 7:473–494, 1988.
21. Janda DH, Loubert P: Basic science and clinical application in the athlete's shoulder. A preventative program focusing on the glenohumeral joint, *Clin Sports Med* 10:955–971, 1991.
22. Jobe FW, Moynes DR, Antonelli DJ: Rotator cuff function during a golf swing, *Am J Sports Med* 14:388–392, 1986.
23. Jobe FW, Pink M: Classification and treatment of shoulder dysfunction in the overhead athlete, *J Orthop Sports Phys Ther* 18:427–432, 1993.
24. Kuriyama S, Fujimaki E, Katagiri T, Uemura S: Anterior dislocation of the shoulder joint sustained through skiing. Arthrographic findings and prognosis, *Am J Sports Med* 12:339–346, 1984.
25. Lo YP, Hsu YC, Chan KM: Epidemiology of shoulder impingement in upper arm sports events, *Br J Sports Med* 24:173–177, 1990.
26. McCann PD, Bigliani LU: Shoulder pain in tennis players, *Sports Med* 17:53–64, 1994.
27. McMaster WC, Troup J: A survey of interfering shoulder pain in United States competitive swimmers, *Am J Sports Med* 21:67–70, 1993.
28. Mendoza FX, Main K: Peripheral nerve injuries of the shoulder in the athlete, *Clin Sports Med* 9:331–342, 1990.
29. Meister K, Andrews JR: Classification and treatment of rotator cuff injuries in the overhand athlete, *J Orthop Sports Phys Ther* 18:413–421, 1993.
30. Miller MD, Cooper DE, Warner JP: Shoulder, In *Review of sports medicine and arthroscopy*, Philadelphia, 1995, WB Saunders Co.
31. Miniaci A, Fowler PJ: Impingement in the athlete, *Clin Sports Med* 12:91–110, 1993.
32. Neviaser TJ: Weight lifting. Risks and injuries to the shoulder, *Clin Sports Med* 10:615–621, 1991.
33. Pforringer W, Smasal V: Aspects of traumatology in ice hockey, *J Sports Sci* 5:327–336, 1987.
34. Pollock RG, Bigliani LU: Recurrent posterior shoulder instability. Diagnosis and treatment, *Clin Orthop* 85–96, 1993.
35. Pollock RG, Duralde XA, Flatow EL, Bigliani LU: The use of arthroscopy in the treatment of resistant frozen shoulder, *Clin Orthop* 30–36, 1994.
36. Richardson AB, Jobe FW, Collins HR: The shoulder in competitive swimming, *Am J Sports Med* 8:159–163, 1980.
37. Richmond DR: Handlebar problems in bicycling, *Clin Sports Med* 13:165–173, 1994.
38. Rockwood CR, Matsen FA, ed: *The Shoulder*, Philadelphia, 1990, W.B. Saunders.
39. Scavenius M, Iversen BF: Nontraumatic clavicular osteolysis in weight lifters, *Am J Sports Med* 20:463–467, 1992.
40. Silliman JF, Hawkins RJ: Current concepts and recent advances in the athlete's shoulder, *Clin Sports Med* 10:693–705, 1991.
41. Smasal V, Pforringer W: Ice hockey injuries. Studies of the highest West German league, *Sportverletz Sportschaden* 1:181–184, 1987.
42. Soslowsky LJ, Flatow EL, Bigliani LU, Mow VC: Articular geometry of the glenohumeral joint, *Clin Orthop* 181–190, 1992.
43. Soslowsky LJ, Flatow EL, Bigliani LU, Pawluk RJ, Ateshian GA, Mow VC: Quantitation of in situ contact areas at the

glenohumeral joint: a biomechanical study, *J Orthop Res* 10:524–534, 1992.

44. Tsai L, Wredmark T, Johansson C, Gibo K, Engstrom B, Tornqvist H: Shoulder function in patients with unoperated anterior shoulder instability, *Am J Sports Med* 19:469–473, 1991.

45. Warren RF: Instability of shoulder in throwing sports, *Instr Course Lect* 34:337–348, 1985.

46. Wilk KE, Arrigo C: Current concepts in the rehabilitation of the athletic shoulder, *J Orthop Sports Phys Ther* 18:365–378, 1993.

CHAPTER 19

THE ELBOW AND FOREARM

Robert T. Goldman
Peter D. McCann

Elbow and forearm injuries are becoming more common as more people participate in throwing and racquet sports. Injuries may involve the bony articulations, muscles, ligaments, tendons, capsule, or nerves, all of which may impair elbow function. The majority of injuries to the elbow and forearm in the athlete are chronic, overuse injuries. These injuries result from repetitive intrinsic and extrinsic overload causing cumulative trauma. In adults, soft tissues, such as ligaments and tendons, become attenuated. In children, apophyses—the weakest link in the immature musculoskeletal system—are susceptible to stress injuries. Early management should be directed toward decreasing pain and inflammation, followed by strengthening and conditioning of the structures surrounding the elbow. Appropriate rehabilitation remains the cornerstone of successful management of overuse injuries of the elbow, facilitating patients' return to activity. Acute injuries to the elbow and forearm, although less common than chronic injuries, also plague the athlete. To fully understand the significance of injuries to the elbow and forearm, functional anatomy, patterns of injury, and current management options will be reviewed.

ELBOW ANATOMY

The elbow is a hinged joint composed of three distinct articulations: the radiocapitellar joint, the ulnohumeral joint, and the proximal radioulnar joint (Fig. 19-1). This unique articulation provides for flexion–extension and forearm rotation (pronation–supination). The normal arc of elbow flexion is 0 to 145°, with considerable individual variation allowing hyperextension or hyperflexion.[14] Forearm pronation averages 80°, and supination averages 85°.[14] The functional elbow range of motion that permits nearly all activities of daily living is 30° to 130° of flexion, 50° of pronation, and 50° of supination.[84]

The carrying angle is defined as the orientation of the forearm in reference to the humerus when the elbow is in full extension. The carrying angle varies as a function of age (smaller in children than adults) and sex (females averaging 3° to 4° more than males). The normal distribution of this angle varies greatly and averages 10° valgus in male subjects and 13° valgus in female subjects.[2]

Elbow stability is composed of three elements: the bony articulations, the capsular and ligamentous structures, and the dynamic contribution of the muscles. Unlike the shoulder, the dynamic contribution of the musculature to elbow stability under normal circumstances is minimal. The articular configuration is the primary stabilizer of the elbow against varus and valgus stress at less than 20° and more than 120° of flexion.[111] Between these extremes, stability is mainly provided by the fibrous and synovial capsule, which is thickened medially and laterally to form the collateral ligament complexes.

The ulnar or medial collateral ligament complex consists of three distinct structures: the anterior oblique, posterior oblique, and transverse ligaments (Fig. 19-2). The anterior oblique ligament is a thick, discrete band with parallel fibers originating from the medial epicondyle and inserting onto the medial aspect of the coronoid process. The results of various sectioning studies have shown that the anterior oblique ligament is the primary stabilizer of the elbow against valgus stress.[83,107] The posterior oblique ligament is a fan-shaped thickening of the capsule best defined with the elbow flexed at 90°. This ligament originates from the medial epicondyle and inserts onto the medial margin of the semilunar notch. The transverse ligament, which does not appear to have any effect on elbow stability, originates from the medial olecranon and inserts onto the inferior medial aspect of the coronoid process.

The radial or lateral collateral ligament complex provides varus stability to the elbow joint and is composed of four structures. The *radial collateral ligament* originates from the lateral epicondyle and inserts into the annular ligament. The *lateral ulnar collateral ligament* originates from the lateral epicondyle and inserts onto the crista supinatoris of the ulna. Rupture of this

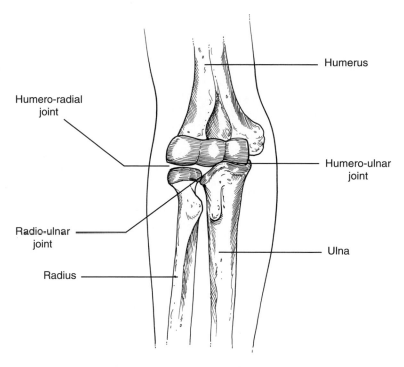

Fig. 19-1. Bony anatomy of the elbow.

ligament has been determined to be the primary lesion in posterolateral rotatory instability of the elbow.[94] The *annular ligament* and the *accessory collateral ligament* ensure the proper articulation of the proximal radioulnar joint but contribute little to varus stability of the elbow.[78]

Although providing minimal stability in the static situation, the flexor–pronator muscle group of the forearm functions as a secondary dynamic stabilizer of the elbow against valgus stress. Likewise, the anconeus muscle provides secondary dynamic stability against varus stress.[104]

OVERUSE INJURIES

Overuse injuries are caused by repetitive intrinsic or extrinsic overload, or both, resulting in microtrauma to soft tissues such as ligaments or tendons (Table 19-1). Intrinsic overload is the force from muscular contraction, concentric or eccentric, that can lead to tendinitis or muscular injury. Extrinsic overload is a tensile overload caused by excessive joint torque forces stressing the soft tissue and resulting in stretching and eventual disruption. Extrinsic overload also may be attributed to compression causing abrasion or impingement. Microrupture

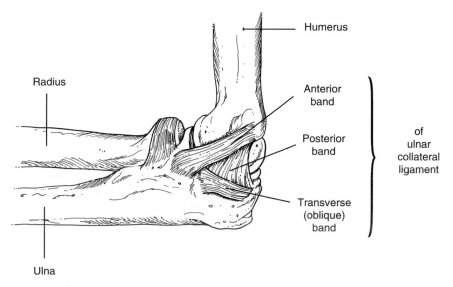

Fig. 19-2. Medial collateral ligament complex of the elbow.

Table 19-1. Sports that commonly produce elbow injuries[108]

Sport	Common injury
Racquet sports	Lateral epicondylitis with backhand
Golf	Medial epicondylitis on downswing with trailing arm
	Lateral epicondylitis at impact with leading arm
Basketball	Posterior compartment with follow-through on jump shot
Waterskiing	Valgus extension overload of posterior compartment with trick skiing
Bowling	Flexor–pronator soreness
Baseball	Valgus stress of pitching medial traction, lateral compression, posterior abutment
Volleyball	Valgus stress at impact of spiking
Football	Valgus stress with throwing a pass; hyperextension and dislocation, and olecranon bursitis with direct trauma
Gymnastics	Radiocapitellar overload and posterior impingement with weight-bearing on extended elbow
Weight training	Ulnar collateral ligament sprain, ulnar nerve irritation
Field events	
Shotput	Posterior impingement with follow through
Javelin	Valgus–extension overload of throwing; medial traction posterior abutment, lateral compression
Canoeing, kayaking	Distal bicipital tendinitis
Archery	Extensor muscle fatigue, lateral epicondylitis of bow arm
Rock climbing	Brachialis or distal biceps tendinitis

From Safran MR: Elbow injuries in athletes: A review, *Clin Orthop* 310:1994.

of soft tissues results in compromise by an imperfect healing process. In children, as apophyses undergo ossification, they are susceptible to stress injuries, resulting in local inflammation, irregular ossification patterns, overgrowth, and pain.

Management of overuse injuries should always start with prevention. Prevention should include education, overall flexibility, strengthening and endurance, proper warm-up and stretching, and avoidance of fatigue. Proper mechanics and equipment are also important.

Once an athlete develops an overuse injury, an aggressive nonoperative program should be started. The acronym PRICEMM[104] can be used to remember the modalities. First, **p**rotect the elbow from further injury. **R**est the elbow from the offending event, but allow the athlete to continue maintaining cardiovascular fitness. **I**ce, **c**ompression with an elastic bandage, and **e**levation are mainstays of nonoperative management. Nonsteroidal anti-inflammatory **m**edications are successful at relieving the pain and inflammation. Several **m**odalities, such as transcutaneous electrical stimulation and ultrasound, have proven helpful as well.[88] A rehabilita-

tion program should be instituted after the acute symptoms have resolved, with a gradual return to activity.

If a quality rehabilitation program is not successful and the patient has constant pain or persistent pain that affects activity, surgery may be indicated. The common features of the many surgical techniques used to manage overuse injuries include identification and excision of the pathologic tissue and reconstruction using normal tissue to close the defect. Healthy scar tissue can form that can withstand the repetitive stresses that the weakened, abnormal tissue could not. After the surgery, the repaired tissue is protected, and gradual postoperative rehabilitation is performed before the patient returns to sports activity.

TENDINOPATHIES

Lateral Epicondylitis—"Tennis Elbow"

Lateral epicondylitis is arguably the most common source of elbow pain in the general population. It occurs 7 to 20 times more frequently than medial epicondylitis.[27] It was first described more than 100 years ago in a tennis player,[72] but has since been described in association with many other athletic and nonathletic endeavors. The typical patient is a recreational tennis player aged 35 to 50 years who plays three to four times a week. They are usually inadequately conditioned and often use poor technique. Advanced tennis players who warm up, use good technique, and are well conditioned rarely suffer from lateral epicondylitis.[90]

Lateral epicondylitis is a chronic tendinitis of the extensor muscles, primarily the extensor carpi radialis brevis, caused by overuse in intensity and duration. It has been shown that 50% of club tennis players older than aged 30 years have experienced symptoms characteristic of lateral epicondylitis at least once.[89] One half of these players noted minor symptoms with a duration of less than 6 months, whereas the other half had major symptoms lasting an average of 2.5 years. Several factors have been associated with this problem: heavier, stiffer, more tightly strung racquets; incorrect grip size; inexperience; and poor backhand technique.

Lateral epicondylitis presents as lateral elbow pain that has an insidious onset beginning with pain after vigorous activity and progressing to pain during the activity. On examination, there is pain with passive wrist flexion and with active wrist extension. There often is point tenderness 1 to 2 cm distal to the lateral epicondyle. Grasping or pinching with the wrist extended (coffee cup test) usually reproduces pain at the point of tenderness.[27] Radiographic results are frequently normal, although 22% of patients will have evidence of a spur at the lateral epicondyle or calcification of the common extensor tendon.[88] The differential diagnosis of lateral epicondylitis includes radial tunnel syndrome (compression neuropathy of the posterior interosseous nerve), localized intraarticular pathology, or subtle instability of the radiocapitellar joint.

Surgical pathology reveals that the extensor carpi radialis brevis tendon is implicated as the source of pain and pathologic change.[90] Surrounding extensor tendons may be involved as well. Initial management is nonoperative (PRICEMM) and is often successful. Proper technique and equipment modifications, such as reduced racquet string tension and a cushioned grip, are useful adjuncts.[28] A counterforce brace has also been useful in managing tennis elbow. These braces are 5- to 6-cm wide nonelastic bands that are applied to encircle the forearm just below the elbow. A number of theories have been presented to explain how the brace works. Essentially, the brace causes a change in the sequence and direction of muscle pull, which decreases the force of muscle contraction by shortening the effective length of the muscle.[44]

If the initial nonoperative management is ineffective after 3 to 4 weeks, injection with xylocaine, 1%, with methylprednisolone just below the extensor carpi radialis brevis origin may be indicated. Some authors recommend no more than three injections in this area per year because they may cause further degeneration of the tendon and subsequent rupture.[86]

If nonoperative management fails to return the athlete to his or her usual activities by 3 to 4 months, which occurs in approximately 10% of patients, Nirschl[88] recommends surgical intervention. Others wait up to 1 year before considering surgical treatment.[86] Many surgical procedures have been described for management of refractory lateral epicondylitis. Procedure of choice is surgical excision of the torn, scarred portion of the tendon and any granulation tissue.[90] One may elect to repair the remaining tendon back to the lateral epicondyle after first drilling the bone to enhance the local blood supply. Once full range of motion is achieved after surgery, a graduated exercise program is initiated. Tennis can usually be resumed after 3 months when adequate strength has returned and little or no pain remains. Of those patients who underwent surgical management for refractory tennis elbow, 85% returned to full activities without pain, 12% improved but still had residual pain with vigorous activities, and 3% showed no improvement.[90]

Medial Epicondylitis

Medial epicondylitis is a tendinitis of the flexor–pronator muscle group. This condition primarily involves the pronator teres and flexor carpi radialis muscles, with occasional involvement of the flexor carpi ulnaris.[66] These two muscles are susceptible to inflammation and injury because they span two joints (wrist and elbow). Excessive valgus forces combined with repetitive flexor forearm muscle pull can produce an overuse syndrome in the common flexor origin. Athletic activities producing this condition include baseball, golf, and racquet sports.

Patients complaining of medial epicondylitis describe aching pain in the medial forearm musculature, originating from the medial epicondyle. These patients occasionally note swelling of the medial elbow and weakness of grip strength related to pain. The pain usually worsens with throwing, serving, or hitting with a forearm stroke. On examination, patients have pain slightly distal and lateral to the medial epicondyle, which increases with resisted wrist flexion and forearm pronation. Conditions that may be mistaken for medial epicondylitis include acute injuries, such as disruption of the common flexor muscle origin with a throwing injury, or rupture of the medial collateral ligament.[104] These entities usually can be differentiated by careful physical examination. Varying degrees of ulnar neuropathy can be seen either separate from or together with medial epicondylitis.[88] This may result from local inflammation or edema from the injured flexor–pronator muscle group, causing a compression neuropathy in the region of the cubital tunnel. Electromyography may be used to distinguish ulnar neuropathy from medial epicondylitis. Radiographs of patients with medial epicondylitis usually appear normal, although medial ulnar traction spurs may be present.

Management of medial epicondylitis is similar to that of lateral epicondylitis. The basic principles (PRICEMM) act to relieve the acute and chronic inflammatory symptoms. After the initial symptoms resolve, a therapy program aimed at gradually increasing flexibility, strength, and endurance is initiated. A counterforce brace has been used in the management of medial epicondylitis, but it has not proved to be as successful as in lateral epicondylitis.[86] A gradual resumption in play is recommended when symptoms have subsided, generally 6 to 12 weeks after injury. For refractory cases, after 4 to 6 weeks of treatment, a local corticosteroid injection may be helpful. Care must be taken not to inject directly into the tendon or ulnar nerve because of risk of damage to these structures.

Indication for surgical management of medial epicondylitis is persistent pain at the medial elbow, unresponsive to a well-managed rehabilitation program for 6 to 12 months.[53] Intraarticular pathology and neurologic dysfunction must be ruled out. Various surgical techniques have been described to manage medial epicondylitis, but most result in significant flexor–pronator strength deficits that may be debilitating to an athlete. In performing any procedure for medial epicondylitis, care must be taken to prevent injury to the ulnar nerve and medial collateral ligament. The recommended technique[112] involves incising the common flexor tendon off the epicondyle, débriding the abnormal tissue from the undersurface of the flexor–pronator mass, and then suturing the tendon back to the epicondyle, which should be abraded to provide an adequate blood supply for healing. The patient is usually splinted for 7 to 10 days, after which gentle active elbow, wrist, and hand range of motion exercises are begun. At 4 to 6 weeks, a progressive strengthening program begins with return to activity generally attained 4 months after surgery. In a review of 35 patients treated surgically, a successful result was obtained in 97% of patients, with all athletically active patients returning to their sport.[112] It should be emphasized that over 90% of patients obtain complete relief of their symptoms with a structured nonoperative treatment regimen.[53]

Distal Biceps Tendon Avulsion

Avulsion of the distal biceps tendon is an uncommon injury, with 97% of biceps tendon ruptures occurring proximally.[5] Almost all cases in the literature have been in men with an average age at rupture being 50 years. Approximately 80% of ruptures occur in the dominant extremity, with bilateral cases being extremely rare.[10]

The mechanism of injury is sudden or prolonged contracture of the biceps against high-load resistance.[85] The elbow is usually flexed at 90°. The onset is sudden, although there may be a history of prodromal symptoms resulting from degenerative changes within the tendon. The tear usually occurs at the tendoosseous junction and notably leaves no stump tendon at the bicipital tuberosity.[91]

When rupture occurs, the patient usually experiences a popping or tearing sensation and presents with acute pain in the antecubital fossa. Clinical findings include tenderness, swelling, and mild-to-moderate ecchymosis in the antecubital region. The distal biceps tendon retracts proximally and is not palpable after a complete rupture. There is usually marked weakness of forearm supination and elbow flexion, although sometimes weakness may be mild because of the intact supinator and brachialis muscles. It is unusual to see radiographic evidence of avulsion fragments from the bicipital tuberosity. Partial distal biceps tendon ruptures are very rare and usually go on to complete rupture if not managed.[15]

Management of a ruptured distal biceps tendon in the athlete is surgical. The goal is to restore supination and flexion power to the elbow and forearm through anatomic repair of the tendon to the radial tuberosity. Nonoperative management can be expected to yield strength deficits of 30% in flexion and 40% in supination, whereas immediate repairs result in near normal strength.[81] Traditionally, the distal biceps tendon rupture is repaired primarily using the two-incision Boyd-Anderson technique.[16] This technique reduces the risk of radial nerve palsy. Others have reported successful repair through a single anterior extensile incision.[70,91]

After repair of the avulsed distal biceps tendon, the elbow is immobilized in 90° of flexion with a neutral or supinated forearm. A gradual range of motion and strengthening program is initiated 6 to 8 weeks after surgery. Unprotected heavy lifting should not be allowed for 6 months. Morrey has reported 97% flexion strength and 95% supination strength in patients with repairs performed within 2 weeks of injury.[85] The results of repair of chronic ruptures are not as satisfactory.

Distal Triceps Tendon Avulsion

Triceps tendon avulsion is a rare injury, perhaps the least common of all tendon ruptures.[5] Nearly 75% of the ruptures reported in the literature occurred in male subjects. The mean age at injury is 25 years, with a range of 7 to 72 years.[8] Dominant and nondominant extremities appear to be injured with equal frequency.

Most avulsions of the distal triceps tendon result from indirect trauma, usually a fall onto the outstretched upper extremity. This imparts a deceleration stress on an already contracted triceps, resulting in distal avulsion at the tendoosseous insertion.[39] The same mechanism of injury may result in olecranon fractures. The avulsed

tendon usually retracts with or without a piece of bone from proximal olecranon. Some of these injuries may result from a direct blow to the elbow. Additionally, spontaneous avulsion of the distal triceps tendon has been reported in patients with hyperparathyroidism, Marfan syndrome, systemic lupus erythematosus, and in those prescribed systemic steroids.[81]

On clinical examination, patients with a distal triceps tendon avulsion have pain and swelling at the posterior aspect of the elbow. A palpable depression just proximal to the olecranon may be noted. Ecchymosis is usually present several days after injury. Testing of elbow extension strength is important to determine whether the tear is partial or complete. Loss of active extension of the elbow signifies a complete tear of the triceps tendon.[39] Radiographs should be performed in all suspected cases. Avulsed flecks of bone from the olecranon have been demonstrated in approximately 83% of patients.[8,39,108]

Management of distal triceps tendon avulsion is surgical repair to restore extension strength. If full active elbow extension is demonstrated on physical examination, the injury is partial and can be followed without surgical repair.[39] For complete tears, the accepted method of repair is reattachment of the avulsed triceps tendon to the olecranon with nonabsorbable sutures through drill holes in bone.[39,108] If a large fragment of the olecranon is avulsed, open reduction and internal fixation are indicated. In cases of delayed reconstruction, an inverted tongue of triceps fascia can be used as a turned-down flap for repair.[48]

After surgery, the elbow is immobilized in 30° to 45° of flexion for 2 to 4 weeks before a graduated range of motion and strengthening program is begun. An extension night splint is used for the first 3 months after repair. Patients may return to active contact sports when maximum motion and extension strength have been obtained, usually at 6 months after surgery. Generally, excellent extension strength is restored after surgical repair.

OLECRANON BURSITIS

The function of the olecranon bursa is to allow the skin to glide freely over the bony prominence of the olecranon. It is a closed sac, lined by synovium, that is interposed between the skin and triceps tendon and olecranon process. The bursa does not communicate with the elbow joint, except in patients with rheumatoid arthritis.[105] The olecranon bursa is not present at birth and is first seen in children aged 7 to 10 years.[24] The size of the bursa increases with age until adulthood.

Traumatic olecranon bursitis is the most common condition affecting the olecranon bursa.[105] In the athlete, traumatic episodes may result in an acute inflammatory response. The bursal walls become thickened and edematous, and the bursal-lining cells produce excess fluid. If the trauma is severe enough to disrupt vessels, the bursa will contain frank blood. Repeated episodes of lesser trauma give rise to a chronic inflammatory process with persistent effusions.

Septic olecranon bursitis commonly occurs in athletes.[47] The source of infection may be from superficial skin breaks, which may seem innocuous. Other sources include coexisting dermatitis, acne lesions colonized with bacteria, or hematogenous sources. Trauma is the most frequently implicated predisposing factor. Steroid injections have also been found to precipitate septic bursitis. By far the most common infecting organism is *Staphylococcus aureus*, with β-hemolytic *Streptococcus* and other *Staphylococcus* species seen as well.[106]

The most common cause of olecranon bursitis is trauma, with the history of a single event or multiple lesser traumas to the tip of the elbow frequently found. Soft-tissue swelling is always present, and careful examination can determine whether the swelling is the thickened bursa, fluid within the bursa, or both. If the process is chronic, nodules consisting of fibrin can be felt within the bursa.[105] Radiographic evaluation may show soft-tissue swelling. Olecranon spurs or calcium deposits may be seen in older patients (Fig. 19-3).

The problem with evaluating olecranon bursitis occurs in the athlete who has a history of either acute or repetitive trauma with a tender, swollen olecranon bursa and overlying skin that is red, warm, and edematous. This is a common presentation in athletes, such as football players who play on artificial surfaces without elbow pads[65] or wrestlers who have mat trauma. The physician must determine whether this is an infectious process. Whenever septic bursitis is a possible diagnosis, sterile aspiration of the bursal fluid for analysis by Gram stain and culture is essential.

In most instances of traumatic olecranon bursitis, the bursa is enlarged, minimally tender, and nontense. Management is symptomatic with rest, ice, and compression. Nonsteroidal anti-inflammatory drugs may be of some benefit. If there is fluid in the bursa, it may be aspirated, and a compression dressing applied. It is not necessary to interrupt athletic participation. It is probably best to protect the bursa with an elbow pad.

In the acute traumatic event in which there is blood in the bursa and limited elbow range of motion, sterile aspiration to evacuate the blood followed by a compression dressing and frequent icing may decrease the chances of progression to chronic bursitis.[105] Blood or fluid may continue to reaccumulate, necessitating additional aspirations. Occasionally, instilling a small amount of corticosteroid after aspiration may minimize the inflammatory process.[65]

When the bursitis is chronic and disabling with inclusion bodies present, it is unlikely that resolution will occur without surgery. Surgery usually consists of complete bursal excision with a small portion of the underlying bone at the tip of the olecranon.[105] It is important to keep the skin flap as thick as possible and to avoid injuring the ulnar nerve. The elbow should be splinted in 45° to 60° of flexion for 10 days to allow wound healing. Range of motion exercises are begun, combined with bicep and tricep-strengthening exercises. Athletic participation can resume in 4 to 6 weeks. Elbow pads should be used until all tenderness has subsided.

When septic bursitis is suspected, fluid should be aspirated and cultures obtained. The elbow should be splinted, and frequent heat treatments instituted. If there are no systemic signs of infection and little cellulitis, oral broad-spectrum antibiotics are administered. If significant clinical improvement ensues over the next 2 to 3 days, the treatment is continued; if not, the bursa should be opened and drained, and intravenous antibiotics used.[47] The duration of antibiotic therapy has not been clearly delineated and is usually based on the clinical response of the patient. Return to athletics is attempted only after there is full resolution of all symptoms from the septic bursitis. If there is a recurrence, the bursa should be excised completely.

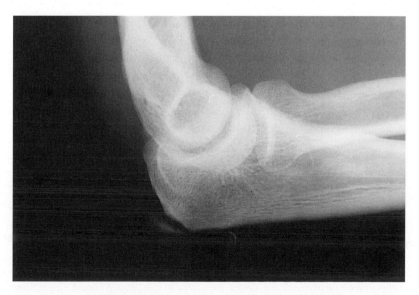

Fig. 19-3. Olecranon spur causing olecranon bursitis.

THROWING INJURIES

Biomechanics and Pathophysiology

The pitching motion, which is seen in many sports, can be broken down into different phases to facilitate a better understanding of the motion (Fig. 19-4). The terms *wind-up, early cocking, late cocking, arm acceleration, arm deceleration,* and *follow-through* are used to delineate the phases in the analysis of throwing. With the use of video and electromyography analysis, the kinetics and kinematics of throwing can be determined. The elbow is flexed at about 85° during the wind-up and cocking phases. It is then rapidly extended during early acceleration until ball release. Forces acting on the elbow include valgus torque and tensioning of the medial elbow structures, reaching a maximum at late cocking; extension torque during acceleration; and flexion and varus torque after ball release.[34]

Injury to the elbow usually occurs during the acceleration phase of throwing. At late cocking, a large forward force is generated by the shoulder musculature to bring the upper arm forward and create acceleration. Because the forearm and hand lag behind, a considerable valgus force is generated at the elbow, with peak angular velocities reaching more than 4500° per second.[96] These large forces are absorbed by the supporting structures on the medial side of the elbow. If the forces generated exceed the tensile strength of the ulnar collateral ligament, microtears will occur. If throwing continues in the presence of injury, attenuation and eventual rupture of the ligament will result. At the same time, considerable compression forces are placed on the lateral side of the elbow. This force is primarily absorbed by the cartilaginous

surfaces of the radial head and the capitellum, leading to microfractures, osteochondritis dissecans, and loose body formation.[29]

As acceleration of the arm continues, the triceps forcefully contract and the elbow rapidly extends as the thrown object is released. Normally, this force is absorbed by the anterior capsular structures and bicep and brachialis muscles. If the elbow is slightly subluxated in a valgus position, because of insufficiency of the ulnar collateral ligament, impaction of the posterior medial olecranon in the olecranon fossa results as extension occurs.[114] Over time, this impaction can lead to chondromalacia and osteophyte formation, producing pain during the follow-through phase of throwing. Pitching-related injuries to the elbow can be classified as medial tension overload, lateral compression, and extensor overload.

Medial Tension Injuries

Medial tension injuries result from repetitive dynamic stress during the late cocking and acceleration phases of throwing, with injury to the ulnar collateral ligament, flexor–pronator muscle group, and the ulnar nerve most common.[42] Symptoms occur predominantly in baseball pitchers but are also observed in other sports. Pain is usually observed during forced extension and valgus strain during the acceleration phase. The pitcher is usually effective for two or three innings and then suffers a gradual loss of control, especially early release, which causes him or her to throw high. Often, a pitcher compensates by snapping the elbow in an attempt to gain speed, but this snapping usually causes further loss of

Biomechanics

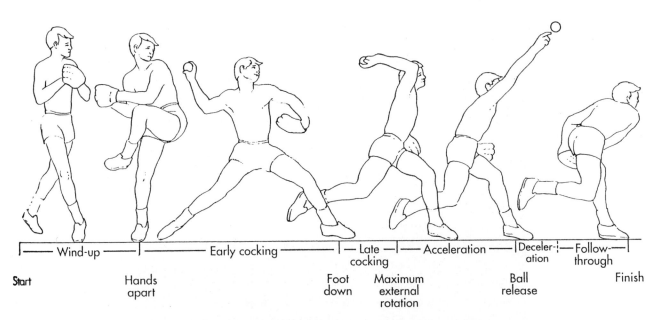

Fig. 19-4. Illustration of the six phases of pitching. From DiGiovine NM, Jobe FW, Pink M, et al: An electromyographic analysis of the upper extremity in pitching. *J Should Elbow Surg* 1:15-25, 1992.

control. Pain is localized to the medial aspect of the elbow and the olecranon process. In addition to examining the elbow, careful attention should be paid to the flexibility of the shoulder. Restricted shoulder range of motion alters the normal throwing mechanics and places increased valgus stress on the elbow, resulting in medial elbow pain.[78]

Valgus stress testing of the elbow is performed by placing the patient's hand against the side of the examiner's body, with the elbow held at 30° of flexion to relax the bony restraints. The examiner uses one hand to apply valgus stress to the patient's elbow while the other hand palpates the medial side of the elbow. The examination is done with the patient supine and repeated with the patient prone to allow direct visualization of the medial side of the elbow.

Routine anteroposterior and lateral radiographs of the elbow should be obtained to check for evidence of loose bodies, bone spurs, or calcification of the ulnar collateral ligament. Valgus stress radiographs can be obtained to further document valgus subluxation, but a normal stress view does not rule out the diagnosis. Magnetic resonance imaging and computed tomography also have been used in the evaluation of medial tension injuries, but their application in this setting is not yet defined.

The anterior oblique band of the ulnar collateral ligament is the most important stabilizing structure of the elbow-resisting valgus force, absorbing up to 55% of the valgus load to the flexed elbow.[82] Patients who present with problems referable to the ulnar collateral ligament often have had recurrent pain and tenderness for months along the medial aspect of the elbow. In some patients, a sudden valgus stress that exceeds the tensile strength of the ligament can cause an acute rupture of the ligament. This rupture is associated with sharp pain, swelling, and ecchymosis at the medial aspect of the elbow. More commonly, a slow deterioration in function of the elbow occurs, accompanied by increasing pain and loss of control. Instability to valgus stress testing is present in all patients. Radiographs are used to rule out loose bodies and other bony pathology. Occasionally, a calcified ulnar collateral ligament is seen in patients with chronic symptoms.[55]

Management for most patients with ulnar collateral ligament injuries is nonoperative (PRICEMM). After the acute symptoms resolve, range of motion exercises are begun. The athlete may resume a throwing program after complete resolution of pain and restoration of motion. Progressive velocity and endurance are allowed with careful supervision. Patients who continue to have ongoing pain or cannot throw effectively after 6 months of this management are candidates for operative intervention. Options include ligament repair or reconstruction.

For acute ligament ruptures, direct repair may be considered by suturing the torn ligament directly to the bone or through drill holes.[92] Patients are then splinted for 10 days and placed in a single axis elbow brace, allowing flexion and extension but preventing valgus stress. Results of this management indicate that 50% of patients can return to their previous level of athletic participation.

Ulnar collateral ligament reconstruction has been recommended in the acute and chronic setting. Jobe[55] advocates use of a free tendon graft of palmaris longus, plantaris, or lateral Achilles tendon. In this technique, the free tendon graft is passed through drill holes in the medial epicondyle and ulna at the anatomic sites of ligament attachment. This provides a functional substitute for the anterior bundle of the ulnar collateral ligament. The ulnar nerve is protected during this procedure and transposed anteriorly at closure. After initial immobilization, patients are begun on active range of motion exercises with a hinged brace. Strengthening begins within 4 to 6 weeks, and a throwing program is initiated after 4 months. In Jobe's initial experience, 11 of the 16 major league baseball players who had a reconstruction returned to play major league baseball.

Ulnar collateral ligament reconstruction is the current recommended procedure for athletes who wish to remain at a highly competitive level of participation.[55] For less-competitive athletes, reconstruction may not be indicated because valgus instability of the elbow appears to cause little disability in activities of daily living.[63] Good functional results have been reported in patients treated nonoperatively.[57]

The flexor–pronator musculature provides dynamic support for the static stabilizing structures on the medial side of the elbow. This muscle group also flexes the wrist and pronates the forearm during throwing. Continued activity beyond the limits of fatigue can result in injury to the muscle and ulnar collateral ligament complex. Rupture of the flexor–pronator group has been reported in throwing athletes.[92]

Injury to the flexor–pronator muscle group is associated with pain and swelling along the medial aspect of the elbow and is exacerbated by extending the wrist and elbow. Minor injuries usually persist for 24 to 48 hours and may be relieved by ice, rest, and nonsteroidal anti-inflammatory medications. More severe injuries can lead to scarring and fibrosis, with resultant loss of elbow or wrist extension.

Occasionally, patients with ulnar collateral ligament insufficiency demonstrate ulnar neuritis. Ulnar neuritis may result from three etiologic factors: traction, friction, or compression.[41] Traction injuries are believed to occur secondary to valgus stress loading during pitching. Compression injuries result from impingement secondary to adhesions, calcification in the soft tissues, osteophytes, or hypertrophy of the flexor muscles of the forearm. Friction injury may occur in the subluxating nerve, which is abraded across the medial epicondyle as the elbow is rapidly flexed and extended during the normal act of pitching. A Tinel sign may be present as 40% of patients with ulnar collateral ligament insufficiency develop ulnar neuritis. Examination usually reveals tenderness along the course of the nerve at the elbow and motor and sensory changes along the distribution of the nerve. Electromyography may be helpful in confirmation of the diagnosis. Submuscular transposition of the nerve is recommended if nonoperative management fails to alleviate the symptoms.

Lateral Compression Injuries— Osteochondritis Dissecans

Lateral compression injuries occur in the throwing elbow as a result of the compression forces in the lateral compartment during the late cocking and acceleration phases and as a result of shearing forces during the deceleration phase of throwing.[61] This condition is usually seen in adolescents as traumatic osteochondritis dissecans of the radiohumeral joint. Osteochondritis dissecans may lead to debilitating osteoarthritis of the lateral elbow in the adult.

In the adult thrower, significant lateral compartment changes are rarely seen because of the debilitating nature of osteochondritis dissecans. Significant injuries of this type usually end careers before the onset of adulthood. Although the exact etiology of osteochondritis dissecans is unknown, the current theory is that it is a lesion resulting from vascular insufficiency caused by repetitive trauma.[12] The capitellar epiphyseal blood supply is tenuous, with end arterioles terminating at the subchondral plate. Repetitive valgus overload results in trauma to this vulnerable epiphysis, causing differing degrees of disruption of the vascular supply and resultant bone death and fragmentation. This lesion has also been found in a young gymnast.[7]

The typical clinical scenario of osteochondritis dissecans is a throwing athlete in the second decade of life, complaining of insidious onset of lateral elbow pain, reduced throwing effectiveness and distance, a flexion contracture of more than 15°, and occasional swelling, catching, or locking. Results of early radiographs may be normal, although, with time, islands of subchondral bone demarcated by a surrounding rarefied zone can be seen, and frequently loose bodies will be present. Computed tomography and magnetic resonance imaging are often helpful in defining the extent of the lesion.

Management of osteochondritis dissecans of the radiocapitellar joint is based on whether the overlying cartilage is intact.[12] This can be determined by arthrotomy, computed tomography arthrography, or arthroscopy if plain films do not show free fragments. If the overlying cartilage is intact, management is immobilization until most pain has resolved and then begin active range of motion exercises without applying any forceful stresses across the elbow. Although symptoms will usually subside with rest alone, throwing is contraindicated for at least 6 months because the healing process is slow. Once full range of motion, strength, and endurance have been achieved, gradual return to throwing is allowed if the patient remains asymptomatic. Sequential radiographs are used to follow the evolution of the lesion, although in many instances radiographic abnormalities persist.

If pain and flexion contracture persist for more than 6 weeks after immobilization or if loose bodies and fragmentation are present, surgery is recommended. O'Driscoll[93] has reported excellent results using arthroscopy to remove loose bodies caused by osteochondritis dissecans and to débride flaps of articular cartilage. Indelicato[52] recommends reattaching large fragments with screws, wires, or biodegradable pins after drilling the bed to enhance vascularity. Smaller fragments are removed. Although patients reported subjective improvement, normal motion was rare.

In the adult, valgus stresses in the face of an incompetent ulnar collateral ligament result in a radiocapitellar overload syndrome.[104] This repetitive increased force leads to radial head abutment against the capitellum, resulting in chondromalacia and eventual degeneration. Osteochondral fractures and loose body formation eventually result. Patients complain of pain, catching, clicking, or locking of the elbow. Patients may have palpable loose bodies and crepitus with motion. Management consisted of removal of loose bodies, either arthroscopically or open. Loose bodies usually recur if the athlete resumes throwing, especially if valgus laxity persists.

Extension Overload Injuries

A combination of valgus and extension forces in the acceleration and deceleration phases of throwing results in chronic changes of the posterior compartment of the elbow.[78] Loose bodies causing catching, locking, and restricted range of motion are the most common lesions of the posterior compartment of the elbow. Inflammatory lesions resulting from triceps tendinitis are also seen. The valgus–extension overload syndrome is a common final pathway for most posterior elbow problems.

As repetitive valgus forces lead to attenuation of the ulnar collateral ligament, posteromedial olecranon impingement occurs within the olecranon fossa.[114] The tip of the olecranon abuts against the olecranon fossa and causes local inflammation, and if inflammation persists, eventually chondromalacia, osteophytes, and loose bodies form (Fig. 19-5). Pain is typically experienced in the posterior compartment during the acceleration phase of throwing. Loss of control and early ball release secondary to pain usually occur after two to three innings. Symptoms are reproduced with forced extension and valgus strain to the elbow. An axial radiographic view with the elbow flexed may reveal posteromedial osteophytes on the olecranon.

Management for the early phases of the valgus–extension overload syndrome include nonsteroidal anti-inflammatory drugs and strengthening of the flexor–pronator muscle group to protect the joint. When posteromedial osteophytes or loose bodies are present, physical therapy is not curative.[114] Arthroscopy can be used to remove loose bodies and burr down osteophytes. Arthrotomy has traditionally been used with good results.[52] Open excision of the tip and medial aspect of the olecranon is performed and any loose bodies are removed. This will allow most throwers to return to their previous level of activity. The problem may recur because of the associated laxity of the ulnar collateral ligament, but the osteophytes usually take years to reform.

Stress fracture of the olecranon is an uncommon source of pain in the throwing athlete. It usually occurs at the tip of the olecranon and results from the repetitive snap of full extension.[110] If symptoms do not resolve with nonoperative treatment (PRICEMM), management should consist of excising the tip fragment or internally fixing the olecranon if the fragment is large.

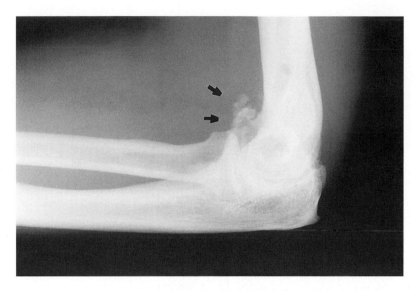

Fig. 19-5. Loose bodies in elbow joint.

NEUROPATHIES

Entrapment neuropathies of the elbow and forearm involve three major nerves (median, radial, and ulnar) that cross the elbow to innervate the musculature and provide sensation to the forearm and hand. In the athlete, most of these conditions follow direct contusion of the tissues that overlie peripheral nerves in vulnerable anatomic areas. Vigorous, repetitive athletic activity that produces inflammation and tissue-swelling can also lead to nerve compression, especially in closed passages or tunnels. The pathophysiology of entrapment neuropathy involves ionic, mechanical, and vascular injury. Obstruction of venous return from the nerve secondary to inflammation initially may cause venous congestion in the vascular plexuses, resulting in anoxia and dilatation of the small vessels in the nerve.[99] Endoneurial edema ensues, increasing the effect of the initial compression, which further slows venous return. With anoxia, fibroblasts proliferate within the nerve, resulting in permanent scarring, which further inhibits nerve circulation.

When a portion of the axon is rendered ischemic, the axioplasmic transport system is also affected.[37] The integrity of the cell membrane is disrupted, and the efficiency of the sodium pump decreases. This decrease eventually leads to a loss of conduction and transmission along the nerve fiber. The segment of the axon rendered ischemic through local external or internal compression reacts by vascular mechanisms and by ionic disruption to further deteriorate nerve function. Although most entrapment neuropathies partially, if not completely, resolve after decompression, in some chronic situations, nerve dysfunction may be irreversible.

Median Nerve Entrapment— Pronator Syndrome

In the arm, the median nerve is intimately related to the brachial artery, first lying lateral to it. At the elbow, the median nerve crosses the artery anteriorly and comes to lie medially in the antecubital fossa. At the elbow, the median nerve leaves the brachial artery to pass between the two heads of the pronator teres muscle and beneath the tendinous arch of the flexor digitorum superficialis. The nerve passes distally into the forearm between the flexor digitorum superficialis and the flexor digitorum profundus muscles.

There are four sites of potential compression (Fig. 19-6), all of which may produce signs and symptoms of pronator syndrome.[37] The first of these is compression of the median nerve at the distal third of the humerus beneath the supracondyloid process at the ligament of Struthers. A second site of potential compression occurs at the lacertus fibrosis, which passes from the bicipital tendon to the flexor muscle mass and courses across the median nerve at the level of the elbow joint. A third site of potential compression is within the hypertrophied pronator teres muscle or between its two heads. Finally, the median nerve can be compressed at the tendinous arch of the flexor digitorum superficialis muscle, which is a firm and sharp-free border beneath which the nerve passes. Occasionally, an abnormal fibrous band may extend from either head of the pronator teres to the tendinous arch and become an additional source of compression.

Pronator syndrome presents with pain in the proximal volar surface of the forearm that generally increases with activity. The symptoms are often vague, with a fatigue-like pain described by many patients. Repetitive, strenuous motions often provoke the symptoms, which usually develop insidiously. In addition, there may be reduced sensibility or paresthesias in the radial three and a half digits of the hand. The absence of these neurologic findings does not preclude this condition.[21]

On examination, patients with pronator syndrome have aggravation of their symptoms with resisted pronation of their forearm.[99] Direct pressure over the proximal portion of the pronator teres, approximately 4 cm distal to the antebrachial crease, while exerting moderate resis-

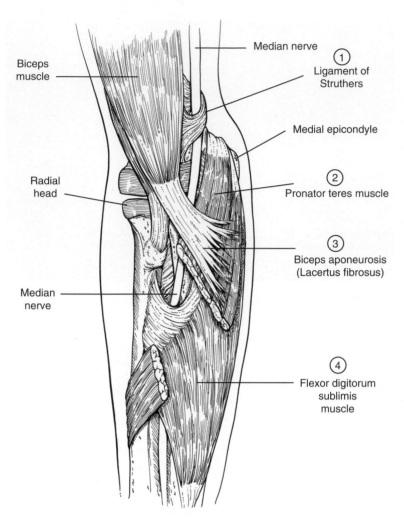

Biceps muscle

Radial head

Median nerve

Median nerve

① Ligament of Struthers

Medial epicondyle

② Pronator teres muscle

③ Biceps aponeurosis (Lacertus fibrosus)

④ Flexor digitorum sublimis muscle

Fig. 19-6. Four sites of potential compression of the median nerve that may produce median nerve entrapment in the elbow and forearm.

tance to pronation may be a more reliable test. If the ligament of Struthers is the site of compression, flexion of the elbow against resistance between 120° and 135° of flexion may aggravate the symptoms. If the arch of the flexor digitorum superficialis is involved in compression, resisted flexion of the superficialis muscle of the middle finger or passive stretching of the finger and wrist flexors may elicit symptoms. A Tinel sign is usually present at the site of compression.

Distal neurovascular function is generally intact, although a careful motor examination is important to distinguish pronator syndrome from anterior interosseous nerve compression. This branch of the median nerve is exclusively motor and controls the flexor digitorum profundus of the index finger, the flexor pollicis longus, and the pronator quadratus muscles. A characteristic posture of pinch is noted with compression of the anterior interosseous branch of the median nerve.[99] This posture consists of hyperextension of the distal interphalangeal joint of the index finger and hyperextension of the interphalangeal joint of the thumb as one attempts a pinch. Electromyography and nerve conduction studies have had

disappointing results in diagnosing pronator syndrome and in differentiating the various sites of compression of the median nerve.[21] Therefore, clinical history and physical examination are the mainstays for accurate diagnosis.

Management of median nerve entrapment should be nonoperative for at least 6 weeks. The regimen should consist of splinting and nonsteroidal anti-inflammatory drugs with curtailment of all weight-lifting activities. Surgical decompression is reserved for severe or refractory cases. The operative management for pronator syndrome consists of a detailed exploration of the median nerve in the proximal forearm.[37] If a supracondyloid process (found in 1% of the general population) is present, it should be explored, and the ligament of Struthers released. The median nerve is then followed distally to the lacertus fibrosis, which should be routinely divided. The nerve is then traced as it enters the forearm between the two heads of the pronator teres muscle. The superficial head is elevated and divided along the course of its fibers to decompress and explore the median nerve. The flexor digitorum superficialis arch is incised, completing the distal extent of exploration for pronator syndrome. Further dissection distally may be necessary to decompress the anterior interosseous branch of the nerve. After surgery, the patient is splinted in neutral rotation for a few days. Active range of motion exercises are begun within 1 week, with restricted pronation for 3 weeks.

Radial Nerve Entrapment—
Radial Tunnel Syndrome

Compression neuropathies of the radial nerve occur in predictable areas along the course of the nerve.[38] The radial nerve pierces the lateral intermuscular septum to proceed from the posterior to anterior compartment of the humerus. The septum is a common cause of nerve compression, especially during open reduction and internal fixation of humerus fractures. As the nerve proceeds to the level of the radiocapitellar joint, it divides into its major branches: the posterior interosseous and superficial radial nerves. At this level, the nerve enters the radial tunnel, which is situated between the brachioradialis and brachialis in the distal arm to the distal edge of the supinator in the forearm. In the radial tunnel, the posterior interosseous nerve passes between the two heads of the supinator muscle, the proximal edge of which is called the arcade of Frohse. The superficial radial nerve passes superficial to the supinator muscle and is covered anteriorly by the brachioradialis muscle.

There are four sites of compression within the radial tunnel (Fig. 19-7). The first site consists of fibrous bands lying anterior to the radial head at the entrance to the radial tunnel. The second site occurs at a fan-shaped group of vessels called the leash of Henry, which lies across the radial nerve and supplies the brachioradialis and extensor carpi radialis longus muscles. The third site of potential compression occurs at the tendinous margin of the extensor carpi radialis brevis near the supinator muscle. The fourth site of compression is the most common and occurs as the radial nerve enters the supinator muscle through the arcade of Frohse.

Athletes presenting with radial tunnel syndrome have often performed repetitive rotatory movements of the forearm in conjunction with their sport, such as tennis.[69] Most people with this syndrome are manual laborers performing pronation and supination movements. The patient usually complains of pain well localized to the extensor mass just below the elbow and that is aching in character. Forearm pronation, often with wrist flexion, intensifies the pain. Night pain and pain after physical exertion are also seen. Differentiation between radial tunnel syndrome and lateral epicondylitis may be

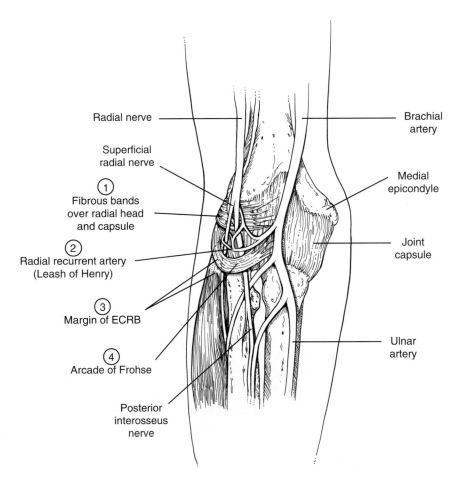

Fig. 19-7. Four sites of potential compression of the radial nerve at the elbow causing radial nerve entrapment.

difficult but can be determined by careful physical examination.[69]

Examination of the patient with radial tunnel syndrome reveals three pathognomonic signs.[102] First, tenderness to palpation is most severe over the radial nerve palpated through the mobile wad muscle mass just distal to the radial head. Pain can occasionally be localized down into the forearm. Second, resisted extension of the middle finger with the elbow extended produces pain at the site of tenderness. This pain results from compression by a fascial extension from the extensor carpi radialis brevis. The third sign is pain on resisted supination of the extended forearm. This pain is distinguished from pain localized to the lateral epicondyle. Electromyography findings are unreliable, and a normal electrophysiologic finding does not exclude the diagnosis of radial tunnel syndrome.[99] In the athlete suspected of having radial tunnel syndrome, diagnostic blocks with small amounts of lidocaine, 1%, can be administered at various points along the radial nerve. If pain is relieved and accompanied by a deep radial nerve palsy and a complementary injection more proximal in the region of the lateral epicondyle does not relieve the patient's symptoms, the diagnosis of radial tunnel syndrome is made.

In the acute stage, radial tunnel syndrome should be managed with rest, splinting, and nonsteroidal anti-inflammatory drugs for at least 2 months. Surgery is reserved for refractory cases not responding to conservative management. The radial tunnel can be decompressed through an anterolateral approach.[99] In this way, the radial nerve can be evaluated from above the elbow through the radial tunnel to the distal end of the supinator. The leash of vessels are ligated, and the fibrous margin of the extensor carpi radialis brevis over the radial nerve should be incised. The dissection continues to the arcade of Frohse, where the deep branch of the radial nerve dives into the substance of the supinator muscle. Division of the supinator muscle allows visualization of the radial nerve to its point of arborization. After surgery, the patient is immobilized for 1 week and then begun on range of motion exercises. A strengthening program is begun after restoration of motion. If the nerve has been damaged, recovery may take 3 to 4 months.

Ulnar Nerve Entrapment— Cubital Tunnel Syndrome

Ulnar neuropathy at the elbow can be related to a number of etiologic factors. Most commonly in the athlete, the ulnar nerve is compressed or stretched at the elbow or proximal forearm.[99] The nerve is particularly vulnerable as it passes subcutaneously under a thick band of fascia around the medial epicondyle and in the area where it passes between the two heads of the flexor carpi ulnaris muscle. The majority of athletic events that result in cubital tunnel syndrome involve throwing or racquet sports.[54]

The ulnar nerve passes from the anterior to posterior compartment of the arm by penetrating through a fibrous thickening called the ligament of Struthers, located approximately 8 cm above the medial epicondyle (Fig. 19-8). The ligament of Struthers is the most proximal source of ulnar nerve entrapment. The ulnar nerve then courses posteriorly to the medial epicondyle and enters the cubital tunnel. The roof of the tunnel is

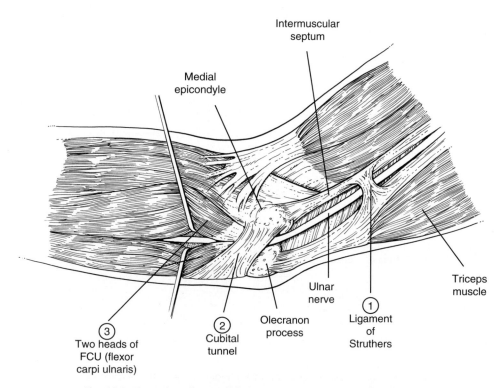

Fig. 19-8. Three sites of potential ulnar nerve entrapment at the elbow.

formed by a ligament that extends from the medial epicondyle to the medial border of the olecranon process. The remaining boundaries of the tunnel are the ulnar collateral ligament, the medial edge of the trochlea, and the medial epicondylar groove. After exiting the cubital tunnel, the ulnar nerve continues into the forearm between the two heads of the flexor carpi ulnaris muscle.

The ulnar nerve is a mobile structure, elongating and moving medially during elbow flexion.[6] Therefore, tethering of the nerve by scar tissue interferes with its mobility and adversely affects its function. Additionally, during flexion, the volume of the cubital tunnel is reduced because of changes in surrounding ligaments.[113]

The pathophysiology of ulnar neuritis in the throwing athlete usually involves a traction injury caused by a cubitus valgus deformity.[54] The considerable tension forces generated on the medial side of the elbow increase the possibility of a traction neuritis. Hypermobility of the ulnar nerve, secondary to either congenital or developmental laxity of soft tissue constraints, may cause subluxation or dislocation of the nerve anterior to the medial epicondyle.[25] This subluxation or dislocation will result in a friction neuritis, which appears to affect baseball pitchers more than any other athlete. Compression secondary to hypertrophy of the confluence of the flexor carpi ulnaris heads can also occur in baseball pitchers.[45] Ischemic changes may occur in the ulnar nerve with marked elbow flexion and wrist extension. Intraneural pressure may increase up to six times by causing physiologic stretch of the nerve and additional external compression.[97]

The clinical findings of ulnar neuritis at the elbow involve pain at the medial side of the proximal forearm, which may radiate proximally or distally. This pain may be accompanied by paresthesias, dysesthesias, or anesthesia in the ring and middle fingers. These findings usually precede any detectable motor weakness of the hand.[99] Muscle wasting of the ulnar intrinsic muscles of the hand is a late finding, but not uncommon. Clumsiness or heaviness of the hand and fingers, especially after pitching a few innings, may be a primary complaint. The athlete with a subluxating or dislocating ulnar nerve may complain of a painful snapping or popping sensation when the elbow is rapidly flexed and extended, with sharp pain radiating into the forearm and hand.[25]

An important localizing physical finding on examination is a positive Tinel sign on percussion of the nerve at the elbow.[38] The ulnar nerve may also be manually subluxated or dislocated from the ulnar groove.[25] The nerve may feel thickened and be tender to palpation. The elbow flexion test may increase or incite symptoms of ulnar nerve compression at the elbow.[22] Both elbows are fully flexed with full extension of the wrists to maximize compressive and tensile forces on the nerve. Patients note numbness and tingling throughout the distribution of the ulnar nerve. The rapid onset and resolution of symptoms make this a useful and reliable test for cubital tunnel syndrome.

Radiographs should be taken to rule out bone spurs or intraarticular abnormality, which may cause impingement of the ulnar nerve. Electrodiagnostic studies may aid in diagnosis; nerve conduction velocities reduced by more than 33% across the elbow suggest cubital tunnel syndrome.[99] Other anatomic areas of ulnar nerve compression, such as cervical ribs and Guyon's canal, must also be ruled out by careful history and examination.[54]

Nonoperative management of ulnar neuritis consists of minimizing the pressure increases that occur about the ulnar nerve with elbow flexion or direct contact.[32] The pressure is minimized by the use of elbow pads and splinting the elbow at 90°. Icing the area may prevent edema and subsequent inflammation that may result in scarring. Approximately 50% of patients with mild ulnar neuritis can expect to recover with this management. In patients whose symptoms are unrelieved after 4 to 6 weeks or who have evidence of motor weakness, intrinsic atrophy, or significant loss of sensation, surgical decompression of the ulnar nerve may be necessary.

There are four basic operative procedures that are performed for ulnar neuropathy at the elbow. They are simple decompression, subcutaneous anterior transposition, submuscular anterior transposition, and medial epicondylectomy.

Decompression of the ulnar nerve is a simple procedure applicable only if there is localized compression of the nerve by the aponeurosis between the heads of the flexor carpi ulnaris.[40] This compression can be seen at surgery by an indentation in the nerve and prestenotic swelling at the site of compression. If any other abnormality is noted, one of the other procedures should be performed.

Anterior transposition of the nerve is the most common procedure performed for cubital tunnel syndrome.[67] The advantage of this procedure is that all pathology is correctable because the nerve is transposed anterior to the medial epicondyle. The nerve is first identified proximally at the level of the ligament of Struthers. Any nerve entrapment is identified and decompressed. The ulnar nerve is traced distally behind the medial epicondyle, where it is released from its tunnel. The aponeurosis and heads of the flexor carpi ulnaris are divided to complete the decompression. The nerve is then elevated from its bed and transposed anteriorly. The nerve can be left in a subcutaneous position or placed in a submuscular position after elevating the flexor muscles from the medial epicondyle. The flexor origin is next reattached to the epicondyle. After surgery, patients are placed in a splint for 7 to 10 days, after which they are gently mobilized. When the nerve is transposed submuscularly, strengthening is begun after 3 to 4 weeks to allow for adequate tissue healing. The submuscular position affords greater protection of the nerve, and excellent results are achieved with this technique in more than 80% of patients.[32] This technique also has the lowest recurrence rate.

Medial epicondylectomy has been used in the past with fair results.[62] The ulnar nerve is not exposed and, therefore, is at minimal risk of damage. The theory behind this technique is that tension on the nerve as it passes behind the medial epicondyle is removed after excision. This removal of tension will allow the nerve to slide forward and seek its optimum position and tension.

Potential disadvantages include missing additional sites of compression, creating new sources of compression as the nerve slides anteriorly, and disrupting the origin of the flexor muscle mass. This procedure is rarely performed today for ulnar neuritis.

ELBOW DISLOCATION

Elbow dislocation in the athlete is not a common injury, having an incidence of 0.1% of all athletic injuries.[30] The mechanism of injury is usually a posterolateral rotatory directed force with a fall on the outstretched hand. O'Driscoll et al[95] have suggested that extension and a varus stress can disrupt the lateral collateral ligament complex, allowing a perched dislocation. Further forces rotate the forearm and allow a complete dislocation. Others have suggested that with hyperextension, the olecranon impinges on the olecranon fossa, thus levering the ulna and radius from their capsular and ligamentous constraints.[87]

Elbow dislocations can be classified according to the position of the olecranon in reference to the distal humerus. Posterior dislocations (direct, medial, or lateral) are the most common (Fig. 19-9). Anterior dislocations are rare and can occur in young patients, in whom hyperextension allows the olecranon to slide under the trochlea.[13] Divergent dislocations also are rare and require tearing of the interosseous membrane, annular ligament, and distal radioulnar joint capsule.[31]

When complete elbow dislocation occurs, the medial collateral ligament complex is usually disrupted.[95] The anterior capsule and brachialis muscle are also torn or significantly stretched. Others have suggested that the lateral collateral ligament structures must also be disrupted.[57] The most common injuries associated with complete elbow dislocation include radial head and neck fractures (10%), avulsion of the medial or lateral epicondyles (12%), and coronoid fractures (10%).[79] Neurovascular injuries, although uncommon, are potentially devastating. The brachial artery can be injured during dislocation or relocation.[1] The median nerve may become entrapped in the joint after elbow reduction.[98] Injuries to the ulnar nerve and occasionally to the radial nerve may occur.

Although elbow dislocations may be diagnosed clinically, swelling often obscures the bony landmarks about the elbow. Radiographic examination is essential to make the diagnosis of elbow dislocation and to assess associated fractures. The radiographs will also define the type and direction of dislocation. Assessment of the extremity for neurovascular injury is mandatory before reduction.

The goal of management of any elbow dislocation is the restoration of articular alignment as expeditiously and atraumatically as possible. Although an elbow dislocation can often be reduced without any anesthetic, if several hours have elapsed and soft-tissue swelling and spasm have occurred, a general or regional anesthetic may be necessary to minimize the required force. Multiple attempts at reduction should be avoided because the potential to create additional soft tissue and muscle trauma will increase, thus predisposing to ectopic bone.[109]

Several techniques have been described for reduction of the dislocated elbow. The most predictable technique is that of gentle traction applied to the extended forearm with countertraction on the humerus.[46] The olecranon is then manipulated distally and anteriorly until the coronoid clears the trochlea of the humerus. Residual medial or lateral displacement can be corrected, followed by gentle flexion of the forearm. The reduction is often appreciated by a palpable and occasionally audible "clunk." In the anterior dislocation, one has to flex the elbow to unlock the olecranon from the front of the humerus. Divergent dislocations need separate reductions of each bone. After a manuever is performed, reduction is confirmed by radiographs and clinical examination. The elbow should be ranged from full extension

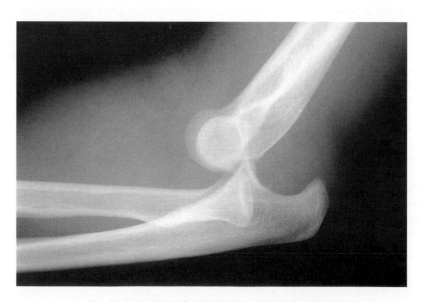

Fig. 19-9. Radiograph of posterior elbow dislocation.

to full flexion to ensure that no block to motion exists and to document any instability in the plane of motion. After a posterior dislocation, instability usually occurs in extension. In addition, the elbow should be subjected to varus and valgus stress in full extension and moderate flexion to check for instability.

Irreducible elbow dislocations are uncommon. They are usually seen with associated fractures[33] or resulting from buttonholing through muscle or fascia.[43] Rarely, a bone fragment or avulsed medial epicondyle may become interposed in the joint, preventing complete reduction. Irreducible dislocations, incomplete reductions, and chronic dislocations usually require open reduction. Brachial artery and median nerve injuries after reduction attempts may require open reduction and exploration if function does not promptly return.

After reduction of simple elbow dislocations, careful evaluation of the neurovascular status is necessary for 24 to 48 hours. The elbow should be splinted in a safe zone (at least 90° of flexion) for 7 to 10 days, after which active range of motion exercises are begun. A hinged brace with a controlled extension block should be used in patients demonstrating instability on examination. This brace will protect the collateral ligaments and prevent subluxation on extension. After 3 weeks, the extension block can be decreased, and full range of motion can be obtained in 6 to 8 weeks.

In uncomplicated cases, 50% of patients will have a normal range of motion.[58] Some will develop a flexion contracture of up to 15°, especially if they are immoblized longer than 3 weeks. In dislocations with associated injuries, the results are much poorer, with flexion contractures more than 30° being common.[58] Complications after elbow dislocation include recurrent instability, stiffness, myositis ossificans, and neurovascular dysfunction.

For the athlete, a devastating complication is recurrent elbow instability. Although uncommon, it is more likely when the initial dislocation occurs in children or adolescents.[115] Although recurrent dislocation is an obvious diagnosis, recurrent subluxation may be more subtle. O'Driscoll et al[94] have described the examination technique, which is analogous to the pivot shift test of the knee, used to diagnose recurrent instability of the elbow. The elbow is extended with valgus stress and then supinated, causing the radial head to roll below the capitellum and the ulna to externally rotate on the trochlea. With elbow flexion and pronation, a clunk is felt as the elbow reduces. The deficiency allowing this instability is believed to result from an incompetent lateral ulnar collateral ligament.[94] Others have postulated that an attenuated medial collateral ligament or failure of the anterior capsule to heal may lead to recurrent elbow instability.[115] O'Driscoll et al[94] recommend reconstructing the lateral ulnar collateral ligament with a tendon graft to manage recurrent elbow instability.

Residual stiffness tends to increase with associated injuries, prolonged immobilization, and formation of heterotopic ossification. Some have investigated loss of motion and correlated it with the type of dislocation. Josefsson et al[58] thought that loss of motion was greater with lateral or posterolateral dislocations and that motion loss was greater in adults than in children. An extension turnbuckle splint is used to treat these patients, although results are unpredictable. Occasionally, open capsular releases are required to regain motion in severe cases.

Ectopic bone is frequently seen with elbow fracture–dislocations. Innocuous ectopic calcification, which occurs in ligaments or capsule, must be distinguished from true myositis ossificans, which can be a devastating complication. Myositis ossificans is associated with multiple attempts at reduction or may occur after surgical intervention.[109] It usually causes pain, swelling, and severely restricted range of motion. Seventy percent of patients with myositis ossificans show some improvement with nonoperative treatment.[109] The remainder of patients may require surgery to remove the painful, persistent mass. Surgery is performed only after the lesion is mature, at least 6 months after the injury.[103] A bone scan may be used to distinguish between the active (immature) lesion and the inactive (mature) lesion. Additionally, the sedimentation rate and alkaline phosphatase activity should be normal when the lesion is mature. Patients should be treated with indomethacin after surgery for 3 to 6 months to retard new bone formation, which recurs in two thirds of patients.[101]

Vascular injury is uncommon after elbow dislocation. The brachial artery is vulnerable to injury and must be assessed carefully before and after reduction. A pulseless distal extremity may result from vascular disruption or spasm. An arteriogram can differentiate between disruption, intimal tear, and spasm.[1] Surgical repair is usually required for complete vascular compromise. Collateral circulation around the elbow may provide the extremity with adequate blood supply, eliminating the need for surgical intervention. Compartment syndrome after elbow dislocation has been reported within the first 24 to 48 hours and must not be overlooked after elbow reduction.[68] Neurologic injuries may occur in up to 20% of elbow dislocations.[68] These are primarily traction injuries to the ulnar nerve caused by valgus stretch or mechanical compression of the median nerve either before or after closed reduction. Rarely, the radial nerve is injured. Neurologic injuries may take 3 to 6 months to resolve completely. If the ulnar and median nerves are both injured, it is likely the brachial artery is injured.

FRACTURES OF THE ELBOW AND FOREARM

Fractures of the elbow and forearm that result from participation in sports are classified the same way as fractures in any posttraumatic injury. The majority of these fractures result from direct trauma, but occasionally may occur from indirect activities, such as a fall on an outstretched arm or twisting motion to the elbow. Basic principles of management include adequate immobilization, elevation, and icing of the affected extremity. Radiographic evaluation includes anteroposterior and lateral views visualizing the joints above and below the injury, comparison views of the contralateral extremity (especially in the pediatric population), and additional tests such as oblique radiographs, tomograms, computed tomography, and magnetic resonance imaging if deemed necessary for diagnosis. It is extremely important to obtain anatomic restoration of the osseous structures involved to prevent limitation of motion and function. Stable fixation of fractures is important to allow early motion and use of the extremity. Most serious injuries about the elbow leave a residual flexion deformity, usually ranging between 5° and 15°, despite meticulous management and early range of motion. Although this is acceptable for normal activities of daily living, this limitation can be career-ending for an athlete requiring full flexion and extension of the elbow. Detailed classification and management of various fractures about the elbow and forearm are covered in many orthopedic fracture textbooks. In the following section, common fractures of the elbow and forearm and their management will be briefly discussed.

Distal Humerus Fractures

Because of the complex anatomy of these fractures, they are very difficult to manage. These injuries have a propensity for posttraumatic and postoperative stiffness. One third of all fractures about the elbow involve the distal humerus and most commonly occur in children aged 5 to 10 years.[59] Many classifications exist based on anatomy and fracture pattern. Broadly, these fractures can be classified as extracapsular (epicondylar fractures), supracondylar, and intraarticular (unicondylar, bicondylar, capitellum, and trochlea fractures).

Epicondylar fractures are all extracapsular, with medial epicondyle fractures more common than lateral epicondyle fractures. These injuries are rare in adults. Medial epicondyle fractures occur in young throwing athletes, who subject their elbows to high valgus stresses.[11] The fractures can be acute (undisplaced or displaced) or chronic (little leaguer's elbow). In adults, these injuries may result from direct trauma.[11] Medial epicondyle fractures may occur secondary to elbow dislocation and may spontaneously reduce on relocation.[50] The acceptable amount of displacement for medial epicondyle fractures is 2 to 3 mm, with some authors recommending up to 1 cm.[50] Management for undisplaced or minimally displaced fractures is immobilization for 10 days with the elbow flexed to 90° and the forearm pronated and wrist flexed to reduce flexor pull. Displaced or incarcerated fragments can be reduced manually or managed with open reduction and internal fixation. Early motion is mandatory to avoid stiffness. There is a high incidence of ulnar nerve symptoms with medial epicondyle fractures.[20]

Fractures of the lateral epicondyle are very rare and are secondary to varus stress at the elbow or a direct blow.[20] Most are managed by immobilizing the elbow at 90° of flexion with the forearm supinated and wrist extended to minimize the extensor pull. They rarely need open reduction and internal fixation.

Supracondylar fractures are the second-most common fracture in children aged 5 to 10 years.[59] The fractures occur during a fall on the outstretched hand with a flexed elbow and, therefore, are usually of an exten-

sion pattern. These injuries can be associated with injuries to the brachial artery and median, radial, or ulnar nerves.[50] A careful neurovascular examination is mandatory before and after reduction. Management involves closed reduction if possible. This reduction is done by extending the forearm, applying traction, and then flexing the joint to lock the distal fragment onto the end of the humerus. The arm is immobilized in flexion with careful monitoring of the neurovascular status. Other modes of management include traction, closed reduction and percutaneous pinning, and open reduction and internal fixation for very unstable fractures. Complications include neurovascular injury and malalignment. Displaced supracondylar fractures in adults usually require open reduction and internal fixation.

Medial and lateral condyle fractures account for 5% of all distal humerus fractures.[20] Lateral condyle fractures are more common than medial condyle fractures. These fractures can be divided into two types based on whether the lateral wall of the trochlea remains attached to the humerus (type I) or attached to the fracture fragment (type II).[76] These fractures usually result from falling on an outstretched hand with a varus or valgus force to the elbow.[50] Collateral ligament injuries may be associated with these fractures.[59] The neurovascular status of the extremity must be evaluated before reduction. Although these injuries are intraarticular, closed management has been advocated in the past.[77] If successfully reduced, these fractures must be immobilized for 4 to 6 weeks. More recently, open reduction and internal fixation has been advocated, even for minimally displaced fractures.[20] This will allow early mobilization of the elbow and quicker return of function. In the event reduction cannot be achieved, overhead traction can be considered. Complications of these fractures and their management include malunion, nonunion, avascular necrosis, cubitus varus or valgus deformity, and restricted range of motion.

Bicondylar fractures are the most common type of distal humerus fracture in the adult.[20] The injury occurs when the olecranon acts as a wedge driven into the trochlea, forcing the fracture proximally into the humerus.[50] The elbow must be flexed more than 90° for a bicondylar fracture to be produced.[51] If the elbow is flexed less than 90°, an olecranon fracture will result instead. Up to 50% of these fractures are open injuries. Many classifications exist based on fracture pattern, separation of fragments, and comminution. Closed reduction and casting has lost popularity because of the very high incidence of stiffness.[59] Traction followed by immobilization has been advocated by some.[64] "Bag of bones" treatment has been used for highly comminuted fractures in elderly, osteopenic patients by placing the elbow in a sling and instituting early mobilization.[19] Currently, open reduction and internal fixation is ideally advocated, using either a transolecranon or triceps-splitting approach.[50] After surgery, these patients are mobilized as soon as possible. Complications include delayed union, nonunion, ankylosis, myositis ossificans, and ulnar neuritis.[20,59]

Capitellum fractures account for 6% of all distal humerus fractures.[20] They are associated with radial head fractures and posterior elbow dislocations. The mechanism of injury is a shear force in the coronal plane displacing the capitellum from the lateral condyle of the humerus.[50] These fractures are classified as two types: type I (Hahn-Steinthal) is a complete fracture of the capitellum, and type II (Kocher-Lorenz) is a shear fracture of the articular surface shell with a thin layer of subchondral bone. Diagnosis of these fractures can be difficult, with lateral radiographs being particularly helpful. Sometimes a positive fat pad sign on a radiograph is the only clue to a fracture.[20] Management of type I fractures is open reduction and internal fixation through a lateral approach if the fragment is displaced.[50] In most cases of type II fractures, excision of the fragments is necessary because fixation is difficult.[50] In all cases, early postoperative motion is necessary for successful outcome. Complications include loss of motion, especially when fragments have been excised; avascular necrosis of the capitellum; and nonunion.[20,59] Avascular necrosis and nonunion may require delayed excision.

Isolated fractures of the trochlea are rare.[50] Small fragments should be excised, and early range of motion instituted. For larger fragments, open reduction and internal fixation is necessary. Care must be taken to prevent injury to the ulnar nerve during operative exposure.

Radial Head Fractures

Approximately 20% of all elbow trauma and 33% of elbow fractures involve fractures of the radial head.[80] Ten percent are associated with elbow dislocations, and 10% of elbow dislocations have associated radial head fractures. Fifteen percent to 20% of radial head fractures involve the radial neck, especially in children. Fractures of the radial head are most frequently caused by direct longitudinal loading, usually from a fall on the outstretched hand.[50] This effect is compounded with valgus stresses. Radial head fractures may be associated with injury to the ulnar collateral ligament complex resulting from the valgus stress. Any injury that causes an elbow dislocation may also cause a radial head fracture.

The most widely used classification of radial head fractures (Fig. 19-10) is that of Mason:[73] type I are undisplaced; type II are displaced; type III are comminuted; and type IV[56] are any of the previous associated with an elbow dislocation. Distal radioulnar joint injuries are important to identify in association with radial head fractures because excision of the radial head may allow proximal subluxation of the radius, resulting in wrist pathology. This is called the Essex-Lopresti lesion.[36]

Anteroposterior and lateral view radiographs are usually sufficient to diagnose a radial head fracture. Occasionally, a radiocapitellar view or tomography is necessary to delineate the fracture.[50] Aspiration of the hemarthrosis and injection of lidocaine, 1%, will allow a complete examination of the elbow to assess if there is a mechanical block to motion.[59] If the patient has pain on the medial aspect of the elbow as well, ulnar collateral ligament injury must be suspected. Pain at the wrist is suspicious for associated distal radioulnar joint injury.

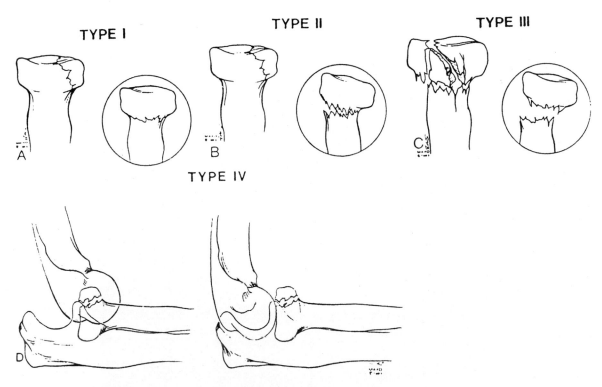

Fig. 19-10. Mason classification of radial head fractures. From Morrey BF: Radial head fractures. In Morrey BF, ed: *The elbow and its disorders*, Philadelphia, 1985, WB Saunders.

Management options vary for the type of fracture and the associated injuries. For undisplaced type I fractures, hematoma may be aspirated to reduce the pain and swelling.[49] This is therapeutic and diagnostic to decide if there is blockage to motion. Patients are treated with a sling for comfort, and early motion is begun. Ninety percent will do well, but 10% will lose some motion, especially extension.

Management of type II fractures depends on the stability of the fracture pattern. If stable, early motion should be attempted. If unstable and surgery is not elected, immobilization should be maintained for 2 to 3 weeks. If surgery is elected and the fragment is small, excision of the fragment may be performed. If the fragment involves more than 30% of the radial head or is displaced more than 3 mm, open reduction and internal fixation or radial head excision proximal to the annular ligament may be performed.[80]

Type III fractures are usually managed with radial head excision.[80] In patients with proximal migration of the radius resulting from concomitant distal radioulnar joint injury, preservation of the radial head is important. If the radial head is excised, consideration should be given to inserting a silicone radial head prosthesis to act as a spacer, although this is not predictable in preventing proximal translation of the radius.[71]

In type IV fractures, management consists primarily of reducing the elbow dislocation and then dealing with the radial head fracture. Because the radial head is a secondary stabilizer of the elbow to valgus stress, excision may lead to gross instability of the elbow because of the injured medial collateral ligament complex.[50] If the radial head is excised, a silicone prosthesis may be inserted to act as a buttress. The elbow should be protected in a hinged orthosis with an extension stop. This orthosis allows early motion but protects against valgus stress and recurrent dislocation during capsular healing. Flexion contractures of 15° to 30° and reduced rotation of 25° to 50° are not uncommon. Delayed excision of the radial head may be performed to improve pain and motion.[18]

Olecranon Fractures

Fractures of the olecranon (Fig. 19-11) occur in response to three main types of injury.[50] Direct trauma resulting from a fall on the point of the elbow or a direct blow to the olecranon often results in a comminuted fracture. Indirect trauma, such as a fall on the outstretched hand with the elbow flexed accompanied by a strong contraction of the triceps, can result in an oblique or transverse fracture through the olecranon. Finally, a combination of direct and indirect forces may act to produce displaced, comminuted fractures. In cases of extreme violence, a fracture–dislocation may occur.

All fractures of the olecranon have an intraarticular component. Inability to extend the elbow actively against gravity is the most important sign to be elicited on examination. This inability indicates the discontinuity of the triceps mechanism. The presence or absence of this sign determines management for these fractures. Ulnar nerve injuries may accompany this fracture.[50] Anteroposterior and particularly lateral radiographs are necessary to evaluate the extent of these fractures.

Olecranon fractures can be classified as undisplaced (<2 mm, no separation on flexion, and able to extend against gravity) or displaced.[26] Displaced fractures can be further divided into avulsion fractures, oblique and transverse fractures, comminuted fractures, and fracture–dislocations. Management is based on this classification.

Undisplaced fractures are best managed by immobilization in a long-arm cast with the elbow in 45° to 90° of flexion.[23] The cast can be removed after 3 weeks to allow protected range of motion exercises, avoiding flexion past 90° until union is complete at 6 to 8 weeks. Displaced fractures require open reduction and internal fixation or primary excision.[50] The goals of surgery are to maintain extension power of the elbow, to avoid incon-

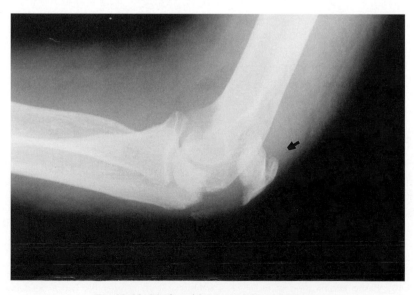

Fig. 19-11. Displaced fracture of the olecranon.

gruity of the articular surface, to restore stability of the elbow, and to prevent stiffness of the joint. For transverse and stable oblique fractures, tension band wiring or intramedullary fixation is the preferred management.[23] Comminuted and other unstable fractures can be managed with neutralization plates and screws. Excision of the proximal fragment and repair of the triceps tendon to the remaining olecranon can be used for tip avulsion fractures or comminuted fractures in osteoporotic patients.[50] Up to 80% of the olecranon can be removed without producing instability of the elbow joint.[74]

A complication after olecranon fracture is loss of motion in 50% of patients.[35] Posttraumatic arthritis develops in 20% to 30% of patients, especially in the event of articular cartilage damage and bone loss, and nonunion occurs in 5% of olecranon fractures. Treatment of young, active patients with a nonunion should be open reduction and internal fixation with bone grafting at the fracture site. Excision of the ununited proximal fragment with reattachment of the triceps is performed in older patients.[50]

Coronoid Process Fractures

Coronoid process fractures occur in 2% to 10% of elbow dislocations.[59] There are three types: type I is a tip avulsion; type II involves less than 50% of the coronoid, and type III involves more than 50% of the coronoid.[100] All may be associated with other fractures of the elbow. Management addresses the fracture and the dislocation. After the dislocation is reduced, type I fractures can be managed like a simple dislocation with early range of motion. Types II and III are similarly managed if the elbow is stable. If the elbow is unstable, type II and type III coronoid fractures may require open reduction and internal fixation.[59]

Fractures of the Shafts of the Radius and Ulna

The radius and ulna are relatively parallel bones articulating proximally and distally. The ulna acts as a fixed strut around which the bowed radius rotates in pronation and supination.[3] Between the two shafts lies the interosseous membrane that separates the two compartments of the forearm and provides for longitudinal support of the radius if the radial head is resected.[3] If satisfactory functional results are to be achieved in the management of fractures of the forearm, length, axial alignment, rotational alignment, and normal radial bow must be restored. Therefore, open reduction and internal fixation are recommended for most displaced diaphyseal fractures of the forearm in adults.[60]

Fracture of the radius and ulna, or "both bones fracture," usually results from some type of direct blow to the forearm.[3] Occasionally, a fall on the outstretched arm will cause a fracture to both bones. These fractures are almost always displaced because of the extreme force necessary to break both bones. Patients with this injury have pain, deformity, and loss of function of the forearm and hand. Soft-tissue damage and swelling always accompanies this fracture. Compartment syndrome and neurovascular damage is occasionally seen and should be ruled out in all cases.[3] Anteroposterior and lateral radio-graphs will show the pattern of fracture and the degree of comminution. Elbow and wrist films are necessary to assess associated injuries. Management of undisplaced fractures of the radius and ulna, although rare, is cast immobilization with frequent radiographic follow-up evaluations to check for displacement.[3] Displaced fractures in children can be treated with closed reduction and casting, but this injury in adults is usually managed by open reduction and internal fixation with plates and screws or intramedullary nails. Bone grafting may be necessary in cases with significant comminution. Most studies examining compression plating of "both bones" forearm fractures report union rates of more than 95%, with excellent functional results.[4] Plates may be removed 18 months after healing, but the extremity should be protected for 6 weeks with a splint to prevent fracture through a screw hole. Complications of open reduction and internal fixation of forearm fractures include nonunion, malunion, neurovascular injury, compartment syndrome, and synostosis.

Fracture of the ulna alone, or "nightstick fracture," is fairly common and results from a direct blow to the ulna.[3] Injury to the proximal and distal radioulnar joints must be ruled out. Undisplaced fractures can be managed with a long-arm cast or functional brace with frequent radiographic evaluation to assess displacement. Displaced fractures (>10° of angulation or more than 50% translation) should be managed with open reduction and internal fixation with compression plating.[60]

A Monteggia fracture is a fracture of the proximal third of the ulna, with an associated dislocation of the radial head.[3] The most common type is anterior dislocation, but posterior and lateral dislocations are also seen. The mechanism of injury varies depending on the type of lesion and direction of dislocation. A fall on the outstretched hand with the forearm in pronation or a direct blow to the posterior aspect of the elbow may result in a Monteggia fracture.[3] The forearm externally rotates, and the ulna acts as a fulcrum to dislocate the radial head anteriorly. A posterior radial head dislocation may be caused by supination rotational forces, and a lateral dislocation may result from a direct blow to the inner aspect of the elbow.[3] Frequently, the posterior interosseous nerve is injured in a Monteggia fracture.[17] Anteroposterior and lateral radiographs are mandatory to avoid missing the radial head injury. Treatment differs depending on the patient's age. In children, Monteggia fractures can successfully be managed by closed reduction and cast immobilization.[9] In adults, closed reduction of the radial head and open reduction and internal fixation of the ulna fracture is the management of choice.[3] Positioning of the elbow and forearm is important after surgery. In cases of anterior and lateral radial head dislocations, the elbow should be held in 110° of flexion with the forearm in supination for 6 weeks to prevent redislocation of the radial head.[3] When the radial head has dislocated posteriorly, the elbow should be maintained in 70° of flexion with the forearm pronated for 6 weeks.[3] Complications of Monteggia fractures include nonunion, malunion, posterior interosseous nerve palsy, and redislocation of the radial head.[3]

Isolated fractures of the radius usually occur in the proximal two-thirds of the shaft and are not common. Most injuries severe enough to fracture the radius at this level will also fracture the ulna.[3] When this fracture is undisplaced, the forearm should be immobilized in a long-arm cast in supination. Radiographs should be taken frequently because this fracture tends to displace. Displaced fractures can be managed with compression plating or intramedullary nail fixation with care to maintain the normal radial bow.

A Galeazzi fracture (Fig. 19-12) is a solitary fracture of the radius at the junction of the middle and distal thirds and is associated with a dislocation or subluxation of the distal radioulnar joint.[60] The injury to the radioulnar joint may be purely ligamentous, or the ulnar styloid may be avulsed. The mechanism of injury is a direct blow to the dorsolateral side of the wrist or a fall on the outstretched hand combined with pronation of the forearm.[75] There is usually prominence of the head of the ulna, with tenderness over the distal radioulnar joint. Neurovascular damage is rare. Optimal results are obtained by compression plating of the radius fracture anteriorly.[60] Anatomic fixation of the radius will usually result in reduction of the distal radioulnar joint. If this joint is still subluxed, closed reduction and percutaneous pinning may be performed. After surgery, patients should be splinted in supination for 6 weeks. The most common complication of a Galeazzi fracture is angula-

tion of the fracture and subluxation or dislocation of the distal radioulnar joint.[3]

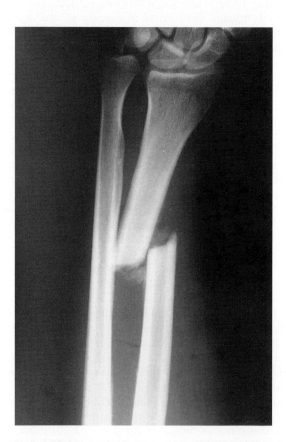

Fig. 19-12. Radiograph of a fracture at the junction of the middle and distal thirds of the radius associated with subluxation of the distal radioulnar joint (Galeazzi fracture).

REFERENCES

1. Amsallem JL, Blankstein A, Bass A, Horoszowski H: Brachial artery injury: a complication of posterior elbow dislocation, *Orthop Rev* 15:61–64, 1986.
2. An KN, Morrey BF, Chao EYS: Carrying angle of the human elbow joint, *J Orthop Res* 1:369–378, 1984.
3. Anderson LD, Meyer FN: Fractures of the shafts of the radius and ulna. In Rockwood CA, Green DP, Bucholz RW, eds: Fractures in adults, New York, 1991, JB Lippincott.
4. Anderson LD, Sisk TD, Tooms RE, Park WI: Compression plate fixation in acute diaphyseal fractures of the radius and ulna, *J Bone Joint Surg* 57A:287–297, 1975.
5. Anzel SH, Covey KW, Weiner AD, Lipscomb PR: Disruption of muscles and tendons: an analysis of 1014 cases, *Surgery* 45:406–412, 1959.
6. Apfelberg PB, Larson SJ: Dynamic anatomy of the ulnar nerve at the elbow, *Plast Reconstr Surg* 51:76–81, 1973.
7. Aronen JG: Problems of the upper extremity in gymnastics, *Clin Sports Med* 4:61–71, 1985.
8. Bach BR, Warren RF, Wickiewicz TL: Triceps rupture: a case report and literature review, *Am J Sports Med* 15:285–289, 1987.
9. Bado JL: The Monteggia lesion, *Clin Orthop* 50:71–86, 1967.
10. Baker BE, Bierwagen D: Rupture of the distal tendon of the biceps brachii: operative vs. non–operative treatment, *J Bone Joint Surg* 67A:414–417, 1985.
11. Bernstein SM, King JD, Sanderson RA: Fractures of the medial epicondyles of the humerus, *Contemp Orthop* 3:637–642, 1981.
12. Bianco AJ: Osteochondritis dissecans. In: Morrey BF, ed: *The elbow and its disorders*, Philadelphia, 1985, WB Saunders.
13. Blatz DJ: Anterior dislocation of the elbow. Findings in a case of Ehlers–Danlos syndrome, *Orthop Rev* 10:129, 1981.
14. Boone DC, Azen SP: Normal range of motion of joints in male subjects, *J Bone Joint Surg* 61A:756–759, 1979.
15. Bourne MH, Morrey BF: Partial rupture of the distal biceps tendon, *Clin Orthop* 271:143–148, 1991.
16. Boyd HB, Anderson LD: A method for reinsertion of the distal biceps brachii tendon, *J Bone Joint Surg* 43A:1041–1043, 1961.
17. Boyd HB, Boals JC: The Monteggia lesion. A review of 159 cases, *Clin Orthop* 66:94–100, 1969.
18. Broberg MA, Morrey BF: Results of delayed excision of the radial head after fracture, *J Bone Joint Surg* 68A:669–674, 1986.
19. Brown RF, Morgan RG: Intercondylar T–shaped fractures of the humerus, *J Bone Joint Surg* 53B:425–428, 1971.
20. Bryan RS, Morrey BF: Fractures of the distal humerus. In Morrey BF, ed: *The elbow and its disorders*, Philadelphia, 1985, WB Saunders.
21. Buchthal F, Rosenfalck A, Trojaborg W: Electrophysiological findings in entrapment of the median nerve to wrist and elbow, *J Neurol Neurosurg Psychiatry* 37:340, 1974.
22. Buehler MJ, Thayer DT: The elbow flexion test—a clinical test for cubital tunnel syndrome, *Clin Orthop* 233:213, 1988.
23. Cabanela ME: Fractures of the proximal ulna and olecranon. In Morrey BF, ed: *The elbow and its disorders*, Philadelphia, 1985, WB Saunders.
24. Chen J, Alk D, Eventov I, Weintroub S: Development of the olecranon bursa: an anatomic cadaveric study, *Acta Orthop Scand* 58:408–409, 1987.

25. Childress HM: Recurrent ulnar nerve dislocation at the elbow, *Clin Orthop* 180:168–173, 1975.

26. Colton CL: Fractures of the olecranon in adults: classification and management, *Injury* 5:121–129, 1973.

27. Coonrad RW: Tendinopathies at the elbow, *Instruct Course Lect* 40:25–32, 1991.

28. Coonrad RW: Tennis elbow, *Instruct Course Lect* 35:94–101, 1986.

29. DeHaven KE, Evarts CM: Throwing injuries of the elbow in athletes, *Orthop Clin North Am* 4:801–808, 1973.

30. DeHaven KE, Lintner DM: Athletic injuries: comparison by age, sport, and gender, *Am J Sports Med* 14:218–224, 1986.

31. DeLee JC: Transverse divergent dislocation of the elbow in a child, *J Bone Joint Surg* 63A:322, 1981.

32. Dellon AL: Review of treatment results for ulnar nerve entrapment at the elbow, *J Hand Surg* 11:199–205, 1986.

33. Devadoss A: Irreducible posterior dislocation of the elbow, *Br Med J* 3:659, 1967.

34. DiGiovine NM, Jobe FW, Pink M, Perry J: An electromyographic analysis of the upper extremity in pitching, *J Should Elbow Surg* 1:15–25, 1992.

35. Eriksson E, Sahlen O, Sandahl U: Late results of conservative and surgical treatment of fracture of the olecranon, *Acta Chir Scand* 113:153–166, 1957.

36. Essex–Lopresti P: Fractures of the radial head with distal radial–ulnar dislocations, *J Bone Joint Surg* 33B:244–247, 1951.

37. Eversmann WW: Compression entrapment neuropathies of the upper extremity, *J Hand Surg* 8:759–766, 1983.

38. Eversmann WW: Entrapment and compression neuropathies. In Green DP, ed: *Operative hand surgery*, New York, 1988, Churchill Livingstone.

39. Farrar EC, Lippert FG: Avulsion of the triceps tendon, *Clin Orthop* 161:242–246, 1981.

40. Feindel W, Stratford J: The role of the cubital tunnel in tardy ulnar nerve palsy, *Can J Surg* 1:287–300, 1958.

41. Glousman RE: Ulnar nerve problems in the athlete's elbow, *Clin Sports Med* 9:365–377, 1990.

42. Glousman RE, Barron J, Jobe FW, Perry J, Pink M: An electromyographic analysis of the elbow in normal and injured pitchers with medial collateral ligament insufficiency, *Am J Sports Med* 20:311–317, 1992.

43. Greiss M, Messias R: Irreducible posterolateral elbow dislocation: a case report, *Acta Orthop Scand* 58:421–422, 1987.

44. Groppel JL, Nirschl RP: A mechanical and electromyographical analysis of the effects of various joint counterforce braces on the tennis player, *Am J Sports Med* 14:195–200, 1986.

45. Hang Y: Tardy ulnar neuritis in a little league baseball pitcher, *Am J Sports Med* 9:244–246, 1981.

46. Hankin FM: Posterior dislocation of the elbow: a simplified method of closed reduction, *Clin Orthop* 190:254–256, 1985.

47. Ho G, Tice AD, Kaplan SR: Septic bursitis in the prepatellar and olecranon bursae, *Ann Intern Med* 89:21–27, 1978.

48. Holder SF, Grana WA: Complete triceps tendon avulsion, *Orthopedics* 9:1581–1582, 1986.

49. Holdsworth BJ, Clement DA, Rothwell PN: Fractures of the radial head—the benefit of aspiration: a prospective controlled trial, *Injury* 18:44–47, 1987.

50. Hotchkiss RN, Green DP: Fractures and dislocations of the elbow. In Rockwood CA, Green DP, Bucholz RW, eds: *Fractures in adults*, New York, 1991, JB Lippincott.

51. Hurley JA: Complicated elbow fractures in athletes, *Clin Sports Med* 9:39–57, 1990.

52. Indelicato PA, Jobe FW, Kerlan RK, Carter VS, Shields CL, Lombardo SJ: Correctable elbow lesions in professional baseball players, *Am J Sports Med* 7:72, 1979.

53. Jobe FW, Ciccotti MG: Lateral and medial epicondylitis of the elbow, *J Am Acad Orthop Surg* 2:1–8, 1994.

54. Jobe FW, Fanton GS: Nerve injuries. In Morrey BF, ed: *The elbow and its disorders*, Philadelphia, 1985, WB Saunders.

55. Jobe FW, Stark H, Lombardo SJ: Reconstruction of the ulnar collateral ligament in athletes, *J Bone Joint Surg* 68A:1158–1163, 1986.

56. Johnston GW: A follow-up of one hundred cases of fracture of the radial head with a review of the literature, *Ulster Med J* 31:51–56, 1962.

57. Josefsson PO, Gentz CP, Johnell O, Wendeberg B: Surgical vs. non–surgical treatment of ligamentous injuries following dislocation of the elbow joint: a prospective randomized study, *J Bone Joint Surg* 89A:605–608, 1987.

58. Josefsson PO, Johnell O, Gentz CP: Long-term sequelae of simple dislocation of the elbow, *J Bone Joint Surg* 66A:927–930, 1984.

59. Jupiter JB, Mehne DK: Trauma to the adult elbow and fractures of the distal humerus, In Browner BD, Jupiter JB, Levine AM, eds: *Skeletal trauma*, Philadelphia, 1992, WB Saunders.

60. Kellam JF, Jupiter JB: Diaphyseal fractures of the forearm, In Browner BD, Jupiter JB, Levine AM, eds: *Skeletal trauma*, Philadelphia, 1992, WB Saunders.

61. King JW, Brelsford HJ, Tullos HS: Analysis of the pitching arm of the professional baseball pitcher, *Clin Orthop* 67:116–123, 1969.

62. King T, Morgan FP: Late results of removing the medial humeral condyle for traumatic ulnar neuritis, *J Bone Joint Surg* 41B:51–55, 1959.

63. Kuroda S, Sakamaki K: Ulnar collateral ligament tears of the elbow joint, *Clin Orthop* 218:266–271, 1986.

64. Lansinger O, Mare K: Intercondylar T fractures of the humerus in adults, *Acta Orthop Traumatol Surg* 100:37, 1982.

65. Larson R, Osternig LR: Traumatic bursitis and artificial turf, *Am J Sports Med* 2:183–188, 1974.

66. Leach RE, Miller JK: Lateral and medial epicondylitis of the elbow, *Clin Sports Med* 6:259–272, 1987.

67. Leffert RD: Anterior submuscular transposition of the ulnar nerve by the Learmonth technique, *J Hand Surg* 7:147–155, 1982.

68. Linscheid RL: Elbow dislocations. In Morrey BF, ed: *The elbow and its disorders*, Philadelphia, 1985, WB Saunders.

69. Lister GD, Belsole RB, Kleinert HE: The radial tunnel syndrome, *J Hand Surg* 4:52–59, 1979.

70. Louis DS, Hankin FM, Eckinrode JF, Smith PA, Wojtys EM: Distal biceps bracchi tendon avulsion: a simplified method of operative repair, *Am J Sports Med* 14:234–236, 1986.

71. Mackay I, Fitzgerald B, Miller JH: Silastic replacement of the head of the radius in trauma, *J Bone Joint Surg* 61B:494–497, 1979.

72. Major HP: Lawn-tennis elbow, *BMJ* 2:557, 1883.

73. Mason ML: Some observations on fractures of the head of the radius with a review of one hundred cases, *Br J Surg* 42:123–132, 1954.

74. McKeever FM, Buck RM: Fracture of the olecranon process of the ulna, *JAMA* 135:1–5, 1947.

75. Mikic ZD: Galeazzi fracture dislocations, *J Bone Joint Surg* 57A:1071–1080, 1975.

76. Milch H: Fractures of the external humeral condyle, *JAMA* 160:529–539, 1956.

77. Milch H: Fractures and fracture dislocations of the humeral condyles, *J Trauma* 4:592–607, 1964.

78. Miller CD, Savoie FH: Valgus extension injuries of the elbow in the throwing athlete, *J Am Acad Orthop Surg* 2:261–269, 1994.

79. Morrey BF: Elbow dislocation in the athlete. In DeLee JC, Drez D, eds: *Orthopaedic sports medicine*, Philadelphia, 1994, WB Saunders.

80. Morrey BF: Radial head fracture. In Morrey BF, ed: *The elbow and its disorders*, Philadelphia, 1985, WB Saunders.

81. Morrey BF: Tendon injuries about the elbow. In Morrey BF, ed: *The elbow and its disorders*, Philadelphia, 1985, WB Saunders.

82. Morrey BF, An KN: Articular and ligamentous contributions to the stability of the elbow joint, *Am J Sports Med* 11:315–319, 1983.

83. Morrey BF, An KN: Functional anatomy of the ligaments of the elbow, *Clin Orthop* 201:84–90, 1985.

84. Morrey BF, Askew LJ, An KN, Chao EYS: A biomechanical study of normal elbow motion, *J Bone Joint Surg* 63A:872–877, 1981.

85. Morrey BF, Askew LJ, An KN, Dobyns JH: Rupture of the distal tendon of the biceps brachii: a biomechanical study, *J Bone Joint Surg* 67A:418–421, 1985.

86. Morrey BF, Regan WD: Tendinopathies about the elbow. In DeLee JC, Drez D, eds: *Orthopaedic sports medicine*, Philadelphia, 1994, WB Saunders.

87. Neviaser JS, Wickstrom JK: Dislocations of the elbow: a retrospective study of 115 patients, *South Med J* 70:172–173, 1977.

88. Nirschl RP: Muscle and tendon trauma: tennis elbow. In Morrey BF, ed: *The elbow and its disorders*, Philadelphia, 1985, WB Saunders.

89. Nirschl RP: Tennis elbow, *Orthop Clin North Am* 4:787–800, 1973.

90. Nirschl RP, Pettrone FA: Tennis elbow—the surgical treatment of lateral epicondylitis, *J Bone Joint Surg* 61A:832–839, 1979.

91. Norman WH: Repair of avulsion of insertion of biceps brachii tendon, *Clin Orthop* 193:189–194, 1985.

92. Norwood LA, Shook JA, Andrews JR: Acute medial elbow ruptures, *Am J Sports Med* 9:16–19, 1981.

93. O'Driscoll SW: Arthroscopy of the elbow, *J Bone Joint Surg* 74A:84–94, 1992.

94. O'Driscoll SW, Bell DF, Morrey BF: Posterolateral rotatory instability of the elbow, *J Bone Joint Surg* 73A:440–446, 1991.

95. O'Driscoll SW, Morrey BF, An KN: Elbow dislocation and subluxation: a spectrum of instability, *Clin Orthop* 280:186, 1992.

96. Pappas AM, Zawacki RM, Sullivan TJ: Biomechanics of baseball pitching: a preliminary report, *Am J Sports Med* 13:216–222, 1985.

97. Pechan J, Julius I: The pressure measurement in the ulnar nerve: a contribution to the pathophysiology of the cubital tunnel syndrome, *J Biomech* 8:75–79, 1975.

98. Pritchard DJ, Linscheid RL, Svien HJ: Intra–articular median nerve entrapment with dislocation of the elbow, *Clin Orthop* 90:100–103, 1973.

99. Regan WD, Morrey BF: Entrapment neuropathies about the elbow. In DeLee JC, Drez D, eds: *Orthopaedic sports medicine*, Philadelphia, 1994, WB Saunders.

100. Regan WD, Morrey BF: Fractures of the coronoid process of the ulna, *J Bone Joint Surg* 71A:1348–1354, 1989.

101. Ritter ME, Gioe TJ: The effect of indomethicin on para-articular ectopic ossification following total hip arthroplasty, *Clin Orthop* 167:113, 1982.

102. Ritts ED, Wood MB, Linscheid RL: Radial tunnel syndrome: a ten year surgical experience, *Clin Orthop* 279:201–205, 1987.

103. Roberts JB, Pankratz DG: The surgical treatment of heterotopic ossification of the elbow following long-term coma, *J Bone Joint Surg* 61:760–763, 1979.

104. Safran MR: Elbow injuries in athletes: a review, *Clin Orthop* 310:257–277, 1995.

105. Singer KM, Butters KP: Olecranon bursitis. In DeLee JC, Drez D, eds: *Orthopaedic sports medicine*, Philadelphia, 1994, WB Saunders.

106. Soderquist B, Hedstrom SA: Predisposing factors, bacteriology, and antibiotic therapy in 35 cases of septic bursitis, *Scand J Infect Dis* 18:305–311, 1986.

107. Sojbjerg JO, Ovesen J, Nielsen S: Experimental elbow instability after transection of the medial collateral ligament, *Clin Orthop* 218:186–190, 1987.

108. Tarsney FF: Rupture and avulsion of the triceps, *Clin Orthop* 83:177–183, 1972.

109. Thompson HC, Garcia A: Myositis ossificans: aftermath of elbow injuries, *Clin Orthop* 50:129–134, 1967.

110. Tullos HS, Erwin WD, Woods GW, Wukasch DC, Cooley DA, King JW: Unusual lesions of the pitching arm, *Clin Orthop* 88:169, 1972.

111. Tullos HS, Schwab G, Bennett JB, Woods GW: Factors influencing elbow instability, *Instruct Course Lect* 30:185–199, 1981.

112. Vangsness CT, Jobe FW: Surgical treatment of medial epicondylitis: results in 35 elbows, *J Bone Joint Surg* 73B:409–411, 1991.

113. Wadsworth TG: The external compression syndrome of the ulnar nerve at the cubital tunnel, *Clin Orthop* 124:189–204, 1977.

114. Wilson FD, Andrews JR, Blackburn TA, McCluskey G: Valgus extension overload in the pitching elbow, *Am J Sports Med* 11:83–87, 1983.

115. Zeier FG: Recurrent traumatic elbow dislocation, *Clin Orthop* 169:211–214, 1982.

CHAPTER 20

THE WRIST

Melvin P. Rosenwasser
Robert H. Wilson

Although approximately 25% of all athletic injuries occur in the hand and wrist,[1] the understanding of wrist injuries in athletes has lagged behind other anatomic areas, such as the knee and shoulder. Generally, participants in organized sports are predisposed to chronic or repetitive injury.[57] The dilemma in managing these common afflictions is the controversy regarding the criteria for normal wrist anatomy, motion, and function.[30] The bony anatomy provides structure, and there is little debate about its function. But the intricate intrinsic and extrinsic ligaments, which are responsible for stability and function, have been subject to differing interpretations.[24,72] Extrinsic tendons to the hand must cross the wrist dorsally or palmarward, restrained by a retinacular system. Lastly, neural supply to the hand crosses the wrist in the protective compartments of the carpal tunnel and Guyon's canal.

ANATOMY

Carpal Bones

The wrist consists of eight small bones that articulate tightly into a compact, mobile structure (Fig. 20-1). The carpal bones consist of the proximal row (scaphoid, lunate, and triquetrum), the distal row (trapezium, trapezoid, capitate, and hamate), and the pisiform. They possess sufficient strength to sustain enormous forces. There is very little space between them. Some are nearly completely covered by cartilage. There are no primary insertions of tendons to the carpal bones, but the distal row may receive secondary insertions.

The capitate is the largest carpal bone and the keystone of the entire carpus. It articulates with the long finger metacarpal, providing the longitudinal axis for the wrist. Injury to the capitate often leads to nonunion or avascular necrosis.[2,43] It is the first carpal bone to ossify in the developing child. The other carpal bones will then begin to ossify in a sequential, counterclockwise pattern with the hamate next in line.

The scaphoid is the most commonly injured bone. It has an odd shape, much like a twisted peanut shell. It has a peculiar pattern of blood supply that depends on

the dorsal radial artery vessels,[2] which enter into the distal end of the bone and leave the proximal end vulnerable to osteonecrosis if that blood supply is interrupted by fracture.

One to two capsular branches of the radial artery supply blood to the lunate. Like the name, the lunate has the shape of a crescent moon when viewed laterally, and it and the scaphoid articulate with the radius to form the radiocarpal joint.

Along with the scaphoid and lunate, the triquetrum completes the proximal row. It is an infrequent site of injury, well protected by the soft tissues, pisiform, and triangular fibrocartilage. Bony and soft-tissue injury to the ulnar carpus is often misunderstood and misdiagnosed, such as pisiform fracture or pisotriquetral injury.

Although included as a carpal bone, the pisiform is actually a large sesamoid of the flexor carpi ulnaris ensheathed in tendoligamentous tissue. It rests palmarly, on the triquetrum and does not bear axial weight like the rest of the carpus.

The hamate bone has an odd configuration by its wedge shape and palmarly projecting "hook." This structure forms a strut between the carpal tunnel and Guyon's canal and provides stable insertions for the ligaments that span these tunnels for the important neurovascular structures. The hook of the hamate is subject to injury because of its projection palmarward either from direct blow or avulsion resulting from its strong ligamentous attachment.

The trapezium and trapezoid comprise the carpal articulations with the thumb and index fingers. Whereas the thumb carpometacarpal joint enjoys a great deal of motion (flexion, extension, adduction, abduction, pronation, and supination), the index carpometacarpal joint is allowed limited radial and ulnar deviation. The deep, opposing "saddle-shaped" surfaces at the trapeziometacarpal articulation account for its universal joint motion.

The distal radius provides the junction of the forearm and wrist. The congruous scaphoid and lunate facets give the radiocarpal joint bony stability (Fig. 20-2). Yet, slight alteration of the articular relationship (2 mm of displace-

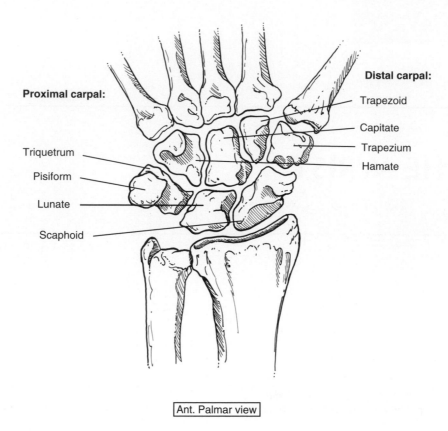

Ant. Palmar view

Fig. 20-1. Wrist bones. The carpal bones consist of the proximal row (scaphoid, lunate, and triquetrum), the distal row (trapezium, trapezoid, capitate, and hamate), and the pisiform.

ment) can lead to abnormal force distribution and wear.[34] The sigmoid notch is an articular groove on the ulnar side of the distal radius that allows the radius to rotate around the ulna. Lister's tubercle is a bony projection on the dorsal radius that functions as a pulley for the extensor pollicis longus (EPL).

Injury to the carpal bones occurs less frequently in the immature skeleton. However, the active physeal growth center of the distal radius is commonly injured. It is responsible for 80% of radial longitudinal growth. There is substantial remodeling potential for many fractures occurring near the physis; however, there is also a significant risk of growth disturbance in displaced, crushed, or chronically injured distal radial epiphyses.[39]

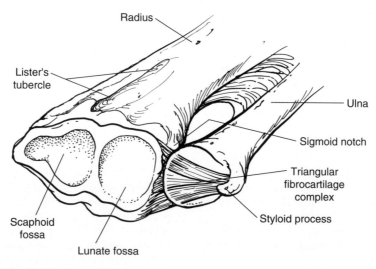

Fig. 20-2. The distal radius articulates with the carpus through the scaphoid and lunate facets. It articulates with the distal ulna via the sigmoid notch. The triangular fibrocartilage complex inserts into ulnar border of the radial articular surface.

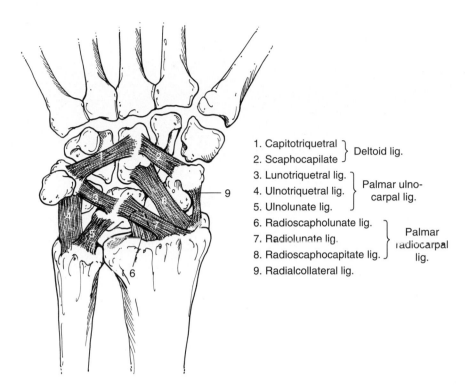

1. Capitotriquetral ⎫ Deltoid lig.
2. Scaphocapilate ⎭
3. Lunotriquetral lig. ⎫
4. Ulnotriquetral lig. ⎬ Palmar ulno-carpal lig.
5. Ulnolunate lig. ⎭
6. Radioscapholunate lig. ⎫
7. Radiolunate lig. ⎬ Palmar radiocarpal lig.
8. Radioscaphocapitate lig. ⎭
9. Radialcollateral lig.

Fig. 20-3. The palmar extrinsic ligaments of the wrist include the radiolunate, radioscapholunate, radioscaphocapitate, radial collateral, ulnolunate, lunotriquetral, and V or deltoid.

Carpal Ligaments

EXTRINSIC. The wrist possesses a complex array of fibrous linkages or ligaments.[41,70] The ligaments control the complex motion of the carpus as an intercalated link between the forearm and hand. Most ligaments provide a connection between the carpal bones and the distal radius and ulna. These extrinsic ligaments are confluent with the wrist capsule. Collateral and dorsal ligament support is relatively weak, yet the palmar ligaments are the strongest and most critical. Taleisnik[71] has described the radial palmar ligaments as the radioscaphocapitate (radiocapitate), radiolunate (long radiolunate), and radioscapholunate (short radiolunate) (Fig. 20-3).[71] Besides being the primary stabilizer of the scaphoid proximal pole, the radioscapholunate ligament serves as a mesentery for blood supply. Lastly, the V-shaped deltoid ligament is responsible for maintaining midcarpal stability, and its components include scaphocapitate and capitotriquetral bands.

INTRINSIC. The interosseous ligaments provide strong linkages between the carpal bones within the wrist capsule. The scapholunate ligament is important in maintaining proximal row stability and normal wrist kinematics, and it is the most commonly injured interosseous ligament. Of similar significance is the lunotriquetral ligament. Lunotriquetral injuries are less common and may be difficult to detect, particularly if there is no radiographic evidence of instability.

Triangular Fibrocartilage Complex

Although the ulnar articular surface area is small, the ulnar carpus is supported by the triangular fibrocartilage complex (TFCC) (Fig. 20-4).[50] The TFCC consists of the triangular fibrocartilage (TFC) with palmar and dorsal radioulnar ligaments, which provide strong ligamentous support for the distal radioulnar joint and a stable articular surface for the ulnocarpal joint. This structure experiences significant stress in rotation and deviation of the wrist. The substantial palmar ulnocarpal ligament completes the TFCC; it provides stability with power grip. There is a fibrocartilaginous meniscal homologue in a minority of patients that may have some load-bearing function.

Dorsal Soft Tissue

TENDONS. The dorsal tendons that cross the wrist originate from extensor muscles of the forearm that animate the wrist and hand. At the distal radius, the extensor retinaculum protects the tendons while ensheathing them in a complex pulley system that prevents bowstringing. The extensor retinaculum divides the traversing tendons into six compartments (Fig. 20-5). The first and most radial compartment connects the abductor pollicis longus (APL) and extensor pollicis brevis (EPB) tendons to the thumb. The extensor carpi radialis longus and brevis (ECRL, ECRB) are in the second compartment. They are powerful wrist extensors. Lister's tubercle forms the radial border of the third compartment, and it serves as a fulcrum for the EPL as it courses radially toward the thumb. The EPL dorsally and the APB and EPB palmarly serve as the border for the anatomic "snuff-box" (Fig. 20-6). The scaphoid and radial artery are palpable in this area. The large fourth compartment includes the extensor indicis proprius (EIP) and the extensor digitorum communis (EDC) tendons, and compartments five and

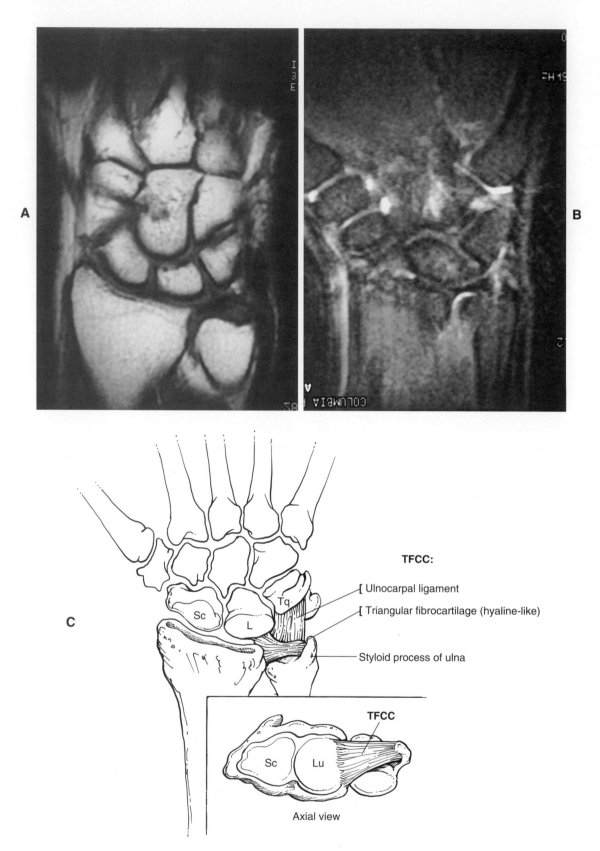

Fig. 20-4. The triangular fibrocartilage complex consists of the ulnocarpal ligament and triangular fibrocartilage primarily. These structures are very important for the stability of the ulnar side of the wrist. **A** and **B,** Coronal MRI of ligamentous anatomy of the ulnar wrist. **C,** Coronal and axial diagrams of TFCC components.

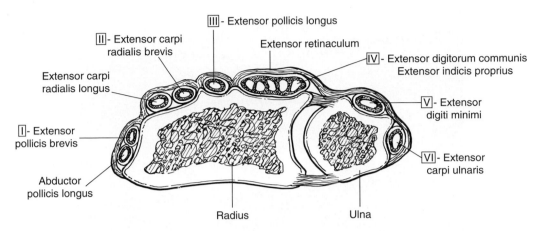

Fig. 20-5. This axial section near the articular level of the distal radius demonstrates the six retinacular compartments that house the extensor tendons: I—abductor pollicis longus and extensor pollicis brevis, II—extensor carpi radialis longus and extensor carpi radialis brevis, III—extensor pollicis longus, IV—extensor digitorum communis and extensor indicis proprius, V—extensor digit minimi, and VI—extensor carpi ulnaris.

six contain the extensor digiti minimi (EDM) and extensor carpi ulnaris (ECU), respectively. The ECU is confined within the dorsal distal ulnar groove by strong ligamentous attachments.

Palmar Soft Tissue

TENDONS. The flexor carpi radialis (FCR) and flexor carpi ulnaris (FCU) are the primary wrist flexors. The FCR travels within the confined space of its long fibro-osseous sheath.[7] It inserts into the index metacarpal primarily, with secondary slips to the long finger metacarpal and the trapezium. The stronger FCU inserts proximally onto the pisiform and has no fibrous sheath. The palmaris longus becomes confluent with the palmar fascia. This vestigial structure may help cup the palm. It

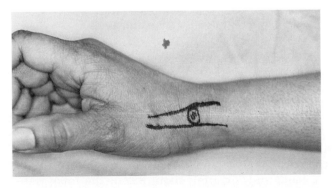

Fig. 20-6. The "anatomic snuffbox" is easily viewed in this wrist. The dorsal boundary is the extensor pollicis longus, and the extensor pollicis brevis and abductor pollicis longus provide the palmar boundary. The proximal boundary is the radial styloid (not demarcated). The scaphoid (S) can be palpated in this region.

is absent in 12% to 15% of the population, and it is valuable as a donor for tendon grafting and reconstructive procedures.

Neurovascular

DORSAL NERVES. Sensory innervation to the dorsal hand is provided by branches from the superficial radial nerve and the dorsal sensory branch of the ulnar nerve, and innervating the wrist capsule are the terminal fibers of the posterior interosseous nerve.

CARPAL TUNNEL. The carpal tunnel is the passageway for the median nerve and nine digital flexors. It protects the median nerve and functions as a pulley for the flexor digitorum profundus (FDP), flexor digitorum superficialis (FDS), and flexor pollicis longus (FPL) tendons. The superficial boundary is the thick, fibrous transverse carpal ligament spanning from the scaphoid tubercle to the hamate hook. The carpal bones form an arc to create its floor and sides. The tendons are covered with a synovial bursa at this level, which aids in tendon lubrication and nutrition. The median nerve is located superficially and slightly radial (Fig. 20-7). It provides sensation for most of the palm and radial three and one-half fingers. Motor branches innervate the thenar muscles and two radial lumbricals. Eight to 10 centimeters proximal to the carpal tunnel, the median nerve gives off a palmar cutaneous branch that supplies sensation to the thenar eminence.

GUYON'S CANAL. The ulnar nerve and artery enter the hand through Guyon's canal. Its borders consist of the volar carpal ligament, palmarward; the hamate hook, radially; and the pisiform, ulnarly. The transverse carpal ligament makes up the floor of this structure. The ulnar nerve innervates all of the intrinsic muscles of the hand, excluding the thenar muscles and the radial lumbricals. It does supply the deep head of

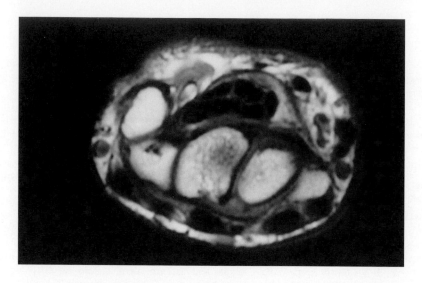

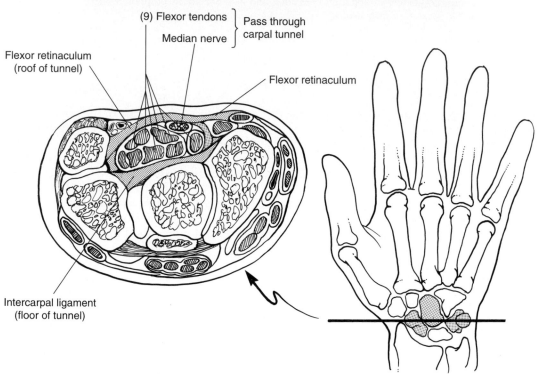

Fig. 20-7. The axial magnetic resonance imaging section of the proximal palm shows the carpal tunnel contents. The median nerve lies radial and superficial and produces a different signal than the flexor tendons.

the flexor pollicis brevis as well. Sensation to the ulnar one and one-half fingers is supplied via the ulnar nerve. Guyon's canal protects the neurovascular structures, but the ulnar side of the hand is often subject to direct trauma, which may lead to arterial injury.[22]

BIOMECHANICS

Kinematics

Normal wrist range of motion is 80° of flexion and 70° of extension. Radial and ulnar deviations are 20° and 30°, respectively (Fig. 20-8). Motion occurs at the radiocarpal joint and between the proximal and distal rows (mid-

carpal joint).[29] Patients may function well with little wrist motion, but this ability would not apply to athletic activities requiring flexibility of the wrist.

Kinetics

The wrist is important in transmitting forces between the hand and forearm. About 85° of the force transfers through the radius when the wrist is in neutral position.[17] The percentage decreases with wrist pronation or ulnar deviation. The strong radiocarpal ligaments must allow wrist motion and stability when it is loaded. Disruption of one or more of the ligamen-

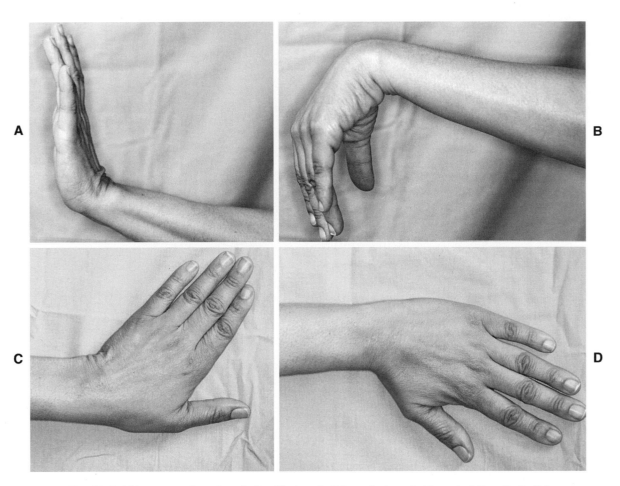

Fig. 20-8. Wrist range of motion. **A,** Dorsiflexion. **B,** Palmar flexion. **C,** Ulnar deviation. **D,** Radial deviation.

tous structures can lead to instability or malalignment. The altered kinematics may lead to pain, carpal collapse, and arthritis.

EVALUATION

History

The history of the injury and details of the chief complaint are extremely important. Obvious problems, such as acute fractures, tendon ruptures, and major nerve lacerations create no diagnostic dilemmas. However, many sports injuries are categorized under the generic diagnosis of "wrist sprain."[6] Focal pain, which is reproducible, may indicate certain structural problems, therefore, it is extremely important to specify the location, severity, and chronicity of the complaint. The examiner must indicate the dominant extremity, specific sport, and energy that caused the injury. The patient should report previous injuries, provocative activities, and any confounding medical conditions or predisposing factors.

Physical Examination

On the playing field, the physical examination may be limited to inspection and palpation. The examiner should look for symmetry and alignment. A fracture or dislocation may be obvious. The examiner should check the integrity of the skin for possible lacerations, contusions, or punctures because open fractures are surgical emergencies, and any pain, swelling, alignment, and color changes should be noted. The neurologic and vascular examinations must be done completely and documented well so later examiners can assess progression. The sensory examination requires testing the autonomous zones of the median (index finger pad), ulnar (small finger pad), and radial (dorsal first web space) nerves. Motor function may be difficult to assess because of pain, but the examiner can palpate muscle group contraction in each territory. Radial and ulnar pulses should be assessed as well as capillary filling. The Allen test is used to evaluate radial and ulnar artery patency and the adequacy of collateralization between the radial and ulnar circulation. The test is performed by compressing the ulnar and radial arteries and exsanguinating the hand, usually by asking the patient to make a tight fist. Upon opening the palm, the entire palmar surface of the hand should be blanched. The examiner should release the compression on one artery and check for swiftness, intensity, and area of color return and sequentially repeat to check the other vessel.

In nonacute conditions, the examiner must carefully determine the location of the complaint. The history, physical examination, plain radiographs, and more sophisticated imaging, such as arthrography, computed tomography, and magnetic resonance imaging, can assist in confirming a diagnosis.

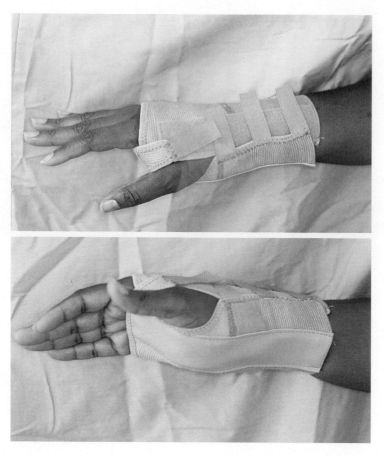

Fig. 20-9. Wrist splint. A prefabricated device can provide some limited stability.

Immediate Management

Immobilization plays a key role in patient comfort.[45] A firm splinting device is useful while waiting for a complete evaluation, including radiographs (Fig. 20-9). A neurovascular examination is mandatory. Elevation and ice are measures that can control swelling and reduce pain.

Imaging

Radiography remains the initial imaging modality for wrist conditions.[43] The standard series are anteroposterior, lateral, and oblique projections (Fig. 20-10).[6] Magnetic resonance imaging is ideal for evaluating bone vascularity and soft-tissue integrity. Arthrography has been useful for evaluation of the intercarpal ligaments and the TFCC. Bone scintigraphy is useful for the diagnosis of occult fractures.[69] Computed tomography has a limited role in chronic conditions, but it can be useful in assessing fracture patterns and assessing progress to bony union, particularly in scaphoid fractures.

CLASSIFICATION

Burton has classified upper extremity conditions according to tissue type and location.[9] The present description will organize wrist injuries into categories relevant to the mechanism of injury,[45] including overuse, excessive loading, trauma, and neurovascular. Addi-

tional specific disorders that are common to athletes will be described.

Overuse

Most sports injuries are the result of chronic, repetitive soft-tissue overload, fatigue, and resultant failure.[16,70] During rugged athletic activity, tendinous, ligamentous, and synovial structures suffer microscopic trauma. Collagen fibers in the tendon or ligament may fail under excessive tension. The soft-tissue healing process includes an inflammatory stage, a reparative stage, and, lastly, a remodeling stage.[31,55] If the tissues are not afforded the time to completely heal, they will be even more susceptible to reinjury, leading to inflammation and pain. When a soft tissue, such as synovium, remains chronically in the inflammatory stage, it may undergo fibrosis and have limited potential for complete remodelling.

Most wrist overuse problems are related to tendons, especially as they pass through the limited space of a tendon sheath, under a retinaculum, or near their bony insertion. Activities that require high wrist torques cause most of the overuse injuries, including racquet sports, gymnastics, wrestling, and rowing. Conservative management allows the tissue to heal with rest while maintaining mobility, and can be facilitated with oral anti-inflammatory medications. Local peritendinous corticosteroid injection may be helpful as well. A careful, gradual return to activity will

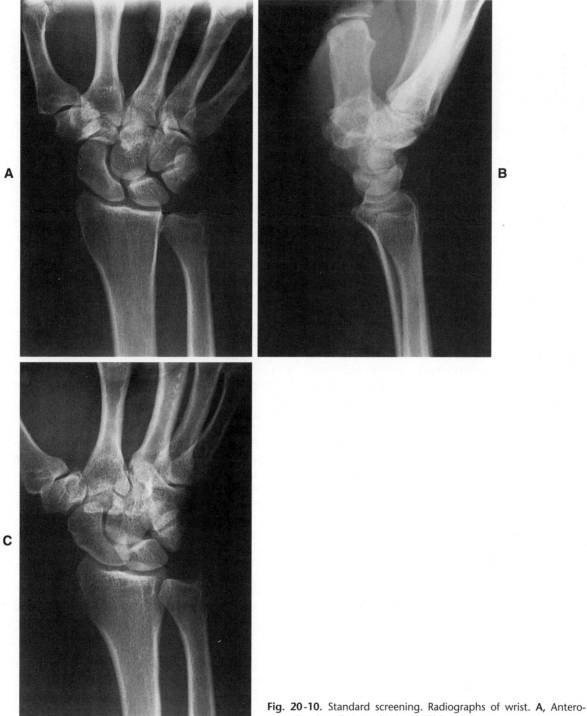

Fig. 20-10. Standard screening. Radiographs of wrist. **A,** Anteroposterior view. **B,** Lateral view. **C,** Oblique view.

help prevent atrophy and weakness.[48] Some of these enthetic disorders do not respond to this approach, and in some cases, surgical management may be considered.

TENDON

First Dorsal Compartment. Tenosynovitis of the first dorsal compartment is common in women of middle age or postpartum.[70] However, it is also seen in athletes of both sexes. The APL and EPB reside in the first dorsal compartment. Patients will complain of ex-

quisite pain with passive wrist ulnar deviation or active thumb extension, and grip will be painful.

On examination, patients may have swelling proximal to the radial styloid. On palpation, the extensor sheath can be firm, almost nodular. A ganglion cyst may be present within the tendon sheath. Tenderness can be consistently localized proximal to the radial styloid, directly over the tendon sheath. The Finklestein test will produce marked discomfort (Fig. 20-11).[18] This test is

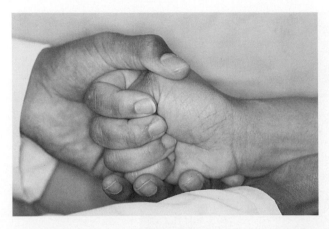

Fig. 20-11. The Finklestein test is performed by ulnarly deviating the wrist with the thumb in the adducted position. This test may cause significant discomfort.

performed by positioning the thumb fully adducted within the palm and then ulnarly deviating the wrist, which causes painful excursion of the involved tendons.

Initial management is splinting. The splint should provide firm support for the wrist and thumb, while keeping them in a functional position. The splint can be removed for periods of nonstressful exercise, and nonsteroidal anti-inflammatory medication may facilitate resolution of the process. Corticosteroid injection is very useful and may effect a cure. These treatments may fail in patients with chronic injury with significant fibrosis and thickening of the sheath. Also, an anatomic variant such as a partition within the compartment often fails conservative management. Those patients may be cured by surgical release.

Intersection Syndrome. Intersection syndrome is a rare condition.[26] The APL and EPB muscles cross the ECRL and ECRB tendons several centimeters proximal to the extensor retinaculum (Fig. 20-12). Patients may develop pain and swelling over this area, particularly with activity. Some patients will note audible crepitus during wrist flexion and extension. The pathophysiology is unclear but may be the result of bursitis, ECRL and ECRB tenosynovitis, or APL and EPB muscular hypertrophy or degeneration. Nevertheless, it is a problem related to excessive friction between contacting soft tissues. Intersection syndrome has been described in oarsmen, weightlifters, skiers,[51] and racquetball players.[66]

Initial management includes rest, splinting, and therapeutic modalities. Nonsteroidal anti-inflammatory medication and corticosteroid injection augment the conservative protocol. After the inflammatory process has resolved, reconditioning can help decrease the chances of recurrence. If there is no improvement, surgical decompression and débridement should be considered.

Extensor Pollicis Longus Tendinitis. Often, the EPL is affected by rheumatoid arthritis or distal radius fractures. The tendon is subject to late rupture in both conditions. Rarely does overuse lead to EPL tenosynovitis and rupture, but it has been reported in squash players and drummers.[31]

Initial symptoms include pain with thumb extension localized over Lister's tubercle. Pain can radiate proximally as well. The history and radiographs should rule out a previous distal radius fracture. EPL muscle hypertrophy in its dorsal compartment is a postulated etiology of the condition known as "drummer boy's palsy."[49] Management consists of rest, splinting, and nonsteroidal anti-inflammatory medications. Steroid injections should be avoided for fear of hastening a rupture. Surgery includes decompression with translocation of the EPL out of Lister's canal.

Extensor Carpi Ulnaris. Athletes who heavily load the wrist, such as rowers, are prone to ECU tendinitis. Participants of racquet sports are affected as well.[49] Patients describe pain on the dorsal and ulnar side of the wrist. As already noted, there are many structures tightly packed into this region, and many confounding diagnoses, such as TFCC or distal radioulnar joint injuries, must be considered. A distinctive feature of ECU tendinitis includes crepitation on wrist motion. A targeted lidocaine injection may confirm the diagnosis. Management consists of splinting and nonsteroidal anti-inflammatory medication with a gradual return to activity.

Other Extensor Tendinitis. Overuse tenosynovitis of the EDC or EDM tendon occurs uncommonly. Symptoms related to these tendons are more likely the result of direct trauma or preexisting systemic disease. However, swelling may indicate a mass effect in an enclosed space. A lesion such as a ganglion cyst, anomalous muscle,[3,33] or tumor must be ruled out.

Flexor Carpi Radialis. Flexor carpi radialis tendinitis is becoming more frequently recognized. The FCR is confined to a tight fibrous sheath as it courses across the wrist toward the index metacarpal. Chronic repetitive wrist motion can cause irritation of the synovial sheath, leading to inflammation.[20] Inflammation can also be secondary to adjacent scaphotrapezial arthritis. Pain localized over the FCR tendon is elicited with passive extension and resisted flexion. Synovitis may present as swelling just proximal to the wrist crease. Long-standing disease may cause adhesions within the fibrous sheath.

Rest, splinting, and nonsteroidal anti-inflammatory medication are the initial management protocols. Steroid injection is often required and very successful. Surgery includes release of the entire sheath.[21]

Flexor Carpi Ulnaris. The FCU may be influenced by the same activities that cause FCR tendinitis. Participants in racquet sports and golf are more commonly affected.[49] Tenderness is palpated more distally, near the insertion into the pisiform. Pisotriquetral arthritis must be ruled out either radiographically or by physical examination. Rest and splinting are usually successful in relieving symptoms. Surgical management includes resection of the pisiform with possible FCU lengthening but is rarely indicated.

LIGAMENT. Chronic ulnar-sided wrist pain should raise suspicion about a TFCC injury.[25] Complaints will range from dorsal wrist pain ("sprained wrist") to inability to hold a racquet. These patients may present with symptoms similar to ulnar-sided tendinitis. Studies have demonstrated chronic TFC perforations associated with a positive ulnar variance and with aging in asymptomatic patients (Fig. 20-13). Healthy subjects may possess

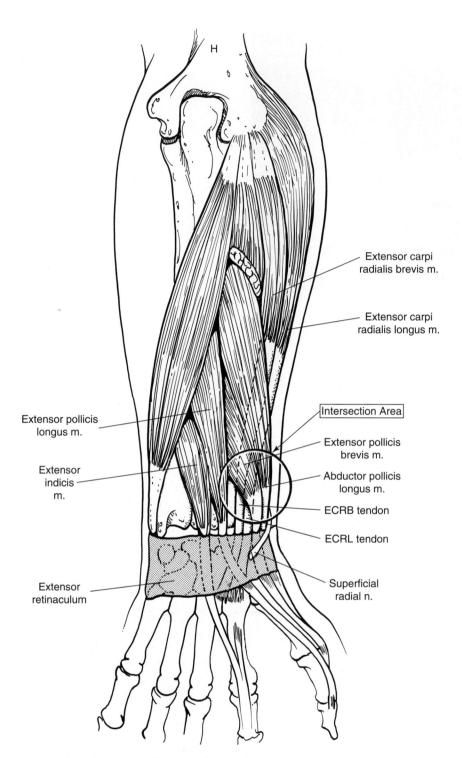

H

Extensor carpi
radialis brevis m.

Extensor carpi
radialis longus m.

Intersection Area

Extensor pollicis
longus m.

Extensor pollicis
brevis m.

Abductor pollicis
longus m.

Extensor
indicis
m.

ECRB tendon

ECRL tendon

Extensor
retinaculum

Superficial
radial n.

Fig. 20-12. The affected site of the intersection syndrome is located at the crossing of the abductor pollicis longus and extensor pollicis brevis over the extensor carpi radialis longus and brevis.

asymptomatic TFC tears, however, a tear is probably abnormal in patients less than 30 years with neutral ulnar variance. Degenerative TFC injuries do not cause distal radioulnar instability.

If TFC injury is suspected, the diagnosis may be confirmed by arthrography or magnetic resonance imaging. Magnetic resonance imaging is highly sensitive in soft-tissue assessment but may not be specific.[32] Arthroscopy

is useful in skilled hands because of its diagnostic benefit and potential therapeutic indications. Tears can be visualized, and if stable, débrided with arthroscopic instruments.[75] The TFCC may require repair if there is instability of the ulnar carpus. Arthroscopy may be the most economical and efficient way to diagnose and potentially manage ulnar wrist pain that has not responded to prolonged conservative therapy.

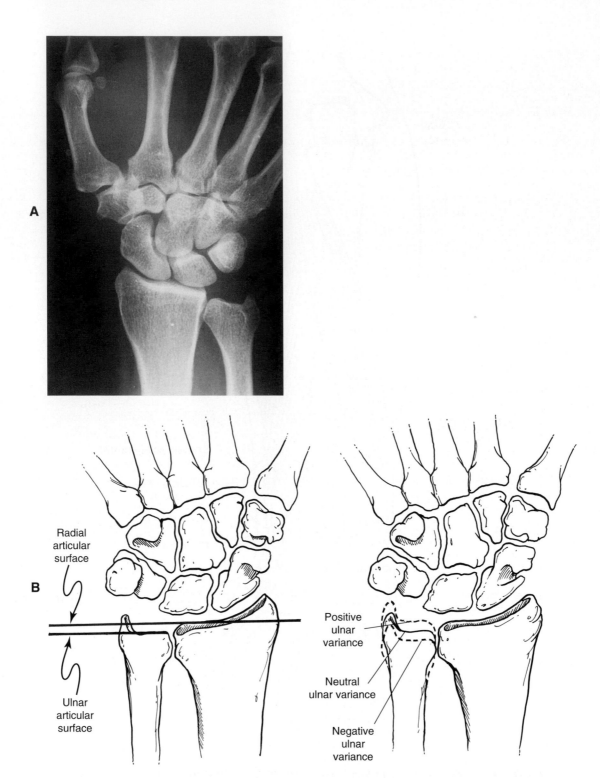

Fig. 20-13. Radiograph demonstrating ulnar variance. **A,** Ulnar variance is measured by drawing a tangential line across the articular edge of the radius and by observing the relative level of the distal ulnar articular edge. **B,** When the line is flush with ulnar articular edge, this is considered neutral ulnar variance. If the line is distal, negative ulnar variance; and if proximal, positive ulnar variance. This measurement must be in the neutral rotation position or it may be unreliable.

Load-Bearing Injury

Sports requiring the use of the upper extremity as a load-bearing structure will have participants who suffer such injuries. These injuries occur primarily to gymnasts and weightlifters. These athletes place exceptional compressive and rotational forces on the wrist.[41] Most gymnasts will suffer symptoms at some point during their training and competition.[38] Their conditions usually have a chronic component, particularly if serious training and competition is begun before skeletal maturity.

DORSAL WRIST PAIN. Gymnasts may complain of diffuse dorsal wrist pain with swelling and warmth. This problem is familiar to most gymnasts and has been called "wrist capsulitis" and "wrist pain syndrome"[38] in the literature. It is hypothesized that the chronically loaded dorsiflexed wrist sustains repetitive impaction trauma to the capsule or synovium, creating the diffuse inflammation and swelling.[15] Another possible cause of pain is perineural fibrosis about the posterior interosseous nerve that innervates the dorsal wrist capsule. These patients may benefit from therapeutic modalities, such as ice, ultrasound, and taping, and brief periods of rest.

DISTAL RADIAL EPIPHYSIS STRESS FRACTURE. Previous studies have shown that young gymnasts may suffer chronic injuries to the distal radial epiphysis.[73] Patients present with symptoms of radially sided wrist pain and tenderness. Radiographs may reveal widening of the physis, cystic metaphyseal changes, and a "beaked effect" of the distal aspect of the epiphysis.[63] It is believed that these changes reflect a stress fracture or reaction. Repeated trauma may result in early physeal closure and eventual positive ulnar variance.[40] There have been reports of partial physeal closure, mimicking "Madelung's deformity" at the distal forearm.[74] The best treatment for these young athletes is rest with a gradual return to gymnastics once symptoms have resolved. Patients without radiographic changes may return within weeks, and those who have changes may require up to 6 months of inactivity.

ULNAR IMPACTION SYNDROME. A published report on college gymnasts has shown a high incidence of positive ulnar variance.[38] It was postulated that this syndrome may result from a ephyseal injury caused by excessive compressive forces on the maturing distal radius as noted above. Later, patients may suffer from chronic symptoms associated with continued gymnastics, such as the pommel horse and parallel bars. This long ulna may cause tears of the TFC and chondromalacia of the lunate and triquetrum.[15] Patients with ulnocarpal abutment and degenerative changes often require a joint-leveling procedure, such as ulna shortening, to decompress this area.

Trauma

TENDON

Rupture. Acute tendon rupture occurs occasionally at the tendon insertion distally more on the extensor side (mallet fingers) than the flexor side (jersey finger; FDP ring avulsion). However, intrasubstance tendon rupture at the level of the wrist is uncommon in healthy athletes. If documented, an investigation into preexisting local or systemic conditions should follow.

Extensor Carpi Ulnaris Dislocation. With forceful hypersupination and ulnar deviation, the ECU may rupture its ulnar septum and subluxate from its groove.[58] This injury has been reported in golfers, tennis players, weightlifters, basketball players, and bronco riders. Patients may present with an acute injury or with complaints of chronic painful "clicking" and "snapping" associated with wrist rotation. The diagnosis can be made by careful examination over the ECU groove. Acute cases may be managed with reduction and immobilization for several weeks, and chronic cases may require surgical reconstruction of the ECU tendon sheath.[62]

LIGAMENT

Scapholunate Ligament. Interosseous ligaments stabilize the proximal carpal row bones for normal kinematic function.[30] A high-loading force on the dorsiflexed wrist may cause ligament disruption. The scapholunate ligament is most commonly affected.[11] Some patients may be predisposed to ligament attenuation and rupture even with trivial insults. Some authors believe the radioscapholunate ligament can be ruptured along with the scapholunate, causing more severe instability.[72] This condition is called dorsal intercalated segmental instability and leads to an alteration in the loading pattern on the radius and scaphoid, causing accelerated cartilage wear.

Patients may present with an acute injury or chronic symptoms of pain, swelling, and crepitus. Pain is located dorsoradially over the scapholunate interval. Watson[75] has described a provocative test that consists of stabilizing and extending the distal pole of the scaphoid and then flexing and radially deviating the wrist (Fig. 20-14), which will produce a subluxation at the radioscaphoid articulation. Pain constitutes a positive test result.

Normal radiographic alignment on standard views may suggest a dynamic instability.[72] Gapping and rotation between the scaphoid and lunate is consistent with a static instability. The posteroanterior clenched fist or loaded view accentuates the gap or may demonstrate a dynamic instability. The scaphoid flexes and radially deviates. This displacement is evaluated by measuring the scapholunate angle (Fig. 20-15). The normal scapholunate angle range is 30° to 60°, with an average of 47°. An angle of more than 70° is deemed abnormal. It is not uncommon that while investigating an unrelated wrist or hand problem, a relatively asymptomatic scapholunate instability may be detected. It is important to obtain comparable radiographs of the opposite wrist in those patients.

In most cases, nonsurgical management is unsatisfactory. The surgical protocol is based on the individual surgeon's training, experience, and preference. Those choices are affected by chronicity and the degree of arthritis. At present, no single procedure can be confidently advocated.

Lunotriquetral Ligament. Lunotriquetral instability is less common than scapholunate instability and is difficult to confirm.[8] The mechanism of injury is often a fall with a torquing component. Patients complain of dorsoulnar wrist pain. Often, these injuries are managed as a "sprain" and do not present to the physician acutely. The provocative tests as described by Reagan et al.[59] ("ballottement") and Kleinmann[24] ("shear") help to reproduce pain symptoms (Fig. 20-16). The tests are performed by stabilizing the lunate with one hand and attempting translation of the triquetrum palmarly and dorsally with the other. Lateral radiographs may demonstrate a scapholunate angle of less than 30°, only if there is a static deformity. An arthrogram may be nondiagnos-

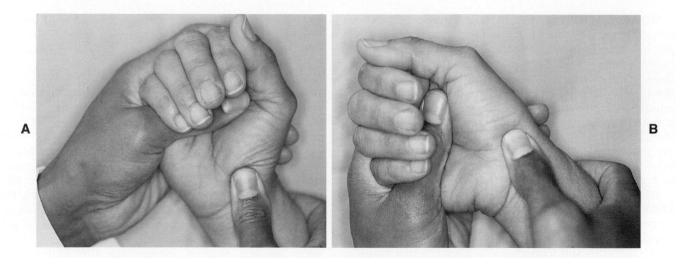

Fig. 20-14. Scaphoid shift test. The test is performed by **(A)** stabilizing the scaphoid tubercle in the ulnarly deviated wrist, then **(B)** maintaining a dorsiflexon force while radially deviating the wrist. Scaphoid subluxation may be appreciated during the examination. Pain indicates a positive test result.

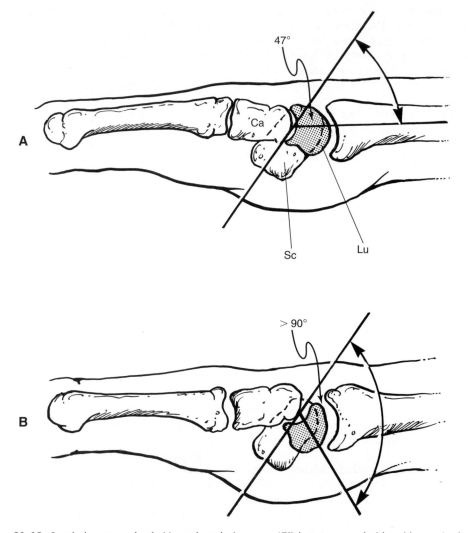

Fig. 20-15. Scapholunate angle. **A,** Normal angle (average 47°) between scaphoid and lunate in the lateral projection. **B,** Abnormal palmar flexion of the scaphoid in relation to the dorsiflexed lunate, thereby creating an increased scapholunate angle.

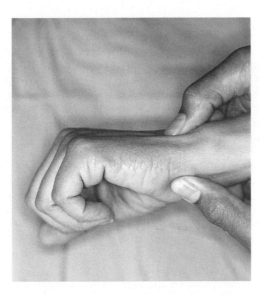

Fig. 20-16. Ballottement test. The lunate is stabilized with one hand while dorsal and palmar translation of the triquetrum is attempted by the other by applying a dorsally directed force on the pisiform prominence. Translation or pain are positive findings of lunotriquetral abnormality.

tic, but magnetic resonance imaging is becoming the most sensitive, accurate test.

Immobilization should be tried first, especially in acute cases. Chronic cases may not respond to splints, injections, or nonsteroidal anti-inflammatory medicine. Lunotriquetral arthrodesis is preferred over lunotriquetral ligament reconstruction.[24,43]

Arcuate Ligament. Patients with midcarpal instability complain of a bothersome and at times painful "trick" or "clunking" wrist.[36] They may be able to demonstrate this problem voluntarily. The patient will hold the wrist in radial deviation, and with ulnar deviation, there will be an abrupt translation. This instability pattern occurs as a result of repetitive loading of the ligamentous link between the proximal and distal rows.[24,36] It can also occur with congenital ligamentous laxity. On cineradiography, the translation appears to be taking place at the triquetrohamate articulation. Painful midcarpal instability may be managed with arthrodesis, which limits motion, or ligament reconstruction, which may not provide durable stabilization for the long term. Instability at the midcarpal joint that is not painful should be managed by observation.

Triangular Fibrocartilage Complex. Many racquet, rowing, and batting sports require strong wrist action for effective performance.[49] Participants may suffer acute injuries or overuse syndromes on the ulnar side of the wrist. Wrist hyperrotation can cause tearing of the palmar or dorsal radioulnar band of the triangular fibrocartilage, leading to radioulnar instability. A fall may overload the TFC and produce intrasubstance tears or perforations of the load-bearing cushion or "disc." Patients will complain of pain that intensifies with loading and twisting. Applying compression across the ulnar side of the wrist is a good

test. The "shuck" test for radioulnar translation can be performed. Also, extremes of rotation may cause crepitus or "snapping," which is indicative of instability. With instability, the distal ulna may be prominent dorsally.

Radiographs may reveal a positive ulnar variance, which is associated with TFC injuries. However, diagnosis of actual tears requires arthrography and, more recently, magnetic resonance imaging. Management of TFC injuries depends on chronicity and location, peripheral or central. An initial splinting or casting is often indicated. Failures of this approach may require arthrotomy or arthroscopy with either TFC repair or débridement.[44] Results can be predictable if the presenting complaint truly correlates with a radiographic or arthroscopic abnormality.

BONE

Scaphoid. The scaphoid is the most commonly fractured carpal bone.[37,64] The fracture typically is the result of a significant fall or blunt trauma (Fig. 20-17). Often, the injury is misinterpreted as a bad "wrist sprain." Athletes may continue to perform in their sport while the discomfort becomes tolerable. Frequently, the injury is detected late as a malaligned nonunion when the athlete suffers a second injury or develops posttraumatic wrist osteoarthritis known as scapholunate advanced collapse

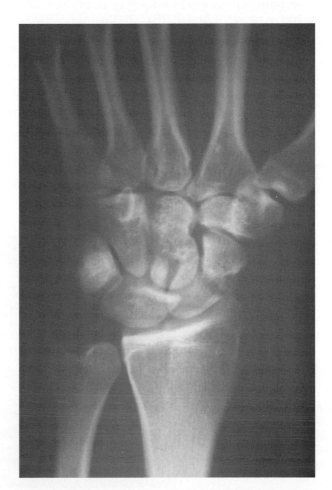

Fig. 20-17. Transverse fracture of the scaphoid waist caused by fall onto the outstretched palm.

(or SLAC wrist). Contact sports with frequent falls like football, basketball,[12,77] and hockey will cause a high rate of scaphoid fractures.

Clinically, patients will complain of pain and tenderness localized to the anatomic snuffbox. Axial loading of the thumb provokes pain. Swelling may be mild to minimal. All injuries with localizing pain to the scaphoid area require radiographs. Serial plain radiographs and computed tomograms may demonstrate a fracture in subtle cases. Patients with a suspicious clinical examination should be treated with splinting, even if results of radiographs are negative. Often, it takes 1 to 2 weeks before the fracture line resorbs, and it can be seen with imaging. A bone scan may also confirm the diagnosis in the early postinjury period (1 to 2 weeks). There have been few reports of scaphoid stress fracture in gymnasts diagnosed by bone scan.[27,39] Magnetic resonance imaging is a highly sensitive test for fracture definition and assessment of vascularity to the vulnerable scaphoid proximal pole.

Scaphoid fractures, especially when displaced, may take 3 to 6 months to heal, if at all.[60] Surgery is indicated for displaced, angulated, or nonunited fractures. Anatomic reduction and stable fixation enhances function and carpal kinematics.

Hamate. Hamate body fractures are uncommon, but the prominent hook can be injured by an avulsion of the transverse carpal ligament (Fig. 20-18). Also, direct or repetitive trauma,[53] particularly by the force of a baseball bat or tennis racquet,[68] can lead to injury. Palpation directly over the hook, which is located in the hypothenar eminence, elicits pain. Carpal tunnel radiographs may demonstrate a fracture. Plain or computed tomography shows the base of the hook in better detail. Bone scintigraphy is less specific but useful.

For acute injuries, initial management is cast immobilization to enhance healing. Frequently, the patient reports the second injury, and a nonunion is detected. Excision of the ununited fragment allows the fastest return

to play. Associated complications with hamate hook nonunions include flexor digitorum profundus tendon to the small finger rupture and ulnar neuropathy.

Trapezoid. Body fracture of the trapezoid is not a reported sports injury, although osteochondral injury to the carpometacarpal joint of the index finger may occur during forceful radial and ulnar deviation in activities such as baseball batting.

Trapezium. Trapezium body fractures have been reported in cyclists,[2] but generally are rare. The mechanism is usually axial trauma while the hands rest on the handle bars. The trapezial ridge is seldom fractured, but the fracture can be easily missed. Patients will complain of pain just distal to the scaphoid tuberosity within the thenar eminence. Radiographs using the carpal tunnel view may show a fracture of the ridge. Special trapezium views are needed to examine the body appropriately.

Acute cases can be managed with protective immobilization. Chronic trapezial ridge fractures that are persistently symptomatic are appropriately managed by excision of the painful ridge.

Triquetrum. The body of the triquetrum is fractured infrequently.[2] Palmarly, it is protected by the pisiform. Avulsion fractures of the dorsal surface may occur with wrist hyperextension and impingement on the hamate. Radiographically, a small fleck of bone will be seen lying dorsal to the triquetrum on the lateral projection. Patients may be treated with immobilization for a few weeks until they are comfortable. Surgery is usually not indicated, even if dorsal carpal bossing or prominence occurs.

Pisiform. Similar to the hamate, pisiform fractures result from direct trauma on the ulnar side of the palm and usually are nondisplaced. They may also result from fatigue failure. Accepted management is immobilization and protection until healing. Sometimes an osteochondral fracture will occur, resulting in chronic arthritic

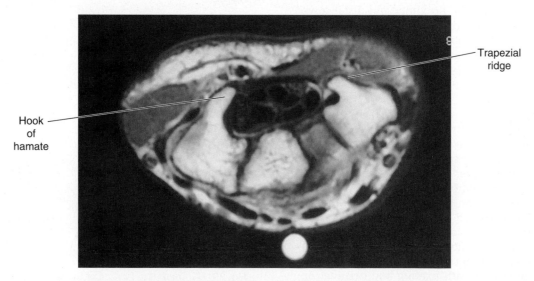

Fig. 20-18. This computed tomography image of the distal carpal row demonstrates the palmar projections of the trapezial ridge radially and the hamate hook ulnarly.

symptoms. Surgery is indicated if painful symptoms persist. In those cases, excision of the pisiform is curative, and return to function is routine.[52]

Capitate. Capitate fractures result from violent trauma and are most often associated with other carpal injuries. They are commonly missed fractures initially. Nondisplaced fractures can be managed by immobilization. A vulnerable blood supply to the head of the capitate may predispose to avascular necrosis and nonunion. Displaced fractures and nonunion require surgery.

Distal Radius. Distal radius fractures are most common in the elderly population but are frequently seen in younger athletes as a result of severe trauma to the wrist. The mechanism of injury is via direct or indirect high-energy forces through extremes of wrist motion. Patients will have severe pain with swelling, ecchymosis, and deformity. Radiographs will demonstrate the anatomy of the fracture (Fig. 20-19). Comminution, intraarticular extension, angulation, and shortening are criteria that help predict the success or failure of a closed reduction.[34] Displaced distal radius fractures require immediate attention with reduction and immobilization, followed by elevation and ice to control swelling. Neuromuscular assessment is essential before and after initial treatment. High kinetic energy injuries with resultant comminution may require external fixation to affect and maintain a satisfactory alignment.

Ulnar Styloid. Fractures of the ulnar styloid may accompany distal radius fractures or be seen in isolation. Distal fractures or avulsions can be followed conservatively if there is distal radioulnar stability.[14] Ulnar styloid basal fractures can be destabilizing to the ulnar carpus because the TFCC originates there. If fracture is symptomatic and unstable, it may require open reduction and internal fixation or bony excision with reattachment of the TFC to the ulnar stump.

CARTILAGE. Injuries to the cartilaginous surfaces of the wrist are difficult to image even with modern techniques such as magnetic resonance imaging because of tissue resolution limitations. Arthroscopy has become the most reliable way to visualize the injury and can be used for management via débridement (Fig. 20-20).[32] It has been reported that more than 50% of patients with chronic wrist pain treated using arthroscopy will demonstrate cartilage lesions.[76]

The athlete may complain of a traumatic injury with persistent pain or recurrent locking. Symptoms consistent with inflammation or synovitis may linger. It is important to carefully obtain a history from these patients to identify those who may have an intraarticular process consistent with an acute injury or even chronic chondromalacia.

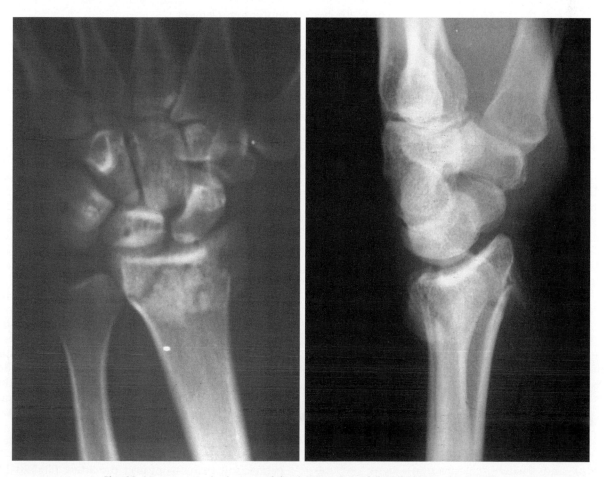

Fig. 20-19. Intraarticular fracture of distal radius after a fall while playing basketball.

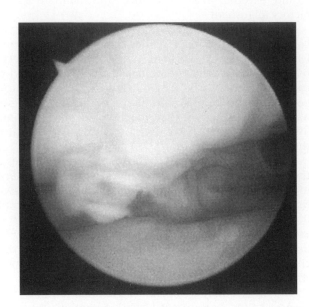

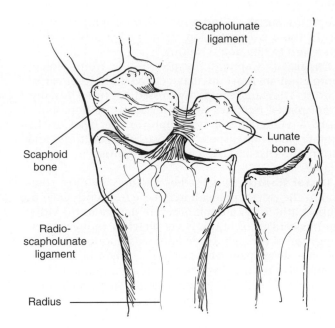

Fig 20-20. Arthroscopic view of radiocarpal articulation, notably the intact scapholunate ligament in this patient.

Perilunate and Lunate Dislocation. It is important not to overlook the perilunate dislocation. Typically, a patient falls violently and sprains his or her wrist. A brief glance at the radiographs does not show a bony abnormality. But if viewed carefully, there is a dorsal dislocation of the capitate from the lunate on the lateral projection. This injury is serious, and open or closed reduction is mandatory.[2]

Hyperextension with severe loading of the wrist may cause this palmar lunate dislocation or perilunate dislocation with or without an associated scaphoid fracture (trans-scaphoid perilunate dislocation) (Fig. 20-21). These injuries should be considered as a continuum caused by the same mechanism of injury.[42] They must be addressed surgically by reduction and internal fixation.

Radioulnar. Radioulnar dislocation can result from a significant TFCC tear. This dislocation is discussed under acute ligament trauma. Proper management includes reduction and maintenance of position by immobilization or surgical repair.

NEUROLOGIC

Carpal Tunnel Syndrome. The carpal tunnel is a conduit for the finger flexors and median nerve. Because of its limited space, it is a common site of nerve entrapment.[4] Athletes develop carpal tunnel complaints because of repetitive wrist and hand usage. Likewise, an anatomic variant, the lumbrical muscles, may be more proximally sited in the carpal tunnel, creating a mass effect. Median nerve compression has been reported in racquetball players,[35] golfers,. and rock climbers.[65] The features include intermittent numbness and paresthesias in the palmar aspect of the radial three and one-half fingers. Symptoms are exacerbated by activity and may include night pain, paresthesia, or numbness.[54] The Tinel (irritation) and Phalen (compression) signs are frequently positive. More advanced findings are persistent

sensory changes and thenar weakness or atrophy. Nerve conduction studies help to quantify the degree of nerve impairment. Electromyography assists in documenting motor involvement.

It is reasonable to attempt conservative measures in mild cases. Rest, splints, and anti-inflammatory medications can be effective. Chronic or more severe disease is definitively managed with surgical release. Open carpal tunnel release may have fewer complications than endoscopic release and allows for excision of inflamed or hypertrophic synovium when indicated.

Ulnar Tunnel Syndrome. The ulnar nerve can be traumatized by direct repetitive pressure or trauma. The primary symptom is numbness and tingling on the palmar aspect of the ulnar one and one-half fingers. Cyclists may develop a "handle-bar palsy"[19,67] by chronic pressure on the ulnar nerve as it traverses Guyon's canal. Nerve conduction velocities and electromyography identify the sensory and motor components of the nerve injury. Symptoms should resolve with inactivity. Padding of the handlebars or gloves will help protect the nerve from repeated insults.[61]

Contusion. Actual nerve contusions occur primarily on the wrist dorsum. Athletes involved in contact sports suffer these injuries. Blunt trauma directed over the sensory branches of the radial or ulnar nerve causes paresthesias in their respective distributions, which is usually transient. Persistent paresthesia or pain over the dorsoradial or dorsoulnar aspect of the hand warrants immediate follow-up evaluation, with possible requirement for exploration.

VASCULAR

Ulnar Artery. The ulnar artery is vulnerable to injury at Guyon's canal. At that level, there is very little palmar soft tissue to protect the artery (Fig. 20-22). The palmar fascia does not cover the hypothenar area, leav-

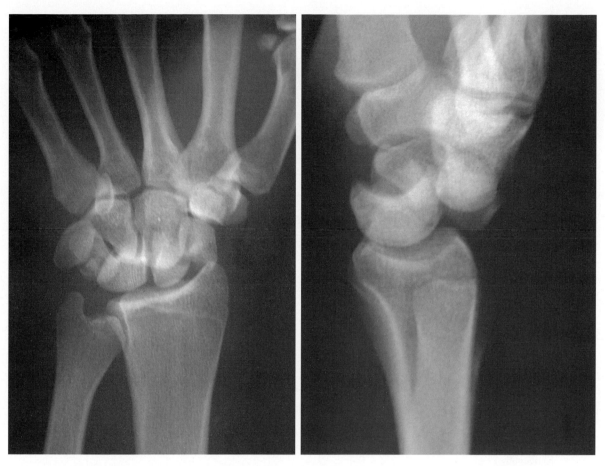

Fig. 20-21. Severe injury of the wrist defined as having a perilunate dislocation (best viewed in the lateral projection) compounded with a scaphoid waist fracture.

ing the palmaris brevis, if present, as the only true protection. Cyclists, handball players, and racquet sport participants sustain significant blunt trauma directly over the artery. Patients present with pain and possible ulnar nerve symptoms.[5] Raynaud's phenomenon, cold intolerance, and ischemic changes in the ulnar fingers may be documented.[10] Also, a pulsatile mass or bruit may be present if there is an aneurysm.

Thrombosis, aneurysm,[29] or vascular spasm can occur. Results of the Allen test may be positive in these patients.[56] Angiographic studies confirm the diagnosis. Suitable management is usually resection of the involved segment of artery, if hemodynamically tolerated. Otherwise, the condition demands some form of vascular reconstruction.

MISCELLANEOUS

Ganglion Cyst. A ganglion cyst is the most common soft-tissue mass found about the wrist. It can be a source of recurrent discomfort.[78] Patients will complain of an enlarging, mobile mass on the wrist dorsum. In contact sports, it may rupture and then slowly return. Occasionally, the cyst will be less prominent but cause significant tenderness. Sometimes it will occur palmarly, adjacent to the radial artery. The cyst originates from synovial tissue and is filled with a gelatinous substance. The dorsal scapholunate ligament is the most common origin for the dorsal gan-

glion and the radioscaphoid joint is most common for the volar ganglion.

Management will vary according to the symptoms and size of the cyst. Extremely large or symptomatic ganglion cysts can be carefully excised. Otherwise, they can be observed or aspirated, although there is a high recurrence rate with aspiration.

Carpometacarpal Bossing. Often seen in middle-aged women, carpometacarpal bossing is usually a painless firm mass over the hand dorsum at the base of the index metacarpal. It corresponds to osteophyte formation around the joint as a consequence of tendon insertion pull[13] or arthritis. Often, this "mass" is confused with other dorsal wrist lesions, such as the ganglion cyst, but it is more firm and immobile. Painless lesions can be observed. Painful lesions can be injected first, and then managed with excision of the spurring and joint débridement. If that fails, carpometacarpal arthrodesis should be considered.

Arthrosis and Chondromalacia. "Racquet player's pisiform" has been described;[28] it occurs in racquet sports participants. Patients complain of ulnar-sided wrist pain associated with firm grip and twisting while using the racquet. Tenderness can be localized over the pisiform bone in the hypothenar eminence. It is postulated that there is abnormal movement of the pisiform in relation to the trapezium. Cineradiography may confirm the abnormal motion. Early management is rest and adminis-

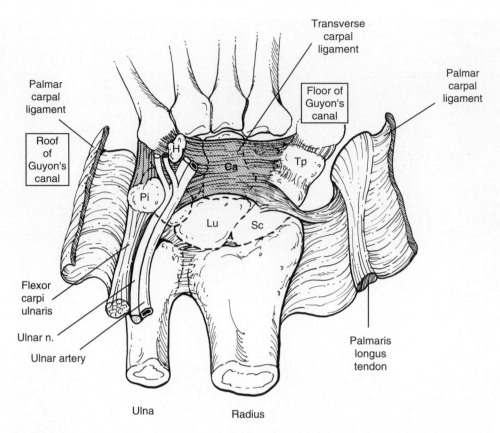

Fig. 20-22. The ulnar nerve and artery traverse Guyon's canal. There is a bony protection on the radial (hamate) and ulnar (pisiform) aspects, but only soft-tissue protection (volar carpal ligament) palmarly.

tration of anti-inflammatory medications followed by surgical excision for refractory cases.[52]

Avascular Necrosis. Avascular necrosis may affect individual carpal bones. The etiology of such entities is unclear, however, repetitive trauma or loading may have a role. The scaphoid, lunate, and capitate are particularly susceptible to avascular necrosis. The blood supply to these bones is as abundant as to any other. The problem is that inflow is limited to a few vessels. Depending on the sport, the wrist is subject to significant loading, which can create stress fractures, thereby damaging the blood supply.[47]

Avascular necrosis of the lunate, or Kienböck's disease, is the most common osteochondrosis seen in the general population. A slightly shortened ulna relative to the radius is a predisposing factor.[23] Avascular necrosis of the capitate is rare, although it has been reported in gymnasts.[46] Preiser's disease (scaphoid avascular necrosis) is very rare and not related to athletics.

Generally, these patients will complain of pain and stiffness, resulting from chronic synovitis. Swelling may be present, and point tenderness may be localized over the affected bone. Management for these lesions is varied and beyond the scope of this chapter. The concept is to avoid activity that will destroy the normal structure of the weakened, avascular bone and allow it to heal. Persistent pain or loss of normal architecture warrants reconstructive procedures.

SUMMARY

Clearly, wrist injury occurs in many athletic activities. When evaluating an athlete with wrist pain, it is important to understand the complex anatomy. Grasping the history and mechanism of injury will aid in classifying the problem. Most conditions result from overuse and can be managed conservatively. The key to appropriate management is the correct diagnosis. If a careful history and meticulous physical examination are complemented by specific modern imaging techniques, diagnoses that are more specific than "wrist sprain" will allow the provider and athlete to understand and treat this complex area, the wrist.

REFERENCES

1. Amadio PC: Epidemiology of hand and wrist injuries in sports, *Hand Clin* 6(3):379–381, 1990.
2. Amadio PC, Taleisnik J: Fractures of the carpal bones. In Green DP, ed: *Operative hand surgery,* New York, 1993, Churchill Livingstone Inc.
3. Ambrose J, Goldstone R: Anomalous extensor digiti minimi proprius causing tunnel syndrome in the dorsal compartment, *J Bone Joint Surg* 57A:706–707, 1975.
4. Aulicino PL: Neurovascular injuries in the hands of athletes, *Hand Clin* 6(3):455–466, 1990.
5. Axe MJ, McClain EJ: Complete involvement of the ulnar nerve secondary to an ulnar artery aneurysm, *Am J Sports Med* 14:178–180, 1986.

6. Beckenbaugh RD: Accurate evaluation and management of the painful wrist following injury, *Orthop Clin North Am* 15:289–305, 1984.

7. Bishop AT, Gabel G, Carmichael SW: Flexor carpi radialis tendinitis. Part I: operative anatomy, *J Bone Joint Surg* 76A(7):1009–1014, 1994.

8. Brown DE, Lichtman DM: The evaluation of chronic wrist pain, *Orthop Clin North Am* 15:183–192, 1984.

9. Burton RI: Overview for athletic upper extremity injuries, *AAOS Instr Course Lect* 34:297–299, 1985.

10. Conn J Jr, Bergan JJ, Bell JL: Hypothenar hammer syndrome: posttraumatic digital ischemia, *Surgery* 68:122–128, 1970.

11. Culver JE: Instabilities of the wrist, *Clin Sports Med* 5(4):725, 1986.

12. Culver JE, Anderson TE: Fractures of the hand and wrist in the athlete, *Clin Sports Med* 11:101, 1992.

13. Cuono CB, Watson HK: The carpal boss: surgical treatment and etiological considerations, *Plast Reconstr Surg* 63:88, 1979.

14. Dell PC: Traumatic disorders of the distal radioulnar joint, *Clin Sports Med* 11:141–159, 1992.

15. Dobyns JH, Gabel GT: Gymnast's wrist, *Hand Clin* 6(3):493–505, 1990.

16. Dobyns JH, Sim FH, Linscheid RL: Sports stress syndromes of the hand and wrist, *Am J Sports Med* 6:236–253, 1978.

17. Ekenstam FW, Palmer AK, Glisson RR: The load on the radius and ulna at different positions of the wrist and forearm: a cadaver study, *Acta Orthop Scand* 55:363–365, 1984.

18. Finklestein H: Stenosing tendovaginitis at the radial styloid process, *J Bone Joint Surg* 12A:509, 1930.

19. Finelli PF: Handlebar palsy, *N Engl J Med* 292:702, 1975.

20. Fitton JM, Shea FW, Goldie W: Lesions of the flexor carpi radialis tendon and sheath causing pain in the wrist, *J Bone Joint Surg* 50:359–363, 1968.

21. Gabel G, Bishop AT, Wood MB: Flexor carpi radialis tendinitis. Part II: results of operative treatment, *J Bone Joint Surg* 76A(7):1015–1018, 1994.

22. Gelberman RH, Panagis JS, Taleisnik J, et al: The arterial anatomy of the human carpus I: the extraosseous vascularity, *J Hand Surg* 8:367, 1983.

23. Gelberman RH, Salamon PB, Jurist JM, Posch JL: Ulnar variance in Kienböck's disease, *J Hand Surg* 5:272–278, 1980.

24. Green DP: Carpal dislocations and instabilities. In Green DP, ed: *Operative hand surgery*, New York, 1993, Churchill Livingstone Inc.

25. Green DP: The sore wrist without a fracture, *AAOS Instr Course Lect* 34:300–313, 1985.

26. Grundberg AB, Reagan DS: Pathologic anatomy of the forearm: intersection syndrome. *J Hand Surg* 10:299–302, 1985.

27. Hanks GA, Kalenak A, Bowman LS, Sebaestianelli WJ: Stress fractures of the carpal scaphoid: a report of four cases, *J Bone Joint Surg* 71A:938–941, 1989.

28. Helal B: Racquet player's pisiform, *Hand* 10(1):87–90, 1978.

29. Ho PK, Dellon AL, Wilgis EFS: True aneurysms of the hand resulting from athletic injury, *Am J Sports Med* 13:136–137, 1985.

30. Kauer JMG: The mechanism of the carpal joint, *Clin Orthop* 202:16–26, 1986.

31. Kiefhaber TR, Stern PJ: Upper extremity tendinitis and overuse syndromes in the athlete, *Clin Sports Med* 11(1):39–55, 1992.

32. Koman LA, Mooney JF III, Poehling GG: Fractures and ligamentous injuries of the wrist, *Hand Clin* 6(3):477–491, 1990.

33. Kushner SH, Gellman H, Bindiger A: Extensor digitorum brevis manus—an unusual cause of exercise induced wrist pain, *Am J Sports Med* 17:440–441, 1989.

34. Knirk JL, Jupiter JB: Intra-articular fractures of the distal radius in young adults, *J Bone Joint Surg* 68A:647, 1986.

35. Layfer LF, Jones JV: Hand paresthesias after racquetball, *Ill Med J* 152:190, 1977.

36. Lichtman DM, Schneider JR, Swafford AR, et al: Ulnar midcarpal instability—clinical and laboratory analysis, *J Hand Surg* 6:515, 1981.

37. Linscheid RL, Dobyns JH: Athletic injuries of the wrist, *Clin Orthop* 198:141–151, 1985.

38. Mandlebaum BR, Bartolozzi AR, Davis CA, Teurlings L, Bragonier B: Wrist pain syndrome in the gymnast, *Am J Sports Med* 17(3):305–317, 1989.

39. Manzione M, Pizzutillo PD: Stress fracture of the scaphoid waist, *Am J Sports Med* 9:268–269, 1981.

40. Markiewitz AD, Andrish JT: Hand and wrist injuries in the preadolescent and adolescent athlete, *Clin Sports Med* 11(1):203–225, 1992.

41. Markoff KL, Shapiro MS, Mandlebaum BR, Teurlings L: Wrist loading patterns during pommel horse exercises, *J Biomech* 23:1001–1011, 1990.

42. Mayfield JK, Johnson RP, Kilcoyne RF: Carpal dislocations, pathomechanics, and progressive perilunar instability, *J Hand Surg* 5:226, 1980.

43. McCue FC III, Bruce JF Jr: Chapter 18. In DeLee JC, Drez Jr D, eds: *The wrist in orthopaedic sports medicine*, Philadelphia, 1994, WB Saunders Co.

44. Melone CP Jr, Nathan R: Traumatic disruption of the triangular fibrocartilage complex, *Clin Orthop* 275:65–73, 1992.

45. Mirabello SC, Loeb PE, Andrews JR: The wrist: field evaluation and treatment, *Clin Sports Med* 11(1):1–25, 1992.

46. Murakami S, Nakajima H: Aseptic necrosis of the capitate bone, *Am J Sports Med* 12(2):170–173, 1984.

47. Nakamura R, Imaeda T, Suzuki K, Miura T: Sports-related Kienböck's disease, *Am J Sports Med* 19:88–91, 1991.

48. O'Neil DB, Micheli LJ: Overuse injuries in the young athlete, *Clin Sports Med* 7(3):591–610, 1988.

49. Osterman AL, Moskow L, Low DW: Soft-tissue injuries of the hand and wrist in racquet sports, *Clin Sports Med* 7(2):329–348, 1988.

50. Palmer AK, Werner FW: The triangular fibrocartilage complex of the wrist—anatomy and function, *J Hand Surg* 6:153, 1981.

51. Palmer DH, Lane-Larsen CL: Helicopter skiing wrist injuries. A case report of "bugaboo forearm," *Am J Sports Med* 22(1):148–149, 1994.

52. Palmieri TJ: Pisiform area pain treatment by pisiform excision, *J Hand Surg* 7:477–480, 1982.

53. Parker RD, Berkowitz MS, Brahms MA, et al: Hook of the hamate fractures in athletes, *Am J Sports Med* 14:517, 1986.

54. Phalen GS: The carpal tunnel syndrome: seventeen years experience in diagnosis and treatment of 654 hands, *J Bone Joint Surg* 48A:211–228, 1966.

55. Pitner MA: Pathophysiology of overuse injuries in the hand and wrist, *Hand Clin* 6(3):355–364, 1990.

56. Porubsky GL, Brown SI, Urbaniak JR: Ulnar artery thrombosis: a sports related injury, *Am J Sports Med* 14:170–175, 1986.

57. Primiano GA, Lee RL: Sports related distal upper extremity injuries, *Orthop Rev* 13(9):61, 1984.

58. Rayan GM: Recurrent dislocation of the extensor carpi ulnaris in athletes, *Am J Sports Med* 11(3):183, 1983.

59. Reagan DS, Linscheid RL, Dobyns JH: Lunotriquetral sprains, *J Hand Surg* 9A:502–514, 1984.

60. Reister JN, Baker BE, Mosher JF, Lowe D: A review of scaphoid healing in competitive athletes, *Am J Sports Med* 13:159–161, 1985.

61. Rettig AC: Neurovascular injuries in the wrists and hands of athletes, *Clin Sports Med* 9:389–418, 1990.

62. Rowland SA: Acute traumatic subluxation of the extensor carpi ulnaris tendon at the wrist, *J Hand Surg* 11A:809–811, 1986.

63. Roy S, Caine D, Singer KM: Stress changes of the distal radial epiphysis in young gymnasts, *Am J Sports Med* 13(5):301–308, 1985.

64. Russe O: Fracture of the carpal navicular, *J Bone Joint Surg* 47A:759, 1960.

65. Shea KG, Shea OF, Meals RA: Manual demands and consequences of rock climbing, *J Hand Surg* 17A(2):200–205, 1992.

66. Silko GJ, Cullen PT: Indoor racquet sports injuries, *Am Fam Phys* 50(2):374–380, 383–384, 1994.

67. Smail DF: Handlebar palsy, *N Engl J Med* 292:322, 1975.

68. Stark HH, Jobe FW, Boyes JH, et al: Fracture of the hook of the hamate in athletes, *J Bone Joint Surg* 59A:575–582, 1977.

69. Stein F, Miale A Jr, Stein A: Enhanced diagnosis of hand and wrist disorders by triple phase radionuclide bone imaging, *Bull Hosp Joint Dis* 44:477, 1984.

70. Stern PJ: Tendinitis, overuse syndromes, and tendon injuries, *Hand Clin* 6(3):467–476, 1990.

71. Taleisnik J: The ligaments of the wrist, *J Hand Surg* 1:110–118, 1976.

72. Taleisnik J: Wrist: anatomy, function, and injury, *AAOS Instr Course Lect* 27:61–87, 1978.

73. Tolat AR, Sanderson PL, De Smet L, Stanley JK: The gymnast's wrist: acquired positive ulnar variance following chronic epiphyseal injury, *J Hand Surg* 17B(6):678–681, 1992.

74. Vender MI, Watson HK: Acquired Madelung-like deformity in a gymnast, *J Hand Surg* 13A(1):19–21, 1988.

75. Watson HK, Ashmead DIV, Makhloof MU: Examination of the scaphoid. *J Hand Surg* 13A:657, 1988.

76. Whipple TL: The role of arthroscopy in the treatment of wrist injuries in the athlete, *Clin Sports Med* 11:227–238, 1992.

77. Wilson RL, McGinty LD: Common hand and wrist injuries in basketball players, *Clin Sports Med* 12(2):265–291, 1993.

78. Wood MB, Dobyns JH: Sports-related extra-articular wrist syndromes, *Clin Orthop* 202:93–102, 1986.

CHAPTER 21

THE HAND

Martin A. Posner

By virtue of its dominant role in many sports activities, the hand is vulnerable to a wide variety of injuries. Most involve abrasions, contusions, and minor skin lacerations, which generally do not seriously impact the athletes' ability to continue sports participation. However, every injury should be evaluated because of the possibility of a more serious injury to underlying structures. The involvement of athletic trainers and therapists is important in this regard because they often provide the initial evaluation, particularly with injuries in organized sports at the high school and college level. This chapter will discuss the primary care of injuries to muscle–tendon units, ligaments, and bones.

MUSCLE–TENDON INJURIES

A muscle–tendon injury is a strain that results either from a single forceful contraction of the muscle against resistance *(overexertion)* or a sudden stretch of the muscle beyond its normal extensile range *(overstretching)*. A muscle injury can also be caused by direct trauma, such as a sharp blow to the extremity. The muscles in the upper arm and forearm are most frequently injured in this fashion, although the intrinsic hand muscles can be similarly injured because closed trauma to the dorsal aspect of the hand is common. When trauma to the hand is severe, there may be hemorrhage within an intrinsic muscle(s), which can lead to fibrosis and contracture. Early recognition is important, and as soon as the acute swelling subsides, stretching exercises are encouraged to restore the injured muscle(s) to its normal length. To accomplish this, the joints are moved in directions opposite from the normal action of the intrinsic muscles, which flex the metacarpophalangeal joints and extend the interphalangeal joints. The exercises are done in either of two methods: the metacarpophalangeal joint is passively held in extension and the proximal interphalangeal joint is actively and passively flexed, or both interphalangeal joints are maintained in complete flexion, usually with the aid of an elastic strap wrapped around the proximal and distal segments of the finger, and the metacarpophalangeal joint is actively and passively extended.

Regarding strains, the most frequently injured sites are the muscle belly, its musculotendinous junction, or the tendon at its bony insertion. Rarely is the tendon itself damaged unless it is diseased, as may occur when chronically inflamed. *Overexertion* injuries commonly affect the extrinsic muscles in the upper arm and forearm or the intrinsic muscles in the hand with activities that involve forceful and sustained gripping, such as required when playing golf or tennis. *Overstretching* injuries are generally confined to the extrinsic muscles. Regardless of etiology, all strains are categorized as *first, second,* or *third degree.*

A *first degree* or *mild strain* does not compromise strength or mobility of the muscle–tendon unit. Although there may be some localized tenderness and swelling, there is rarely any ecchymoses. Management is primarily symptomatic, consisting of application of cold compresses and rest. Recovery can be expected within a few days.

A *second degree* or *moderate strain* indicates actual damage to some part of the muscle–tendon unit, usually a partial tear of the muscle or a partial tear of its musculotendinous junction. Generally, there is greater swelling and ecchymoses and more pain with contraction of the affected muscle–tendon unit than with a first degree injury. Differentiating between first and second degree strains can sometimes be difficult, and if there is any doubt about the diagnosis, it is prudent to manage the injury as the more severe second degree injury. It is important to protect the injured muscle–tendon unit from further damage, which can best be accomplished by splint immobilization. For a sprain of a wrist muscle, tension on the muscle is relieved by splinting the wrist joint in either slight flexion or extension, depending on whether the injury is to a flexor or extensor muscle. The splint is extended to include the fingers or thumb when the injury involves the digital muscle–tendon units. Sports activities should be avoided until pain and swelling subside and until the strength of the injured muscle has been restored, which usually takes several weeks. Second degree strains rarely leave any sequelae, provided that care is taken to prevent any additional damage to the injured muscle–tendon unit.

A *third degree* or *severe strain* indicates rupture of some part of the muscle–tendon unit. Except for ruptures of the distal end of the biceps, third degree strains are rare in the forearm. In the hand, however, they commonly involve the terminal extensor tendons at their insertion into the bases of the distal phalanges, the central extensor tendons over the proximal interphalangeal joints, and the flexor profundi tendons at their insertion into the distal phalanges.

Terminal Extensor Tendon

Ruptures of the terminal extensor tendons are exceedingly common injuries in sports requiring catching or hitting a ball with one's hand (i.e., football, basketball, baseball, and volleyball). Typically, the end of the finger is struck by the ball, which forces the distal interphalangeal joint into acute flexion. Most are closed injuries, and the tendon either tears, or avulses from the distal phalanx with a bony fragment. Swelling and tenderness over the dorsum of the joint may be minimal, but some loss of joint extension will usually be obvious. The flexed deformity of the distal segment is frequently referred to as a "mallet" or "baseball" finger, although a "drop" finger is probably a more accurate and descriptive term.[1] A swan-neck deformity can sometimes develop, with hyperextension at the proximal interphalangeal joint, that can have a more serious impact on finger function than the loss of extension at the distal joint. These deformities most commonly occur in loose-jointed individuals and result from the increase in the extension force on the proximal interphalangeal joint caused by retraction of the injured tendon.

Although terminal extensor tendon injuries are frequently dismissed as trivial, and most are, radiographs of the injured finger are necessary because of the possibility that the distal phalanx has subluxated volarly. A subluxation can develop after two different types of injuries. The first type, which is more common, occurs when the terminal extensor tendon avulses with a fracture fragment that is so large that not only is the tendon attached to it, but also most of both collateral ligaments, which normally provide lateral and dorsal stability to the distal phalanx. The second type of injury follows a hyperextension injury to the distal joint that causes a compression fracture to the dorsal aspect of the distal phalanx, usually more than 50% of its articular surface. Regardless of etiology, a volar subluxation should be reduced and the distal phalanx stabilized in its correct position with a transarticular 0.032-inch Kirschner wire.[63] Failure to restore articular congruity is likely to lead to degenerative arthritis, which can be disabling. A large avulsion fracture fragment is also reduced and fixed with either a Kirschner wire or wire suture.

Because the majority of terminal extensor injuries do not result in any volar subluxation of the distal phalanx, surgery is rarely necessary, and management involves splinting the distal interphalangeal joint in extension for 6 weeks. The splint should never be applied in a manner that hyperextends the distal joint and causes the dorsal skin to blanch because it can lead to ulceration. This would most likely occur immediately after the injury when soft-tissue swelling is most severe. Either a volar or dorsal splint can be used, although a dorsal splint is usually preferred because the tactile surface of the finger remains free (Fig. 21-1). A dorsal splint is also easier to change while keeping the distal joint extended. Maintaining constant extension is important because allowing the joint to flex, even for a moment, damages any tendon healing that has occurred. The athlete should be instructed in the proper technique of changing the splint without inadvertently flexing the distal joint. By pressing the fingertip down on a tabletop, the distal joint will remain extended and the proximal interphalangeal joint will be flexed, providing access to both sides of the finger. In some athletes, particularly professionals whose performance is not compromised by the injury, such as football linemen, it may be unrealistic to expect that they wear the extension splint for many weeks. In these individuals, the joint should be splinted, but only for 1 to 2 weeks, to permit some scarring to develop, which will reduce the risk that the extension lag will worsen. In selected cases, a Kirschner wire can be drilled across the joint in a percutaneous manner to hold it in extension. The proximal interphalangeal joint should never be immobilized, and active range of motions should be encouraged to prevent it from becoming stiff.

Central Extensor Tendon

Injuries to the central tendon over the proximal interphalangeal joint, although not as common as injuries to the terminal extensor tendon, result in more disabling problems. They are caused either by direct trauma to the tendon or by sudden forced flexion of the joint. The central tendon tears, and the head of the proximal phalanx protrudes through the lateral bands, which slip volarly and surround the bone, similar to the edges of a buttonhole surrounding a button, which is the reason the condition is called a *boutonniere deformity*. In France, it has been curiously Anglicized and is referred to as a *buttonhole deformité*. Initially, there may be a paucity of clinical signs, and active extension of the joint may be only minimally restricted, if at all. The diagnosis of these injuries requires a careful physical examination, and an index of suspicion is often helpful. Because the entire joint is usually painful, localizing the area of maximum tenderness is important. If the examination is done in a slow and careful manner, it can usually be determined if the injury is located dorsally over the base of the middle phalanx where the central extensor tendon inserts or over the tendon itself, laterally over one of the collateral ligaments, or volarly. Although any loss of joint mobility should not be ignored, a loss of extension at the proximal interphalangeal joint is not by itself pathognomonic of a central tendon injury. It may indicate damage to the joint capsule (collateral ligament or volar plate), which is a more common injury and from which it must be differentiated. A capsular injury will affect motions limited to the proximal interphalangeal joint, but an injury to

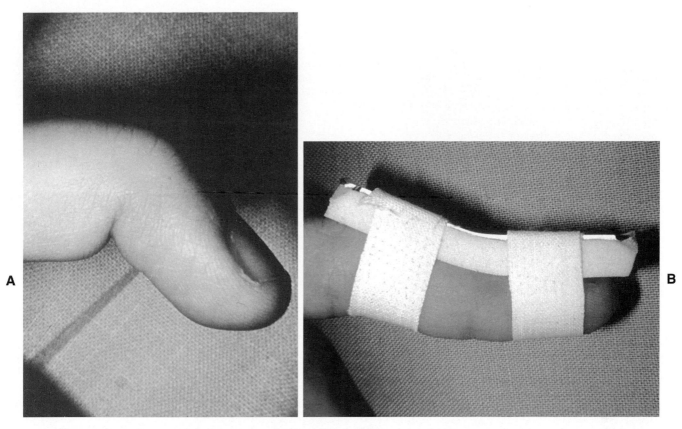

Fig. 21-1. A, Acute injury to the terminal extensor tendon resulted in a 65° "drop" finger deformity, managed **B,** with a dorsal extension splint.

the central tendon will likely affect mobility at both interphalangeal joints. Usually, there will be some limitation of active and passive flexion at the distal joint, even if displacement of the lateral bands over the proximal interphalangeal joint is minimal.[47] Therefore, observing flexion at the distal interphalangeal joint is important in differentiating an injury confined to the capsule of the proximal interphalangeal joint, sometimes referred to as a *pseudoboutonniere deformity,* from an injury to the central extensor tendon, which may also involve the capsule of the joint (Fig. 21-2). Results of radiographs are usually negative unless the central tendon avulses with a fragment from the dorsal base of the middle phalanx, which is a rare occurrence.

Management in the absence of an avulsion fragment is splinting the proximal interphalangeal joint in extension. If there is no loss of extension or only a slight loss, but the dorsal aspect of the joint is tender, an extension splint should still be used. Any suspicion that the central tendon has been injured requires that the joint be splinted in extension. It is better to needlessly splint a finger, reexamine the patient in 1 week, and discontinue the splint if there is no tenderness or loss of mobility than to incorrectly dismiss an injury as trivial and the athlete returns weeks later with fixed joint contractures. When swelling is severe, it may be impossible to splint the proximal interphalangeal joint in full extension. The joint should be splinted in as much extension as possible without causing the patient any undue discomfort. As

swelling subsides, which may take a week, the splint is changed to achieve full joint extension. Extension splinting is maintained for 3 to 4 weeks, followed by intermittent splinting for an additional 2 to 3 weeks during which active range of motion exercises are done. While splinted, the distal interphalangeal joint is left free to permit active and passive flexion to prevent contractures of the oblique retinacular ligaments (Fig. 21-3). In the rare case that the extensor tendon avulsed with a bone fragment, surgery is necessary to reinsert the fragment, which can best be achieved with a wire suture.

FLEXOR PROFUNDUS AVULSION. Avulsion of a flexor profundus tendon is a severe *overstretch injury* that occurs when the muscle contracts forcefully against strong resistance. It typically occurs when a sudden extension force is applied to a finger that is tightly gripping an object. Classically, these injuries are seen in the football or rugby player, who in effort to stop or tackle an opponent, firmly grasps the opponent's jersey. The opponent struggles to pull away, and the athlete's finger gets caught in the jersey and is forcefully hyperextended. The flexor profundus tendon to the ring finger is the most commonly injured of all the profundi because the ring finger has the least amount of independent extension.[17] This lack of extension can easily be observed by placing one's palm and fingers on a flat surface and then extending each finger separately. The limited independent extension of the ring finger, which is often considered a hindrance by musicians, particularly pianists, results

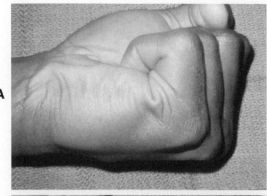

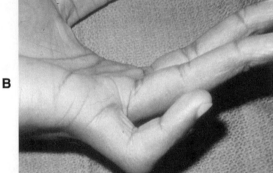

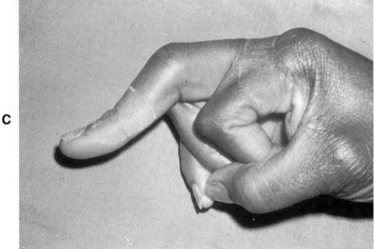

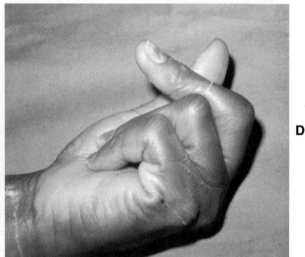

Fig. 21-2. A and **B,** A pseudoboutonniere deformity resulting from scarring of the volar plate. Because there was no damage to the dorsal extensor tendon mechanism, active flexion at the *distal* interphalangeal joint was not affected. **C** and **D,** A boutonniere deformity. The key to the diagnosis was the position of the *distal* interphalangeal joint. Not only was active flexion of the joint limited, it was hyperextended in the resting position.

from the anatomic arrangement of the interconnections between the extensor tendons (the juncturae tendinae) on the dorsal aspect of the hand.[24,25] Two other theories have also been proposed to explain the propensity for rupture of the ring finger profundus: its insertion is slightly weaker than the insertions of the other profundi,[27] and when the metacarpophalangeal and proximal interphalangeal joints of the fingers are flexed with the distal interphalangeal joints extended, the ring finger is the "longest" finger and is, therefore, more exposed to be injured.[6]

Frequently, the seriousness of a profundus avulsion is not immediately apparent to the athlete because there is no obvious deformity like after an injury to the terminal extensor tendon. The athlete may not be aware of any inability to actively flex the distal phalanx until days or even weeks later. The clinical diagnosis of a profundus avulsion should not be difficult because it is the sole flexor of the distal interphalangeal joint. Immediately after the injury, the volar aspect of the finger is often ecchymotic, and there is tenderness at the base of the distal phalanx and over the retracted end of the tendon.

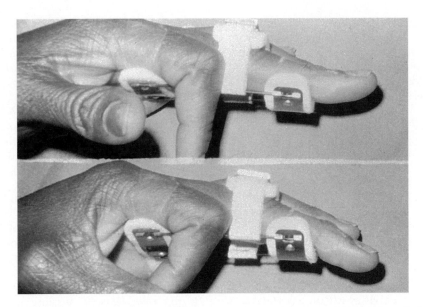

Fig. 21-3. Proper splinting of an acute boutonniere deformity requires that the distal interphalangeal joint be left free to permit active and passive flexion. Usually, a molded splint fabricated by a hand therapist is substituted for this commercially available safety pin splint after the first week, when swelling has subsided.

The tendon can sometimes be palpated, usually in the digit and occasionally in the palm. Active flexion of the proximal interphalangeal joint may be limited if the end of the profundus retracted into the decussation of the flexor superficialis tendon. Radiographs of the injured finger are always necessary, but they can confuse an unsophisticated examiner. They may show a large avulsion fragment from the volar surface of the distal phalanx, which may distract from the more serious tendon injury, or if there is a small bony fragment that retracted with the tendon to the level of the proximal interphalangeal joint, it may be incorrectly interpreted as a chip fracture from that joint.[50]

Flexor profundus avulsions have been classified into three types.[25] In type 1 injuries, both vincula have disrupted, and the tendon retracts into the palm. Generally, this type of tendon avulsion is not associated with any avulsion fracture fragment. In type 2 injuries, the profundus avulsed with a small bone fragment and retracted to the level of the proximal interphalangeal joint. The fragment, which can easily be visualized on a lateral radiograph, provides an excellent key to the location of the tendon end. A type 3 injury is associated with a large bony fragment, which is caught at the A4 pulley of the tendon sheath and is prevented from retracting further proximally. However, a profundus avulsion associated with a large bone fragment to which the tendon was no longer attached and retracted further proximally into the finger has been reported,[23] as well as a profundus avulsion combined with a comminuted fracture of the distal phalanx.[53]

Surgery is necessary for all acute flexor profundus ruptures. When swelling and ecchymosis are severe, surgery should be deferred until the soft-tissue reaction to the injury subsides, which is usually after a few days. Any undue delay, which generally results from the athlete neglecting to seek immediate medical attention, can result in a secondary contracture of the muscle belly, which prevents reinserting the avulsed tendon. Muscle contractures generally develop after 3 weeks, although they can occur earlier the more proximal the tendon retraction. Therefore, a type 1 injury where the tendon has retracted into the palm should be repaired promptly, whereas a type 2 injury is not as urgent because the tendon retraction is less severe. Although surgery should still be carried out promptly for a type 2 injury, repair as late as 4 weeks after the injury may be feasible in cases where the diagnosis was delayed. For the type 3 injury, the large fracture fragment should be reduced and fixed, which will also restore function of the profundus tendon.

For a chronic profundus avulsion, surgery is necessary when function of the flexor superficialis tendon has been compromised by the retracted end of the ruptured profundus. A tendolysis is done in such cases, and the profundus tendon excised. When mobility of the proximal interphalangeal joint is complete, management of a chronic injury is either to accept the loss of flexion at the distal interphalangeal joint, which is justified if the patient has full function of the flexor superficialis tendon and the distal joint is stable (not hyperextensible), or if the distal joint is unstable, to arthrodese it in a functional position of slight flexion. Another management option for a chronic profundus avulsion is a tendon graft through the intact flexor superficialis tendon. However, this option, which may require a staged reconstruction with the preliminary insertion of a silicone rod, places the function of the intact superficialis tendon at significant risk. This risk should be understood by patient and physician. Generally, a tendon graft through an intact flexor superficialis is reserved for young patients in their teenage years or in the rare chronic rupture of a profundus to the little finger because the superficialis tendon of that finger is normally weak and usually does not provide sufficient power of flexion for many grasping activities.

LIGAMENT INJURIES

A *sprain* is an injury that occurs when a ligament is no longer capable of resisting a stress that is applied to it and fails. The magnitude of damage depends on the magnitude of the force and the duration of its application. Similar to muscle–tendon strains, ligament sprains are classified as *first, second,* or *third degree.*

A *first degree* or *mild sprain* does not compromise the ligament's strength. It is generally unnecessary to protect the ligament from further damage, and only symptomatic care and rest are required. The athlete should be able to resume full sports activities within a few days. A *second degree* or *moderate sprain* tears a portion of the ligament and may result in some functional impairment. Although the joint is stable, some laxity can usually be demonstrated when it is stressed. Management is primarily protective to avoid damage to the intact portion of the ligament. The joint is usually immobilized for several weeks, followed by active and resistive exercises to restore mobility and muscle strength. A *third degree* or *severe sprain* is a complete tear of the ligament that usually occurs at either end of its attachments and it may be associated with an avulsion bone fragment. Ligaments that rupture within their substance are rare. Third degree sprains indicate joint instability, and management depends on the ligament that is injured. However, there are two indications when surgery is required. The first is failure to restore articular congruity after closed reduction of a subluxation or dislocation, which would indicate that soft tissues are interposed within the joint, and the second is unstressed instability—the joint fails to remain in alignment with active motions, which indicates that there has been extensive tearing of capsular tissues.

Thumb

CARPOMETACARPAL JOINT (TRAPEZIOMETACARPAL JOINT). The trapeziometacarpal joint is commonly referred to as a "saddle" joint because of its unique configuration. Because of its wide range of motions in three planes (flexion–extension, abduction–adduction, and pronation–supination) it is the most important of the three thumb joints. Although the capsule of the trapeziometacarpal joint permits considerable mobility, it also provides stability, primarily by means of a short, thick ligament between the volar beak of the metacarpal and the contiguous distal portion of the ridge of the trapezium. The ligament has been called the ulnar ligament,[49] and the anterior oblique ligament,[34] but a more appropriate name is the *volar ligament* because it accurately describes its anatomic position. In flexion and pronation (opposition), the volar beak of the metacarpal is closest to the trapezium, whereas in extension and supination, it moves away from the trapezium, a distance limited only by the volar ligament (Fig. 21-4).

Although the vast majority of injuries to the trapeziometacarpal joint are fractures, isolated ligament injuries occur occasionally. An acute dislocation has been referred to as a "Bennett's fracture without a fracture."[32] However, unlike a Bennett's fracture, which is often unstable after reduction and requires internal fixation, a dislocation is usually stable after reduction, and management in a thumb spica cast for 5 to 6 weeks suffices. If the joint remains unstable after reduction, it should be pinned, which can best be accomplished by drilling a 0.032-inch Kirschner wire across the joint in a percutaneous fashion. Because the volar beak of the

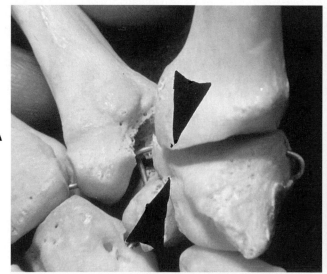
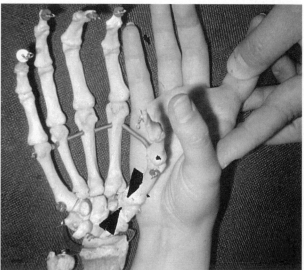

A
B

Fig. 21-4. A, Anatomic view of the trapeziometacarpal joint showing the volar beak of the metacarpal to which is attached the important *volar ligament.* **B,** When the thumb is pronated, the volar beak of the metacarpal and corresponding surface of the trapezium are in close contact.

metacarpal is closest to the trapezium in pronation and flexion, this is the position in which the metacarpal is held while the wire is drilled. The wire is maintained for a minimum of 6 weeks, by which time sufficient scarring should have developed to prevent later joint instability. Surgery for an acute dislocation is indicated only when reduction cannot be achieved, which would indicate interposition of ligamentous tissue.[8] If surgery is required, primary repair of the volar ligament is difficult because of its short length and relative inaccessibility. A more predictable procedure is to reconstruct a new ligament using a strip of the flexor carpi radialis tendon, a technique that is more commonly used for cases of chronic nonarthritic instability.[10]

METACARPOPHALANGEAL JOINT. The metacarpophalangeal joint of the thumb is a condyloid joint like its counterpart in the fingers, but it has several important anatomic differences. The shape of the head of the first metacarpal is less spherical and its articular surface is wider and flatter with more limited cartilage on its dorsal surface than a finger metacarpal.[18] The sesamoids in the thumb are also more constant, and they are intimately connected to the intrinsics, the flexor pollicis brevis radially and the adductor pollicis ulnarly, which is not the situation in the fingers where the sesamoids are not attached to the intrinsics.[15] In addition, the insertions of the intrinsic muscles in the thumb form thicker and stronger tendinous and aponeurotic expansions on both sides of the joint that is seen in the fingers.[2] As a consequence of these differences, the flexion–extension arc of a thumb metacarpophalangeal joint is generally more limited than the metacarpophalangeal joint of a finger. Abduction and adduction motions are definitely more limited, which is consistent with the primary role of the joint, a limited hinge where stability is more important than mobility.

Dorsal Capsule. Anterior dislocation of the metacarpophalangeal joint is a rare injury that tears not only the dorsal capsule but also the extensor pollicis brevis tendon, which is intimately connected to the capsule and inserts with it into the base of the proximal phalanx. Usually the injury occurs in conjunction with a tear of one of the collateral ligaments because the metacarpophalangeal joint is rarely forced in a purely anterior direction. More commonly, it is forced in an anteromedial or anterolateral direction.[51] A pure flexion injury can damage both collateral ligaments, at least their dorsal portions, which normally provide dorsal stability. This injury would be evident if the proximal phalanx remained slightly volarly subluxated after a closed reduction. In such cases, surgery is indicated to repair the torn joint capsule and extensor pollicis brevis tendon. Temporary pin fixation of the joint in complete extension for 6 weeks is also necessary to counteract the normal strong flexion forces on the joint during healing.

Collateral Ligaments. Acute sprains of the collateral ligaments are common, with the ulnar collateral ligament (UCL) injured in about 90% of cases. Although an acute UCL sprain is frequently referred to as a "gamekeeper's thumb," the term actually described a chronic occupational condition in Scottish gamekeepers.[7] A more appropriate term for an acute sprain is a "skier's thumb" because skiing is responsible for most of the injuries.[11,31] The mechanism of injury is a strong abduction force on the joint, whereas an acute radial collateral ligament sprain results from an adduction force, as may occur after a fall on the outstretched hand.

Regardless of which collateral ligament is injured, the diagnosis and proper classification of the sprain depends on a careful examination. The objective is to differentiate a partial sprain, in which joint stability has not been compromised, from a complete tear (third degree sprain), which results in instability and usually requires surgery. Simply observing the thumb in its resting position provides important clues as to the severity of the injury. Ecchymoses indicate tearing of tissues that may include the collateral ligament, and if torn, the metacarpophalangeal joint may actually deviate away from the side of the injured ligament. There is tenderness over the ligament, and an effort should be made to determine if it is located proximally at the origin of the ligament's attachment to the metacarpal head or distally at its insertion into the phalanx. Stability is evaluated by stressing the joint, but before doing so, radiographs are obtained to rule out an intra-articular fracture or epiphyseal plate injury in a skeletally immature child. Ulnar collateral ligaments generally tear at their insertion (90%), and a common radiographic finding is an avulsion bone fragment at that site. Because the fragment is almost always attached to the ligament, the distance that the fragment displaced indicates the distance that the ligament has displaced. Although a displaced fragment is generally associated with an unstable joint, instability can also exist with a nondisplaced fragment. The bone fragment in these rare cases, and usually it is associated with UCL tears, is not the result of an avulsion injury but rather a shear injury (Fig. 21-5). When the proximal phalanx realigns itself after being severely radially deviated at the moment of injury, its ulnar base strikes the metacarpal head, causing a shear fracture to the phalanx.[58] Therefore, joint stability should never be assumed to be intact solely on the basis of a radiograph that shows a nondisplaced fracture fragment.

A variety of imaging studies has been recommended to determine the severity of ligament injuries and the necessity for surgery. The objective is primarily to visualize a lesion described by Stener in 1962,[57] which occurs with some UCL ruptures, interposition of the adductor aponeurosis between the torn ligament and phalanx. Stener properly concluded that ligaments that ruptured in this fashion would never heal unless they were surgically repaired. Although imaging studies such as arthrography,[59] stress arthrography,[3] and magnetic resonance imaging[26] can demonstrate Stener lesions, they are not infallible, and a "negative" study can be misleading because most ruptures of the UCL do not result in Stener lesions yet require surgery. A Stener lesion is a reflection of the severity of the angulation of the proximal phalanx at the moment of injury (Fig. 21-6). It must have exceeded 60° because at that angle the proximal edge of the adductor aponeurosis shifts far enough distal to the base of the proximal phalanx to permit an avulsed UCL

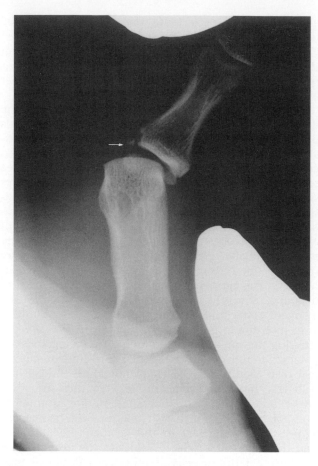

Fig. 21-5. The small nondisplaced fracture fragment (arrow) in this obviously unstable thumb was not the result of an avulsion injury, but rather a shear injury.

to displace outside the aponeurosis after the phalanx realigns itself.[47] Because most UCL ruptures result from injuries that cause less than 60° angulation of the metacarpophalangeal joint, imaging studies should never be the sole criterion for surgery. Rather, the decision should be based on a properly performed stress test.

Opinions vary as to the optimum position for the metacarpophalangeal joint when it is stressed. These positions vary from complete extension,[37,54] to complete flexion,[40] slight flexion,[31] and a combination of flexion and extension.[8,9,57] The rationale for stressing the joint in complete flexion is that because the collateral ligaments are maximally taut in this position, significant angulation of the joint would indicate a third degree sprain. The problem with stressing the joint in flexion is that what may appear to be joint angulation may actually be rotation of the metacarpal at its trapeziometacarpal joint or rotation at the metacarpophalangeal joint itself resulting from laxity of the dorsal capsule, a common finding in loose-jointed individuals who have considerable metacarpophalangeal flexion (Fig. 21-7). The preferred position for stress testing is with the metacarpophalangeal joint in complete extension, and angulation of 30° or more indicates a third degree sprain.[47] A theoretical objection to stressing the joint in complete extension is that a tear of a collateral ligament might go undetected if the accessory collateral ligament, which is normally taut in extension, remains intact. However, this situation has not been observed. Unlike the metacarpophalangeal joints of the fingers, which are normally lax in extension and stable in full flexion, the metacarpophalangeal joint of a thumb must be stable in extension and flexion to function effectively.

Fig. 21-6. A, Thumb instability after rupture of the ulnar collateral ligament. The marked degree of instability of almost 90° indicated that there was probably a Stener lesion. **B,** This was confirmed at surgery (probe on the avulsed ligament, arrow on adductor aponeurosis).

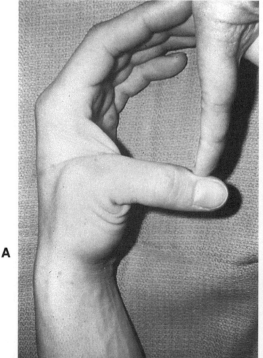

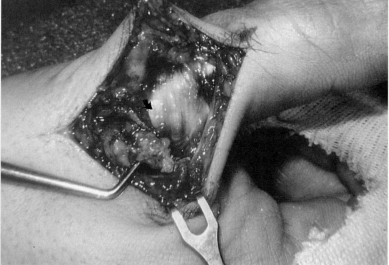

A

B

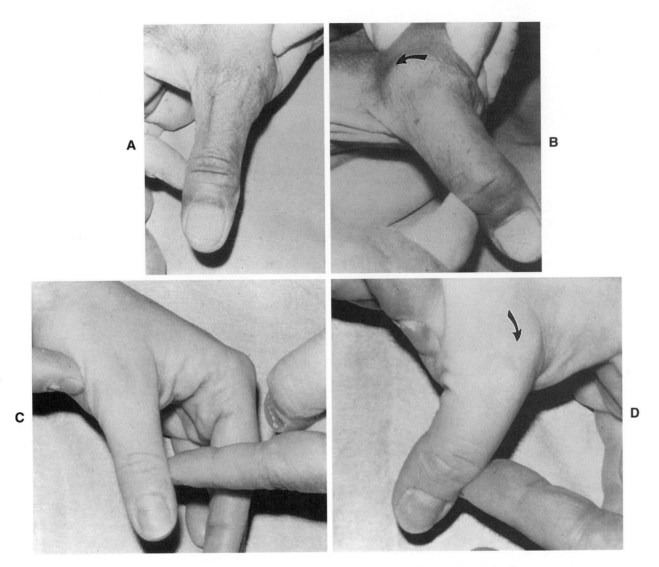

Fig. 21-7. Stress testing two healthy thumbs in extension and flexion. **A** and **B**, The apparent angulation of the metacarpophalangeal joint when stressed in flexion was actually normal rotation occurring at the trapeziometacarpal joint. **C** and **D**, In this thumb, there was also no abnormal angulation at the metacarpophalangeal joint. The joint rotated when stressed in flexion because of normal laxity of its dorsal capsule.

Management for a partial collateral ligament injury is immobilization of the thumb using a palm-based orthosis or a thumb spica cast (Fig. 21-8). Initially, it may be difficult to differentiate between a first and second degree injury, although marked swelling and ecchymoses would be consistent with the more severe sprain. If after the first week the swelling and local tenderness have almost completely resolved, the injury can be considered first degree. The splint or cast can then be discontinued, and active range of motion exercises started. Return to full sport activities can be expected within days, although adhesive taping of the thumb or immobilizing it with a small splint for an additional week or two is recommended. If, however, tenderness persists and if there is slight laxity when stressing the joint, the injury should be considered second degree and thumb immobilization continued for 3 to 4 weeks.

A third degree or complete ligament rupture requires surgery. If surgery is carried out within 3 weeks of the injury, the likelihood of achieving a painfree stable thumb can almost be assured. After surgery, the thumb is immobilized for 4 to 5 weeks. The splint is removed several times each day for active range of motion exercises and discontinued after another week. Resistive exercises to improve muscle strength are important. For the intrinsic muscles, abducting the thumb against the resistance of a rubberband wrapped around it and the palm will strengthen the abductors, and adducting the thumb against the resistance of a sponge within the first web space will strengthen the adductors.

Volar Plate. Dorsal dislocations of the metacarpophalangeal joint are more common than volar dislocations and result from hyperextension injuries that tear the volar plate.[51] The metacarpal head protrudes through the intrinsic muscles that pass on both sides of it and insert on the radial and ulnar sesamoids and respective

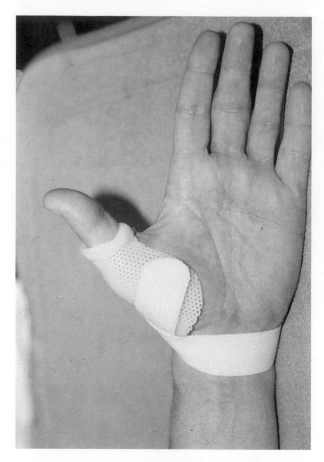

Fig. 21-8. A palm-based thumb splint provides effective immobilization of a thumb metacarpophalangeal joint. When worn under a glove (i.e., skiing), the velcro strap can be removed.

sides of the base of the proximal phalanx. A lateral radiograph will show the dislocation, and the position of the sesamoids will aid in determining the site of the tear in the volar plate. If the sesamoids remain close to the dislocated phalanx, which is the usual situation, the plate has torn proximally and is interposed between the phalanx and dorsal surface of the metacarpal head. A closed reduction should be attempted, generally under regional block anesthesia. Pressure is applied to the base of the phalanx in a distal direction to push it over the metacarpal head. Relaxing the intrinsic muscles and flexor pollicis longus by flexing and adducting the metacarpal is often helpful. Applying severe force to the phalanx must be avoided, particularly in the skeletally immature patient, because it could result in damage to the epiphyseal plate. Some dorsal dislocations are irreducible and require surgery. After reduction, either by closed manipulation or surgery, a dorsal extension block splint is used for several weeks.

INTERPHALANGEAL JOINT. Dislocations of the interphalangeal joint are almost always dorsal and are often compound because the soft tissue envelop around the distal phalanx is firmly anchored by dense, strong skin ligaments. Lateral dislocations are less common than at the distal interphalangeal joints of fingers because the transverse diameter of the condyles of the proximal phalanx in

a thumb are wider than the transverse diameter of the condyles of the middle phalanx in a finger. Careful wound lavage and débridement are important and parental antibiotics should be administered. Occasionally, surgery is necessary when the dislocation is irreducible because of entrapment of the distal phalanx by the volar plate or flexor pollicis longus tendon. Stability after reduction, either closed or open, is excellent, and a dorsal extension block splint is used for several weeks.

Fingers

CARPOMETACARPAL JOINT. Sprains of the carpometacarpal joint(s) are frequently dismissed by athletes as "bone bruises," and treatment is rarely sought until the problem is chronic. Even acute third degree sprains, which are often associated with an avulsion fracture from the base of the metacarpal(s) or the contiguous surface of the carpal bone, are sometimes ignored. Clinically, these injuries are accompanied by local swelling and tenderness, and there is often a bony prominence resulting from dorsal displacement of the metacarpal base. Stability is determined by completely flexing the metacarpophalangeal joint, which locks the metacarpal head, and then, grasping the proximal phalanx, pushing the finger upward and pulling it downward. This maneuver will demonstrate that the second and third carpometacarpal joints are normally rigid, whereas the fourth and fifth carpometacarpal joints have some laxity (about 15° for the fourth and about 30° for the fifth). The laxity of the fourth and fifth carpometacarpal joints is important for maintaining the normal curvature of the distal metacarpal arch when making a fist.

Visualizing a subluxation of any of the carpometacarpal joints requires oblique radiographs to profile the injured joint. Almost all subluxations and dislocations are dorsal, and if recognized early they can easily be reduced by manipulation. However, they have a propensity to displace, particularly the carpometacarpal joints of the index and middle fingers because of contraction of the powerful extensor carpi radialis longus and brevis tendons.[52] Generally, plaster immobilization is inadequate for these injuries, and percutaneous Kirschner wire fixation of the joint is advisable. Care is taken when inserting the wires to avoid injuring the dorsal sensory branches of the radial and ulnar nerves and the extensor tendons. The radiocarpal joint should not be transfixed, and if possible the midcarpal joint also should be left free. A volar wrist splint is applied, which is removed several times daily for active range of motion exercises. The Kirschner wires, which are generally left out of the skin, are removed after 8 weeks. Despite prolonged immobilization, later subluxations can occur, and follow-up observations are required for at least 6 to 9 months.

Most carpometacarpal sprains are not seen until the condition is chronic and the athlete has a significant disability. This chronic condition is common in amateur and professional boxers, particularly when the instability affects the carpometacarpal joints of the index and/or middle fingers—joints that are normally rigid and comprise the solid base for the longitudinal arch of the hand. As the condition worsens, the athlete experiences increasing pain and swelling that persist for progressively longer periods of time after each successive bout. When the athlete realizes that he is unable to continue with his sport, surgery is warranted. Arthrodesis is the most effective procedure, even for the normally mobile fourth and fifth carpometacarpal joints, provided they are fused in sufficient flexion to maintain the normal curvature of the transverse metacarpal arch.

METACARPOPHALANGEAL JOINT

Dorsal Capsule. Direct trauma to the knuckle usually causes a contusion to the soft tissues including the extensor tendon. Sometimes the sagittal fibers are injured, although sudden torsion on the finger is more likely the mechanism of injury than direct trauma. The extensor tendon displaces, usually in an ulnar direction because the radial sagittal fibers are more commonly injured than the ulnar sagittal fibers. If direct trauma is severe, such as a hard blow to the knuckle or repetitive blows during a single episode as may occur in boxing or karate, the dorsal joint capsule can also rupture.[46] Generally, these injuries are not diagnosed until there is a chronic problem. Clinically, the most significant finding is a palpable defect in the joint capsule, which would not be present if the injury was confined to the tendon or its dorsal hood mechanism. Surgery is usually necessary, and the capsule can always be repaired, regardless of the chronicity of the injury, because of the manner in which it tears. Invariably, the tear is in a longitudinal direction, and although the two edges of the capsule may be retracted, they can be brought together for repair.

Collateral Ligaments. Unlike the thumb, collateral ligament injuries of the finger metacarpophalangeal joints are rare for several reasons. Each joint is protected by its recessed position in the palm, is supported by an adjacent finger(s), and in extension can easily deviate when a laterally directed force is applied to it. However, when that same force is applied to the joint when flexed, it is likely to cause ligamentous damage because in that position the ligaments are normally taut and do not permit lateral deviation. After a collateral ligament injury, the patient will complain of pain in the general area of the knuckle but will rarely localize it to the ligament itself, which is a reason these injuries are often overlooked. Clinically, there will be tenderness over the injured ligament. The radial collateral ligaments of the ring and little fingers are most commonly injured because these two fingers are most prone to be forcefully deviated ulnarly when in flexed positions. Stability is tested by stressing the joint in complete flexion (Fig. 21-9). For a first or second degree injury, rest and splinting the joint are effective, but for a third degree injury surgery is usually necessary, particularly when there is gross instability. In some patients, the finger will deviate ulnarly simply by the effect of gravity (Fig. 21-10). At surgery, the ligament, which tears with equal frequency at its metacarpal and phalangeal attachments, is reinserted into the bone.

Volar Plate. Tears of the volar plate result from sudden hyperextension of the metacarpophalangeal joint. The plate tears at its proximal membranous attachment to the neck of the metacarpal and displaces dorsally with the proximal phalanx, to which it remains attached. The metacarpophalangeal joint of the index finger is most frequently dislocated, followed by the metacarpophalangeal joint of the little finger. Usually, dorsal dislocations cannot be reduced by closed manipulation because, in addition to the volar plate that is displaced behind the metacarpal head, there are structures on both sides of the metacarpal head that entrap it. This anatomic entrapment resembles a child's Chinese finger-

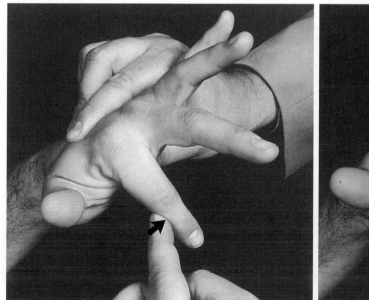
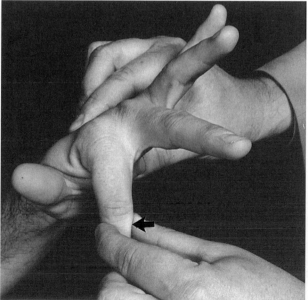

Fig. 21-9. A and **B,** Unlike the metacarpophalangeal joint of the thumb, evaluating stability of the collateral ligaments of a finger metacarpophalangeal joint requires stressing the joint in full flexion.

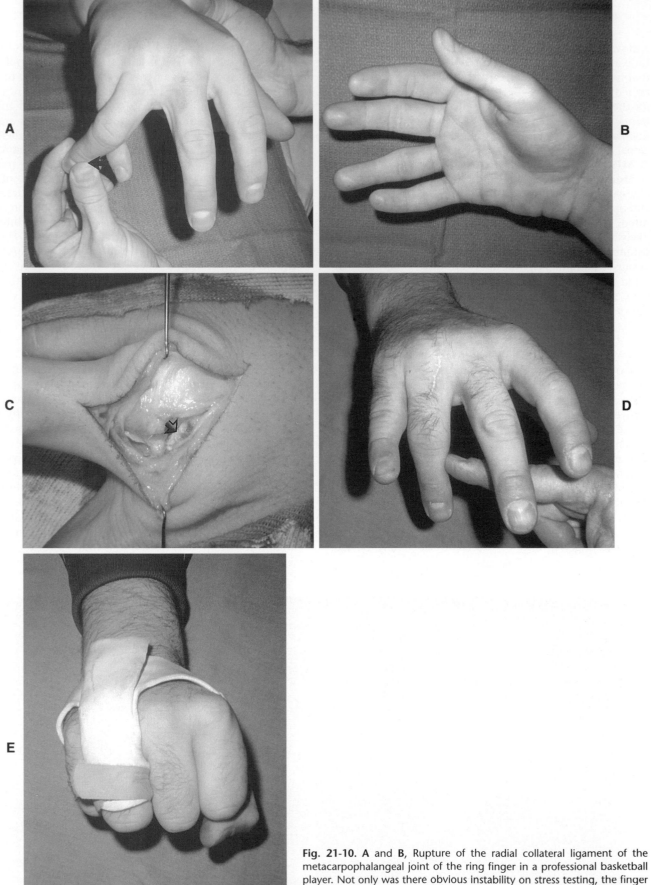

Fig. 21-10. A and **B**, Rupture of the radial collateral ligament of the metacarpophalangeal joint of the ring finger in a professional basketball player. Not only was there obvious instability on stress testing, the finger deviated ulnarly in the resting position. **C**, At surgery, the ligament (arrow) was completely torn. **D** and **E**, After surgery, stability was restored. To facilitate his early return to playing, the athlete wore a protective dorsal splint, which did not interfere with handling the ball, but prevented the finger from deviating ulnarly.

trap; the more traction placed on the finger, the tighter the structures become, and the more difficult the reduction. It is for this reason that these dislocations have been referred to as "complex" dislocations.[19]

When the metacarpophalangeal joint of the index finger is dislocated, the finger is flexed at both interphalangeal joints, hyperextended at its metacarpophalangeal joint, and slightly deviated toward the adjacent fingers. The palmar skin is dimpled or puckered at the proximal palmar crease, which is an important diagnostic clue. Dorsally, a defect can usually be palpated just proximal to the base of the dislocated phalanx. When the joint is subluxated rather than dislocated, there is no lateral deviation of the finger, and the articular surface of the proximal phalanx, which may be hyperextended as much as 90°, still is in contact with the dorsal surface of the metacarpal head.[15] Radiographs of a subluxation or dislocation will show widening of the joint space on the anteroposterior view. The lateral view in a complex dislocation will show the sesamoids to be within the joint because they remain attached to the volar plate, which displaced with the phalanx.[36,61]

The classical surgical approach is volar, and the incision must be carried out with great care because the neurovascular bundle (radial neurovascular bundle for the index finger and ulnar neurovascular bundle for the little finger) is tented over the metacarpal head and can be cut inadvertently. Because of this risk, a dorsal surgical approach is preferred. A longitudinal incision is made in the joint capsule, and the volar plate, which is the structure primarily responsible for preventing reduction, is levered back to its normal position. After surgery, active flexion exercises are begun immediately because there is an inverse relationship between the duration of immobilization and the ultimate mobility of the joint.[29] During the first 2 weeks, a dorsal block splint is worn to protect the joint from hyperextending. If the patient has difficulty regaining active flexion of the metacarpophalangeal joint, a dynamic flexion splint is used. The elastic attached to the cuff over the dorsal aspect of the proximal segment should be of sufficient tension to prevent hyperextension, but it should not prevent full active extension.

PROXIMAL INTERPHALANGEAL JOINTS. Injuries to the proximal interphalangeal joints are among the most common injuries that affect the hand. Many athletes dismiss the injury as a "jammed finger" and neglect to seek treatment. A "jammed finger" is not a medical diagnosis; it neither refers to a specific pathologic condition nor, in most cases, does it accurately describe the mechanism of injury. Fortunately, most are first degree sprains, but occasionally they are third degree sprains or even fracture–dislocations of the joint.

Dorsal Capsule. Injuries to the dorsal capsule are always associated with damage to the central extensor tendon because both structures are intimately connected. Because the tendon is the more important dorsal stabilizer of the joint, management is directed at restoring its function. The most severe injury is a volar dislocation, which results from a violent flexion force on the joint that tears the capsule and central extensor tendon. Reduction is achieved by closed manipulation, which is confirmed on a lateral radiograph. Although primary repair of the tendon has been recommended for these injuries,[30,56] preferred management is extension splinting as used for an acute boutonniere deformity without a dislocation.

Some volar dislocations are caused by a violent torsional injury on the joint. The middle phalanx rotates volarly, which tears the collateral ligament, and the condyle of the proximal phalanx herniates through the extensor mechanism. The lateral band on that side, alone or with the central slip, which remains attached at its insertion, slips volar to the condyle and entraps it.[33,35,45] Radiographs will not show complete volar displacement of the middle phalanx but rather incongruity of the joint surfaces. Because the joint is twisted, the proximal and middle phalanges will project differently: one will appear lateral, whereas the other will appear oblique (Fig. 21-11). A closed reduction should be attempted with the metacarpophalangeal joint flexed to relax the displaced lateral band. The proximal interphalangeal joint is then derotated and extended, and hopefully the lateral band will slip back into its normal position.[8] If this maneuver is not successful, surgery is necessary. Paradoxically, the prognosis is better for this injury, even if surgery is required, than the volar dislocation that is easily reduced. In the irreducible dislocation, the extensor tendon mechanism is displaced, but not disrupted, and active range of motion exercises can begin within 1 week of surgery, whereas in the reducible dislocation, the central tendon is torn, which requires more prolonged immobilization and frequently leads to some permanent loss of mobility.

Collateral Ligament and Volar Plate. Injuries to the collateral ligaments and volar plate almost always occur together, although their severity may differ. A lateral dislocation that completely tears either the radial or ulnar collateral ligament will also tear the volar plate. However, a dorsal dislocation that disrupts the volar plate will not necessarily tear either collateral ligament unless the extension force is also directed radially or ulnarly. Injuries to the collateral ligaments and volar plate are exceedingly common. The majority never receive medical attention, and fortunately, because most are first degree sprains, they rarely cause any residual problem. Even second and third degree sprains may leave the athlete unscathed, although these injuries, particularly when they involve the volar plate, can result in later joint stiffness and cause a significant disability. Commonly, individuals who sustain proximal interphalangeal joint injuries seek treatment because they are more concerned about the swelling that has persisted for weeks or even months than any slight loss of mobility. Swelling after most joint injuries in the hand will persist for many months, and it takes generally up to 18 months until it reaches maximum improvement. Even at that time there will often be some permanent enlargement of the joint, and educating patients to this fact will allay their fears.

After a lateral dislocation, the joint hinges either radially or ulnarly, depending on which ligament remains intact. Generally, the joint hinges ulnarly because most

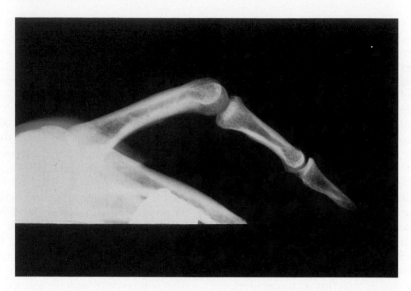

Fig. 21-11. Lateral radiograph of a irreducible volar subluxation of a proximal interphalangeal joint. The key to the diagnosis is not only the incongruity of the joint surfaces, but also its twisted appearance. The radiograph shows a lateral view of the middle phalanx, but an oblique view of the proximal phalanx.

third degree sprains involve the radial collateral ligament. Usually, the dislocation is easily reduced, and often the reduction is carried out immediately after the injury by the athlete who "pulled on the finger." Although the volar plate has also been disrupted, usually at its insertion,[28,48] and only one collateral ligament remains intact, the joint is relatively stable after reduction. Stability results from the normal congruity of the tongue-and-groove configuration of the articular surfaces of the proximal and middle phalanges, and from the compressive effect of the intact flexor and extensor tendon systems. Although many proximal interphalangeal dislocations are never treated and others are simply "buddy taped" to an adjacent finger for 1 to 2 weeks, proper management requires a more careful approach. A radiograph should always be taken to rule out a more serious problem, such as an intra-articular fracture, which will be discussed in a later section. The injured joint is splinted for 2 to 3 weeks in slight flexion. Active range of motion exercises are then begun, and the joint is protected for several more weeks. During this time, "buddy taping" is effective, and, if possible, the injured finger is taped to the finger on the side of the ligament rupture because it will provide better protection. Surgery for the acute dislocation is necessary only in those very rare cases in which reduction cannot be achieved because of interposition of capsular tissue or if there is unstressed instability.

Failure to provide adequate management for the acute dislocation can result in chronic instability, which is generally seen in athletes who report multiple dislocations, none of which ever received any treatment. Clinically, the joint is enlarged on the side of the injured collateral ligament, usually the radial, and on stress testing, there is more than 20° of instability.[20] In mild cases, "buddy taping" during sports activities may suffice, but when there

is a significant disability, surgery is necessary. If possible, the avulsed ligament is reinserted into the proximal phalanx. If, however, there is no recognizable ligamentous tissue, a new ligament must be reconstructed, and in such cases, a portion of the volar plate can be used[12] or one slip of the flexor superficialis tendon.[22]

Regarding the volar plate, it is the primary static restraint limiting extension at the proximal interphalangeal joint. Experimental studies have shown that when an extension force is applied slowly to the joint, the proximal attachments of the plate gradually attenuate.[4] If that extension force continues, the middle phalanx dislocates dorsally with the volar plate, which then becomes trapped over the head of the proximal phalanx and blocks reduction. Because slow hyperextension is a rare mechanism of injury, irreducible dorsal dislocations are exceedingly uncommon.[16,21] Rather, the usual method of injury is rapid loading, which tears the plate at its distal attachments. There are two types of distal ruptures, and each may be associated with a bone chip from the base of the middle phalanx.[4,5] In the type I rupture, the damage is confined to the thin central portion of the plate, and its corner attachments remain intact. Although these injuries can be painful and the joint swells, there is no instability. Overtreatment must be avoided, and immobilization of the joint should not exceed 1 week. Because there is always some bleeding with these injuries, scarring occurs, which can result in a later flexion contracture of the joint. It is, therefore, important to monitor the athlete's condition to ensure that complete joint mobility is restored. A dynamic extension (or flexion) splint is sometimes required if mobility remains restricted after a few weeks. In the type II rupture, which results when the hyperextension force on the joint is more severe, the entire distal attachment of the plate tears, and the lateral capsule also tears between the collateral ligaments and the accessory collateral ligaments. The middle phalanx shifts dorsally hinged on both collateral ligaments. If the split is between the collateral and accessory collateral ligaments, the joint will hyperextend, sometimes as much as 70° to 80°, but the articular surfaces still remain in contact as the middle phalanx articulates with the dorsal aspect of the head of the proximal phalanx. However, when the tears in the lateral capsule are more severe, the middle phalanx will completely dislocate dorsally and produce a bayonet deformity with the proximal phalanx. Closed reduction after these injuries is achieved by simply pushing the base of the middle phalanx over the head of the proximal phalanx. Traction should be avoided because it can entrap soft tissues within the joint and convert a reducible dislocation into an irreducible one.[5] Rarely is there any lateral instability after reduction because the collateral ligaments remain intact. A dorsal block splint is worn for 2 to 3 weeks, which blocks the last 20° to 30° of joint extension, but permits active and passive flexion exercises.

Chronic volar instability is a less common problem than a flexion contracture and is probably related to the poor vascularity at the distal attachment of the volar plate. After a volar plate rupture, particularly if it occurred without a bone fragment, there may be no "fracture bleeding" to cause later scarring.[5,38] In addition, if the joint was not immobilized after injury or if there were multiple injuries, any small clots would have been washed away by the synovial fluid. The distal end of the ruptured plate would therefore fail to scar under such circumstances. Instead, its torn end becomes smooth, similar to the end of an unrepaired flexor tendon that is severed within its digital synovial sheath.

In mild cases of volar instability, a small extension block splint can be used to correct the hyperextended joint. Double-connected rings are also effective because they are light weight and do not interfere with joint flexion. In severe cases, the middle phalanx can get stuck in its hyperextended position, and the patient is unable to flex the finger. For the joint to be flexed, it must first be "unlocked" by passively flexing the middle phalanx. Surgery is often necessary for these problems, and the objective is to construct a constraint that prevents complete joint extension. A variety of surgical procedures have been described, but the most predictable is a tenodesis of the proximal interphalangeal joint using the flexor superficialis tendon.[47]

DISTAL INTERPHALANGEAL JOINT. Stability of the distal interphalangeal joints is greater than the proximal interphalangeal joints because of the short lever arm of the distal phalanx and the insertion of the flexor profundus, which is immediately adjacent to the joint. When dislocations occur, they are usually lateral or dorsal and often compound because of the strong connections that anchor the skin to the bone. Wound lavage and antibiotics are necessary and, as with dislocations of the interphalangeal joint of the thumb, some may be irreducible because of entrapment of the volar plate,[41] flexor tendon,[43] or osteochondral fragment.[60] After reduction, joint stability is excellent, and active range of motion exercises are begun within 2 weeks. Chronic instability is a rare problem.

FRACTURES

Thumb

The most significant fractures of the thumb involve the metacarpal, and they account for 25% of all metacarpal fractures.[42] They distinguish themselves from fractures of the other metacarpals by their potential to cause an adduction contraction and their potential deleterious effect on function of the important trapeziometacarpal joint. The latter problem usually occurs as a result of an intraarticular fracture at the base of the bone of which there are two types: the Bennett's fracture and the Rolando fracture. The Bennett's fracture is an oblique fracture that does not disturb the position of the volar beak of the bone, which is held in place by the intact volar ligament. However, the main portion of the metacarpal often displaces radially and sometimes dorsally because of pull of the abductor pollicis longus tendon. The subluxation component of the fracture is more important than the size of the volar fragment because, if not reduced and articular congruity restored, secondary arthritis is likely. Therefore, a careful radiographic examination is necessary to visualize the articular surface, and if conventional radiographs are inadequate, computed tomography is required. If the fracture is nondisplaced or minimally displaced (less than 2 mm), plaster immobilization with a thumb spica cast will suffice. If there is greater than 2 mm of articular incongruity, the fracture should be reduced and the joint stabilized. The method of reduction is important. As discussed in the section dealing with ligamentous injuries of the trapeziometacarpal joint, the volar beak of the metacarpal is closest to the contiguous surface of the trapezium when the metacarpal is flexed and pronated. It is in this position that the metacarpal is held as a 0.032-inch Kirschner wire is drilled percutaneously across the joint. Pinning the fracture fragment itself is avoided because pressure of the wire tip against it can cause it to shift in position. If an accurate reduction can not be achieved by closed means, operative reduction and internal fixation is required using either a Kirschner wire or a small cortical screw, provided the fracture fragment is of ample size.

A Rolando intraarticular fracture is characterized by its T- or Y-shaped configuration. Because these fractures are more comminuted than Bennett's fractures, restoring articular congruity is more difficult to achieve by closed means, and surgery is usually necessary. Occasionally, an intraarticular fracture of the metacarpal base may be so severely comminuted that skeletal traction is the only feasible method of management.[14,62]

Fingers

The first step in evaluating any fracture is a clinical examination, and its importance cannot be overstated. Observing the relationship of the injured finger to the other fingers at rest and during gentle active motions

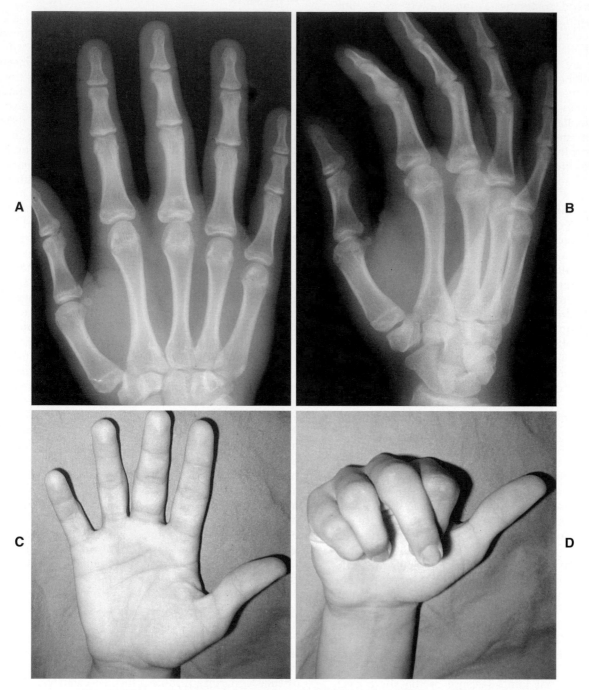

Fig. 21-12. A and **B**, Posterior–anterior and oblique radiographs show what appears to be a nondisplaced fracture through the base of the proximal phalanx of the middle finger. **C** and **D**, Clinically, however, there was obvious malrotation of the finger.

will provide important clues to any abnormal rotation, angulation, or shortening at the fracture site. Not infrequently, the clinical examination is more important than the radiographic examination, and it should always precede it, particularly to assess any rotational deformity of the finger (Fig. 21-12). For each degree of malrotation at the fracture site, as much as 5° of malrotation occurs at the finger tip.[39] A metacarpal fracture that is rotated only 5° can therefore cause 1.5 cm of finger overlap, which is an unacceptable condition that requires correction.

Most metacarpal fractures can be successfully managed by closed reductions. Although circular plaster casts are frequently applied in hospital emergency rooms, they are unnecessary and often troublesome to the patient and to the physician providing follow-up care. Effective immobilization for an acute fracture is more easily provided by applying a padded aluminum splint to the volar surface of the injured finger, which is first bent to conform to the position of the wrist (slight extension) and finger (metacarpophalangeal joint flexion to minimize the risk of a later extension contracture). By sandwiching the aluminum splint between layers of plaster that immobilize the wrist joint, its proximal end will not press into the patient's skin and be an additional source of discomfort. It is important that the splint is bent to conform to the position of the finger and never the reverse. The normal capsular laxity of a metacarpophalangeal joint in extension can permit a malrotated or angulated fracture to appear to be "reduced" if the finger is taped to a splint that has been bent to conform to the desired position of the finger. The improvement in alignment or rotation of the injured finger would be illusory because as soon as the splint is removed, the deformity would be obvious.

With stable fractures, active range of motion exercises can be started within 1 to 2 weeks. The splint is removed several times each day for the exercises, which are carried out in warm water, and then reapplied and worn at all other times. With less stable fractures, the period of immobilization before active exercises are begun is longer, but it should not exceed 3 weeks. If longer immobilization is required, the fracture probably requires some type of internal fixation. Although uninjured fingers are frequently immobilized in the belief that it provides more rigid fixation of the fracture, this practice should be avoided because of its propensity to cause permanent stiffness. If a fracture is so unstable that immobilization of an adjacent finger(s) is contemplated, the fracture should be internally fixed. With each follow-up visit, it is important to not only obtain new radiographs, but also to clinically evaluate the finger for any fracture displacement. Generally, fractures that remain stable after 2 to 3 weeks are unlikely to displace. A more molded splint can then be fabricated by a hand therapist from a thermoplastic material and substituted for the original aluminum and plaster splint. The patient is instructed to remove the splint several times each day for active range of motion exercises, but is to wear it at all other times. The fracture is protected until there is radiographic evidence that healing is complete.

Metacarpal fractures are classified as oblique (spiral), which is the most common type, transverse, or comminuted. Transverse fractures are the least likely to displace once reduced because the fracture fragments can be "locked" together. However, these fractures commonly angulate dorsally with the head of the metacarpal flexed into the palm. Opinions vary as to the degree of angulation that is "acceptable" for each metacarpal. Because the fourth and fifth metacarpals are normally mobile, acceptable angulation for the fourth has been reported to be 20° and for the fifth, 35°.[13,55] These figures should serve only as reference points, and they should not be applied to every patient. Each fracture must be managed on the basis of the demands placed on the athlete's hand in his or her particular sport activity. For the amateur or professional boxer, any angulation of a fractured metacarpal, whether it is the stable second or third or the mobile fourth or fifth, is unacceptable and requires correction. The tremendous compressive force applied to the hand in this sport will likely refracture a metacarpal that is permitted to heal in angulation.

Oblique (spiral) and comminuted fractures are more likely to displace than transverse fractures, and they require close follow-up evaluation, particularly during the first 2 weeks. When there is displacement, internal fixation of the fracture is necessary, and a variety of techniques have been recommended. Kirschner wires are probably used the most frequently, but if the configuration of the fragments permits, cortical screws provide more rigid fixation (Fig. 21-13). Inserting Kirschner wires in a percutaneous fashion down the medullary canal of the bone should be avoided because they can result in scarring of the metacarpophalangeal joint capsule and extensor hood mechanism. They also fail to control rotation.[44]

Phalangeal fractures require as meticulous care as metacarpal fractures, particularly when they are intraarticular. Restoring alignment and articular congruity are the goals of management to minimize later joint stiffness. Many of these fractures require operative reduction and internal fixation. With severely comminuted fractures, such as those that involve the base of the middle phalanx, skeletal traction may be the only feasible treatment.

CONCLUSIONS

The majority of hand injuries are minor and heal without the need for any specific medical attention. However, there are many injuries that if not properly managed can result in significant and permanent disabilities. Therefore, every injury requires a careful evaluation, the importance of which cannot be overstated. Except for fractures, the physical examination is more important than radiographs.

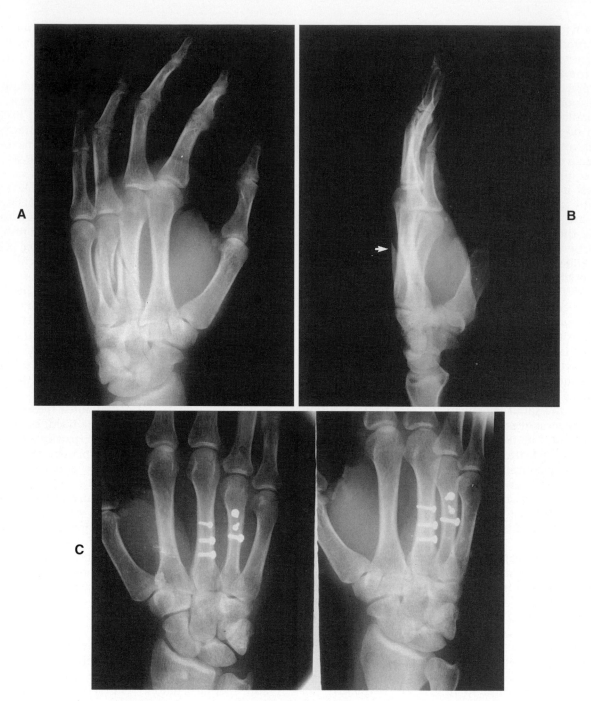

Fig. 21-13. A and **B,** Oblique and spiral fractures of the third and fourth metacarpals. There was significant displacement evident on the lateral radiograph (arrow). **C,** Rigid internal fixation was obtained using 1.5- and 2.0-mm cortical screws.

REFERENCES

1. Abouna JM, Brown H: The treatment of mallet finger: the results of a series of 148 consecutive cases and a review of the literature, *Br J Surg* 55:652, 1968.
2. Aubriot JH: The metacarpophalangeal joint of the thumb. In Tubiana R, ed: *The hand,* vol 1, Philadelphia, 1981, WB Saunders.
3. Bowers WH: Sprains and joint injuries in the hand, *Hand Clin* 2:93, 1986.
4. Bowers WH: The proximal interphalangeal joint. II. A clinical study of hyperextension, *J Hand Surg* 6:77, 1981.
5. Bowers WH, Hurst LC: Gamekeeper's thumb: evaluation by arthrography and stress roentgenography, *J Bone Joint Surg* 59A:519, 1977.
6. Bynum DK, Gilbert JA: Avulsion of the flexor digitorum profundus: anatomic and biomechanical considerations, *J Hand Surg* 13A:222, 1988.
7. Campbell CS: Gamekeeper's thumb, *J Bone Joint Surg* 37B:148, 1955.
8. Dray GJ, Eaton RG: Dislocations and ligament injuries in the digits. In Green DP, ed: *Operative hand surgery,* ed 2, New York, 1988, Churchill Livingstone.
9. Eaton RG: Acute and chronic ligamentous injuries of the

fingers and thumb. In Tubiana R, ed: *The hand*, vol 2, Philadelphia, 1985, WB Saunders.

10. Eaton RG, Littler JW: Ligament reconstruction for the painful thumb carpometacarpal joint, *J Bone Joint Surg* 55A:1655, 1973.
11. Engkvist O, Balkfors B, Lindsjo U: Thumb injuries in downhill skiing, *Int J Sports Med* 3:50, 1982.
12. Faithfull DK: Treatment of chronic instability of the digital joints using a strip of volar plate, *Hand* 13:36, 1981.
13. Flatt AE: *Fractures: care of minor hand injuries*, ed 3, St Louis, 1972, The CV Mosby Co.
14. Gelberman RH, Vance RM, Zakaib GS: Fractures at the base of the thumb. Treatment with oblique traction, *J Bone Joint Surg* 61A:260, 1979.
15. Green DP, Terry GC: Complex dislocation of the metacarpophalangeal joint: corrective pathological anatomy, *J Bone Joint Surg* 55A:1480, 1973.
16. Green S, Posner MA: Irreducible dorsal dislocation of the proximal interphalangeal joint, *J Hand Surg* 10A:85, 1985.
17. Gunter GS: Traumatic avulsion of the insertion of the flexor digitorum profundus, *Aust N Z J Surg* 30:1, 1960.
18. Joseph J: Further studies of the metacarpophalangeal and interphalangeal joints of the thumb, *J Anat* 85:221, 1951.
19. Kaplan EB: Dorsal dislocation of the metacarpophalangeal joint of the index finger, *J Bone Joint Surg* 39A:1081, 1957.
20. Kiefhaber TR, Stern PJ, Grood ES: Lateral stability of the proximal interphalangeal joint, *J Hand Surg* 11A:661, 1986.
21. Kjeldal I: Irreducible compound dorsal dislocation of the proximal interphalangeal joint of a finger, *J Hand Surg* 11B:49, 1986.
22. Lane CS: Reconstruction of the unstable proximal interphalangeal joint: the double superficialis tenodesis, *J Hand Surg* 3:368, 1978.
23. Langa V, Posner MA: Unusual rupture of a flexor profundus tendon, *J Hand Surg* 11A:227, 1986.
24. Leddy JP: Flexor tendon: acute injuries. In Green DP, ed: *Operative hand surgery*, ed 2, New York, 1988, Churchill Livingston.
25. Leddy JP, Packer JT: Avulsion of the profundus insertion in athletes, *J Hand Surg* 2:66, 1977.
26. Louis DS, Buckwater KA: Magnetic resonance imagery of the collateral ligaments of the thumbs, *J Hand Surg* 14A:739, 1989.
27. Manske PR, Lesker PA: Avulsion of the ring finger flexor digitorum profundus: an experimental study, *Hand* 10:52, 1978.
28. McCue FC, Honner R, Johnson MC, Geick JH: Athletic injuries of the proximal interphalangeal joint requiring surgical treatment, *J Bone Joint Surg* 52A:937, 1970.
29. McLaughlin HL: Complex "locked" dislocation of the metacarpophalangeal joints, *J Trauma* 5:683, 1965.
30. Melone CP: Joint injuries of the fingers and thumb, *Emerg Med Clin North Am* 3:319, 1985.
31. Miller RJ: Dislocation and fracture dislocations of the metacarpophalangeal joint of the thumb, *Hand Clin* 4:45, 1988.
32. Moberg E, Stener B: Injuries to the ligaments of the thumb and fingers: diagnosis, treatment and prognosis, *Acta Chir Scand* 106:166, 1953.
33. Murakam Y: Irreducible volar dislocation of the proximal interphalangeal joint of the finger, *Hand* 6:87, 1974.
34. Napier JR: The form and function of the carpometacarpal joint of the thumb, *J Anat* 89:362, 1955.
35. Neviaser RJ, Wilson JN: Interposition of the extensor tendon resulting in persistent subluxation of the proximal interphalangeal joint of the finger, *Clin Orthop* 8:118, 1972.
36. Nutter PD: Interposition of sesamoids into metacarpophalangeal dislocations, *J Bone Joint Surg* 22:730, 1940.
37. O'Brien ET: Fractures of the metacarpals and phalanges. In Green DP, ed: *Operative hand surgery*, ed 2, New York, 1988, Churchill Livingston.
38. Ochiai N, et al: Vascular anatomy of flexor tendons. I. Vascular system and blood supply of the profundus tendon in the digital sheath, *J Hand Surg* 4:321, 1979.
39. Opgrande JD, Westphal SA: Fractures of the hand, *Orthop Clin North Am* 14:669, 1983.
40. Palmar AK, Linscheid RL: Irreducible dorsal dislocation of the distal interphalangeal joint of the finger, *J Hand Surg* 2:406, 1977.
41. Palmar AK, Louis DS: Assessing ulnar instability of the metacarpophalangeal joint of the thumb, *J Hand Surg* 3:542, 1978.
42. Pellegrini UD: Fractures of the base of the thumb, *Hand Clin* 4:87, 1988.
43. Pohl AL: Irreducible dislocation of a distal interphalangeal joint, *Br J Plast Surg* 29:227, 1976.
44. Posner MA: Hand injuries. In Nicholas JA, Hershman EB, Posner MA, ed: *The upper extremity in sports medicine*, ed 3, St Louis, 1995, CV Mosby
45. Posner MA: Injuries to the hand and wrist in athletes, *Orthop Clin North Am* 8:593, 1977.
46. Posner MA, Ambrose L: The boxer's knuckle; dorsal capsule rupture of the metacarpophalangeal joint of a finger, *J Hand Surg* 14A:229, 1989.
47. Posner MA, Wilenski M: Irreducible volar dislocation of the proximal interphalangeal joint of a finger caused by interposition of an intact central slip: a case report, *J Bone Joint Surg* 60A:133, 1978.
48. Redler I, Williams JT: Rupture of a collateral ligament of the proximal interphalangeal joint of the finger: analysis of 18 cases, *J Bone Joint Surg* 49A:322, 1967.
49. Riordan DC, Kaplan EB: The thumb. In Spinner M, ed: *Kaplan's functional and surgical anatomy of the hand*, Philadelphia, 1984, JB Lippincott Co.
50. Schneider LH: Tendon injuries of the hand. In Nicholas JA, Hershman EB, Posner MA, eds: *The upper extremity in sports medicine*, St Louis, 1990, CV Mosby.
51. Sedel L: Dislocation of the carpometacarpal joints. In Tubiana R, ed: *The hand*, vol 2, Philadelphia, 1985, WB Saunders.
52. Sedel L: Dislocation of the metacarpophalangeal joint. In Tubiana R, ed: *The hand*, vol 2, Philadelphia, 1985, WB Saunders.
53. Smith JH: Avulsion of a profundus tendon with simultaneous intraarticular fracture of the distal phalanx: case report, *J Hand Surg* 6:600, 1981.
54. Smith RJ: Post-traumatic instability of the metacarpophalangeal joint of the thumb, *J Bone Joint Surg* 59A:14, 1977.
55. Smith RJ, Peimer CA: Injuries to the metacarpal bones and joints, *Adv Surg* 2:341, 1977.
56. Spinner M, Choi BY: Anterior dislocation of the proximal interphalangeal joint: a care of rupture of the central slip of the extensor mechanism, *J Bone Joint Surg* 52A:1329, 1970.
57. Stener B: Acute injuries to the metacarpophalangeal joint of the thumb. In Tubiana R, ed: *The hand,* vol 2, Philadelphia, 1985, WB Saunders.
58. Stener B: Displacement of the ruptured ulnar collateral ligament of the metacarpophalangeal joint of the thumb: a clinical and anatomical study, *J Bone Joint Surg* 44B:869, 1962.
59. Stothard J, Caird DM: Experience with arthrography of the first metacarpophalangeal joint, *Hand* 13:257, 1981.
60. Stripling WD: Displaced intra-articular osteochondral fracture: cause for irreducible dislocation of the distal interphalangeal joint, *J Hand Surg* 7:77, 1982.
61. Sweterlitsch PR, Torg JS, Pollack H: Entrapment of a sesamoid on the index metacarpophalangeal joint: report of two cases, *J Bone Joint Surg* 51A:995, 1969.
62. Thoren L: A new method of extension treatment in Bennett's fracture, *Acta Chir Scand* 110:485, 1956.
63. Webbe MA, Schneider LH: Mallet fractures, *J Bone Joint Surg* 66A:658, 1984.

CHAPTER 22

PELVIS, HIP, AND THIGH

Gregory M. Lieberman
Steven F. Harwin

Although sports injuries of the pelvis, hip, and thigh may not receive the same attention as those of the knee, ankle, and upper extremities, these body regions are equally important to the athlete's performance at all levels of competition and with all types of functions, including throwing activities and running. Older athletes are at increased risk for injuries to the pelvis, hip, and thigh as a result of previous injuries, diminished elasticity, and decreased injury repair mechanisms[51] of a body region that constantly bears a significant amount of stresses with activities of daily living.

The pelvis, hip, and thigh include the largest bone in the body, the femur, and the most powerful and largest muscles, the glutei, the quadriceps, and the hamstrings. They are involved as a link and support system connecting the trunk to the lower extremity for weight bearing, locomotion, and visceral protection. It is obvious that injuries disabling such structures would cause difficulties with sports and activities of daily living. The ability to diagnose and manage injuries of this body region in a timely fashion is of paramount importance to the athlete.

ANATOMY

Understanding the complex anatomy of this region is important to help the practitioner diagnose and manage injuries affecting the pelvis, hip, and thigh. A complete review of the anatomy is beyond the scope of this chapter. A brief overview of the pertinent anatomy, however, is appropriate.

The bony pelvis is composed of the two innominate bones, each of which are composed of three bones: the ilium, the ischium, and the pubis. The three converge at the acetabulum, the pelvic portion of the hip joint. The sacrum and coccyx, which are cradled by the innominate bones, compose the posterior bony pelvis. These articulate posteriorly with the paired innominate bones to form the sacroiliac joint. The innominate bones articulate anteriorly via the pubis and the ischium to form the symphysis pubis. Neither of these joints have any gross

motion across them. There is no muscle action across these joints. However, the entire pelvis is capable of moving as a unit. These motions are anterior–posterior tilt, lateral tilt, and rotation.

The femur, or thigh bone, has a head and neck region that articulates with the acetabulum to form the hip joint, a complex ball and socket joint. It also has a greater and lesser trochanter to which muscles attach. The average angle between the head and the neck is 125° to 135°.[37] The hip is capable of motion in several planes, but most motion occurs in the sagittal plane.[63] Activities of daily living require 100° to 120° of flexion, 20° of abduction, and 20° of external rotation.[43] Sporting activities require more motion.[43] The hip is subjected to significant joint forces of up to three times body weight in the early and late stance phase of walking and up to five times body weight with running.[61,63] The bony configuration, the ligaments, the labrum surrounding the acetabulum, a.nd the muscles surrounding the hip joint contribute to hip joint stability (Fig. 22-1).

There are several major muscle groups affecting pelvis, hip, and thigh motions. The abdominal group—the external obliques, the internal obliques, the transversus abdominis, and the rectus abdominis—is often overlooked regarding this function. They insert on the iliac wing and flex the trunk if the pelvis is fixed or flex the pelvis when the trunk is fixed. They are segmentally innervated.

The three gluteal muscles—the gluteus maximus, medius, and minimus—originate from the posterior and lateral ilium and insert onto the posterior femur and the greater trochanter. The gluteus maximus is the strongest hip joint extensor, which makes it especially important for running and jumping activities. It is innervated by the inferior gluteal nerve. The gluteus medius and minimus are abductors and internal rotators of the hip as is the tensor fascia femoris. Their innervation is derived from the superior gluteal nerve.

The three adductors—the adductor brevis, longus,

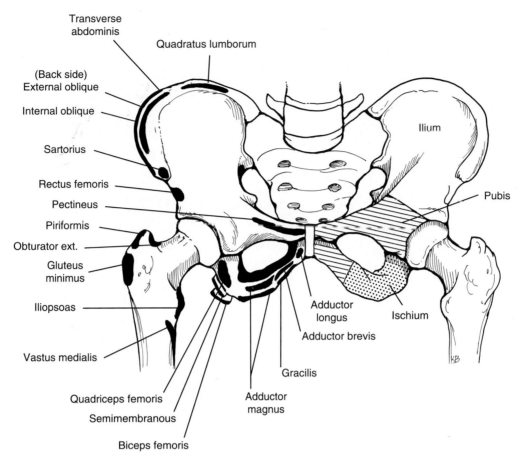

Transverse
abdominis

Quadratus lumborum

(Back side)
External oblique

Internal oblique

Sartorius

Rectus femoris

Pectineus

Piriformis

Obturator ext.

Gluteus
minimus

Iliopsoas

Vastus medialis

Quadriceps femoris

Semimembranous

Biceps femoris

Ilium

Pubis

Adductor
longus

Ischium

Adductor brevis

Gracilis

Adductor
magnus

Fig. 22-1. Diagram of the bony anatomy of the pelvis, hip, and thigh. Also included are selected muscle origins.

and magnus—originate from the pubis and insert onto the medial femur. These muscles adduct the hip and thigh. The gracilis and pectineus are often grouped with the adductors because they share a similar origin. However, the pectineus is actually a minor hip flexor and is innervated by the femoral nerve, whereas the adductors and the gracilis are innervated by the obturator nerve.

The iliopsoas is the primary muscle responsible for hip flexion. It originates from the transverse processes of the lumbar vertebrae and inserts onto the lesser trochanter of the femur. It is important with jumping and uphill running.

The sartorius muscle is a minor hip flexor and external rotator. Its origin is the anterior superior iliac spine of the pelvis, and it inserts onto the proximal medial tibia. Therefore, it crosses two joints and is subject to significant stresses; it is innervated by the femoral nerve.

The short external rotators of the hip include the piriformis, the obturator externus and internus, the superior and inferior gemelli, and the quadratus femoris. The gluteus maximus is the primary external rotator of the hip. As a group, the short external rotators originate from the pelvis about the ischium and insert onto and around the posterior greater trochanter of the femur.

It is simplest to view the thigh as being composed of

two compartments: the anterior and posterior, or flexor and extensor compartments, respectively. The anterior muscles are the quadriceps femoris, composed of the rectus femoris, the vastus medialis, the vastus lateralis, and the vastus intermedius, which is the deepest. The rectus femoris originates from the anterior inferior iliac spine of the pelvis and the anterior acetabulum and inserts via the patella onto the tibial tubercle of the proximal tibia. The other quadriceps muscles originate from the anterior proximal femur and share the same insertion as the rectus femoris. The rectus femoris is a hip flexor. It crosses the hip and knee joints, and, like the sartorius, it is more prone to injury because of greater applied stresses. The quadriceps muscle group is innervated by the femoral nerve.

The posterior thigh compartment contains the hamstring muscles. These are the semimembranosus, the semitendinososus, and the short and long head of the biceps femoris. The hamstrings originate from the ischial tuberosity and insert onto the proximal tibia and fibular head. The semimembranosus has a complex insertion that makes up a significant portion of the supporting posterior medial structures of the knee. The semitendinosus shares a common insertion onto the anterior tibia with the sartorius and the gracilis called the pes anserinus or *goose foot*.

The hamstrings cross the hip and knee joint and are also susceptible to injury because of this relationship.

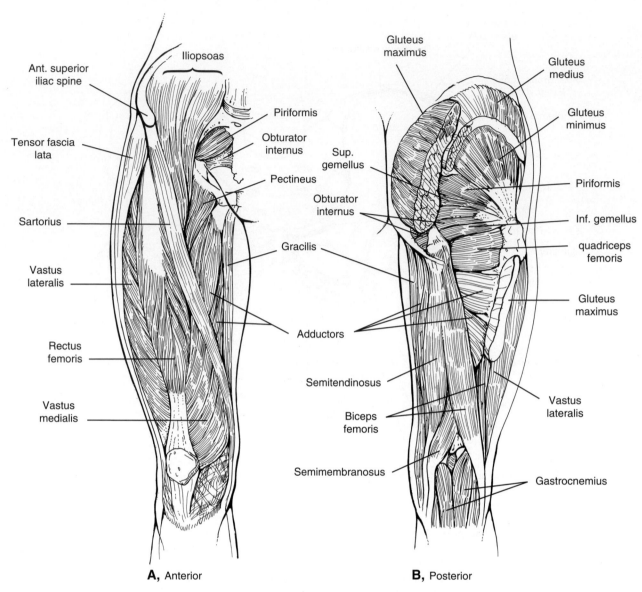

A, Anterior   **B,** Posterior

Fig. 22-2. Diagram of the muscles of the pelvis, hip, and thigh. **A,** Anterior view. **B,** Posterior view.

Primarily, they are hip extensors and knee flexors. However, they also affect rotatory motions to the thigh. The biceps femoris is an external rotator, and the semitendinosus affects internal rotation.[28] The hamstrings are innervated by the tibial division of the sciatic nerve, ex-

cept for the short head of the biceps femoris, which is innervated by the peroneal division of the sciatic nerve (Fig. 22-2 and Table 22-1).

The iliotibial band is the fascial extension of the tensor fascia femoris and the gluteus maximus. It traverses

Table 22-1. Muscle group functions

Muscle	Primary	Secondary
Hip flexors	Iliopsoas	Sartorius, quadriceps
Hip extensors	Gluteus maximus	Hamstrings
Hip abductors and internal rotators	Gluteus medius, gluteus minimus, tensor fascia lata	Gracilis
Hip adductors	Adductor magnus, adductor longus, adductor brevis	Pectineus, posterior gluteus maximus, quadratus femoris, hamstrings
External rotators	Gluteus maximus	Piriformis, biceps femoris, obturator internus and externus, superior and inferior gemelli, quadratus femoris

down the posterior lateral thigh to the lateral intermuscular septum and the vastus lateralis onto the proximal lateral tibia at Gerdy's tubercle.[29] It assists knee flexion and extension, depending on the starting position of the knee.

The major ligaments of the pelvis are those of the sacroiliac joint and those of the symphysis pubis. The suprapubic, the arcuate pubic, and interpubic ligaments support the symphysis pubis. The dorsal and anterior sacroiliac ligaments and the posterior interosseous are the primary ligaments supporting the sacroiliac joint. The sacrospinous and the sacrotuberous ligaments are accessory ligaments of the complex of the sacroiliac joint.

The hip joint has two major ligaments: the iliofemoral anteriorly and the ischiofemoral posteriorly. The pubofemoral is a minor hip joint ligament. These three

ligaments compose the hip capsule, which extends from the acetabulum anteriorly and posteriorly to the proximal femoral neck. The capsule tightens with internal rotation of the hip. The intracapsular blood supply to the femoral head and neck are from the retinacular vessels, which are branches of the medial and lateral circumflex femoral arteries.

The sensory dermatomes of the hip and thigh are important to know and assess during the physical examination. The inner thigh has a distribution of innervation from L1 to L4. The lateral thigh is innervated from L5, and the posterior thigh is innervated from S1 and S2 (Fig. 22-3).[38]

HISTORY AND PHYSICAL EXAMINATION

A time-honored adage of all fields of medicine is certainly applicable to the sports medicine physician—nothing can take the place of a thorough history and physical examination.

Particularly with the pelvis, hip, and thigh, the physical examination should proceed through several sequential steps. Observation of the athlete is the first phase, which includes observation in stance and during gait, looking for deformities, swelling, ecchymosis, and gait abnormalities. An examination with the athlete supine is the next step. Palpation should be performed eliciting asymmetry, tenderness, and spasm. The range of motion of the joints can then be assessed. This assessment must include the hip and the knee and spine. The joints above and below the affected area should be examined. Any contractures should be ruled out, which can be done using the Thomas test whereby both hips are initially flexed, and then one hip is extended. A lack of complete extension indicates a flexion contracture of the hip. Passive straight leg raising should be examined. If the knee begins to flex when the hip is flexed less than 60°, then the hamstrings are tight.

Next, a prone examination is performed and should include observation and palpation. Here, lack of flexion of the knee or hip flexion with attempted full knee flexion indicates tight anterior muscles. This is an Ely test. Finally, the athlete should be fully examined in the lateral decubitus position.

The next step is a radiographic analysis based on the findings elicited during the history and physical examination. Radiographs are a routine part of the examination because it may be difficult to differentiate a sprain from an avulsion fracture, especially in athletes with open growth centers. For pelvic injuries, an anteroposterior radiograph and inlet and outlet views (Fig. 22-4) and oblique, Judet,[44] (Fig. 22-5) views in some combination are necessary. A hip series includes anteroposterior and lateral radiographs, possibly anteroposterior radiographs with internal or external rotation of the hip. The femur requires anteroposterior and lateral radiographs to include the hip and knee joints.

Also, laboratory studies would be indicated based on the working diagnosis arrived at during the previously mentioned work-up.

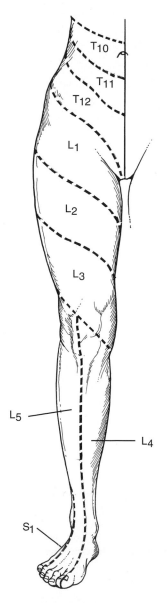

Fig. 22-3. Sensory dermatome innervation of the pelvis, hip, and thigh seen anteriorly.

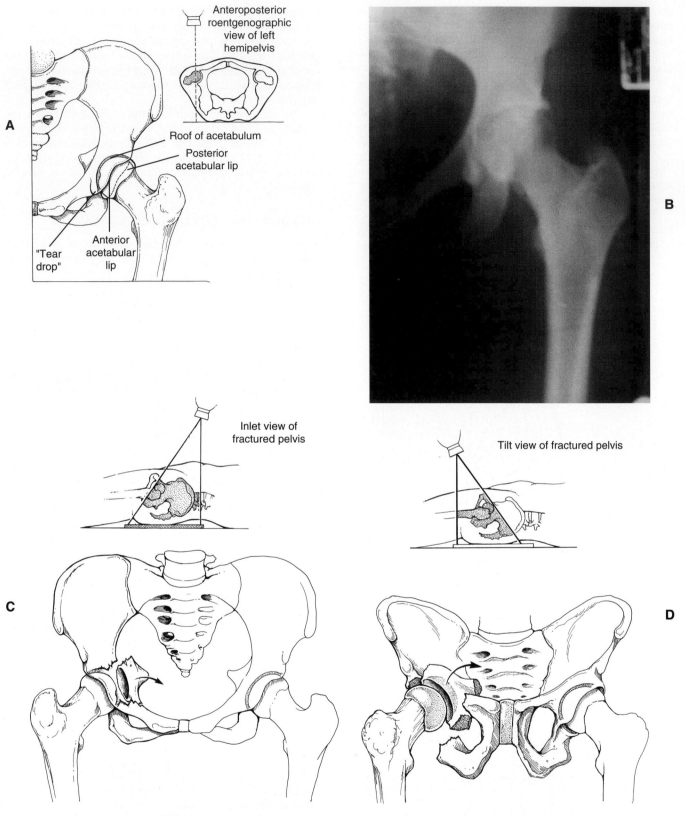

Fig. 22-4. A, Illustration of the technique used for patient positioning for obtaining hemipelvic radiographs. **B,** An anteroposterior radiograph of a hemipelvis. **C,** Illustration of a pelvic inlet view. The same position of the patient as for an anteroposterior view with the x-ray beam angled 25° caudally. **D,** Illustration of a pelvic outlet view. The x-ray beam is angled 35° cephalad.

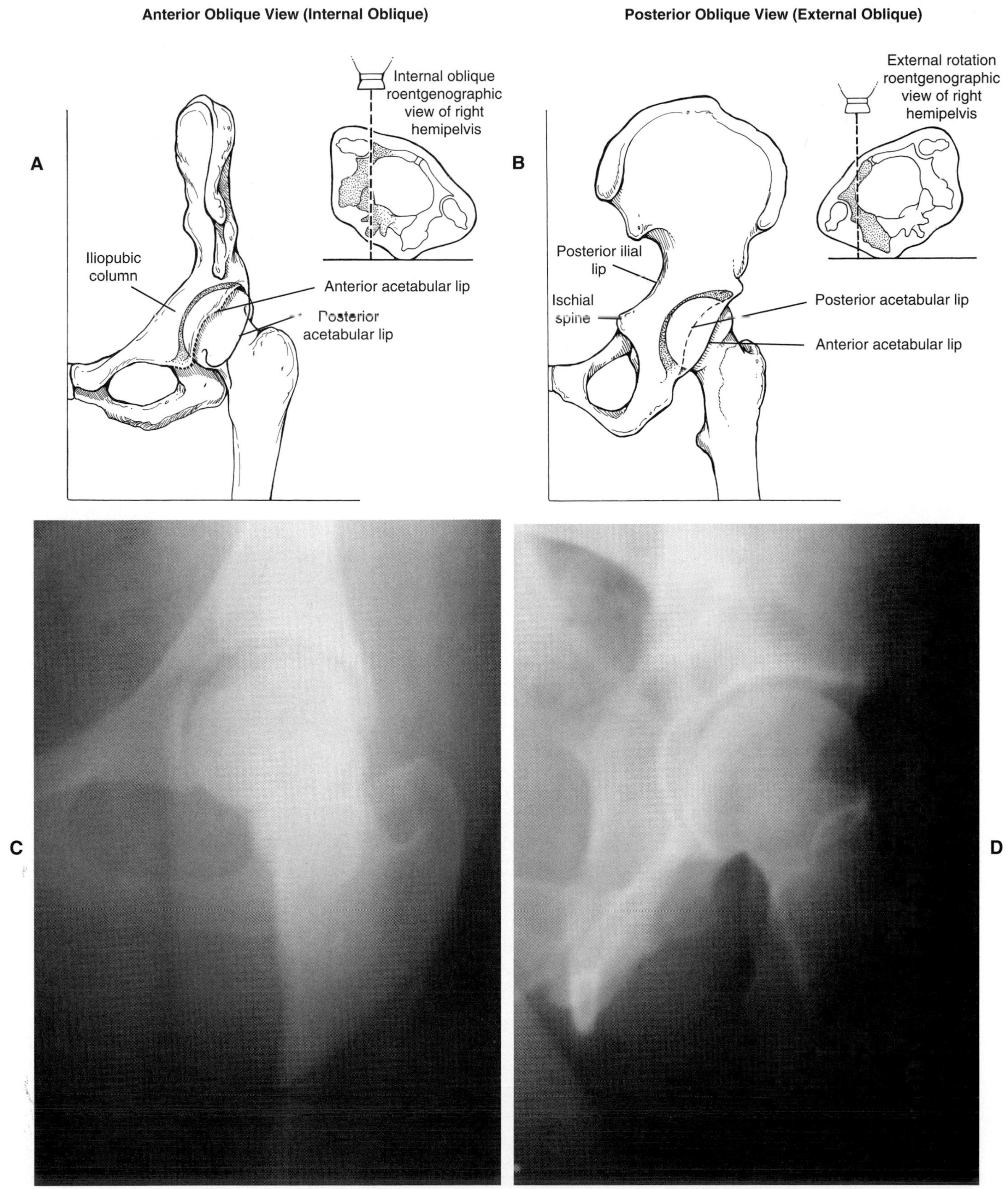

Anterior Oblique View (Internal Oblique)

A

Internal oblique roentgenographic view of right hemipelvis

Iliopubic column

Anterior acetabular lip

Posterior acetabular lip

Posterior Oblique View (External Oblique)

B

External rotation roentgenographic view of right hemipelvis

Posterior ilial lip

Ischial spine

Posterior acetabular lip

Anterior acetabular lip

C

D

Fig. 22-5. Oblique (Judet) views of the pelvis to better view the acetabulum. **A,** Anterior oblique view (internal oblique); an anteroposterior pelvic radiograph with the patient rotated 45° away from the injured side, which the iliopubic column and the posterior acetabular lip. **B,** Posterior oblique view (external oblique). The patient is rotated toward the affected side, which visualizes the posterior column and the anterior acetabular lip. **C,** Radiograph illustrating anterior oblique view. **D,** Radiograph illustrating posterior oblique view.

SOFT TISSUE INJURIES

Contusions

Soft tissue injuries are common in sports in general, but especially in the pelvis, hip, and thigh. Contusions, or bruises, are the most common of these injuries. Contusions can involve any structures from the skin superficially to the bones. Usually, they are of minor severity and are managed symptomatically.[94] However, these injuries often cause hematoma formation.[30] Radiographs of the affected area are necessary to exclude the possibility of a fracture or dislocation.

Contusions of the skin run the gamut of a simple ecchymosis to a more significant "raspberry," where the dermis is scraped, scabbed, rough, and tender. These are caused during sliding activities, especially on artificial turf or hard dirt. Management involves cleansing the area and applying topical antimicrobial agents. With activities, the region must be protected from further injury.

Muscle contusions are very common in the anterior and anterolateral thigh. Specifically, these contusions will involve the sartorius and the rectus femoris and are commonly referred to as the "Charley Horse" injury. They are caused by a significant blunt force being applied directly to the thigh, and may lead to hematoma or heterotopic ossification formation.

Bony contusions are deeper, involve greater force application, and take longer to resolve. The most common locations are the greater trochanter, the ischial tuberosity, the pubic ramus, and the sacrum. These bony areas are more superficial, with less soft-tissue coverings. "Hip pointers" are included among these injuries (Fig. 22-6). This term is confusing, but it typically involves a blunt-force injury to the iliac crest with subperiosteal

hematoma formation.[49] The hip pointer injury includes apophyseal avulsions and fractures and contusions of the iliac crest.[49] With a hip pointer, the athlete experiences difficulty with ambulation and with standing upright secondary to muscle spasm and pain.

In general, the symptoms involved with soft-tissue contusions are localized pain and tenderness acutely, which can become diffuse with time. The patient often will experience decreased range of motion and muscle spasm. Disuse atrophy of the surrounding musculature may ensue if the recovery process is prolonged by symptoms.

Management is similar to that used for all soft tissue injuries. The first component is rest, ice, compression, and elevation. A graduated therapy program then begins and is progressed as the patient tolerates. Later, heat and massage therapies and ultrasound and possibly transcutaneous electrical stimulation are used as adjunctive pain therapeutic modalities.

The first goal of the therapy program is to improve the symptoms. Then, restoring flexibility by stretching the surrounding muscles is instituted. Restoration of power, strength, and speed are the next goals to be attained. Therapy involves a progression from isometric exercises to isotonic exercises to isokinetic and dynamic resistant exercises. Aerobic reconditioning is essential. The final step of therapy is sports-specific rehabilitation (see box titled "Physiotherapy Principles"). Aspirin and nonsteroidal anti-inflammatory drugs (NSAIDs) must be used cautiously because they may increase the bleeding into the soft tissue[30] and aggravate the initial insult. Physiotherapy modalities and regimens will be discussed in greater detail in another chapter.

Return to sports is guided by the athlete's symptoms and objective evidence of functional normalcy including

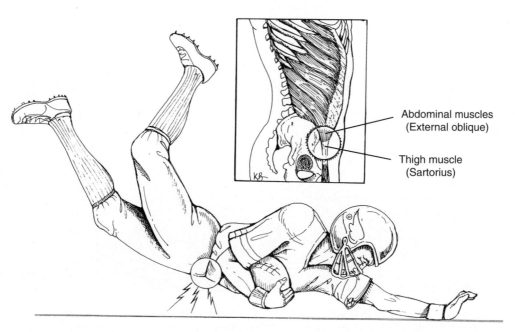

Abdominal muscles
(External oblique)

Thigh muscle
(Sartorius)

Fig. 22-6. Illustration of the mechanism of a hip pointer. A direct blow causes a contusion to the iliac crest.

PHYSIOTHERAPY PRINCIPLES

1. First resolve symtoms*
2. Stretch affected muscles
3. Regain muscle power and strengh and flexibility
4. Regain endurance and aerobic conditioning†
5. Sport-specific training‡

*Rest, ice, NSAIDs, etc.
†When 95% ROM, 75% strength of uninjured leg attained.
‡Sports return when 90% strength of uninjured leg attained.

ETIOLOGY OF MUSCLE INJURIES

Poor flexibility

Poor coordination

Poor warm-up

Muscle strength imbalance

Muscle weakness

Fatigue

Electrolyte imbalance

Poor technique with sports activity

Increased age

coordination, strength, speed, endurance, and painless athletic participation.[30]

Several diagnoses must be considered when a probable soft-tissue contusion is encountered about the pelvis, hip, and thigh in the athlete, e.g., a sciatic nerve contusion. Buttock pain and pain in the sciatic nerve distribution, possibly to the first web space in the foot, would be reported. Also, crush injuries and compartment syndrome must be included in the differential diagnosis with severe soft-tissue injuries. Crush injuries and compartment syndrome involve a rather tense thigh with the mechanism of injury imparting a significant amount of energy to the region. The examining physician must have a high index of suspicion of thigh compartment syndrome because the symptoms may be subtle with pain and sensory abnormalities and only a mildly swollen thigh. If this diagnosis is suspected, compartment pressures must be measured in the offending compartment. If they are within 20 mm Hg of the diastolic pressure, emergent operative release of all offending fascial compartments must be performed.

The most common long term-complications of soft-tissue contusions are bursitis and the formation of heterotopic ossification, or myositis ossificans. Either one of these conditions can significantly prolong and impede an athlete's rehabilitation and return to sporting activities.

MUSCLE INJURIES

Muscle injuries are extremely common in sports, and are the most common athletic injuries of the pelvis, hip, and thigh. They usually are minor strains, which are tears or "pulls" at the musculotendinous junction.[100] It is important for the examining and treating physician to distinguish between partial and complete tears. The mechanism of injury involves violent contractions with forceful stretching of the involved muscle.[23] This contracting and stretching cause increased energy to be absorbed in the muscle, which exceeds its ultimate tensile strength. This same mechanism causes avulsion fractures in skeletally immature athletes because the tendons are stronger than the cartilage growth plate.

Risk factors for muscle injuries include inadequate flexibility and warm-up, muscle strength imbalances, muscle weakness, electrolyte imbalance, and increased age. Preconditioning and stretching to increase blood flow to the muscles and to increase their ability to absorb energy decreases the incidence of muscle injuries (see box above).[80]

Physical therapy regimens are progressed as was previously discussed with soft-tissue contusions. Surgery is warranted only for complete tears.

Hamstrings

The hamstring muscles are the most commonly involved muscular injury of the pelvis, hip, and thigh.[49] The injuries often occur at the musculotendinous junction with forced flexion of the hip with a fully extended knee, or when the hamstrings are maximally stretched. The symptoms are posterior thigh pain, possibly a "pop" being felt, and difficulty ambulating. Sports activities are inhibited, and a defect may be palpated with the athlete prone with the knee flexed against resistance. The symptoms are exacerbated by knee extension while the hip is flexed. The medial hamstrings—the semimembranosus and the semitendinosus—are usually injured during the swing phase of the gait cycle, whereas the lateral hamstrings—the biceps femoris—are injured during the foot take-off phase of the gait cycle.[10] The biceps femoris are the most commonly injured. Hamstring injuries occur primarily in runners because they are antagonists to hip flexion and knee extension, which is an important position of the limb during running. The hamstrings are at increased risk for injury because they cross two joints, the hip and knee joints.

Risk factors for hamstring injuries are poor technique with athletic activities, such as warm-up, stretching, and posture. Poor flexibility, endurance, leg length discrepancy, and muscle strength imbalance will increase the susceptibility to hamstring injuries.[52] These and all muscle injuries are clinically classified according to the degree of symptoms and injury. Symptom severity can increase up to 2 weeks after the injury.[41]

A first degree hamstring injury resolves in a few days with little hemorrhage, no structural damage, and without any objective evidence of functional loss. Second degree injuries are of moderate severity and represent a partial tear of the muscle with some functional loss. A "pop" is usually heard, and structural damage is present. A painful mass may be palpated posteriorly in the muscle

Table 22-2. Muscle injury classification

Degree	Severity	Structural damage	Functional loss	Recovery time
1st	Mild	None	None to mild	Several days
2nd	Moderate	Partial tear	Mild to moderate	1–3 weeks
3rd	Severe	Complete tear	Moderate to severe	Several weeks

belly. Third degree injuries are severe, complete tears, usually occurring near the origin or insertion of the muscle. A mass is also palpable in the muscle belly (Table 22-2).[52]

Radiographs should be taken to rule out an avulsion fracture of the ischial tuberosity.

Return to sports activities is allowed when the isokinetic strength is within 10% of the uninjured side and when the other criteria that were previously discussed with soft-tissue injuries are attained.[52]

Quadriceps Femoris

The quadriceps femoris consists of four muscles, of which only the rectus femoris crosses the hip and knee joints. Maximal activity in this muscle group occurs during the heel-off phase of the gait cycle,[17] which coincides with maximal hamstring activity. The quadriceps also function as a decelerator during the support phase of running.[87] The classification of injuries is similar to that for hamstring injuries, except that knee range of motion is also used as a criterion to classify quadriceps injuries. In a first degree injury, the athlete can flex the knee at least 90°. With a second degree injury, the athlete can flex the knee between 45° and 90°, and a third degree injury limits the athlete's knee flexion to less than 45° (Table 22-3).[41]

The symptoms experienced with quadriceps injuries include pain, spasm, and diminished knee flexion. The limited motion becomes more evident with hip extension if the rectus femoris is primarily involved. The more significantly the motion is restricted, the longer the recovery takes. Hematoma formation is usually evident, but a mass may not be palpable. Radiographic examination is important to rule out a fracture and to assess any heterotopic ossification, especially in chronic injuries.

Complications are relatively common with anterior

Table 22-3. Quadriceps contusion classification

Contusion	Knee motion (°)	Gait	Physical examination
Mild	>90	Normal	Mildly tender
Moderate	45–90	Antalgic	Tender, large thigh
Severe	<45	Antalgic	Very swollen thigh, painful contraction

thigh muscle injuries. The most common is an extensor lag or weakness and decreased knee flexion. Reruptures and heterotopic ossification formation are more common with complete tears.

Therapy progresses as has already been elucidated. Operative repair usually is necessary for complete tears of the lower-to-middle third of the rectus femoris.[41]

Sports activity return is guided by the principles previously stated. Also, the athlete must have painless motion within 10° of the uninjured side.[41]

Adductors

The adductors are injured when the thigh is externally rotated and the hip is abducted.[57] This position places maximal stretch on this muscle group. An injury to the adductors is the "groin pull."[30] It also has been referred to as "horse rider's" strain. This injury is more common in professional and older athletes. The etiology of adductor strains is an imbalance of strength between muscle groups and within the adductor group itself.[57]

Symptomatology includes pain from the groin to the middle medial thigh, especially in the region of the adductor longus tendon. The pain is worsened with hip abduction.[57] A defect or mass may be palpable over the medial thigh if the tear is complete. These injuries are rarely severe, although power deficits up to 25% have been reported with this injury.[58] The differential diagnosis includes an abdominal muscle injury,[89] an avulsion fracture of the pubis, or osteitis pubis. A bone scan is useful in the early detection of the latter two injuries.

Management proceeds as previously mentioned. In addition, an operative tenotomy of the adductor longus has been advocated with chronic injuries.[74] Athletic return is guided by the same parameters as for quadriceps injuries.

Other Muscles

The external oblique muscles can be torn at their insertion onto the iliac crests. This injury results from muscle contraction while the trunk is flexed toward the opposite side. The symptoms include pain and tenderness with flexion toward the contralateral side and difficulty straightening the torso. Management is guided by the symptoms and involves restriction from activities, a protective pad, and possibly abdominal binders.

The iliopsoas can also be injured, especially with muscle contraction when the hip is fixed in extension. The symptoms are deep groin pain or lower abdominal tenderness. Passive external rotation of the hip exacerbates the pain because this position increases the stretch of the iliopsoas.

When the gluteus medius is injured chronically, tendinitis will often ensue. The athlete will experience posterior greater trochanteric pain.

The gracilis is often injured with the adductor muscles. Its symptoms and management are the same as for that muscle group.

MYOSITIS OSSIFICANS TRAUMATICA

Myositis ossificans traumatica is heterotopic ossification that occurs in a muscle belly or periosteum after trauma, particularly blunt trauma. It is second only to

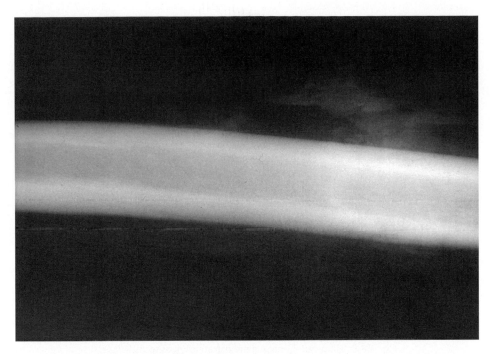

Fig. 22-7. A lateral radiograph of the mid-shaft of the femur demonstrating myositis ossificans traumatica adjacent to, but not connected to, the cortex.

muscle injuries in frequency of injury in the thigh. The thigh is more commonly involved than the hip (Fig. 22-7).

This is a reactive condition[42] secondary to a soft-tissue injury with hematoma formation. Granulation and scar tissue form secondarily,[93] with calcification developing in the affected area in approximately 3 to 4 weeks.[65] Myositis ossificans is usually located deep near muscle origins, especially about fractures and joints.[2] The exact etiology has not been determined.[99] However, athletes with blood dyscrasias may be predisposed to develop this condition with even minor injuries. Risk factors for development of myositis ossificans include a severe injury, reinjury during the early healing stage, delay in management of muscle injury, a previous history of development of myositis, early vigorous physiotherapy, and surgery before maturity of the lesion (see box below). The overall prognosis is usually excellent.[41,53]

RISK FACTORS FOR MYOSITIS OSSIFICANS TRAUMATICA

Severe injury

Reinjury during early recovery phase

Delay in treatment of muscle injury

Previous history of myositis ossificans

Early vigorous massage and heat with physiotherapy

Surgery before lesion maturity

Myositis ossificans traumatica has been reported to occur in up to 20% of military recruits with thigh contusions.[41] It is less common after thigh muscle strains. The diagnosis should be considered in any athlete with a firm mass at the original sight of injury that develops after 3 to 4 weeks.[1] The athlete will present with a painful and sometimes palpable mass that causes a decreased range of motion.[30] The symptoms also include local swelling, tenderness, and possibly erythema and increased local temperature.

Radiographic examination of the affected area is important to exclude a fracture and to sequentially follow the development and maturation of the myositis. However, the radiographs may not be positive for 2 to 4 weeks.[1,49] The growth of the mass on radiographs stabilizes at 6 months. Ultrasonography has been reported to detect early changes in the soft tissues indicative of the development of myositis ossificans (Fig. 22-8).[47]

Myositis ossificans may be confused with a periosteal osteogenic sarcoma. These two entities are distinguished based on the history, radiographic location of the mass, and the histologic analysis. Myositis ossificans has an antecedent traumatic event, and the athlete is usually aged less than 30 years. The mass involves the anterior thigh in the majority of patients and stabilizes at 6 months. The alkaline phosphatase is normal, and the radiographs usually will demonstrate a separation between the cortex of the bone and the mass.

With periosteal osteogenic sarcoma, however, the affected individuals are older without an antecedent traumatic event being elicited in the history. The alkaline phosphatase is elevated, and the mass demonstrates continued growth. On radiographic analysis, the mass is contiguous with the cortex of the bone.[65]

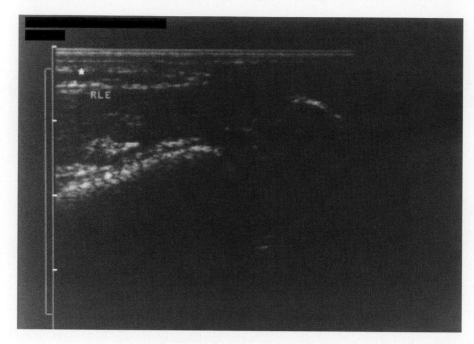

Fig. 22-8. Ultrasound image demonstrating myositis ossificans.

Furthermore, on histologic examination, the abnormal cells are noted at the periphery of the lesion of the sarcoma, whereas they are centrally located with myositis ossificans. The previously mentioned points of differentiation should help avoid performing a biopsy (Table 22-4).[65]

Management is similar to that for other soft-tissue injuries. Bedrest may be necessary if the symptoms are severe. Partial weight-bearing with crutches may be instituted until the pain subsides. NSAIDs should be used cautiously because they can exacerbate the condition by increasing the local bleeding at the injury sight. Massage and manipulation must be avoided because they can increase hematoma formation.[2]

The physiotherapy program begins when the athlete is pain-free. Passive range of motion should be avoided for 4 to 6 months.[30] If the functional return is inhibited by the soft-tissue mass, surgery and excision may be necessary. Surgery and excision should not be performed until the mass matures at 9 to 12 months.[66] If done before, the myositis will recur with greater intensity and quantity. Aspiration and injection of proteolytic enzymes have been used but are better considered experimental modalities at this time.[1,66]

Return to sports is allowed when full strength and agility are obtained, and the athlete can flex the knee 120°.[41] A protective pad over the affected area should be worn.

BURSITIS

The development of a bursitis is very common. Pathology involves an inflammation of the lining, bursa, surrounding bony edges, and joints. The condition is caused by friction from overuse or after trauma from a direct blow to the area that produces an inflammatory response. Classically, the athlete experiences pain that increases with motion and localized tenderness and fullness. Motion is restricted secondary to the pain, and an audible "snapping" may develop if the condition is chronic.

Bursitis usually develops over the ischial tuberosity, iliopectineal region (Fig. 22-9), and the greater trochanter.[66] Ischial bursitis, "benchwarmer's bursitis," is painful when seated and must be differentiated from a hamstring injury.[71] Pain is likely secondary to sciatic nerve irritation.

Iliopectineal bursitis causes anterior hip pain and an antalgic gait. The symptoms are lessened with flexion and external rotation of the hip.[21] With trochanteric bursitis, adduction and external rotation of the hip worsens the symptoms. Risk factors for developing

Table 22-4. Differential diagnosis of myositis ossificans traumatica and osteogenic sarcoma

	Myositis ossificans	Osteogenic sarcoma
Antecedent trauma	+	−
Location of mass	Diaphyseal	Metaphyseal
Status of cortex	Intact	Violated
Histology	Peripheral cells mature	Central cells mature
Symptoms	Pain with activity	Rest and night pain
Size	Decreases with time	Increases with time
Alkaline phosphatase	Normal	Increased

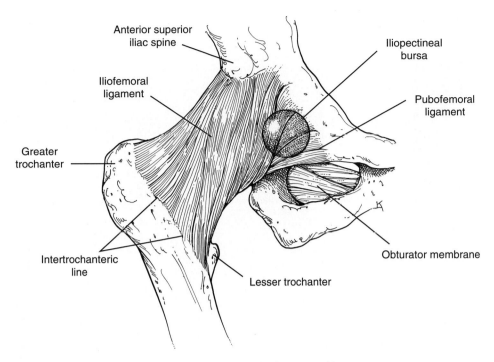

Anterior superior
iliac spine

Iliofemoral
ligament

Greater
trochanter

Intertrochanteric
line

Lesser trochanter

Iliopectineal
bursa

Pubofemoral
ligament

Obturator membrane

Fig. 22-9. Illustration of the iliopectineal bursa.

trochanteric bursitis include a broad pelvis, which is postulated as the reason for the increased incidence in female athletes. Leg-length discrepancy, pronated feet, previous injuries to the area, and abnormal running mechanics, such as the feet crossing the midline, are other factors that increase the likelihood of developing this condition.[30]

Management is similar to that for other soft-tissue injuries. NSAIDs play a major role. Aspiration of the bursa and steroid injection may be beneficial if the symptoms persists. With chronicity of the condition, operative excision or release of the offending bursa may be indicated,[68] but only as a final resort.

SNAPPING HIP SYNDROME

Snapping hip syndrome refers to conditions about the hip that cause an audible or palpable "snapping." In addition, the athlete may experience tenderness or occasional pain, crepitation, and local warmth. The athlete's performance is rarely impaired by this syndrome.

There are intraarticular and extraarticular etiologies for this syndrome.[101] The most common etiology involves the iliotibial band or tensor fascia lata moving over the greater trochanter.[94] It can also involve the iliopsoas tendon gliding over the iliopectineal eminence in the pelvis or the iliofemoral ligament moving over the femoral head.[94] Posteriorly, the long head of the biceps femoris tendon gliding over the ischial tuberosity can cause this syndrome. Loose bodies, labral tears, synovial chondromatosis, bony exostosis, and subluxation of the hip joint can also produce the snapping hip syndrome.[60,101] Furthermore, women with a wide pelvis, prominent trochanter, and ligament laxity are at increased risk for this condition.

Management involves observation and is symptomatically guided. If signs of inflammation are elicited, NSAIDs should be used. Surgery is rare.

OSTEITIS PUBIS

Osteitis pubis is a self-limited[67] condition caused by inflammation and a reactive periostitis leading to bony changes of the symphysis pubis. Histologic analysis demonstrates a nonspecific inflammatory response with bone resorption and fibrous tissue replacement. The etiologies are a continuum along the spectrum of musculoskeletal injuries and include muscle strains with degenerative changes secondary to overuse, avascular necrosis, an osteochondral defect, a fatigue fracture, and an avulsion fracture by the gracilis tendon.[97] The condition has also been seen in postpartum women.

The athlete may experience gradual, insidious groin pain, possibly with radiation to the medial thigh and lower abdomen.[30] Tenderness over the pubis may also be elicited. Muscle spasm may be present, particularly in the rectus abdominis and the adductors. Abduction and resisted adduction and pivoting with sports activities increases the pain. Severe symptoms can cause an antalgic or a waddling gait and a clicking sensation, which is known to occur after surgery on the bladder and prostate.[4]

Radiographic findings take approximately 2 to 3 weeks to appear.[97] The findings include symmetrical bone resorption medially, widening of the symphysis, rarefaction or sclerosis of the symphysis, and possibly cystic changes (Fig. 22-10).[33] If cystic changes are present, the physician must also consider hyperparathyroidism, myelomatosis, sarcoidosis, hemochromatosis, rheumatoid arthritis, and osteomyelitis in the differen-

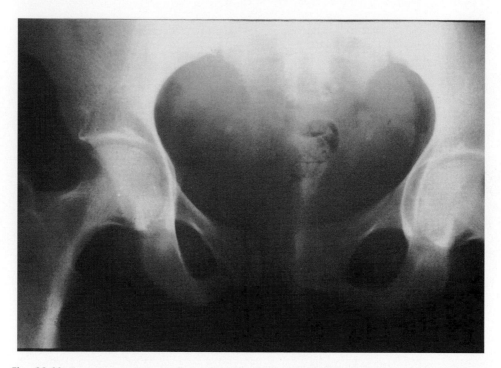

Fig. 22-10. An anteroposterior radiograph of the pelvis demonstrating widening of the symphysis pubis consistent with osteitis pubis.

tial diagnosis.[33] Clinically, the differential diagnosis includes a hernia.

Bone scans demonstrating increased uptake can aid in the early detection of this syndrome.[97] Comparison, weight-bearing views, so-called "flamingo" views, will detect if instability is present. These are taken as two separate radiographs, each one in single leg stance, one with the right leg down and the second with the left leg down. A difference of more than 2 mm in height from a line drawn parallel to the top of the superior pubic ramus on one side of the symphysis pubis to the other is indicative of instability.[7]

Management is symptomatically based. Rest and NSAIDs are the mainstays of treatment. Injection of steroids may also be used. Recalcitrant symptoms may necessitate fusion or debridement of the symphysis.[67,97]

ADDUCTOR CANAL SYNDROME

Another condition that may affect the athlete's thigh is the rare adductor canal syndrome, which involves a disruption or compression[3] of the femoral artery at Hunter's Canal in the middle third of the anterior thigh. This canal is bordered by the vastus medialis anterolaterally, the sartorius medially, and the adductor longus posterolaterally.[29] The femoral artery and vein and the saphenous nerve pass through this space.

The exact etiology of this syndrome is unclear. It is usually caused by direct trauma leading to thrombosis of the femoral artery. However, an abnormal muscle band from the adductor magnus to the vastus medialis has also been implicated.[91]

Symptoms include leg claudication, which worsens with activity and resolves with rest. The physical examination is normal except for absent or diminished pulses. The athlete will have an abnormal response to exercise, with claudication developing, and will have a decreased ankle brachial index.[91] When the saphenous nerve is affected by the syndrome, the athlete will experience anterior and medial knee pain and possibly dysesthesias.[77] In this case, the symptoms will resolve with injection of a local anaesthetic.

The diagnostic work-up includes pulse volume recordings[50] or arteriography[91] to diagnose arterial abnormalities. The Doppler ankle brachial index can be used as a noninvasive screening test. If results are abnormal, arteriography must be performed. If the superficial femoral artery is determined to be occluded, operative intervention to bypass this lesion is necessary. When recovered, a protective pad for the region should be used during sports participation.

FRACTURES

Pelvis

Pelvic fractures result from very high energy forces in young patients and from lower energy injuries in elderly athletes (Fig. 22-11). Pelvic fractures are rarely incurred by the athlete. The mechanism of injury is either a direct or rotational force application to the pelvis. Collision sports, such as football or rugby, can cause this injury. Other high risk sports include hang gliding, auto racing, and snowmobiling. A thorough physical examination is necessary to assess the neu-

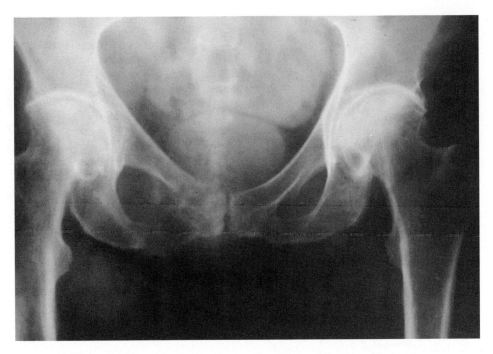

Fig. 22-11. An anteroposterior radiograph of the pelvis demonstrating superior and inferior pubic rami fractures on the right side.

rovascular status of the limbs and to exclude any visceral damage to the gastrointestinal or genitourinary tracts; 10% to 30% of pelvic fractures have these associated injuries.[9]

Pelvic fractures are classified as either stable or unstable. One-third of all pelvic fractures are unstable.[9] Stable fractures are single bone fractures that do not involve displacement of the fracture or disruption of the pelvic ring. They are caused by a direct blow to the affected bone. Management is symptomatically guided. A fracture of the iliac wing, sacrum, coccyx, and ischium are examples of stable fractures (Fig. 22-12). With these single bone fractures, it is essential that the examining physician exclude the possibility of second fracture site in the pelvic ring, indicating potential instability. Three classic examination maneuvers are performed to assess instability. First, posterior pressure is applied to the iliac crests, and then lateral-to-medial pressure is applied. Finally, downward pressure on the symphysis pubis is performed. Excessive pain or gross motion may indicate an unstable injury pattern.[45] Even in the most experienced hands, pelvic fractures are difficult to assess by physical examination alone.

Unstable pelvis or acetabular fractures less commonly result from sports activities.[94] Unstable fractures include displaced fractures, fractures with dislocations, or joint separations (Fig. 22-13). Accurate reduction of these fractures and maintenance of the reduction are imperative.

Radiographic analysis must include anteroposterior, lateral, inlet and outlet views, and oblique views of the pelvis. Analgesics and appropriate intravenous hydration or blood products are the initial mainstays of treatment. Additional management is guided by the fracture type.

Protected weight-bearing is begun when tolerated if the fracture is stable or after operative fixation of unstable fractures.

Hip

Hip fractures also rarely result from athletic participation. The mechanism of injury involves a high energy trauma being applied to the femoral shaft, a rotational force application to the proximal femur, especially in an older patient, or a direct blow to the greater trochanter. Symptoms are severe groin pain. The athlete is unable to bear weight unless the fracture is an impacted subcapital hip fracture or a rare greenstick fracture, occurring in a skeletally immature athlete. With displacement, the leg is held in an externally rotated and shortened position. With nondisplaced fractures, the athlete holds the leg externally rotated because this position is comfortable. Attempts at motion are resisted secondary to pain (Fig. 22-14 on page 322).

Management is urgent reduction to attain anatomic union because the athlete cannot function well with a significant leg-length discrepancy or rotational malalignment. Disruption of the blood supply to the femoral head with ensuing avascular necrosis[21] can be devastating and may occur even with prompt intervention. Skeletally immature athletes may develop premature growth-plate closure, causing a varus deformity as a result of this injury.

The classification of hip injuries in skeletally immature patients is based on location in relation to the growth plate. Commonly, the athlete affected is aged 11 to 13 years.[72] A type I fracture is transepiphyseal; type II is transcervical; type III is cervicotrochanteric; and type

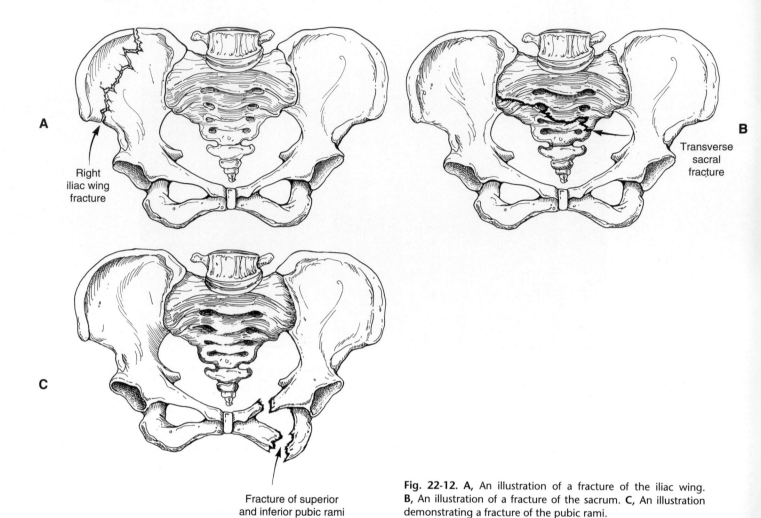

Right iliac wing fracture

Transverse sacral fracture

Fracture of superior and inferior pubic rami

Fig. 22-12. A, An illustration of a fracture of the iliac wing. **B,** An illustration of a fracture of the sacrum. **C,** An illustration demonstrating a fracture of the pubic rami.

IV is an intertrochanteric fracture (Fig. 22-15). Surgery is indicated for type I and II fractures and for a type III fracture if it is displaced. The type IV fracture can be managed with traction and spica casting in the very young skeletally immature athlete.[13] The adolescent will need operative fixation.

Potential complications from hip fractures can occur in up to 60% of patients.[85] Avascular necrosis of the femoral head may occur in up to one-third of hip fractures. The chance of developing avascular necrosis depends on fracture location and the amount of displacement. The rate with a type I fracture is 100%; with type II fracture, the incidence is 15% to 50%; and with a type III fracture, the reported incidence is 30% to 40%.[40] Avascular necrosis rarely develops with intertrochanteric fractures. Varus deformity secondary to physeal injury can also occur.

Coccyx

Fractures of the coccyx do not commonly result from sports activities. These fractures are sustained when the athlete falls in a seated position or by a direct blow.[30] Symptoms include lower spine and buttock pain that is worse when seated. The pain is localized over the coccyx either externally or internally elicited by a rectal examination. Radiographs should be taken although they may be difficult to interpret because of the overlying bowel gas patterns. Management is symptomatically guided with NSAIDs or analgesics and donut pads while seated. Warm sitz baths may reduce local muscle spasm. Sports activities are begun when the athlete is pain-free. A protective pad should be used over the coccyx. A painful ununited fracture may require operative excision.

Avulsion

Avulsion fractures more commonly occur in skeletally immature athletes because the tendons are stronger than the cartilaginous growth centers. However, adults can sustain this injury, too. The age range of patients affected is reported to be from 14 to 25 years of age.[96] In the skeletally immature athlete, these fractures occur at secondary growth centers, apophyses, which become separated from the underlying bone. The fractures occur before the secondary ossification centers appear on radiographs. The fractures do not displace widely secondary to the surrounding thick periosteum. The mechanism of injury involves a very strong muscular contraction against the weaker cartilage apophysis (Fig. 22-16 on page 324).[58] Radiographic analysis is

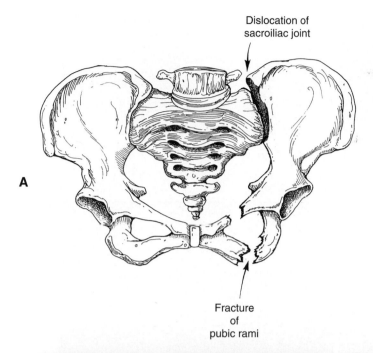

Dislocation of sacroiliac joint

Fracture of pubic rami

A

Fig. 22-13. A, An illustration of an unstable Malgaigne fracture, which involves two vertical fractures on the same side of the pelvis with a dislocation of sacrolliac joint. **B,** A CAT scan demonstrating the normal relationship between the acetabulum and the femoral head. **C,** A CAT scan showing a fracture of the acetabulum with disruption of the normal congruity between the acetabulum and the femoral head with medial wall fracture.

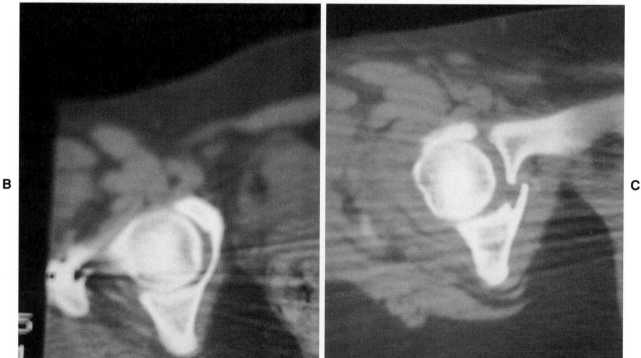

B

C

used to exclude apophysitis, which is an inflammation of the secondary growth centers and causes similar symptoms to avulsion fractures.

Symptoms include localized pain, tenderness, swelling, and sometimes ecchymosis. The functional limitations depend on the specific muscle involved. Radiographs of the affected location must be taken along with comparison views of the uninjured side. Management is symptomatically guided with positioning to relieve the tension of the offending muscle. Protected weight-bearing and a graduated therapy program ensue as the symptoms subside. Usually, these fractures can be managed nonop-

eratively. Some authors recommend operative fixation in competitive athletes to avoid late onset functional disability.[83]

ILIAC CREST. Iliac crest avulsion fractures result from a twisting injury while the trunk is abducted. The iliac crest fuses at age 16 years in boys and at age 14 in girls. It fuses beginning on the anterolateral crest and progressing to the posterior crest.[75] Pain to palpation over the iliac crest that worsens with resisted abduction is a characteristic finding with this avulsion fracture. Oblique radiographs and comparison views are needed to diagnose this condition.[27] Management involves par-

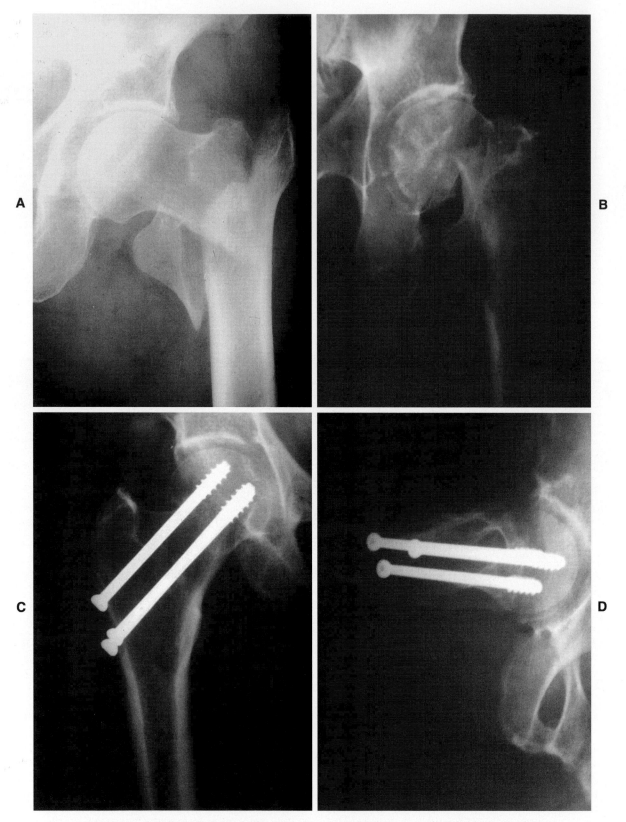

Fig. 22-14. Radiographic examples of intertrochanteric and femoral neck hip fractures. **A,** Three-part intertrochanteric fracture. **B,** Femoral neck fracture. **C,** Anteroposterior view after open reduction and internal fixation with cannulated lag screws for a nondisplaced femoral neck fracture. **D,** Lateral view.

Pediatric hip fracture classifications

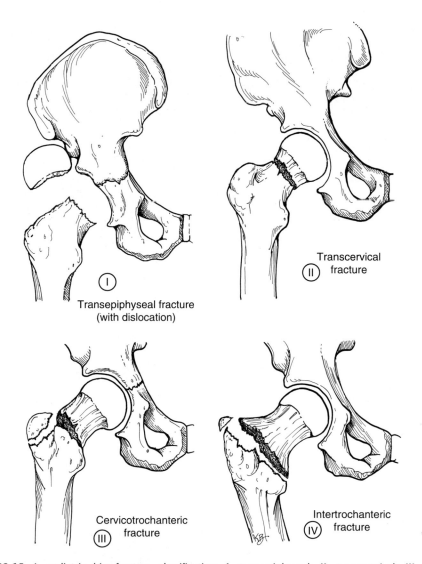

Fig. 22-15. A pediatric hip fracture classification. **I**, transepiphyseal; **II**, transcervical; **III**, cervicotrochanteric; and **IV**, intertrochanteric.

tial weight-bearing with crutches for 5 to 7 days with analgesics as needed. The symptoms will resolve within 4 to 6 weeks. At that time, the weight-bearing status can be advanced, and sporting activities resumed as symptoms resolve.

ANTERIOR SUPERIOR AND ANTERIOR INFE-RIOR ILIAC SPINE. The sartorius is the muscle that causes an anterior superior iliac spine avulsion fracture, which is more common in running and jumping sports.[21] Active flexion and passive extension of the hip worsen the symptoms. The avulsed fragment may be palpated in some patients.

The direct head of the rectus femoris causes anterior inferior iliac spine avulsions (Fig. 22-17), which are less common than anterior superior iliac spine avulsions because less stresses are borne here and because this apophysis fuses at an earlier age.[73] Localized pain and weakness with hip flexion are experienced by the athlete. Active hip flexion exacerbates the symptoms. Radiographs of

comparison views are needed. An accessory ossicle of the acetabulum, a normal variant, should be excluded. If present, it often will be noted bilaterally. Management is similar to that for other avulsion fractures.

ISCHIAL APOPHYSIS. Avulsion fractures of the ischial apophysis are also called "hurdler's" fractures. The hamstrings are responsible for this avulsion fracture, which occurs at a later age because the ischial apophysis fuses when the athlete is aged 20 to 25 years.[13] This fracture occurs when the hamstrings strongly contract while the pelvis is fixed and flexed and the knee is extended. The patient experiences substantial disability and difficulty with prolonged sitting and pain when the thigh is flexed with the knee extended. A controversy exists regarding conservative management versus excising the fragment. A 68% rate of ununited fractures has been reported.[58] Most orthopedists would only consider operative excision for exuberant, painful callus formation.

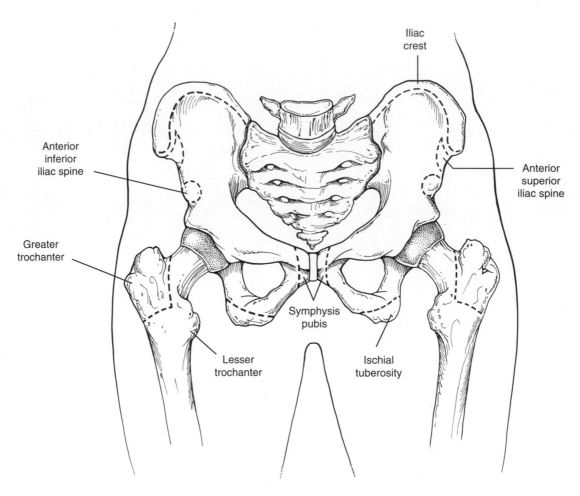

Fig. 22-16. Diagram of potential areas of avulsion fractures from the pelvic apophyses.

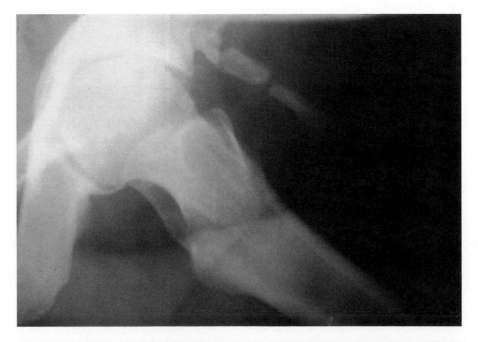

Fig. 22-17. A skeletally mature individual sustained an avulsion fracture of the anterior inferior iliac spine from the pull of the rectus, which is seen on a lateral radiograph as a late finding with calcification of the proximal rectus muscle.

GREATER AND LESSER TROCHANTER AND ACETABULAR LIP. Avulsion fractures of the greater and lesser trochanter are very rare, accounting for only 1% of all hip injuries.[58] Still more rare is the acetabula lip avulsion fracture (Fig. 22-18).

Avulsions of the lesser trochanter are caused by the pull of the iliopsoas muscle. Eighty-five percent of these fractures occur when the athlete is aged less than 20 years.[16] The patient will experience anteromedial thigh pain and difficulty elevating the leg with the knee extended. The athlete holds the thigh flexed and adducted. The radiograph must be taken in slight external rotation of the hip to demonstrate the fracture. Management is the same as for other avulsion fractures.

Greater trochanter avulsion fractures are caused by the pull of the abductor muscles (Fig. 22-19). Acetabular lip avulsions are caused by the forceful pull of the hip capsule.

Stress Fractures

The etiology of stress fractures is not fully elucidated. However, they involve a progressive imbalance between the force absorbed by the bone and the ability of the bone to withstand this force. Thus, they involve an imbalance between the degree of force application and the bone strength.[22] It has been postulated that repeated

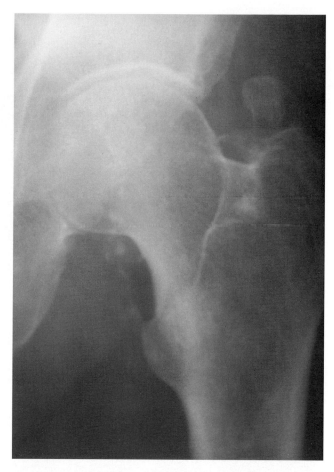

Fig. 22-19. A radiograph demonstrating an avulsion fracture of the greater trochanter, which is caused by the pull from the abductor muscles.

submaximal stress causes muscle fatigue,[11,31] as the constant bending of a coat hanger will weaken it. This fatigue allows excessive force to be transferred to bone that may be greater than the capacity of the bone to absorb such force. There is a 2% incidence of stress fractures of the proximal thigh in the general population.[54]

Stress fractures are diagnosed first by bone scans and later by radiographic changes.

PELVIC. The pubic rami is the most common bone of this region to be afflicted by stress fractures. Although the incidence of this fracture is low in athletes in general, long distance runners are more susceptible to this injury. The difference in tensile muscle forces and gait are the main reasons why women are more commonly affected than men.[69] The patient experiences inguinal or peroneal pain and an antalgic gait. Weight-bearing capacity may be diminished because of pain. A "standing sign" is indicative of this injury, that is, the inability to stand on the affected limb without support.[62] A bone scan can aid in the early detection of this entity if the clinician has a high index of suspicion (Fig. 22-20).[24,25] Radiographic findings are usually positive after several weeks. Activity should be restricted for several months, depending on the radiographic evidence of healing and the symptoms. Supportive taping or strapping may be used adjunctively.

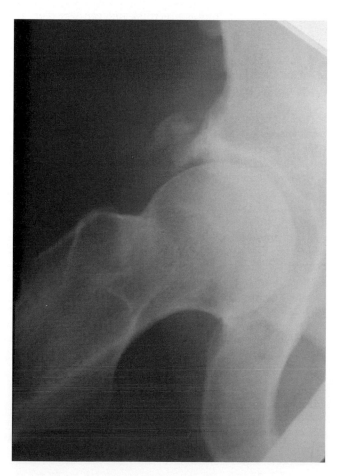

Fig. 22-18. A skeletally mature individual sustained an avulsion fracture of the anterior acetabular lip from the pull of the hip capsule and the acetabular labrum.

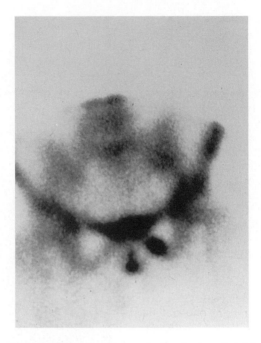

Fig. 22-20. A technetium-labeled bone scan demonstrating increased uptake in the left inferior pubic ramus consistent with a stress fracture.

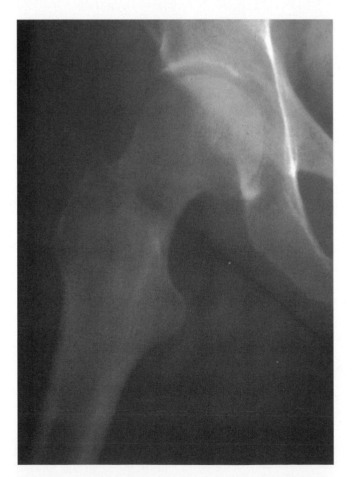

Fig. 22-21. An anteroposterior radiograph of the hip showing a femoral neck stress fracture at inferior femoral neck.

FEMORAL NECK. Femoral neck stress fractures are more common in military recruits and runners (Fig. 22-21).[31,59] The proposed etiology is the loss of shock absorption with muscle fatigue.[6] Training errors, poor footwear, and poor running surfaces may contribute to the development of this condition. Coxa vara will increase athletes' susceptibility to developing femoral neck stress fractures[30] because of the changes in biomechanical stresses incurred at the hip with this condition. There are two main types: a transverse fracture that begins at the superior femoral neck, and a compression type that develops at the inferior femoral neck. The transverse type is potentially unstable and more likely to displace.[21] Compression-type fractures are more common in younger athletes.

Results of bone scans are positive earlier than radiographs. Tomograms and computed tomographic scans or magnetic resonance imaging may also be useful to help diagnose this condition. These stress fractures have been classified according to Blickenstaff based on the radiographic findings.[6] A type I fracture has callus evident, but no fracture line is visible. These fractures are managed with rest. A type II stress fracture has a fracture line present on radiographs but is not displaced. Management involves either casting or operative fixation. A type III fracture is displaced and necessitates operative fixation. There are more complications with a type III fracture (Table 22-5).

Table 22-5. Femoral neck stress fracture classification

Type	Callus	Fracture on radiograph	Treatment
I	+	−	Rest
II	+	+, nondisplaced	Cast vs. operative
III	+	+, displaced	Operative

The symptoms include pain in the groin, thigh, or knee that is worsened with weight-bearing. An antalgic gait is present, and motion is decreased, particularly internal rotation of the hip. If the diagnosis is uncertain, an athlete should have an initial radiograph taken and be empirically treated with rest and not allowed to bear weight on the extremity for 1 week. Radiographs are re-peated and a bone scan is done. If results of both are negative, they are repeated in 1 week. Again, if they are both negative, a new diagnosis should be entertained. Patients who have a positive bone scan with a negative radiograph should be treated as a "stress reaction" with protected weight-bearing (Fig. 22-22).[22]

There is potential for serious complications such as

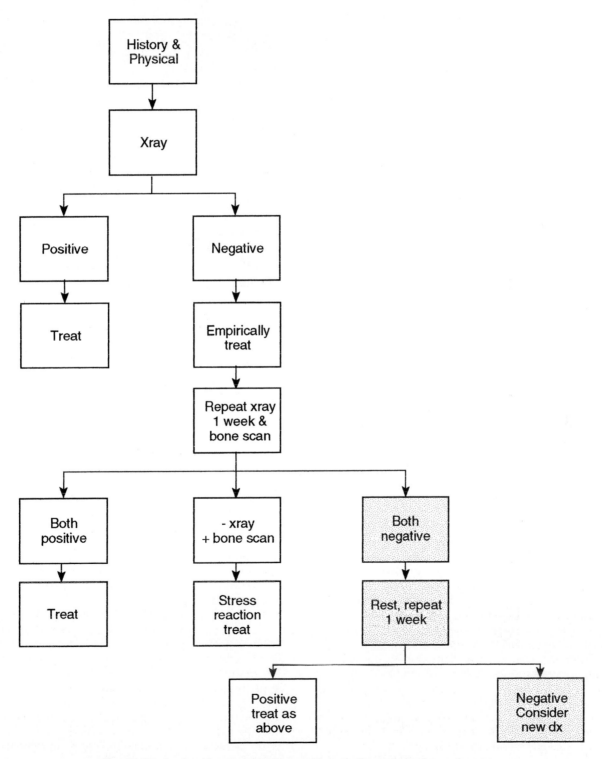

Fig. 22-22. An algorithm to guide the practitioner in the work-up of stress fractures.

avascular necrosis, nonunion, and varus deformity, especially with displacement. The athlete can resume activities when radiographs demonstrate full healing and when the bone scan does not show increased activity. The indication for surgery includes undisplaced fractures that do not heal with conservative management or ones that continue to cause pain even with cessation of activities.[56]

FEMORAL SHAFT. Stress fractures can occur anywhere along the femoral shaft;[70] most commonly they occur at the junction of the proximal and middle third of the femur. Runners are the most susceptible to sustaining this injury, and the incidence is related to training intensity.[20] Osteoporosis[15] and external rotation of the hip beyond 65° increases the risk of developing this stress fracture.[26]

The symptoms include insidious thigh or groin pain that is usually described as aching. Occasionally, the pain may be acute. Swelling and diminished motion are common. Any activity increases the pain, whereas rest relieves the symptoms.

The radiographic findings are delayed.[6,81,98] Bone scans can demonstrate early increased uptake along the femoral shaft.[8] The radiographs should be repeated every 3 months to evaluate the healing process. The physician must be cognizant of the nutrient artery penetrating the femoral cortex, which can be mistaken for a fracture.

Management includes partial weight-bearing for 1 to 4 weeks and cessation of athletic activities.[32,54] Once the athlete is pain-free, then full weight-bearing is begun. These fractures usually heal in 4 to 8 weeks.[21] During this period, a phased rehabilitation program is instituted. Sports activities can be resumed after 8 to 16 weeks.

The diagnosis of femoral periostitis must be considered; it is an overuse syndrome that affects the mid-thigh at the adductor insertion. It was first reported in female military recruits, particularly those who were noted to overstride with sports activities.[70] Bone scan will demonstrate linear uptake in the upper half to middle third of the femur. It commonly occurs bilaterally and can occur with femoral shaft stress fractures.[81]

HIP DISLOCATIONS

Hip dislocations rarely result from participation in athletics (Fig. 22-23). However, with the recent hip dislocations sustained by two professional football players, Bo Jackson of the Los Angeles Raiders and Mike Sherrard of the New York Giants, there is more awareness of this condition in the athlete. The mechanism of injury involves either falling on a flexed knee or a direct force application along the length of the femur, as would occur against the dashboard in a vehicular accident (Fig. 22-24).

These injuries are surgical emergencies that necessitate immediate reduction of the dislocated joint. It is important to minimize any vascular disruption to the femoral head and injury to the sciatic nerve. If the blood supply is disrupted, avascular necrosis will certainly leave the athlete disabled in activities of daily living and sporting activities. The neurovascular status of the extremity must also be assessed acutely, and the athlete must be immobilized and transported emergently to a hospital.

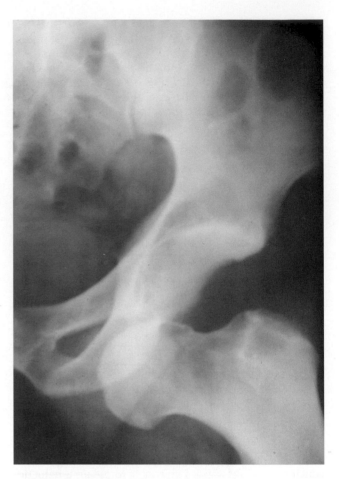

Fig. 22-23. An anteroposterior view of the left hip demonstrating an inferior dislocation of the hip. A lateral radiograph would determine if this was an anterior or posterior hip dislocation.

Symptoms include extreme pain that is worsened with any motion. The athlete is unable to bear weight and is completely immobile. Muscle spasm is present, and motion is restricted secondary to pain. Posterior dislocations are more common than anterior ones.[92] The leg is held in a flexed, adducted, and internally rotated position. Concurrent sciatic nerve injury must be excluded. With anterior dislocations, the leg is flexed, abducted, and externally rotated. Sometimes the femoral head can be palpated anteriorly.[18] Femoral nerve injuries must be excluded (Fig. 22-25).

A child is likely to sustain a hip dislocation without an associated fracture of the acetabulum. Adolescents and adults, however, often sustain a fracture of the acetabulum with hip dislocations.

A thorough neurologic examination and radiographs of the hip joint, including anteroposterior, lateral, and oblique, Judet[44] images, must be performed before attempting a reduction maneuver on the hip, preferably under anesthesia. Once the hip is relocated, a CAT scan may be performed to exclude any intraarticular fragments remaining in the joint. Also, the stability of the hip joint and the neurovascular status of the limb must be assessed after the reduction of the joint. If the joint is unstable after the reduction and a fracture is present, operative fixa-

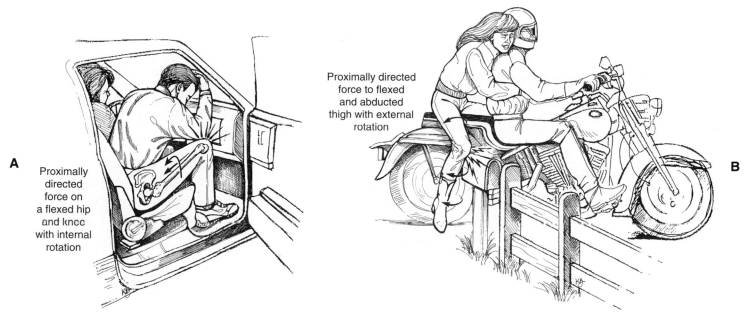

Fig. 22-24. Illustration of the mechanism causing hip dislocations. **A,** Posterior dislocation. **B,** Anterior dislocation.

tion is required. Concurrent knee ligament injuries can be assessed once the hip is reduced into position.

Avascular necrosis is a potential complication of hip dislocations (Fig. 22-26). The incidence rate is between 10% and 20%[76] and is directly related to the time delay in reducing the dislocation. The goal is to obtain a reduction as soon as possible and certainly within 24 hours. Avascular necrosis can take up to 2 years to become apparent.

There is no correlation between early weight-bearing and the development of avascular necrosis.[85]

After a stable reduction, the leg is placed in skin traction until the pain and muscle spasm subsides. Range of motion exercises can be instituted subsequently. Full weight-bearing should be delayed for 3 to 4 weeks[85] until the soft tissues have had time to heal. Sports return is allowed when full motion, agility, and strength are re-

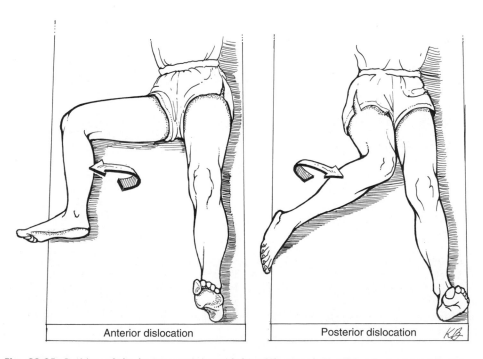

Fig. 22-25. Position of the lower extremity with hip dislocations. **A,** With anterior hip dislocations, the leg is held in a flexed, abducted, and externally rotated position. **B,** With posterior dislocations, the leg is shortened, adducted, and internally rotated.

gained. Radiographic evaluation should be followed every 3 months for 1 year and then every 6 months for 2 years.[18]

SLIPPED CAPITAL FEMORAL EPIPHYSIS

A slipped capital femoral epiphysis is the most common hip disorder in adolescents.[88] The etiology is not fully elucidated, however, it may involve hormonal factors, genetic factors, or mechanical factors. Patients afflicted are usually aged 10 to 15 years and at the time of the growth spurt, which is why it has been postulated that an increase in growth hormone relative to sex hormone may be causative because it decreases the shear strength of the physeal plate.[35] More than 50% of affected children are in the ninety-fifth or greater percentile in

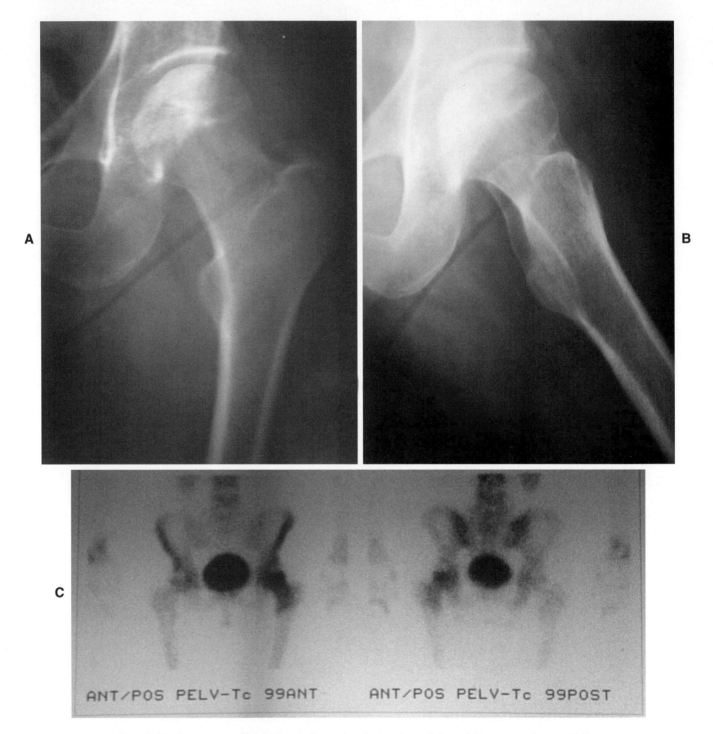

Fig. 22-26. A, An anteroposterior radiograph of the hip demonstrating avascular necrosis. **B,** The same hip as seen on a lateral radiograph. **C,** A bone scan of the hip demonstrating changes consistent with avascular necrosis.

Continued.

Fig. 22-26, cont'd. D, A magnetic resonance imaging scan showing avascular necrosis. **E,** An anteroposterior radiograph of the hip demonstrating advanced changes secondary to avascular necrosis.

D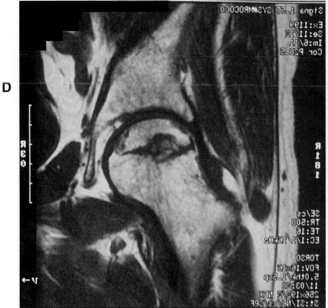

E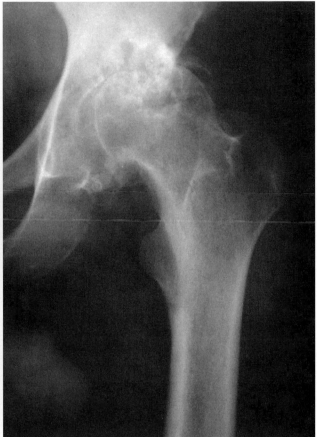

weight for their age.[46] Boys are more commonly affected than girls.[5] African-American males are the group with the highest incidence.[55]

The symptoms include groin, anteromedial thigh, and possibly knee pain. Motion is usually restricted, especially internal rotation of the hip. An antalgic, external rotation gait is seen. In chronic cases, thigh atrophy and a shortened limb can be observed.

Radiographs, including anteroposterior and lateral views and possibly frog lateral views, are used to diagnose this condition. Sometimes this condition is only demonstrated on one radiographic view (Fig. 22-27). The affected side should be compared with the contralateral side. The capital epiphysis is seen to displace posteriorly and downward, whereas the femoral neck displaces upward and anteriorly.

A slipped capital femoral epiphysis is classified as either acute, acute on chronic, or chronic. Further

Table 22-6. Slipped capital femoral epiphysis classification

Type	Epiphyseal width involvement (%)
I	<33
II	33–50
III	>50

classification requires a lateral radiograph of the hip. A type I involves a slip of less than one-third the width of the femoral epiphysis. Type II involves a 33% to 50% slip, and a type III, severe, slip involves more than 50% of the width of the femoral epiphysis (Table 22-6).[55]

Management is operative fixation of the slipped femoral epiphysis. In the preslip phase, with only irregularity and widening of the physis evident on radiographs, *in situ* operative fixation is recommended.[5] Crutch use and non–weight-bearing is recommended. Weight-bearing is begun at 6 weeks. A displaced epiphysis may require reduction before fixation.

LEGG-CALVÉ-PERTHES DISEASE

Legg-Calvé-Perthes disease is a self-limited, noninflammatory condition that causes avascular necrosis to develop in the hip of patients usually aged 4 to 8 years (Fig. 22-28).[88] This condition must be suspected in any child aged less than 12 years with hip pain.[55] The etiology, although uncertain, may involve a vascular insult to the femoral head. Antecedent trauma has been noted in 25% of children with Legg-Calvé-Perthes.[85]

The symptoms of Legg-Calvé-Perthes involve groin, hip, anteromedial, and thigh pain. Knee pain alone has been noted to be present 15% of the time.[55] The patient will also experience muscle spasm, an antalgic gait, and

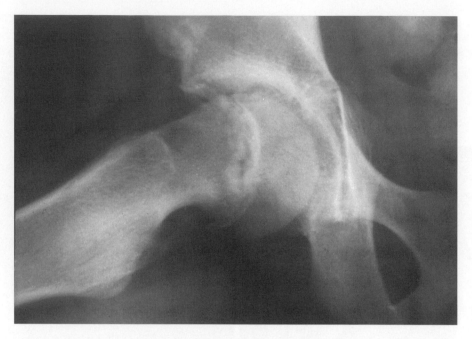

Fig. 22-27. A frog lateral view of the hip demonstrating a slipped capital femoral epiphysis, which is the best view to visualize minimal slips of the capital epiphysis.

decreased hip motion, especially internal rotation. Chronically, this condition can cause the development of a flexion and adduction contracture of the hip.[88]

Management involves regaining full motion of the hip; specifically, the gluteus medius and maximus and quadriceps must be reconditioned.[55] Anti-inflammatory medications and bedrest may help reduce the pain and increase the motion. Traction may also be necessary. The goal of management is containment of the femoral head within the acetabulum, either by bracing or surgical osteotomy.[88] If the patient wears a brace, he or she is weaned from it, and full activities are allowed when the femoral head demonstrates reossification on radiographs.[55]

A poor prognosis with Legg-Calvé-Perthes is associ-

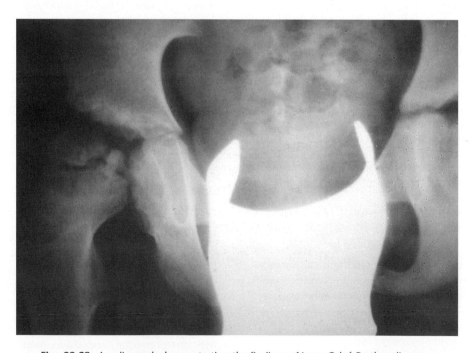

Fig. 22-28. A radiograph demonstrating the findings of Legg-Calvé-Perthes disease.

ated with the affected child aged more than 8 years, the majority of the femoral head being involved and premature physeal closure.[55]

TRANSIENT SYNOVITIS OF THE HIP

Transient synovitis is a self-limited, rapidly resolving inflammation of the hip joint. It is the most common cause of hip pain in children,[55] particularly those aged less than 10 years. The etiology may be viral, allergic, or posttraumatic.[55] It is a diagnosis of exclusion, requiring that the physician have a high index of suspicion. Other diagnostic tests must be performed to exclude slipped capital femoral epiphysis, Legg-Calvé-Perthes disease, or arthritis.

The child experiences inguinal, thigh, or knee pain. Motion at the hip is painful, and the child will guard against it. If the child will ambulate, an antalgic gait will be observed. Management involves bedrest, possibly with traction. The child will usually recover in 48 hours.[55] Activities are resumed gradually because early return to activities has been shown to cause recurrences.[36] This condition will precede Legg-Calvé-Perthes disease up to 10% of the time.[88]

ACETABULAR LABRAL TEARS

Acetabular labral tears are an unusual cause of mechanical hip pain. A high index of suspicion is necessary to reach this diagnosis. The athlete will experience a sharp, catching pain in the groin that radiates into the anterior thigh, particularly with rotation of the hip while arising from a seated position.[39] A feeling of "giving way" is sometimes encountered. A palpable and audible click may be elicited with extension and internal rotation of the hip mimicking "snapping hip syndrome."

Arthrography will demonstrate a filling defect.[85] Magnetic resonance imaging and arthroscopy can diagnose this condition. Injection of a local anesthetic can be therapeutic and diagnostic. This condition is treated nonoperatively with physiotherapy and analgesics as needed. Arthroscopic or open operative excision may be necessary for the athlete with recurrent symptoms, despite conservative treatment modalities.

MISCELLANEOUS

Sacroiliac Joint Pain

There are great stresses borne across the sacroiliac in the young athlete, which are controlled by the supporting ligaments.[85] Pain in this region is caused by sudden twisting motions, improper weightlifting, or a fall on the buttocks. Runners with short legs and poor running mechanics are susceptible to developing sacroiliac joint pain.[85]

Symptoms involve localized pain and tenderness. A positive Lasègue test can be elicited, which is straight leg raising with forced passive dorsiflexion of the foot increasing the pain. Results of a Gaenslen test may also be positive. This test involves the athlete lying on the unaffected side and flexing the hip while the injured hip is extended. An increase in pain in the sacroiliac joint is encountered. The condition is managed symptomatically. Abdominal

strengthening and postural exercises are part of the rehabilitation protocol. An abdominal constricting band or sacral corset may help alleviate the pain. NSAIDs, and, rarely, local injections, can be helpful.

Pelvic Floor Myalgia

Pelvic floor myalgia is an unusual condition of increased tension involving the muscles and fascia of the pelvic cavity and causing pain.[84] It includes "levator ani syndrome," "piriformis syndrome," "anorectal pain," and "coccygodynia." The main muscles affected are the levator ani, coccygeus, and piriformis. The coccygeus and levator ani compose the pelvic diaphragm that surrounds the excretory and reproductive sphincters.

The signs and symptoms include back and leg pain, a heavy feeling in the pelvis, possibly pain with bowel movements, constipation, rectal pain, and dyspareunia.[86] A rectal examination will elicit pain. Management is guided by the symptoms, and include deep heat, mobilization of the sacrococcygeal joint, stretching, relaxation, and abdominal strengthening.[86]

SUMMARY

There are many causes of pelvic, hip, and thigh pain in athletes. In addition to the entities discussed in this chapter, the practitioner must always consider metabolic bone diseases, neoplasms, infections, and inflammatory conditions (see box below).[85]

With these entities in mind and guided by a thorough

ETIOLOGY OF HIP PAIN

Primary pelvis or hip
   Pathology
   Injury

Referred pain
   Lumbar sacral spine
   Pelvic viscera

Inflammatory conditions
   Ankylosing spondylitis
   Reiter's syndrome
   Spondylosis
   Monoarticular arthritides

Infectious conditions
   Osteomyelitis
   Septic arthritis

Neoplasms
   Osteoid osteoma
   Metastatic lesions

Metabolic bone disorders
   Paget's disease
   Endocrine disorders

history and physical examination, the sports medicine physician will be well armed to diagnose and begin the treatment of the athletes afflicted with injuries to the pelvis, hip, and thigh.

REFERENCES

1. American Academy of Orthopaedic Surgeons, eds: *Athletic training and sports medicine*, Chicago, 1984, American Academy of Orthopaedic Surgeons.
2. Antao NA: Myositis ossificans of the hip in a professional soccer player, *Am J Sports Med* 16:82, 1988.
3. Balaji MR, DeWeese JA: Adductor canal outlet syndrome, *JAMA* 245:167–170, 1981.
4. Beer E: Periostitis and osteitis of the symphysis pubis following suprapubic cystotomies, *J Urol* 20:233, 1928.
5. Bianco AJ Jr: Treatment of slipping of the capital femoral epiphysis, *Clin Orthop* 48:103, 1966.
6. Blickenstaff LP, Morris JM: Fatigue fracture of the femoral neck, *J Bone Joint Surg* 48A:1031–1046, 1966.
7. Bowerman JW: *Radiology and injury in sport*, New York, 1977, Appleton-Century-Crofts.
8. Brunet ME, Hontas RB: The thigh. In DeLee JC, Drez D Jr, eds: *Orthopaedic sports medicine*, Philadelphia, 1994, WB Saunders.
9. Burgess AR, Tile M: Fractures of the pelvis. In Rockwood CA Jr, Green DP, Bucholz RW, eds: *Fractures in adults*, Philadelphia, 1991, JB Lippincott.
10. Burkett LN: Investigation into hamstring strains: the case of the hybrid muscle. *J Sports Med* 3:228–231, 1976.
11. Butler JE, Eggert AW: Fracture of the iliac crest apophysis: an unusual hip pointer, *J Sports Med* 3:192, 1975.
12. Canale ST, Bourland WL: Fracture of the neck and intertrochanteric region of the femur in children, *J Bone Joint Surg* 59A:431, 1977.
13. Canale ST, King RE: Pelvic and hip fractures. In Rockwood CA Jr, Wilkins KE, King RE, eds: *Fractures in children*, Philadelphia, 1991, JB Lippincott.
14. Colonna PC: Fractures of the neck of the femur in children, *Am J Surg* 6:793, 1929.
15. Cook SD, et al: Trabecular bone density in menstrual function in women runners, *Am J Sports Med* 15:503–507, 1987.
16. DeLee JC: Fractures and dislocations of the hip. In Rockwood CA Jr, Green DP, Bucholz RW, eds: *Fractures in adults*, Phladelphia, 1991, JB Lippincott.
17. Elliott BC, Blanksby BA: The synchronization of muscle activity and body segment movements during a running cycle, *Med Sci Sports Exerc* 11:322–327, 1979.
18. Epstein HC: Traumatic dislocations of the hip, *Clin Orthop* 92:116, 1973.
19. Eriksson E, Arvidsson I, Arvidsson H: Diagnostic and operative arthroscopy of the hip, *Orthopaedics* 9(2):169–176, 1986.
20. Fitch KD: Stress fractures of the lower limbs in runners, *Aust Fam Phys* 13:511–515, 1984.
21. Fox JM: Thigh. In Nicholas JA, Hershman, EB, eds: *The lower extremity and spine in sports medicine*, St. Louis, 1986, CV Mosby.
22. Fullerton LR, Snowdy HA: Femoral neck stress fractures, *Am J Sports Med* 16:365, 1988.
23. Garrett WE, et al: Biomechanical comparison of stimulated and nonstimulated muscle pulled to failure, *Am J Sports Med* 15:448, 1987.
24. Garrick JG, et al: Early diagnosis of stress fractures and their precursors, *J Bone Joint Surg* 58A:733, 1976.
25. Geslien GE, et al: Early detection of stress fractures using ^{99}mTc-polyphosphate, *Radiology* 121:683, 1976.
26. Giladi M, et al: External rotation of the hip: a predictor of risk for stress fractures, *Clin Orthop* 216:131–134, 1987.
27. Godshall RW, Hansen CA: Incomplete avulsion of a portion of the iliac epiphysis: an injury to young athletes, *J Bone Joint Surg* 55A:1301, 1973.
28. Grant JCB: In Anderson JE, ed: *Grant's atlas of anatomy*, Ed 8, Baltimore, 1983, Williams & Wilkins.
29. Gray AH: *Anatomy of the human body*, Philadelphia, 1959, Lea & Febiger.
30. Gross ML, Nasser S, Finerman GAM: In DeLee JC, Drez D Jr, eds: *Orthopaedic sports medicine*, Philadelphia, 1994, WB Saunders.
31. Hajek MR, Noble HB: Stress fractures of the femoral neck in runners, *Am J Sports Med* 10:112, 1982.
32. Hallel T, Amit S, Sega D: Fatigue fractures of the tibial and femoral shaft in soldiers, *Clin Orthop* 118: 35–43, 1976.
33. Hanson PG, Angevine M, Juhl JH: Osteitis pubis in sports activities, *Phys Sports Med* 6:111, 1978.
34. Harris NH, Murray RO: Lesions of the symphysis in athletes, *BMJ* 4:211, 1974.
35. Harris WR: The endocrine basis for slipping of the upper femoral epiphysis, *J Bone Joint Surg* 32B:5, 1950.
36. Hermel MB, Albert SM: Transient synovitis of the hip, *Clin Orthop* 22:21, 1962.
37. Hollingshead WH: *Anatomy for surgeons, the back and limbs*, vol 3, Philadelphia, 1958, Harper & Row.
38. Hoppenfeld S: *Orthopaedic neurology*, Philadelphia, 1977, JB Lippincott.
39. Ikeda T, et al: Torn acetabular labrum in young patients. Arthroscopic diagnosis and management, *J Bone Joint Surg* 70B(1):13–16, 1988.
40. Ingram AJ, Bachynski B: Fractures of the hip in children. Treatment and results, *J Bone Joint Surg* 35A:867, 1953.
41. Jackson DW, Feagin JA: Quadriceps contusions in young athletes: relation of severity of injury to treatment and prognosis, *J Bone Joint Surg* 55A:95–105, 1973.
42. Jeffreys TE: Pseudomalignant osseous tumor of soft tissue, *J Bone Joint Surg* 48B:488, 1966.
43. Johnson RC, Schmidt GL: Hip motion measurements for selected activities of daily living, *Clin Orthop* 72:205, 1970.
44. Judet R, Judet J, LeTournel E: Fractures of the acetabulum: classification and surgical approaches for open reduction, *J Bone Joint Surg* 46A:1615, 1964.
45. Kane WJ: Fractures of the pelvis. In Rockwood CA Jr, Green DP, eds: *Fractures in adults*, Philadelphia, 1984, JB Lippincott.
46. Kelsey JL, Acheson DM, Keggi KJ: The body build of patients with slipped capital femoral epiphysis, *Am J Dis Child* 124:276, 1972.
47. Kirkpatrick JS, Koman LA, Rovere GD: The role of ultrasound in the early diagnosis of myositis ossificans: a case report, *Am J Sports Med* 15:179–181, 1987.
48. Komi PV, Burskirk ER: Effect of eccentric and concentric muscle conditioning on tension and electric activity of human muscle, *Ergonomics* 15:417–434, 1972.
49. Kulund DN: *The injured athlete*, Philadelphia, 1982, JB Lippincott.
50. Lee BY, LaPointe DG, Madden JL: The adductor canal syndrome: description of a case with quantification of arterial pulsatile blood flow, *Am J Surg* 123:617–620, 1972.
51. Levinthal DH: Sports injuries in persons over 30 years of age, *Postgrad Med* 28:121, 1960.
52. Liemohn W: Factors related to hamstring strains, *J Sports Med* 18:71–76, 1978.
53. Lipscomb AB, Thomas ED, Johnston RK: Treatment of myositis ossificans traumatica in athletes, *Am J Sports Med* 4:111–120, 1976.
54. Lombardo SJ, Benson DW: Stress fractures of the femur in runners, *Am J Sports Med* 10:219–227, 1982.
55. MacEwen GD, Bunnell WP, Ramsey PL: The hip. In Lovell

WW, Winter RB, eds: *Pediatric orthopaedics*, Philadelphia, 1993, JB Lippincott.

56. McBryde AM Jr: Stress fractures in athletes, *J Sports Med* 3:212, 1975.

57. Merrifield HH, Cowan RFJ: Groin strain injuries in ice hockey, *J Sports Med* 1(2):41–42, 1973.

58. Metzmaker JN, Pappas AM: Avulsion fractures of the pelvis, *Am J SportsMed* 13:349, 1985.

59. Meurmann KOA, Elfving S: Stress fractures in soldiers: a multifocal bone disorder, *Radiology* 134:483, 1980.

60. Micheli LJ: Overuse injuries in children's sports: the growth factor, *Orthop Clin North Am* 14:337–361, 1983.

61. Morris JM: Biomechanical aspects of the hip joint, *Orthop Clin North Am* 2:33, 1971.

62. Noakes TD, Smith JA, Lindenberg G: Pelvic stress fractures in long distance runners, *Am J Sports Med* 13:120, 1985.

63. Nordin M, Frankel VH: Biomechanics of the hip. In Frankel VH, Burstein AH, eds: *Orthopaedic biomechanics*, Philadelphia, 1970, Lea & Febiger.

64. Norfray JF, et al: Early confirmation of stress fractures in joggers, *JAMA* 243:1647–1649, 1980.

65. Norman A, Dorfman HD: Juxtacortical circumscribed myositis ossificans: evolution and radiographic features, *Radiology* 96:301, 1970.

66. O'Donoghue DH: *Treatment of injuries to athletes*, ed 4. Philadelphia, 1984, WB Saunders.

67. Olerud S, Gerusten S: Chronic pubic symphysiolysis, *J Bone Joint Surg* 56A:799, 1974.

68. O'Neil DB, Micheli LJ: Overuse injuries in young athletes, *Clin Sports Med* 7:591, 1988.

69. Pavlov H, et al: Stress fractures of the pubic ramus, *J Bone Joint Surg* 64A:1020, 1982.

70. Provost RA, Morris JM: Fatigue fracture of the femoral shaft, *J Bone Joint Surg* 51A:487–498, 1969.

71. Puranen J, Orava S: The hamstring syndrome, *Am J Sports Med* 16:517, 1988.

72. Ratliff AHC: Fractures of the neck of the femur in children, *J Bone Joint Surg* 44B:528, 1962.

73. Reed MH: Pelvic fractures in children, *J Can Assoc Radiol* 27:255, 1976.

74. Renstrom PA, Peterson L: Groin injuries in athletes, *Br J Sports Med* 14:30–36, 1980.

75. Risser JC: The iliac apophysis: an invaluable sign in the management of scoliosis, *Clin Orthop* 11:111, 1958.

76. Robertson RC, Peterson HA: Traumatic dislocations of the hip in children: review of Mayo Clinic series. In Harris WH, ed: *The Hip*, St. Louis, 1974, CV Mosby.

77. Romanoff ME, et al: Saphenous nerve entrapment at the adductor canal, *Am J Sports Med* 17:478–481, 1989.

78. Rupani HD, et al: Three-phase radionuclide bone imaging in sports medicine, *Radiology* 156:187–196, 1985.

79. Rydell N: Biomechanics of the hip joint, *Clin Orthop* 92:6, 1973.

80. Safran MR, et al: The role of warm-up in muscular injury and prevention, *Am J Sports Med* 16:123, 1988.

81. Savoca C: Stress fractures: a classification of the earliest radiographic signs, *Radiology* 100:519–524, 1971.

82. Scharberg JE, Harper MC, Allen WC: The snapping hip syndrome, *Am J Sports Med* 12:361, 1984.

83. Schlonsky J, Olix ML: Functional disability following avulsion fracture of the ischial epiphysis, *J Bone Joint Surg* 54A:641, 1972.

84. Segura JW, Opitz JL, Greene LF: Prostatosis, prostatitis or pelvic floor tension myalgia? *J Urol* 122 (2):168–169, 1979.

85. Sim FH, Scott HG: Injuries of the pelvis and hip in athletes. In Nicholas JA, Hershmann EB, eds: *The Lower Extremity and Spine in Sports Medicine*, St. Louis, 1986, CV Mosby.

86. Sinaki M, Merritt JL, Stillwell GK: Tension myalgia of the pelvic floor, *Mayo Clin Proc* 52:717, 1977.

87. Slocum DB, James SL: Biomechanics of running, *JAMA* 205:721–728, 1968.

88. Tachdjian MO: *Pediatric orthopaedics*, vol 1. Philadelphia, 1972, WB Saunders.

89. Taylor DC, et al: Groin pain in athletes due to abdominal musculature abnormalities, *Am J Sports Med* 13:239–242, 1991.

90. Trueta J, Harrison MHM: The normal vascular anatomy of the femoral head in adult man, *J Bone Joint Surg* 35B:442, 1953.

91. Verta MJ, Vitello J, Fuller J: Adductor canal compression syndrome, *Arch Surg* 119:345–346, 1984.

92. Walsh ZT, Micheli LJ: Hip dislocation in a high school football player, *Phys Sports Med* 17:112, 1989.

93. Walton M, Rothwell AG: Reactions of thigh tissues of sheep to blunt trauma, *Clin Orthop* 176:273–281, 1983.

94. Waters PM, Millis MB: Hip and pelvic injuries in the young athlete, *Clin Sports Med* 7:513, 1988.

95. Watson-Jones R: Dislocations and fracture—dislocations of the pelvis, *Br J Surg* 25:773, 1938.

96. Watts HG: Fractures of the pelvis in children, *Orthop Clin North Am* 7:615, 1976.

97. Wiley JJ: Traumatic osteitis pubis: the gracilis syndrome, *Am J Sports Med* 11:360, 1983.

98. Wilson E: Stress fractures, *Radiology* 92:481–486, 1969.

99. Zaccalini PS, Urist MR: Traumatic periosteal proliferations in rabbits: the enigma of experimental myositis ossificans traumatica, *J Trauma* 4:344, 1964.

100. Zarins B, Ciullo JV: Acute muscle and tendon injuries in athletes, *Clin Sports* 2:167–182, 1983.

101. Zoltan DJ, Clancy WG, Keene JS: A new operative approach to snapping hip and refractory trochanteric bursitis in athletes, *Am J Sports Med* 14:201, 1986.

CHAPTER 23

KNEE INJURIES

David Diduch
Giles Scuderi
W. Norman Scott

The knee is the most frequently injured joint managed in sports medicine.[100] Twenty percent of all football-related injuries involve the knee, including an estimated 42 anterior cruciate ligament tears per 1000 players per year.[37] In addition, skiing accounts for at least one anterior cruciate tear per day at major ski areas.[26] Yet, with advancements in surgical and therapeutic techniques, knee injuries are increasingly treatable toward a return to full participation. The primary care physician frequently must evaluate overuse injuries and acute "sprains and strains," both of which can often involve significant intraarticular pathology. Therefore, the treating physician must be completely comfortable with his or her ability to diagnose most common knee injuries, have an understanding of treatment algorithms, and know when it is appropriate to refer the patient to a surgical specialist. This chapter will help to provide the primary care physician with the diagnostic tools for evaluating the majority of knee injuries often resulting from sports activities. It will also help to provide an understanding of the anatomy as it relates to the biomechanics of the joint and common mechanisms of injury. Lastly, the chapter will offer readily available algorithms for appropriate diagnostic work-ups, therapeutic intervention, and indications for referral.

ANATOMY

The knee is composed of three distinct and partially separated joint compartments: the medial and lateral femorotibial joints and the patellofemoral joint. In addition, the proximal tibiofibular joint is included in the knee but is rarely involved in sports-related injuries. Articular cartilage, primarily type II collagen with a high water content, covers each of these joint compartments and provides lubricated gliding surfaces for knee motion. Softening and early "wear and tear" of this surface is referred to as *chondromalacia*. Frank erosion is technically

arthritis. Virtually every adult has at least some degree of wear and tear of these surfaces, but most are minimally symptomatic. Localized traumatic defects of the articular surface are termed *cartilage fractures* or *osteochondral defects* if they involve a "divot" of subchondral bone. A preexisting dysvascular contribution to the etiology of the osteochondral defect confers the term *osteochondritis dissecans*, although the exact etiology most often cannot be determined.

The shapes of the bony articulations provide very little inherent stability to the knee joint, unlike the hip "ball and socket" model. Proper function depends on intact ligamentous structures. Very substantial cruciate ligaments cross in the center of the knee joint. Although they are intraarticular, a surrounding synovial sleeve makes them technically extrasynovial. The anterior cruciate ligament (ACL) is on average 11 mm wide × 38 mm long, originating on the posteromedial part of the lateral femoral condyle (Figs. 23-1, 23-2).[97] It runs distally in an anteromedial direction to a rather long attachment site on the tibial plateau between the tibial spines (Fig. 23-3). An easy way to remember this orientation is that the direction mimics one's hand in a pocket. The ACL functions as the main stabilizer to resist anterior translation, especially when the knee is in the extended position.[36] The ACL is a secondary stabilizer to excessive varus or valgus stress, to rotation, and to hyperextension.

The posterior cruciate ligament (PCL) is slightly larger at 38 mm × 13 mm and up to 50% stronger than the ACL.[47] It originates from a broad attachment site on the lateral side of the medial femoral condyle and runs distally in a posterior–lateral direction to insert on the back of the tibia approximately 1 cm below the articular surface. Accessory meniscofemoral ligaments often run either anterior (Ligament of Humphrey) or posterior (Ligament of Wrisberg) to the PCL from the femur to the lateral meniscus rim. Up to 50% of the

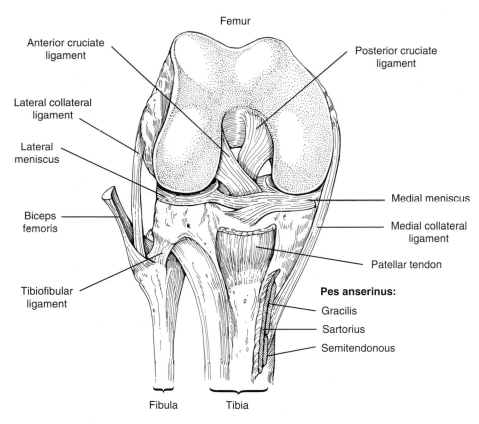

Fig. 23-1. Anterior view of the knee.

size of the PCL, usually (71% of knees) at least one of these accessory ligaments is present, but rarely (6% of knees) both are present.[19,47] The PCL is the main stabilizer to posterior translation of the knee, especially in flexion. It serves as a secondary stabilizer to varus or valgus stress.

The collateral ligaments on either side of the knee are the main stabilizers to side-to-side stresses. The medial collateral, or tibial collateral, ligament (MCL) consists of a stronger superficial layer and a deep layer, which attaches to the medial meniscus. The superficial MCL originates from the medial femoral epicondyle and inserts almost 5 cm below the joint line on the medial tibia. Just posterior and confluent with the superficial MCL is the

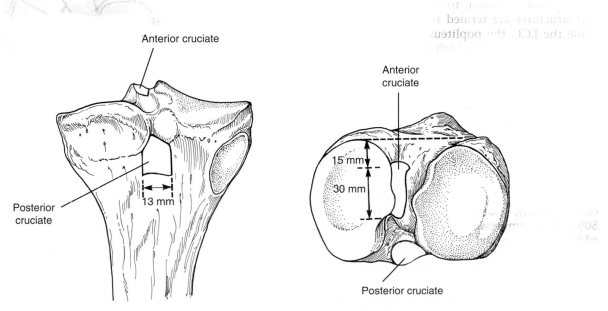

Fig. 23-2. Attachment sites of the anterior and posterior cruciate ligaments on the tibia.

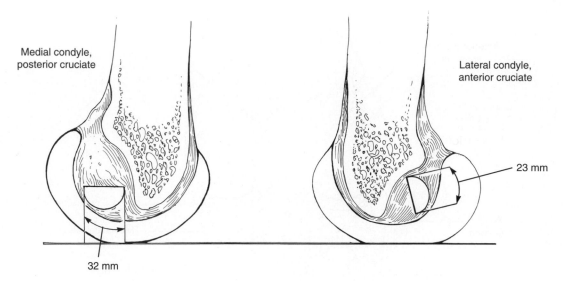

Fig. 23-3. Origin of the anterior and posterior cruciate ligaments on the femur.

posterior oblique ligament. More of a combination of capsule and supporting retinacular layers, including the insertion of the semimembranosus tendon, than a clearly defined ligament, the posterior oblique ligament is taut in extension and is important in resisting valgus stress and external rotation. Completing the medial structures is the pes anserinus, the common insertion of the sartorius, gracilis, and semitendinosus on the antero-medial tibia.

The lateral collateral, or fibular collateral, ligament (LCL) consists of a single layer and runs from the lateral femoral epicondyle to the fibular head (Fig. 23-4). Superficial to the LCL is the iliotibial band, the fascial continuation of the fascia lata from the lateral hip and thigh, attaching to the anterolateral tibia at Gerdy's tubercle. Because of its muscular origin, the iliotibial band acts as a dynamic stabilizer and, along with the LCL, a static stabilizer, to varus stress. The posterolateral structures are termed the *arcuate complex* and include the LCL, the popliteus muscle and tendon, and the arcuate ligament, which is a thickening of the posterolateral capsule. These structures function to resist varus and internal rotation of the tibia. Deep to all of these structures is the knee joint capsule, surrounding the entire joint with an inner layer of synovium. This synovial layer produces the synovial fluid that is essential to joint lubrication and nutrition for articular and meniscal cartilage.

The medial and lateral menisci are wedge-shaped, semicircular structures composed primarily of type I cartilage (fibrocartilage). The collagen fibers are oriented circumferentially, allowing the menisci to absorb 40% to 50% of the compressive forces across the knee joint.[77] In addition, the menisci act as secondary stabilizers to anteroposterior-directed forces by way of increasing the conformity between the rounded femoral and relatively flat tibial articular surfaces. The vascular supply is restricted to the outer third of the meniscal width, a signif-

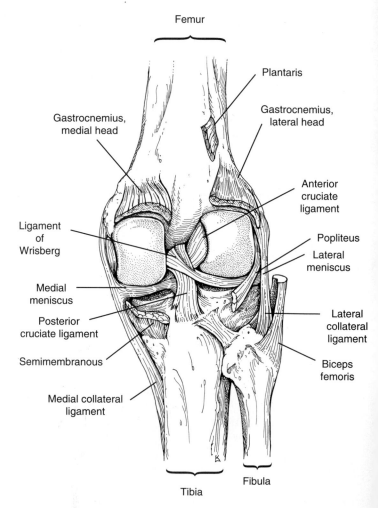

Fig. 23-4. Posterior view of the knee.

icant factor in the inability of most meniscal tears to heal.

CLINICAL EVALUATION

History

As with much of medicine, a thorough history regarding knee injuries often makes the diagnosis (Fig. 23-5). For acute injuries, careful attention should be paid to determining the mechanism of injury. Did the knee suffer a twisting injury, often indicating a meniscal or ACL tear? Was this a contact (i.e., clip in football) or noncontact (i.e., change in direction in basketball) injury? What caused the force, from what direction, of what magnitude, and in what position was the patient's leg at the time of injury? Answers to these questions will often suggest a mechanism putting specific structures under stress, such as a valgus force causing injury to the MCL and ACL.

An audible "pop" often signifies an acute tear of the ACL or sometimes a meniscal tear. The extent and onset of swelling is a helpful sign. A knee that swells rapidly over minutes to a couple of hours suggests a hemarthrosis, as seen with a cruciate ligament tear, patella dislocation, or intraarticular bony injury. An ef-

fusion that develops over several hours to the next day suggests a meniscal tear. Other important questions include knowledge about previous symptoms, injuries, and treatments to the affected knee and whether the athlete was able to continue sports participation after the acute injury.

Chronic injuries require additional questions regarding the nature of the training regimen, including mileage or duration and intervals, stretching, shoe wear, surfaces, and recent changes in the routine. Onset of symptoms and precipitating activities and whether the athlete had any self-administered relief are also important.

Physical Examination

OBSERVATION AND PALPATION. An initial evaluation should determine the specific location of pain and any associated crepitus that may be associated with a fracture. A gentle varus and valgus and anteroposterior stress will elicit any gross instability that precludes further examination modalities and necessitates immediate splint stabilization and transfer for orthopedic evaluation. The presence of an intraarticular effusion can be determined by a fullness in the suprapatellar pouch, a fullness surrounding the patella oblit-

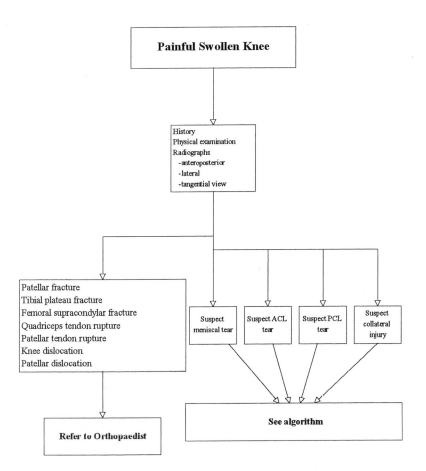

Fig. 23-5. Algorithm for the acutely swollen knee. *Adapted from the AAOS National Orthopedic Leadership Conference 1995.*

erating the usual depressed contour on slight flexion, and possibly the presence of a fluid wave from side to side. A large effusion will result in a ballotable patella that "floats" above its articulating femoral trochlea, making contact only when a posteriorly directed force is applied to bounce the patella up and down (Fig. 23-6). Effusions can be rated as grade 1 (slight), grade 2 (mild lift-off of patella), grade 3 (ballottable patella), or grade 4 (tense). In contrast to an intraarticular effusion, extraarticular soft-tissue swelling is more localized and superficial, usually overriding a bony prominence as with prepatellar bursitis. Chronic intraarticular synovitis, as is seen with arthritic knees, has a boggy texture that cannot be "milked" to other knee compartments.

PATELLA AND EXTENSOR MECHANISM EVALUATION. In the absence of an acute fracture, all patients must be able to actively extend the knee to demonstrate an intact extensor mechanism. One useful method is to have the patient raise the extended leg off the table. Patients need to be coaxed through pain. Inability to extend the knee indicates rupture of the quadriceps tendon or patella tendon, or fracture of the patella and requires immediate referral to an orthopedic surgeon for reconstruction. Often a palpable, painful defect can be determined at the site of disruption. Assuming an intact extensor mechanism, one can determine the active range of motion, from a normal 5° of hyperextension to a maximum of 135° of flexion (Fig. 23-7). Attention

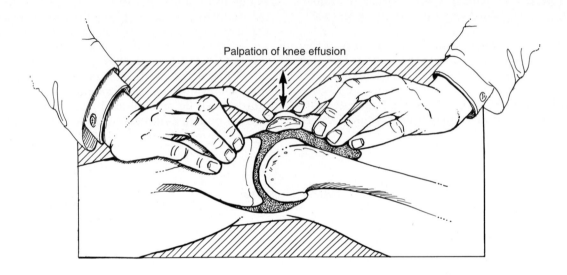

Palpation of knee effusion

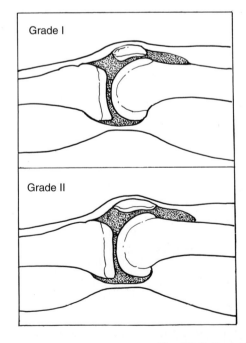

Grade I

Grade II

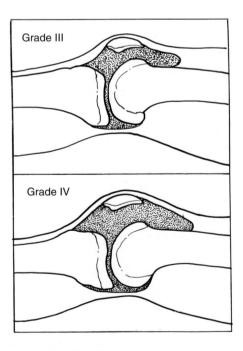

Grade III

Grade IV

Fig. 23-6. Knee effusions, graded from I to IV.

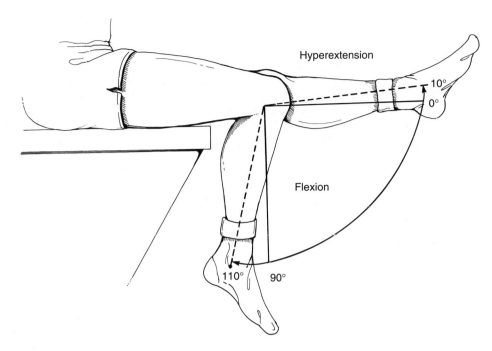

Fig. 23-7. Normal knee range of motion is from 5° to 10° of hyperextension to 135° of flexion.

can also be directed toward any degree of quadriceps atrophy, easily measured circumferentially at a common reference point (i.e., 10 cm) above the patella in extension.

Patella tracking in the femoral sulcus groove can be assessed by observation and palpation through a range of motion. Gentle medial-to-lateral pressure against the medial side of the patella during the passive arc of motion represents the "apprehension test" for patella subluxation. A positive test result elicits discomfort and a sensation of impending dislocation laterally. A recent patella dislocation will demonstrate medial retinacular tenderness and an effusion. A knee with a large Q angle is considered anatomically predisposed to patella tracking problems because the quadriceps muscle vector pulls in a more lateral direction. The Q angle is measured in extension as the intersection of lines drawn from the anterior–superior iliac spine to the center of the patella and a second line from the center of the patella to the tibial tubercle (Fig. 23-8). Normal Q angles in men are 8° to 10° and in women from 10° to 20°.[3] Anterior knee pain can be effectively localized to the patellofemoral articulation by provocative palpation of the undersurface of the patella. In extension with the quadriceps relaxed, the patella can be gently subluxed medially and laterally, affording an opportunity to palpate the articular side with the thumb (Fig. 23-9). Tenderness suggests chondromalacia-type problems. Additionally, the lateral retinaculum adjacent to the patella can be palpated for tight, fibrous bands, which prevent the usual medial displacement on attempted medial subluxation. These bands may cause lateral tilt or track-

ing of the patella in the femoral sulcus, leading to chondromalacia-type symptoms or patella subluxation and dislocation.

MENISCUS EVALUATION. Medial or lateral joint line tenderness is very useful to identify meniscal tears. Firm palpation is directed over the meniscal rim with the knee flexed 90° either over the examining table or supine. A knee inflamed from degenerative arthritis or recent injury can give false-positive results. Other examination techniques seek to mechanically impinge the torn flap of meniscal tissue between moving articular surfaces, which is essentially the cause of symptomatic knee buckling or giving way that patients report in the history. The Steinmann test is performed with the knee relaxed and flexed 90° off the side of the table. While stabilizing the calf with one hand, the opposite hand grasps the foot and sharply internally and externally rotates the leg (Fig. 23-10). Pain at the joint line suggests a meniscal tear. The McMurray test is performed in the supine position by grasping the heel with one hand while stabilizing the leg with the other hand on the thigh and simultaneously palpating the medial and lateral joint lines. In full flexion, a valgus, external rotation force is applied to the foot, which is then brought into varus, internal rotation. A modification of this test involves moving from full flexion to extension while applying valgus, external rotation and then varus, internal rotation (Fig. 23-11). A positive test result is indicated by joint line pain or a palpable click.[98] The Apley test, a variation of the McMurray test, is performed in the prone position with the knee flexed 90° (Fig. 23-12 on p. 344). While grasping the foot, the tibia is axially loaded to compress the menisci while simultaneously internally and externally rotating

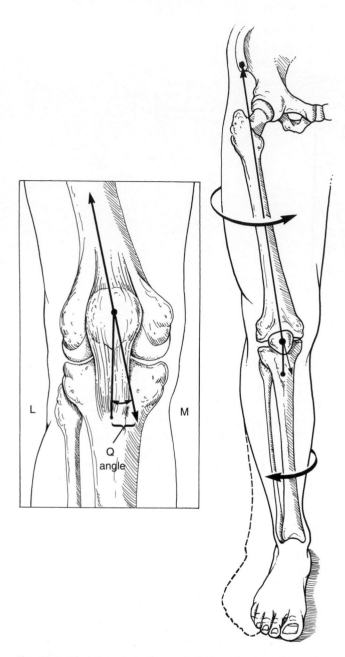

Fig. 23-8. The Q angle is the angle formed by lines drawn from the anterior superior iliac spine to the center of the patella and from the center of the patella to the tibial tubercle.

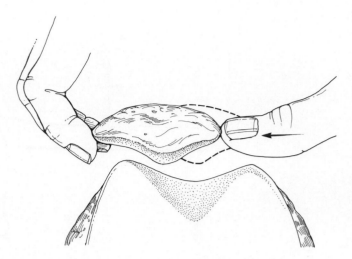

Fig. 23-9. The inferior surface of the patella is palpated for tenderness after being subluxed with the opposite hand.

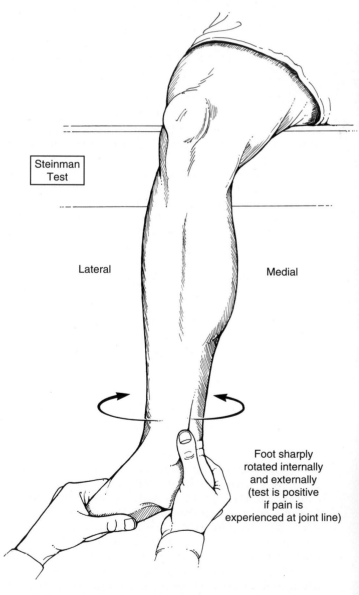

Steinman Test

Lateral

Medial

Foot sharply rotated internally and externally (test is positive if pain is experienced at joint line)

Fig. 23-10. The Steinmann test for meniscal tears. A positive test result is demonstrated by joint line pain with sharp rotation.

the leg. Again, a palpable click or joint line pain represents a positive test result. False-positive tests resulting from ligamentous or soft-tissue pain can be differentiated from meniscal pain by repeating the test while distracting the leg to unload the meniscus, which should result in the absence of pain or click.

COLLATERAL LIGAMENT EVALUATION. The collateral ligaments on either side of the knee are evaluated by stress examinations. The valgus stress test assesses the MCL and supporting structures (Fig. 23-13). With the knee in 30° of flexion, a gentle valgus stress is applied to the knee by grasping the ankle with one hand and applying stabilizing pressure to the lateral

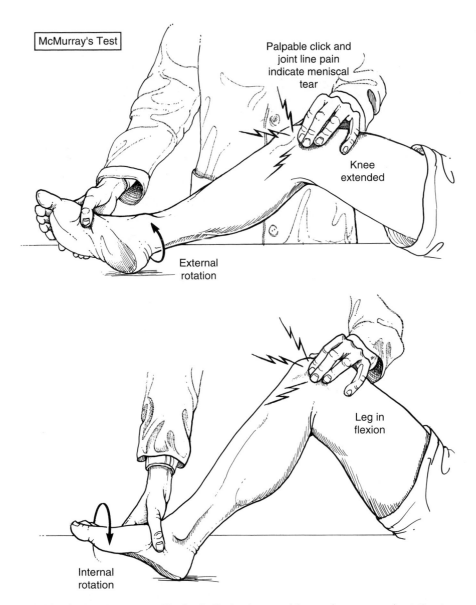

McMurray's Test

Palpable click and
joint line pain
indicate meniscal
tear

Knee
extended

External
rotation

Leg in
flexion

Internal
rotation

Fig. 23-11. The McMurray test. The leg in flexion is moved from valgus, external rotation to varus, internal rotation. Alternatively, the knee can be extended during the maneuver. A meniscal tear is suspected with a palpable click or joint line pain.

thigh with the opposite hand. It is important to perform the test in slight flexion to relax the posterior capsule and effectively isolate stress to the MCL. In full extension, the tight posterior capsule will give a false-negative test result. The test can be repeated in full extension to demonstrate additional laxity of the posterior oblique ligament and posteromedial capsule and possibly tears of the ACL or PCL. Specifically, instability to valgus stress at 30° of knee flexion indicates isolated MCL injury; instability at 0° implies MCL and posteromedial capsule injury; and laxity at −10° of hyperextension suggests MCL, posteromedial capsule, and posterior oblique ligament injury and possibly PCL or ACL tears.

The varus stress test is performed in similar fashion, in 30° of flexion to isolate the LCL, and in full extension and hyperextension to assess secondary stabilizers (Fig. 23-14). Instability to varus stress at 30° of flexion suggests isolated LCL injury; instability at 0° suggests LCL and lateral capsular injury; and instability at −10° (hyperextension) implies LCL, lateral capsule, and arcuate complex injury and possibly a PCL tear.

With varus and valgus stress tests, a positive result is graded as grade 1: up to 5 mm of opening, grade 2: 6 to 10 mm of opening, or grade 3: 11 to 15 mm of opening. It is important with these and all stress examinations to perform the test on the healthy, contralateral leg to differentiate any component of physiologic laxity. If the examiner has difficulty controlling a very large leg, optional variations of the varus or valgus stress test involve cradling the lower leg under the examiner's arm, while applying stress just below the knee with the hands (Fig.

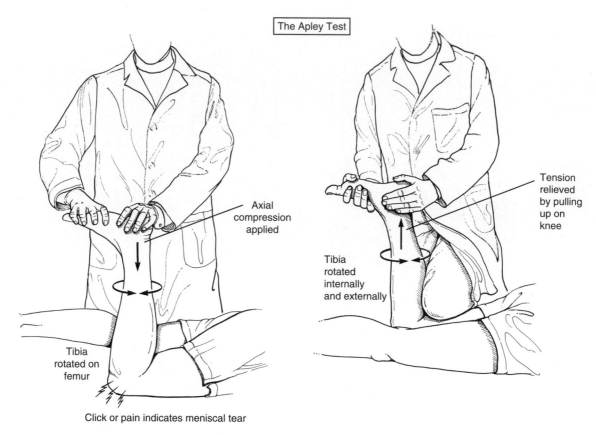

The Apley Test

Axial compression applied

Tibia rotated on femur

Click or pain indicates meniscal tear

Tension relieved by pulling up on knee

Tibia rotated internally and externally

Fig. 23-12. The Apley test. The knee is axially loaded with the patient prone while subjected to internal and external rotation. Pain or palpable click suggest a meniscal tear. Distraction of the knee should relieve the symptoms.

23-15). Alternatively, the leg can be swung partially off the side of the table with the thigh supported and stabilized with one hand while the other hand applies stress at the ankle.

ANTERIOR CRUCIATE LIGAMENT EVALUATION. Numerous tests have been described for ACL instability. The most sensitive and the easiest to perform in the presence of a painful, acutely swollen knee is the Lachman test.[86] With the knee in 20° to 30° of flexion, the leg is grasped with one hand and stabilized at the distal thigh with the other hand. Muscle relaxation is critical to accurate test results. An anteriorly directed force is applied to the proximal tibia to stress the ACL (Fig. 23-16). Anterior displacement compared with the normal contralateral leg is graded as 1+ (0 to 5 mm), 2+ (6 to 10 mm), or 3+ (11 to 15 mm). Additionally, one can comment on whether the endpoint is firm or soft. For problems with a large leg, one may perform the same test with the patient prone.

The anterior drawer test also assesses the integrity of the ACL by an anteriorly directed force on the leg (Fig. 23-17). The patient is supine with the knees flexed to 90°, and the examiner sits on the patient's feet to stabilize the leg. Both hands grasp behind the proximal calf, palpating the hamstring tendons to ensure relaxation, and an anteriorly directed force is applied. Anterior translation is again assessed as 1 to 3+ with a firm or

soft endpoint. The test can be repeated with the foot fixed in an internally or externally rotated position to test the integrity of the posterolateral or posteromedial capsules, respectively.

Several additional tests have been described to evaluate the rotational component of ACL instability, termed *anterolateral rotatory instability*. This rotatory instability better reflects the functional giving way episode experienced by patients than the straight anterior instability tested by the anterior drawer and Lachman tests. The most commonly used of these tests is the pivot shift test of MacIntosh.[31] With the patient supine, the examiner grasps the ankle with one hand while placing the opposite hand laterally at the knee behind the fibular head, directing pressure anteriorly (Fig. 23-18). With the knee extended, the leg is internally rotated, and a valgus force applied. In this position, the tibia is subluxed anteriorly in an ACL-deficient knee. As the knee is flexed, the iliotibial band tightens and reduces the tibia posteriorly to its normal position with a palpable clunk if the test result is positive. This reduction clunk can be graded 1 (glide), 2 (shift), or 3 (shift and clunk or momentary locking). The Losee test is similar to the pivot shift test except the leg begins in an externally rotated, flexed position and is moved into extension. In this case, the examiner looks for a jump into an anteriorly subluxed position. The flexion–rotation drawer test is a combination

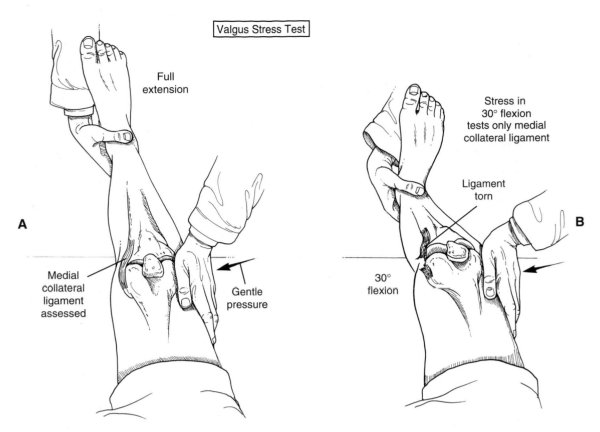

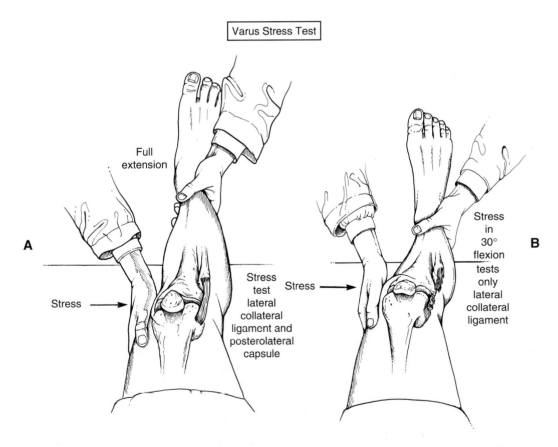

Fig. 23-13. The valgus stress test is performed at full extension to assess secondary restraints **(A)** and at 30° of flexion to assess the medial collateral ligament **(B)**.

Fig. 23-14. The varus stress test is performed at full extension to assess secondary restraints **(A)** and at 30° of flexion to assess the lateral collateral ligament **(B)**.

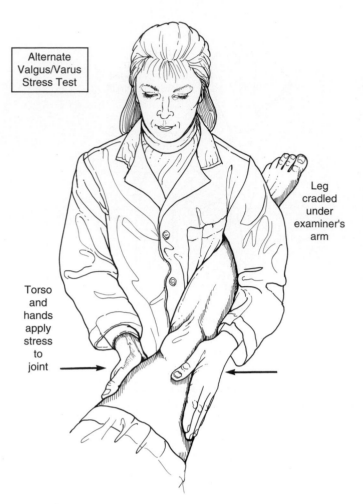

Alternate
Valgus/Varus
Stress Test

Leg
cradled
under
examiner's
arm

Torso
and
hands
apply
stress
to
joint

Fig. 23-15. An alternative method of performing varus and valgus stress testing is with the leg cradled under the examiner's arm while the torso and hands apply the stress.

of the Lachman and pivot shift tests (Fig. 23-19). Both hands are placed behind the calf to sublux the tibia anteriorly in extension while the leg is stabilized by cradling the ankle under the arm. Flexing the knee to 45° results in a palpable clunk as the tibia reduces posteriorly.

POSTERIOR CRUCIATE LIGAMENT EVALUATION. Tests for PCL disruption in general are less sensitive than those developed for ACL tears. The posterior sag sign is noted by flexing both knees to 90° and observing the contour from the side (Fig. 23-20). A PCL-deficient knee will sag posteriorly, resulting in a less prominent tibial tubercle compared with the opposite knee. The examiner can perform the posterior drawer test by applying posteriorly directed pressure to the tibial tubercle to further demonstrate the degree of laxity. The posterior translation is graded as 1 to 3 + as previously described with documentation of endpoint resistance. One potential difficulty in evaluating the PCL is determining the neutral starting position of the tibia in relation to the femoral condyles, which can be determined by the quadriceps active test. The patient is asked to contract the quadriceps with the knee in 90° of flexion while the examiner stabilizes the foot (Fig. 23-21). A posteriorly subluxed tibia caused by PCL laxity will reduce to a neutral position on quadriceps contraction. This reference point can then be used to perform a posterior Lachman test in 30° of flexion (Fig. 23-22). Another useful reference for quantification is to compare the anterior border of the tibia with that of the femoral condyles. Normally, the tibia is 5 mm anterior to the femoral condyles. If the tibia is flush with the condyles on the posterior drawer or Lachman test, this corresponds to 5 to 10 mm of posterior displacement (2 +). An endpoint anterior to the condyles is less than 5 mm (1 +), and an endpoint posterior to the condyles is more than 10 mm (3 +). Comparison with the contralateral, uninvolved knee is critical.

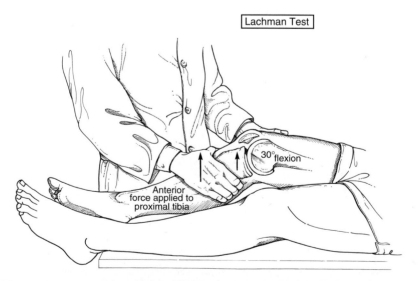

Lachman Test

30° flexion

Anterior
force applied to
proximal tibia

Fig. 23-16. The Lachman test is performed at 30° of flexion with an anteriorly directed force applied to the proximal tibia while the opposite hand stabilizes the thigh.

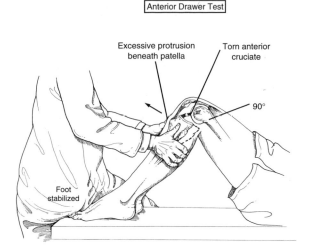

Anterior Drawer Test

Excessive protrusion beneath patella

Torn anterior cruciate

90°

Foot stabilized

Fig. 23-17. The anterior drawer test is performed at 90° of flexion with an anteriorly directed force applied to the proximal tibia.

IMAGING STUDIES

At the initial evaluation of an injured knee, the standard radiographic evaluation should include a standing anteroposterior view, a lateral view, a tunnel view, and a merchant view. The standing anteroposterior view is useful because it allows evaluation of the loaded knee joint and permits measurement of knee alignment. The tunnel view in 30° of flexion demonstrates the intercondylar notch, and delineates the posterior femoral condyles, which may have an osteochondral defect (Fig. 23-23 on p. 350). If a fracture is suspected, additional oblique views can be obtained. Stress views in varus and valgus can be helpful in diagnosing occult physeal fractures in the skeletally immature patient, but they have little role in routine evaluation of ligamentous injuries in the adult.

The sunrise or merchant view is obtained with the patient supine and the knee flexed 45°, with the x-ray beam 30° from horizontal and directed distally toward the cassette (Fig. 23-24 on p. 350). This view demonstrates the alignment of the patellofemoral joint and is used to determine subluxation or tilt of the patella. Other axial

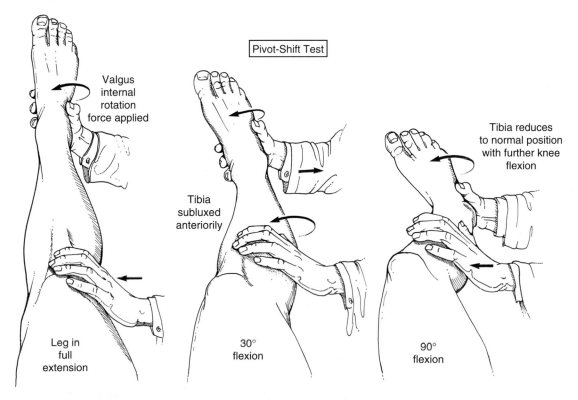

Pivot-Shift Test

Valgus internal rotation force applied

Tibia reduces to normal position with further knee flexion

Tibia subluxed anteriorly

Leg in full extension

30° flexion

90° flexion

Fig. 23-18. The pivot shift test begins in extension with a valgus, internal rotation force applied to the leg. In this position, the tibia is subluxed anteriorly. As the knee is flexed, the tibia subluxes posteriorly to its normal position, and a clunk is seen and felt by the examiner.

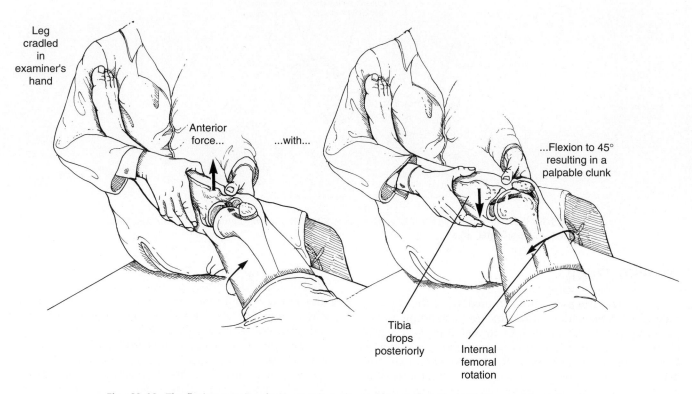

Flexion-Rotation Drawer Test

Leg cradled in examiner's hand

Anterior force...

...with...

...Flexion to 45° resulting in a palpable clunk

Tibia drops posteriorly

Internal femoral rotation

Fig. 23-19. The flexion-rotation drawer test is performed by cradling the leg in the examiner's hands with an anteriorly directed force to sublux the tibia anteriorly. Flexion to 45° results in a palpable clunk as the tibia reduces posteriorly.

views of the patella have been popularized, including the Laurin and Hughston views. Bipartite patella, a normal anatomic variant, can be visualized on the merchant view or on the anteroposterior projection (Fig. 23-25). These well-corticated bony fragments usually are bilateral

and occur at the superolateral pole. They are the result of accessory, ununited ossification centers.[66,78]

Before the advent of magnetic resonance imaging (MRI), arthrograms were helpful in diagnosing meniscal or cruciate ligament pathology with an accuracy of 60%

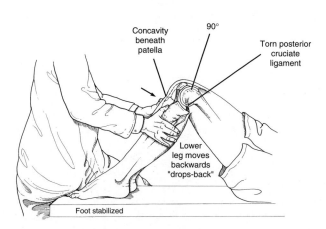

Posterior Drawer Test

Concavity beneath patella

90°

Torn posterior cruciate ligament

Lower leg moves backwards "drops-back"

Foot stabilized

Fig. 23-20. Posterior cruciate ligament deficiency results in a posterior sag in the resting position, which can be appreciated at 90° of flexion by comparing the contour of the anterior knee with the opposite side. Further posteriorly directed force produces the posterior drawer test to assess the extent of laxity.

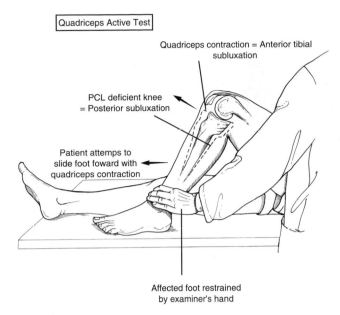

Quadriceps Active Test

Quadriceps contraction = Anterior tibial subluxation

PCL deficient knee = Posterior subluxation

Patient attemps to slide foot foward with quadriceps contraction

Affected foot restrained by examiner's hand

Fig. 23-21. The quadriceps active test is performed with the knee flexed 90° and the examiner stabilizing the foot on the table. In the posterior cruciate ligament-deficient knee, the tibia is at a posteriorly subluxed starting point. Active contraction of the quadriceps causes a forward translation of the tibia to a neutral position.

to 87%.[40] Currently, MRI has become the diagnostic procedure of choice for assessment of intraarticular knee pathology. Accuracy for diagnosing intraarticular pathology ranges from 88% to 97%[12,28] and offers the advantage of providing additional information about the collateral ligaments and bone. Normal meniscal and ligamentous tissue is relatively dark and homogeneous on T1- and T2-weighted images because of the low water and fat content (Fig. 23-26). Findings on MRI compatable with a meniscal tear include change in the usual dark meniscal signal to lighter signal, consistent with in-

terposed joint fluid. Early intrasubstance degeneration is radiographically a grade 1 signal, whereas an intrasubstance tear extending up to but not through the meniscal surface represents a grade 2 signal. Complete tears through the meniscal surface are termed grade 3 signals (Fig. 23-27 on p. 352). Meniscal degeneration, as opposed to a complete tear, often requires arthroscopic confirmation. Cruciate ligament tears are identified by disruption in the normal dark ligament signal with bright joint fluid (Fig. 23-28 on p. 352). Failure to adequately visualize the ACL may be technique-related, re-

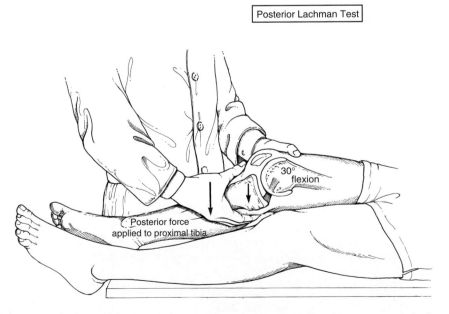

Posterior Lachman Test

30° flexion

Posterior force applied to proximal tibia

Fig. 23-22. The posterior Lachman test is performed with the knee flexed 30°. A posteriorly directed force is applied to the tibia and translation and endpoint assessed.

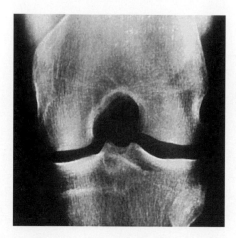

Fig. 23-23. Standing anteroposterior tunnel or notch view of the knee.

sulting from the oblique course of the ligament, or may represent a tear. Therefore, it is important to look in the anteroposterior and lateral projections for the ACL and PCL images. Bone bruises are seen in conjunction with an acute ACL tear 56% to 85% of the time.[33,54] These are usually seen on the distal aspect of the lateral femoral condyle and the posterior lateral tibia (Fig. 23-29).

MENISCAL INJURIES

Meniscal tears usually result from a twisting mechanism in either a contact or noncontact activity. The shear force of the twisting event mechanically catches the meniscus between the femoral condyle and tibial articular surface, creating the tear. Because the medial meniscus is less mobile than the lateral meniscus, it has a greater chance of becoming entrapped between the condyles, resulting in a higher incidence of medial

meniscal tears. Although most meniscal injuries result from an acute traumatic event, the patient may relate a relatively minor precipitating event, such as squatting down or getting up from a chair, which correlates with a meniscus with preexisting, intrasubstance degenerative changes. This can appear as grade 1 or 2 signals on MRI scans, indicating damage within the meniscus not extending to the surface of the meniscus. Acute tears in a previously normal meniscus may be associated with collateral or cruciate ligament injuries. Because symptoms from associated ligamentous injuries usually overshadow meniscal symptoms, meniscal tears should always be entertained with a high index of suspicion.

The patient with an acute meniscal tear usually relates moderate pain that gradually subsides, allowing the individual to ambulate with a slight limp and possibly even to continue play in some cases. A joint effusion usually occurs over the ensuing 24 hours and may be slight to moderate. With large, displaced, bucket-handle–type tears, the torn fragment will get trapped between the femoral condyle and tibial plateau, preventing full knee extension. Bucket-handle–type tears are more common on the medial side compared with the lateral side and result in the classic locked knee, which necessitates early referral to an orthopedist for arthroscopy to restore motion.

Most patients with meniscal tears will have full motion and present days to weeks after the initiating event with a history of painful locking, catching, or giving way, especially with twisting movements, which reflects the torn meniscal fragment being mechanically caught between the condyles. It is this mechanical impingement that causes abrasion and arthritic changes of the articular surfaces. Therefore, arthroscopic débridement or repair of the tear is usually recommended, even if symptoms at present may be minimal.

The physical examination reflects tenderness to palpation along the joint line overlying the tear. Provocative

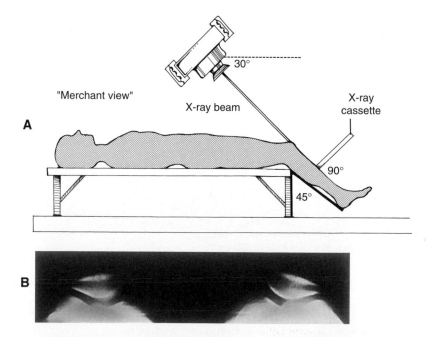

Fig. 23-24. A, Technique for obtaining the merchant view of the patella. **B,** Representative normal radiographic merchant view.

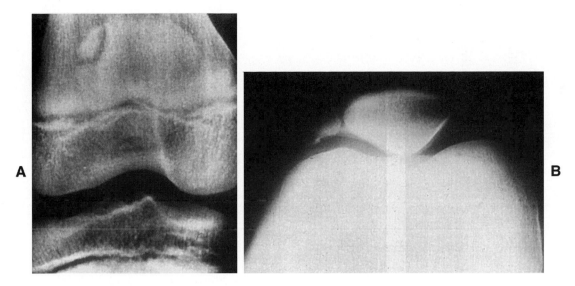

Fig. 23-25. Bipartite patella is demonstrated on anteroposterior **(A)** and merchant **(B)** views of the knee. A well-corticated, separate fragment forms the superolateral pole of the patella.

maneuvers to recreate impingement of the torn fragment are helpful in confirming the diagnosis. These include Steinmann's test, McMurray's test, or the Apley test. Localization of a palpable click and associated pain is helpful but not specific. Loose bodies and impinging synovial soft tissue should be entertained in the difficult diagnosis because they can give false-positive results. As previously stated, MRI evaluation is more than 90% accurate in diagnosing meniscal pathology (Fig. 23-27). One should, however, interpret the MRI findings in the context of the history and examination because an MRI often identifies grade 1 or 2 changes in asymptomatic individuals who do not require intervention.[48,69] Clinically asymptomatic discoid menisci represent a congenital anomaly that may not require intervention in the absence of a tear.

A treatment algorithm for suspected meniscal pathology is presented in Figure 23-30. Initial history and physical examination is usually accompanied by plain radiographs to exclude bony pathology, such as osteochondritis dissecans or a loose osteochondral fragment. If the examination suggests associated ligamentous instability, early referral to an orthopedist is appropriate. Otherwise, initial treatment with ice, a brief period of rest, and a short course of nonsteroidal anti-inflammatory medications (NSAIDs) is indicated. Failure to respond to nonoperative therapy or repeated episodes of catching or giving way suggests a meniscal tear, which should be referred to an orthopedic surgeon. These types of meniscal lesions are successfully managed with arthroscopic surgery. Most tears require débridement to a stable rim. Tears in the peripheral one third or red zone potentially have an adequate blood supply to attempt meniscal repair. Degenerative type patterns, radial tears, horizontal cleavage tears, or tears more than 4 cm in length generally do not heal and are usually addressed by a partial menisectomy. Performing a meniscal repair in conjunction with a cruciate reconstruction has been shown to enhance healing, possibly because of the beneficial healing properties of the bloody, postoperative effusion and subsequent clot. Meniscal repairs in the face of an unsta-

ble knee usually fail and are not recommended. The underlying theme in addressing meniscal pathology at arthroscopy is to retain as much of the meniscus as possible to help prevent future arthritic changes.

After arthroscopic surgery, patients should aggressively rehabilitate the knee to restore motion and strength. Most patients are able to restore quadriceps strength with a cycling program and progressive, resistive exercises with light weights.[11] Other patients who lack individual motivation may benefit from a supervised physical therapy program. Return to sports depends on restoration of full range of motion and equal strength, usually obtained in 3 to 6 weeks. Office work can be resumed immediately as pain permits.

LIGAMENTOUS INJURIES

Collateral Ligament Injuries
Collateral ligament injuries often result from a direct injury. A medially directed force against the lateral side of

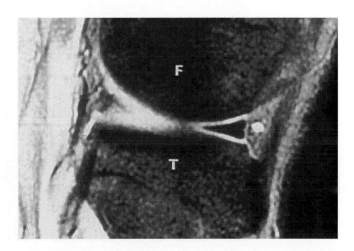

Fig. 23-26. Magnetic resonance imaging of normal meniscus is illustrated on T2-weighted view.

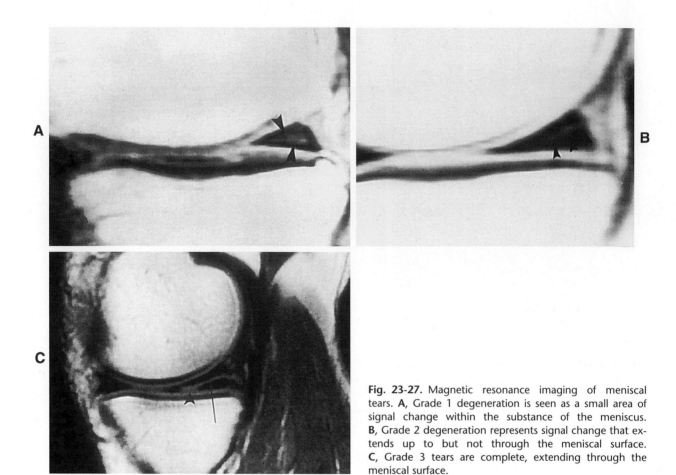

Fig. 23-27. Magnetic resonance imaging of meniscal tears. **A,** Grade 1 degeneration is seen as a small area of signal change within the substance of the meniscus. **B,** Grade 2 degeneration represents signal change that extends up to but not through the meniscal surface. **C,** Grade 3 tears are complete, extending through the meniscal surface.

the knee, as occurs from a clip or tackle in football, creates a valgus-deforming force that injures the medial structures. If no rotational component is involved, an isolated MCL injury may occur. Additional rotational force is more likely to result in an associated meniscal tear and ACL injury. Likewise, a laterally directed force against the medial side of the knee can result in injury to the LCL and supporting lateral structures. Injury to the LCL is less common than injury to the medial side. Noncontact injuries can also result from deceleration or

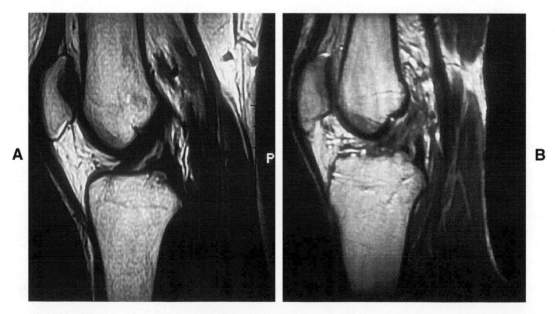

Fig. 23-28. Magnetic resonance imaging of a healthy anterior cruciate ligament **(A),** and a completely torn anterior cruciate ligament **(B).**

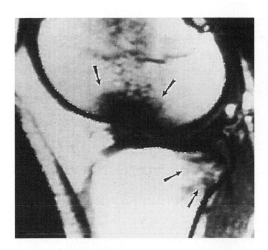

Fig. 23-29. Magnetic resonance imaging of the knee demonstrating the contrasting dark signal characteristic of a bone bruise in the lateral femoral condyle adjacent to the articular surface and extending proximally into the cancellous bone. Corresponding lesion can be seen in the posterolateral tibia.

pivot mechanisms. The addition of rotational forces to the noncontact mechanism results in an increased incidence of ACL injuries.

Varus and valgus stress testing is performed at 30° of flexion, full extension or 0°, and hyperextension. Laxity only in flexion suggests isolated collateral ligament injury, whereas laxity at full extension suggests additional injury to the posteromedial or posterolateral capsule. Laxity in hyperextension may imply injury to the posterior oblique ligament medially or the arcuate ligamentous complex laterally and possibly injury to the PCL or ACL, depending on the magnitude of force. Laxity to varus or valgus stress should be compared with the opposite, noninvolved knee. In less severe injuries, laxity may not be present, but the patient will report pain on stress of the involved collateral ligament.

Patients usually localize pain well to either side of the knee, although, if an associated cruciate ligament injury is present, these intraarticular symptoms will dominate the examination. With significantly lax knees, the patient may complain of giving way and a sense of instability. Swelling, if present, may be localized to one side of the knee. Tenderness along the course of the collateral ligament or at the femoral origin or tibial insertion is a helpful finding.

Plain radiographs are helpful to rule out osseous abnormalities, including avulsion fractures or growth plate injuries that often mimic collateral injuries in skeletally immature patients. Chronic MCL injuries can demonstrate calcification along the course of the ligament (Pellegrini-Stieda sign). Stress films can be helpful if a physeal fracture is suspected. Otherwise, MRI is best to delineate collateral ligament injuries and any associated pathology. The normal low signal ligament is interrupted by the high signal of edema and hemorrhage (Fig. 23-31).

Collateral ligament injuries, like all ligament sprains, are graded as first degree if microscopic disruption of collagen fibers is present without gross elongation or any clinically detectable laxity.[76] Pain on stress testing and local tenderness and swelling are the dominant findings.

Meniscal Injury

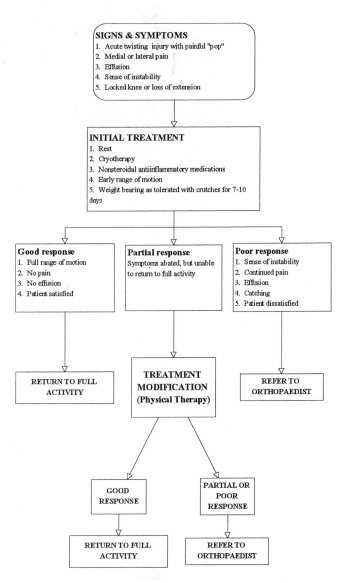

Fig. 23-30. Suspected meniscal tear algorithm. *Adapted from the AAOS National Orthopedic Leadership Conference 1995.*

Management consists of ice and rest as needed, with early range of motion exercises (Fig. 23-32). Bracing is generally not needed unless used purely for increased patient comfort during the first several days. An off-the-shelf knee immobilizer is adequate. It is important to encourage motion to prevent the rapid onset of stiffness that can occur with a brace. A neoprene knee sleeve that permits full motion gives patients a feeling of support and is preferred. Return to sports is usually within 6 to 8 weeks of injury.

A second degree sprain represents macroscopic, partial tearing of the ligament with clinically detectable elongation of 0.5 to 1 cm on stress testing. Pain with stress testing, local tenderness, and swelling are more pronounced. Grade II collateral injuries can also be managed symptomatically with brace immobilization only temporarily (less than 5 days) as needed for patient comfort. Thereafter, a hinged knee brace permitting motion is recommended only if the patient has significant pain. Cane or

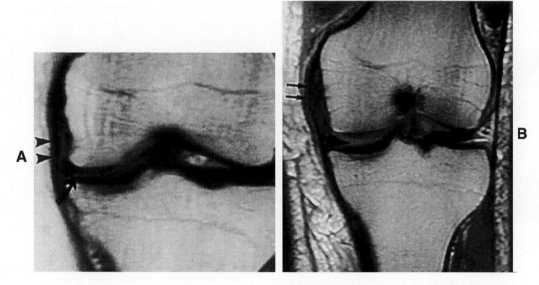

Fig. 23-31. Magnetic resonance imaging of intact **(A)** and torn **(B)** medial collateral ligament (arrows).

crutch support for the first week may facilitate ambulation. Cryotherapy and a short course of NSAIDs may be helpful as the patient works to achieve a full range of motion. Once motion has been obtained, isometric, isotonic, and eventually isokinetic progressive resistive exercises are performed for quadriceps strengthening under physical therapist supervision. Once equal strength is achieved and pain is absent to stress test or palpation, the athlete may return to competitive sports, usually 6 to 8 weeks after injury. Vague, nagging pain can sometimes persist for 3 to 6 months.

A third degree collateral ligament sprain is a complete disruption with more than 1 cm of joint line opening on stress examination. Pain on stress testing may be disproportionately low because no fibers are actually being stressed in a completely torn ligament. Tenderness along the ligament is significant, and a large effusion is also present resulting from the associated capsular disruption. A high level of suspicion should be maintained for concomitant ACL injury.

Management is an initial period of immobilization followed by early motion protected by a hinged knee brace. Physical therapy for motion and strengthening is recommended. Full return to activities generally occurs 2 and 3 months after injury, when the patient achieves 90% strength of the opposite side and can perform an agility program similar to that required in the athlete's sport. Patient comfort and athletic performance are better indicators of readiness to return to sport than a specified time period.[38] A small amount of residual laxity is common and does not appear to be a functional problem. Patients may wear the hinged knee brace up to 6 months during return to activites, and pain with activities even with the brace frequently persists for that length of time.

Previous recommendations for operative management of grade III collateral ligament tears are less popular, and nonoperative management appears to provide comparable results in terms of stability without surgical morbid-

ity and with an earlier return to sports participation.[39] Current recommendations for combined injuries of the ACL and MCL are to manage the MCL injury nonoperatively.[79] A delay of 4 to 8 weeks allows the initial inflammatory phase of healing to subside and full motion to be restored. This delays allows adequate and predictable healing of the MCL with less risk of stiffness after ACL reconstruction than if both ligaments were reconstructed. All grade II and grade III collateral ligament tears should be referred to an orthopedist because there is a very high incidence of associated knee pathology with collateral ligament injuries.

Anterior Cruciate Ligament

ACL tears are becoming increasingly common, with an incidence of 250,000 cases per year in the United States.[42] Women experience up to a sevenfold increase in ACL tears compared with men in competitive sports.[97] This increase perhaps results from anatomic variations of a tighter intercondylar notch, which theoretically could shear the ligament.[70] Women also tend to be more ligamentously lax, which may put the knee at increased risk for injury. As surgical techniques improve and become more predictable, the management of ACL injuries has shifted toward early surgical reconstruction. Understanding of the natural history of the ACL-deficient knee has also influenced decision-making.

The ACL is often torn during running sports when the foot is planted and the knee twists when changing directions. Alternatively, the ACL can be torn by contact to the lateral knee with a valgus, external rotation force; by hyperextension; or rarely by varus, internal rotation force. Classically, the athlete feels a "pop" in the knee, is unable to continue to participate, feels the knee is unsteady, and complains of significant pain. The swelling, secondary to an intraarticular effusion, usually occurs quickly over a few hours. Aspiration is generally reserved for large, tense effusions to provide pain relief. The find-

Collateral Ligament Injury

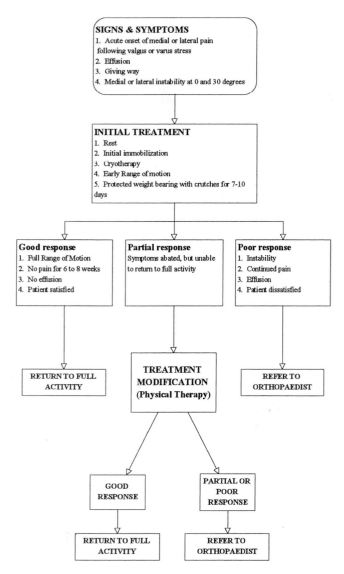

Fig. 23-32. Treatment algorithm for collateral ligament injuries. *Adapted from the AAOS National Orthopedic Leadership Conference 1995.*

ing of a hemarthrosis is very helpful, but somewhat nonspecific, and could be found for an osteochondral fracture, a patellar dislocation, a peripheral meniscal tear, or an intraarticular fracture.

The examination of an acute ACL tear is most productive immediately after the injury on the field or court before the onset of swelling. Otherwise, the subsequent pain and swelling obscure a clear examination and make diagnosis more difficult. Examination techniques include a Lachman test at 30° and, if the patient's pain and range of motion permit, an anterior drawer test at 90° to assess anterior translation of the tibia with respect to the femur. A pivot shift maneuver (or one of its variations) is diagnostic if present. The findings are compared with the contralateral normal knee, because laxity may represent a normal, physiologic variant. Careful attention should also be directed to any possible associated collateral liga-

ment injuries or meniscal tears. Meniscal tears in association with an acute ACL and MCL injury occur more often on the lateral side than on the medial side (Fig. 23-33). Additionally, grade II MCL injuries result in a higher incidence of meniscal tears (71%) than seen with grade III MCL injuries (51%),[79] which may result from a distractive mechanism of injury associated with grade III MCL tears as opposed to a compressive mechanism for grade II MCL tears.

Although standard radiographs are of limited value in diagnosing a torn ACL, they provide useful information and should be performed routinely. It would not be unusual to note an avulsion of the tibial spine, a Segond fracture, or an intraarticular fracture.[73] MRI is the imaging modality of choice to supplement the physical examination and to provide supportive information about related structures (Fig. 23-34). Because partial tears of the ACL are very difficult to assess on clinical examination and by MRI, arthroscopic visualization remains the gold standard for diagnosis.

Although no study has shown conclusively that ACL tears directly lead to arthritis, a number of studies confirm that ACL-deficient knees progress to further meniscal and articular surface injuries. Finsterbush et al.[27] showed a 33% incidence of additional intraarticular injuries over 28 months after an isolated ACL tear. Irvine and Glasgow[41] showed an 86% incidence of meniscal tears at an average of 3 years after injury. Other studies have shown that the variable that best correlates with arthritic changes and pain in an ACL-injured knee is meniscal injury.[58,94] Therefore, reconstructing the ACL to help preserve the menisci theoretically should help prevent arthritic changes. Unfortunately, no prospective, randomized, blinded study has successfully proven that reconstruction of the torn ACL will prevent arthritis. However, there is general agreement in the orthopedic community that young persons should have ACL reconstructions to minimize future knee injury and to maintain the level of activities. "Young" is a relative term and level of activity may be more important as a person ages. In general, the physician can advise an athlete that if he or she is willing to discontinue sports that involve running, jumping, or pivoting activities, he or she may be content without a reconstruction. Episodes of giving way with activities of daily living would be a strong indication for reconstruction, regardless of a person's athletic activities. Giving way episodes with whatever sports activities a person chooses is another indication to reconstruct the ACL to prevent further knee injury. If a person wants to remain more active than walking-, biking-, and swimming-type activities, a reconstruction is warranted, even if that person is somewhat older (i.e., aged 40 to 50 years). An excellent natural history and outcome study by Daniel[22] showed that the best predictors of a late reconstruction for an ACL tear were preinjury hours more than 200 per year of sports requiring cutting, jumping, pivoting, and a significant degree of laxity compared with the opposite knee by KT-1000 arthrometer measurement. A KT-1000 measurement on the manual maximum test that is 3 mm different than the opposite, uninvolved side is considered abnormal.[20] A side-to-side difference more than 7 mm

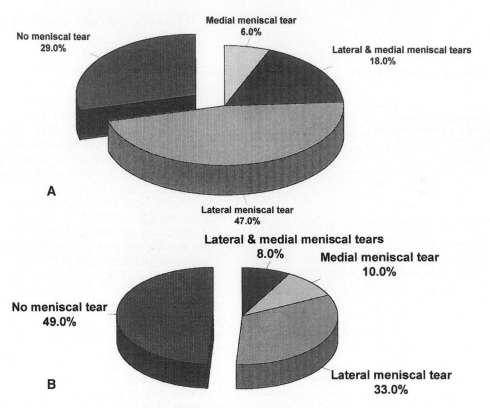

Fig. 23-33. **A,** Distribution of meniscal tears in patients with an acute tear of anterior cruciate ligament and an associated grade II sprain of the medial collateral ligament. **B,** Distribution of meniscal tears in patients with an acute injury of the anterior cruciate ligament and an associated grade III sprain of the medial collateral ligament. From Shelbourne KD, Patel DK: Management of combined injuries of the anterior cruciate ligament and medial collateral ligament, *J Bone Joint Surg* 77A:800, 1995.

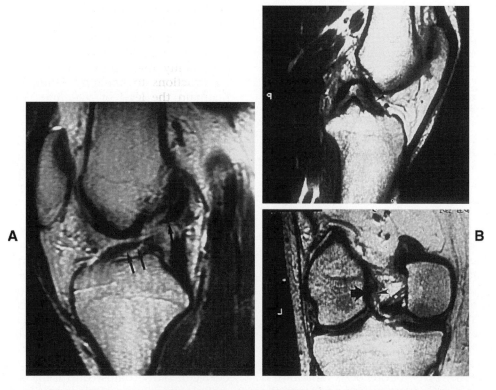

Fig. 23-34. **A,** Magnetic resonance imaging of complete anterior cruciate ligament tear demonstrates bright edema signal within the ligament fibers and poor visualization of fiber continuity. **B,** Partial tear on magnetic resonance imaging is seen as interposed edema with fiber continuity.

Table 23-1. Surgical risk factors

KT-1000 manual maximum, side-to-side difference (mm)	Sports hours per year, level I or II sports		
	< 50 hr	50–199 hr	>200 hr
<5	Low	Low	Moderate
5–7	Low	Moderate	High
>7	Moderate	High	High

puts the athlete at a high risk for needing late reconstruction because of repeated giving way episodes. This information is summarized in Table 23-1.[21,22] Level I sports include basketball, football, and soccer and involve jumping, pivoting, and hard cutting. Level II sports include baseball, racket sports, and skiing and involve less jumping or hard cutting.

Current reconstruction techniques use the arthroscopic approach. These endoscopic techniques implant a ligament substitute in the normal femoral and tibial attachment sites of the ACL. The graft choices for ligament substitution include the central one third bone–patella tendon–bone autograft or allograft, autograft hamstring tendons, allograft achilles tendon, or artificial ligament substitutes. Allograft tendons are most useful for revision situations or in older individuals whose patella tendon may be relatively weak because of age-related degenerative changes. If an allograft is chosen, the patient needs to be counseled regarding disease transmission. Artificial ligament substitutes have shown failure rates in excess of 50% and are not recommended.[43,97] Today's gold standard is the central third bone–patella tendon–bone autograft. With this endoscopic technique, aside from the arthroscopic portals, the only incision necessary is an approximately 6-cm anterior incision used to harvest the bone–patella tendon–bone graft (Fig. 23-35). Arthroscopically positioned guides enable the surgeon to prepare the femoral and tibial tunnels, which are necessary to pass and secure the graft. In this manner, the graft is positioned in the knee along the course of the native ACL (Fig. 23-36).[43] Various options for rigid graft fixation allow immediate motion and weight-bearing for rapid rehabilitation.[50] After an initial period of exercises to restore motion, therapy focuses on strengthening and eventually proprioceptive, agility, and sports-specific activities. In general, rehabilitation programs have become increasingly aggressive, with most athletes now returning to sports by 6 to 8 months after surgery.

Nonoperative management of an ACL tear involves physical therapy for restoration of motion and strengthening. Quadriceps muscle conditioning should ideally be a life-long endeavor. Most athletes can return to sports without surgery by 6 weeks, assuming they have achieved 90% of the strength of the uninvolved knee. The use of a brace provides largely subjective benefit and is controversial, but most athletes seem to prefer their use. The proposed mechanisms by which a brace works

include mechanical constraint of joint motion, although this has only been documented at low loads and has not been shown to be effective at the high loads involved with sports. Also, a brace provides a proprioceptive feedback mechanism, serving as a "reminder" to the athlete to avoid positions that may result in a giving way episode.[49,50] If an athlete suffers giving way episodes with sports, one can assume that this places the knee at significant risk for further meniscal and articular cartilage injury, and one should recommend reconstruction.

Any meniscal tear initially present may be repairable, and every attempt should be made to preserve the meniscus. Healing rates are improved from roughly 50% to 93% when performed in conjunction with an ACL reconstruction.[14] This increased rate of healing results from restoration of the normal knee biomechanics, the beneficial healing effects of a postoperative hemarthrosis, including the associated fibrin clot and growth factors, and the lack of degeneration in the meniscus before acute injury.[7,15] Healing rates of meniscal repair in the ACL-deficient knee in the absence of cruciate reconstruction fall off to approximately 30%.[93]

An important component in the nonoperative management of the ACL-deficient knee is counseling the athlete for activity modification. Avoiding activities involving jumping, twisting, pivoting, or cutting is generally necessary for nonoperative management to succeed. If an athlete is not willing to make these modifications, reconstruction should be recommended. This approach to ACL tear management is summarized in the algorithm in Figure 23-37.

Partial tears of the ACL occur in 10% to 28% of all ligament injuries and can be confusing for prognosis and management considerations.[59,92] The amount of ligament torn cannot be accurately assessed by MRI, and arthroscopic visualization and probing can also be misleading and subjective. Progression of a partial tear to a functionally complete ligament tear occurs 38% to 56% of the time, with ligaments 25% torn rarely progressing, 50% torn progressing 50% of the time, and 75% torn progressing 86% of the time.[51,60] Current recommendations involve the same lifestyle modifications used for decision-making for a complete tear and any history or examination evidence of recurrent instability. If an athlete reports no giving way episodes during activities, has a stable examination, and has less than 50% of the ligament torn at arthroscopy, nonoperative treatment is chosen. However, if the patient has laxity on examination or by history, reconstruction is warranted because the partial tear is functionally a complete tear.[43]

Posterior Cruciate Ligament Injuries

PCL injuries occur less often than ACL tears, with an incidence of 3% to 20% of all knee ligament injuries.[18,19] Often these injuries go undetected, as demonstrated by a 2% incidence in asymptomatic collegiate football players.[65] With the advent of MRI, an increasing number of these injuries are being recognized earlier.

The mechanism of injury usually involves a posteriorly directed force against the proximal tibia while the

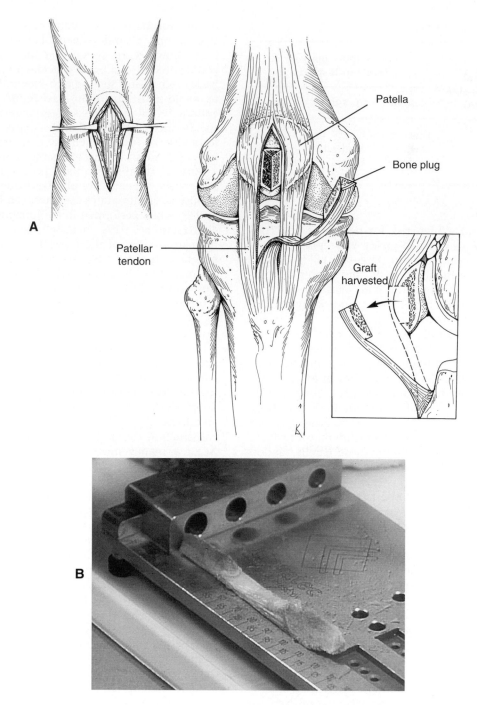

Fig. 23-35. Patella tendon autograft for anterior cruciate ligament reconstruction. **A,** The middle third of the patella tendon is harvested with attached bone plugs from the patella and tibial ends. **B,** Photograph of the patella tendon autograft.

knee is flexed. A fall directly on the knee with the foot plantar flexed causes such posterior displacement. Another common etiology is striking the dashboard against the knee in a motor vehicle accident. PCL injuries have been documented to occur in 44% of major trauma patients with acute hemarthroses.[24] Hyperflexion, possibly with internal rotation, can also cause an isolated PCL tear.[84] Other mechanisms usually involve injury to other ligamentous structures, including extreme varus or valgus injury with combined collateral ligament tears and hyperextension with associated ACL tear.[19,44] One should

be suspicious of a knee dislocation if multiple ligaments are injured or if the mechanism involves hyperextension. Any suspicion of a knee dislocation demands immediate orthopedic and vascular evaluation.

The posterior drawer test performed at 90° of flexion is the most helpful test in the physical examination to determine the status of the PCL.[77,90] Normally, the anterior surface of the tibial condyles rests approximately 10 mm anterior to the anterior surface of the femoral condyles, providing a useful reference for displacement with a posterior force. Displacement up to 5 mm is a

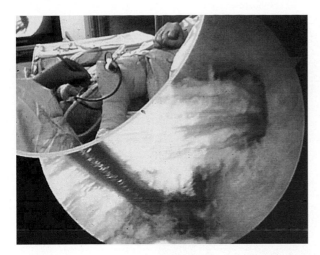

Fig. 23-36. The bone-patella tendon-bone autograft is passed through tunnels drilled with arthroscopic guides to reproduce the orientation of the native anterior cruciate ligament. Fixation of the bone plugs is achieved with interference fit screws within the tunnel or screw and suture combinations.

grade I injury, with the tibial condyles remaining anterior to the femoral condyles. When the tibia and femur are flush, this implies posterior translation of 5 to 10 mm, consistent with a grade II injury. Displacement of the anterior surface of the tibia further posteriorly (more than 10 mm) than the anterior surface of the femoral condyles implies a grade III injury.[90] A posterior sag sign and a positive quadriceps active test are other useful tests for confirming the diagnosis. The posterior Lachman test is somewhat more difficult to use because the proper starting point can be difficult to determine, sometimes giving the false impression of anterior laxity if the posteriorly subluxed starting point is not appreciated. Assessment of the quality of the endpoint to stress and looking for a posterior sag can help avoid this confusion, as can comparison with the healthy knee. Additionally, the KT-2000 arthrometer is very useful to quantitate the degree of posterior laxity and for management decision-making similar to the ACL-deficient knee (Fig. 23-38).

Anterior Cruciate Ligament Injury

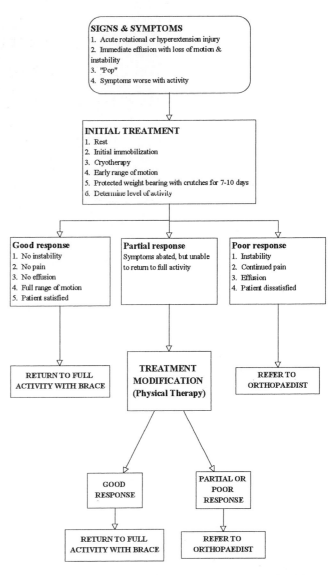

Fig. 23-37. Anterior cruciate ligament tear treatment algorithm.

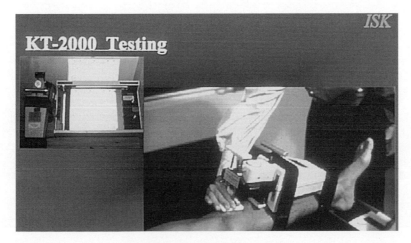

Fig. 23-38. KT-2000 arthrometer.

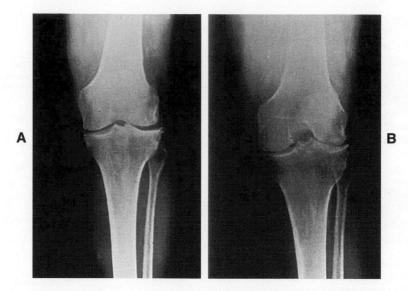

Fig. 23-39. Standing anteroposterior radiograph of the knee **(A)** shows moderate joint space narrowing that is much more evident on the standing, flexed posteroanterior view **(B)**.

An important determination in selecting management options involves the assessment of associated injuries, including the posterolateral corner. Comparing external rotation, posterior translation, and varus laxity with the contralateral knee is useful in assessing injury to the posterolateral corner. Increased external rotation, varus angulation, and posterior translation at 30° and 90° suggests injury to the PCL and the posterolateral corner. However, when the increased rotation, laxity, and translation at 30° decreases at 90° of flexion, the examiner should suspect an isolated injury to the posterolateral corner.[32] Alternatively, injury to the posterolateral corner can be diagnosed by increased passive external rotation of the tibia relative to the femur with the patient prone on the examining table.[19]

Plain radiographs are helpful to look for bony avulsions, which occur in greater frequency in PCL injuries than in ACL injuries. In the chronic PCL-deficient knee, radiographs should be obtained in the standing, weight-bearing mode if possible to assess any degenerative changes that will affect management choices. An additional anteroposterior weight-bearing view with the knee in 45° of flexion often better demonstrates degenerative changes (Fig. 23-39). These degenerative, unstable knees often are in varus alignment and best evaluated on long-length standing films. MRI is the most reliable imaging study to confirm injury to the PCL (Fig. 23-40). The accuracy rate for visualizing a PCL injury is the best of all intraarticular structures and has been shown to be 98% to 100%.[28,35] Because of the posterior orientation of the PCL and its inferior attachment site on the tibial plateau, arthroscopy can yield false-negative results without additional posteromedial portal visualization.[25]

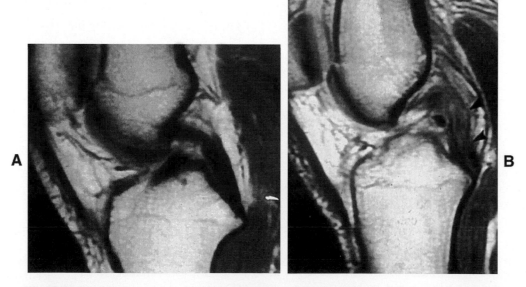

Fig. 23-40. Magnetic resonance imaging of healthy **(A)** and torn **(B)** posterior cruciate ligament. The ligament signal is interrupted by edema with nonhomogeneous fiber appearance.

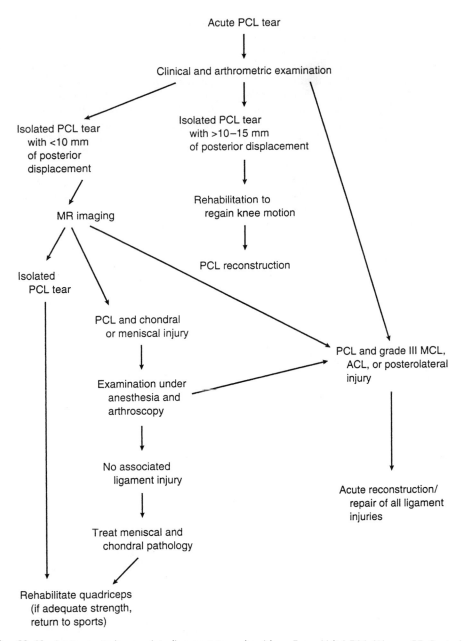

Fig. 23-41. Acute posterior cruciate ligament tear algorithm. From Veltri DM, Warren RF: Posterior cruciate ligament injuries, *J Am Acad Orthop Surg* 1:73, 1993.

Knowledgeable management recommendations for PCL injuries depends on an understanding of the natural history of this injury. Parolie and Bergfeld[65] emphasized quadriceps rehabilitation until strength was equal to the opposite side. With nonoperative treatment, these authors noted that 84% of their athletes had returned to sports and were able to continue to participate for an average of 6.2 years, although only 68% performed at their previous levels.[65] The influence of combined ligamentous injuries has been previously reported, as these patients had significantly worse functional results than those with isolated PCL injuries.[85] Other authors have demonstrated progressive degenerative changes with chronic pain. Clancy[16,17] has confirmed the progression of arthritic changes in the PCL-deficient knee, as substantiated by radiographic evaluation, nuclear imaging, and arthroscopy. Degenerative changes were also confirmed by Keller,[45] who noted a 65%

incidence of arthritic changes and a 90% incidence of pain at 6 years. Based on these observations, the nonoperative management of PCL injuries is currently undergoing scrutiny, however, no good prospective study documents that reconstruction prevents arthritic changes.

Current consensus is to manage acute, isolated PCL tears with less than 10 mm of posterior translation on posterior drawer nonoperatively,[25,77,90] which involves quadriceps rehabilitation using closed kinetic-chain exercises, such as squats and leg presses. Open kinetic-chain extension exercises (e.g., seated knee extensions with weights) are to be avoided because of increased pressure on the patellofemoral joint, a common source of pain in the PCL-deficient knee resulting from increased posterior tibial translation.[90] The athlete may return to sports after achieving at least 90% of equal strength, usually within 3 to 4 weeks. Any associated meniscal or chondral injury warrants arthroscopic management if symptomatic. Acute PCL injuries combined with other ligament injuries or if associated with more than 10 mm of posterior translation should be considered for surgical reconstruction. Reconstruction of associated posterolateral, collateral, and ACL injuries is generally recommended. This approach to PCL injuries is summarized in the algorithm from Veltri and Warren (Fig. 23-41 on p. 361).[90]

Chronic PCL tears focus on the presence or absence of associated posterolateral instability and whether posterior translation is more than 10 mm. An initial trial of quadriceps rehabilitation is attempted to improve symptoms, but if unsuccessful, a reconstruction of the PCL is warranted. This assumes that significant radiographic degenerative changes and varus malalignment are not present, in which case a valgus high tibial osteotomy may be indicated. Management of the chronic PCL-deficient knee is summarized in an algorithm in Figure 23-42.[90]

PCL reconstruction is technically more demanding than ACL surgery, primarily because of the posterior location of the PCL and proximity to neurovascular structures. The principles are similar, with arthroscopic-assisted placement of tunnels in the tibia and femur to pass a graft in the position of the native PCL. Because of the longer overall length needed for the graft and common patellofemoral complaints with a chronically posteriorly subluxed knee, many surgeons are using alternatives to the central third–patella tendon autograft. Popular choices include Achilles tendon or patella tendon allograft or, less commonly, hamstring tendons. The Achilles tendon allograft is the most popular because of its additional intrinsic strength and ease in passing through the bone tunnels. Results have generally been good, with Clancy[16] reporting all 10 of acute tears and 11 of 13 chronic tears reconstructed with good or excellent results at 2 years. Fanelli[25] has reported similar results.

An avulsion of the PCL occurs more commonly than the ACL, and can be managed nonoperatively by cast immobilization with good results only if the fragment is truly nondisplaced. Displaced fragments reduced and fixed surgically generally yield excellent results (Fig. 23-43), and anatomic reapproximation is the procedure of choice.[1,9,23,52,64,67,87,89] Small fragments not amenable to screw fixation can be treated nonoperatively if there is less than 10 mm of posterior laxity. However, more than 10 mm of laxity warrants reconstruction. This management algorithm is found in Figure 23-44.[90]

KNEE DISLOCATIONS

Knee dislocations are relatively infrequent events that result from significant trauma to the knee, usually as a result of motor vehicle accidents or falls, but can also occur in contact sports, such as hyperextension in a football

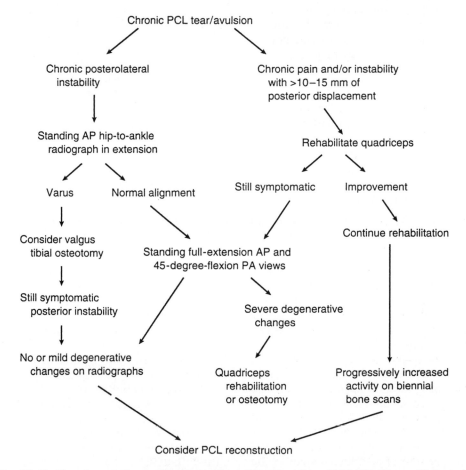

Fig. 23-42. Chronic posterior cruciate ligament tear algorithm. From Veltri DM, Warren RF: Posterior cruciate ligament injuries, *J Am Acad Orthop Surg* 1:74, 1993.

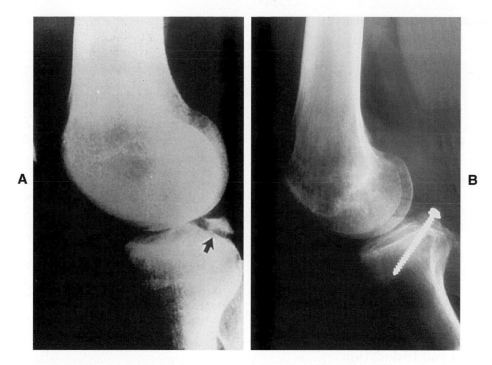

Fig. 23-43. A, Posterior cruciate ligament avulsion fracture from the tibial insertion. **B,** After open reduction and internal fixation.

tackle. Dislocation results in major ligamentous injury, usually tearing ACL and PCL, collateral ligaments, and capsular structures.[96] Perhaps more importantly, arterial injury occurs in knee dislocations with a frequency of 29% to 40%.[34,81,88] Intimal arterial injury may be present even in the face of initially intact pedal pulses.[55,80] Therefore, arteriograms or Doppler examinations are essentially mandatory in the acute knee dislocation. Additionally, neurologic injuries occur in 9% to 49% of knee dislocations with recovery rates ranging from 13% to 80%.[6] Because of the significant risk of neurovascular and extensive ligamentous injury, immediate referral to an orthopedist with access to vascular surgery evaluation is mandatory. Arterial repair is necessary within the first 6 to 8 hours to minimize the risk of amputation. Risk of compartment syndrome necessitating fasciotomy also increases with prolonged limb ischemia (Fig. 23-45).

Management consists of immediate closed reduction on the playing field or at the scene of the accident, followed by splinting. Often the reduction has occurred spontaneously before physician evaluation, and one must be suspicious for dislocation if the examination demonstrates multiple ligamentous injuries or popliteal fossa tenderness and ecchymosis. Open reduction is often necessary for posterolateral dislocations because of interposition of the joint capsule preventing closed reduction.[46,68] Surgical reconstruction of ligamentous injuries should be performed in cases requiring open reduction or open vascular repair. Ligament reconstruction should be delayed if limb ischemia or a tenuous vascular repair precludes early intervention. Current orthopedic opinion favors early reconstruction of all ligamentous injuries, with primary repair of bony avulsions if possible, or using autograft or allograft techniques.[82,95]

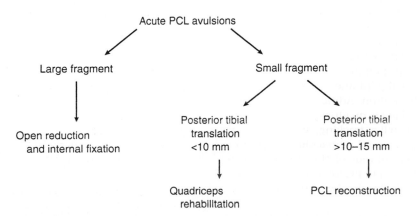

Fig. 23-44. Posterior cruciate ligament avulsion algorithm. From Veltri DM, Warren RF: Posterior cruciate ligament injuries, *J Am Acad Orthop Surg* 1:71, 1993.

Knee Dislocation Algorithm

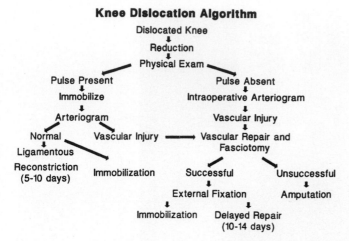

Fig. 23-45. Management algorithm for knee dislocations. From Montgomery et al: Orthopedic management of knee dislocations, *Am J Knee Surg* 8(3): 97-103, 1995.

PATELLOFEMORAL JOINT

Patella Subluxation and Dislocation

Anterior knee pain can be a frustrating complaint for the physician and the patient. The exact etiology is often elusive, and nonoperative management may take an extensive period of time before symptoms improve. Surgical intervention can also be frustrating because of the lack of predictability for achieving good results. Sources of pain include malalignment, chondromalacia patella, osteoarthritis, osteochondral fractures, synovial plicae, bursitis, tendonitis, patella subluxation or dislocation, and others. Merchant's classification of patellofemoral disorders demonstrates an extensive list of possible etiologies (Table 23-2).[56] A thorough understanding of the anatomy as it relates to the biomechanics of the patellofemoral joint can help the physician considerably when confronted with this common complaint.

The extensor mechanism includes the quadriceps musculature, the quadriceps and patellar tendons, the patella, and the femoral sulcus. The Q angle (see Fig. 23-8), measured by the angle made from the anterior–superior iliac spine to the patella and from the patella to the tibial tubercle, reflects the vector of the extensor mechanism. An abnormal Q angle more than 10° in men and more than 20° in women should be put in context with the rest of the history and physical examination. The underlying assumption is that an abnormally high Q angle with a more laterally directed quadriceps pull places excessive pressure on the lateral patellofemoral joint and predisposes to subluxation and possibly dislocation. Additionally, an imbalance in the medial and lateral quadriceps muscle forces may accentuate lateral patellar tracking, which may be further impacted by a tight lateral retinaculum. Anatomic variations in the shape or contour of the femoral sulcus and patella are also influential in disorders of the extensor mechanism. Patella height has also been shown to be a contributing factor.[2,72,74]

One of the most severe injuries to the extensor mechanism is a patellar dislocation. The athlete with a patellar dislocation describes a dramatic event, resulting in a

Table 23-2. Merchant classification of patellofemoral disorders

Trauma (conditions caused by trauma in the otherwise healthy knee)
  Acute trauma
    Contusion (924.11)
    Fracture
      Patella (822)
      Femoral trochlea (821.2)
      Proximal tibial epiphysis (tubercle) (823.0)
    Dislocation (rare in the healthy knee) (836.3)
    Rupture
      Quadriceps tendon (843.8)
      Patellar tendon (844.8)
  Repetitive trauma (overuse syndromes)
    Patellar tendinitis ("jumper's knee") (726.64)
    Quadriceps tendinitis (726.69)
    Peripatellar tendinitis (e.g., anterior knee pain of the adolescent caused by hamstring contracture) (726.699)
    Prepatellar bursitis ("housemaid's knee") (726.65)
    Apophysitis
      Osgood-Schlatter's disease (732.43)
      Sinding-Larsen-Johanssen's disease (732.42)
  Late effects of trauma (905)
    Posttraumatic chondromalacia patellae
    Posttraumatic patellofemoral arthritis
    Anterior fat pad syndrome (posttraumatic fibrosis)
    Reflex sympathetic dystrophy of the patella
    Patellar osseous dystrophy
    Acquired patella infera (718.366)
    Acquired quadriceps fibrosis
Patellofemoral dysplasia
  Lateral patellar compression syndrome (LPCS) (718.365)
    Secondary chondromalacia patellae (717.7)
    Secondary patellofemoral arthritis (715.289)
  Chronic subluxation of the patella (CSP) (718.364)
    Secondary chondromalacia patellae (717.7)
    Secondary patellofemoral arthritis (715.289)
  Recurrent dislocation of the patella (RDP) (718.361)
    Associated fractures (822)
      Osteochondral (intraarticular)
      Avulsion (extraarticular)
    Secondary chondromalacia patellae (717.7)
    Secondary patellofemoral arthritis (715.289)
  Chronic dislocation of the patella (718.362)
    Developmental
    Acquired
Idiopathic chondromalacia patellae (717.7)
Osteochondritis dissecans
  Patella (732.704)
  Femoral trochlea (732.703)
Synovial plicae (727.8916) (anatomic variants made symptomatic by acute or repetitive trauma)
  Pathologic medial patellar plica ("shelf") (727.89161)
  Pathologic suprapatellar plica (727.89165)
  Pathologic lateral patellar plica (727.89165)
Iatrogenic disorders
  Iatrogenic medial patellar compression sybdrome
  Iatrogenic chronic medial subluxation of the patella
  Iatrogenic patella infera (718.366)

Orthopaedic ICD-9-CM Expanded Diagnostic Codes in parentheses.
From Merchant AC: Clinical classification of patellofemoral disorders, *Sports Med Arthroscopy Rev* 2:26-27, 1994.

knee with a bizarre appearance because of the laterally displaced patella and significant pain. The patella dislocates laterally as a result of a sudden quadriceps contraction with the knee in partial flexion, often with a twisting component, causing the patella to displace over the lateral femoral condyle. Many times, the patella will spontaneously reduce as the patient straightens the leg, producing a palpable and audible clunk. Other times, the patella remains dislocated and requires closed reduction by medical personnel. The reduction involves slowly, but forcefully extending the knee, often with associated analgesia. A large, painful, bloody effusion quickly develops secondary to disruption of the medial retinaculum. The patient is reluctant to flex the knee but must be coaxed to perform a straight leg raise against resistance to document an intact extensor mechanism. Tenderness is greatest over the medial retinaculum.

Once reduced, plain radiographs, including a merchant or sunrise view of the patella, should be obtained to look for any osteochondral fracture and possibly loose body from the undersurface of the patella (Fig. 23-46). The merchant view is obtained with the knee in 45° of flexion with the x-ray beam directed caudally at an angle 30° from the plane of the femur (Fig. 23-24). Also, the articular congruence of the patellofemoral articulation can be measured by drawing lines between the lowest point on the femoral sulcus and the highest points on the medial (AC) and lateral (AB) femoral condyles (Fig. 23-47). This sulcus angle is bisected to provide a reference for the patella position (AO). The lowest point on the femoral sulcus is then connected to the lowest point on the articular surface of the patella (AD) to create the congruence angle. An angle medial to the bisector reference line (AO) is considered to be negative, and an angle lateral to the bisector reference line (AO) is positive. The patella apex or central ridge should lie at or medial to the bisector of the sulcus angle, the normal congruence angle being −6°. If the ridge is displaced laterally with a congruence angle more than 4°, the patella is considered subluxed.[30,66]

This merchant view also demonstrates lateral tilt, with a disproportionately widened medial patellofemoral joint space as compared with the lateral. Variability in

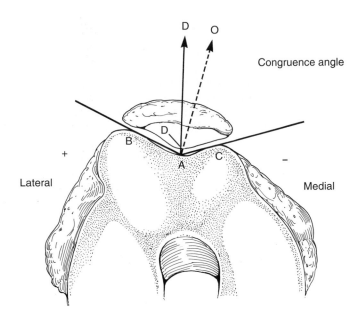

Fig. 23-47. The congruence angle of the patellofemoral joint as seen on the merchant view.

bony morphology makes this assessment of tilt less reproducible. Chronic complaints of patella instability can be further evaluated if necessary with computed tomography scans at 15°, 30°, and 45° of knee flexion to demonstrate abnormal tracking sometimes not evident on standard merchant views. Assessment of patella height can be performed on the lateral radiograph using the Insall-Salvatti ratio (Fig. 23-48). The ratio of the length of the patella tendon divided by the length of the

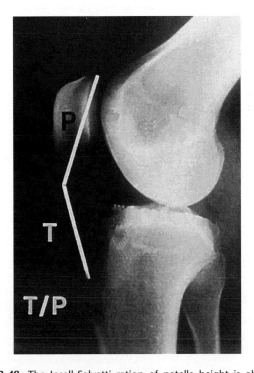

Fig. 23-48. The Insall-Salvatti ration of patella height is obtained from the lateral radiograph. The length of the patella tendon as measured on its deep or posterior surface (*T*) is divided by the length of the patella (*P*). The ratio of T/P is 1.02 ± 0.13.

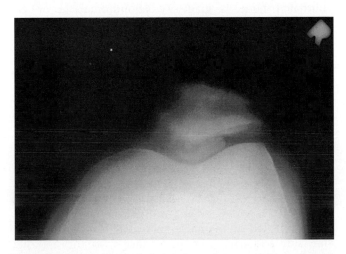

Fig. 23-46. Osteochondral fracture from the articular surface of the patella (arrow).

patella is 1.02 ± 0.13. Variation more than 20% is considered abnormal and evidence of patella baja or alta.[2] Another method of determining patella height has been described by Caton and Linclau.[72]

An athlete with a reduced patella dislocation should be immobilized in extension and referred to an orthopedist. Cryotherapy is recommended for the initial period of swelling and weight-bearing can be to tolerance. Evidence of an osteochondral fracture or loose body warrants arthroscopic surgery for fixation or removal, depending on the size and degree of comminution of the fragment. If the medial retinaculum is torn, it can be surgically repaired with imbrication at the same time. If the athlete reports a chronic history of repeated dislocations or if the patella is displaced laterally or tilted on the merchant view, then a medial proximal realignment with a lateral retinacular release are indicated.[74] In the absence of a fracture in an acute dislocation, MRI can help delineate the extent of pathology. Negative MRI evaluation without patella malalignment on merchant view can be managed with simple immobilization in extension in a knee immobilizer for 1 to 2 weeks until swelling and pain subside. Physical therapy to restore motion and, most importantly, for medial quadriceps strengthening should be instituted. This approach to the acute patella dislocation is summarized in the algorithm in Figure 23-49.[29]

Recurrent episodes of patella subluxation can be elicited during patient history as a sensation of the patella slipping laterally with associated giving way of the knee. Pain is usually temporary and swelling mild if present. Physical examination may reveal a tight lateral retinaculum on attempted medial mobilization of the patella or on attempted lifting of the tilted patella to horizontal (Fig. 23-50). Passively ranging the knee with laterally directed pressure against the medial border of the patella—the patella apprehension test—may reproduce a sensation of impending dislocation and pain. Plain radiographs, including a merchant view, rule out osteochondral injury and look for tilt or radiographic subluxation, which may be separate or combined as shown in Figure 23-51.

Management of patella subluxation should initially be nonoperative with quadriceps strengthening exercises, especially the vastus medialis. Usually, it is beneficial for the athlete to begin these exercises under the supervision of a physical therapist or an athletic trainer. The athlete should be prevented from flexion beyond 90° because it creates excessive contact pressures on the patellofemoral articulation. A patella-stabilizing brace may be of some benefit. Recently, McConnell taping has become popular in centralizing the patella.[53,99] This technique has variable success because of the difficulty with patient compliance. If the athlete fails an extensive course of therapy, with documented evidence of quadriceps strengthening, he or she may be a candidate for a lateral retinacular release and possibly a proximal patellar realignment.[75] One must be certain, however, that the patient truly participated in a supervised physical therapy program without improvement before choosing operative intervention.

Patellofemoral Syndrome and Chondromalacia

Malalignment and acute or repetitive trauma can lead to degenerative changes on the articular surface of the patella and of the femoral sulcus. Softening and early erosive changes are referred to as chondromalacia. Chondromalacia has been graded by clinical and microscopic appearance by Outerbridge.[63] Grade I chondromalacia is edema, softening, and possibly some blister lesions. Grade II chondromalacia has chondral fissures extending down to subchondral bone, and grade III has chondral fibrillation and further thinning or wear. Further erosion to eburnated bone is grade IV chondromalacia or osteoarthritis.[91] Often the exact etiology is difficult to establish, but a careful history may elicit overuse activities, especially high impact activities or activities that necessitate repetitive knee flexion. These activities include running, step machines, squats, or weights beyond 90° of flexion. Maintaining the knee for long periods in a bent position, such as seated in a theatre or on a plane, aggravates symptoms because the extensor mechanism is under tension, compressing the patella against the femur.

The athlete will localize pain diffusely to the anterior knee on history, often describing an aching that increases with activity. Crepitus or cracking noises may be felt or heard during a range of motion, also nonspecific findings. Tenderness on the undersurface of the patella can be elicited by manually subluxing the patella to either side and palpating the surface with the opposite hand, which is a more specific finding. Careful attention should be made to determine any anatomic predisposition to instability or malalignment, including determin-

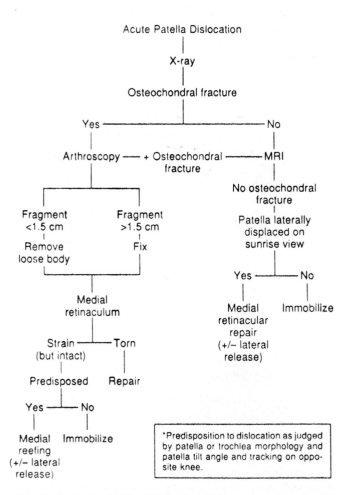

Fig. 23-49. Acute patella dislocation algorithm. From Fox JM, Del Pizzo W, eds: *The patellofemoral joint*, New York, 1993, McGraw-Hill.

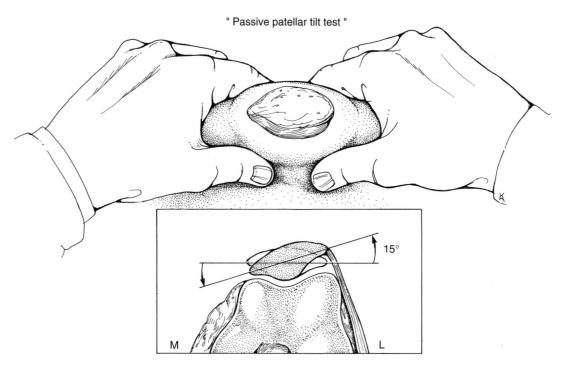

" Passive patellar tilt test "

Fig. 23-50. Passive patella tilt test. In full extension, one should be able to lift the lateral border of the patella beyond horizontal. Inability to do so may indicate a tight lateral retinaculum.

ing any history of dislocation or subluxation or trauma. A tight lateral retinaculum can be identified on attempted medial subluxation and tilt to neutral. If there is no evidence of subluxation or dislocation on history or examination but tenderness on the undersurface of the patella exists with normal alignment, the athlete has lateral patellar compression syndrome (Fig. 23-52). This is a radiographic diagnosis (abnormal patellar tilt without subluxation) and a clinical diagnosis (tight lateral retinaculum, normal mobility, normal Q angle).[57]

Initial management should be nonoperative to include activity modification. Impact activities are to be restricted to recreational status (done on occasion for "fun" but not on a regular basis for conditioning), which would include running, step machines, or aerobics. An aggressive conditioning program for quadriceps strengthening should be performed in nonimpact fashion and include such activities as an exercise bicycle, cross-country ski machine, or swimming for aerobic conditioning. Ice is used for pain and swelling control after work-outs and as needed. Short courses of NSAIDs are used on occasion. If after 6 to 12 weeks of documented rehabilitation and activity modification no benefit is seen, arthroscopic débridement and possibly lateral release may be indicated. The majority of patients do not require surgery for this diagnosis and improve if adequate effort is invested in nonoperative therapy.

Extensor Mechanism Disruptions

Ruptures of the patella or quadriceps tendons are more common in middle-aged or older patients than in young athletes. The patient will note sudden, dramatic pain often in association with an audible "pop." The individual is unable to walk without assistance or a brace. A large, bloody effusion is almost immediate. Radiographs con-

firm the effusion and usually demonstrate a high-riding patella—patella alta—for patella tendon rupture, or possibly a low-lying patella—patella baja—for a quadriceps tendon rupture (Fig. 23-53). On examination, the patient is unable to actively extend the knee against gravity or any resistance. Other injuries can be misinterpreted as an extensor mechanism disruption if the patient cannot be coaxed through the pain to perform a straight leg raise off of the table. If the swelling is not too severe, one can appreciate a palpable, tender defect in either the quadriceps or patella tendon, which is accentuated by attempts at lifting the leg. Ruptures most often occur in close proximity to the attachment to the patella on either side.[8]

Management of extensor mechanism disruptions is surgical anatomic repair, possibly with augmentation.[71] For this reason, the athlete should be placed in a knee immobilizer in extension with a gentle compressive wrap and ice to help control swelling. Consultation with an orthopedic surgeon should be obtained as soon as possible. Delays in reconstruction more than a few days make repair significantly more difficult because of progressive retraction of tendon ends.

TENDONITIS AND BURSITIS

Patella Tendonitis (Jumper's Knee)

Patella tendonitis is a diagnosis consistent with overuse or repetitive trauma to the extensor mechanism of the knee, which commonly results from jumping or running sports, such as basketball and volleyball. Athletes will present with anterior knee pain and intermittent swelling. On examination, tenderness localizes to the patellar tendon, primarily at its origin on the inferior pole of the patella. Tenderness is most easily appreciated

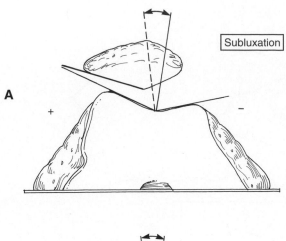

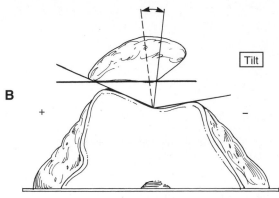

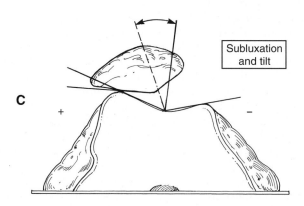

Fig. 23-51. Patella tracking abnormalities include subluxation **(A)**, lateral tilt **(B)**, or both **(C)**.

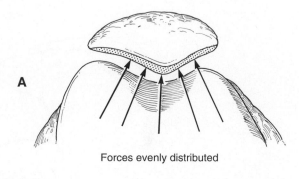

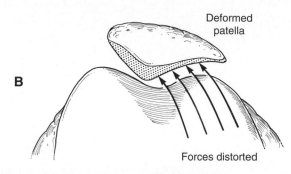

Fig. 23-52. A, Normal equal distribution of contact forces across the patellofemoral joint. **B**, In lateral patella compression syndrome, the forces are unevenly distributed toward the lateral facet, resulting in deformation and thinning of the articular cartilage.

short courses of NSAIDs are helpful adjuncts. Local steroid injections are to be avoided because they have been shown to cause tendon degeneration and potential rupture. Nonoperative treatment is successful in roughly 90% of patients.[83] A patellar tendon strap can be of sub-

with the knee in extension.[57] Radiographic evaluation is helpful in visualizing any bony abnormality, such as elongation or fragmentation of the inferior pole of the patella, periosteal reactive bone, or calcification within the patella tendon.[8] MRI is reserved for recalcitrant cases and is helpful in diagnosing tendon degeneration (Fig. 23-54).

Nonoperative management is directed toward a period of rest to allow symptoms to subside, followed by activity modification that limits high-impact sports. Stretching of the quadriceps and hamstrings is helpful, as is a strengthening program. Isokinetic and plyometric exercises aggravate symptoms and should be avoided.[57] Short arc quadriceps strengthening exercises are performed within the painless range of motion. Ice and

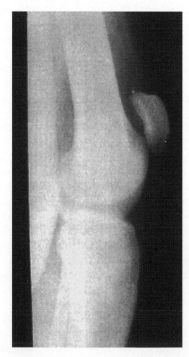

Fig. 23-53. Extensor mechanism disruption results in an acute hemarthrosis, and for patella tendon rupture results in a high-riding patella.

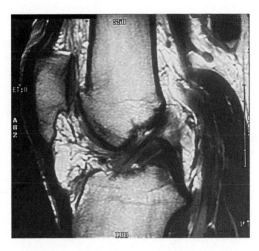

Fig. 23-54. Chronic patella tendonitis may demonstrate elongation of the patella inferior pole or calcification within the tendon (arrow).

jective benefit as the athlete returns to sports. Rarely is operative intervention to remove a portion of degenerative tendon or the lower pole of the patella necessary.

Iliotibial Band Syndrome

Iliotibial band friction syndrome is a descriptive diagnosis for another overuse syndrome involving repetitive friction between the iliotibial band and the lateral femoral condyle. Runners and cyclists most commonly experience these symptoms. Tenderness and pain are localized to the iliotibial band overlying the lateral femoral epicondyle. This area is palpated during knee range of motion. Tenderness is maximal at 30° of flexion.[57] Pain can also be elicited by having the patient lie on the contralateral side while attempting to abduct the leg in extension. Resisting abduction exacerbates pain over the lateral femoral epicondyle and can be enhanced by palpation.

Nonoperative management includes rest and modification of the training routine. Runners are instructed to shorten their distance and stride length as needed to stop symptoms. Ice and occasional short courses of NSAIDs can be helpful. Stretching exercises are recommended with a gradual return to sports-specific training. Rarely, steroid injections are useful for recalcitrant cases. For those unusual cases that fail to respond to a supervised nonoperative program, operative intervention is considered to partially release a small portion of the posterior iliotibial band.

Bursitis

The bursae are synovial-lined cavities normally containing a thin film of fluid that overlie bony prominences around the knee (Fig. 23-55A). Bursae reduce friction during knee motion. Repetitive trauma from overuse or, more commonly, chronic irritation results in local inflammation and fluid collection within the bursa. The prepatellar bursa is the most commonly affected and is termed "housemaid's knee" (Fig. 23-55B). Inflammation can occur from repetitive kneeling or a direct blow. Pene-

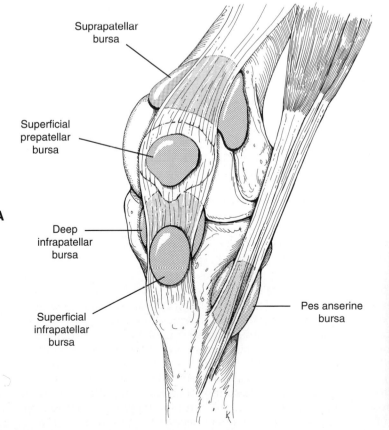

A

Suprapatellar bursa

Superficial prepatellar bursa

Deep infrapatellar bursa

Superficial infrapatellar bursa

Pes anserine bursa

Fig. 23-55. A, Bursae around the knee. **B,** Markedly swollen prepatellar bursa.

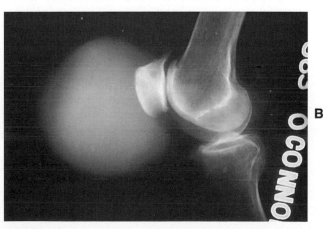

B

trating trauma to the prepatellar region can result in a septic bursitis caused by innoculation with skin flora.

Inferior to the patella are the superficial and deep infrapatellar bursae. Chronic kneeling or acute trauma can cause inflammation of these bursae. Bursitis here is often difficult to distinguish from patellar tendonitis or intraarticular pathology. Under the common insertion of the sartorius, semitendonosis, and gracilis tendons, termed the *pes anserinus,* is the pes anserinus bursa. Overuse activities, such as running, can produce inflammation here, but this is perhaps overdiagnosed as a misinterpretation of meniscal or other intraarticular pathology. An additional bursa rests under the semimembranosis tendon attachment on the proximal tibia, but it is not often inflamed.

Patients present with swelling, pain, and tenderness well localized to the inflamed bursa. The history of chronic irritating activities is usually obtained. Swelling can be dramatic, but it is always confined to the general area of the inflamed bursa. For prepatellar bursitis, the bony contours of the patella are obscured, unlike an intraarticular effusion. Weight-bearing or gentle range of motion does not significantly increase pain, although the patient will note tightness and secondary pain as flexion is increased, which helps distinguish bursitis from septic intraarticular arthritis, which is markedly painful to any range of motion or weight-bearing.

Management is directed at stopping the irritating activity—such as kneeling. Ice and short courses of NSAIDs are used. A gentle compressive wrap can help reduce swelling. Occasionally, a period of immobilization in a knee immobilizer brace is necessary. Aspiration can be performed diagnostically and therapeutically.[77] Drainage relieves distention and, as a result, pain. Septic bursitis is managed with aspiration and antibiotics. Advanced or resistant cases can be improved more rapidly with local incision and drainage in the outpatient setting. Chronic, recurrent cases rarely require surgical excision of the chronically thickened bursa.

SYNOVIAL PLICA

Plicae are normal synovial septums that can sometimes become inflamed and symptomatic. The suprapatellar plica traverses the suprapatellar pouch. The infrapatellar plica, or ligamentum mucosum, loosely connects the fat pad to the superior part of the intercondylar notch. The medial patellar plica and the less common lateral patellar plica run obliquely from the respective sides of the suprapatellar pouch to the anterior fat pad (Fig. 23-56). The incidence of plica as an anatomic structure in the population ranges 20% to 60%.[77]

Athletes complain of vague anterior knee pain often associated with overuse activities, such as running or biking. Symptoms may occur only after a period of exercise as the synovium becomes progressively irritated. Patients may complain of clicking or catching, sometimes occurring at a specific point during flexion as the inflamed plica snaps over the femoral condyle. Sometimes this snapping plica can be palpated and usually is tender. The medial patellar plica is most commonly involved as it becomes inflamed by rub-

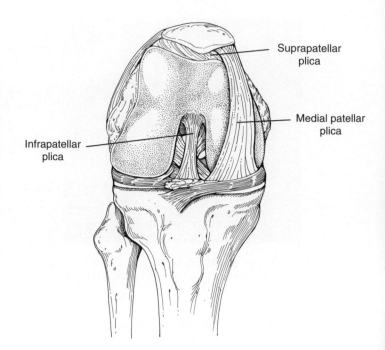

Fig. 23-56. Synovial plicae of the knee.

bing over the medial femoral condyle. The mere existance of a plica is not diagnostic because it is a normal structure. In the absence of irritation, other causes should be ruled out.

Management is initially nonoperative and directed toward rest and cessation of the irritating activity. Ice and a short course of NSAIDs can be helpful. Arthroscopy confirms the diagnosis in recalcitrant cases by visualizing a thickened and inflamed synovial band rubbing over the adjacent femoral condyle, sometimes with a matching abraded bony lesion. Arthroscopic resection of the plica is easily performed and effective in 70% to 92% of patients.[77]

OSGOOD-SCHLATTER APOPHYSITIS

The proximal tibial growth plate slopes distally in the anterior portion to lie beneath the attachment of the patella tendon on the tibial tubercle. Excessive activity can create a traction apophysitis at the tendon insertion. Osgood-Schlatter apophysitis occurs in active, growing adolescents, usually boys. Athletes present with activity-related pain, swelling, and tenderness localized to the tibial tubercle. Findings are bilateral in 20% to 30% of cases.[57] Radiographs in chronic cases show thickening of the patella tendon, soft-tissue swelling, and sometimes fragmentation of the tibial tubercle (Fig. 23-57).

Rest and activity modification are recommended until symptoms subside. Nonoperative management is almost always successful. Advanced apophysitis essentially represents a stress fracture, and significant symptoms not responding to rest should be reason to immobilize the knee. Symptoms are also limited to the duration of skeletal growth. Occasionally, chronic symptoms caused by painful ossicles in the tendon respond to excision, although surgery is rarely necessary. In even more rare in-

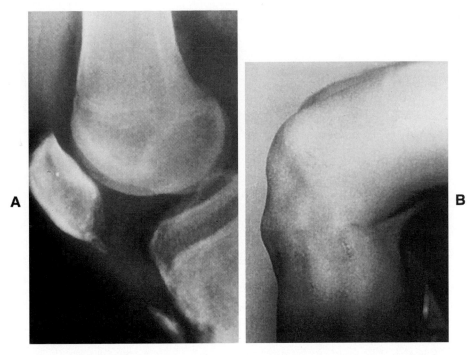

Fig. 23-57. A, Radiograph of Osgood-Schlatter disease demonstrating thickening of patella tendon, fragmentation of the tibial tubercle, and soft tissue swelling. **B,** Clinical picture of bony prominence anteriorly at the tibial tubercle.

stances, continued activity or acute trauma can result in an avulsion fracture of the tibial tubercle, which requires surgical repair.

OSTEOCHONDRITIS DISSECANS

Osteochondritis dissecans is separation of a fragment of subchondral bone with its overlying articular cartilage, leaving a "divot" in the remaining bone. The etiology is likely traumatic, especially in young patients, but is not clear. The most common location is the lateral aspect of the medial femoral condyle, and less often it occurs in the central portion of the lateral femoral condyle (Fig. 23-58).[4,5] An anteroposterior tunnel or notch view can help visualize the lesion (Fig. 23-59). Osteochondritis dissecans occurs during the second to fourth decades, most often in adolescents.[4,77] The osteochondral fragment can be classified by appearance at arthroscopy as intact (grade I), early separation (grade II), partial detachment (grade III), or loose fragment (grade IV).[13]

Patients usually complain of vague, poorly localized knee pain that increases with weight-bearing or activity. Plain radiographs to include the notch or tunnel view are usually sufficient, but MRI can add information about the subchondral extent of the lesion. However, the only precise way to assess stability of the fragment is by arthroscopic probing. Large or loose lesions present with a knee effusion, tenderness, and mechanical symptoms of locking, catching, or giving way.

Patients with osteochondritis dissecans should be examined by an orthopedic surgeon. Prognosis is strongly related to size and displacement of the lesion and age of the patient. Young patients (boys aged less

than 14 years and girls aged less than 12 years) generally do well, and the fragment is less likely to displace and require fixation.[57] Smaller fragments and loose bodies causing mechanical symptoms are removed arthroscopically. Large fragments, especially those larger than 25% of the joint surface area, should be fixed in place.[5,13] Metal pins or screws are being replaced in favor of biodegradable pins as the fixation method of choice. Cartilage autograft transplantation is considered experimental and has recently been reported.[10] Arthroscopic drilling of the crater in unrepairable cases promotes proliferation of fibrocartilage in young patients and may give partial relief of symptoms, but it tends to deteriorate with time.

PROXIMAL TIBIOFIBULAR JOINT DISLOCATIONS

The proximal tibiofibular joint is a synovial joint surrounded by a thickened capsule, allowing little significant motion between the tibia and fibular head. Proximal tibiofibular joint dislocations are rare injuries that can occur as an isolated injury or in conjunction with other injuries in major trauma to the knee. When an isolated injury, the dislocation most often occurs with the knee in flexion and subjected to a twisting mechanism. The LCL attaches to the fibular head and acts to stabilize the proximal tibiofibular joint when the collateral ligament is tight in knee extension. On flexion, the collateral ligament is relatively relaxed, allowing the dislocation to occur given sufficient twisting force.

Ogden[61,62] classified proximal tibiofibular dislocations into three types based on direction of fibular displacement. Anterolateral dislocation is the most common, followed by posteromedial, and superior. Sublux-

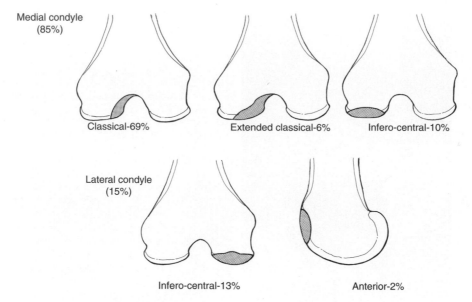

Medial condyle (85%)

Classical-69%   Extended classical-6%   Infero-central-10%

Lateral condyle (15%)

Infero-central-13%   Anterior-2%

Fig. 23-58. Locations of osteochondritis dissecans on the distal femur.

ation of the joint can also occur in ligamentously lax individuals, including those with connective tissue disorders, such as Ehlers-Danlos syndrome. The diagnosis is frequently missed when it occurs in conjunction with other major knee trauma. Comparison radiographic views of the opposite knee are helpful when the diagnosis is in doubt. Plain films are generally sufficient (Fig. 23-60). Patients complain of pain and tenderness localized to the proximal fibula that is increased with movement of the fibular head. Flexing the knee helps to relax the collateral ligament to allow stressing the joint.

Management involves closed reduction of the dislocation by applying manual pressure over the fibular head in a direction that will achieve reduction. Flexion of the knee is beneficial to relax the collateral ligament, and muscle relaxation is often neces-

sary. An audible snap is often heard on reduction. Non–weight-bearing with crutches for 2 weeks is followed by eventual return to full activities, usually by 6 weeks. Rarely, closed reduction is not possible or cannot be maintained. In these cases, surgical management may include internal fixation with Kirschner wires or resection of the proximal fibular head. Arthrodesis can lead to later ankle discomfort and is not generally recommended. Peroneal nerve palsies can occur in roughly 5% of patients, especially in cases of posterior fibular dislocation. Resection of the fibular head can be helpful in patients with peroneal nerve symptoms.[95]

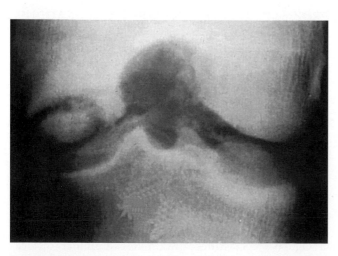

Fig. 23-59. Anteroposterior tunnel or notch view demonstrating osteochondritis dissecans of the medial femoral condyle.

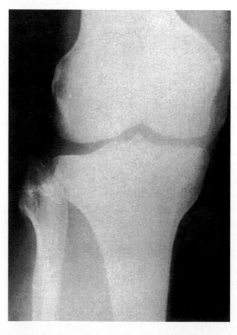

Fig. 23-60. Proximal tibiofibular joint dislocation.

REFERENCES

1. Abbott LC, Saunders JB, Bosh FC, Anderson CE: Injuries to the ligaments of the knee joint, *J Bone Joint Surg* 16A:503, 1944.
2. Aglietti P, Buzzi R, Insall JN: Disorders of the patellofemoral joint. In Insall JI, ed: *Surgery of the knee*, ed 2. New York, 1993, Churchill-Livingston.
3. Aglietti P, Insall JN, Cerulli G: Patella pain and incongruence, *Clin Orthop* 176:217, 1983.
4. Aichroth PM: Osteochondritis dissecans of the knee, *J Bone Joint Surg* 53B:440, 1971.
5. Aichroth PM: Osteochondritis dissecans. In Insall JN ed: *Surgery of the Knee,* ed 2. New York, 1993, Churchill-Livingston.
6. Alicea J, Scuderi GS: Knee dislocations. In Tria F, ed: *Ligaments of the knee,* New York, Churchill-Livingston, pp. 261-274.
7. Belzer JP, Cannon WD Jr: Meniscus tears: treatment in the stable and unstable knee, *J AAOS* 1:41, 1993.
8. Bono J, Haas S, Scuderi GR: Traumatic maladies of the extensor mechanism. In Scuderi GR, ed: *The patella,* New York, 1995, Springer Verlag.
9. Brenn JJ: Avulsion injuries of the posterior cruciate ligament, *Clin Orthop* 18:157, 1960.
10. Brittberg M, Lindahl A, Nilsson A, Ohlsson C, Isaksson O, Peterson L: Treatment of deep cartilage defects in the knee with autologous chondrocyte transplantation, *N Engl J Med* 331:889, 1994.
11. Bullock D, Scuderi GR: Getting your patient back in action after a meniscal tear, *J Musc Med* 11(5):68, 1994.
12. Burk DL, Mitchell DG, Rifkin MD, et al: Recent advances in the MRI of the knee, *Radiol Clin North Am* 28(1):379, 1990.
13. Burks RT, Butorac RB: Injuries and diseases of articular surfaces of the knee. In Scott WN, ed: *The knee,* St. Louis, 1994, Mosby.
14. Cannon WD Jr, Vittori JM: The incidence of healing in arthroscopic meniscal repairs in ACL reconstructed knees versus stable knees, *Am J Sports Med* 20:176, 1992.
15. Cannon WD Jr, Vittori JM: Meniscal repair. In Aichroth PM, Cannon WD Jr, eds: *Knee surgery: current practice,* New York, 1992, Raven Press.
16. Clancy WG, Shelbourne KD, Zoellner GB, et al: Treatment of knee joint instability secondary to rupture of the posterior cruciate ligament, *J Bone Joint Surg* 65A:310, 1983.
17. Clancy WG: Repair and reconstruction of the posterior cruciate ligament. In Chapman MW ed: *Operative orthopedics,* 3:1651, 1988.
18. Clendenin MB, DeLee JC, Hechman JD: Interstitial tears of the posterior cruciate ligament of the knee, *Orthopedics* 3:764, 1980.
19. Cooper DE, Warren RF, Warner JP: The posterior cruciate ligament and posterolateral structures of the knee: anatomy, function, and patterns of injury. *American Academy of Orthopedic Surgeons, Instructional Course Lectures,* 40:249, 1991.
20. Daniel DM: Principles of knee ligament surgery. In Daniel DM, Akeson WH, O'Connor J, eds: *Knee ligaments: structure, function, injury, and repair,* New York, 1990, Raven Press.
21. Daniel DM, Fithian DC: Current concepts: indications for anterior cruciate ligament surgery, *Arthroscopy* 10(4):434, 1994.
22. Daniel DM, Stone ML, Dobson BE, Fithian DC, Rossman DJ, Kaufman KR: Fate of the ACL-injured patient, *Am J Sports Med* 22:632, 1994.
23. Drucker MM, Wynne GF: Avulsion of the posterior cruciate ligament from its femoral attachment, *J Trauma* 15:616, 1975.
24. Fanelli GC: Posterior cruciate ligament injuries in trauma patients, *Arthroscopy* 9(3):291, 1993.
25. Fanelli GC, Giannotti BF, Edson CJ: The posterior cruciate ligament, arthroscopic evaluation and treatment, *Arthroscopy* 10(6):673, 1994.
26. Feagin JA, Lambert KL, Cunningham RR, et al: Consideration of the anterior cruciate ligament injury in skiing. *Clin Orthop* 216:13, 1987.
27. Finsterbush A, Frankl U, Matan Y, Mann G: Secondary damage to the knee after isolated injury of the anterior cruciate ligament, *Am J Sports Med* 18:47, 1990.
28. Fischer SP, Fox JM, DelPizzo W, Friedman MJ, Snyder SJ, Ferkel RD: Accuracy of diagnosis from MRI of the knee, *J Bone Joint Surg* 73A:2, 1991.
29. Fox JM, DelPizzo W, eds: *The patellofemoral joint,* New York, 1991, McGraw Hill.
30. Fulkerson JP: Patellofemoral pain disorders: evaluation and management. *J AAOS* 2:124, 1994.
31. Galway RD, Beaupre A, MacIntosh DL: Pivot shift: a clinical sign of symptomatic anterior cruciate insufficiency, *J Bone Joint Surg* 54B:763, 1972.
32. Gollehon DL, Torzilli PA, Warren RF: The role of the posterolateral and cruciate ligaments in the stability of the human knee, *J Bone Joint Surg* 69A:233, 1987.
33. Graf BK, Cook DA, DeSmet AA, Keene JS: Bone bruises on MRI evaluation of ACL injuries, *Am J Sports Med* 21:220, 1993.
34. Green NE, Allen BL: Vascular injuries associated with dislocation of the knee, *J Bone Joint Surg* 59A:236, 1977.
35. Gross ML, Grover JS, Bassett LW, Seeger LL, Finerman GA: Magnetic resonance imaging of the posterior cruciate ligament, *Am J Sports Med* 20:732, 1992.
36. Guan Y, Butler DL, Dormer SG, et al: Contribution of ACL subunits during anterior drawer in the human knee, *Trans Orthop* 16:589, 1991.
37. Hewson GF, Mendini RA, Wang JB: Prophylactic knee bracing in college football. *Am J Sports Med* 14:262, 1986.
38. Indelicato PA: Isolated MCL injuries in the knee, *J AAOS* 3:9, 1995.
39. Indelicato PA: Non-operative treatment of complete tears of the medial collateral ligament of the knee, *J Bone Joint Surg* 65A:323, 1983.
40. Ireland J, Trickey EL, Stoker DJ: Arthroscopy and arthrography of the knee, *J Bone Joint Surg* 62B:3, 1980.
41. Irvine GB, Glasgow MMS: The natural history of the meniscus in anterior cruciate insufficiency, *J Bone Joint Surg* 74B:403, 1992.
42. Johnson D, Warner JJP: Diagnosis for ACL surgery, *Clin Sports Med* 12:671, 1993.
43. Johnson RJ, Beynnon BD, Nichols CE, Renstrom PA: Current concepts review: the treatment of injuries of the ACL, *J Bone Joint Surg* 74A:140, 1992.
44. Kannus P, Bergfeld J, Jarvinen M, et al: Injuries to the posterior cruciate ligament of the knee, *Sports Med* 12:110, 1991.
45. Keller PM, Shelbourne KD, McCarroll JR, Rettig AC: Non-operatively treated isolated posterior cruciate ligament injuries, *Am J Sports Med* 12:132, 1993.
46. Kennedy JC: Complete dislocation of the knee joint, *J Bone Joint Surg* 45A:889, 1963.
47. Kennedy JC, Hawkins RJ, Willis RB, Danylchuck KD: Tension studies of human knee ligaments, *J Bone Joint Surg* 58A:350, 1976.
48. Kornick J, Trefelner E, McCarthy S, Lange R, Lynch K, Jokl P: Meniscal abnormalities in the asymptomatic population at magnetic resonance imaging, *Radiology* 177:463, 1990.
49. Lance EP, Paulos LE: Knee bracing, *J Am Acad Orthop Surg* 2:281, 1994.

50. Larson RL, Taillon M: Anterior cruciate ligament insufficiency: principles of treatment *J Am Acad Othop Surg* 2:26, 1994.

51. Lehnert M, Eisenschenk A, Zellner A: Results of conservative treatment of partial tears of the ACL, *Int Orthop* 17:219, 1993.

52. Lee HG: Avulsion fractures of the tibial attachments of the cruciate ligaments, *J Bone Joint Surg* 19:460, 1937.

53. Maurer SS, Carlin G, Butters R, Scuderi GR: Rehabilitation of the patellofemoral joint, in Scuderi GR, ed: *The patella*, New York, 1995, Springer Verlag.

54. McCauley TR, Moses M, Kier R, Lynch JK, Bartin JW, Jokl P: Magnetic resonance diagnosis of tears of the anterior cruciate ligament of the knee, *Am J Radiol* 162:115, 1994.

55. McCoy GF, Hannon DG, Barr RJ, Templeton J: Vascular injury associated with low velocity dislocation of the knee joint, *J Bone Joint Surg* 69B:285, 1987.

56. Merchant AC: Clinical classification of patellofemoral disorders, *Sports Med Arthroscopy* 2:26-27, 1994.

57. Miller MD, Cooper DE, Warner JJP: The knee. *Review of sports medicine and arthroscopy*, Philadelphia, 1995, WB Saunders.

58. Noyes FR, Mooar P, Matthews DS, Butler DL: The symptomatic anterior cruciate deficient knee, *J Bone Joint Surg* 65A:154, 1983.

59. Noyes FR, Mooar P, Moorman III CT: Partial tear of the ACL: progression to complete ligament deficiency, *J Bone Joint Surg* 71B:825, 1989.

60. Noyes FR, Mooar LA, Moorman III CT, McGinniss GH: Partial tears of the anterior cruciate ligament, *J Bone Joint Surg* 71B:825, 1989.

61. Ogden JA: Subluxation and dislocation of the proximal tibio-fibular joint, *J Bone Joint Surg* 56A:145, 1974.

62. Ogden JA: Subluxation of the proximal fibula, *Radiology* 105:547, 1972.

63. Outerbridge RE: The etiology of chondromalacia patella, *J Bone Joint Surg* 43B:752, 1961.

64. Palmer I: On the injuries to the ligaments of the knee joint, *Acta Chir Scand Suppl* 81:3, 1938.

65. Parolie JM, Bergfeld JA: Long term results of nonoperative treatment of isolated posterior cruciate ligament injuries in the athlete, *Am J Sports Med* 14:35, 1986.

66. Pavlov H: Radiographic examination. In Insall JN, ed: *Surgery of The Knee*, ed 2. New York, 1993, Churchill Livingston.

67. Pringle JH: Avulsion of the spine of the tibia, *Ann Surg* 46:169, 1907.

68. Quinlan AG, Sharrard WJW: Posterolateral dislocation of the knee with capsular interposition, *J Bone Joint Surg* 40B:660, 1958.

69. Raunest J, Hotzinger H, Burrig KF: MRI and arthroscopy in the detection of meniscal degenerations: correlation of arthroscopy and MRI with histology findings, *Arthroscopy* 10:634, 1994.

70. Scuderi GR: The femoral intercondylar roof angle: radiographic and MRI measurement. *Am J Knee Surg* 6:10, 1993.

71. Scuderi GR: Patellar and quadriceps tendon disruptions. In Scott WN, ed: *The knee*, St. Louis, 1994, Mosby.

72. Scuderi GR: Radiographic assessment of patella length, thickness and height, *Med Sci Sports Exerc* 24(Suppl 5):147, 1992.

73. Scuderi GR: The segond fracture. *Am J Knee Surg* 4(1):32, 1991.

74. Scuderi GR: The surgical management of patellar instability. In Scuderi GR, ed: *The Patella*, New York, 1995, Springer Verlag.

75. Scuderi GR: Surgical treatment for patellar instability. *Orthop Clin North Am* 23:619, 1992.

76. Scuderi GR, Scott WN: Classification of ligament injuries. In Insall JN, ed: *Surgery of the knee,* New York, 1993, Churchill Livingston.

77. Scuderi GR, Scott WN, Insall JN: Knee injuries. In Rockwood, Green, eds: *Fractures in Adults,* ed 4. Philadelphia, JB Lippincott, pp. 2001-2126.

78. Scuderi GR, Scuderi DM: Patellar fragmentation. *Am J Knee Surg* 7:125, 1994.

79. Shelbourne KD, Patel DV: Management of combined injuries of the anterior cruciate and medial collateral ligaments, *J Bone Joint Surg* 77A:800, 1995.

80. Shelbourne KD, Porter DA, Clingman JA, et al: Low velocity knee dislocations, *Orthop Rev* 20:995, 1991.

81. Shields L, Mitral M, Cave EF: Complete dislocation of the knee: experience at the Massachusetts General Hospital, *J Trauma* 9:192, 1969.

82. Sisto DJ, Warren RF: Complete knee dislocation, *Clin Orthop* 198:94, 1985.

83. Stanish WD, Curwin S, Rubinovich RM: Tendonitis: the analysis and treatment for running, *Clin Sports Med* 4:21, 1985.

84. Stanish WO, Rubinovich M, Armason T, Lapenskie G: Posterior cruciate ligament tears in wrestlers, *Can J Appl Sports Sci* 4:173, 1986.

85. Torg JS, Barton TM, Pavlov H, et al: Natural history of the PCL deficient knee, *Clin Orthop* 246:208, 1989.

86. Torg JS, Conrad W, Kalen V: Clinical diagnosis of ACL instability in the athlete, *Am J Sports Med* 4:84, 1976.

87. Toriso T: Avulsion fracture of the tibial attachment of the posterior cruciate ligament, *Clin Orthop* 143:107, 1979.

88. Treiman GS, Yellin AE, Weaver FA, et al: Examination of the patient with a knee dislocation: the case for selective arteriography, *Arch Surg* 127:1056, 1992.

89. Trickey EL: Rupture of the posterior cruciate ligament of the knee, *J Bone Joint Surg* 50B:334, 1968.

90. Veltri DM, Warren RF: Isolated and combined posterior cruciate ligament injuries, *J Am Acad Orthop Surg* 1:67, 1993.

91. Vigorita VJ, Morgan D: Pathology of the patella, In Scuderi GR, ed: *The patella*, New York, 1995, Springer Verlag.

92. Warner JJP, Warren RF, Cooper DE: Management of acute anterior cruciate ligament injuries, *AAOS Inst Course Lect* XL:201, 1991.

93. Warren RF: Meniscectomy and repair in the ACL deficient patient, *Clin Orthop* 252:55, 1990.

94. Warren RF, Friederich NF, Muller W, Jackson RW, James PH, Henning CE, Lynch MA: Degenerative arthritis of the knee following anterior cruciate ligament injury, *Orthop Trans* 13(3):546, 1989.

95. Windsor RE: Knee dislocations. In Insall JN, ed: *Surgery of the knee,* ed 2. New York, 1993, Churchill Livingstone.

96. Windsor RE: Soft tissue disorders. In Insall JN, ed: *Surgery of the knee,* ed 2. New York, 1993, Churchill Livingstone.

97. Woztzs EM: *The ACL deficient knee,* Rosemont, Il, 1994, AAOS Monograph Series.

98. Yormak JH, Scuderi GR: Physical examination of the knee. In Tria F, ed: *Ligaments of the knee,* New York, 1995, Churchill Livingstone.

99. Zappala F, Taffel C, Scuderi GR: Rehabilitation of the patellofemoral joint, *Orthop Clin North Am* 23:555, 1992.

100. Zarins B, Adams M: Knee injuries in sports, *N Engl J Med* 318:950, 1988.

CHAPTER 24

THE LEG

Stephen P. Geary
Michael A. Kelly

Sports-related acute and chronic injuries are common in the leg. Patients with these problems are frequently seen in the primary care and sports medicine specialty setting. It is, therefore, relevant for any clinician who evaluates athletes to be familiar with the more common problems. Many of these clinical entities are overuse phenomena. Proper training techniques should be emphasized in the preventative and therapeutic scenario. An adequate warm-up period and stretching is particularly important in the aging population when physiologic soft-tissue resiliency is decreasing. The maintenance of a consistent baseline conditioning program, gradual increases in activity, and appropriate shoe wear are part of the basics to be emphasized.

COMPARTMENT SYNDROME

Compartment syndrome is a condition of increased tissue pressure within a closed fascial space that leads to decreased microvascular perfusion and can potentially cause irreversible damage to the soft-tissue contents of the closed space. Clinical recognition of compartment syndrome is attributed to Richard von Volkmann based on his 1881 description of posttraumatic irreversible forearm contractures, which he believed to be of ischemic origin.[90] In the leg, this condition is more common in the anterior and deep posterior compartments where there are less compliant fascial boundaries (Fig. 24-1).

Compartment syndrome can be classified as acute or chronic, and each has different etiologies and presentations. Acute compartment syndrome can be caused by fractures, muscle rupture, soft-tissue trauma, arterial injury, limb compression, constrictive dressings or casts, and burns. Chronic compartment syndrome is usually an exertional phenomenon, such as that seen in long distance runners and military recruits. Exertional compartment syndrome can occur with exercise-induced increases in muscle volume in an otherwise healthy compartment. Compartments with isolated fascial defects may lead to muscle herniation, predisposing to exertional compartment syndrome.[23]

Pathophysiology

Compartment syndrome develops when pressure is raised within a limited space. The pathophysiology of compartment syndrome is progressive ischemia to muscle and nerve as tissue compartment pressure overcomes capillary perfusion pressure. This ischemic insult creates a vicious cycle of progressive cellular swelling and increasing compartment pressure, resulting in decreasing microvascular perfusion. Compartment syndrome can occur with any process that increases the volume in a noncompliant compartment, such as hemorrhage, fractures, and iatrogenic infusions. Increased capillary permeability may also lead to intrinsic compartmental swelling, which may be associated with burns, soft-tissue trauma, reperfusion after repair of vascular injuries, embolectomy, and operative tourniquet use. Additionally, any process reducing the volume of a compartment may initiate this process, including extrinsic compression with prolonged limb compression, as in the drug-overdosed or comatose patient, and with tight dressings or casts. The acute sequelae of compartment syndrome can include electrolyte abnormalities, rhabdomyolysis, cardiac arrhythmia, renal failure, and even death. The chronic sequelae can result in fibrosis of muscle, fixed contractures, and a nonfunctional limb.

The development of a compartment syndrome depends on the magnitude of pressure elevation and the duration of increased pressure. Therefore, a compartment syndrome can occur rapidly with significant pressure elevations or have a gradual onset with prolonged moderate elevations of pressure. Interference with muscle perfusion and nerve conduction becomes progressively severe with the duration of applied pressure.[78] Canine studies have demonstrated peroneal nerve conduction velocity begins to change after 8 hours of pressure elevation to 30 mm Hg in the anterior compartments of the leg.[77,78] If higher pressures are applied, these conduction velocity changes have been observed to occur sooner. When tissue pressure elevates to within 10 to 20 mm Hg of diastolic pressure microvascular ischemia occurs.[91,92] Muscle necrosis may ensue when tissue pressure elevates to 40 to 50 mm

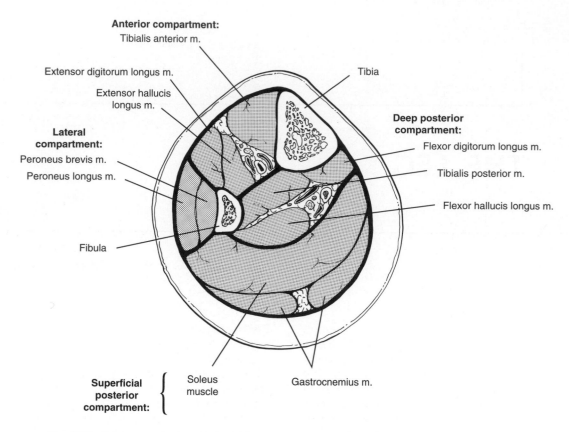

Fig. 24-1. Four compartments of the leg: transverse section through middle section of left leg. Redrawn from Mubarak SJ, Owen CA: Double incision fasciotomy of the leg for decompression in compartment syndromes, *J Bone Joint Surg* 59A:184, 1977.

Hg.[91,92] It is critical to understand that the development of a compartment syndrome depends on multiple factors and tissue compartment pressure. These factors include systemic blood pressure, particularly diastolic; bleeding; increased capillary permeability; and the presence of external compression.

Anatomy

The leg is divided into four fascial compartments: the anterior, lateral, superficial posterior, and deep posterior compartments. These are anatomic spaces bounded by dense fascia and osseous borders. Pertinent anatomy of each compartment includes the major neurovascular structures in each compartment (Fig. 24-1). The deep peroneal nerve lies in the anterior compartment; the posterior tibial nerve lies in the deep posterior compartment; the superficial peroneal nerve lies in the lateral compartment; and the sural nerve lies in the superficial posterior compartment. Evaluation for compartment syndrome includes localizing symptoms to the involved muscles and an assessment of the distal sensory component of the involved nerve.

Diagnosis

ACUTE COMPARTMENT SYNDROME. It is important to differentiate acute compartment syndrome from chronic exertional compartment syndrome. Acute compartment syndrome is nonreversible by definition because compartment pressure remains elevated above physiologic limits. The diagnosis of acute compartment

syndrome may be subtle. Clinical suspicion is critical. Rarely an acute compartment syndrome has been reported with extreme exertional overuse, ankle fractures or sprains, crush injuries, and with medical illnesses including influenza B virus and sickle cell trait.[1,7,14,33,57,68] In the athlete, compartment syndrome is more commonly seen with tibial fracture and muscle rupture.[2] The patient presents with a history of injury, progressive severe unrelenting pain in the involved compartments of the leg, localized swelling with exquisite tenderness to palpation, and exacerbation of pain with dynamic attempted use of the involved muscle group on motor examination (active or passive stretch). Acute compartment syndrome is usually a secondary diagnosis of a primary inciting event. The pain seen in acute compartment syndrome is usually well out of proportion to that of the primary diagnosis. Historically, compartment syndrome was associated with "the five Ps": pain, pallor, paresthesias, paralysis, and pulselessness. However, these may be misleading.[70] Early, the most reproducible finding is severe pain. Later, the sensory examination is often remarkable for dysesthesias in the involved compartment's neural component. The arterial examination is most often normal, eliminating any large vessel occlusive process. Although acute compartment syndrome is a clinical diagnosis, direct measurement of compartment pressures should be obtained to further confirm the diagnosis; this may be performed with surgical consultation.

A simple method of directly measuring compartment pressures has been described by Whitesides.[91] Compartment pressure can be measured using an intravenous catheter and tubing, a three-way stopcock, a syringe, and a mercury manometer. Pressure measurements are made when the inflow saline–air meniscus is in a steady state with the compartment, applying digital pressure on the syringe (Fig. 24-2). More recently, a continuous infusion technique has been described for continuous monitoring of intracompartmental pressures and to prevent catheter plugging.[41] More sophisticated and commercially available monitoring devices include the wick, slit, and the solid-state transducer intracompartmental catheters.[45,59,78] These devices allow for rapid, simple measurement of intracompartmental pressures. Additionally, they can be used for continuous monitoring during exercise and may assist in evaluating the dynamic pressures involved in chronic exertional compartment syndrome. Direct compartment pressure measurement of more than 30 mm Hg with positive clinical findings is typically diagnostic of acute compartment syndrome.[59,76,77]

CHRONIC EXERTIONAL COMPARTMENT SYNDROME. Chronic exertional compartment syndrome is a reversible event. During strenuous exercise, there can be a 20% increase in muscle volume.[71] When fascial boundaries limit muscle expansion, the compartment pressure will rise. Rest usually allows compartment pressure to decrease. Therefore, the athlete, usually a runner, presents with leg pain brought on by exercise and relieved by rest. Pain is initially dull, occuring in the muscle mass after exercise. With continued overuse, progression of the process can cause symptoms to linger for an increased period of time after running, even into the next day. Bilateral involvement has been reported in up to 82% of patients.[19] Approximately 80% of cases involve either the anterior compartment or the deep posterior compartment.[18,69] There may be associated compartment swelling and dysesthesias from nerve compression within the involved compartment, typically, the plantar aspect of the foot in a deep posterior compartment syndrome or on the dorsum of the foot in an anterior compartment syndrome. Results of the physical examination are often normal. However, there may be increased fullness and tenderness of the involved muscle after exercise. Fascial hernias have been found in up to 39% of patients with anterolateral compartment syndrome.[23] The diagnosis of chronic exertional compartment syndrome relies on the objective measurement of compartment pressures, which are measured at rest and after activity. Normal muscle tissue pressures range from 0 to 14 mm Hg at rest.[61] The generally accepted guidelines for the diagnosis of chronic exertional compartment syndrome include any of the following: (1) a preexercise pressure more than 15 mm Hg, (2) a 1-minute postexercise pressure more than 30 mm Hg, and (3) a prolonged return of pressure to baseline levels (a 5-minute postexercise pressure more than or equal to 20 mm Hg).[69] Again, the wick-type catheters are useful for monitoring.

Management

Management of acute compartment syndrome is immediate fasciotomy. Fasciotomy is a surgical procedure that involves longitudinally incising the entire length of the dense fascial lining of a muscle compartment, releasing the compartment. In the acute setting, all four compartments of the lower extremity are released via one or two skin incisions, which are closed on a delayed basis, usually after a few days. Persistently symptomatic chronic exertional compartment syndrome is managed by elective fasciotomy of the involved compartment.

MEDIAL TIBIAL STRESS SYNDROME

The term *shin splint syndrome* describes multiple clinical entities without clearly defining location or etiology. Therefore, shin splints is a term not generally useful as a medical diagnosis and has recently fallen out of favor. The more appropriate term is *medial tibial syndrome* or *medial tibial stress syndrome*.[2] Tibial periostitis has been proposed as the more specific diagnosis to explain this clinical entity based on the pathophysiology. However, this label creates some confusion regarding location because tibial periostitis can occur at the origin of the soleus, tibialis posterior, and uncommonly at the tibialis anterior muscle. The differential diagnosis of medial tibial stress syndrome primarily revolves around tibial stress fracture and chronic exertional compartment syndrome.

Presentation

Patients with medial tibial syndrome present with gradually progressive pain over the posteromedial border of the tibia at the middle and distal thirds. Initially, pain may be present on the initiation of an activity and resolve with continued exertion. As this exercise syndrome progresses, the pain may change from a dull ache to a more severe pattern and fail to resolve throughout the course of the activity. The process may progress to limit athletic activity and the activities of daily living. As with all overuse injuries, significant changes in activity, footwear, terrain, surface, mileage, or intensity of workouts can predispose to the development of medial tibial syndrome. This syndrome accounts for about 13% of injuries in a runners' clinic and 4% of new military recruits.[3,34]

Clinical Evaluation and Diagnosis

The physical examination is remarkable for tenderness along the posteromedial edge of the middle and distal thirds of the tibia. This tenderness typically is not well localized but extends over approximately one third of the length of the posteromedial border of the tibia. Minimal swelling may be present, but no specific mass is seen. The pain may be recreated with resistance to active plantar and dorsiflexion of the foot. Results of neurovascular examination of the extremity should be normal. The differential diagnosis includes tibial stress fracture, the findings of which are typically more localized with specific point tenderness. Compartment pressure measurements during activity may be performed to evaluate exertional compartment syndrome in the vague clinical

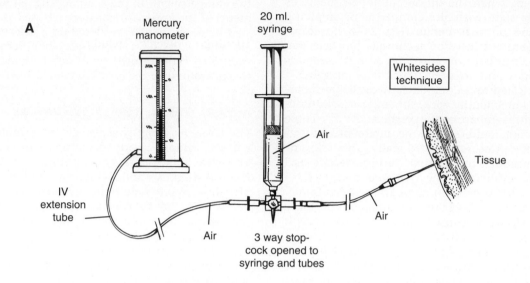

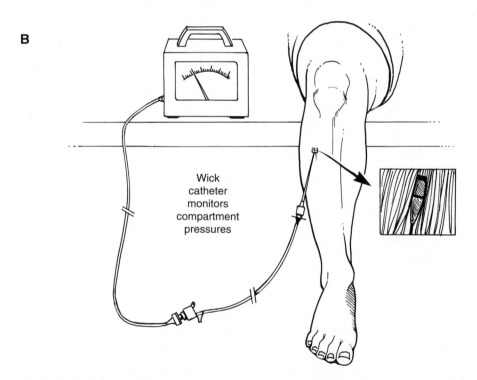

Fig. 24-2. Technique of Whitesides et al. for determination of tissue pressure. **A,** Tissue pressure is measured by determining amount of pressure within closed system required to overcome pressure within closed compartment and inject minute amount of saline. **B,** Use of wick catheter for monitoring compartment pressures. **A** from Whitesides T Jr, et al: Tissue perfusion measurements as a determinant for the need of fasciotomy, *Clin Orthop* 113:43, 1975.

situation.[58] Routine radiographs should be obtained. Although radiographs are typically normal, there may be an associated hypertrophy of the posterior cortex and subperiosteal lucency and scalloping of the medial tibia. Additionally, there may be a periosteal reaction, which must be differentiated from stress fracture as the diagnosis. Serial radiographs may be helpful.

A bone scan can be the definitive study in the evaluation and diagnosis of medial tibial stress syndrome, particularly in the differentiation from stress fracture of the tibia. The typical findings of three-phase radionuclide imaging involve increased uptake that can extend from one-third to three-fourths of the length of the tibia, which correlates with periostitis of the soleus and posterior tibialis muscle origins. In tibial stress fractures, uptake is usually well localized, intense, round, and fusiform about the tibia and can be positive on any or all three phases of the bone scan. Radionuclide activity rarely extends beyond 20% of the length of the tibia with stress fractures.[80] Complete scintigraphic evaluation should include medial and lateral views to localize the site of periostitis in medial tibial syndrome. Tomographic views can help to precisely localize a tibial stress fracture.

Pathophysiology

The soleus and its dense fascia, the tibialis posterior, and the flexor digitorum longus muscle originate along the posteromedial border of the middle and distal thirds of the tibia. The forces transmitted through these muscles with chronic overuse result in a periosteal reaction from microtearing of Sharpey's fibers at the interdigitation of muscle and bone. The reactive inflammation causes a periostitis along this interface.

Biomechanical evaluation, including gait analysis studies, has revealed the association of excessive foot pronation with medial tibial stress syndrome. In normal running, the initial contact at foot strike is on the lateral aspect of the foot, and the tibia rotates externally. As the stance phase progresses, the body comes over the foot, and the tibia rotates internally. There is a compensatory eversion of the subtalar joint, which results in pronation of the foot. This position is typical of the foot before heel lift. Eversion of the subtalar joint and foot pronation help dissipate forces at foot impact and allow adaptation to running on varying terrain. The medial soleus functions in inversion of the subtalar joint. Therefore, with normal running and foot pronation, there is a lengthening or eccentric contraction of the soleus. Excessive pronation applies increased stress and strain on the supporting musculature. Additionally, a tight heel cord has been observed in association with medial tibial stress syndrome.

Management and Rehabilitation

Initial management of medial tibial stress syndrome is rest. Abstaining from the offending activity from a few days to several weeks allows the inflammation at the musculofascial origins to subside. No management combinations have been shown to work better than rest alone. Ice locally, heel cord stretching, and anti-inflammatory medications are used as well. Rest need not be absolute, but rather individualized depending on the intensity, mileage, and terrain of the athlete's workout. Review of the athlete's training habits and a clear understanding of the problem are helpful during treatment.

Prevention requires the eradication of associated training problems including poor shoes, excessive mileage, and hard training surfaces. Custom-made semi-rigid orthotics may be used to control excessive pronation. As with all overuse syndromes, the maintenance of an adequate strengthening and flexibility program remains crucial to prevention and reinjury.

STRESS FRACTURES OF THE TIBIA AND FIBULA

Stress fractures are overuse injuries of bone to the point of biomechanical failure and are also called "fatigue fractures."[56] Originally described as "march fractures" in the metatarsals of German soldiers in the 19th century, stress fractures were not reported in athletes until 1939.[10,74] In athletes, the tibia is the most common site of involvement.[17,20,25,28,29,31,42,43] In runners, the incidence ranges from 4%[65] to more than 15%.[42] Women runners have been found to have up to 12 times the risk for stress fractures than men.[6,65] Other factors associated with increased risk include increasing age, poor fitness, non–black race, menstrual irregularities, and narrow tibial width.[6,26,38,50] Stress fractures can occur in all regions of the tibia and may be multiple.[2,11,53,60,63] The most frequent site for tibial stress fractures is controversial, with authors reporting fractures in the proximal, central, and distal thirds of the tibia.[39,40,51,52,64,65,67,79,88] Rarely, the injury can be on the tension side of the tibia occurring in the central third at the anterior cortex and displaying more ominous biologic behavior.[8,30,66,67] Development of stress fractures is most commonly associated with an increased mileage and intensity of running. Hyperpronation and tibia vara predispose the athlete to stress fractures.[42,88]

Pathophysiology

Current theory is that repetitive cyclic loading induces remodeling through increased osteonal activity, which is outpaced by impact-stimulated periosteal resorption. The cortex is weakened until the threshold for disruption is surpassed, resulting in a stress fracture. Histopathologically, stress induces a vascular response in bone with an increased number of erythrocytes, resulting in vascular congestion and thrombosis. This response initiates osteoclastic resorption, which precedes osteoblastic and periosteal new bone formation.[37] Normally, stress-induced remodeling leads to cortical hypertrophy and increased mineralization, outpacing any resorption. The cortex is weakened with repetitive stress as resorption cavities and reactive periosteal callus form. Cortical fracture occurs when these stresses overload this weakened cortex. Stress fractures occur most commonly posteromedially on the compression side of the bone.[16,83] Because these compression-type stress fractures develop slowly, there is ample time for bone remodeling and cortical hypertrophy. Less commonly, stress fractures can occur in the middle third of the tibia anteriorly on the tension side. The prognosis for this fracture is more ominous and unpredictable, with an increased incidence of delayed union.[40,73] It is sometimes described as the "dreaded black line." The tension-type stress fracture is more commonly seen in athletes who engage in repetitive jumping activities, such gymnastics, basketball, and ballet.[40,73]

Clinical Evaluation and Diagnosis

Typical of overuse syndromes, the athlete with a stress fracture presents with leg pain. There may be a history of a change in training habits including mileage, a change in training surface, or inadequate shoe wear. The pain is well localized. In the early stages, it occurs at the end of activity and is relieved with rest. As the

process progresses, pain may be present with any impact activity, including walking. Unlike medial tibial stress syndrome, a short period of rest usually does not relieve the symptoms. Physical examination is remarkable for localized point tenderness along the tibia. There also may be a dense tender soft-tissue mass or local warmth associated with the callus. Less often, there is also pain at the involved site with percussion of the tibia.

Results of early radiographs may be normal. Later, radiographic changes may include periosteal new bone formation, subperiosteal resorption, endosteal thickening, cortical hypertrophy, and a radiolucent line (Figs. 24-3, 24-4). However, these findings are variable and can be subtle. Initially only 50% of the patients with stress fractures will have positive radiographic results.[62,72] These fractures are usually transverse, al-

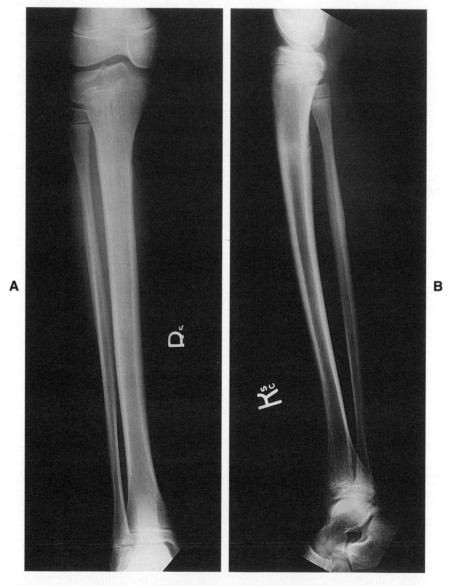

Fig. 24-3. Anteroposterior (**A**) and lateral (**B**) radiographs demonstrating early presentation of stress fracture in proximal third of tibia. Subtle fracture changes are noted.

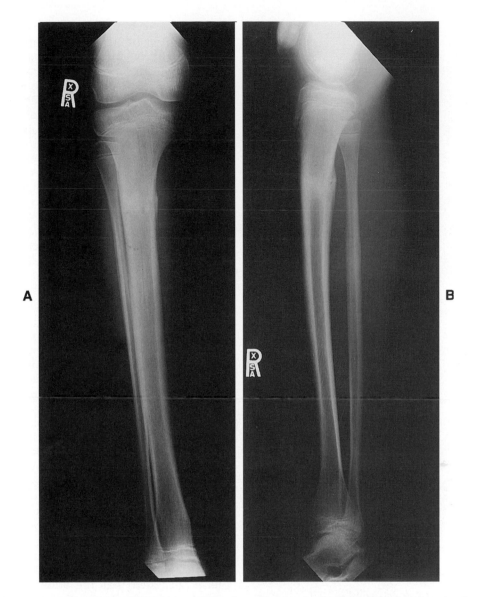

Fig. 24-4. Anteroposterior (**A**) and lateral (**B**) radiographs of same tibial stress fractures 4 weeks after presentation. Fracture callus and periosseal new bone are present at fracture site.

though, longitudinal stress fractures of the tibia have been reported.[12,55]

The most sensitive indicator of a stress fracture is the three-phase technetium bone scan, which may be positive in 2 to 7 days after presentation. A negative bone scan virtually excludes the diagnosis of stress fracture. The three-phase technetium bone scan is essentially 100% sensitive for stress fractures during the time of symptoms.[48,62,63,79,80,95] The bone scan reveals a well-localized area of intensely increased radionuclide activity (Fig. 24-5). Stress fractures may be positive in any or all phases of the bone scan, which may be indicative of accelerated remodeling early with more diffuse uptake or a more sharply marginated area of activity late with a healing fracture. Early stress remodeling and late healing may only be positive on the delayed images. When symptoms peak with an increased hy-

peremia, bone turnover, and repair, results of the bone scan can become positive in all three phases.[40,80] It is important to realize that stress fractures may be positive on delayed images for more than 12 months, even with the resolution of symptoms and an athlete's return to activity.[60] Likewise, multifocal synchronous areas of increased scintigraphic uptake are common in the lower extremity; up to 50% of patients with a positive bone scan correlating to a specific site of pain will have increased uptake in other areas from accelerated bone remodeling.[42,47,60,63]

Stress fractures of the fibula represent the sixth-most common site overall.[42] This injury is usually seen in long distance runners and typically occurs 3 to 7 cm above the lateral malleolus.[21] Proximal fibular stress fractures are rare. There are similar findings to tibial stress fractures in the history, physical examination, and in imag-

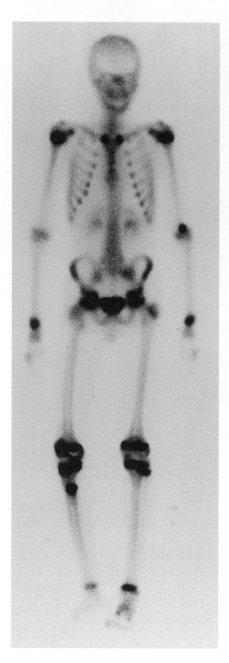

Fig. 24-5. Bone scan depicting focal changes in proximal third (right) tibia consistent with tibial stress fracture.

ing evaluation. Fibular stress fractures have also been reported in association with tibiofibular synostosis.

Management

On diagnosing a tibial or fibular stress fracture, the inciting impact activity should be stopped. The period of impact-free time must allow adequate repair and remodeling. Increased rates of delayed union or nonunion up to 10% may occur if these activities are not sufficiently curtailed.[65] There is usually complete resolution of compression-type tibial stress fractures after 6 to 8 weeks of relative rest. The return to full training activities may take 3 months.

Effective communication between the athlete and physician regarding an understanding of the diagnosis and activity modification during treatment is imperative. An effective treatment regimen for the more common posteromedial compression-type tibial stress fracture is a two-phase protocol.[13] Phase one includes cessation of running and local pain control with local physiotherapy, ice massage, and possibly a short course of nonsteriodal anti-inflammatory medication. Casting or bracing is rarely needed, and weight-bearing for daily activities is permitted. Running is stopped. During this period, alternative aerobic, strengthening, and flexibility activities are prescribed, which can be achieved with cycling, swimming, and water running. The second phase begins when the athlete has been pain-free for at least 2 weeks with any impact activity. At that time, activities are gradually progressed. If symptoms persist or recur, these impact activities are tapered or stopped. The recurrence rates of stress fractures approach 10% at either the original or metachronous site.[27,49,65] Therefore, the importance of maintaining cardiorespiratory, strengthening, and flexibility exercises and a graded return to impact activity cannot be over emphasized. The average time to return to full activity may be 3 months. Management of fibular stress fractures involves a similar two-phase protocol with healing usually in 4 to 8 weeks.

The less common anterior tibial stress fracture occurring on the tension side of the bone seen in repetitive jumping athletes requires special attention. This side stress fracture is prone to delayed union, nonunion, and potentially fracture displacement because of its poor biomechanics located on the tension side of the tibia.[9] Thus, this notorious overuse injury should be managed with prolonged immobilization.[40,73] Initially, a short-leg non–weight-bearing cast is used, followed by a walking cast or cast-brace as the examination and radiographs demonstrate healing. Some physicians have suggested that the addition of pulsed external electromagnetic stimulation may facilitate healing, which may take 3 to 6 months.[73] When closed treatments of tibial and fibular stress fractures fail, surgical alternatives may be considered, including excision and bone grafting, drilling of the lesion, and internal fixation.[30,35] The role of early surgical intervention has yet to be defined. However, prophylactic intramedullary internal fixation has been used successfully to treat the professional-level athlete.[5] Surgical takedown of tibiofibular synostosis associated with recalcitrant fibular stress fracture has been performed to successfully achieve union.[35]

TEAR OF THE MEDIAL HEAD OF THE GASTROCNEMIUS

Acute tears of the medial head of the gastrocnemious muscle typically occur in the middle-aged individual during recreational athletics and have been referred to as "tennis leg."[22] Usually the tear occurs at the time of maximal force during running, jumping, or a sharp change of direction. Patients describe a sudden acute pain in the calf and often a feeling of having been struck in the calf. Pain, swelling, and ecchymosis usually progressively increase during the following 24 to 48 hours. This condition has been commonly misinterpreted as a rupture of the plantaris tendon. Although historically this diagnosis was common, there is no significant evidence in the literature to substantiate a diagnosis of isolated rupture of the plantaris tendon.[15,32,36,81]

Anatomy and Pathophysiology

The gastrocnemius muscle is comprised of a lateral and medial head. Both originate from the femoral condyles and posterior capsule with the muscle mass tapering distally into a broad aponeurosis before blending with the deeper soleus tendon to form the Achilles tendon, which inserts onto the posterior tuberosity of the calcaneus. The medial head of the gastrocnemius muscle has some unique and important differences from the lateral head that may predispose it to rupture.[89] The medial head is a larger muscle mass, originates more superiorly on the femur, and has a more oblique fiber orientation than the vertically directed lateral head. Additionally, the gastrocnemius muscle fibers are fast-twitch fibers compared with the soleus, which is primarily slow twitch.[85] The gastrocnemius muscle has been described as a "short action" muscle, making it uniquely vulnerable to overstretch and rupture.[22] It crosses two joints, the knee and the ankle, which makes it prone to injury.[4] Rupture of the medial head occurs with a high-force eccentric muscle contraction, which often occurs during the mechanism of combined extension of the knee and forced ankle dorsiflexion as may occur during tennis, jogging, or landing from a jump.[2,54,71,82,89] Rupture usually occurs at the musculotendinous junction.[46,54,86,89] Decreased elasticity, dysvascular changes, and atrophy seen with aging or disease reduce the threshold force, causing myotendinous rupture.[93,94]

Clinical Evaluation and Diagnosis

The patient usually gives a history of sudden pain in the calf while running, cutting, accelerating, or stopping. Often, there is a feeling of having been hit in the calf or the sensation of a "pop." Swelling and pain in the calf usually progressively worsen during the next 24 hours. Ecchymosis of the entire leg can be significant and is usually maximal after a few days. These signs vary with severity of injury. There is usually localized tenderness of the musculotendinous junction. Over time, a palpable defect may be present. The foot rests most comfortably in an equinus position. The Achilles mechanism must be intact with active plantar flexion of the ankle and passive ankle plantar flexion on compression of the calf (Thompson test). There is guarding to standing toe raising and pain with active or passive dorsiflexion of the ankle. Results of the sensory and vascular examinations are normal. Radiographic findings are normal. The diagnosis can usually be made on clinical evaluation. Magnetic resonance imaging can demonstrate tears of the medial head of the gastrocnemius, but these are rarely repaired.[86]

Differential diagnosis includes acute deep vein thromboembolism, acute compartment syndrome, and popliteal cyst rupture. Clinical history may prove helpful in establishing the diagnosis. Doppler ultrasound and the gold standard venogram may be used to evaluate suspected deep venous thromboembolism. Rupture of the medial head of the gastrocnemius can be confused with thromboembolism and managed with anticoagulants, causing complications from increased bleeding from the torn muscle and possible compartment syndrome.[44] It is important to be aware that deep venous thrombosis has been reported as a complication of rupture of the medial head of the gastrocnemius muscle and both may coexist.[75,84] Compartment syndrome presents with severe progressive pain out of proportion to the injury, exacerbation of pain with passive dorsiflexion of the ankle or toes, a palpably tense and tender calf, and eventually paresthesias. Acute compartment syndrome may occur after rupture of the medial head of the gastrocnemius muscle but is rare.[4,87] If present, this condition requires emergency surgical decompression. Direct compartment measurements may be performed to rule out this diagnosis. Popliteal cyst rupture is usually seen in patients with inflammatory arthritis. The diagnosis may be difficult, and magnetic resonance imaging is helpful in establishing the diagnosis.

Management

Management for tears of the medial head of the gastrocnemius muscle is nonoperative. An associated compartment syndrome is managed by fasciotomy. Many nonoperative protocols have yielded good results for management of medial gastrocnemius ruptures.[24,36,54] Acutely, ice and elevation are recommended to minimize pain and swelling. Ankle motion is initiated as tolerated. A short course of nonsteroidal anti-inflammatory medication is prescribed, and analgesics are administered as needed providing there are no contraindications. Crutches are useful, and a heel lift in the shoe may be used for a brief period.[22] An aggressive rehabilitation program is initiated within 48 to 72 hours when the bleeding has stopped. Such a program has resulted in a full rehabilitation of 85% of patients by 2 weeks in a study of 720 patients.[54] Passive stretching of the calf using a towel or elastic band is performed with the knee extended. This program progresses to standing stretch exercises of the calf as tolerated. Similarly, strengthening progresses from isometric ankle dorsiflexion and plantarflexion to resistance exercises. These can be performed as active resistance exercises with an elastic band and toe raises against progressive resistance or weight. Evaluation with isokinetic plantarflexion strength testing may be helpful in recommending return to competitive activities. It is not uncommon that these injuries may require 6 weeks of rehabilitation before return to sports, especially in the nonprofessional athlete.

To avoid recurrence or new injury, prevention should be emphasized. Prevention involves increasing the warm-up period and stretching and maintaining a consistent strength and conditioning program, which is especially important in this population at an age when musculotendinous is decreasing. Stretching exercises of the hamstrings, gastrocnemius muscle groups, and the Achilles tendon are crucial.

REFERENCES

1. Amundson DE: The spectrum of heat related injury with compartment syndrome, *Milit Med* 154(9):450–452, 1989.
2. Andrish JT: *The leg in orthopaedic sports medicine,* vol 2. St. Louis, 1993, Mosby.
3. Andrish JT, Bergfeld JA, Walheim J: A prospective study of the management of shin splints, *J Bone Joint Surg* 56:1697–1700, 1974.
4. Anouchi Y, Parker R, Seitz W: Posterior compartment syndrome of the calf resulting from misdiagnosis of a rupture of the medial head of the gastrocnemius, *J Trauma* 27(6):678–680, 1987.
5. Barrick EF, Jackson CB: Prophylactic intramedullary fixation of the tibia for stress fracture in a professional athlete, *J Orthop Trauma* 6(2):241–244, 1992.
6. Barrow GW, Saha S: Menstrual irregularity and stress fractures in collegiate female distance runners, *Am J Sports Med* 16(3):209–216, 1988.
7. Blaiser D, Barry RJ, Weaver T: Force march-induced peroneal compartment syndrome, *Clin Orthop* 284:189–192, 1992.
8. Blank S: Transverse tibial stress fractures: a special problem, *Am J Sports Med* 15:597–602, 1987.
9. Brahms MA, Fumich RM, Ippolito VD: A typical stress fracture of the tibia in a professional athlete, *Am J Sports Med* 8:131–132, 1980.
10. Briethaupt MD: Zur pathologie des menschlichen Fusses, *Med Zeitung* 24:169, 1855.
11. Burrows HJ: Fatigue fracture of the middle third of the tibia in ballet dancers, *J Bone Joint Surg* 38:83–94, 1956.
12. Clayer M, Krishnan J, Lee WK, Tamblyn P: Longitudinal stress fractures of the tibia, *Clin Radiol* 46(6):401–404, 1992.
13. Clement DB: Tibial stress syndrome in athletes, *Am J Sports Med* 2:81–85, 1974.
14. Cook T, Brown D, Roe J: Hypokalemia, hypophosphatemia and compartment syndrome of the leg after downhill skiing on moguls, *J Emerg Med* 11(6):709–715, 1993.
15. Daffner RH: Anterior tibial striations, *AJR Am J Roentgenol* 143(3):651–653, 1984.
16. Daffner RH, Martinez S, Gehweiler JA: Stress fractures of the proximal tibia in runners, *Radiology* 142:63–65, 1982.
17. Darby RE: Stress fractures of the os calcis, *JAMA* 200:131–132, 1967.
18. Davey J, Rorabeck C, Fowler P: The tibialis posterior muscle compartment, *Am J Sports Med* 12(5):391–397, 1984.
19. Detmer DE, Sharp K, Sufit RL, Girdley FM: Chronic compartment syndrome: diagnosis, management and outcomes, *Am J Sports Med* 13:162, 1985.
20. Devas MB: Stress fractures in athletes, *Proc R Soc Med* 62:933–937, 1969.
21. Devas MB, Sweetnam R: Stress fractures of the fibula, *J Bone Joint Surg* 38B:818–829, 1956.
22. Froimson A: Tennis leg, *JAMA* 209:415–416, 1969.
23. Fronek J, Mubarak SJ, Hargens AR, et al: Management of chronic exertional anterior compartment syndrome of the lower extremity, *Clin Orthop* 220:217, 1987.
24. Gecha S, Torg E: Knee injuries in tennis, *Clin Sports Med* 7(2):435–452, 1988.
25. Giladi M, Ahronson Z, Stein M, et al: Unusual distribution and onset of stress fractures in soldiers, *Clin Orthop* 192:142–146, 1985.
26. Gilandi M, Milgrom C, Simkin A, Stein M, Kashtan H, Margulies J, Rand N, Chisin R, Steinberg R, Aharonson Z, Kedem R, Frankel V: Stress fractures and tibial bone width, *J Bone Joint Surg* 69B:326–329, 1987.
27. Giladi M, Ziv Y, Aharonson Z, Nli E, Danon Y: Comparison between radiography, bone scan and ultrasound in the diagnosis of stress fractures, *Milit Med* 149:459–461, 1984.
28. Gilbert RS, Johnson HA: Stress fractures in military recruits: a review of twelve years experience, *Milit Med* 131:716–721, 1966.
29. Greaney RB, Gerber FH, Laughlin RL: Distribution and natural history of stress fractures in U.S. Marine recruits, *Radiology* 146:338–346, 1983.
30. Green NE, Rogers RA, Lipscomb AB: Nonunions of stress fractures of the tibia, *Am J Sports Med* 13(3):171–176, 1985.
31. Hallel T, Amit S, Segal D: Fatigue fractures of tibia and femoral shafts in soldiers, *Clin Orthop* 118:35–43, 1976.
32. Helms CA, Fritz RC, Garvin GJ: Plantaris muscle injury: evaluation with MR imaging, *Radiology* 195(1):201–203, 1995.
33. Hieb LD, Alexander AH: Bilateral anterior and lateral compartment syndromes in a patient with sickle-cell trait. A case report and a review of the literature, *Clin Orthop* 228:190–193, 1988.
34. James SL, Bates BT, Ostering LR: Injuries to runners, *Am J Sports Med* 6(2):40–50, 1978.
35. Kottmeier SA, Hanks GA, Kalenak A: Fibular stress fracture associated with distal tibiofibular synostosis in an athlete, *Clin Orthop* 281:195–198, 1992.
36. Leach R: Leg and foot injuries in racquet sports, *Clin Sports Med* 7(2):359–370, 1988.
37. Li G, Zhang S, Chen G, et al: Radiographic and histologic analysis of stress fracture in rabbit tibias, *Am J Sports Med* 13:285–294, 1985.
38. Margulies J, Simkin A, Leichter I, Bivas A, Steinberg R, Giladi M, Stein M, Kashtan H, Milgrom C: Effect of intense physical activity on the bone-mineral content in the lower limbs of young adults, *J Bone Joint Surg* 68A(7):1090–1093, 1986.
39. Martire JR: Differentiating stress fractures from periostitis: the finer points of bone scans, *Phys Sports Med* 22(10):71–81, 1994.
40. Martire JR: The role of nuclear medicine bone scans in evaluating pain in athletic injuries, *Clin Sports Med* 6(4):713–737, 1987.
41. Matsen F, Winquist R, Krugmire R: Diagnosis and management of compartmental syndromes, *J Bone Joint Surg* 62A:286–291, 1980.
42. Matheson GO, Clement DB, McKenzie DC, et al: Scintigraphic uptake of 99m Tc at non-painful sites in athletes with stress fractures: the concept of bone strain, *Sports Med* 4:65–75, 1987.
43. Matheson GO, Clement DB, McKenzie DC, Taunton JE, Lloyd-Smith DR, Macintyre JG: Stress fractures in athletes: a study of 320 cases, *Am J Sports Med* 15(1):46–58, 1987.
44. McClure JG: Gastrocnemius musculotendinous rupture: a condition confused with thrombophlebitis, *South Med J* 77:1143, 1984.
45. McDermott A, Marble A, Yabsley R, Phillip M: Monitoring dynamic anterior compartment pressures during exercise, *Am J Sports Med* 10(2):83–89, 1982.
46. Menz MJ, Lucas GL: Magnetic resonance imaging of a rupture of the medial head of the gastrocnemius muscle, *J Bone Joint Surg* 73:1260–1262, 1991.
47. Milgrom C, Chisin R, Giladi M, et al: Multiple stress fractures, *Clin Orthop* 192:174–179, 1985.
48. Milgrom C, Chisin R, Giladi M, Stein M, Kashtan H, Margulies J, Atlan H: Negative bone scans in impending tibial stress fractures, *Am J Sports Med* 12(4):488–491, 1984.
49. Milgrom C, Giladi M, Chisin R, Dizian R: The long term follow-up of soldiers with stress fractures, *Am J Sports Med* 13(6):398–400, 1985.
50. Milgrom C, Giladi M, Simkin A, Rand N, Kedem R, Kashtan H, Stein M: An analysis of the biomechanical mechanism of tibial stress fractures among Israeli infantry recruits, *Clin Orthop* 231:216–221, 1988.

51. Milgrom C, Giladi M, Stein M, Kashtan H, Margulies JY, Chisin R, Steinberg R, Aharonson Z: Stress fractures in military recruits, *J Bone Joint Surg* 67B:732–735, 1985.

52. Milgrom C, Giladi M, Stein M, Kashtan H, Margulies J, Chisin R, Steinberg R, Swissa A, Aharonson Z: Medial tibial pain, *Clin Orthop* 213:167–171, 1986.

53. Miller EH, Schneider HJ, Bronson JL, et al: A new consideration in athletic injuries: the classical ballet dancer, *Clin Orthop* 111:181–191, 1975.

54. Miller WA: Rupture of the musculotendinous juncture of the medial head of the gastrocnemius muscle, *Am J Sports Med* 5:191–193, 1977.

55. Miniaci A, McLaren AC, Haddad RG: Longitudinal stress fractures of the tibia, *Can Assoc Radiol J* 39(3):221–223, 1988.

56. Morris JM, Blickenstaff LD: *Fatigue fractures: a clinical study,* Springfield, IL, 1967.

57. Moyer RA, Boden BP, Marchetto PA, Kleinbart F, Kelly JD: Acute compartment syndrome of the lower extremity secondary to noncontact injury, *Foot and Ankle* 14(9):534–537, 1993.

58. Mubarak SJ, Gould RN, Lee YF, et al: The medial tibial stress syndrome, *Am J Sports Med* 10:201–205, 1982.

59. Mubarak S, Hargens A: *Compartment syndromes and Volkmann's contractures,* Philadelphia, 1981, WB Saunders.

60. Nielsen MB, Hansen K, Hlmer P, Dyrbe M: Tibial periosteal reactions in soldiers, *Acta Orthop Scand* 62(6):531–534, 1991.

61. Nkele C, Aindow J, Grant L: Study of the pressure of the normal anterior tibial compartment in different age groups using the slit-catheter method, *J Bone Joint Surg* 70A:98, 1988.

62. Norfray J, Schlachter L, Kernahan W, Arenson D, Smith S, Roth I, Schlefman B: Early confirmation of stress fractures in joggers, *JAMA* 243(16):1647–1649, 1980.

63. Nussbaum AR, Treves ST, Micheli L: Bone stress lesions in ballet dancers: scintigraphic assessment, *AJR Am J Roentgenol* 150(4):851–855, 1988.

64. Orava S: Stress fractures, *Br J Sports Med* 14:40–44, 1980.

65. Orava S, Hulkko A: Stress fractures in athletes, *Int J Sports Med* 8:221–226, 1987.

66. Orava S, Hulkko A: Stress fractures of the mid-tibial shaft, *Acta Orthop Scand* 55:35–37, 1984.

67. Orava S, Puranen J, Ala-Ketola L: Stress fractures caused by physical exercise, *Acta Orthop Scand* 49:19–27, 1978.

68. Paletta CE, Lynch R, Knutsen AP: Rhabdomyolysis and lower extremity compartment syndrome due to influenza B virus, *Ann Plast Surg* 30:272–273, 1993.

69. Pedowitz R, Hargens A, Mubarak S, Gershuni D: Modified criteria for the abjective diagnosis of chronic compartment syndrome of the leg, *Am J Sports Med* 18(1):35–40, 1990.

70. Pellegrini VD, Evarts CM: *Complications in Rockwood and Green's fractures in adults,* 1991, Philadelphia, JB Lippincott.

71. Phillips BB: Traumatic disorders. In *Campbell's operative orthopaedics,* ed 8. St. Louis, Mosby.

72. Prather JL, Nusynowitz ML, Snowdy NA: Scintigraphic findings in stress fractures, *J Bone Joint Surg* 59A:869–874, 1977.

73. Rettig AC, Shelbourn KD, McCarroll JR, et al: The natural history and treatment of delayed union stress fractures of the anterior cortex of the tibia, *Am J Sports Med* 16:250–255, 1988.

74. Roberts SM, Vogt EC: Pseudofracture of the tibia, *J Bone Joint Surg* 21(4):891–901, 1939.

75. Robinson N: Spontaneous rupture of the gastrocnemius muscle presenting as acute thrombophlebitis, *Am Surg* 38(7):385–388, 1972.

76. Rorabeck CA: A practical approach to compartmental syndrome, *AAOS Instr Course Lect* 32:102–113, 1983.

77. Rorabeck CH, Castle GSP, Hardie R, Logan J: Compartmental pressure measurements: an experimental investigation using the slit catheter, *J Trauma* 21:446–449, 1991.

78. Rorabeck CH, Clarke KM: The pathophysiology of the anterior tibial compartment syndrome, *J Trauma* 18:299, 1978.

79. Roub L, Gumerman L, Hanley E, Williams-Clark M, Goodman M, Hebert D: Bone stress: a radionuclide imaging perspective, *Radiology* 132:431–438, 1979.

80. Rupani MD, Molder LE, Espinola DA: The three-phase of radionuclide bone imaging in sports medicine, *Radiology* 156:187–196, 1985.

81. Severance H, Bassett F: Rupture of the plantaris—Does it exist? *J Bone Joint Surg* 64(9):1387–1388, 1982.

82. Shields CL, Redix L, Brewster CE: Acute tears of the gastrocnemius, *Foot Ankle* 5:186–190, 1985.

83. Singer M, Maudsley RH: Fatigue fractures in the lower tibia, *J Bone Joint Surg* 36B:647–649, 1954.

84. Slawski DP: Deep venous thrombosis complicating rupture of the medial head of the gastrocnemius muscle, *J Orthop Trauma* 8(3):263–264, 1994.

85. Smith MJ: Muscle fiber types, *Orthop Clin North Am* 14:403–411, 1983.

86. Speer KP, Lohnes J, Garrett WE: Radiographic imaging of muscle strain injury, *Am J Sports Med* 21(1):89–95, 1993.

87. Straehley D, Jones W: Acute compartment syndrome following tear of the medial head of the gastrocnemius muscle, *Am J Sports Med* 14(1):96–99, 1986.

88. Sullivan D, Warren RF, Pavlov H, Kelman G: Stress fractures in 51 runners, *Clin Orthop* 187:188–192, 1984.

89. Sutro C, Sutro W: The medial head of the gastrocnemius: a review of the basis for partial rupture and for intermittent claudication, *Bull Hosp Joint Dis Orthop Inst* 45(2):150–157, 1985.

90. Volkman R: Die ischaemischen muskellamungen und kontrakturen, *Zentrabl Chir* 8:801, 1881.

91. Whitesides TE, Haney TC, Morimoto K, Harada H: Tissue perfusion measurements as a determinant for the need of fasciotomy, *Clin Orthop* 113:43, 1975.

92. Whitesides TE, Harada, H, Morimoto K: The response of skeletal muscle to temporary ischemia: an experimental study, *J Bone Joint Surg* 53A:1027, 1971.

93. Zarins B, Ciullo JV: Acute muscle and tendon injuries in athletes, *Clin Sports Med* 2:167–182, 1983.

94. Zarins B, Ciullo JV: Biomechanics of the musculotendinous unity: relation to athletic performance and injuries, *Clin Sports Med* 2:71–86, 1983.

95. Zwas S, Elkanovitch R, Frank G: Interpretation and classification of bone scintigraphic findings in stress fractures, *N Nucl Med* 28(4):452–457, 1987.

CHAPTER 25

THE FOOT AND ANKLE

Cherise M. Dyal
Francesca M. Thompson

EVALUATION

Examination of patients presenting with foot and ankle complaints begins with a thorough history followed by a systematic physical examination. Consistency is key to appropriate diagnosis and avoidance of overlooking signs. The clinician should develop a format that he or she is comfortable with and apply the format to every patient.

Past medical, surgical, and family history should be obtained to elucidate any systemic or inherited disorders that may be related to the current problem. A familiarity with the patient's medications and allergies should be attained because treatment with medications on primary contact for a foot or ankle disorder often occurs. A history of previous problems with the foot or ankle and previous treatment is essential. Historical evaluation must include background information on the patient's lifestyle and preferred athletic activities. Most importantly, the physician must ascertain why the patient is presenting to the office at this time. Although many deformities might be observed, only one may be problematic and require treatment.

The history must include a thorough account of all symptoms and their duration. Exacerbating and alleviating factors must be elucidated, and the quality and timing of complaints is key. Is the pain present at rest or only with activity? What activities specifically? Only at night? On awakening? On all ambulation or when landing from a jump? All of these questions must be answered. Previous management of the problem should also be addressed.

Determining the mechanism of injury will assist in appropriate diagnosis and management. Did immediate swelling occur, or did it develop gradually? Could the patient walk or did he or she need to be carried away? Did the patient hear or feel any popping or snapping or crunching? Did the patient notice any deformity? When did the injury occur, and how was it immediately managed? What has the patient's level of activity been since the injury?

A complete physical examination requires access to both feet and ankles and visualization of the patient from the knees down. One order of evaluation that will avoid overlooking any problems is inspection, palpation, neurovascular assessment, functional evaluation, and observation of gait. Once these have been evaluated, special clinical tests are performed to determine specific disorders. When conducting the evaluation, it is often helpful to divide the foot into regions of the hindfoot, midfoot, and forefoot.

Inspection must include observation of the involved and uninvolved extremities and should occur while the patient is seated and standing if possible. It is ideal to have the patient directly in front of the seated examiner. The patient should be asked to stand on a stepstool of medium height facing the physician and then with his or her back turned. Notation of any deformity, swelling, ecchymosis, or erythema is made. The skin is evaluated for its coloring and quality. Blisters or calluses are noted. Any maceration, laceration, or break in skin integrity is observed. Alignment of the feet and any clawing, hammering, or malleting of the toes is assessed. The integrity of the medial longitudinal arch and hindfoot alignment is assessed. Congenital and acquired deformities and bony prominences are noted. The toenails are inspected for their quality, subungual discoloration, and the presence of infection.

Palpation of the feet and ankles is then carried out. From this point, it is usually best to evaluate the uninvolved side first so that the patient knows what to expect and to give the physician an idea of what normal is for that patient. Local areas of tenderness or warmth are identified. The surrounding soft tissues and bony prominences are palpated for tenderness and crepitus. Systematic evaluation of the joints, ligaments, and tendons (along their courses and with passive and active movement) is performed.

The foot and ankle should be assessed by region while palpating. In the forefoot, the toes, sesamoids, metatarsal heads and shafts dorsally and plantarly, and the fat pads should be felt as well as all articulations for warmth and tenderness. The webspaces should be palpated for areas of fullness or pain as felt in a neuroma. Corns and calluses should be assessed for tenderness.

In the midfoot, the navicular, talar head, cuboid, and

cuneiforms and all of their articulations should be palpated for prominences and ligamentous and tendon insertional tenderness. The medial longitudinal arch and underlying plantar fascia should be palpated.

In the hindfoot, the plantar aspect of the heel should be assessed for integrity and tenderness. The tuberosities of the calcaneus (posterior and medial) must be felt. The insertion of the Achilles tendon is evaluated. The superficial Achilles bursa (lying between the skin and the posterior aspect of the tendon) and the retrocalcaneal bursa (lying between the anterior surface of the tendon and the posterior aspect of the calcaneus) are palpated. The calcaneus is compressed to elucidate possible stress fractures.

The ankle should be evaluated anteriorly, posteriorly, medially, and laterally. The medial and lateral malleoli and the ligaments and the insertions of the medial and lateral collateral ligament complexes are palpated. The anterior ankle joint is palpated through the anteromedial and anterolateral clear spaces in neutral, dorsiflexion, and plantarflexion. Tenderness and effusion are noted: the anterior tibial tendon (ATT), extensor hallucis longus (EHL), and extensor digitorum longus (EDL) are palpated as they cross the anterior ankle[3] to their insertions and as the ankle and toes are passively and actively ranged. The peroneal tendons are assessed along their course behind the lateral malleolus and to their insertions. The posterior tibial tendon (PTT), flexor hallucis longus (FHL), and flexor digitorum longus (FDL) are palpated as they pass behind the medial malleolus and into their insertions. Any tendinous tenderness, subluxation, dislocation, or snapping are noted. Anteriorly, the dome of the talus is palpated as the foot is plantarflexed and inverted. Posteriorly, the back of the talus or an os trigonum[11] is palpated. The anterior–inferior tibiofibular joint and the surrounding ligamentous structures are palpated.

At this stage, a neurovascular assessment is carried out. Observation of foot coloring, and capillary refill, and pedal edema should be done. Attempts should be made to palpate the posterior tibial artery as it lies between the FHL and FDL behind the medial malleolus. This artery is the major arterial supplier of the foot, and its importance must not be overlooked. The dorsal pedis arterial pulse may be palpable on the dorsum of the foot between the EHL and EDL tendons between the first and second metatarsals. It is absent 12% to 15% of the time.[5] Absence of palpable pulses may necessitate Doppler evaluation.

Sensation is assessed in each region of innervation. The deep peroneal nerve (a branch of the common peroneal nerve) innervates the first webspace. The posterior tibial nerve innervates the sole of the foot. The dorsomedial aspect of the foot is supplied by the saphenous nerve (a terminal branch of the femoral nerve). The dorsum of the foot is innervated by the superficial peroneal nerve (a branch of the common peroneal nerve) through the medial and intermediate dorsal cutaneous nerves. The sural nerve (formed from an anastomosis of the common peroneal and medial sural nerves) supplies the dorsolateral aspect of the foot. Vibratory sensation should also be evaluated to identify any neuropathies. Deep tendon reflexes at the ankle should be tested to elucidate any spinal abnormality.

Muscle testing should be performed, and muscle strength should be graded using the standard 0/5 to 5/5 scale. Muscles may be grouped into dorsiflexors, plantarflexors, invertors, and evertors. At this point, functional assessment should begin.

The dorsiflexors of the foot and ankle include the EHL, extensor hallucis brevis (EHB), EDL, extensor digitorum brevis (EDB), and tibialis anterior. Dorsiflexion and the strength of the great toe at its tip and metatarsophalangeal joint should be assessed to evaluate the EHL and EHB, respectively. To test the EHL functionally, the patient should heel walk in neutral and the tendon as it inserts into the great toe should be observed. To test integrity of the EDL and EDB, the patient should dorsiflex the toes and then test against resistance. Functional assessment of the EDL requires the patient to heel walk without inversion or eversion, and the tendon as it stands out and fans out to the toes should be observed. To isolate the tibialis anterior, the patient should attempt to touch a finger that is positioned to require dorsiflexion and inversion. Once the patient has done this, an attempt is made to plantarflex and evert the foot forcefully. Functional assessment requires the patient to heel walk with inverted feet.

Plantarflexors of the foot and ankle include the gastrocnemius–soleus complex, which terminates in the Achilles tendon, FHL, and FDL. Forceful plantarflexion will assess the gastrocnemius–soleus complex. Asking the patient to toe walk and hop on the ball of the foot provides functional assessment. To evaluate the FHL, the patient should try to curl his or her great toe and then apply resistance. Observation of a smooth toe-off during ambulation provides functional assessment. The FDL is assessed by asking the patient to curl his or her toes against resistance.

The invertor of the foot and ankle is the tibialis posterior muscle. To test the muscle in isolation, a patient is asked to evert the foot and then invert it against resistance (Fig. 25-1), which prevents the use of the anterior tibialis.

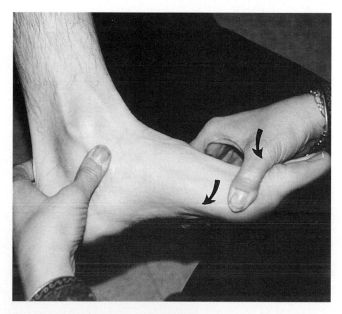

Fig. 25-1. Testing posterior tibialis strength. Note the patient's foot in eversion initially, and inverting against resistance from this position.

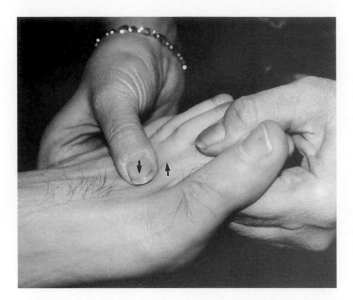

Fig. 25-2. Vertical stress test for metatarsophalangeal stability. One of the examiner's hands stabilizes the metatarsal head, whereas the other grasps the proximal phalanx. Examiner attempts to displace the proximal phalanx dorsally. A positive test result is the ability to displace dorsally while reproducing symptoms.

Once the patient is in this position, the examiner resists the motion. Functional assessment requires the patient to plantarflex and invert while the tendon is palpated along its course behind the medial malleolus and into the navicular tubercle. The patient should single-stance toe raise and the heel observed for inversion to assess its function.

The peroneus longus and brevis are the evertors of the foot. They are tested by asking the patient to touch a finger whose placement requires plantarflexion and eversion. Resistance is then provided by the examiner, who attempts to invert and dorsiflex the foot. Functional assessment is performed by asking the patient to walk on

the medial aspect of the feet. Observation is made for prominence of the tendons.

Functional evaluation is continued by assessing the range of motion and stability of each joint in the foot and ankle and comparing it with the opposite side. Differences between the extremities are actually more important than the absolute ranges because there is a large variation among individuals. Motion should be assessed actively and passively, and any pain during range of motion should be noted. The first metatarsophalangeal joint usually can achieve 45° of flexion and 70° to 90° of extension. The first interphalangeal (IP) joint can flex to 90°, and no extension is possible. The lesser toes can achieve 50° to 60° of extension and 30° of flexion at the metatarsophalangeal joints. IP motion can range to 65° of flexion without any extension. Stability of the lesser metatarsophalangeal joints should be assessed by stabilizing the metatarsal and attempting to translate the toe superiorly (Fig. 25-2).

In the forefoot, adduction and abduction are possible and occur across the talonavicular and calcaneocuboid joints. To assess them, the examiner must stabilize the calcaneus in neutral and move the forefoot medially (adduction) and laterally (abduction). Twenty degrees of adduction and 10° of abduction is usually possible.

Hindfoot motion is assessed through subtalar motion. Inversion (at least 5°) and eversion (at least 5°) are possible. To evaluate this motion, the tibia is stabilized, and the calcaneus is gripped and inverted and everted.

Next, ankle motion is evaluated. It is important not to mistakenly include forefoot motion in this assessment. To test pure ankle range of motion, the forefoot should be adducted fully and the calcaneus grasped to stabilize the subtalar joint. Approximately 20° of dorsiflexion and 50° of plantarflexion are possible. While the ankle is being assessed, its stability should be determined. To test the stability of the deltoid ligament, the patient's foot should be everted while the tibia and calcaneus are stabilized. The ankle should be observed for opening. To as-

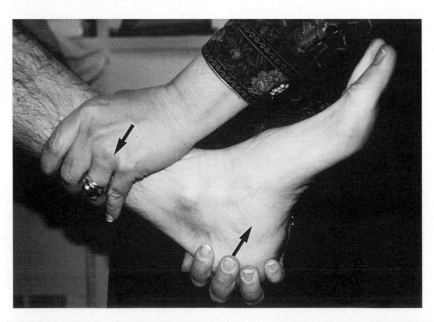

Fig. 25-3. The anterior drawer test. One of the examiner's hands grasps the distal tibia, whereas the other hand grasps the patient's heel and attempts to displace the foot anteriorly.

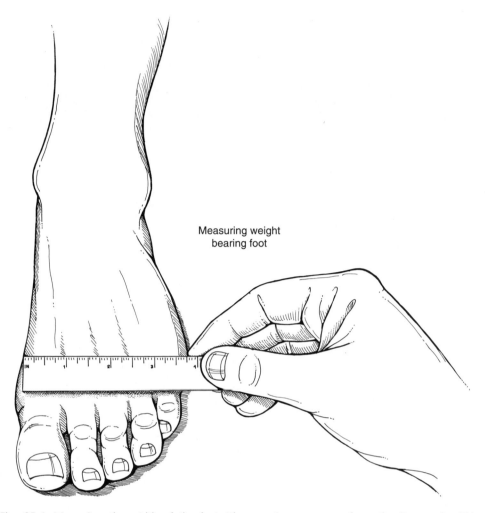

Measuring weight
bearing foot

Fig. 25-4. Measuring the width of the foot. The examiner measures from the first to the fifth metatarsal while the patient is weight-bearing.

sess the integrity of the anterior talofibular ligament (ATFL), the foot should be inverted while in plantarflexion and determined if this elicits pain. If the talus gaps open and rocks in the mortise, the ATFL and the calcaneofibular (CFL) ligaments are stretched or torn.

The anterior drawer test assesses gross ankle instability (Fig. 25-3). A positive test result indicates a tear of the ATFL and possibly the CFL. The tibia should be grasped and stabilized with one hand while the other hand grasps the calcaneus and attempts to pull it (and the talus with it) forward. A positive test result is when the examiner is able to pull the talus forward. The test is graded as a 1+, 2+, or 3+, depending on the degree of instability.

Finally, the patient's gait is observed. The examiner is watching for limping and pain. Abnormal patterns of weight-bearing are assessed. Motion in swing and stance phases are noted. Motor weakness is determined. For real clues to the patient's typical gait patterns, the shoes should be inspected for patterns of wear on the soles and sides, the pattern of creases across the dorsum, and for deformities where bony prominences have worn the shoe. Measuring the width of the feet and the shoes allows an assessment of appropriateness of the patient's shoe wear (Figs. 25-4, 25-5).

ANKLE INSTABILITY

Sprain

The most common foot and ankle injury is the ankle sprain. A sprain is defined as a stretching or tearing of the ligaments, which contrasts with a strain, which is defined as an injury to a muscle or tendon. An understanding of the anatomy of the bony structures and the medial and lateral ligament complexes of the ankle is essential for understanding the pathology, mechanism, and management of ankle sprains and chronic instability.

The ankle joint is the articulation of the talus with the tibia and fibula. At the level of the ankle, the tibia and fibula are joined by the syndesmotic ligament, which is composed of the anterior tibiofibular and posterior tibiofibular ligaments. The medial ligament complex is composed of the deltoid ligament. The deltoid ligament has a superficial portion comprised of the tibionavicular, calcaneotibal, and posterior talotibial ligaments and a deep portion. The deep deltoid ligament is formed from the deep anterior talotibial and deep posterior talotibial ligaments. The medial side of the ankle has more inherent stability than the lateral side, making eversion injury less common.

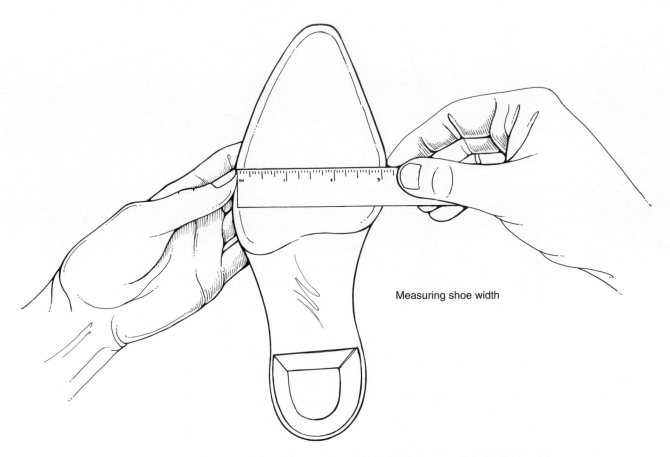

Measuring shoe width

Fig. 25-5. Measuring the patient's shoe. The examiner uses a ruler to measure the widest part of the patient's shoe and demonstrates to the patient the discrepancy of the patient's 4''-foot and the 3''-shoe.

The lateral ligament complex is formed from three anatomically distinct ligaments: the ATFL, the CFL, and the posterior talofibular ligament (PTFL). Inversion injuries to the ankle occur more frequently because of the less inherent stability of this side.

Sprains occur as the foot is brought into sudden uncontrolled inversion or eversion resulting from falls, blunt trauma, or uneven surfaces. The fibers of the ligamentous complexes stretch, and if motion is not controlled, they may tear partially or completely. As noted previously, the majority of injuries result from inversion (95%). These injuries are graded in increasing order of severity from I to III based on anatomic, physical, and radiographic findings.[4,7] Grade I sprain is a mild stretch with no instability. Anatomically, the ATFL may be partially torn, but the CFL and PTFL are intact. These ankles have a negative anterior drawer test and normal radiographs. A grade II sprain exhibits some instability. The AFTL is torn, but the CFL and PTFL are intact. There is a 1 to 2+ drawer sign (3 to 5 mm) and moderate talar tilt and drawer on plain radiographs and stress radiographs. A grade III sprain demonstrates gross instability. The AFTL and CFL are torn (the PTFL is rarely torn, except in cases of massive trauma). There is a 3+ drawer sign (> 5 mm of anterior displacement) and marked talar tilt and drawer on stress radiographs.

Diagnosis of the sprained ankle is based on history, physical examination, and, if indicated, radiographs. Acutely, these patients present with history of injury, pain, swelling that may be localized or diffuse, difficulty ambulating, and potential ecchymosis. Physical examination, which includes anterior drawer testing, usually reveals the absence of bony tenderness but the presence of pain along the injured ligaments. The examiner must be careful to palpate proximally along the leg and distally in the foot for concurrent injuries. The presence of any bony tenderness indicates the need for radiographs, which should include three views of the ankle: weight-bearing anteroposterior, lateral, and non–weight-bearing mortise views (taken with the leg and foot in internal rotation). If bony tenderness is elicited in the foot, weight-bearing anteroposterior and lateral radiographs and non–weight-bearing oblique views are appropriate. If there is proximal leg tenderness, anteroposterior and lateral views of the tibia and fibula are necessary to rule out Maisonneuve fractures. If instability is noted as indicated by a positive drawer sign, referral to an orthopedist for possible stress radiographs is appropriate. Radiographs are evaluated for fractures, dislocations, anterior drawer, and asymmetric talar tilt (> 10° difference).

Medial ankle sprains involving the deltoid ligament occur rarely and result from eversion. Partial tears of the anterior fibers of the deltoid are more common than isolated complete ruptures. If in doubt of stability, a weight-bearing anteroposterior radiograph of the contralateral ankle is appropriate.

Initial management of grade I and II sprains consists of

rest, ice, compression, and elevation—the acronym RICE. This management is usually followed by immediate weight-bearing in an aircast, ankle sleeve, or controlled ankle motion (CAM) walker and crutches. Early rehabilitation (1 to 3 weeks after injury) includes range of motion exercises, peroneal strengthening, and proprioception training for 4 to 6 weeks. Follow-up evaluation 1 week after injury is suggested to check for hidden injuries.

Management of Grade III sprains remains controversial. Initial management as outlined previously is one choice. Some physicians believe cast immobilization in dorsiflexion is most appropriate. These injuries are best referred for orthopedic management. Primary repair is only indicated in the professional ballet dancer or athlete who cannot perform with these injuries. Once the patient can return to activity, he or she should be braced or taped during athletic participation until his or her lower extremity strength is fully restored.

PERSISTENT PAIN AFTER MANAGEMENT OF ANKLE SPRAINS. Occasionally, the physician is faced with a patient who complains of persistent pain despite appropriate initial treatment. These patients can be extremely difficult to treat, and many possible etiologies exist. The most common cause of chronic complaints results from untreated peroneal weakness. The physical examination will reveal this readily (Fig. 25-6), and if this weakness is found, a course of rehabilitation concentrating on peroneal strengthening is appropriate (Fig. 25-7) (see box).

If, however, the peroneals are strong, there are several possible causes of chronic pain. The "high ankle sprain" is an injury of the anterior tibiofibular ligament. Although these injuries do heal, the recovery is much longer, and patience on the part of the patient and the physician is in order. Other potential causes include loss of subtalar motion, medial or lateral talar dome fractures, avulsion fractures of the fibula, a fracture of the anterior process of the calcaneus, other talar fractures (lateral, posterior, or anterior processes), previously asymptomatic accessory ossicles (os trigonum or os subfibulare), peroneal tendon pathology including tears or tendinitis, FHL tears or tendinitis, cuboid subluxation, sinus tarsi syndrome, or subtalar instability. Occasionally, anterolateral ankle impingement of the soft tissue is the cause. In these patients, pain may result from a thickened distal slip of the anteroinferior tibiofibular ligament[1] or from scar tissue and synovitis in the anterolateral gutter of the ankle.[2] Abnormalities, such as tarsal coalition, rheumatoid arthritis, nerve entrapment or neuropraxia, and tumors, must not be overlooked as potential causes. These patients require consultation with an orthopedist for further evaluation. The orthopedist may recommend additional imaging studies; in certain patients, a bone scan or computed tomography may be more appropriate than magnetic resonance imaging. It is best to allow the orthopedist to determine the most appropriate imaging studies.

RECURRENT ANKLE SPRAINS. Recurrent ankle sprains most commonly result from ligament stretching secondary to ATFL or CFL tears or generalized ligamentous laxity. Associated injuries include peroneal or posterior tibial tendon abnormality, osteochondritis dissecans,

PERONEAL STRENGTHENING EXERCISES

Props required
Sofa with padded arm rest, no end table

Canvas bag with wide handle

Weights (soup or juice cans can be used)

Instructions
Lie on the side on the sofa with the injured side up. Put the injured ankle on the arm rest so that the bone on the inside is fully supported by the arm rest. Hang the bag with the weights on the foot, which is slightly hanging over the edge. The bag will fall off the foot if the foot is too far off the arm rest.

Keeping the toes pointed way down like a ballet dancer and the ankle on the arm rest, lift the bag directly up with the foot only, toward the ceiling, and hold for 5 seconds. Relax and lower the bag, then lift again. Do not pull toes and ankle up (dorsiflexion); concentrate on keeping the toes and ankle pointed down.

How often
Two sessions a day, 25 lifts per session, 5 seconds each lift. Start with 3 pounds in the bag the first week. Add 3 pounds per week until the weight is up to 15 pounds (at the start of the fifth week). Do not advance faster. Stay at the 15-pound level indefinitely.

What if it hurts?
Reread the instructions. If the exercise is being done correctly, decrease number of lifts or weight until there is no pain. Return to physician if the pain persists after a couple of weeks.

degenerative disease, tarsal coalition, synovitis, or loose bodies. Once conservative treatment has failed, these patients may require surgical ligamentous reconstruction.

SYNDESMOTIC LIGAMENT INJURIES. When evaluating the acutely injured ankle, the clinician must be aware of the potential for syndesmotic ligament injury. Although these injuries are relatively uncommon, they can result from an athletic injury, especially in the football player. Physical examination is key in this diagnosis because radiographic results are often normal. In addition to the standard examination, the squeeze test and external rotation stress test should be performed.

For the squeeze test, the tibia and fibula are squeezed together in the mid-calf, and pain in the ankle region indicates syndesmotic injury. The external rotation stress test is positive if there is pain in the syndesmotic area with external rotation stress applied with the knee flexed to 90° and the ankle in a neutral position. A diastasis of the tibia and fibula on radiographs would also indicate syndesmotic rupture.

Initial management for stable injuries is RICE with weight-bearing as tolerated. Rehabilitation includes range of motion, strengthening, and pain modalities as for a lateral ankle sprain. However, the physician and pa-

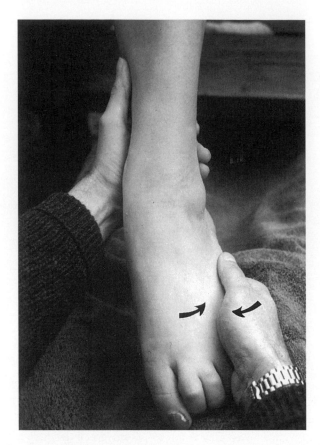

Fig. 25-6. Testing peroneal strength. The patient begins in a position of plantarflexion and eversion, and the examiner attempts to break the patient's held position. The examiner's ability to invert the foot signifies peroneal weakness.

tient should expect a prolonged recovery time. If the injury is unstable and diastasis is noted, the patient should be referred to an orthopedist for reduction, potential surgical removal of soft tissue from the distal tibiofibular joint, or placement of a syndesmotic screw and cast immobilization.

TENDON ABNORMALITIES ABOUT THE FOOT AND ANKLE

General Considerations

When considering tendon abnormalities, a brief review of tendon anatomy and terminology of pathology is helpful. The tendon itself is surrounded by the paratenon or outer sheath. Tendon inflammation and degeneration can be divided into three categories. *Paratenonitis* refers to inflammation of the paratenon only. It is marked by pain, local tenderness, swelling, warmth, and crepitus. *Tendinosis* is intratendinous degeneration secondary to aging, vascular compromise, or repetitive microtrauma in the absence of paratenonitis. In this case, there is usually a palpable swelling or nodule within the substance of the tendon. Tendinosis frequently occurs without any other signs or symptoms and can be a precursor to partial or complete tendon ruptures. Finally, there is *paratenonitis with tendinosis*, in which inflammation of the paratenon occurs in the presence of intratendinous degeneration. This condition is marked by pain, local tenderness, warmth, crepitus, and a palpable tendon nodule.

Achilles Tendinitis and Bursitis

Achilles tendinitis is the most common tendinitis and is frequently seen in athletes, runners particularly. It is often secondary to overuse or sudden increase in activity, but it may also be seen in patients with cavus feet (especially those with prominent posterosuperior prominences on their calcanei), tight hamstrings, tight Achilles tendons, and hindfoot varus. Patients present with pain, swelling, local tenderness, warmth, and crepitus along the distal 7.5 to 10 cm of the Achilles tendon.

Insertional Achilles tendinitis localizes to the posterior heel near the insertion into the calcaneal tuberosity. Point tenderness over the tendon and a decrease in passive dorsiflexion are often found. Although radiographs are not always necessary, they may show calcifications in the tendon in the face of tendinosis. Management is initially rest, nonsteroidal antiinflammatory drugs, ice, contrast baths, and heel lifts. Once comfort is achieved, stretching exercises and modification of activities are begun. Steroid injections are to be avoided because they can lead to tendon rupture.

Insertional Achilles tendinitis must be differentiated from superficial Achilles bursitis and retrocalcaneal bursitis. The superficial Achilles bursa lies between the skin and the posterior aspect of the Achilles tendon in about 50% of the population. Ill-fitting shoes can rub against the upper edge of the heel and cause irritation and inflammation of this bursa with associated thickening of the skin and callus formation. Soft-tissue swelling superficial to the tendon indicates this condition. Management includes shoe modification, nonsteroidal antiinflammatory drugs, and a heel lift.

The retrocalcaneal bursa is horseshoe-shaped and lies between the posterior aspect of the calcaneus and the anterior edge of the Achilles tendon. Inflammation can result from pressure from the shoe counter or systemic inflammatory disease as in rheumatoid or psoriatic arthritis, Reiter's syndrome, or gout. Although this condition also presents as posterior heel pain with swelling, warmth, and pain with dorsiflexion, the tenderness is localized between the calcaneus and the Achilles tendon. A localized lidocaine injection can be diagnostic. Management consists of rest, nonsteroidal anti-inflammatory drugs, ice, shoe modifications to relieve pressure (like a backless clog or cutting a "V" out over the irritated bursa), and a heel lift. Stretching and activity modification are appropriate.

When a patient presents with insertional tendinitis or retrocalcaneal bursitis and when an abnormally prominent superior posterolateral calcaneus is present, this condition is known as Haglund's syndrome. This anatomic variation can lead to chronic Achilles tendinitis. The initial treatment is as indicated previously, but refractory cases should be referred for possible surgical resection of the deformity. In the case of tendinitis or bursitis refractory to initial management, cast immobilization and months of conservative care or surgical intervention can be considered, but recovery time is prolonged.

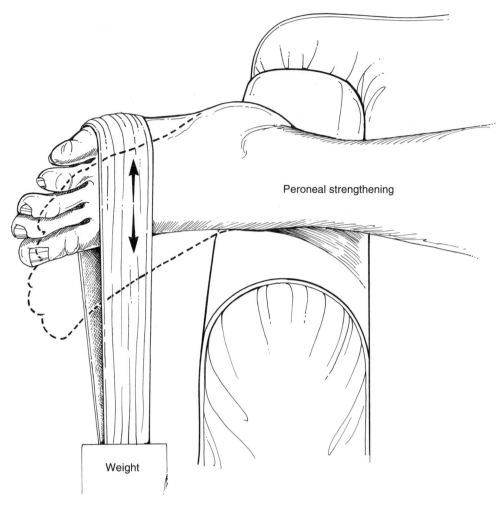

Peroneal strengthening

Weight

Fig. 25-7. Peroneal strengthening exercises. The patient rests with the medial ankle supported by the end of a couch and a bag with the appropriate weights suspended from the forefoot. The patient then raises the bag by everting the foot: 25 lifts, 5 seconds per lift, twice a day.

Achilles Tendon Ruptures

Chronic tendinosis can lead to ruptures of the Achilles tendon, especially in those aged 40 to 50 years or in the weekend athlete. Other risk factors for rupture include tight Achilles tendon, weakness of the gastrocnemius–soleus complex, congenitally small Achilles tendon, and overuse. Patients present with complaints of sudden pain, swelling, and marked weakness or inability to plantarflex. They often report hearing a popping sound and a feeling of being struck in the lower calf by an unseen object or person. Patients have usually been playing football, soccer, basketball, or running. Rupture is rare in those aged less than 20 years in whom it usually results from extreme mechanical overload. Ruptures typically occur 2 to 6 cm proximal to the insertion in the calcaneus.

Physical examination reveals the patient unable to walk on his or her toes with a palpable defect in the tendon. With the patient prone and his or her feet hanging off the table, the position of the feet is observed for differences in resting tension (Fig. 25-8). The Thompson test, or calf squeeze test, is performed with the patient prone on the examining table with the feet hanging over the edge. The superficial calf is squeezed, and the ankle is observed for plantarflexion. The absence of plan-

tarflexion when the calf is squeezed is considered a positive test result.

Management is controversial. Options include no treatment, cast immobilization in the equinus position, and operative repair. Risks and benefits of each option must be considered for each patient. In the patient who is very old, sick, or inactive no treatment may be best, but in most patients active enough to sustain these injuries, some treatment is reasonable. Casting alone has a decreased morbidity, greater residual weakness, and a higher rerupture rate. Surgery leads to more power and lower incidence of rerupture, but increased morbidity from potential surgical complications like infection and skin slough. If surgery is elected in addition to primary repair (if possible), many techniques have been described. It must be understood that casting will be necessary after surgery until tendon healing occurs so that both methods of treatment require an equivalent rehabilitation time, which is about 6 months, before active contact sports can be resumed.

Peroneal Tendinitis and Ruptures

The peroneus longus and brevis tendons lie in a common tendon sheath proximal to the lateral malleolus,

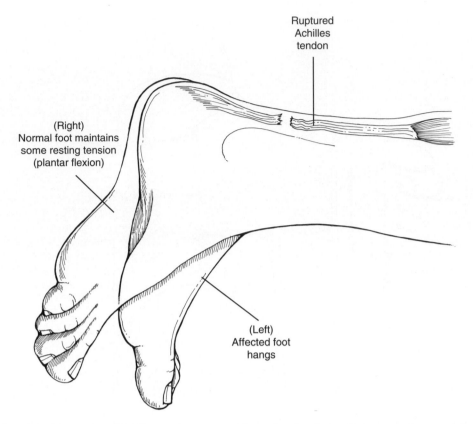

Ruptured
Achilles
tendon

(Right)
Normal foot maintains
some resting tension
(plantar flexion)

(Left)
Affected foot
hangs

Fig. 25-8. Observation of Achilles tendon rupture. The patient is asked to lie prone on the examining table with feet hanging off the end. The intact leg retains inherent plantarflexion, whereas on the injured side, the foot hangs straight down with gravity.

pass posterior to the lateral malleolus, and then run in individual sheaths distal to this. The brevis runs anterior to the longus and inserts in the base of the fifth metatarsal. The longus runs inferior to the trochlear process and takes a sharp turn medially under the cuboid to insert on the base of the first metatarsal. Peroneal tendinitis can occur after sudden forceful plantarflexion and inversion of the ankle, overuse, or can accompany ankle sprains. More commonly, it is associated with chronic ankle instability or occurs after traumatic peroneal subluxation or dislocation. Peroneal tendinitis presents as pain and swelling behind the lateral malleolus and along the course of the tendons. Pain with active and resisted eversion is present. Initial management includes rest, ice, nonsteroidal antiinflammatory drugs, and, in severe cases, immobilization. Refractory cases may require operative intervention.

As with other tendons, peroneal tendinitis can lead to degenerative partial tears or ruptures. Rupture can also occur secondary to trauma or steroid injections. Attritional tears are usually longitudinal and occur more commonly in the brevis. Patients present with pain and swelling along the course of the tendons. Examination will reveal pain with passive inversion or resisted eversion. Acute ruptures occur after a sudden inversion or dorsiflexion injury as the peroneals contract to prevent further inversion or dorsiflexion.

Signs and symptoms are the same as in tendinitis; a defect is rarely palpable. Initial management includes ice, rest, nonsteroidal anti-inflammatory drugs, and immobilization.

Peroneal Subluxation and Dislocation

Subluxation and dislocation of the peroneal tendons can occur, although relatively uncommon. It can be associated with injuries sustained during skiing (when the ski tips dig into the snow as the body is thrust forward downhill), basketball, waterskiing, dancing, ice skating, or gymnastics. Although the mechanism of injury is debated most examiners believe it occurs with forced dorsiflexion and eversion and violent peroneal contraction. A snapping or popping is heard or felt, and pain is located behind the lateral malleolus, distinguishing this from an ankle sprain. Swelling and ecchymosis frequently occur, and if the condition becomes chronic, the patient complains of snapping of the tendons over the malleolus and ankle instability. Radiographic results are usually normal, but if a part of the fibula is avulsed off with the retinaculum, it may be seen on radiograph. Magnetic resonance imaging is the diagnostic test of choice. Management consists of cast immobilization in the plantar-flexed position if the tendons are stably reduced. Persistent dislocations are managed with surgical repair or reconstruction of the retinaculum through soft tissue or bony procedures.

Posterior Tibial Tendinitis and Rupture

As the primary invertor of the heel and adductor of the forefoot, the PTT is subject to great mechanical stress. Dysfunction of the PTT occurs as a spectrum of changes, beginning with synovitis and progressing through tendonitis, tendinosis, and flexible and ultimately rigid flatfoot deformity. Patients are rarely aged less than 40 years and present with complaints of pain and swelling along the course of the tendon and inability to ambulate comfortably and participate in athletics. In later stages, patients note a progressive flattening of the arch. Physical examination reveals tenderness over the tendon sheath, swelling, possible tendon thickening, heel valgus, and unilateral flatfoot. Inversion weakness is found, and single-footed toe raising is painful or impossible. Decreased or no heel inversion occurs with toe raising, and observation of the patient from behind may reveal more toes visible on the affected side ("too many toes sign") (Fig. 25-9). As eversion progresses to cause impingement of the calcaneus on the fibula, some patients complain of lateral ankle pain.

History may reveal a traumatic episode with gradual decline in function and endurance. When tendinosis leads to rupture, it is usually between the navicular insertion and the malleolus in the zone of critical hypovascularity. Results of weight-bearing lateral radiographs of the foot are usually normal initially but later reveal a decreased longitudinal arch and ultimately may show arthritic changes. Magnetic resonance imaging is diagnostic but usually unnecessary because the diagnosis can be made on clinical examination.

Initial management in the absence of deformity consists of RICE, nonsteroidal anti-inflammatory drugs for at least 2 weeks around the clock, and restriction from athletic activities. If initial management is successful, physical therapy for stretching and strengthening with a gradual return to sports and longitudinal arch supports in the athletic shoe are appropriate. If initial management fails, therapy for pain modalities and immobilization in a cast or brace for 4 to 6 weeks should be attempted. Steroid injections should be avoided because they cause tendon rupture. Once this phase of management has proven unsuccessful, the patient should be evaluated to determine need for synovectomy (in the early stages), tendon transfer, and potentially arch reconstruction (in the presence of flexible deformity) or arthrodesis (if there is fixed deformity or in the older or obese patient). For patients unsuited to surgical reconstruction, a molded, customized ankle–foot orthosis that slips inside a lace up shoe can prevent further foot collapse and relieve pain.

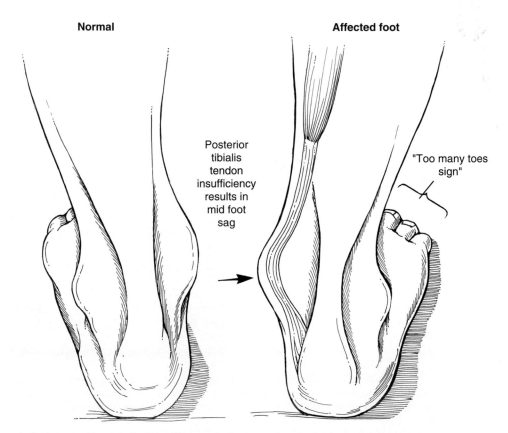

Normal

Posterior tibialis tendon insufficiency results in mid foot sag

Affected foot

"Too many toes sign"

Fig. 25-9. "Too many toes sign." Observation of the patient from behind reveals more toes visible on the side with the posterior tibial tendon insuffiency.

Posterior Tibial Tendon Subluxation and Dislocation

Subluxation and dislocation of the PTT is extremely rare, and few cases have been reported in the English literature.[9] Patients are usually aged 16 to 50 years and present with a history of a twisting injury to the ankle and possibly a pop or snap followed by medial ankle pain and swelling (anterior or posterior). If the condition is recurrent, popping can be felt by the patient as the tendon dislocates and spontaneously is reduced. There is medial ankle tenderness and dysfunction of the PTT. The

tendon may be palpable anterior to the medial malleolus. Magnetic resonance imaging will reveal the tendon subluxed or dislocated from its position behind the malleolus (Fig. 25-10). Conservative management, such as immobilization, is usually unsuccessful, and patients need referral for surgical repair.

Flexor Hallucis Longus, Flexor Hallucis Brevis, and Anterior Tibial Tendon Pathology

Tendinitis and rupture of the remaining tendons are rare in the general population. The FHL passes behind

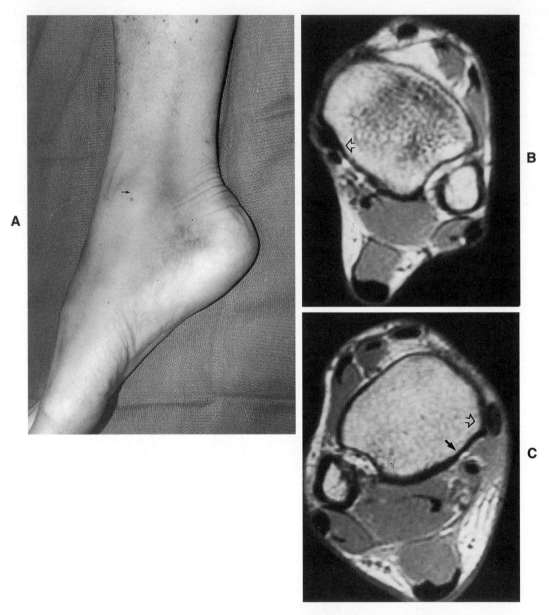

Fig. 25-10. Posterior tibial tendon dislocation. **A,** Photograph of the foot and ankle after posterior tibial tendon dislocation. Note the ecchymosis and anterior position of the dislocated tendon (solid arrow). **B,** Magnetic resonance imaging of the normal position of the posterior tibial tendon just anterior to the flexor digitorum longus tendon (open arrow). **C,** Magnetic resonance imaging of the dislocated posterior tibial tendon in its anterior position. Note soft tissue grey area anterior to the flexor digitorum longus tendon (solid arrow). *Courtesy of W. G. Hamilton, MD.*

the medial malleolus with the PTT and the FDL and is subject to tendinitis, stenosis, and inflammation at the point of entry to the tarsal tunnel. This condition can lead to posteromedial ankle pain and snapping or triggering of the tendon (hallux saltans). Through tendinosis, partial ruptures occur. Most frequently affected are ballet dancers and athletes whose sports require repetitive push off. Patients will have pain on palpation of the FHL in the tarsal tunnel and pain with resisted and passive plantarflexion of the great toe. Initial management is rest, ice, and nonsteroidal anti-inflammatory drugs. Steroid injections are avoided. If conservative management fails, surgical decompression is appropriate.

Flexor hallucis brevis (FHB) rupture is very rare and is indicated by pain under the first metatarsophalangeal joint (Fig. 25-11). Radiographs will reveal proximal migration of one or both sesamoids. Conservative management with rest, ice, nonsteroidal anti-inflammatory drugs, and metatarsal pads to relieve the pressure of weight-bearing is appropriate.

Anterior tibial tendon problems are infrequent because of low mechanical demands. Tendinitis and rupture can occur and present with anterior ankle pain, swelling, and tenderness. Management is usually successful and consists of rest, ice, and nonsteroidal anti-inflammatory drugs. Rupture or avulsion is marked by foot drop. Surgical repair is the treatment of choice.

OVERUSE SYNDROMES

Heel Pain

Plantar heel pain is one of the most common foot complaints. Unfortunately, the etiology is not always clear. A variety of disorders can produce plantar heel pain, including heel pain syndrome (also known as proximal plantar fasciitis), plantar fasciitis (or distal plantar fasciitis), nerve entrapment, heel pad atrophy, inferior or subcalcaneal bursitis, stress fracture of the calcaneus, rheumatoid arthritis, Reiter's syndrome, psoriatic arthritis, ankylosing spondylitis, gout and pseudogout, diabetes, and infection. Diagnosis and management depend on a very careful history and physical examination.

The most common cause of plantar heel pain is heel pain syndrome (HPS) or proximal plantar fasciitis. Patients are usually middle-aged and overweight and present with unilateral heel pain that is worst in the morning. Their first steps are excruciatingly painful, and increased sports activity exacerbates the symptoms, although pain often improves over the course of the day. Physical examination reveals pain with palpation of the medial tubercle of the calcaneus, which is the insertion of the plantar fascia. Pain is believed to be caused by microtears, hemorrhage, and degeneration of the plantar fascia at its insertion. Radiographic results are usually normal but may show a calcaneal spur in the area. It is important to understand that the spur is not the cause of pain because only 50% of patients with HPS have a spur,

and 15% of the general asymptomatic population has a spur.

Management consists of rest, heel cord stretching exercises, cushioned heels, nonsteroidal anti-inflammatory drugs, and activity modification. Steroid injections may exacerbate symptoms and lead to plantar fascia rupture or heel pad atrophy. Recovery time is prolonged and may take several months. Recalcitrant cases may be managed with night splinting to keep the foot out of equinus during sleep, physical therapy for deep friction massage, stretching and pain modalities, and potentially cast immobilization for 3 to 4 weeks. Ninety-five percent of patients improve with these measures. Surgery is considered a last resort and only after a minimum of 6 to 12 months of treatment. Barring any other abnormality, surgery usually consists of open partial plantar fascia release. The role of endoscopic release has not yet been established and has a high complication rate, the most intractable of which is dorsolateral midfoot pain secondary to collapse of the plantar arch.

Distal plantar fasciitis also presents as heel and arch pain. It occurs less frequently than HPS. On physical examination, tenderness is elicited with palpation of the plantar fascia in its midsubstance. Dorsiflexion of the toes makes the plantar fascia more taut and can elicit pain. Management is as for HPS.

Fat pad atrophy can also cause heel pain. Onset is gradual, but steroid injections may contribute to this condition. Patients complain of pain after excessive walking in hard soles rather than morning pain. Physical examination will reveal the atrophy. Heel cushions and centralizing heel cups are the treatments of choice.

Subcalcaneal bursitis is an inflammation of the bursa lying between the plantar aspect of the calcaneus and the skin secondary to trauma. Patients complain of well-localized nonradiating pain. Palpation of the heel on the posterior plantar surface rather than the medial tubercle elicits pain. Management consists of a heel pad, cup, or cut-out to relieve pressure. Nonsteroidal anti-inflamatory drugs may be helpful in decreasing inflammation. Deep friction massage may be helpful.

When the plantar heel pain is located on the medial border of the foot along the calcaneus' medial wall, it may result from compression of the first branch of the lateral plantar nerve, which supplies the abductor digiti quinti muscle. Palpation along the medial aspect of the calcaneus at the origin of the abductor hallucis muscle reproduces the patient's pain. A positive Tinel's sign (tapping over the nerve causes tingling along its course) is diagnostic but not always present. Initial management is aimed at relieving pressure on the nerve through shoe modifications, heel cushions, and arch supports. Nonsteroidal anti-inflammatory drugs are helpful, and steroid injections may be of benefit. When initial management fails, surgical decompression is appropriate.

Traumatic plantar fascia rupture can occur when the foot is in the push-off position. The patient complains of sudden onset of pain and often hears a pop or snap. Ecchymosis and swelling are noted, and tenderness with palpation and great toe dorsiflexion are present. A defect

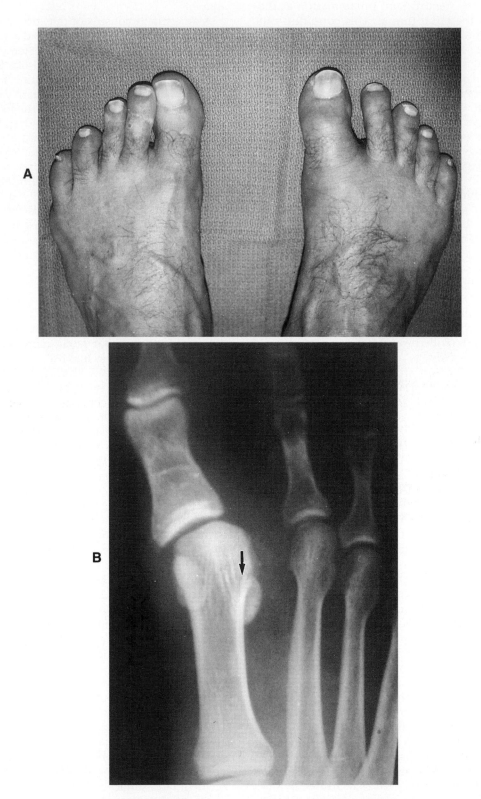

Fig. 25-11. Flexor hallucis brevis (FHB) rupture. **A**, Photograph showing varus deformity of the great toe after rupture of the lateral head of the FHB. **B**, Radiograph of FHB rupture. Note the proximal migration of the lateral sesamoid. *Courtesy of W. G. Hamilton, MD.*

may be palpated. The patient should be advised of a prolonged recovery time of 3 to 6 months. Management is immobilization for 2 weeks followed by physical therapy and protected weight-bearing and flexible longitudinal arch supports in a lace-up shoe.

Calcaneal stress fracture must also be ruled out. History usually reveals onset of sudden unremitting heel pain. Physical examination will reveal pain on compression of the calcaneus between the examiner's hands. Initial radiographs will probably be normal, and a bone scan may be necessary for early diagnosis. Radiographs taken 4 to 6 weeks after fracture will reveal a dense bony fracture line. Management is with ice, rest, and elevation. Activity modification with reduction of impact exercises should be instituted until the patient is pain-free.

Bilateral heel pain or migratory pain should make the clinician suspicious of a seronegative spondyloarthropathy. A rheumatology evaluation should be sought.

Sesamoiditis and Sesamoid Bursitis

The sesamoids lie beneath the head of the first metatarsal, wrapped within the flexor hallucis brevis tendon. Sesamoiditis is very common in athletes, especially runners and barefooted dancers. Cavus feet predispose to this condition. Patients present with pain beneath the first metatarsal head, which is increased during toe off. Physical examination will reveal tenderness to sesamoid palpation, swelling, and decreased range of motion. If the medial sesamoid is enlarged, an intractable plantar keratosis may be present just beneath it.

Sesamoiditis should be distinguished from sesamoid bursitis. A bursa lies between the sesamoids and skin in 30% of the population. With overuse, this bursa can also become inflamed, leading to pain, swelling, and erythema. Sesamoiditis may be thought of as one stage of a spectrum of disease beginning with bursitis, then sesamoiditis, osteochondritis, osteomalacia, degeneration, and finally fracture.

Radiographs are often negative, and conservative management begins with activity modification, metatarsal bars or pads to unweight the area, nonsteroidal antiinflammatory drugs, low-heeled shoes, rocker bottom soles, and taping of the great toe to reduce dorsiflexion (Fig. 25-12). In the absence of a fracture, cortisone injection may be used. Symptoms unresponsive to 6 to 12 months of conservative therapy indicate the need for orthopedic evaluation to assess the need for sesamoid shaving or excision.

Second Metatarsophalangeal Joint Instability

Patients may present with a complaint of vague, persistent pain beneath the second metatarsal head and potential swelling of the toe with medial or dorsal deviation. A diagnosis of second metatarsophalangeal joint instability and associated synovitis must be ruled out.[13] This condition usually occurs in joggers, tennis players, bicyclists, power or long distance walkers, and ballet dancers. History reveals an insidious onset of gradually increasing pain and potential toe deviation. Systemic arthritis should be ruled out. The physical examination will usually show pain to palpation of the plantar aspect

of the second metatarsophalangeal joint and possibly an associated bunion deformity that exacerbates the problem. A diagnostic test is the vertical stress or drawer test, in which the base of the proximal phalanx is grasped and an attempt is made to translate the toe dorsally (see Fig. 25-2). Successful subluxation is a positive test result, and this usually reproduces the patient's pain. Initial management is taping of the toe into the resting position or use of a commercial toe retainer (Fig. 25-13). Metatarsal pads and modification of the shoes to add a rocker bottom (to allow the patient to roll over the toe) is appropriate. Nonsteroidal anti-inflammatory drugs and perhaps a steroid injection into the second metatarsophalangeal joint to manage the synovitis may be attempted. If conservative measures fail, surgical management of the joint is necessary. The untreated toe is more apt to progress to a spontaneous metatarsophalangeal dislocation with an associated severe hammertoe.

Stress Fractures

It is not uncommon for patients who participate in vigorous repetitive impact training to present with complaints of localized pain and possibly swelling on the dorsum of the foot in the absence of any remembered trauma. Physical examination will reveal very localized pain over one specific point on a bone, although deformity and crepitus will be absent. Radiographs should be taken in three planes: anteroposterior, lateral, and oblique. Radiographs may initially be negative, but may show callus 3 to 4 weeks later. Localized bony tenderness can be evaluated with a bone scan in the professional athlete, the results of which will often be positive. These results should be interpreted as indicating a stress reaction or stress fracture. Nonprofessional athletes may be treated symptomatically with a postoperative shoe and radiographs taken again 3 to 4 weeks later.

Stress fractures occur most commonly at the base of the second or third metatarsal (Fig. 25-14 on p. 402), the navicular, the talus, the cuneiform, the metaphyseal and diaphyseal junction in the proximal fifth metatarsal (Jones fracture) (Fig. 25-15 on p. 403), the sesamoid, the calcaneus, and the distal fibula. Bone failure results from repetitive loading but may also be caused by bony insufficiency in young female athletes with anorexia or older perimenopausal women. If radiographs are repeated at 3 to 4 weeks, they will often show signs of callus formation (healing bone).

Most stress fractures are managed with rest, ice, elevation, and a hard-soled shoe and usually heal in 4 to 6 weeks. Exceptions are stress fractures of the navicular, which require 6 to 8 weeks wearing a non–weight-bearing cast and potentially open reduction and bone grafting with internal fixation if radiographs show sclerosis. Jones stress fractures require prolonged non–weight-bearing cast immobilization (some up to 20 weeks) and may require bone grafting and screw fixation for delayed unions or nonunions, which are not uncommon. Sesamoid stress fractures also require prolonged immobilization or activity restriction for definitive healing and may require currettage and grafting or excision if not responsive to conservative management.

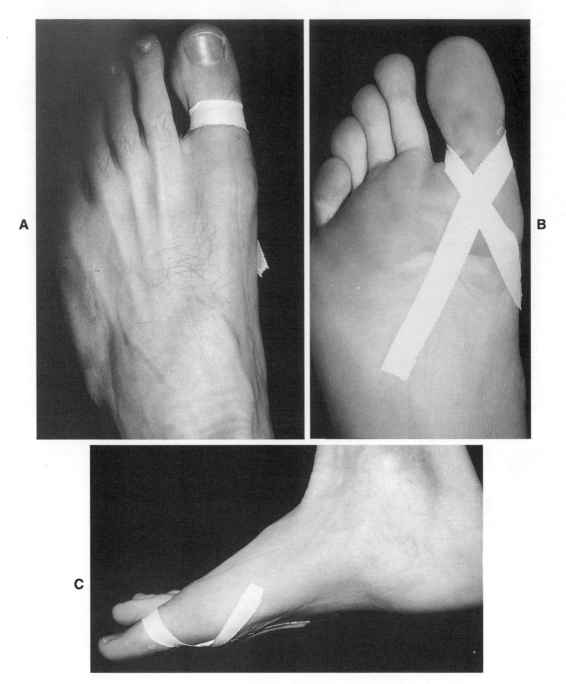

Fig. 25-12. Taping of the great toe for sesamoiditis or turf toe. Visualization from the dorsal (**A**), plantar (**B**), and medial (**C**) aspects of the foot. Note toe is slightly plantarflexed.

FRACTURES AND DISLOCATIONS

General Considerations

Fractures of the foot and ankle are quite common, and adequate management requires careful diagnosis of the extent of the injury. Radiographs in three planes of view are crucial. For the foot, this includes anteroposterior, lateral (weight-bearing if possible), and oblique views. To evaluate the ankle, anteroposterior, lateral, and mortise views are required. The goal of fracture management is to achieve a plantigrade foot capable of pain-free weight-bearing.

When considering fractures, the clinician must assess the degree of displacement. Nondisplaced fractures maintain their anatomic alignment with minimal or no separation of the fragments. Displaced fractures have fragments that are malaligned or significantly separated. Intraarticular fractures involve fracture lines that extend into the articular surface. Extraarticular fractures occur outside of the articular surface. Management of most forefoot injuries by primary care physicians is appropriate, whereas management of mid-foot and hind-foot injuries usually requires consultation with an orthopedist for definitive care.

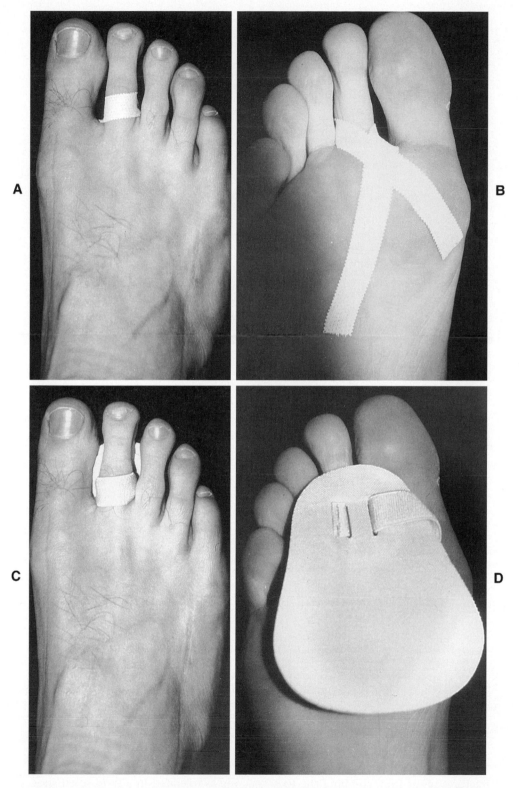

Fig. 25-13. Management of second metatarsophalangeal instability. Taping of the toe from the dorsal (**A**) and plantar (**B**) aspect. Use of a commercial toe retainer (**C** and **D**).

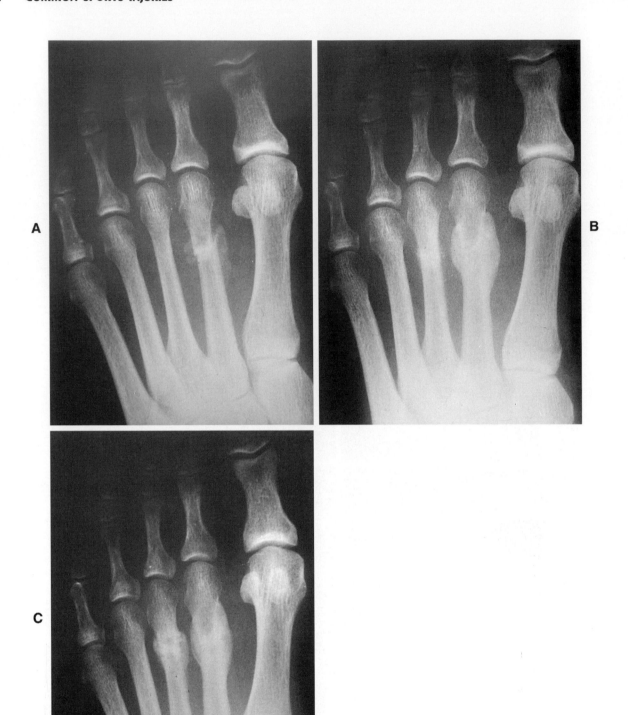

Fig. 25-14. Stress fractures at the second and third metatarsal. **A**, Initial radiographs reveal the second, but not the third, metatarsal stress fracture. **B**, Later radiographs reveal a small amount of callous formation at the site of the third metatarsal fracture. **C**, Exuberant callous formation is now seen at the second and the third metatarsals.

Phalangeal Fractures

Most phalangeal fractures result from stubbing the toes, but blunt trauma from objects dropped on the feet is also a significant mechanism. The proximal phalanx is most commonly fractured. If the fracture is extraarticular and nondisplaced, it may be taped to the adjacent toe ("buddy taped"), and the patient is allowed weight-bear-ing as tolerated in a hard-soled shoe. Comfort is usually achieved after 3 weeks. Displaced fractures are reduced through manipulation and buddy taped for approxi-mately 3 weeks until the pain subsides. The fifth toe is best stabilized with a "pinky toe sling" of ½"-tape around the foot (Fig. 25-16).

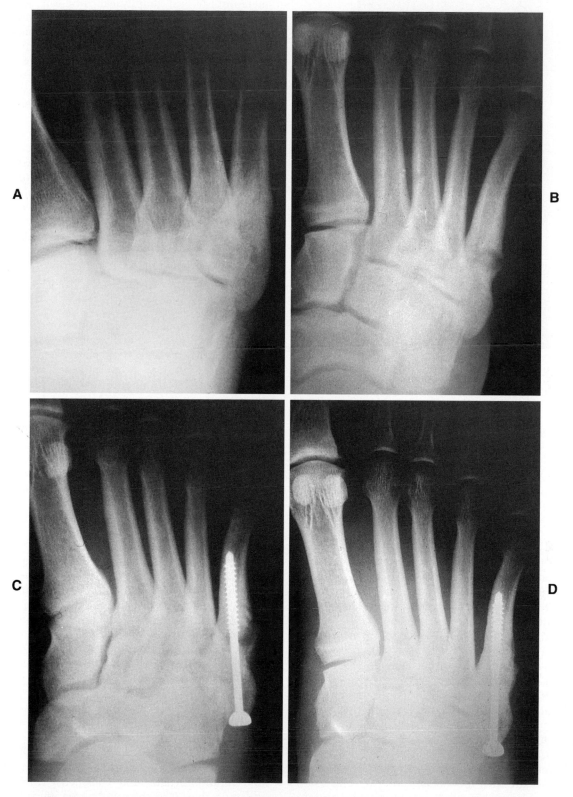

Fig. 25-15. Jones stress fracture. **A,** Stress reaction. **B,** Frank fracture. **C,** Immediate postoperative radiograph showing bone grafting and intramedullary screw fixation. **D,** Follow-up radiograph.

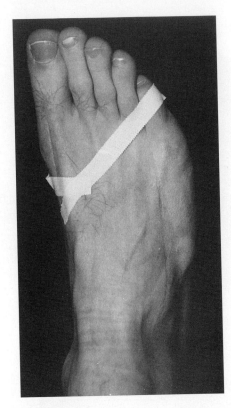

Fig. 25-16. Pinky toe sling affords better stabilization of the fifth toe than buddy taping.

Intraarticular fractures usually require open reduction and internal fixation to avoid posttraumatic arthritis and joint subluxation. All open fractures (fractures with open wounds allowing communication of the bone with the outside environment) require irrigation and débridement and reduction. Patients with open fractures should be referred to an orthopedist.

Metatarsal Fractures

Fractures of the metatarsal usually involve the neck or shaft. Metatarsal head fractures are rare and require reduction of the articular surface and fixation with wires if the reduction is unstable. Single nondisplaced metatarsal neck or shaft fractures may be managed with weight-bearing as tolerated in a hard-soled shoe; two or more nondisplaced metatarsal fractures should be placed in a well-molded and padded cast that extends beyond the toes for 4 to 6 weeks. Displaced fractures require reduction if the fracture will heal with significant dorsal or plantar angulation. If the reduction is stable, the fracture can be managed as outlined previously. If the fracture is unstable, if multiple metartarsals are fractured, or if the first metatarsal is fractured and displaced, open reduction and internal fixation are required.

Fractures of the fifth metatarsal can also occur as an avulsion of the tuberosity or at the metaphyseal and diaphyseal junction. Avulsion fractures occur as the foot is placed in sudden inversion and the peroneus brevis contracts violently to prevent this, resulting in avulsion of the tuberosity to which the tendon is attached. These fractures are managed with a soft bulky dressing,

ice, and elevation followed by weight-bearing as tolerated in a hard-soled shoe. Fractures occurring at the metaphyseal and diaphyseal junction are known as Jones fractures and have a high rate of delayed union and nonunion (25%). In the general population, these fractures are managed in non–weight-bearing casts for 8 to 12 weeks or longer until the fracture site is pain-free, indicating healing. In the athlete with delayed union or an acute displaced Jones fracture, open reduction and internal fixation with an intramedullary screw is appropriate.

Dislocations

Dislocations usually occur at the metatarsophalangeal joint, but they can also occur at the proximal and distal interphalangeal joints. Most can easily be reduced with manipulation, and once reduced, the toes should be buddy taped for 1 to 2 weeks. Occasionally, a dislocation will be irreducible, which is usually secondary to the metatarsal head becoming trapped in the plantar soft tissues. With irreducible or chronic dislocation, open reduction and stabilization will be required.

Turf Toe

Turf toe is a hyperextension injury of the first metatarsophalangeal joint associated with play on artificial turf. Patients present with first metatarsophalangeal joint pain. Physical examination reveals tenderness with localized swelling and decreased range of motion. Injury can range from a mild sprain to tearing of the capsuloligamentous complex with dislocation and first metatarsal head fracture. Initial management consists of rest, ice, elevation, nonsteroidal anti-inflammatory drugs, taping in slight plantarflexion, and contrast baths (Fig. 25-12). Return to normal and athletic activities should be gradual. Surgical repair of the capsule and excision of loose fragments may be necessary in cases of severe injury.

Sesamoid Fractures

Fractures of the medial and lateral sesamoids can occur and require prolonged recovery time (3 to 6 months). Care must be taken to differentiate fractured sesamoids from multipartite ones in which the bone forms from two or more ununited ossification centers. Bipartite sesamoids are usually divided transversely with smooth edges. The fractured sesamoid has jagged uneven edges. Treatment requires cast immobilization followed by shoe modifications to unweight the area until the foot is no longer painful. If symptoms persist after 6 to 12 months excision can be considered.

Midfoot and Hindfoot Fractures and Dislocations

Midfoot (the three cuneiforms, navicular, and cuboid) and hindfoot (talus and calcaneus) fractures are less common than forefoot injuries. Significant force is necessary to injure these structures, and because of this, in addition to evaluating for obvious fractures and dislocation, the clinician must be aware of the risk of compartment syndrome. In addition to the three standard views, special radiographic views, bone scans, and computed tomography scans may also be required. Initial management is ice, elevation, and splinting for immobilization. If casting is required immediately after injury, care must be taken to bivalve (split) the cast to allow for swelling and decrease the chance of compartment syndrome. Any fracture with significant displacement will require reduction and possibly internal fixation. Because of the significant force required for these injuries to occur and the need for anatomic reduction and often surgical intervention, patients with these injuries should be referred to an orthopedist for definitive care.

Cuboid fractures usually occur as chip fractures with minimal displacement and can be managed with weight-bearing casting for approximately 4 to 6 weeks. The exception is the so-called "nutcracker" fracture, which is a compression of the lateral border of the cuboid that shortens the lateral column of the foot. In the face of significant shortening or displacement, open reduction and restoration of length with bone grafting is required. Cuboid subluxation as a result of inversion injury has been known to occur but is rare, and radiographic evidence may be subtle (Fig. 25-17). Subluxation is more common in the ballet dancer,[8] who notes midfoot lateral pain and has problems "working through the foot." Traumatic dislocations require open reduction and internal fixation, whereas in dancers these fractures are best treated by experienced physical therapists.

Navicular fractures can be classified as avulsion fractures of the dorsal lip, body fractures, and tuberosity fractures. Lip avulsion fractures occur with inversion injury and usually can be managed with cast immobilization for 4 to 6 weeks. Fractures of the body require anatomic reduction to avoid posttraumatic arthritis and deformity. Even with proper management, prognosis is poor, and patients should be warned of the high rate of complications. Tuberosity fractures are often small and result from sudden eversion injury as the posterior tibial tendon contracts to prevent additional eversion. These injuries must be differentiated from an accessory navicular fracture, which is not a traumatic condition (Fig. 25-18). Immobilization for 4 to 6 weeks is appropriate, with excision being necessary if a painful nonunion occurs. Associated fractures of the cuboid are common and must be considered.

Cuneiform fractures are rare as isolated injuries, and much more commonly occur in association with tarsometatarsal (Lisfranc) fracture–dislocations. These injuries occur as significant forces pass through the hyperplantarflexed foot, disrupting ligamentous structures and fracturing the metatarsal bases and tarsal bones. Because of the high degree of trauma necessary to cause these injuries, compartment syndromes and open injuries are common. Prognosis is very poor if these injuries are missed or if anatomic reduction is not achieved and maintained. Bilateral weight-bearing anteroposterior radiographs, bone scans, and computed tomography scans may be necessary to make the diagnosis in subtle cases. Management usually requires open reduction and internal fixation, followed by cast immobilization. Clues to Lisfranc injuries are (Fig. 25-19): (1) loss of alignment of the medial border of the second metatarsal with the medial border of the first cuneiform on anteroposterior radiograph, (2) loss of alignment of the first and second metatarsals dorsal borders with the dorsal borders of the first and second cuneiforms, respectively, on lateral radiographs; and (3) loss of alignment of the medial border of the fourth metatarsal with the medial border of the cuboid on oblique radiographs.[6]

Talar fractures occur with significant traumatic force in dorsiflexion. Fractures can occur in the body (very poor prognosis), the neck (significant risk of avascular necrosis), and as osteochondral fragments of the talar dome. Associ-

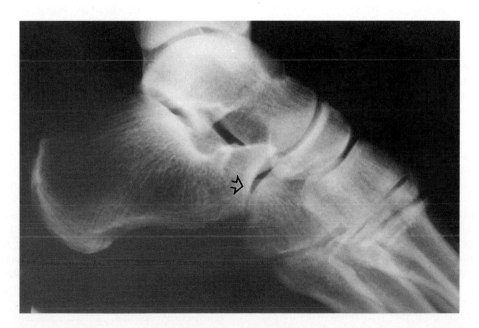

Fig. 25-17. Lateral radiograph revealing cuboid subluxation. Note the incongruity of the joint. *Courtesy of W. G. Hamilton, MD.*

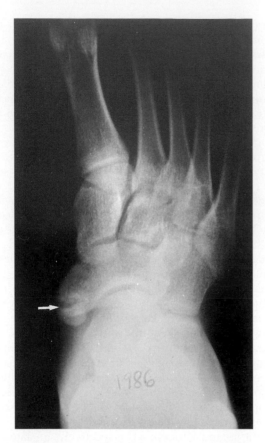

Fig. 25-18. Accessory navicular. An accessory navicular is often mistaken for a fracture of the navicular.

ated injuries are common because of the high energy necessary to cause talar fractures. Standard radiographs may be insufficient for diagnosis, and special views (Broden's view of the subtalar joint) or computed tomography scans may be necessary. Management requires anatomic reduction, fixation if necessary, and immobilization.

Calcaneal fractures are very common. Axial loading is the usual mechanism of injury, but distraction forces that avulse the tuberosity of the calcaneus into which the Achilles tendon inserts can also cause fracture. In addition to standard radiographs, Broden's and Harris (axial heel) views and computed tomography scans are necessary for evaluation. Management depends on the fracture pattern and level of expertise of the clinician. Nondisplaced avulsion fractures of the posterior tuberosity may be managed with immobilization, whereas displaced fractures will require open reduction and internal fixation. In general, nondisplaced fractures are managed with bulky dressings, range of motion exercises and non–weight-bearing for 6 weeks. Displaced fractures with large fragments are managed with open reduction and internal fixation. Severely comminuted fractures that defy open reduction and internal fixation may be managed with primary arthrodesis or, more commonly, non–weight-bearing for 12 weeks with early motion. Subtalar or triple arthrodesis can be performed in those who are very symptomatic 12 to 18 months after injury.

Compartment Syndrome

Compartment syndrome is defined as a neurovascular or muscular injury secondary to high pressure within a confined space. Definitive diagnosis is made by directly measuring the intracompartmental pressures. Unlike in other parts of the body, the signs and symptoms of compartment syndrome in the foot are not classic, but the diagnosis should be suspected with significant trauma, especially crush injuries, tense swelling, and severe pain. Definitive management requires release of the pressure through fasciotomies of the foot compartments. Untreated compartment syndrome can lead to hypesthesia, clawing, and stiffness of the toes.

Ankle Fractures

Fractures of the ankle are very common and result from a variety of mechanisms. Isolated medial malleolus fractures can result from blunt trauma or inversion injuries in association with lateral ligament complex sprain or tear. Eversion injuries can lead to isolated lateral fibular fractures or fractures associated with deltoid ligament injury or rupture. Bimalleolar fractures refer to fractures of the medial and lateral malleoli. Trimalleolar fractures are fractures of the medial and lateral malleoli plus the posterior malleolus of the tibia.

Initial management requires ice, elevation, and immediate reduction of severely displaced feet to reduce the risk of skin slough and compartment syndrome. The three standard views of the ankle are required. Management requires anatomic reduction and maintenance of the symmetry of the ankle joint. Open reduction and internal fixation is required with any displacement of the fracture fragments more than 2 mm, open injuries, or incongruence of the ankle joint.

NERVE ENTRAPMENT SYNDROMES ABOUT THE FOOT AND ANKLE

Morton's (Interdigital) Neuroma

The most common nerve entrapment syndrome in the foot and ankle is Morton's, or interdigital, neuroma. It occurs when the interdigital nerve, which is formed from medial or lateral plantar branches of the tibial nerve, becomes compressed beneath the deep transverse metatarsal ligament. Rather than a classical neuroma, it is a perineural fibrosis consistent with nerve compression. It occurs more frequently in women, probably secondary to ill-fitting shoes,[12] and presents as lancinating pain in the toes that may radiate up the leg. Paresthesias may be present in the adjacent sides of the involved toes. Pain is usually relieved by rest and removal of shoes. Morton's neuromas is most common in the third webspace; involvement in the second webspace is less frequent, and first and fourth webspace neuromas are rare as are multiple simultaneous webspace neuromas. Compression of the webspace will usually reproduce the pain, and a click (Mulder's click) may be felt on compression of the foot as the webspace is pressed. Diagnosis is confirmed when injection of lidocaine into the webspace relieves symptoms. Initial management consists of metatarsal pads to unweight the area, shoe modification to lower heels and wider toe boxes, and nonsteroidal

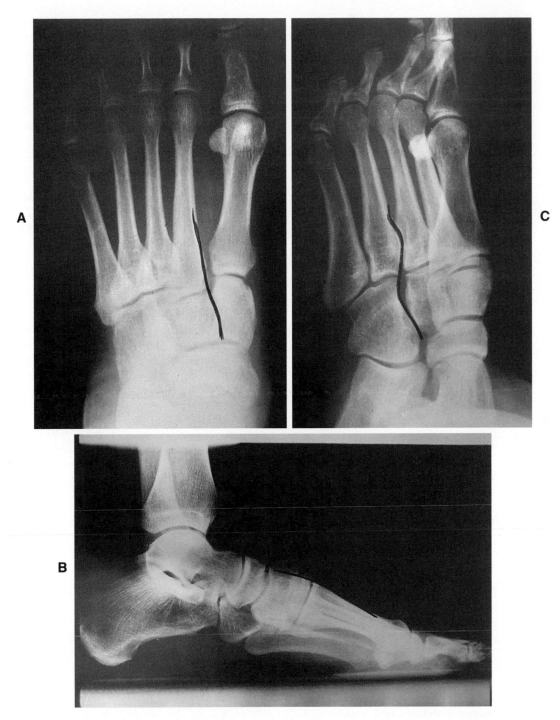

Fig. 25-19. Normal relationships of the metatarsal and cuneiform bones. **A,** Anteroposterior radiograph. **B,** Lateral radiograph. **C,** Oblique radiograph.

anti-inflammatory drugs. Injection of steroids into the webspace may lead to long-term relief (Fig. 25-20). Excision is appropriate for symptoms recalcitrant to conservative management, but patients should be aware of a 10% to 15% incidence of recurrence.

Other Nerve Entrapment Syndromes

Other nerve entrapment syndromes can occur in the foot and ankle, but they are rare and usually occur secondary to trauma, inflammation, or compression beneath anatomic retinacula. Entrapment of the posterior tibial nerve in the tarsal tunnel is known as tarsal tunnel syndrome. The deep peroneal nerve may become entrapped beneath the superior or inferior ankle retinacula or under the EHB tendon. The superficial peroneal nerve can be compressed secondary to muscle herniation or under the edge of the deep crural fascia. The sural nerve is usually compressed with calcaneal or fifth metatarsal

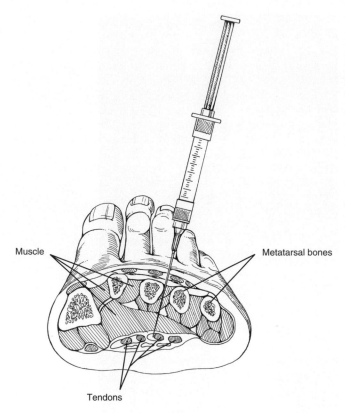

Muscle

Metatarsal bones

Tendons

Fig. 25-20. Injection of the webspace in Morton's neuroma. The needle is directed into the webspace and beneath the deep transverse metatarsal ligament to infiltrate the area surrounding the interdigital nerve.

fractures. The saphenous nerve usually impinges on the fascial edge.

Symptoms are usually pain of a burning or tingling nature, which is worse with activity, hypesthesia, or paresthesias in the dermatomal distribution, and intrinsic motor weakness in the case of the posterior tibial nerve compression. Physical examination will reveal a positive Tinel's sign and decreased sensation. Electrodiagnostic testing may be necessary to make the diagnosis. Initial management includes nonsteroidal anti-inflammatory drugs, rest, shoe modifications, and orthoses to relieve stretch on the nerves. A steroid injection may be of benefit. If conservative management fails, surgical release of compressing structures and neurolysis is appropriate.

TOENAILS

Ingrown Toenails

Proper toenail care requires trimming of the nails straight across with smooth edges to avoid snagging of the nail on shoes and socks. With improper toenail trimming or in patients with C-shaped incurved nails, ingrown toenails can develop and lead to irritation or infection. Initial management involves warm soaks and nail training by placing a wisp of cotton under the nail edge to get the nail to grow appropriately. If infection is present, soaks,

oral antibiotics, and parital or complete excision of the nail, depending on the extent of the infection, are appropriate. With advanced recurrent ingrowth, surgical ablation of the nail and matrix is necessary.

Blue Toenails (Joggers Nail or Tennis Toenail)

Blue or black painless discoloration can occur under the nail of the longest toe from repetitive trauma (start and stop running). The cause is usually a chronic subungual hematoma that will resolve slowly. Management involves shoe modifications with metatarsal pads, tighter vamps, warm soaks, and rest. If the discoloration is the result of sudden blunt trauma, the discoloration is caused by an acute subungual hematoma, which usually becomes progressively more painful. Evacuation of the hematoma is the treatment of choice.

Fungal Infections (Onychomycosis)

Onychomycosis is extremely common in adults and presents with thickening and splitting of the nail, accompanied by whitish discoloration. The infections are usually caused by dermatophytes, with *Trichophyton rubrum* being the most common fungus. Diagnosis is made by the characteristic appearance and potassium hydroxide examination of nail samples. Cultures should be taken if necessary.

There are four types of fungal nail infections. The distal subungual variety is the most common. Proximal subungual infection is rare. Both are managed with naftifine hydrochloride, 1%, gel or oral griseofulvin if severe, although management can take up to 18 months. Griseofulvin can, however, cause hepatic damage. White superficial onychomycosis is caused by *Trichophyton mentagrophytes* and is managed by scraping of the nail surface and proper nail care. *Candida onychomycosis* usually occurs in the diabetic population and management requires meticulous drying of nails to prevent *Pseudomonas* superinfection, soaks with acetic acid, and naftifine hydrochloride, 1%, gel.

SKIN PROBLEMS

Athlete's Foot (*Tinea pedis*)

Athlete's foot is a common condition caused by a superficial fungal infection. As in fungal infections of the nails, the dermatophytes *T. rubrum* and *T. mentagrophytes* are most commonly responsible. Diagnosis is usually based on history and physical examination but may be confirmed by placing skin in potassium hydroxide for microscopic evaluation or culturing. Management is initially with tolnaflate, which is a topical fungistatic antifungal. If the skin is macerated and has oozing areas, wet soaks or potassium permanganate solution is appropriate until skin heals, followed by antifungals. Resistance to topical management may require oral griseofulvin or ketoconazole and probably should be managed by dermatology consultation.

Plantar Warts

Warts are keratotic lesions on the plantar aspect of the foot caused by papilloma virus. Patients present with complaints of painful calluses on weight-bearing areas.

They are differentiated from seed corns (caused by invagination of the dermal layer) by the appearance of punctate areas of bleeding with trimming. Plantar warts are very resistant to management, and may be self-limited. Management involves trimming, keratolytics, and shoe modifications for comfort. Freezing with nitrogen or excision may be done for multiple warts or those unresponsive to conservative management. The more invasive the treatment, the greater the risk of trading a self-limited condition for a painful plantar iatrogenic scar that would be permanent.

Hyperhidrosis (Excessive Sweating)

Hyperhidrosis can occur as the temperature in the shoe or sneaker increases, which can lead to an increased incidence of infection and foot odor. Modification of sock and shoe wear may be helpful. Topical solutions of aluminum chloride, 20%, may also be used at bedtime, and the feet can be wrapped in plastic wrap.

FOREFOOT ABNORMALITIES

Hallux Valgus (Bunions)

Hallux valgus deformity, more commonly known as bunions, is a lateral deviation of the great toe. Although the etiology is unclear, it appears to be associated with heredity and tight shoes. The condition is more common in women (believed to result from inappropriate shoe wear). Patients present with complaints of pain, occasionally bursitis over the prominent medial eminence, and difficulty finding comfortable shoes. Physical examination will reveal deformity, possibly tenderness, bursitis, great toe pronation, associated lesser toe deformities, calluses, neuromas, or corns.

Evaluation requires weight-bearing radiographs in the standard three views. A sesamoid view directed tangentially to the plantar surface of the first metatarsal head can aid in assessing sesamoid displacement. Measuring the first and second intermetatarsal angle, which normally is approximately 9°, and the hallux valgus angle (obtained by longitudinally bisecting the proximal phalanx and the first metatarsal), which is normally approximately 15°, helps to assess the degree of deformity.

Initial management should be conservative. Shoe modifications to a wider toe box, lower heels, and soft leather with flexible soles is often helpful. The patient should avoid seams or stitching in the toe box overlying the bunion. Drainage of a painful bursa is appropriate. If excessive pronation of the first toe is present, an orthosis may be helpful. Patients must be made to understand that surgery should be reserved for painful bunions. The athlete, in particular, must be aware that return to a high performance level after surgery may be impossible. Professional dancers should never have their bunions corrected until they are ready to retire; even so, they must be aware that they may lose the ability to relevé.

Hallux Rigidus

Hallux rigidus is painful loss of motion of the first metatarsophalangeal joint. Although trauma may be one cause, it usually results from arthritic changes in the joint, particularly, the dorsal portion. Patients complain of pain, especially during push-off activities. Physical examination reveals decreased range of motion and pain with passive motion. Swelling may be present. Radiographs often reveal dorsal osteophytes on the metatarsal head and base of the proximal phalanx. Initial management involves shoe modification to a stiff sole. A steel shank may be added to the shoe or sneaker. A rocker bottom may be placed on shoes as a last conservative effort. If these measures fail, surgery to excise the dorsal metatarsal head or arthrodesis is appropriate.

Lesser Toe Deformities

Clawtoes are defined as dorsiflexion of the metatarsophalangeal joints associated with flexion at the proximal and distal interphalangeal joints. Hammertoes are flexed at the proximal interphalangeal joint. Mallet toes are defined as flexion of the distal interphalangeal joints. These deformities can either be fixed (rigid) or flexible. They are usually associated with painful callus formation on the dorsum of the flexed joints and the toe tips. The second toe is most commonly involved. Hammertoes and mallet toes usually result from wearing tight shoes. Clawing represents a muscle imbalance with weak intrinsic muscles.

Clawtoes should initially be managed with modifications to the shoes (high toe boxes). Hammertoes and mallet toes should be managed with toe crests to elevate the tips of rigid toes or toe taping or commercial toe retainers if the deformity is flexible. Surgical correction should be contemplated if conservative measures fail and if there is jeopardy of the skin integrity. Painless toe deformities with intact skin do not require surgery.

A bunionette is a painful lateral prominence of the fifth metatarsal head. The prominence may result from an abnormally large head, lateral flaring of the metatarsal shaft, or a large intermetatarsal angle between the fourth and fifth metatarsals. The prominence is irritated by shoe wear, and as with hallux valgus deformities, pain, bursitis, and callosities develop. Management is aimed at pain relief with wider shoes of soft material. Orthoses for excessive pronation, as with hallux valgus, may be helpful. Surgery, if necessary, is aimed at correction of the underlying deformity.

Metatarsalgia

Metatarsalgia is pain beneath the metatarsal heads. Its cause are many, including clawing, fat pad atrophy, instability, synovitis, neuromas, inflammatory disease, tight Achilles tendons, and a long second metatarsal (especially in runners). History and physical examination lead to the underlying cause. Management is aimed at relieving underlying pathology as has been detailed previously.

REFERENCES

1. Basset FA, et al: Talar impingement by the anteroinferior tibiofibular ligament, *J Bone Joint Surg* 72A:55–59, 1990.
2. Ferkel RD, et al: Arthroscopic treatment of anterolateral

impingement of the ankle, *Am J Sports Med* 19:440–446, 1991.

3. Hamilton WG: Surgical anatomy of the foot and ankle, *CIBA Clin Symp*, vol 37. New Jersey, 1985, CIBA-GEIGY.

4. Hamilton WG: Current concepts in the the treatment of acute and chronic lateral ankle instability. In *Sports medicine and arthroscopy review*, vol 2. New York, 1994, Raven Press.

5. Hoppenfeld S: Physical examination of the foot and ankle. In *Physical examination of the spine and extremities*, New York, 1976, Appleton-Century-Crofts.

6. Lutter LD, et al., eds: *Orthopaedic knowledge update: foot and ankle*, Rosemont, IL, 1994, American Academy of Orthopaedic Surgeons.

7. Mann RA, Coughlin MJ, eds: *Surgery of the foot and ankle*, ed 6, 2 vols. St. Louis, 1993, Mosby.

8. Marshall P, Hamilton WG: Cuboid subluxation in ballet dancers, *Am J Sports Med* 20:169–175, 1992.

9. Ouzounian TJ, Myerson MS: Dislocation of the posterior tibial tendon, *Foot Ankle* 13:215–219, 1991.

10. Sammarco GA, ed: *Foot and ankle manual*, Philadelphia, 1991, Lea & Febiger.

11. Sarrafian S: *Anatomy of the foot and ankle: descriptive topographic, functional*, Philadelphia, 1993, JB Lippincott.

12. Thompson FM, Coughlin MJ: The high price of high fashion footwear, *J Bone Joint Surg* 76A:1586–1593, 1994.

13. Thompson FM, Hamilton WG: Problems of the second metatarsophalangeal joint, *Orthopedics* 10:83–89, 1987.

THE PEDIATRIC ATHLETE

CHAPTER 26

THE LOWER EXTREMITY

Peter G. Gerbino, II
Lyle J. Micheli

Primary care of the pediatric athlete can be a challenging endeavor. The pediatric population sustains many of the same injuries as adults and, in addition, is at risk for other types of injuries. Because of the physeal growth centers and the physiology of growth itself, many more and potentially serious injuries may occur in this population. The physes not only add diagnostic possibilities, they also make treatment more difficult because they must be protected. Conversely, children generally heal more quickly and more completely, which permits early, focused intervention and achieves better results.

Understanding the types of injury that can occur is the first step in effective management. We must then apply our knowledge of pertinent risk factors to arrive at a specific diagnosis. Treatment, rehabilitation, and prevention are only effective if the proper diagnosis has been made. In this chapter we will examine all these variables as they pertain to the lower extremity. Types of injuries, risk factors, diagnosis, treatment, rehabilitation, and prevention will be explored. In addition, three problems that can be particularly frustrating—acute knee effusion, patellofemoral pain, and shin splints—receive special attention. Management algorithms have been provided for these problems.

TYPES OF INJURY

Trauma

In the lower extremity, the athlete can sustain acute macrotrauma or repetitive microtrauma. Trauma can result in fractures, dislocations, muscle-tendon tears, ligament tears, and contusions. Fractures and dislocations can be fairly straightforward to manage, but certain of these, patella subluxation for example, can be more challenging to correct. In acute trauma, the greatest pitfall is failure to diagnose. We must remain vigilant in our treatment of subtle physeal injuries and internal derangements that frequently are misdiagnosed as contusions, sprains, or strains.

Overuse

All mechanical structures will eventually fail if loaded cyclically for a long enough period of time. The mechanical structures in the young athlete include bone, cartilage, muscles, tendons, and the specialized ligaments, cartilages, and bone of joints. Cyclic loading overuse leads to different problems in each of these structures. In many respects, thinking broadly about the tissue involved and its overuse risk factors will lead to more efficacious management than will affixing a syndrome name to the problem.

BONE. Cyclic loading of diaphyseal long bones will lead to stress or fatigue fracture. Bone follows well understood mechanical properties of anisotropic materials for crack propagation.[7] Before the fracture occurs, however, the bone undergoing such loads will respond metabolically. In response to Wolff's Law, the stressed bone thickens and strengthens.[22] When the ability of the bone to remodel is outpaced by the loading stresses, microfracture and inflammation occur.[7] Inflammation metabolites eventually cause pain, which is the only warning sign of an impending stress fracture. Ignoring or misdiagnosing this pain can result in a much longer recovery period than if addressed early. A young ballerina ignored pain under her left hallux for several weeks before she was suddenly no longer able to bear weight. Radiographs and Tc99m bone scan confirmed a medial sesamoid stress fracture and also showed increased uptake in both femurs, both tibiae, and both ankles (Fig. 26-1). Only the sesamoid had been painful.

JOINTS. Joints are special places where bone, articular cartilage, meniscal cartilage, ligaments, and joint fluid interact. Overuse in a joint can result in joint inflammation, effusion, pain, and eventually degeneration. Pain in a joint can originate at torn or irritated synovium, capsules, retinacula, or ligaments. Mechanical deformation from a torn labrum or meniscus, osteochondral fragment, or excess fluid can indirectly produce

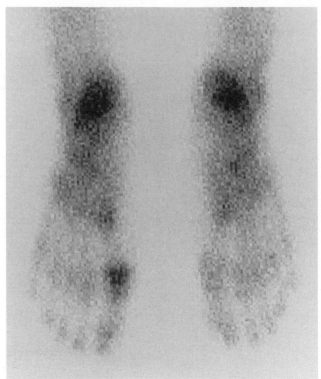
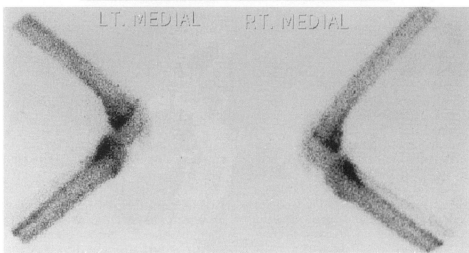

Fig. 26-1. Bone scan of an 18-year-old ballerina with painful stress fracture of the left medial sesamoid. The additional areas of increased uptake in both ankles, femurs, and tibiae were asymptomatic but mildly tender to palpation. In the presence of pain, each of these other areas would have been diagnosed as a stress fracture rather than a bone stress reaction.

pain. Finally, metabolic products from articular cartilage breakdown or synovitis may directly cause pain.[5]

GROWTH CARTILAGE. In addition to articular cartilage, there is physeal and apophyseal growth cartilage in the young athlete. Both of these growth cartilages are subject to overuse injury. Cyclic loading can lead to traction apophysitis, apophyseal disruption, or physeal fracture.

MUSCLE AND TENDONS. Supervised maximal use of muscles leads to hypertrophy and increased fiber size.[2] Unsupervised weight-training can lead to muscle tears and scarring.[14] Scarring can cause shortening and exacer-

bate the tightness that accompanies axial skeleton growth.

Tendons rarely become directly inflamed in children. More common is apophyseal injury or bursitis from excess friction. When muscles and tendons are overused, all risk factors for that injury must be identified and corrected.

RISK FACTORS

Epidemiologic studies of children's overuse injuries have identified several intrinsic and extrinsic risk factors (Table 26-1).[37]

Table 26-1. Risk factors associated with overuse injuries in the young athlete

Intrinsic	Extrinsic
Growth	Training or technique error
Anatomic malalignment	Improper footwear or gear
Muscle-tendon imbalance	Playing surface
Psychological factors	Nutrition
Associated disease state	Cultural deconditioning

Not sex (yet)

Intrinsic Growth

In children, growth and growth spurts are major risk factors for overuse injury of the lower extremity. As the axial skeleton grows, the soft tissues are passively stretched. In a growth spurt, this can cause pathological tightness and several types of overuse injury.

Anatomic Malalignment

In the lower extremity, anatomic malalignment can result in several types of injury. In a given child, a common malalignment such as pes planus or patella alta may never lead to pathology. In some athletes, however, these types of conditions can lead to relative overuse. For example, a young runner may be able to increase his or her mileage 10% per week normally. If the child has flat feet, 10% per week may be overuse and result in patellofemoral pain or another injury. A list of anatomic malalignments and some of their possible sequelae is provided in Table 26-2.

Muscle-Tendon Imbalance

Overdevelopment of one muscle group without development of its antagonists can result in overuse injury. An extremely common occurrence in young basketball players is patellofemoral pain and overuse exacerbated by tight, weak hamstrings. Stretching the hamstrings may be all that is needed to end the knee pain. Unfortunately, the recent trend to more single-sport athleticism[44] and the lack of cross-training results in more muscle-tendon imbalance problems.

Psychologic Factors

The mind-body interaction always has a role in illness. In trauma or overuse injury, this interplay may seem less, but not always. Reflex sympathetic dystrophy (RSD), especially around the knee, was virtually unknown in teenage athletes until several investigators began reporting this phenomenon, especially in young women.[16,41,49] As in adult RSD, early aggressive treatment with physical therapy and sympathetic blockade leads to better results. Surgical intervention may exacerbate the problem.

Associated Disease State

Genetic or developmental anomalies and diseases can alter risk for overuse injury. Osteochondritis dissecans, Legg-Calvé-Perthes disease, and slipped capital femoral epiphysis are examples of tissue injury resulting from activity that normally would not be overuse. Although it may be many years before these conditions are completely understood, it is helpful to think of them in terms of at-risk patients with suboptimal tissues.

Extrinsic Training or Technique Error

Training error is usually too much too soon of mileage, weight-lifting, etc. It can also be poor technique, such as running on only one side of the road, effectively duplicating leg length discrepancy. Increasing training 10% per week seems to be optimal for avoiding overuse injuries in an otherwise healthy child.[36]

Improper Footwear or Gear

The wrong running shoes can lead to foot, knee, hip, or back pain. Manufacturers work to improve impact absorption quality of shoes while decreasing their weight.[8] Similarly, the wrong gear for a given athlete can precipitate an overuse injury. For example, large adult-size soccer balls led to many lower extremity injuries in children, and we now have balls of several sizes and weights for different aged children.

Playing Surface

The hardness of the playing surface is causally related to early season shin splints and patellofemoral syndrome.[29] Traction qualities also factor into injury risk calculation. A comparison of natural grass to Astroturf showed significantly higher knee injury rates on the Astroturf.[43]

Table 26-2. Common anatomic malalignments and possible resulting sequelae from overuse

Malalignment	Injuries	Prevention
Increased femoral anteversion	Hip pain, knee pain, snapping hip	Stretching Activity modification
Leg length inequality	Unilateral shin splints, patellofemoral stress, back pain	Heel lift
Internal tibial torsion	Knee pain	Orthotics
Patellar maltracking	Patellofemoral stress, subluxation	Selective VMO strengthening
Patella alta	Patellofemoral stress, subluxation	Bracing, VMO strengthening
Pes planus	Knee pain	Orthotics

Nutrition

Intensive research to find performance enhancing nutrition is underway by manufacturers. More important, however, is the lack of certain nutrients that some children have or the radical dietary practices of other children. All children, but especially females, may be calcium, vitamin D, and iron deficient.[61] Wrestlers may severely restrict fluid intake to make weight and have been shown to develop morphological changes as a result.[55] Drug and substance abuse can be placed in this category as well. Use of diuretics or anabolic steroids may directly and indirectly increase risk for overuse injury.[59]

Cultural Deconditioning

Twenty years ago, children engaged in free-play (usually out-of-doors) when they were not at school. Now that time is increasingly occupied with sedentary watching of television and playing with computers and video games.[45] Pediatric obesity is increasing.[23] These factors create "weekend warriors" of children with all the overuse injuries formerly seen only in their parents.

SPECIFIC LOWER EXTREMITY INJURIES

Hip and Pelvis

Acute trauma about the hip and pelvis in the young athlete is common. Most injuries are contusions and minor muscle strains, but more serious injuries can occur. The most common of these is apophysis avulsion. This can easily be confused with a muscle strain but tends to resolve more slowly. Specific avulsions include sartorius pull-off at the anterosuperior iliac spine or rectus femoris avulsion at the anteroinferior iliac spine. The iliopsoas tendon may avulse the lesser trochanter, and the abdominal obliques may avulse their insertion on the ilium. All will occur as a result of a sudden force and are tender to palpation at the apophysis. Radiographs will show a widened apophyseal clear space and possibly soft tissue swelling. Iliopsoas avulsion may result in extensive swelling and ecchymosis of the medial thigh.

Treatment is rest, application of ice, and gentle stretching of the involved muscles until resolution of symptoms in 4 to 6 weeks. Rarely will operative repair be required. Rehabilitation involves continued stretching of the involved muscles and, most important, stretching of the antagonist muscles. Prevention requires adequate warm-up and stretching and identifying at-risk athletes. These are children in a growth spurt with generalized lower extremity tightness.

Hip and pelvis fractures and dislocations occasionally occur. These require stabilization and transport to a trauma center for emergent care by the orthopedic traumatologist.

Overuse injuries about the hip and pelvis are also common. Any of the sites of traumatic apophyseal avulsions may present as a chronic apophysitis. Diagnosis is similar to that of the avulsion, except that the radiographs may be normal. If necessary, a Te99 bone scan may be done and comparison made to the contralateral apophysis for relative increased uptake on the injured side. Treatment, rehabilitation, and prevention are similar to that for avulsions.

Tendinitis and bursitis occur about the hip. A snapping hip may be caused by the iliopsoas tendon, rectus femoris, or fascia lata. Trochanteric bursitis and snapping fascia lata may be the result of tight adductors and relative overuse of the abductors. Stretching the adductors and fascia lata in combination with taking anti-inflammatories may be effective, but corticosteroid injection of the trochanteric bursa may be necessary. Refractory cases may require surgical release.

Snapping psoas and rectus femoris tendons typically occur with hip flexion and external rotation maneuvers. The risk factors seem to be tight posterior capsule and lax anterior hip capsule. Primary treatment is rest and stretching of the psoas, quadriceps, hamstrings, and posterior hip capsule. Corticosteroid injection of the tendon sheath may be successful, but tendon recession or release may be necessary.

Stress fracture of the femoral neck occurs in young runners. Inguinal pain that persists warrants further investigation. Bone scan may be necessary to confirm the diagnosis. Treatment consists of decreasing activities until symptoms resolve and slowly returning to activities.

Slipped capital femoral epiphysis occurs most commonly in preadolescent boys that tend to be overweight and during a growth spurt. Evidence exists that this phy-

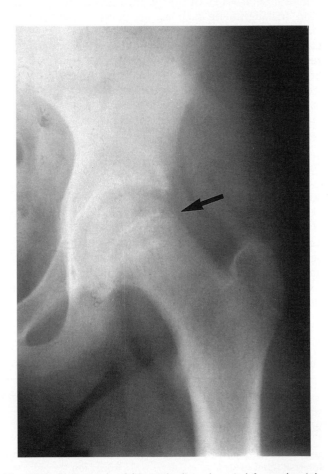

Fig. 26-2. Radiograph of hip with slipped capital femoral epiphysis. The range of injury is from pre-slip (physeal injury without epiphyseal movement) to mild (⅓ head diameter slip), moderate (⅓ to ½ diameter slip), to severe (greater than ½ diameter slip). This would be graded as mild.

seal stress fracture occurs as a result of several factors including genetic predisposition, hormonal influence, and orientation of the physis itself.[32] A large acute slip will be apparent on plain radiographs. Plain films will be negative in a preslip. Fig. 26-2 shows the different grades of slip, from preslip to severe. Bone scan may show increased uptake compared with the contralateral physis. MRI may show fluid changes about the physis.[56] Treatment depends upon the extent of the problem. Because of the consequences of a displaced physeal fracture, aggressive treatment is warranted. The child should be placed on crutches, and if the diagnosis is confirmed, hospitalization and transphyseal fixation is required. The contralateral hip should be thoroughly investigated because there is a 15% to 30% incidence of bilaterality.[32]

Legg-Calvé-Perthes disease results in avascular necrosis of portions of the femoral head. Fig. 26-3 shows the radiographs of the progression of head necrosis. If diagnosed early and treated with decreased weightbearing, the head will reconstitute without serious sequelae.[42] Risk factors include low birth weight, male sex, and certain socioeconomic backgrounds.[33] Athletic participation is not necessary for the condition to occur. In a predisposed individual, however, athletic activity may amplify the problem.

Thigh and Femur

Acute trauma to the thigh will result in contusion, muscle tears, or femur fracture. Contusions are treated with rest, ice, compression, and elevation (RICE), and one must ensure that myositis ossifans does not develop. There is some evidence that oral nonsteroidal anti-inflammatories (NSAIDs) may help decrease myositis ossificans formation if given after 2 to 3 days of icing.[60]

Muscle strains (tears) occur with both concentric and eccentric muscle loading. Both the electrophysiological status of the muscle (e.g., amount of preexercise stretching) and the rate of muscle fiber loading appear to be causally related to these injuries. After RICE treatment, gentle stretching to maintain flexibility during healing is required. Full recovery can be expected in 4 to 6 weeks.

Overuse injury in the thigh is limited to occasional femur stress fractures. These can occur in runners, ballerinas, and other young athletes who place repetitive demands upon their lower extremities. Modifying the inciting activity will result in resolution of symptoms in a matter of weeks. Stretching the hamstrings and quadriceps may prevent recurrence. Water therapy has been extremely helpful in keeping these athletes in condition while allowing the stress fracture to heal.[30] It is essential to avoid dismissing inguinal or thigh pain as "growing pains."

Knee

The knee sustains more injuries than any other joint. It is useful to think of the knee in terms of its three articulating regions: the patellofemoral joint, the medial compartment, and the lateral compartment. Severe trauma can produce fracture of the femur, patella, or tibia, and may even cause dislocation of the tibia from the femur, a

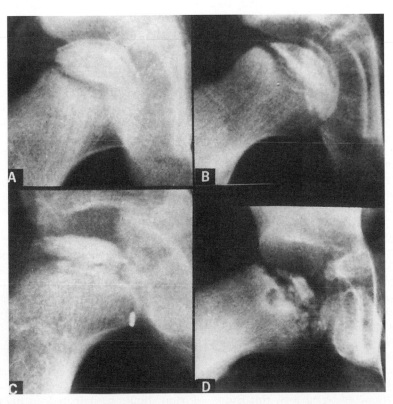

Fig. 26-3. Radiographs of the progression of necrosis in Legg-Calvés-Perthes disease. The final stage **(D)** is fragmentation of the epiphysis with incongruity of the joint.

condition requiring thorough assessment of anterial patency after reduction. These topics are beyond the scope of this chapter, and the reader is directed to any of the standard orthopedic fracture texts for additional information. All require urgent (or in the case of dislocation-emergent) orthopedic consultation.

Trauma may also result in patella dislocation, ligament injuries, meniscal tears, and osteochondral fracture. Acute knee trauma in a young athlete is a frequent occurrence, and primary care clinicians caring for these athletes should be comfortable in its management. A diagnosis of "knee sprain" in a young athlete does not address the specific injury and may delay or circumvent appropriate care.

HISTORY. In the vast majority of knee injuries, the history alone will lead to the correct diagnosis. An athlete with a twisting injury to the knee resulting in a "pop" with rapid swelling and inability to continue playing has most likely torn the anterior cruciate ligament (ACL). We know that there is a high incidence of meniscal tear associated with ACL tear,[3] and so this tearing should be sought. This same type of injury without a distinctive "pop" or with more gradual swelling may be the result of a partial ACL tear or simply a meniscal tear.

Nonpainful giving way commonly indicates ACL laxity. Painful giving way may indicate patella subluxation. Locking of the knee, defined as inability to fully extend the joint, is caused by mechanical obstruction. Effusion may limit the final 10° of extension because of discomfort, but a torn meniscus flap, osteochondral fragment, or ACL stump may lock the knee at 30° or 40° of flexion. An acutely locked knee requires urgent referral to the sports medicine orthopedist. This type of internal derangement can only be managed operatively. Forcing the knee into extension (such as would occur by use of a knee immobilizer) can extend a meniscal tear or produce articular cartilage damage. A posterior splint with the knee in a comfortable position is far safer.

A pure varus or valgus stress may result in lateral or medial collateral ligament tear. These injuries may be isolated or occur with meniscus, cruciate, or osteochondral injury. A direct trauma to the knee followed by a "pop" and then another "pop" should be suspect for patellar dislocation and reduction. Before beginning the physical exam, the history should have led the examiner to be searching for patellofemoral, cruciate ligament, meniscal, and/or collateral ligament pathology.

PHYSICAL EXAMINATION. Much can be gained by simple inspection of the injured knee. The contralateral knee is almost always available for comparison. A large effusion will not be overlooked, but a small effusion might. A subtle fullness on either side of the injured-side patellar tendon might be the only finding. If the patient holds his knee in a position of flexion, this may indicate effusion or a locked knee.

Examination of the knee with posttraumatic effusion in a young athlete is directed by the history. If ACL tear is suspected, the ACL patency is examined last, as guarding may prevent further examination. Similarly, if patellofemoral injury is suspected by history, this is examined last to minimize pain. Whatever order of examination is chosen, the patellofemoral mechanism, medial structures, lateral structures, and cruciates need to be individually assessed.

An acute, posttraumatic effusion is always presumed to be hemarthrosis. Hemarthrosis may be caused by ligament tear, peripheral meniscus tear, patellar retinaculum tear, or fracture. Of these, only collateral ligament tears are usually treated nonoperatively. All other sources of acute hemarthrosis require consideration of surgical intervention and should be referred to a sports medicine orthopaedist within 48 hours. Some confusion exists regarding the differentiation between effusion and edema. Effusion is always symmetric, versus edema, which is more superficial and focal. Edema may be caused by contusion, collateral ligament tears, bursitis, local infection, or other focal conditions. Traumatic effusion is caused by internal derangement. Range of motion, varus and valgus laxity at 30° of flexion, and Lachman's or 30° anterior drawer tests should be performed. Joint line tenderness may be the only indicator of meniscal tear. McMurray's test[34] will be positive for large tears but may be negative for smaller ones. Internal and external tibial rotation with the knee in full flexion stresses the posterior meniscal horns and can aid with meniscal tear diagnosis. The pivot shift[18] assesses the ACL and posterolateral capsule. Tests for the PCL include the sag,[9] reverse drawer,[9] and quad active test.[11] All these tests are the same in children as in adults and are performed similarly. If the effusion prevents one or more tests, aspiration with or without lidocaine injection can be performed.

Required radiographs are the same as for an adult. Anteroposterior, lateral, tunnel, and skyline views demonstrate all compartments and bony structures. A tibial eminence avulsion is an ACL tear equivalent and will be seen best on the tunnel view.[35] A lateral capsular sign (Segond fracture) indicates ACL tear.[25]

A strong case can be made for obtaining radiographs in a child before the detailed ligamentous exam is performed. A tibial eminence fracture may be nondisplaced until a Lachman's or pivot shift test displaces it. A knee may be locked because of a displaced osteochondral fracture fragment making range of motion testing contraindicated. For these same reasons, care must be taken when ordering radiographs for a locked knee. The technologist may try to force the knee into full extension to obtain a standard AP. Instructions should be given to the technician specifying what positions are possible with the particular knee. Fig. 26-4 provides an algorithm for assessment of posttraumatic effusion. Note that MRI is not mandatory and is used to solve diagnostic dilemmas. A primary care provider who has diagnosed an acute traumatic effusion has ample evidence of internal derangement by the effusion alone to obtain orthopaedic consultation. The surgeon may or may not require MRI to classify the injury.

Physical examination of the patellofemoral mechanism requires assessing each portion of the mechanism (Fig. 26-5). As in the adult, the quadriceps tendon, patella, medial and lateral retinaculae, and patellar tendon should be palpated. In the child, the tibial tubercle apophysis and distal pole of the patella should also be

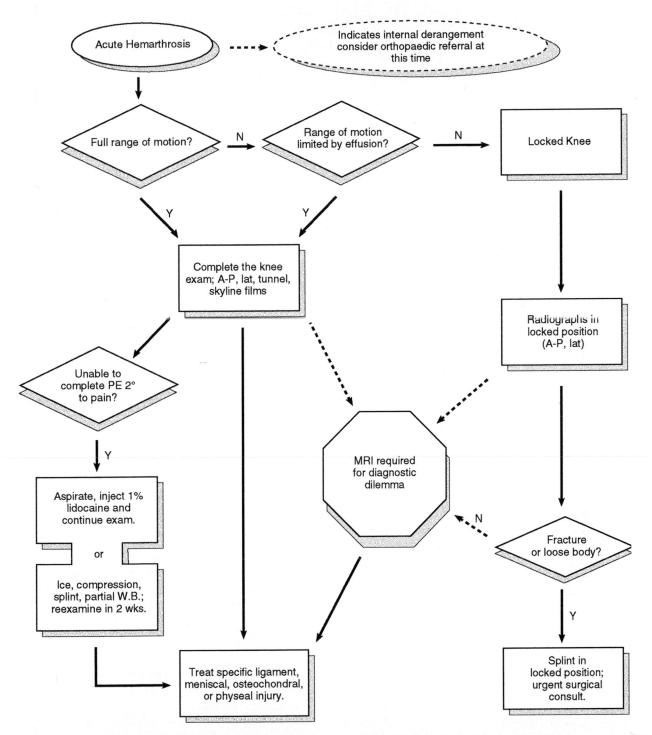

Fig. 26-4. Algorithm for management of a traumatic effusion of the knee. Traumatic effusion is always presumed to be hemarthrosis, indicating internal derangement and requiring surgical consideration.

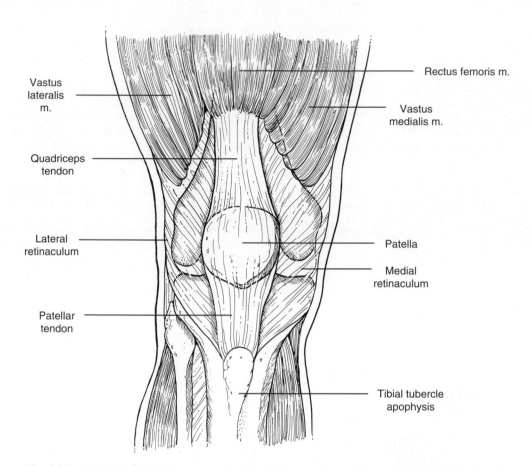

Fig. 26-5. Anatomy of the extensor mechanism. Each component of the system is evaluated for its contribution to patellofemoral pain or dysfunction.

assessed. Dynamic tracking of the patella is evaluated. Hemarthrosis with a medial retinacular defect and pain indicates patella subluxation or dislocation. An acutely enlarged, painful tibial tubercle may indicate avulsion fracture.

TREATMENT. Locked knee, for whatever reason, is referred to the sports medicine orthopaedist for prompt operative treatment. Non-weight-bearing in a posterior splint with the knee in its locked position is appropriate. The nonsteroidal anti-inflammatory may prolong bleeding and swelling and so is not a good option for initial pain relief.

An acute effusion also warrants orthopaedic evaluation. As the effusion resolves over several weeks, the quadriceps muscles atrophy, altering the patellofemoral mechanics and making rehabilitation more difficult. Meniscal tears almost always require arthroscopic treatment. A reparable meniscus may become irreparable if the child further damages the torn portion during the delay. ACL tears may or may not require reconstruction, but they always require thorough evaluation and rehabilitation. A free osteochondral fragment must be replaced or removed promptly to avoid further chondral injury.

Patella dislocation, tibial tubercle avulsion, and tibial eminence avulsions may or may not require surgical intervention. Treatment recommendations are constantly evolving and depend upon several variables.[19,24,28,35] All require orthopedic evaluation.

Rehabilitation after traumatic knee injury is quite spe-cific depending upon the injury. This field is also constantly evolving, and in the past 10 years we have seen ACL reconstruction rehabilitation change dramatically. It was once felt that 6 weeks of immobilization in flexion and 1 year of physical therapy was required to achieve optimal results.[46] Now most surgeons utilize immediate postoperative continuous passive motion and full activities within 6 to 9 months.[47]

Prevention is yet another area in which exciting progress has been made. Several studies have now clearly demonstrated that prophylactic knee bracing does not affect ACL injury rates.[6] This has resulted in considerable cost saving to youth sports teams. Recent and ongoing research into the variables which may predispose certain athletes to ACL tears is generating hypotheses which may aid in preventing some of these injuries.[52,53]

OVERUSE KNEE INJURIES. Overuse injuries about the knee in the young athlete usually result in extensor mechanism problems. The single other entity which may be regarded as an overuse injury in this age group is osteochondritis dissecans.

Osteochondritis Dissecans. By definition, osteo-chondritis dissecans (OCD) is an osteochondral lesion of unknown etiology that may or may not result in knee pain. It is most commonly found on the medial femoral condyle weightbearing surface but may also be found on the lateral femoral condyle. A vascular insult to a portion of the condyle leads to avascular necrosis, possible fracture along the line of necrosis, and possible separation of the fragment.[20] Early in the process there is no pain or point tenderness, and radiographs of the knee or knees may only show a mottled appearance of the condyle, which indicates increased vascularity. Continued running and jumping can lead to the avascular lesion that may or may not separate from the femur (Fig. 26-6). MRI shows more detail (Fig. 26-7).

Treatment depends upon the stage of disease. If there is not a discrete lesion on imaging studies, simple rest will relieve symptoms and eventually result in normal condyle architecture. Achieving relative rest in this population may be difficult and require casting in extension simply to slow down the child. Focal lesions may require immobilization in extension or arthroscopic drilling if stable. Displaced or loose fragments require internal fixation with pins or screws. All efforts should be made to restore normal condylar architecture, and even long-standing free fragments can be successfully replaced in the young athlete, although they may have to be reshaped to fit the original defect.

Extensor Mechanism. Overuse injuries to the exten-

sor mechanism can occur anywhere from the quadriceps to the tibial tubercle. Two force vectors are responsible for virtually all extensor mechanism problems. The first is the anteroposterior (AP) joint force. This force is proportional to the forces generated by the quadriceps muscles. These forces can be concentric, as in a jump, or eccentric, as in deceleration following a jump when landing. Tight hamstrings and/or quadriceps, such as typically occur during the growth spurts, exacerbate the problem. The cyclic loading of running, jumping, and other vigorous knee extension can lead to partial tendon avulsion at the distal pole of the patella (Sinding-Larsen-Johansson syndrome) (Fig. 26-8) or at the tibial tubercle (Osgood-Schlatter's disease) (Fig. 26-9). The patellar tendon itself may become inflamed or painful on rare occasions.

More difficult to diagnose and treat is peripatellar pain from AP force overload. The source of pain in this condition has remained elusive but is felt to be the medial and lateral patellar retinaculi and possibly the patellar subchondral bone itself.[12,17] The history will reveal pain with stair-climbing, after prolonged sitting, or after sports activities. Rarely is there pain during the activity.

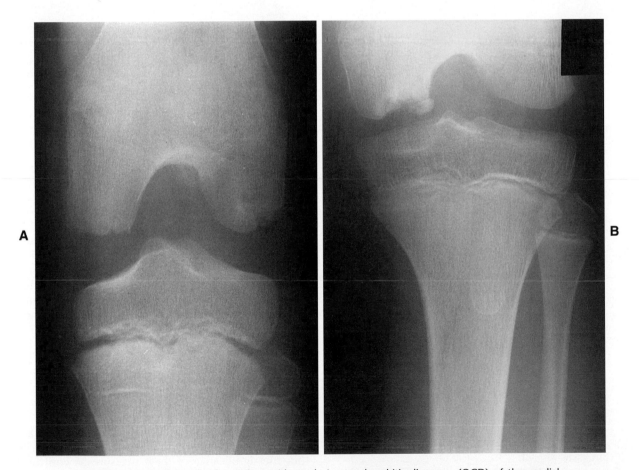

Fig. 26-6. A, Radiograph of a patient with grade I osteochondritis dissecans (OCD) of the medial femoral condyle and grade II OCD of the lateral condyle. The appearance of the medial condyle can be associated with an asymptomatic as well as exquisitely tender knee. The process is felt to be localized osteomalacia from stress-induced hypervascularity. When the process becomes painful, subchondral microfractures are felt to have occurred. The lateral condyle with grade II OCD shows the avascular region. No displacement of the fragment is present. **B,** Grade III OCD with displacement of the osteochondral fragment.

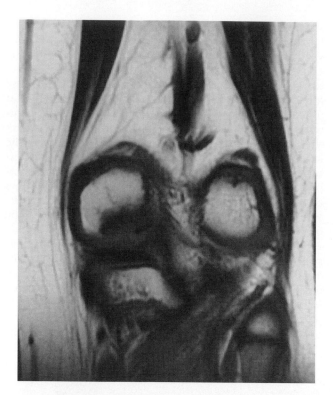

Fig. 26-7. Magnetic resonance image of the grade III OCD in **Fig. 26-4B** showing extensive edema or hypervascularity in the bone surrounding the areas of the defect.

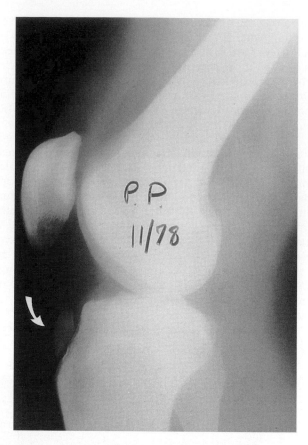

Fig. 26-9. Osgood-Schlatter's apophysitis tibial tubercle. Note apophyseal widening and tubercle enlargement.

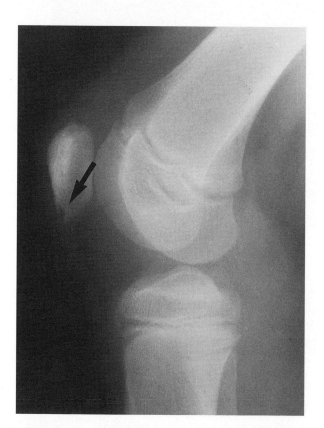

Fig. 26-8. Sinding-Larsen-Johansson apophysitis of the distal pole of the patella.

Instead of point tenderness at the tendon or its insertion, there is diffuse tenderness along one or both sides of the patella and increased symptoms with the patella apprehension test[15] or with AP loading of the patella.

A second force vector that frequently leads to patellofemoral pain is excessive lateral pull of the quadriceps as opposed to medial pull. The more severe cases of lateral tracking will lead to recurrent subluxation or dislocation of the patella. The history may be similar to AP overload, but physical exam will demonstrate more lateral retinacular tenderness and will usually demonstrate lateral tracking and decreased patella mobility. If there is also medial retinaculum tenderness, care should be taken to check for a painful medial plica palpable as a tender medial band on flexion-extension. Excessive lateral tracking may pull a previously normal plica into the medial femoral condyle, causing thickening and eventually fibrosis and inflammation.

A large quadriceps or Q-angle and varus-valgus anomalies of the knee may influence patellofemoral stresses, but the significance of these measures is controversial.[15] Evidence of excessive lateral compression may be demonstrated on the skyline view radiograph, but these films are difficult to standardize in a nonresearch setting and, at best, give a static view of a dynamic problem.[13] The box on p. 423 lists risk factors associated with both types of patellofemoral stress overload.

RISK FACTORS ASSOCIATED WITH EXTENSOR MECHANISM PAIN FROM ANTEROPOSTERIOR AND LATERAL FORCE OVERLOAD

Normal alignment with excessive joint reaction forces
Extrinsic
   Traning error

   Hard playing surface

   Poor footwear

Intrinsic
   Anatomic malalignment (patella alta or infera)

   Muscle-tendon imbalance (tight hamstrings and/or quadriceps)

Laterally tracking patella
Extrinsic
   Training error ("whip kick" associated with breast stroke)

Intrinsic
   Muscle-tendon imbalance (overdeveloped lateral quads or underdeveloped vastus medialis obliquus)

   Anatomic malalignment (internal tibial torsion, genu valgum, increased Q-angle, pes planus)

Of special interest is patella alta, a growth spurt-related phenomenon in which the patellar tendon portion of the extensor mechanism elongates more than the quadriceps tendon portion. This leaves the patella higher in the femoral sulcus with increased distal pole compressive forces and greater risk for lateral subluxation in extension. Patella alta is a condition that can exacerbate both AP and lateral patellofemoral stress overload.

Treatment of patellofemoral stress syndrome is based upon the specific etiology. With normal tracking and AP overload, emphasis is on hamstring stretching, quad stretching, and decreased running, jumping, and stair-climbing. Symptoms should resolve over several weeks. For lateral tracking, AP forces can be decreased, but emphasis is on selective vastus medialis obliquus strengthening to dynamically pull the patella medially.[40] Braces which centralize the patella are sometimes helpful.[48] Bands which alter the fulcrum of the patellofemoral mechanism may help.[31]

Despite adequate physical therapy and bracing, it is not always possible to relieve symptoms in a laterally tracking patella. Arthroscopic lateral retinacular release may be necessary to achieve balanced, centralized tracking.[38] For more severe tracking problems or recurrent subluxation or dislocations, lateral release is combined with medial reefing and possible tibial tubercle repositioning.[10] In any of these procedures, the goal is to visualize corrected, centralized tracking during the operation. If true chondromalacia of the retropatellar surface

has already developed, it may not be possible to restore the knee to a totally pain-free status.

Other extensor mechanism problems include isolated medial plica syndrome, usually caused by a direct medial blow,[27] and the apophysitises Sinding-Larsen-Johansson syndrome and Osgood-Schlatter's disease. Apophysitis is treated precisely the same as normal tracking patellar overload with hamstring and quadriceps stretching, local application of ice acutely and then heat subsequently, and relative rest of the mechanism to restore the pain-free state. As in osteochondritis dissecans, it is occasionally necessary to immobilize overactive youngsters in a cylinder cast to achieve relative rest.

A blow to the medial knee may produce inflammation and tenderness in a previously normal medial plica. Examination may elicit a tender focal band of tissue snapping over the medial femoral condyle during knee flexion-extension. If this does not resolve with massage and oral anti-inflammatories, arthroscopic debridement is necessary. Occasionally corticosteroid injection into the thickened plica tissue may be effective. An algorithm for evaluation and treatment of patellofemoral pain is presented in Fig. 26-10. Repeat examinations may be necessary to fully understand the particular risk factors and etiology.

Other Knee Overuse Problems. When the quadriceps are tight relative to the hamstrings and there is selective adductor or abductor overuse, pes anserinrus or iliotibial band bursitis may occur. The pes attachment on the anterior medial tibia is tender to palpation, and there may be palpable fluctuance of the underlying bursa. Similarly, the iliotibial band may be tender laterally, and pain may be exacerbated by adduction stretching of the lateral thigh soft tissues.

Treatment for either condition consists of oral anti-inflammatories, postexercise ice massage, and gentle passive stretching of the affected structures as well as the antagonist structures. Any relative muscle strength or tightness imbalance should be corrected. Other identified risk factors need to be eliminated or modified. If symptoms persist, the bursa can be injected with a corticosteroid.

Lower Leg

Acute trauma to the leg usually results in contusion but occasionally will cause fracture. Contusions are treated with rest, ice, compression, and elevation for the first 48 to 72 hours. NSAIDs may decrease the incidence of myositis ossificans, but starting them immediately may prolong bleeding and increase swelling.

Tibial fractures in children rarely require surgical management. Physeal injury must be considered, and if a non-displaced Salter-Harris Type I physeal fracture is suspected (point tenderness at the physis and a normal x-ray), it is better to treat it aggressively with casting until the pain resolves. The low energy type of tibial fracture that young athletes sustain are readily treated with casting and subsequent rehabilitation. All fractures should be referred to the orthopaedist. Any acute trauma can result in excessive swelling to the point where venous outflow is blocked. This condition is tibial com-

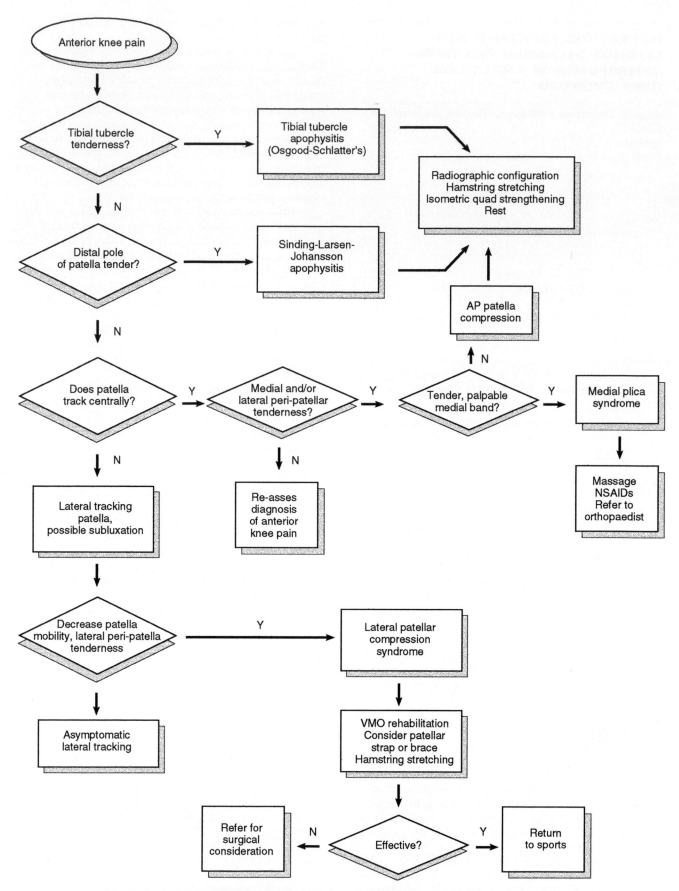

Fig. 26-10. Algorithm for evaluation and management of knee extensor mechanism pain. Focused treatment based on specific etiology will prevent recurrence.

partment syndrome and must be arrested immediately before tissue necrosis occurs. Any posttraumatic extremity that is swollen and elicits *pain to passive motion of,* for example, a toe, should be immediately referred to compartment syndrome evaluation of the classic five Ps: pain, pallor, paresthesias, pulselessness, and paralysis. Only pain is present before permanent damage has occurred.

Overuse injuries of the leg have been collectively referred to as "shin splints" and are actually one of three types of injury. Lower leg pain may be caused by periostitis, stress fracture, or diffuse compartment swelling. Distinguishing among these conditions is an important skill and requires precise history, physical examination, and imaging studies.

A young athlete with leg pain brought on by exercise should be questioned about the nature of the pain. The pain of exertional compartment syndrome is debilitating pain that intensifies as the workout progresses. The pain usually dissipates over several minutes after cessation of activity. Stress fractures and periostitis tend to cause pain continuously during the activity. Symptoms may intensify over a period of days to weeks, but not usually within an exercise period. Discriminating between stress fracture and periostitis is more difficult, especially since periostitis frequently precedes a stress fracture. Fibular point tenderness is usually a stress fracture or impending stress fracture. Tibia pain may be focal or diffuse and may occur medially or laterally. Focal pain is more likely to be stress fracture, diffuse pain periostitis. Indirect, three-point bending forces applied to the tibia may increase stress fracture pain but should not increase periostitis symptoms. Young runners classically develop a stress fracture of the distal fibula just proximal to the ankle syndesmosis after increasing their mileage.[57] Lateral tibial periostitis arises from tibialis anterior overuse, and medial periostitis from tibialis posterior (predominantly) overuse.[54]

Resisted ankle dorsiflexion exacerbates lateral tibial periostitis, and resisted pronation and eversion exacerbates medial tibial periostitis. A tight Achilles tendon and strong gastrocsoleus muscles frequently accompany lateral tibial periostitis. Imaging studies for tibial periostitis and stress fractures begin with plain radiographs. Early on, these will be normal, but after 3 or more weeks, diffuse (periostitis) or focal (stress fracture) periosteal reaction may be present. It may be necessary to obtain imaging confirmation of either diagnosis. Some children (or their parents) will be non-compliant without hard evidence, and treatment will vary depending on the precise etiology. A Te99 bone scan will show focal uptake for stress fracture, whereas in periostitis there is diffuse activity (Fig. 26-11). MRI has shown fluid changes associated with both conditions in different patterns.[54] If the sensitivity and specificity of MRI are eventually found to be comparable to bone scan, this may become the diagnostic tool of choice.

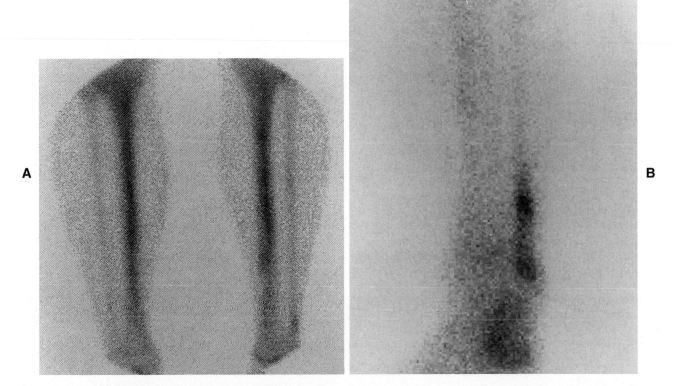

Fig. 26-11. A, Periostitis of both tibiae in a runner. Isotope uptake is all among anterior tibiae, as is tenderness. **B,** Fibular stress fracture showing focal uptake by Tc99m bone scan. Indirect force on fibula elicits pain.

Relative rest is employed for the treatment of periostitis and stress fractures. Stress fractures will usually heal following 4 to 6 weeks of painless ambulation. Casting is not necessary unless an overt fracture occurs or the child cannot be rested any other way. Once again, NSAIDs may not be optimal pain relievers for stress fractures because their antiprostaglandin effects theoretically slow bone healing. Once pain and point tenderness have resolved, the child can progress as tolerated to his or her activities. Training error is the most common risk factor for stress fracture, and applying the "10% increase per week" limit on training should prevent recurrence.

In addition to relative rest, periostitis requires identification of risk factors and specific physical therapy. Lateral tibial periostitis is exacerbated by running hills or stairs, by a tight Achilles tendon, or by other situations requiring overuse of the tibialis anterior for ankle dorsiflexion. Likewise, poor running shoes, concrete surfaces, and activities demanding more shock absorption from pronation will overstress the tibialis posterior. These risk factors can be the major cause of medial tibial periostitis. Stretching the gastrocsoleus complex, avoiding repetitive dorsiflexion, and ice massage after activity will aid healing of lateral symptoms. Orthotics help with medial periostitis. Surgery is never indicated for these conditions.

If exertional compartment syndrome is suspected, an exercise stress test is done by having the patient exercise until symptoms occur. The anterior, lateral, posterior, deep posterior, and posterior tibial compartments are palpated for tenderness. Objective tests require taking compartment pressure measurements at rest and at 1 and 2 minutes after exercise. A compartment pressure 30 to 40 mmHg above resting pressure at 1 minute after exercise is abnormal.[1]

A condition that presents similarly to exertional compartment syndrome is muscle hernia through a fascial defect in the leg. A fascial defect may be palpable, and compartment pressures may be elevated after exercise.

Both exertional compartment syndrome and fascial hernia are treated the same. Conservative attempts can be made at deep myofascial massage and slow increase of running distance to avoid the painful threshold. If these treatments fail, and they frequently do, the fascia must be released. In contrast with posttraumatic compartment syndrome, the skin does not have to be widely incised and left open. Only the affected compartments need to be released, and early return to activities is necessary to avoid "bridging" scar formation along the line of release. Operative release is rarely necessary in children and is only done after a positive compartment stress test.

Most fascia hernias are felt to result from high compartment pressures, so closure of the defect will exacerbate the problem. Occasionally, a traumatic fascial defect can be repaired without resulting in exertional compartment syndrome, but this is risky. Full release as in exertional compartment syndrome is typically required. An algorithm for diagnosis and management of shin splints is presented in Fig. 26-12.

Foot and Ankle

Trauma to the juvenile athlete about the foot and ankle can cause fracture, dislocation, physeal injury, or ligament sprains. The common inversion ankle injury which causes anterior talofibular ligament tears in the adult commonly results in a nondisplaced Salter-Harris Type I physeal fracture of the distal fibula in the immature athlete. Radiographs are normal. Physical examination elicits tenderness at the distal fibula and possibly also to the lateral ligaments. Experimental work is being done with MRI to identify these injuries,[51] but at present the diagnosis remains a clinical one. In an inversion ankle sprain of any magnitude, the distal fibula itself should not be tender. If it is, physeal fracture must be presumed and treated with 3 weeks of casting with partial weightbearing. If at 3 weeks the tenderness is gone, physical therapy may be begun to restore motion, peroneal strength, and ankle proprioception. If symptoms persist, further casting is required. Follow-up radiographs may be necessary at 3 to 6 month intervals to watch for premature physeal closure.

Routine ankle sprains are treated as adult injuries with the RICE routine initially, followed as quickly as possible (within days) with weightbearing as tolerated. A stirrup Aircast (Summit, New Jersey) splint is helpful in restoring crutch-free ambulation within 1 to 2 weeks. Physical therapy is also begun immediately, and full competition is permitted once symmetrical proprioception and balance have returned. Prophylactic taping does have a place in competition and during the recuperation period.[21]

One possible complication of ankle sprain is chondral or osteochondral injury of the talar dome. This usually occurs on the anterolateral corner or centromedial ridge of the dome. The youngster may complain of ankle sprain that never resolves or may not ever recall a sprain. Physical examination will elicit point tenderness on the talar dome anterolaterally with the foot in plantarflexion, or there may be anterior or posterior tenderness medially on the dome. Radiographs will be normal or show a small osteochondral injury to either corner (Fig. 26-13). MRI will show much more extensive damage to the talus (Fig. 26-14). Treatment is by arthroscopic debridement and drilling. Occasionally, a fragment will be large enough to repair, but this is unusual. A medial injury frequently requires a small posterior arthrotomy to excise the symptomatic chondral flap. Despite this treatment, permanent ankle pain can result.

An ankle sprain that is slow to heal may also be what the trainers call a "high" ankle sprain. This is a tear of the anterior tibiofibular syndesmosis ligament and can take 8 to 12 weeks or longer to resolve. Tenderness is found at the area of syndesmosis just proximal to the ankle joint, and mediolateral compression of the leg above the ankle will be painful. If widening of the syndesmosis is seen on the mortise view of the ankle, AP and lateral views of the entire leg must be obtained to rule out a proximal fibular fracture (Maisonneuve's fracture) (Fig. 26-15). Complete syndesmosis disruptions require operative repair with transmalleolar screw fixation. Partial tears require up to 12 weeks of immobilization and protected weight training.

Management of fractures about the ankle requires de-

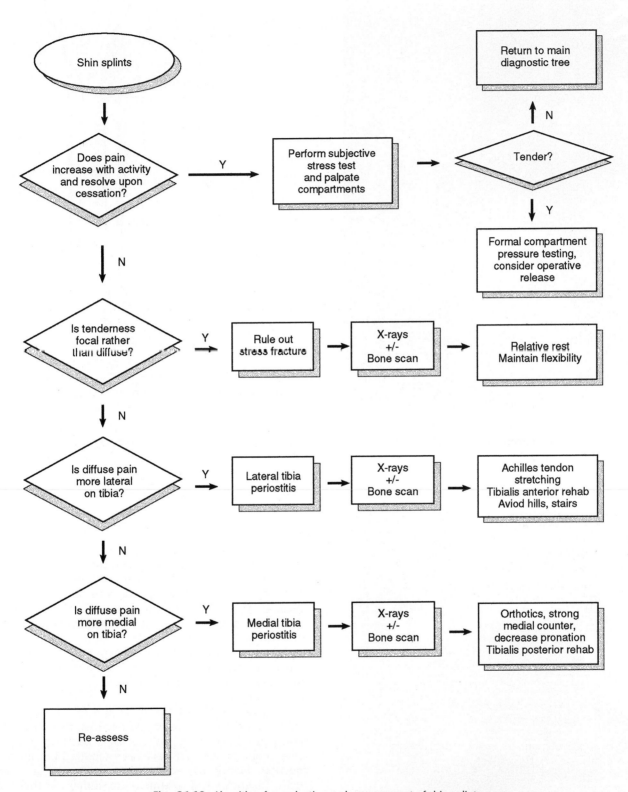

Fig. 26-12. Algorithm for evaluation and management of shin splints.

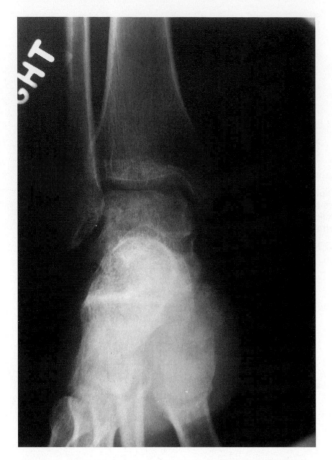

Fig. 26-13. Osteochondral injury to the medial talar dome in an adult. Note the disuse osteopenia that resulted from prolonged immobilization.

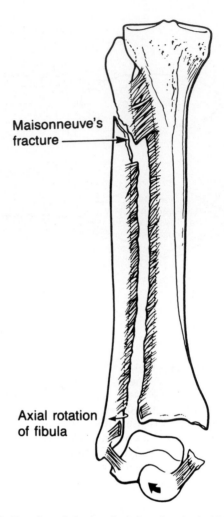

Fig. 26-15. Drawing of the leg depicting the classic Maisonneuve proximal fibula fracture and its mechanism of injury.

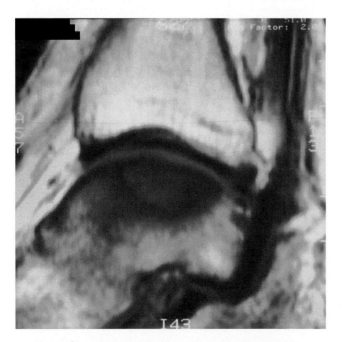

Fig. 26-14. MRI of a talar dome osteochondritis dissecans lesion.

tailed knowledge of the bony and soft tissue anatomy. A fracture may appear relatively innocuous on radiographs but may have interposed periosteum preventing proper healing. Medial malleolus and juvenile Tillaux fractures are such examples.[4] Both usually require open reduction and internal fixation.

In the foot, eversion trauma may cause fracture of the navicular apophysis leading to painful accessory navicular. These may heal and become nontender or can require excision.

Overuse injuries in the ankle and foot include stress fracture, apophysitis, avascular necrosis, plantar fasciitis, and painful accessory ossicle. Stress fractures of almost every bone of the foot have been reported but most frequently include the sesamoids, metatarsals, and calcaneus. Diagnosis and treatment are similar to other lower extremity stress fractures. Prevention entails identifying and eliminating risk factors.

As in the knee, muscle-tendon overuse in the child produces apophysitis rather than tendinitis. Most com-

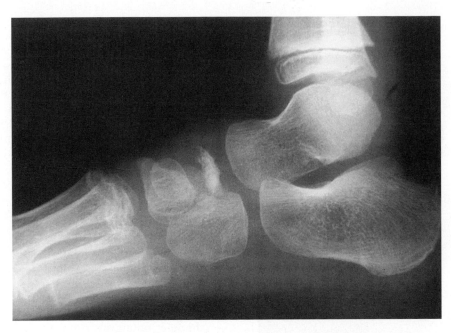

Fig. 26-16. Köhler's avascular necrosis of the tarsal navicular.

mon is Achilles tendon apophysitis at the calcaneal insertion, or Sever's disease. This is felt to be a stress injury to the physis caused by overpull of a tight, strong triceps surae. Avoiding running and jumping will resolve pain and, over time, radiographs will show resolution of the increased opacification of apophysis.

Pain, point tenderness, and opacification of the tarsal navicular are the hallmarks of Köhler's bone disease. Radiographs show opacification and collapse of the navicular (Fig. 26-16) and MRI shows changes consistent with avascular necrosis (AVN). The condition is felt to occur from overuse in predisposed individuals. Even when there is collapse of the navicular, virtually all resolve over eight months with rest of the foot. Casting for 12 weeks may speed healing.[26]

A similar osteochondrosis is Freiberg's infarction, or AVN of the metatarsal head (usually the second metatarsal). Localized pain is the usual complaint, and radiographs typically show opacification and irregularity of the head consistent with AVN (Fig. 26-17). As in Köhler's bone disease, repetitive microtrauma in a predisposed youngster is felt to be causative.[50] Treatment consists of metatarsal padding or orthotics with relative rest. Three to 4 weeks of casting may be required to relieve symptoms. Collapse of a metatarsal head may not resolve spontaneously and harmlessly. In this regard, Freiberg's infarction behaves more like Legg-Calvé-Perthes disease of the hip rather than Köhler's disease. Chronic pain and degenerative arthritis may follow Freiberg's infarction, requiring surgical intervention.

Bony anatomic variations can also lead to overuse problems. In the adolescent foot, these include adoles-

cent bunion, tarsal coalition, and os trigonum. Bunion may be symptomatic in any adolescent, but the demands of competition may exacerbate pain. Initially, treatment consists of footwear modifications and padding, possibly including orthotics. Surgery is reserved for those with persistent symptoms, and many procedures exist for varying amounts of deformity.[58]

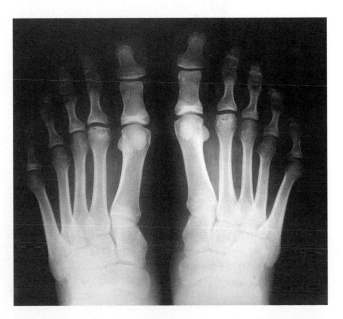

Fig. 26-17. Freiberg's infarction of the second metatarsal head.

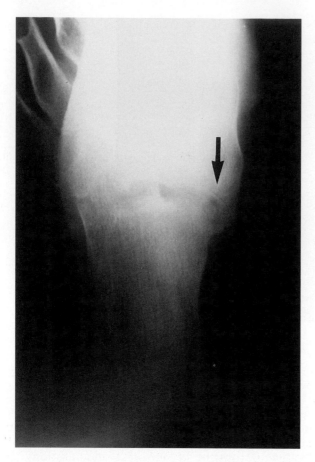

Fig. 26-18. Harris axial view of the heel showing talocalcaneal coalition (*arrow*).

Tarsal coalition encompasses bony or fibrous unions of the calcaneus to the talus or cuboid or of the talus to the navicular. Other coalitions are reported but are less common.[39] In the child, presenting symptoms may be rearfoot pain associated with increased activity. Physical examination will show limited or absent subtalar motion and tenderness in the medial or lateral hindfoot. Pes planus is a common associated finding. Routine radiographs are almost always read as negative, but a Harris axial view can demonstrate a talocalcaneal coalition (Fig. 26-18). Computed tomography in the sagittal and coronal planes will best demonstrate the bony relationships (Fig. 26-19).[62]

Rest and orthotics may resolve symptoms, but permanent correction requires resection of the bony or fibrous bridge. Long-term results of resection are generally good to excellent with much improved motion.[39]

Flat feet are common and not usually symptomatic. Because pronation accounts for some shock absorption during running, lack of effective pronation can be a risk factor for overuse injury. Altering the training schedule, obtaining running shoes with a strong medial counter, and utilizing orthotics to regain some of the shock absorption of controlled pronation can be helpful.

Os trigonum tarsi is a normal variant but becomes symptomatic in ballerinas who must achieve and maintain pointe. In this position, the accessory ossicle impinges the posterior ankle capsule (Fig. 26-20) and, if symptomatic, requires excision.

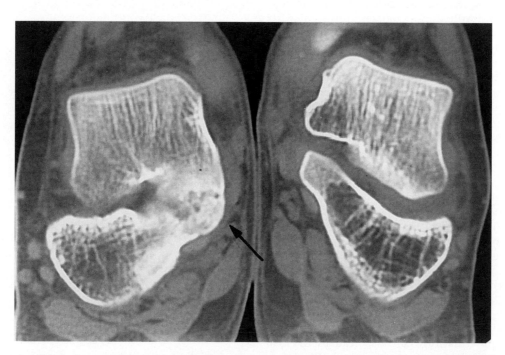

Fig. 26-19. Computerized tomogram shows talocalcaneal coalition with better detail (*arrow*). Contralateral foot has normal talocalcaneal joint.

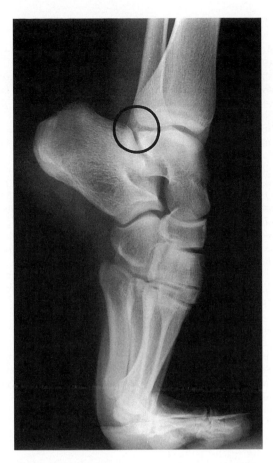

Fig. 26-20. Radiograph of ankle in demi-pointe. Small os trigonum is seen at center of circle and was responsible for painful impingement in maximal plantar flexion.

SUMMARY

Lower extremity injuries in children and adolescents include most of those found in adults and also include the apophysitises, osteochondritises, and physeal injuries. The young athlete has unique risk factors associated with both growth and the different mechanical properties of bone, cartilage, and collagen as compared with the adult. Adequate diagnosis and treatment requires detailed knowledge of these properties and risk factors. Despite the knowledge that youngsters heal readily and generally do not suffer long-term sequelae from imprecise diagnosis, this situation is changing. Single-sport athletes and high demand sports are resulting in more and more debilitating injuries. Identifying risk factors and preventing recurrence is essential to providing quality care.

REFERENCES

1. Abramowitz AJ, Schepsis AA: Chronic exertional compartment syndrome of the lower leg, *Orthop Review* 23(3):219-25, 1994.
2. Andersen P, Henriksson J: Training induced changes in the subgroups of human type II skeletal muscle fibres, *Acta Physiol Scand* 99(1):123-5, 1977.
3. Balkfors B: The course of knee-ligament injuries, *Acta Orthop Scand* 198(Suppl):1-99, 1982.
4. Beaty JH, Linton RC: Medial malleolar fracture in a child. A case report, *J Bone Joint Surg* 70A(8):1254-5, 1988.
5. Bollet AJ: Analgesic and anti-inflammatory drugs in therapy of osteoarthritis, *Semin Arthritis Rheum* 11(1 suppl:130), 1981.
6. Brewster CE, et al: Rehabilitation of the knee. In Nicholas JA, Hershman EB, eds: *The Lower Extremity and Spine in Sports Medicine,* ed 2, St. Louis, 1995, Mosby–Year Book.
7. Carter DR, Hayes WC: Compact bone fatigue damage: a microscopic examination, *Clin Orthop* 127:265-74, 1977.
8. Cavanagh PR: *The Running Shoe Book,* Mountain View, Calif, 1980, Anderson World.
9. Clancy WG Jr, et al: Treatment of knee joint instability secondary to rupture of the posterior cruciate ligament: report of a new procedure, *J Bone Joint Surg* 65A(3):310-22, 1983.
10. Cox JS: Evaluation of the Roux-Elmslie-Trillat procedure for knee extensor realignment, *Am J Sports Med* 19(5):303-10, 1982.
11. Daniel DM, et al: Use of the quadriceps active test to diagnose posterior cruciate-ligament disruption and measure posterior laxity of the knee, *J Bone Joint Surg* 70A(3):386-91, 1988.
12. Darracott J, Vernon-Roberts B: The bony changes in "chondromalacia patellae," *Rheumatol Phys Med* 11(4):175-9, 1971.
13. Delgado-Martins H: A study of the position of the patella using computerized tomography, *J Bone Joint Surg* 61B(4):443-4, 1979.
14. Ebbeling CB, Clarkson PM: Exercise-induced muscle damage and adaptation, *Sports Med* 7(4):207-34, 1989.
15. Fairbank JC, et al: Mechanical factors in the incidence of knee pain in adolescents and young adults, *J Bone Joint Surg* 66B(5):685-93, 1984.
16. Forster RS, Fu FH: Reflex sympathetic dystrophy in children. A case report and review of literature, *Orthopedics* 8(4):475-7, 1985.
17. Fulkerson JP, et al: Histologic evidence of retinacular nerve injury associated with patellofemoral malalignment, *Clin Orthop* 197:196-205, 1985.
18. Galway RD, Beaupre A, MacIntosh DL: Pivot shift: a clinical sign of symptomatic anterior cruciate ligament insufficiency, *J Bone Joint Surg* 54B(4):763, 1972.
19. Garcia A, Neer CS: Isolated fractures of the intercondylar eminence of the tibia, *Am J Surg* 95:593-8, 1958.
20. Garrett JC: Osteochondritis dissecans, *Clin Sports Med* 10(3):569-93, 1991.
21. Garrick JG, Requa RK: Role of external support in prevention of ankle sprains, *Med Sci Sports Exerc* 5(3):200-3, 1973.
22. Goodship AE, Lanyon LE, McFie H: Functional adaptation of bone to increased stress. An experimental study, *J Bone Joint Surg* 61A(4):539-46, 1979.
23. Gortmaker SL, et al: Increasing pediatric obesity in the United States, *Am J Dis Child* 141(5):535-40, 1987.
24. Gronkvist H, Hirsch G, Johansson CL: Fracture of the anterior tibial spine in children, *J Pediatr Orthop* 4(4):465-8, 1984.
25. Hess T, et al: Lateral tibial avulsion fractures and disruptions to the anterior cruciate ligament. A clinical study of their incidence and correlation, *Clin Orthop* 303:193-7, 1994.
26. Ippolito E, Ricciardi-Pollini PT, Falez F: Köhler's disease of the tarsal navicular: long-term follow-up of 12 cases, *J Pediatr Orthop* 4(4):416-7, 1984.
27. Johnson DP, Eastwood DM, Witherow PJ: Symptomatic synovial plicae of the knee, *J Bone Joint Surg* 75A(10):1485-96, 1993.
28. Janarv P, et al: Long-term follow-up of anterior tibial spine fractures in children, *J Pediatr Orthop* 15(1):63-8, 1995.

29. Jones DC, James SL: Overuse injuries of the lower extremity: shin splints, iliotibial band friction syndrome, and exertional compartment syndromes, *Clin Sports Med* 6(2):273-90, 1987.

30. Kelsey DD, Tyson E: A new method of training for the lower extremity using unloading, *J Orthop Sports Phys Ther* 19(4):218-23, 1994.

31. Levine J, Splain S: Use of the infrapatella strap in the treatment of patellofemoral pain, *Clin Orthop* 139:179-81, 1979.

32. Loder RT, Aronson DD, Greenfield ML: The epidemiology of bilateral slipped capital femoral epiphysis. A study of children in Michigan, *J Bone Joint Surg* 75A(8):1141-7, 1993.

33. Loder RT, Schwartz EM, Hensinger RN: Behavioral characteristics of children with Legg-Calvé-Perthes disease. *J Pediatr Orthop* 13(5):598-601, 1993.

34. McMurray TP: The semilunar cartilages, *Br J Med* 29:407, 1942.

35. Meyers MH, McKeever FM: Fracture of the intercondylar eminence of the tibia, *J Bone Joint Surg* 52A(8):1677-84, 1970.

36. Micheli LJ: The child and adolescent, In Harris M et al, eds: *Oxford Textbook of Sports Medicine*, New York, 1994, Oxford University Press.

37. Micheli LJ: The incidence of injuries in children's sports: a medical perspective. In Brown E, Branta CF, eds: *Competitive Sports for Children and Youth: An Overview of Research and Issues*, Champaign, Illinois, 1988, Human Kinetics Publishers.

38. Micheli LJ, Stanitski CL: Lateral patellar retinacular release, *Am J Sports Med* 9(5):330-6, 1981.

39. O'Neill DB, Micheli LJ: Tarsal coalition: a follow-up of adolescent athletes, *Am J Sports Med* 17(4):544-9, 1989.

40. Outerbridge RE, Dunlop JA: The problem of chondromalacia patellae, *Clin Orthop* 110:177-96, 1975.

41. Pillemer FG, Micheli LJ: Psychological considerations in youth sports, *Clin Sports Med* 7(3):679-89, 1988.

42. Poussa M, et al: Prognosis after conservative and operative treatment in Perthes disease, *Clin Orthop* 297:82-6, 1993.

43. Powell JW, Schootman M: A multivariate risk analysis of selected playing surfaces in the National Football League: 1980-1989. An epidemiologic study of knee injuries, *Am J Sports Med* 20(6):686-94, 1992.

44. Requa RK: The scope of the problem: the impact of sports-related injuries. In National Institutes of Health Publication #93-3444: Conference on Sports Injuries in Youth: Surveillance Strategies. Proceedings. April 8-9, 1991, Bethesda, Maryland.

45. Salminen JJ, et al: Leisure time physical activity in the young. Correlation with low-back pain, spinal mobility and trunk muscle strength in 15-year-old school children, *Int J Sports Med* 14(7):406-10, 1993.

46. Shelbourne KD, et al: Arthrofibrosis in acute anterior cruciate ligament reconstruction. The effect of timing of reconstruction and rehabilitation, *Am J Sports Med* 19(4):332, 1991.

47. Shelbourne KD, Wilckens JH: Current concepts in anterior cruciate ligament rehabilitation, *Orthop Review* 19(11):957-64, 1990.

48. Shellock FG, et al: Effect of a patellar realignment brace on patellofemoral relationships: evaluation with kinematic MR imaging, *J Magnetic Resonance Imaging* 4(4):590-4, 1994.

49. Silber TJ, Majd M: Reflex sympathetic dystrophy syndrome in children and adolescents. Report of 18 cases and review of the literature. *Am J Dis Child* 142(12):1325-30, 1988.

50. Smille IS: Freiberg's infraction (Köhler's second disease), *J Bone Joint Surg* 39B:580, 1957.

51. Smith BG, et al: Early MR imaging of lower-extremity physeal fracture-separations: a preliminary report, *J Pediatr Orthop* 14(4):526-33, 1994.

52. Souryal TO, Freeman TR: Intercondylar notch size and anterior cruciate ligament injuries in athletes. A prospective study, *Am J Sports Med* 21(4):535-9, 1993.

53. Souryal TO, Moore HA, Evans JP: Bilaterality in anterior cruciate ligament injuries: associated intercondylar notch stenosis, *Am J Sports Med* 16(5):449-54, 1988.

54. Spaeth HJ, et al: Magnetic resonance imaging detection of early experimental periostitis. Comparison of magnetic resonance imaging, computed tomography, and plain radiography with histopathologic correlation, *Investigative Radiol* 26(4):304-8, 1991.

55. Steen SN, Brownell KD: Patterns of weight loss and regain in wrestlers: has the tradition changed? *Med Sci Sports Exerc* 22(6):762-8, 1990.

56. Stover B, et al: Early changes in the hip joint following epiphysiolysis of the femoral head. Results of an MRT study, *Radiologe* 34(1):46-51, 1994.

57. Sullivan D, et al: Stress fractures in 51 runners, *Clin Orthop* 187:188-92, 1984.

58. Trott A: Hallux valgus in the adolescent, *AAOS Instructional Course Lect* 21:262, 1975.

59. Wagner JC: Enhancement of athletic performance with drugs. An overview, *Sports Med* 12(4):250-65, 1991.

60. Wahlstrom O, et al: Heterotopic bone formation prevented by diclofenac. Prospective study of 100 hip arthroplasties, *Acta Orthop Scand* 62(5):419-21, 1991.

61. Warren MP: Excessive dieting and exercise: the dangers for young athletes, *J Musculoskel Med* 4:31-40, 1987.

62. Wechsler RJ, et al: Tarsal coalition: depiction and characterization with CT and MR imaging, *Radiology* 193(2):447-52, 1994.

CHAPTER 27

THE UPPER EXTREMITY

Laura Forese

Children and adolescents are engaging in sports in greater numbers than ever before, and unfortunately, along with the positive benefits of athletic endeavor, they are also experiencing sports injuries in greater numbers. The upper extremity is the site of many problems for the young athlete. Certain sports predispose the immature upper extremity to injury, but virtually all sports (as well as free play) expose the young athlete to the dangers of falls that can lead to fractures. The sports related upper extremity disorders can be broken down into two major categories: overuse injuries and fractures and dislocations.

For the purposes of general classification, the pediatric upper extremity will be divided into five anatomic areas: hand, wrist, elbow, shoulder, and clavicle, and each will be addressed for both overuse injuries and typical fractures and dislocations. Because this is not a comprehensive text on trauma, only selected fractures and dislocations will be discussed.

GENERAL PRINCIPLES

It is trite but true that children and adolescents are not simply small versions of adults. The importance of the growing musculoskeletal system cannot be overemphasized. Growth plate injuries are common and may have important sequelae. Ligamentous injuries, in contrast, are much less common because of the relative strength of soft tissues compared to immature bone.

Children may have real difficulty localizing pain or other symptoms. Children and adolescents may also underestimate the importance of reporting pain, especially if they believe that this may keep them out of sports and other play activities. Careful attention must be paid to the physical examination of the child with a sports injury. Comparison must always be made with the uninvolved side.

Radiographs can be confusing in the immature skeleton, therefore it is critical that comparison views

of the contralateral extremity be used. CT scans and MRIs may be necessary to image the osteocartilaginous structures.

Overuse injuries arise because of repetitive microtrauma to the growing skeleton.[7] Rest is often the treatment of choice. Children and adolescents are often at the mercy of adults who establish and supervise training regimens and athletic events. It is critical that appropriate technique be used and that strict guidelines about rest be observed, even before an injury occurs.[15,23]

HAND

General Examination

The hand is commonly injured in all athletes, including children and adolescents. Close attention must be paid to the examination of the hand in an injury. Radiographs, although often necessary, do not take the place of a careful examination because there are many soft tissue injuries that occur. Injured joints must be assessed for stability in all directions, and tendon avulsions must be specifically ruled out. Any limitation of motion, either active or passive, demands a radiograph. As in all fractures, it is critical to obtain at least two radiographs—a true anteroposterior and a true lateral—of the area in question. Oblique views are not sufficient. In general, pediatric injuries are treated conservatively with good results. Poor results are often due to late diagnosis.[21]

Fractures and Dislocations

FDP AVULSION. Avulsion of the flexor digitorum profundus tendon off of the distal phalanx is often called a "jersey finger," because a player catches the fingertip in another player's jersey while trying to tackle him. Bony injury is rare in this problem, and it can often go undetected because the only deficit is inability to actively flex at the distal interphalangeal joint.[14] The most common digit involved is the ring finger. Surgical repair is indicated to reattach the tendon as soon as possible. Late repair may be impossible (Fig. 27-1).

MALLET FINGER. In distinction to the flexor digitorum profundus avulsion is the mallet finger, which results from an injury around the insertion of the extensor tendon. Depending on the forces involved and the age of the athlete, this injury can produce a fracture, an avulsion of the tendon, or a tendon disruption.[9] Unless there is a fractured piece large enough to reduce and pin back, the treatment is immobilization in extension at the distal interphalangeal joint (Fig. 27-2).

JAMMED FINGER. A jammed finger is the result of a significant force on the extended finger, which causes pain and swelling at the proximal interphalangeal joint. There is no bony or ligamentous injury, and the joint is stable. After other problems are ruled out, the jammed finger is protected with rest and a slow return to range of motion and full activity. The joint may remain persistently sore for many months, and the swollen appearance around this joint may never fully resolve.

METACARPAL AND PHALANGEAL FRACTURES AND DISLOCATIONS. A full discussion of all the different types of metacarpal and phalangeal frac-

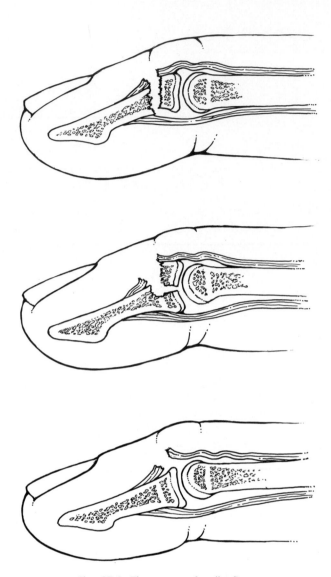

Fig. 27-2. Three types of mallet finger.

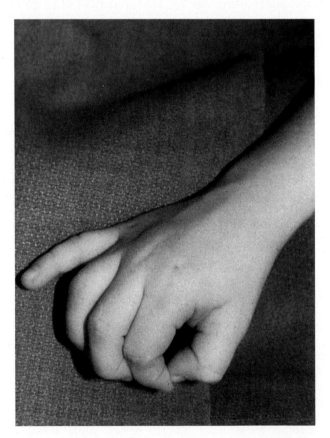

Fig. 27-1. This child avulsed the FDP of the fifth finger while playing on the sports field.

tures and dislocations is far beyond the scope of this text, however, there are some important general principles for the primary care provider. At least two radiographs at right angles to each other are critically important because of the problems with malunion. A fracture that appears adequately reduced on an anteroposterior view and on an oblique view may be significantly displaced on the lateral view. A rotatory deformity of just a small amount can cause real problems of overlapping of the fingers with the hand closed. As with most fractures in children, closed methods are usually sufficient, however, open reductions are sometimes indicated, and an early diagnosis and treatment plan is far superior to a late one (Fig. 27-3).

Dislocations are often easily reduced by a well meaning person or by the child or adolescent himself on the playing field. However, the dislocation still requires a careful physical examination, including testing of range of motion and stability of the ligamentous complex. Ra-

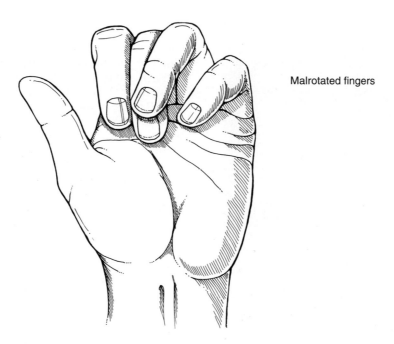

Malrotated fingers

Fig. 27-3. Malrotated fingers as a result of malunion of a phalanx fracture.

diographs are also necessary to rule out any associated bony injury. Some dislocations are not reducible by closed methods, and thus persistent reduction attempts are not appropriate.

OVERUSE INJURIES. There are no specific overuse injuries of the hand in children and adolescents.

WRIST

General Examination

It can be difficult to sort out the site of injury in the wrist because of the close anatomic relationship of the structures. Again, a careful examination of the contralateral wrist area is necessary. The centers of ossification of the carpal bones and the distal radius and ulna do not all have the same timing of ossification, so radiographs can be misleading. Comparison views are highly recommended.

Fractures and Dislocations

SCAPHOID FRACTURES. The scaphoid is by far the most commonly injured of the carpal bones in children and adolescents. This injury usually results from a fall on the outstretched hand. Unfortunately, this injury often goes unnoticed even when radiographs are taken because radiographs are often negative. If any doubt exists, especially in the presence of tenderness in the snuff-box, the child should be casted. Although most pediatric scaphoid fractures heal with immobilization, some will go onto nonunion, particularly if untreated.[6] Displaced fractures and nonunions often require surgical intervention.

RADIUS AND ULNA FRACTURES. It is usually not difficult to diagnose a fracture of the radius and/or ulna. The mechanism of injury is also from a fall on the outstretched hand, and the child is usually exquisitely tender at the site of the fracture. A complete fracture of either or both bones typically has an obvious deformity. There are few indications for surgical intervention in radius and ulna fractures in children. Most of them can be treated quite successfully with closed reduction and casting or splinting. While distal radius growth plate fractures are common, they rarely lead to any significant problem with subsequent growth arrest.

Of note is the torus (or buckle) fracture, which is a cortical compression without significant displacement. Torus fractures can go completely unnoticed and are often only mildly painful. Often the diagnosis is delayed because of the lack of symptoms. These fractures do not require reduction and are often treated with simple splinting for comfort.

Overuse Injuries

DISTAL RADIUS INJURY. A repetitive stress response that has been seen in gymnasts is overuse syndrome in the distal radius.[22] The patients complained of pain particularly with weightbearing on the hand and placement of the wrist in dorsiflexion. Radiographs may be slow to show the findings that are typical of stress changes to the open growth plates: cystic changes and widening of the growth plate.[20] The suggestion has been made that those who are treated prior to radiographic changes will recover faster. The treatment has been rest and typically, the patients recover completely. There is no evidence of sequelae in those who rest (Fig. 27-4).

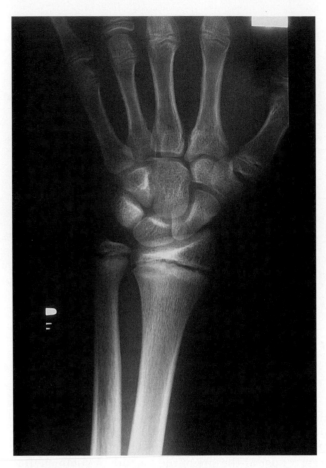

Fig. 27-4. This child, a competitive gymnast, had chronic wrist pain and tenderness over the growth plate that responded to rest and modified activity.

ELBOW

General Examination

Much of the elbow anatomy is palpable, and an examination should include careful inspection and palpation in an attempt to pinpoint the exact area of pain (Fig. 27-5). Full range of motion is from 0° of flexion to over 130° of flexion. People with laxity actually have hyperextension of the elbow beyond 0° of flexion. This full range of motion is not actually necessary for most activities, and an athlete can easily hide a somewhat limited range of motion. The ulnar nerve is in close proximity to the bony structures and must be carefully assessed.

The immature elbow is a particularly vulnerable joint in throwing sports and in gymnastics. In baseball, there are throws that are particularly damaging to the elbow, and in gymnastics the elbow is a weight-bearing joint.[10] The elbow is easily fractured when a child falls because of the anatomy. Common in these sports is the presence of chronic pain.

Fractures and Dislocations

Dislocation of the elbow is particularly rare in children.[11] Unfortunately, fractures about the elbow are common. The mechanism of injury can vary with the specific type of elbow fracture, however, most are from falls onto the arm or the outstretched hand. Because there is so much osteocartilaginous tissue around the elbow, radiographs can be deceptive or at least difficult to interpret. Unlike the principles of treatment for many other upper extremity fractures discussed here, fractures around the elbow in children and adolescents often require open or closed surgical reduction with percutaneous pinning to prevent displacement. This is due to the significant forces around the elbow that tend

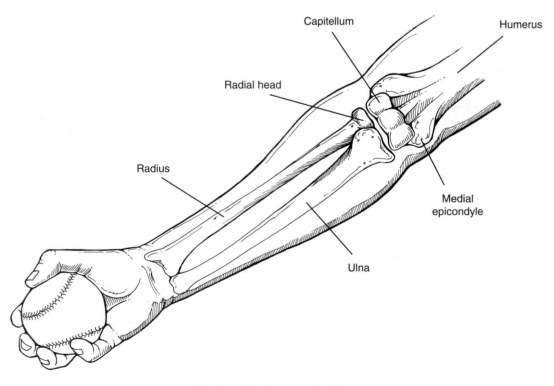

Fig. 27-5. Anatomy of the elbow.

to displace fractures, which could result in functional and cosmetic problems in the future (Fig. 27-6).

Overuse Injuries

LITTLE LEAGUE ELBOW. Little league elbow, although first described as an avulsion of the ossification center of the medial epicondyle, is actually a constellation of problems with the immature elbow that can occur singly or in combination as a result of the forces in throwing.[3,8,18] The lateral and the medial sides of the elbow are affected differently in this condition. The medial side is subjected to valgus stresses, while the lateral side is subjected to compression.[7] Different problems occur in the elbow at different stages in the child's life because of the changing pattern of fusion and ossification in the elbow.

On the medial side, epicondylitis is the result of overuse in the child's elbow but responds rapidly to rest and does not cause any significant problems.[17] As the child grows into adolescence, the medial epicondyle may actually pull off as a fracture. This will often heal without problem as long as the offending activity ceases.[25] If the mass goes on to nonunion, this may require surgical intervention. The older adolescent and young adult are less prone to bony injury and more likely to sustain muscle injury on the medial side of the elbow.

On the lateral side of the elbow, the radial head and the capitellum are at risk. Avascular necrosis may occur in these structures, and there may even be the formation of loose bodies.[7]

The major treatment for all of these injuries is rest and, of course, changes in training once the athlete has recovered enough to return to activity.[26] Prevention is even more effective than treatment, and it is for this reason that there should be some restrictions on the numbers of innings pitched in a given week.

SHOULDER

General Examination

In distinction to the next section on clavicle, here, the shoulder is meant to be the glenohumeral joint. Range of motion should of course be tested in relationship to the unaffected side. Forward elevation is a key motion to the shoulder. It is tested by bringing the arm out from the body in a position roughly between straight ahead and straight out to the side. External rotation can be tested by keeping the elbow at the side and bringing the hand away from the body. Internal rotation is tested by how far up the back the hand can be brought.

Fractures and Dislocations

Fractures of the humerus are usually obvious to the observer and the examiner. As in most other fractures of the upper extremity in children and adolescents, the mechanism of injury is often a fall on the outstretched hand. Operative intervention is rarely indicated in proximal and midshaft humerus fractures (distal humerus fractures are included in the section on elbow). Even major displacement can be expected to remodel in children, and so a closed reduction or no reduction is usually all that is necessary (Fig. 27-7).

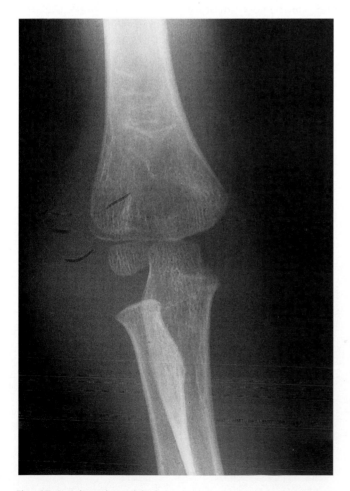

Fig. 27-6. A lateral condyle fracture that required pinning to prevent malunion or nonunion.

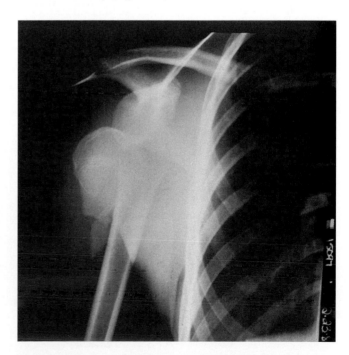

Fig. 27-7. A fracture sustained on the football field that did require some manipulative reduction.

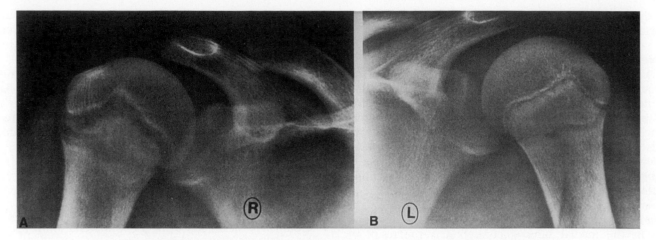

Fig. 27-8. Widening of the growth plate on the right in this ball player. (From Busch M, in Morrissey RT: *Pediatric Orthopaedics,* 3d ed, Philadelphia, 1990, JB Lippincott Co.)

Dislocation of the glenohumeral joint occurs in adolescents in much the same way that it occurs in adults. The shoulder has the least stability of all the major joints because it has soft tissue rather than bony stability. This is in direct contrast to the hip, for instance, where the bony stability is much more important and hence there are many fewer hip dislocations than shoulder dislocations. This injury is not common in children who tend to sustain fractures rather than dislocations, but as children age into adolescence and then into young adulthood, the shoulder becomes more vulnerable. Anterior dislocation is far more common than posterior dislocation; a typical scenario is for the basketball player to go up for a rebound with the arm overhead and to have it forced backwards. The humeral head then dislocates anteriorly.

Treatment is by reduction, which should not be attempted without radiographs to rule out any associated bony pathology. The first dislocation is usually treated by immobilization after the reduction and rest for several weeks, followed by a rehabilitation program that strengthens the shoulder musculature. Some athletes have no further problems after a single dislocation. Unfortunately, many young athletes go on to recurrent dislocations, which can be a major problem.[13] Although recurrent dislocations are often easily reduced, even by the athlete himself on the playing field, the instability in the joint can be very uncomfortable and may make the athlete extremely apprehensive. Surgery may be the only option for these athletes in order to compete.

Overuse Injuries

LITTLE LEAGUE SHOULDER. Little League shoulder is a well recognized term, although it appears to mean different things to different authors.[5] It is a classic overuse injury in which the immature skeleton responds to constant low levels of stress from pitching with changes at the growth plate.[24] Although this syndrome is called Little League shoulder because of the high incidence in pitchers in organized activity, a similar syndrome has also been described in tennis players.[12] The mechanism of injury appears to be the repetitive rota-

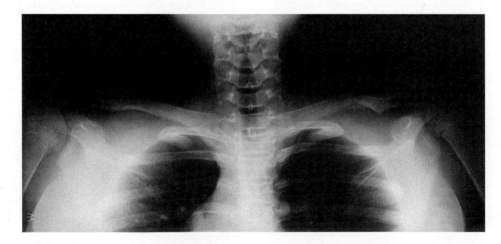

Fig. 27-9. A typical midshaft clavical fracture with early healing.

tional motion. Afflicted children and adolescents have pain and some mild loss of range of motion, which seems to respond rapidly to cessation of pitching and rest.[2] Potential injury to the site of future growth is what causes concern in this syndrome, but there do not appear to be cases of actual growth problems (Fig. 27-8).

IMPINGEMENT SYNDROME. Impingement is a syndrome where the supraspinatus tendon (part of the rotator cuff) is progressively irritated by rubbing on the undersurface of the acromion. This is brought about by forward elevation activities, precisely those that are used in certain swimming and tennis strokes and overhead throwing.

While the impingement is in the initial stages of pain with forward elevation, rest is once again the treatment of choice. Modification of training practices may be critical to getting the athlete back to competition.[19] Full range of motion must also be regained. Acromioplasty, the surgical removal of some offending bone from the undersurface of the acromion, is sometimes necessary if conservative care does not resolve the problem.

CLAVICLE

General Examination
Because the clavicle is subcutaneous, palpation of the bone is relatively easy. Examination of the sternoclavicular joint, however, can be deceptive because it may be difficult to assess which side is more prominent. In a typical midshaft clavicle injury, the fracture can be both seen and felt, and the bone ends may even be tenting the muscles and skin. Close attention must be paid to any respiratory symptoms such as shortness of breath or painful respiration and any neurovascular symptoms, as this may signal respiratory compromise due to pressure from the clavicle on the great vessels or the brachial plexus.

Fractures and Dislocations
Midshaft clavicle fractures are among the most common injuries for children and adolescents. The typical cause is a fall on the outstretched hand. The clavicle has tremendous potential to remodel and therefore is virtually always treated closed, often with just a sling or a figure of eight bandage that attempts to keep the fracture reduced. These fractures lay down abundant callus and thus a bump is often visible and palpable long after healing has taken place. An exception to closed treatment is the case where the bone ends have become fixed in muscle and are not reducible closed. Another rare exception is a fracture that is causing pressure on the brachial plexus, which may also have to be treated by open reduction and perhaps internal fixation (Fig. 27-9).

Sternoclavicular injuries are much less common than fractures of the midshaft or the distal portion of the clavicle. A significant force is usually required to cause injury that will present with pain at the junction of the sternum and clavicle. Dislocations of this joint in the immature skeleton are virtually unheard of since the growth plate does not close until the late teens or early twenties. Instead, an epiphyseal fracture occurs. Radiographic confirmation is notoriously difficult to obtain with plain ra-

diographs, so other imaging such as a CT scan or MRI may be necessary. Treatment, other than rest, is rarely necessary unless there is some compression of the great vessels.

At the distal end of the clavicle, fractures also occur, especially through the distal growth plate or metaphysis. The mechanism of injury is typically a fall directly on the point of the shoulder. This is the equivalent of an acromioclavicular separation in an adult. In the mid to late teens, acromioclavicular separation can occur and this should be treated as adult injury. The treatment for most distal clavicle injuries is rest, typically a sling, for those injuries that are non- to minimally displaced. Even those with moderate displacement are often treated with observation because of the remodeling potential of the clavicle. Fractures with major or fixed displacement and those causing neurovascular symptoms may require more extensive, operative treatment.

Overuse Injuries
Osteolysis can occur in the distal clavicle, particularly in weightlifters, although this has not been documented in children.[4] The cause of the osteolysis has not been determined, but the lesion typically responds to changes in overhead lifting and rest. Rest is obviously the fastest way to recovery, however, some have suggested moving the hands closer to each other in overhead lifting as a way to allow the lifter to continue training.

CONCLUSION

Fractures and related trauma of the upper extremity in children and adolescents are common place occurrences. We expect those falls and are often aware of the potential sequelae. The overuse injuries to the upper extremity are less common and receive much less attention in print and in the training of health care professionals.

Children and adolescents who participate in sports, particularly organized sports, are directed by parents and coaches to perform certain training and practice activities. It is incumbent upon those adults to pay careful attention to time spent on certain stressful activities and to allow adequate periods of rest. No child or adolescent is aided by being told to work through the pain. In the upper extremity, the consequences of not resting an overused joint or of missing a fracture can be devastating.

REFERENCES

1. Aronen JG: Problems of the upper extremity in gymnasts, *Clin Sports Med* 4:61–71, 1985.
2. Barnett LS: Little league shoulder syndrome: proximal humeral epiphysiolysis in adolescent baseball pitchers, *JBJS* 67A:495–496, 1985.
3. Brogdon BG, Crow NE: Little leaguer's elbow, *AJR* 83:671–685, 1960.
4. Cahill BR: Osteolysis of the distal part of the clavicle in male athletes, *JBJS* 64A:1053–1058, 1982.
5. Cahill BR, Tullos HS, Fain RH: Little league shoulder, *J Sports Med* 2:150–152, 1974.
6. Christodoulou AG, Colton CL: Scaphoid fractures in children, *J Ped Ortho* 6:37–39, 1986.

7. Clain MAR, Hershman EB: Overuse injuries in children and adolescents, *Physician Sports Med* 17:111–123, 1989.

8. DeHaven KE, Evarts CM: Throwing injuries of the elbow in athletes, *Ortho Clin North Am* 4:801–808, 1973.

9. Garcia-Moral CA: Injuries to the Hand and Wrist. In Sullivan JA, Grana WA eds, The Pediatric Athlete. 1988 American Academy of Orthopaedic Surgery.

10. Goldberg MJ: Gymnastic injuries, *Ortho Clin North Am* 11:717–726, 1980.

11. Green N: Fractures and dislocations about the elbow. In Green NE, Swiontkowski MF, eds: *Skeletal Trauma in Children,* Philadelphia, 1994, WB Saunders.

12. Gregg JR, Torg E: Upper extremity injuries in adolescent tennis players, *Clin Sports Med* 7:371–385, 1988.

13. Hovelius L: Anterior dislocation of the shoulder in teenagers and young adults: five year prognosis, *JBJS* 69A:393–399, 1987.

14. Leddy JP, Packer J: Avulsion of the profundus tendon insertion in athletes, *J Hand Surg* 2:66–69, 1977.

15. Meyers JF: Injuries to the shoulder girdle and elbow in the pediatric athlete. In Sullivan JA, Frana WA, eds: American Academy of Orthopaedic Surgeons, 1988.

16. Micheli LJ: Overuse injuries in children's sports: the growth factor, *Ortho Clin North Am* 14:337–360, 1983.

17. Pappas AM: Elbow problems associated with baseball during childhood and adolescence. *CORR* 164:30–41, 1982.

18. Pavlov H, et al: Nonunion of olecranon epiphysis: two cases in adolescent baseball pitchers, *AJR* 136:819–820, 1981.

19. Richardson AB, Jobe FW, Collins HR: The shoulder in competitive swimming, *Am J Sports Med* 8:159–163, 1980.

20. Roy S, Caine D, Singer KM: Stress changes of the distal radial epiphysis in young gymnasts. *Am J Sports Med* 13:301–308, 1985.

21. Ruby LK: Common hand injuries in the athlete, *Ortho Clin NA* 11:819–839, 1980.

22. Simmons BP, Lovallo JL: Hand and wrist injuries in children, *Clin Sports Med* 7:495–512, 1988.

23. Snook GA: Injuries in women's gymnastics, *Am J Sports Med* 7:242–244, 1979.

24. Tibone JE: Shoulder problems of adolescents, *Clin Sports Med* 2:423–7, 1983.

25. Tullos HS, King JW: Lesions of the pitching arm in adolescents, *JAMA* 220:264–271, 1972.

26. Woods GW, Tullos HS, King JW: The throwing arm: elbow joint injuries, *J Sports Med* 1:43–47, 1973.

CHAPTER 28

THE SPINE

Gail S. Chorney

Spinal injuries, whether in the cervical, thoracic, or lumbar spine, are uncommon in children. The etiology of these injuries is age dependent. In the pediatric age group from years 5 to 15, the most common cause is motor vehicle accident. However, the second cause is recreational sports. Football is credited with the largest number of injuries, although gymnastics and wrestling also are associated with spinal injuries. The number and severity of injuries can often be decreased with careful attention to training, supervision, and proper equipment. The use of the trampoline, however, has a high association of catastrophic spinal injury (quadriplegia) that cannot be controlled by supervision or equipment. This has led to the recommendation that the trampoline be discouraged as a training device.[11]

This chapter is concerned with evaluation in the physician's office of back complaints in the pediatric patient. The care of the seriously injured patient with accompanying spinal cord injury on the playing field or ski slope is not dealt with here. In the office, a careful history and physical examination along with the appropriate radiographic studies can lead to a diagnosis and guidelines for treatments and further athletic participation.

HISTORY

Obtaining a history from the pediatric patient is always more difficult than in the adult patient. The type of athletic participation as well as the intensity of training can always be elicited from both child and parent. Many of the issues encountered in the physician's office are of a chronic nature. The child needs to be guided in the history taking to relate the complaints to the specific sport. Direct questions are asked about the location, nature, and timing of the pain. The timing of the pain should be established in relation to practice sessions, games, and the occurrence of the pain when not participating in

sports. Does the pain occur during athletic participation or after the practice session/game is over? Obviously any history of known injury must be obtained. In the older child, the patient can demonstrate which maneuvers in the sport reproduce the complaint. The child may minimize the complaint in order to prevent restriction of activity. The physician must still attempt to form an accurate picture of the child's impaired function, including deterioration in performance and changes in neurologic status.

PHYSICAL EVALUATION AND RADIOGRAPHY

The physical examination should be performed with the child undressed, with a hospital gown for modesty. Regardless of where the complaints are localized, the entire spine as well as the extremities need a complete evaluation. Again, the child will more often minimize the complaints rather than exaggerate them in order to continue athletic participation.

As in every physical examination of a child, the general appearance should be noted. Does the child appear to be in pain or have difficulty raising up from the chair or getting onto the examination table? Is there difficulty in undressing?

Cervical Spine

The cervical spine should be observed for possible kyphosis. The range of motion of the cervical spine is determined as well as the presence of local tenderness in the midline. The cervical spine is more mobile in the young patient than in the adult because of increased ligamentous laxity in the pediatric age group. This increased motion accounts for the pseudo subluxation that can often be seen on a later radiograph. If there is a full, painless range of motion of the cervical spine, the physician need not be alarmed by the pseudo subluxation on the radiograph. The anterior translation is usually seen at C_{2-3} or C_{3-4}. The presence of midline tenderness or restriction of motion in the cervical spine should alert the physician to the possibility of injury to the posterior ligamentous structures. Flexion and extension lateral radiographs of the cervical spine are the appropriate studies to obtain. Since initial radiographs may not be conclusive for instability, suspicion of this injury requires careful follow-up. Contact sports or diving need to be avoided. Minor injuries will resolve with time, with decreased tenderness and restoration of motion. However, persistent midline tenderness and continued loss of motion should alert the primary caregiver to refer the patient on to a specialist for evaluation. Latent instability of the cervical spine requires posterior arthrodesis to protect the patient from possible neurological injury.[9]

A short neck or a restriction of motion in the cervical spine that is not associated with tenderness may be an indication of congenital anomalies of the spine. Anterior-posterior and lateral views of the cervical spine should be obtained. Congenital anomalies of the cervical spine such as fusion of vertebral bodies is known as Klippel-Feil syndrome. Again, participation in contact sports or diving should not be allowed for fear or neurologic injury. The physician must also investigate the child's cardiac and renal status since there is a high incidence of congenital problems in these organ systems that are associated with Klippel-Feil syndrome.

Thoracic Spine

The trunk is then inspected with regard to a possible increase in the thoracic kyphosis. A painless round back in the pediatric patient is usually noted by the parent and not the child. On examination, the physician should view the patient from the front, back, and side to assess the presence of an increased kyphosis. An attempt should be made to passively correct the kyphosis. On a forward bend test, if there is rigidity to the kyphosis, the diagnosis of Scheuermann's round back is suspected. There is frequently a complaint of mild pain. Tight hamstrings are often a physical finding. This diagnosis is confirmed on lateral radiographs of the thoraco-lumbar spine by the presence of wedging of three or more vertebral bodies (Figs. 28-1, 28-2).

Scheuermann's round back is a relatively common complaint in adolescent males. There is an increase in incidence in weight lifters, however. The treatment is bracing, which can decrease pain as well as prevent further deformity. Bracing may allow restoration of the height of the vertebral bodies in the skeletally immature skeleton and thus decrease the deformity. Weight lifting should probably be restricted during the treatment period.[9]

Lumbar Spine

An increase in the thoracic kyphosis is often accompanied by an increase in the lumbar lordosis. In addition, complaints of pain in the lumbar spine are probably the most common complaints of young athletes. Participation in recreational sports does not lead to an increase in mechanical back pain in young people. It also does not decrease the incidence either. Before the diagnosis of me-

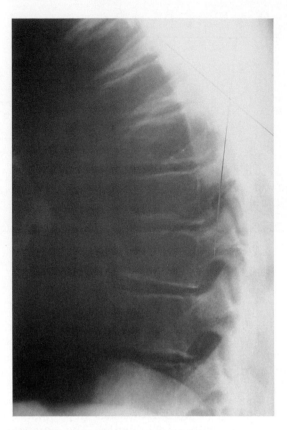

Fig. 28-1. Lateral radiograph of thoracic spine showing minor wedging of three vertebral bodies characteristic of Scheuermann's round back.

chanical back pain is made, the more serious diagnoses of spondylolysis and spondylolisthesis must be ruled out. Micheli has written extensively about these injuries in the gymnast.[7] These injuries should be suspected in young athletes participating in gymnastics or other sports involving repetitive hyperextension of the lumbar spine.

Spondylolisthesis is the slipping forward of one vertebral body on another. The usual location is L_5 on S_1 (Figs. 28-3, 28-4). Spondylolysis is a disruption of the pars interarticularis. It may be unilateral or bilateral. Slippage is not present (Fig. 28-5). There may be simply an elongation of the pars interarticularis rather than a fracture. Congenital dysplasia may be a predisposing factor in addition to the athletic participation.

The physical examination for the above injuries reveals an increase in the lumbar lordosis. The child may not be able to reverse the lordosis on forward bends. There may be midline tenderness to palpation over the lower lumbar spine. Paraspinal muscle spasms may be present if symptoms are severe enough. Forward flexion does not cause discomfort, but extension of the lumbar spine reproduces the symptoms. The child may have difficulty raising from a chair. Pain produced by standing on one leg is indicative of injury to the pars interarticularis on that side. Hamstring tightness is present. The examiner must bear in mind that children are more flexible than adults and that young athletes

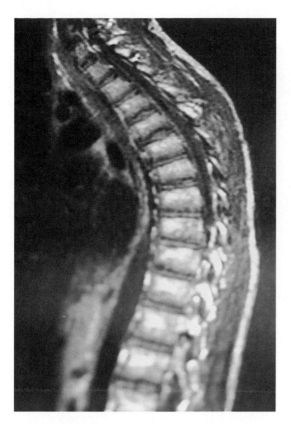

Fig. 28-2. MRI of the spine of the same patient as in Figure 28-1, again showing the minor wedging of vertebral bodies resulting in a kyphosis.

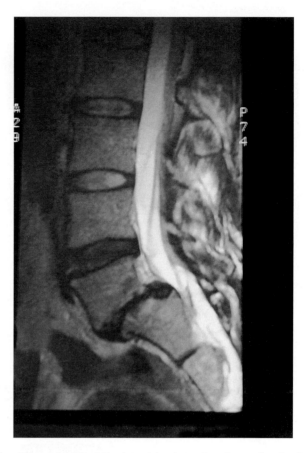

Fig. 28-4. An MRI of the lateral lumbar spine shows the Grade I slippage more dramatically.

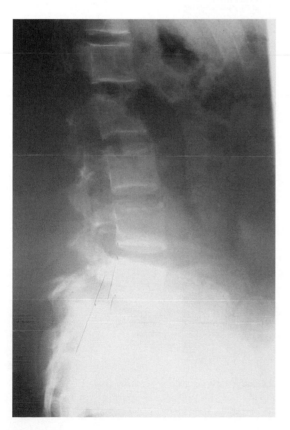

Fig. 28-3. Lateral radiograph of the lumbar-sacral junction showing a Grade I spondylolisthesis of L_5-S_1.

are probably more flexible. Therefore, restrictions in motion may be more subtle. The neurologic examination is normal.[4]

The radiographs to order are the usual standing anterior-posterior and lateral views. Oblique views are needed to demonstrate spondylolysis. However, radiographs may be negative for bony lesions, even the oblique views. A bone scan is often necessary to confirm the diagnosis.

The treatment of spondylolysis is bracing, which rapidly decreases the pain. The brace is a thoracolumbar orthosis. Casts have been used in order to increase compliance. Spondylolysis is a stable lesion, however, and thus continued participation in the sport during the healing process may be an issue. Guidelines for participation may be influenced by pain tolerance and the importance of competition to the young athlete. Usually avoidance of the specific maneuvers that reproduce the pain are suggested.[4,7]

Again, spondylolisthesis is the slippage of one vertebral body on the next lower one. Grading is based on the percentage of the lower body that is now uncovered. The child with a spondylolisthesis of greater than 50% will have a short trunk on physical examination as well as hamstring tightness. The hips may have a flexion contracture secondary to the tilt of the pelvis.

Progression of the slippage occurs early in the presen-

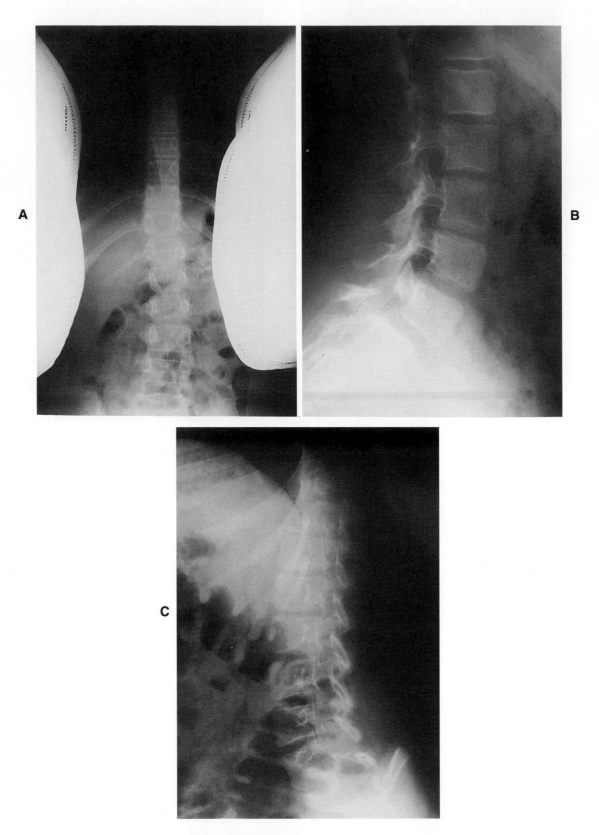

Fig. 28-5. A, The AP radiograph of a patient with a spondylolysis shows a minor scoliosis that is secondary to the pain. **B,** The lateral radiograph shows elongation of the posterior element of L_5. **C,** The oblique view also shows the defect in the pars interarticularis of L_5.

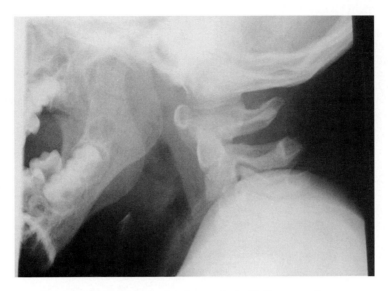

Fig. 28-6. A hypoplastic dens in a patient with Down syndrome.

tation. Therefore, a young child (less than 10 years of age) with a spondylolisthesis should be followed with serial lateral radiographs. Lesions of greater than 50% are treated with a fusion. Any lesions that show progression of a slippage should also be treated with a fusion.

The asymptomatic athlete with less than a 25% spondylolisthesis may participate in sports without restriction. Those symptomatic patients with between 25% and 50% slippage are treated with a brace. The resolution of pain and no progression of slippage is criteria for returning to sports.

Down Syndrome

The athlete with Down syndrome must be carefully evaluated with respect to cervical instability at C_2. Approximately 25% of individuals with Down syndrome demonstrate some level of instability. This instability is secondary to the generalized ligamentous laxity and common occurrence of hypoplasia of the dens or a defect in the posterior ring of C. These children are more difficult to evaluate because of the inability to obtain an accurate history and the increased mobility of their skeletons. In addition, it is much more difficult to obtain adequate flexion-extension lateral radiographs of the cervical spine because of lack of cooperation (Fig. 28-6).

The child with Down syndrome certainly needs initial evaluation prior to athletic participation with a physical examination and radiographs. The child should be followed on a regular basis (every 6 to 12 months). There are no clear-cut guidelines for repeat radiographs. Certainly any changes on clinical examinations should prompt the need for new imaging.

Accurate history taking from a parent or caretaker may elicit signs of atlantoaxial instability. Any signs of decrease in physical tolerance or regression in motor skills should be taken seriously. Changes in gait may represent ataxia.

On the lateral flexion and extension radiographs the atlanto-dens interval is measured. There is no need for concern when this interval is less than 5 mm. Over 9 mm of surgical fusion is necessary. The gray zone between these guidelines is where repeated examinations are a must. Changes in the neurologic examination would necessitate a fusion.

Uncommon Causes of Back Pain

When evaluating a young athlete for back pain, one must remember etiologies unrelated to sports participation. When tumor or infection present as back pain in the pediatric patient, the child may relate the onset of symptoms to minor trauma received during some athletic event. The parents also may assume there is some correlation, particularly in a very active child. The clue to diagnosis is the physical presentation of the child. The child will appear more sickly than one will expect for an injury. The child may be pale and weak. The pain may be out of proportion to the minor injury and does not resolve within the expected time period. Screening radiographs of the spine are necessary. Multiple compression fractures would be indicative of a systemic illness such as leukemia. Destruction of a disc space would suggest infection.

SUMMARY

The primary care physician can detect the more common spine injuries in the young athlete by paying attention to the type of athletic competition and having awareness of the injuries associated with various sports. A careful physical examination will lead to the proper imaging studies. Knowledge of the natural history of the more common problems will help establish guidelines for continues participation in sports.

REFERENCES

1. Blitzer CM, et al: Downhill skiing injuries in children, *Am J Sports Med*, 12(2):142–147, 1984.
2. Burton AK, Tillotson KM: Does leisure sports activity influence lumbar mobility or the risk of low back trouble? *J Spinal Disord* 4(3):329–336, 1991.
3. Cantu RC, Mueller FO: Catastrophic Spine Injuries in Football (1977–1989), *J Spinal Disord* 3(3):227–231, 1990.
4. Ciullo JV, Jackson DW: Pars interarticularis stress reaction. or: Spondylolysis and Spondylolisthesis in gymnasts, *Clin Sports Med* 4(1):95–110, 1985.
5. Hardcastle P, et al: Spinal abnormalities in young fast bowlers, *JBJS* 74B:421–425, 1992.
6. Mann DC, Keen JS, Drummond DS: Unusual Causes of Back Pain in Athletes, *J Spinal Disord* 4(3):337–343, 1991.
7. Micheli LJ: Back Injuries in Gymnastics, *Clin Sports Med* 4(1):85–93, 1985.
8. Oh S: Cervical Injury from Skiing, *Int J Sports Med* 5:268–271, 1984.
9. Pizzutillo PD: Spinal Considerations in the Young Athlete, Instructional Course Lect 42:463–472, 1993.
10. Sward L, et al: Vertebral ring apophysis injury in athletes is the etiology difference in the thoracic and lumbar spine, *Am J Sports Med* 21(6):841–846, 1993.
11. Torg JS, Das M: Trampoline and minitrampoline injuries to the cervical spine, *Clin Sports Med* 4(1):45–60.

REHABILITATION

CHAPTER 29

REHABILITATION TECHNIQUES AND THERAPEUTIC MODALITIES

David A. Gold
Michael Saunders
Gordon Huie

In this chapter, the basic principles for various common techniques and therapeutic modalities in the rehabilitation of a sports medicine patient are discussed. The basic application of these modalities is also described.

In general, after a sports-related injury, the goal of the postinjury therapeutic period is to address pain, inflammation, stiffness, muscle weakness, and muscle spasm. These elements of the injured state can exist individually, but more commonly they are interrelated. Injury causes tissue inflammation, which in turn leads to pain, which may cause muscle spasm and joint stiffness.

Breaking this inflammation-pain-spasm cycle is crucial to a patient's early return to activities. There are certain treatment techniques and therapeutic modalities that can make it a smoother transition. Selection of the appropriate technique or modality is determined by the type of injury, its severity, and the goals of the patient.

The commonly performed treatment techniques available to the patient and therapist are immobilization, mechanical modalities, stretching, and continuous passive motion. The readily available therapeutic strategies are thermotherapy (heat treatments), cryotherapy (cold treatments), and electrical stimulation.

Each of these techniques and modalities is addressed in the following pages of this chapter. Muscle physiology, exact rehabilitation protocols, the specifics of exercise regimens, and the pharmacology of rehabilitation are covered elsewhere in the text.

TREATMENT TECHNIQUES IN REHABILITATION

Immobilization

In sports, as well as in many activities of daily living, injuries to the extremities are quite common. Soft tissue trauma, muscle strains, ligamentous injuries, cartilage damage, and bony fractures are frequently encountered. Immobilization of the affected extremity not only reduces pain, but also prevents further insult until a definitive diagnosis and treatment plan are established. Immobilization can be used to rest an injured or postoperative extremity during the healing phase because it assists in the resolution of swelling and in holding proximate injured tissues still during healing.

In the primary care setting, immobilization is most useful when treating an acutely injured extremity. Depending on the age of the patient, the extremity injured, the tissue involved, and the degree of injury, the use of immobilization will be applied differently.

IMMOBILIZATION FOR SPECIFIC TYPES OF INJURIES. In acute soft tissue contusions there often is muscular injury as well as hematoma formation. Depending on the extent of the injury, extremity immobilization may play a role in the healing process. In a recent study of quadriceps muscle contusions, the authors found that a short course of early immobilization of the knee in flexion assists in returning patients to activity earlier.[1] Most clinicians agree, however, that after a short course of initial immobilization, early motion is essential to avoiding atrophy and joint stiffness.

Muscle strains most often are treated with rest, ice, compression, and elevation in the early periods after an injury. This is usually followed by modalities to reduce pain and swelling, and range-of-motion and strengthening exercises. Immobilization usually is not necessary for this type of injury.

In *ligamentous* injuries such as ankle sprains, the use of immobilization is based on the extent of injury. The goal of immobilization in ligamentous injuries is to assist with pain control and swelling, as well as to prevent additional injury. A padded stirrup-type splint (Fig. 29-1) is useful in treating these injuries. This type of immobilization protects the sprained lateral ligaments but allows for other motions that do not adversely affect the injured tissues (i.e., ankle dorsiflexion and plantar flexion). The immobilization allows for weight-bearing functional rehabilitation without the loss of joint range of motion.

Ligament injuries heal at variable rates and immobilization is prescribed accordingly. The typical healing time required for basic ligamentous sprains varies from three days for minor ankle sprains to eight weeks for moderate to severe sprains.[67]

Immobilization can be used in treating certain types of *cartilage* injuries. Salter fractures in children affect the growing physeal cartilage in varying degrees. Anatomic positioning is vital for appropriate healing. Splints or casts can help in maintaining such position during the healing phase.

Immobilization can play a role in treating other cartilaginous injuries such as osteochondral fractures. After surgical treatment of these injuries, a period of immo-

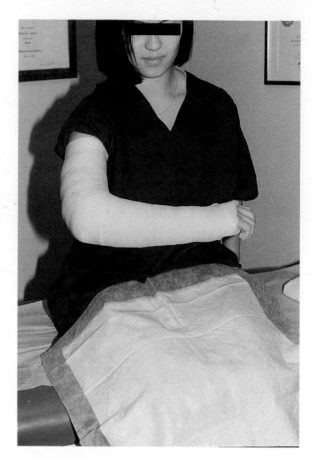

Fig. 29-2. A long arm plaster cast.

bilization is usually necessary to help facilitate early healing.

The most notable use of immobilization is the use of casts (Fig. 29-2) for *fractures*. In general, a period of immobilization is required to maintain alignment and allow for direct bone healing and the formation of fracture callus. The age of the patient, the specific bone fractured, the extent of concomitant soft tissue injury, the need for surgical intervention, and several other factors measure into the type and length of immobilization necessary.

SPECIFIC TYPES OF IMMOBILIZATION. Splinting is similar to cast immobilization except that it is not applied in a circumferential manner. A splint is a rigid device that is applied to one part of an extremity and held in place around the extremity with straps. This allows for easy removal for wound care and other purposes. A splint is usually used for more minor injuries or as an intermediate device between a cast and no immobilization.

A *brace* is a splinting device that spans and stabilizes a joint but may allow for motion of the joint. There are many types of braces available. Braces for the upper extremities include thumb cone splints, wrist splints, elbow immobilizers, and shoulder immobilizers. The spine can be immobilized or protected using thoraco-lumbar-

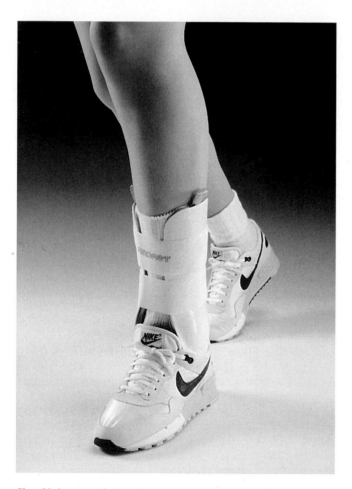

Fig. 29-1. A padded prefabricated ankle stirrup splint. (Courtesy Aircast, Inc.)

sacral orthoses or lumbosacral corsets. Lower extremity braces include hip spica orthoses and various types of knee and ankle splints. Because braces are most commonly used for the knee joint, the following is a discussion of the different types of knee braces. Knee braces can be classified as either prophylactic, functional, or rehabilitative.[76] A *prophylactic knee brace* is designed to protect the knee against or reduce the severity of a sports injury. There is currently no consensus as to whether or not these braces actually achieve this goal. Most of the clinical data on this subject come from studying college athletes.[22,51,62,64] Conflicting conclusions abound, with some studies reporting a protective value for the brace,[62] some studies showing no difference in ligament injury between braced and unbraced players,[22] and some studies suggesting an actual increase in the injury rate among the braced players.[51,64] Teitz and others, for instance, found that braced players had an injury rate of 10.2% compared to 6.2% in the unbraced group.[64] A study by Hewson and others, however, showed no significant difference in the rate of injury between their two groups.[22] Thus the routine use of prophylactic knee braces is limited at this time.[76]

A *functional knee brace* (Fig. 29-3) is designed to provide stability to an unstable knee. These braces, some of which are also called derotational braces, come in several different varieties. Functional knee braces are commonly used for anterior cruciate ligament (ACL)–deficient knees, as well as for some knees after ACL reconstruction, to protect the reconstructed ligament if some level of residual instability persists. The braces are used also during the graft maturation phase of healing, especially in high-profile competitive athletes. A study examining the efficacy of functional knee braces in a group of patients with ACL–deficient knees revealed subjective improvement in 90% and a global improvement of at least one grade of instability when compared to the same knee unbraced.[6] Many other investigators point out, however, that the force applied in objective ligament testing is a fraction of the force applied in normal knee function and in sports participation.[43] It is important to realize that a functional knee brace, although providing some level of added cruciate and collateral ligament stability, is not a reliable substitute for intact ACL.[76] Activity modification, surgical intervention, and a focused physical therapy regimen also play an important role in managing the unstable knee.

The *rehabilitative knee brace* (Fig. 29-4) is a brace with a simple design that protects the injured or postoperative patient from the excesses of motion. It is usually hinged at the joint line with changeable stops to control the extents of flexion and extension. These braces are commonly used after injury or surgery to provide support and stability. Also the brace allows a protected range of motion to help prevent postinjury or postoperative joint stiffness. Smaller, lower-profile models of rehabilitative knee braces are the hinged knee braces designed for protection of collateral ligament injuries.

Patella cut-out neoprene sleeves (Fig. 29-5) provide gentle elastic compression around the knee, theoretically to

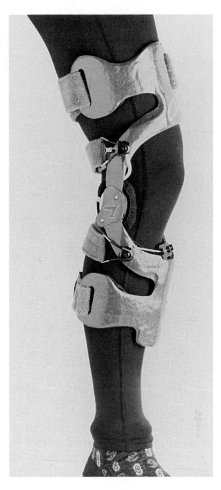

Fig. 29-3. A functional (derotational) knee brace. (Courtesy Sutter Corporation.)

help maintain normal patellar tracking and to provide some proprioceptive feedback and the sensation of additional stability. Some are hinged and some have lateral struts for additional varus-valgus support. The theory that they function to help stabilize the patella throughout the knee range of motion is debatable. A recent study evaluated the effect of a new patellar realignment brace on patellofemoral displacement, using an active-movement kinematic magnetic resonance imager.[55] The study showed that a brace consisting of a neoprene sleeve with a circular silicone and plastic insert to stabilize the patella provided some level of patellofemoral displacement correction in 76% of the knees studied. The radiographic results, however, were not correlated with any clinical data.[55]

Another study compared the effectiveness of a simple elastic knee sleeve, one with a silicone patellar ring, and no brace at all in a population of military recruits with overuse patellofemoral pain.[14] The study concluded that the simple elastic knee sleeve was no more effective than no treatment at all but that it was better than the knee sleeve with the silicone patellar ring.[14]

It is important to remember that immobilization

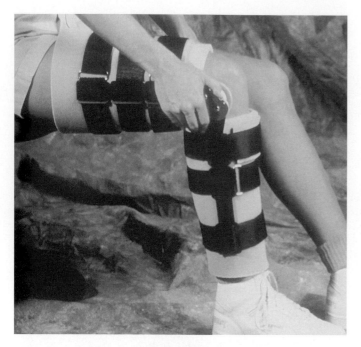

Fig. 29-4. A rehabilitative knee brace. (Courtesy Sutter Corporation.)

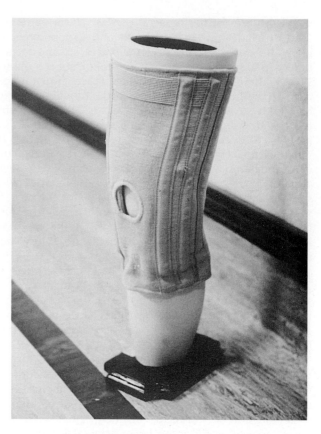

Fig. 29-5. A patella cut-out knee sleeve.

causes some possible deleterious effects to the immobilized tissues. Immobilization can result in muscle atrophy, ligamentous and tendinous stiffening, cartilage dehydration, and osteoporosis.[47] A recent study showed that only nine days of wrist immobilization caused forearm cross-sectional area to decrease by 4.1% and that muscle strength decreased by 29.3% for wrist flexion and 32.5% for extension.[39]

The goal of treatment is to return a patient to the preinjury level of function. It is imperative to take note of potential complications of immobilization so as to most effectively treat a patient. There is a delicate balance between too much and too little immobilization.

Mechanical Modalities

There are several rehabilitation modalities that rely on the mechanical manipulation of tissues. The most commonly used of these are traction and massage.

Traction is used most effectively and efficiently for muscle spasm in the neck or low back, as well as for some spinal nerve impingement conditions.[40] The traction is usually applied in either a continuous mode over the course of 30 to 120 minutes or in an intermittent mode in which the traction is cycled on for 15 to 30 seconds and then released for 5 to 10 seconds. Traction is typically used as an adjunct treatment to other therapeutic modalities.

A recent review of the literature on the efficacy of traction for back and neck pain concluded that most studies are flawed in their design; therefore it remains questionable whether or not traction offers any statistically significant advantage in the management of these conditions.[66] Nonetheless, traction is a commonly employed and popular therapeutic modality.

Massage (Fig. 29-6) is another mechanical modality designed to manually manipulate soft tissues. Most people agree that massage is relaxing and that it feels good, but there is also some science behind its effectiveness. Massage increases local blood circulation, relaxes muscles, and mobilizes and stretches scar tissue.[40] Massage also has been found to reduce levels of creatinine kinase, circulating neutrophil count, and delayed-onset muscle soreness after eccentric exercise, by theoretically interrupting the inflammatory response.[58] Another recent study, however, showed no statistical difference between massage, electrical stimulation, ergometry, and simple rest in reducing delayed onset muscle soreness after exercise.[72] Similarly, Pope in a prospective randomized study, showed that their massage group scored the greatest improvement in extension effort and fatigue time, but that massage offered no significant difference in physical outcome measures, when compared to electrical stimulation or chiropractic spinal manipulation,[48] in treating subacute low back pain. Koes and others found that manual therapy and physiotherapy were effective methods of reducing pain and restoring function in patients with nonspecific back and neck complaints, but they conjectured that much of the improvement was likely due to placebo effects.[27]

Stretching

Stretching is a therapeutic modality usually employed by athletes on their own. Stretching is used to achieve and

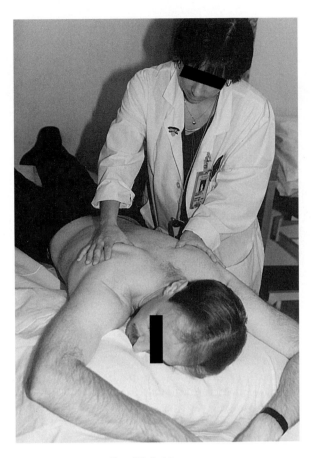

Fig. 29-6. Massage.

maintain maximal joint range of motion and soft tissue excursion. It is most commonly used before participating in sports in the warming-up period, as well as after an injury or surgery to regain passive and active joint range of motion.

The three major types of stretching techniques are static, ballistic, and proprioceptive neuromuscular facilitation (PNF).[68] Static stretching (Fig. 29-7), using a slow and progressive stretch for a period of 10 to 30 seconds, is the most common type used.

Ballistic stretching employs repetitive forceful motions to stretch tissues. An example of ballistic stretching is bouncing forward lunges, with one heel on the ground, designed to stretch the gastrocnemius-soleus-Achilles complex. This technique is less popular than static stretching because it requires more energy and puts the tissues at a higher risk for injury. A recent study comparing static and ballistic stretching found these two techniques to be similar in their ability to increase flexibility.[70]

PNF has been shown to increase the ease and range of extremity motion because it involves alternating muscle contraction with relaxation. Typically, PNF is performed with a therapist, who passively stretches a muscle to its greatest length. The patient then exerts a maximal contraction against resistance, which is followed by additional passive stretching by the therapist.[63] How PNF compares to other stretching techniques remains debatable.[46]

For effectiveness, it is recommended that the local temperature of the tissues be raised before stretching.[68] This can be achieved by some form of light exercise or by the application of heat. Raising the temperature of the soft tissues increases elasticity and optimizes muscle contractions and nerve impulse conductions.[68] A recent study compared passive stretching to no stretching in a small group of patients with short hamstrings. It was found that four weeks of daily home hamstring stretching produced a significant increase in the extensibility and stretching moment tolerated by the hamstrings but that the stretching program did not actually lengthen the muscles nor significantly alter their elasticity.[18]

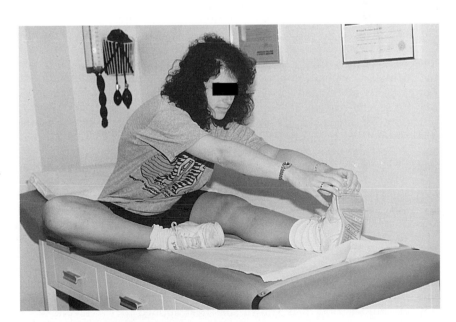

Fig. 29-7. Static stretching of the hamstrings.

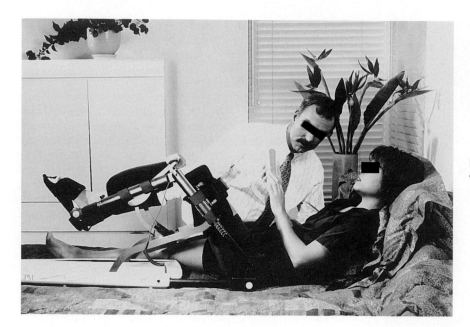

Fig. 29-8. A continuous passive motion machine. (Courtesy Sutter Corporation.)

Continuous Passive Motion

Continuous passive motion (CPM) is a technique designed to provide pure external passive movement to a joint (Fig. 29-8). It was first introduced as a concept in the early 1970s and has since been elaborated and refined. Basic science and clinical studies have validated its use.[52] In addition to playing a role in cartilage, tendon, and ligament healing after injury or surgery,[45,53,75] CPM has been found to increase knee range of motion,[25,34] decrease postoperative swelling,[34] decrease the length of hospital stay,[7,25,71] and decrease the use of narcotic analgesics[7,69] after total knee replacement. Other studies of patients with knee replacements dispute some of these findings.[49]

In animal studies comparing CPM to immobilization, CPM has been shown to increase muscle mass,[16] maintain normal biomechanical properties of tendons,[32] improve joint nutrition,[33,53,57] and prevent joint stiffness.

CPM is commonly used in sports rehabilitation after joint or extremity injury or after surgery when potential stiffness is a major concern. After ACL reconstruction, CPM is often used in the early postoperative period for several reasons: it helps to maintain knee joint nutrition, promotes healing by increasing collagen formation and organization, reduces pain and swelling, and helps achieve and maintain knee range of motion.[19]

THERAPEUTIC MODALITIES IN REHABILITATION

Thermotherapy

Thermotherapy, or heat treatment, has several applications. It is used for pain relief, to improve soft tissue stretching, and to raise the metabolic rate of local tissues. Although the science behind thermotherapy is not fully understood, it is known that heat applied to tissues causes local vasodilatation, which in turn causes analgesia through a variety of mechanisms that serve to raise the pain threshold, decrease muscle spindle activity, and increase local oxygen and other cellular nutrients.[50] It is to be avoided in the treatment of acute injuries, near the eyes, and in areas of abnormal sensation.

There are several ways to apply thermotherapy. Superficial techniques include hydrocollator packs, whirlpool, fluidotherapy, paraffin baths, and infrared heat lamps. Deep techniques include diathermy and ultrasound. Each of these techniques will be reviewed individually.

Hydrocollator packs (Fig. 29-9) are used to apply moist heat. These are composed of a silicone gel wrapped in canvas containers. They are heated in hot water tanks and are able to absorb large amounts of the surrounding heat. They are wrapped in towels before being applied to the affected area, to protect the underlying skin from thermal injury. Hydrocollator packs are used primarily for chronic soft tissue maladies such as muscle spasms, cramps, contusions, and strains. The recommended time of treatment is 15 to 20 minutes.[50]

Whirlpool (Fig. 29-10) is one of the most commonly used therapeutic modalities for applying heat. A whirlpool bath is effective in raising the temperature of the skin and subcutaneous tissues as well as providing gentle fluid massage to the portion of the body immersed in the bath. These effects combine to provide muscle relaxation, increased blood flow, and pain relief. Some of the effects of whirlpool therapy can be augmented by the patient's performing gentle exercises during the treatment.[50] Whirlpool is used primarily for increasing joint range of motion and for treating soft tissue trauma.

Fluidotherapy (Fig. 29-11) is a method of applying heat and massage that involves circulating small solid particles (usually cellulose) in a heated air unit. It compares favorably to other superficial thermotherapy modalities

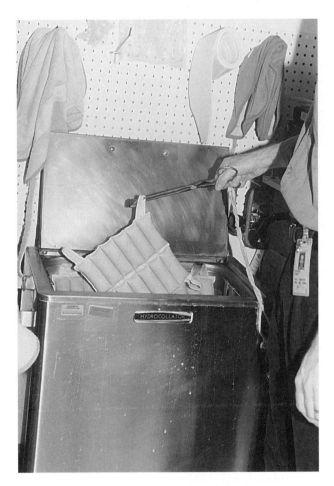

Fig. 29-9. A hydrocollator pack.

in its effectiveness in elevating tissue temperatures.[3] Typically, the affected extremity is exercised in the fluidotherapy unit in an attempt to increase range of motion. There are also units that are designed to treat back problems. A fluidotherapy unit can vary temperature as well as the agitation of the air. It is used to treat muscle spasms, painful soft tissue injuries, and to assist in increasing the range of motion of stiff or injured joints.

Paraffin baths are a very effective way of providing thermotherapy to injured or arthritic hands and feet. This thermotherapy involves immersing the affected extremity into a heated mixture of mineral oil and paraffin wax for a few seconds. After the extremity is removed and the paraffin hardens, the process is repeated several times to form a thick layer. The extremity is then typically soaked in the heated paraffin for about 20 minutes. Another method involves several repetitions of the immersing-hardening cycle followed by wrapping the extremity in a plastic bag and several towels to insulate the heat. The extremity typically is elevated for about 20 minutes and then is exercised. It is important to monitor the patient closely during paraffin treatments because the risk of burns is significantly greater than with other types of thermotherapy.[50] Paraffin baths should not be used for patients with open wounds.

Infrared heat lamps are a relatively inexpensive and simple method of applying superficial heat to a body area. Heat lamps provide a more rapid superficial temperature rise than hydrocollator packs.[50] Surrounding regions not being treated usually are draped off with towels. It is recommended that the treatment area be situated 20 inches from the lamp and that heat be applied for approximately 20 minutes.

Diathermy is a method of applying deep thermotherapy. Diathermy takes advantage of the fact that applying high-frequency electromagnetic current to the skin produces a rise in temperature of deeper tissues. This causes an increase in deep tissue circulation and metabolism as well as a decrease in muscle spasm and pain.[54] Since it is difficult to control and monitor tissue temperature,[65] and since there is a significant degree of variability in the heating patterns produced by different units,[29] diathermy should only be applied by a therapist with expertise in its use. Indications for diathermy include painful inflammatory conditions and osteoarthritis, muscle strains, ligament sprains, tendinopathies, and hematomas.

Diathermy can be applied using shortwave or microwave units. Shortwave diathermy uses radio waves as its power source. It has been shown to be effective in managing pain and swelling, muscle spasm, and joint stiffness,[17] as well as in accelerating wound healing and

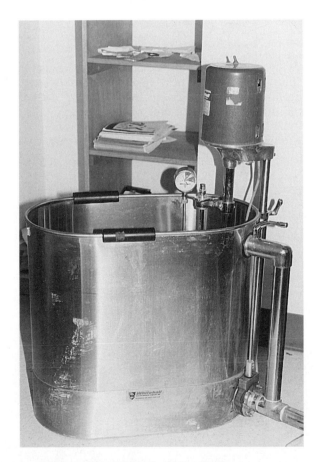

Fig. 29-10. A whirlpool bath.

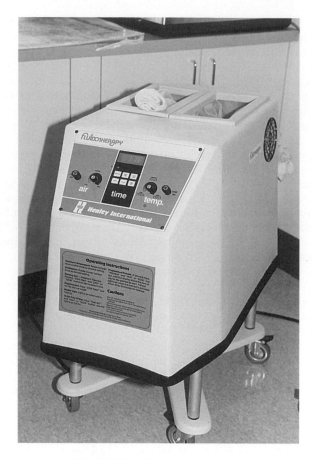

Fig. 29-11. A Fluidotherapy unit.

resolving hematomas.[54] In a recent critical evaluation of the most common physical therapy modalities used for controlling musculoskeletal pain, shortwave diathermy was found to be the one type of heat therapy that had reasonable scientific evidence to support its use.[4]

Microwave diathermy uses higher-frequency electro-magnetic waves than shortwave diathermy, which makes it somewhat more efficient in its energy transmission. Microwave diathermy has been shown to be effective for managing muscle contractures and tenosynovitis,[65] as well as for resolving hematomas.[28]

Ultrasound (Fig. 29-12) is a therapeutic modality that uses high-frequency sound waves to elevate soft tissue temperature. Like other deep heat modalities, ultrasound increases local blood circulation and tissue metabolism. Ultrasound also has been shown to increase cortisol levels in peripheral nerves, which may account for some of its analgesic properties.[54] It is used primarily to treat muscle spasm and pain and, like other forms of heat therapy, is usually avoided in the acute trauma setting. The ultrasound probe is applied to the skin and a glycerin or mineral oil conductive medium is used to facilitate energy transfer. The probe is moved in a circular fashion to prevent any one specific area from being heated too much. Ultrasound has been used successfully to treat numerous maladies including soft tissue pain, muscle spasms, tendon injuries,[50] and back pain.[44,54]

Pulsed ultrasound is a technique that causes primarily nonthermal effects on the treatment tissues, which result in the relief of pain and inflammation. Because there is no significant thermal effect, pulsed ultrasound is sometimes applied in the acute injury setting.[50]

Another application of ultrasound is *phonophoresis*. Phonophoresis is a method of delivering analgesic and anti-inflammatory medication (usually hydrocortisone, lidocaine, or aspirin cream) to local tissues by the use of ultrasound.[50] Cooling the area with ice or heating the area with a hydrocollator pack before phonophoresis have both been shown to improve the absorption and distribution of the applied medicine.[30]

Cryotherapy

Cryotherapy is a commonly employed physical therapy modality that uses the application of cold temperature for treating tissue injuries. Although the science behind

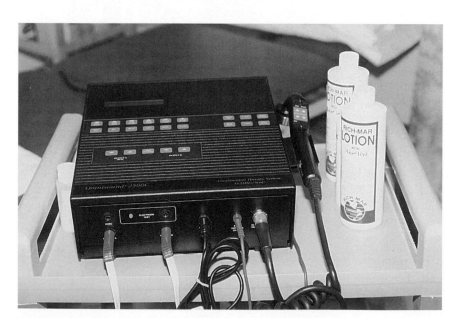

Fig. 29-12. An ultrasound machine and probe.

cryotherapy is not fully understood, it is believed to provide its beneficial effects through mechanisms of vasoconstriction followed by vasodilation, which blocks pain sensory transmission and decreases muscle spasm.

Cryotherapy is particularly useful in the early postinjury period in reducing inflammation, pain, swelling, and muscle spasm.[35,50] Hocutt compared early cryotherapy, late cryotherapy, and heat therapy in the treatment of ankle sprains and found that early cryotherapy was the superior method.[23] As the main component of "RICE" therapy (rest, ice, compression, elevation), ice is used to treat acute musculoskeletal injuries such as sprains, strains, and contusions. Ice decreases swelling, pain, and tissue metabolism, which, in turn, decreases the patient's "down time."

Cryotherapy is commonly used after surgical procedures. Scientific evidence is unclear as to its effectiveness in this setting. Cohn showed that patients receiving cold therapy after anterior cruciate ligament reconstruction required less postoperative pain medication and were converted from injectable to oral pain medication faster than patients not receiving cold therapy.[5] Another study of ACL reconstruction patients, however, showed no difference between those treated and those not treated with cryotherapy with respect to the use of pain medication, length of hospital stay, perceived pain, knee girth, and range of motion.[8] Studies of total knee arthroplasty patients have shown that those given cold compression therapy had significantly less postoperative blood loss, mild improvement in early return of range of motion, and less pain medication requirements than those not receiving cold therapy.[31] A similar study, however, showed no appreciable advantage to a cold compression dressing with respect to range of motion, swelling, wound drainage, or narcotic requirements after total knee arthroplasty.[21]

It has been postulated that the analgesic effect of cryotherapy is probably due to many factors, including an antinociceptive effect on the gate control of pain—a theoretical effect of eliminating or reducing spasm and edema, and of decreasing sensory nerve conduction.[12]

Cold therapy also is useful in the later rehabilitative phase after tissue injury. As in the acute postinjury phase, cooling reduces muscle spasm and sensory nerve conduction in the later rehabilitative phase, which can provide pain relief. Also in the rehabilitative phase, cryotherapy has been shown to be helpful used in conjunction with exercises (cryokinetics).[26]

There are several important contraindications to the use of cold therapy. Absolute contraindications include Raynaud's phenomenon, cardiovascular disease, cryoglobulinemia, and paroxysmal cold hemoglobinuria. Relative contraindications include cold allergy, sensory impairment, and arthritic conditions.[50] Complications of cold therapy include ice burns, frostbite, and nerve palsy.[9]

As in thermotherapy, there are many different ways of applying cryotherapy. These include ice packs, refreezable gel cold packs, chemical cold packs, ice massage, cold compression devices, cold hydrotherapy, and evaporative vapocoolant sprays. In the following pages we review each of these techniques individually.

Ice packs are plastic bags filled with ice. They are inexpensive, readily available, and simple to use. When compared to gel cold packs, chemical cold packs, and a refrigerant gas bladder, ice packs were shown to be superior in their ability to cool deep soft tissues.[36] An ice pack is either simply placed on the affected area or held there with a compressive elastic bandage and the area is elevated. It is recommended that a moist cloth barrier, such as a terry cloth towel, be used between the ice bag and the skin to prevent unwanted "burning" skin reaction. Treatment usually lasts for 15 to 30 minutes.

Refreezable gel cold packs (Fig. 29-13) provide another simple and effective method of applying local cold therapy. They are thin plastic bags containing a flexible refreezable gel. For hygiene reasons, it is recommended that gel cold packs be wrapped in a towel before applica-

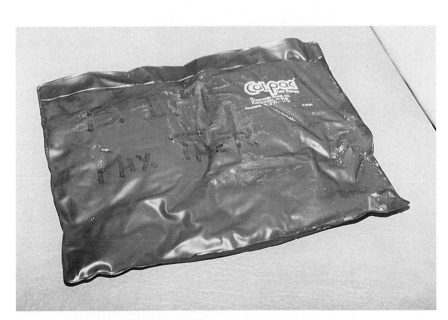

Fig. 29-13. A refreezable gel cold pack.

tion to the skin. Like ice packs, refreezable gel cold packs are often applied in conjunction with compression and elevation and are usually applied for 15 to 30 minutes.

Chemical cold packs involve the mixing of two chemicals to produce an endothermic cooling reaction. These packs are less commonly used because they cool in an inconsistent manner, are relatively expensive, are not reusable, and can cause a chemical burn if the packs leak their contents.[40]

Ice massage involves freezing a paper or Styrofoam cup full of water and then removing the block of ice from the cup and directly massaging it into the treatment area. Massage is usually done for approximately five to ten minutes, until analgesia is achieved. It is most commonly used for back pain and painful inflammatory conditions such as tendinitis. Ice massage compares favorably with electrical stimulation in the treatment of low back pain.[37]

A cold *compression device* (Fig. 29-14) is a commercially manufactured unit composed of a cold substance that is circulated into a sleeve covering and compressing the treatment area. It is an effective method of cooling tissues to assist in pain and edema control. There is con-

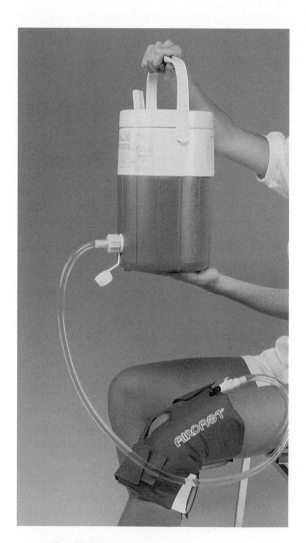

Fig. 29-14. A knee cold compression unit.

flicting evidence as to its usefulness after knee replacement or ligament reconstruction.[5,8,21,31]

Cold hydrotherapy is low-temperature whirlpool treatment, usually in the 55° to 65° F range. Cold hydrotherapy provides excellent contact with and cooling of an affected extremity. It is used most commonly for upper and lower extremity injuries. Cold hydrotherapy is usually avoided in patients with acute postinjury edema since the extremity must be placed in a dependent position in the unit.

Evaporative vapocoolant sprays cool the skin on contact by the rapid evaporation of methyl fluoride or ethyl chloride. They are most commonly used in combination with other therapies to treat myofascial disorders, and to stretch out areas of pain, muscle spasm, and joint stiffness. Typically, the coolant is sprayed onto the affected area and then stretching or massage is begun. It is important to avoid inhaling the vapors and to avoid inducing frostbite.

Electrical Stimulation

Electrical stimulation is used as a rehabilitative therapeutic modality primarily to reduce pain and to assist in muscle strengthening. Although the specific mechanisms of its action have not been entirely made clear, electrical stimulation has been found to be effective in various clinical situations.

In this section, the basic principles behind electrical stimulation as a therapeutic modality are discussed and the most common applications of this technique are described.

PRINCIPLES OF ELECTRICAL STIMULATION. It has been known since the 18th century than an electric current can cause a muscle to contract. This action involves the depolarization of nerve fibers in response to an electrical impulse placed on the surface of the skin. Biologic tissues offer both resistance and variability to current flow because of its nonhomogenous nature. Other determinants of current flow are its wave amplitude, frequency, and wave form.

Electrical stimulation gives the clinician the opportunity to alter the normal electrical characteristics and thus the cellular environment of biologic tissues. Because all tissues contain positively and negatively charged ions, applying electricity can cause these ions to move in such a way as to increase the cellular activity of the tissues. The resulting change in cellular activity can be associated with pain control, involuntary muscle contraction, and injured tissue healing.

For rehabilitative purposes, the electrical current is most commonly applied through surface electrodes connected to an alternating current source. Most current sources offer the clinician the option of varying wave form, pulse width and amplitude, and frequency. These parameters are manipulated to obtain the desired clinical effect.

ELECTRICAL STIMULATION FOR PAIN CONTROL. Upon the description of the gate theory of pain in 1965,[38] scientists began experimenting with electrical stimulation in an attempt to modulate a patient's perception of pain by "closing" the pain "gate." This gave

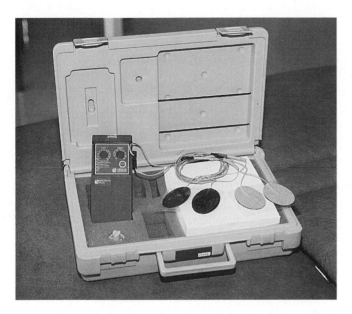

Fig. 29-15. A transcutaneous electric nerve stimulation (TENS) unit.

rise to the development of the transcutaneous electric nerve stimulation (TENS) unit (Fig. 29-15).

Although studies have documented the effectiveness of TENS for pain control, there is little agreement as to the way it works. In fact, although many different types of units exist with the ability to vary multiple parameters, no one particular type of unit or regimen has emerged as being more effective than any other.[24] Nonetheless, several theories have been proposed, including the stimulation of endorphin and enkephalin release,[2] the electrical blocking of afferent pain impulses,[2] and the triggering of a central pain inhibition center.[61]

TENS applies an electrical stimulus in such a way as to inhibit pain fiber nerve transmission and, at the same time, stimulates large afferent fibers, which also theoretically assists in "closing the gate" to pain transmission. Another way of using TENS is to alter the frequency of electrical current so as to induce the release of endogenous opiates, thus helping to control pain.[11]

Although it is difficult to measure the effectiveness of any type of pain control regimen because of the inherent subjectivity involved, there are studies that support the use of TENS for pain control.[60] Although TENS has been used for nearly all types of pain, it is most commonly used as an adjunct treatment for pain that arises from acute trauma and surgical procedures. It has been shown to be effective in improving acute as well as chronic low back pain.[13,54] It is usually applied once daily for 20 minutes for several days' duration, but particular protocols vary depending on the type and location of pain.

TENS is also useful as adjunct therapy when pain is limiting the progression of a global rehabilitation protocol (i.e., ACL reconstruction rehabilitation, shoulder capsular reconstruction rehabilitation). In these situations, especially in the early post-operative period when oral analgesic medication is only partially effective, TENS can provide an additional method of pain control to allow specific rehabilitation goals to be achieved.

Although TENS has been applied in many conditions, few scientific data to support its use in controlling chronic pain syndromes exist.[15] It is also important to remember that there are known contraindications to the use of TENS for pain control.[42] TENS should be avoided in patients with cardiac pacemakers, in those who are pregnant, and in patients with an unclear etiology of pain. TENS applied to the head theoretically can affect seizure threshold and vascular activity and is not recommended. TENS also can be dangerous when applied in the region of the carotid sinus because it can elicit reflex hypotension; thus it is not recommended. TENS should be avoided in an anterior to posterior plane in the transthoracic region because of the possibility of inducing a cardiac arrhythmia.[42]

In general, TENS remains somewhat of an enigma. It is difficult to discern from available scientific data its applicability to any given pain situation. It also remains difficult to pinpoint its actual mechanism of pain modulation. Nonetheless, TENS is commonly and effectively used for acute and postoperative pain and as an adjunct therapy to a rehabilitation protocol that is being slowed by pain.

Another application of electrical stimulation for pain control is the point stimulator. The point stimulator elicits a brain stem response to inhibit pain by a focused, high-intensity, low-frequency current. This type of electrical analgesia has been likened to acupuncture.[40]

ELECTRICAL STIMULATION FOR MUSCLE STRENGTHENING. Since it is known that surface electrical stimulation can elicit muscle contractions, this modality has been used in the rehabilitative strengthening of muscles in the postoperative and postinjury periods when voluntary muscle contraction may be limited. It has also been applied to the strengthening of otherwise-normal muscles.

In the postoperative or postinjury patient population, electrical stimulation can be used to rehabilitate muscles. In general, electrodes are placed in such a way as to excite the motor nerve to the muscle of group of muscles being stimulated. A tetanic muscle contraction is induced and maintained for a period of seconds.

This has been reported to be useful, when combined with a regimen of strengthening exercises, in preventing muscle atrophy and loss of strength after major knee ligament surgery.[10,74] Snyder-Mackler and others found that patients who received electrical stimulation after ACL reconstruction had stronger quadriceps and a more normal gait pattern than those who did not.[59] There are other articles in the literature, however, that show no significant difference in long-lasting strength gains and/or muscle mass when comparing an exercise group with an exercise plus electrical stimulation–group.[56] It also has been suggested that many of the gains made by electrical stimulation are lost after a period of time.

Electrical stimulation has been applied to normal muscles with hopes of building both strength and muscle mass. The main problem encountered in this application is that, typically, the muscle contraction elicited by electrical stimulation is not as strong as the contraction produced by a patient's own maximal voluntary effort. Since strength gains are directly proportional to the ability to contract muscles as strongly as possible, electrical stimulation has only a theoretical role at this time.

OTHER APPLICATIONS OF ELECTRICAL STIMULATION. Electrical current can be used to help deliver certain medications to the tissues beneath the skin. This process, called *iontophoresis*, takes advantage of the ionized nature of certain medications (most commonly salicylates and hydrocortisone). When electrodes are positioned in the appropriate fashion, low-voltage electrical stimulation can actually repel the medication away from the electric source and drive it into the symptomatic tissues. Iontophoresis is most commonly used as an adjunct treatment for acute soft tissue conditions such as muscle strains and contusions, bursitis, and tendinitis. It has also been shown to be useful in treating traumatic myositis ossificans.[73] A recent study showed that dexamethasone iontophoresis significantly decreased the perception of muscle soreness but did not significantly alter maximal muscle contraction, peak torque, or work.[20]

Interferential electrical stimulation is similar to other types of electrical analgesia except in the configuration and type of electrodes used. Essentially, paired biphasic electrodes are used in concert to deliver the current, which allows the current intensity to be lessened but still provide as good or even better therapeutic response.

Electrical stimulation has been studied to assess its applicability to *soft tissue healing*. Although animal studies have been performed, few methods are applicable to human subjects. One clinical study assessing the use of electrical stimulation in ankle sprains showed no significant difference between ankles treated with electrical stimulation and those that were not.[65] The applicability for the routine use of electrical stimulation for soft tissue healing has yet to be determined.

REFERENCES

1. Aronen JA, Chronister R, Ove P, McDevitt ER: Thigh contusions: Minimizing the length of time before return to full athletic activities with early immobilization in 120 degrees of knee flexion. Presented at the American Orthopaedic Society for Sports Medicine Annual Meeting, Sun Valley, Idaho, July 16–19, 1990.
2. Bishop B: Pain: Its physiology and rationale for management, *Phys Ther* 60:13–37, 1980.
3. Borrell RM, Parker R, Henley EJ, Masley D, Repinecz M: Comparison of *in vivo* temperatures produced by hydrotherapy, paraffin wax treatment, and fluidotherapy, *Phys Ther* 60:1273–1276, 1980.
4. Chapman CE: Can the use of physical modalities for pain control be rationalized by the research evidence? *Can J Physiol Pharmacol* 69:704–712, 1991.
5. Cohn BT, Draeger RI, Jackson DW: The effects of cold therapy in the postoperative management of pain in patients undergoing anterior cruciate ligament reconstruction, *Am J Sports Med* 17:344–349, 1989.
6. Colville MR, Lee CL, Ciullo JV: The Lenox Hill Brace: An evaluation of effectiveness in treating knee instability, *Am J Sports Med* 14:257–261, 1986.
7. Colwell CW Jr, Morris BA: The influence of continuous passive motion on the results of total knee arthroplasty, *Clin Orthop* 276:225–228, 1992.
8. Daniel DM, Stone ML, Arendt DL: The effect of cold therapy on pain, swelling, and range of motion after anterior cruciate ligament reconstructive surgery, *Arthroscopy* 10:530–533, 1994.
9. Drez D, Faust DC, Evans JP: Cryotherapy and nerve palsy, *Am J Sports Med* 9:256–257, 1981.
10. Eriksson E, Haggmark T: Comparison of isometric muscle training and electrical stimulation supplementing isometric muscle training in the recovery after major knee ligament surgery: A preliminary report, *Am J Sports Med* 7:169–171, 1979.
11. Eriksson MBE, Sjolund BH, Nielzen S: Long term results of peripheral conditioning stimulation as an analgesic measure in chronic pain, *Pain* 6:335–347, 1979.
12. Ernst E, Fialka V: Ice freezes pain? A review of the clinical effectiveness of analgesic cold therapy, *J Pain Symptom Manage* 9:56–59, 1994.
13. Ersek RA: Low-back pain: Prompt relief with transcutaneous neurostimulation, *Orthop Rev* 5:12–16, 1976.
14. Finestone A, Radin EL, Lev B, Shlamkovitch N, et al: Treatment of overuse patellofemoral pain: Prospective randomized controlled clinical trial in a military setting, *Clin Orthop* 293:208–210, 1993.
15. Fried T, Johnson R, McCracken W: Transcutaneous electrical nerve stimulation: Its role in the control of chronic pain, *Arch Phys Med Rehabil* 65:228–231, 1984.
16. Gebhard JS, Kabo JM, Meals RA: Passive motion: The dose effects on joint stiffness, muscle mass, bone density, and regional swelling. A study in an experimental model following intra-articular injury, *J Bone Joint Surg* 75:1636–1647, 1993.
17. Goats GC: Continuous short-wave (radio-frequency) diathermy, *Br J Sports Med* 23:123–127, 1989.
18. Halberstan JP, Goeken LN: Stretching exercises: Effect on passive extensibility and stiffness in short hamstrings of healthy subjects, *Arch Phys Med Rehabil* 75:976–981, 1994.
19. Halling AH, Howard ME, Cawley PW: Rehabilitation of anterior cruciate ligament injuries, *Clin Sports Med* 12:329–348, 1993.
20. Hasson SM, Wible CL, Reich M: Dexamethasone iontophoresis: Effect on delayed muscle soreness and muscle function, *Can J Sports Sci* 17:8–13, 1992.
21. Healy WL, Seidman J, Pfeifer BA, Brown DG: Cold compressive dressing after total knee arthroplasty, *Clin Orthop* 229:143–146, 1994.
22. Hewson GR Jr, Mendini RA, Wong JB: Prophylactic knee bracing in college football, *Am J Sports Med* 14:262–266, 1986.
23. Hocutt JE Jr, Jaffe R, Rylander CR, Beebe JK: Cryotherapy in ankle sprains, *Am J Sports Med* 10:316–319, 1982.
24. Jensen JE, Etheridge GL, Hazelrigg G: Effectiveness of transcutaneous electrical neural stimulation in the treatment of pain. Recommendations for use in the treatment of sports injuries, *Sports Med* 3:79–88, 1986.
25. Johnson DP: The effect of continuous passive motion on wound-healing and joint mobility after knee arthroplasty, *J Bone Joint Surg* 72:421–426, 1990.
26. Knight KL Londeree BR: Comparison of blood flow in the ankle of uninjured subjects during therapeutic applications of heat, cold, and exercise, *Med Sci Sports Exerc* 12:76–80, 1980.
27. Koes BW, Bouter LM, van Mameren H, et al: The effectiveness of manual therapy, physiotherapy, and treatment by the general practitioner for nonspecific back and neck complaints. A randomized clinical trial, *Spine* 17:28–35, 1992.

28. Lehmann JF, Dundore DE, Esselman PC, Nelp WB: Microwave diathermy: Effects on experimental muscle hematoma resolution, *Arch Phys Med Rehabil* 64:127–129, 1983.

29. Lehmann JF, McDougall JA, Guy AW, Warren CG, Esselman PC: Heating patterns produced by shortwave diathermy applicators in tissue substitute models, *Arch Phys Med Rehabil* 64:575–577, 1983.

30. Lehman JF, Warren CG, Scham SM: Therapeutic heat and cold, *Clin Orthop* 99:207–245, 1974.

31. Levy AS, Marmar E: The role of cold compression dressings in the postoperative treatment of total knee arthroplasty, *Clin Orthop* 297:174–178, 1993.

32. Loitz BJ, Zernicke RF, Vailas AC, Kody MH, Meals RA: Effect of short-term immobilization versus continuous passive motion on the biomechanical and biochemical properties of the rabbit tendon, *Clin Orthop* 244:265–271, 1989.

33. McDonough AL: Effects of immobilization and exercise on articular cartilage—a review of literature, *J Orthop Sports Phys Ther* 3:2–4, 1981.

34. McInnes J, Larson MG, Daltroy LH: A controlled evaluation of continuous passive motion in patients undergoing total knee arthroplasty, *JAMA* 268:1423–1428, 1992.

35. McMaster WC: A literary review on ice therapy in injuries, *Am J Sports Med* 5:124–126, 1977.

36. McMaster WC, Liddle S, Waugh TR: Laboratory evaluation of various cold therapy modalities, *Am J Sports Med* 6:291–294, 1978.

37. Melzack R, Jeans ME, Stratford JG, Monks RC: Ice massage and transcutaneous electrical stimulation: Comparison of treatment for low-back pain, *Pain* 9:209–217, 1980.

38. Melzack R, Wall PD: Pain mechanisms: A new theory, *Science* 150:971–979, 1965.

39. Miles MP, Clarkson PM, Bean M: Muscle function at the wrist following nine days of immobilization and suspension, *Med Sci Sports Exerc* 26:615–623, 1994.

40. American Academy of Orthopaedic Surgeons: Modalities. In *Athletic Training and Sports Medicine,* ed 2, Rosemont, Ill, 1991, The Academy.

41. Namba RS, Kabo JM, Dorey FJ, Meals RA: Continuous passive motion versus immobilization. The effect on posttraumatic joint stiffness, *Clin Orthop* 267:218–223, 1991.

42. Neuromuscular stimulation. Presented at The International Academy of Physio Therapeutics, Electrotherapy and Ultrasound Update, November 19–20, 1994.

43. Noyes FR, Grood ES, Butler DL, Malek M: Clinical laxity tests and functional stability of the knee: Biomechanical concepts, *Clin Orthop* 146:84–89, 1980.

44. Nwuga VC: Ultrasound in the treatment of back pain resulting from prolapsed intervertebral disc, *Arth Phys Med Rehabil* 64:88–89, 1983.

45. O'Driscoll SW, Salter RB: The induction of neochondrogenesis in free intraarticular periosteal autografts under the influence of continuous passive motion, *J Bone Joint Surg* 66:1248–1257, 1984.

46. Osternig LR, Robertson R, Troxel R, Hansen P: Muscle activation during proprioceptive neuromuscular facilitation stretching techniques, *Am J Phys Med* 66:298–307, 1987.

47. Paulos LE, Grauer JD: Exercise. In DeLee JC, Drez D, editors: *Orthopaedic sports medicine: principles and practice,* Philadelphia, 1994, W.B. Saunders.

48. Pope MH, Phillips RB, Haugh LD: A prospective randomized three-week trial of spinal manipulation, transcutaneous muscle stimulation, massage and corset in the treatment of subacute low back pain, *Spine* 19:2571–2577, 1994.

49. Ritter MA, Gandolf VS, Holston KS: Continuous passive motion versus physical therapy in total knee arthroplasty, *Clin Orthop* 244:239–243, 1989.

50. Rivenburgh DW: Physical modalities in the treatment of tendon injuries, *Clin Sports Med* 11:645–659, 1992.

51. Rovere GD, Haupt HA, Yates CS: Prophylactic knee bracing in college football, *Am J Sports Med* 15:111–116, 1987.

52. Salter RB: The biologic concept of continuous passive motion of synovial joints. The first 18 years of basic research and its clinical application, *Clin Orthop* 242:12–25, 1989.

53. Salter RB, Simmonds DF, Malcolm BW, et al: The biological effect of continuous passive motion on the healing of full thickness defects in articular cartilage, *J Bone Joint Surg* 62:1232–1251, 1980.

54. Santiesteban AJ: The role of physical agents in the treatment of spine pain, *Clin Orthop* 179:24–30, 1983.

55. Shellock FG, Mink JH, Deutsch AL: Effect of a patellar realignment brace on patellofemoral relationships: Evaluation with kinematic MR imaging, *J Magn Reson Imaging* 4:590–594, 1994.

56. Sisk TD, Stalka SW, Deering MB, Griffen JW: Effect of electrical stimulation on quadriceps strength after reconstructive surgery of the anterior cruciate ligament, *Am J Sports Med* 13:215–220, 1985.

57. Skyhar MJ, Danzig LA, Hargens AR, Akeson WH: Nutrition of the anterior cruciate ligament. Effects of continuous passive motion, *Am J Sports Med* 13:415–418, 1985.

58. Smith LL, Keating MN, Holbert D: The effects of athletic massage on delayed onset muscle soreness, creatinine kinase, and neutrophil count: A preliminary report, *J Orthop Sports Phys Ther* 19:93–99, 1994.

59. Snyder-Mackler L, Ladin Z, Schepsis AA, Young JC: Electrical stimulation of the thigh muscles after reconstruction of the anterior cruciate ligament, *J Bone Joint Surg* 73:1025–1036, 1991.

60. Solomon RA, Vienstein MC, Long DM: Reduction of postoperative pain and narcotic use by transcutaneous electrical nerve stimulation, *Surgery* 87:142–146, 1980.

61. Soric R, Devlin M: Transcutaneous electrical nerve stimulation: Practical aspects and applications, *Postgrad Med* 78:101–107, 1985.

62. Taft TN, Hunter S, Fundurbeck CH Jr: Preventative lateral knee bracing in football. Presented at the American Orthopaedic Society for Sports Medicine Annual Meeting, Nashville, Tennessee, July 2, 1985.

63. Tanigawa MC: Comparison of the hold-relax procedure and passive mobilization on increasing muscle length, *Phys Ther* 52:725–735, 1972.

64. Teitz CC, Hermanson BK, Kronmal RA, Diehr PH: Evaluation of the use of braces to prevent injury to the knee in collegiate football players, *J Bone Joint Surg* 69:2–9, 1987.

65. American Academy of Orthopaedic Surgeons: Therapeutic modalities in sports medicine. In Griffin LY, editor: *Orthopaedic knowledge update: Sports medicine,* Rosemont, Ill, 1994, AAOS.

66. van der Heijden GJ, Beurskens AJ, Koes BW: The efficacy of traction for back and neck pain: A systematic, blinded review of randomized clinical trial methods, *Phys Ther* 75:93–104, 1995.

67. Vegso JJ: Ankle sprain: Nonoperative management. In Torg JS, Shephard RJ, editors: *Current therapy in sports medicine,* ed 3, St. Louis, 1995, Mosby–Year Book.

68. Vegso JJ: Principles of stretching. In Torg JS, Shephard RJ, editors: *Current therapy in sports medicine,* ed 3, St. Louis, 1995, Mosby–Year Book.

69. Walker RH, Morris BA, Angulo DL: Postoperative use of continuous passive motion, transcutaneous electrical nerve stimulation, and continuous cooling pad following total knee arthroplasty, *J Arthroplasty* 6:151–156, 1991.

70. Wallin D, Ekblom B, Graham R, Nordenborg T: Improve-

ment of muscle flexibility: A comparison between two techniques, *Am J Sports Med* 13:263–268, 1985.

71. Wasilewski SA, Woods LC, Togerson WR Jr., Healy WL: Value of continuous passive motion in total knee arthroplasty, *Orthopaedics* 13:291–295, 1990.

72. Weber MD, Servedio FJ, Woodall WR: The effects of three modalities on delayed onset muscle soreness, *J Orthop Sports Phys Ther* 20:236–242, 1994.

73. Wieder DL: Treatment of traumatic myositis ossificans with acetic acid iontophoresis, *Phys Ther* 72:133–137, 1992.

74. Wigerstad-Lossing I, Grimby G, Jonsson T: Effects of electrical muscle stimulation combined with voluntary contractions after knee ligament surgery, *Med Sci Sports Exerc* 20:93–98, 1988.

75. Williams JM, Moran M, Thonar EJ, Salter RB: Continuous passive motion stimulates repair of rabbit knee articular cartilage after matrix proteoglycan loss, *Clin Orthop*, 304: 252–262, 1994.

76. Wirth MA, DeLee JC: The history and classification of knee braces, *Clin Sports Med* 9:731–741, 1990.

CHAPTER 30

THE LOWER EXTREMITY

Robert S. Gotlin

The appendicular and axial skeleton are the lattice that maintains the stability of our upright posture. Through the highly sophisticated coordination of the neuromusculoskeletal system, the appendicular skeleton, comprising the upper and lower extremities, and the axial skeleton, comprising the vertebral column and pelvis, form the biomechanical structures that allow purposeful movement. Every one of our actions is a process of patterned, programmed, and skillfully regulated information processed through the central nervous system. A delicate blend of force production and absorption allows our lower extremity muscles to propel our bodies.

Particularly vulnerable to injury, the lower extremities constantly accept forces from the environment. Just as a force is produced by the body onto the surface below as a person makes foot-to-floor contact, an equal force is produced by the surface (ground reactive) onto the body above. Rehabilitation programs must include both force production (acceleration) and force absorption (deceleration) strategies. The lower extremities—hip, thigh, knee, leg, ankle, and feet—are closely related in functional activities and must all be considered when we focus on a specific disability. Although the emphasis in treating injuries of the lower extremities initially is on the joint or region involved, the ultimate rehabilitation program emphasizes training the entire lower limb. Our obligation as clinicians is not merely to treat dysfunction but also to determine its etiology. A thorough biomechanical analysis of the specific motions required by an injured athlete's sport is very helpful in customizing a rehabilitation program. In our training, the development of skill is the goal. The components of skill are many and the techniques for achieving it varied.

Coordination, stability, force production, and force absorption are four key elements to mastering a task. All play an important role in various levels of activities, and each must be addressed as part of skill training. It is our experience that success is not fully appreciated unless this is accomplished.

Coordination, as described in motor learning, integrates the nervous system's ability to regulate the interaction of agonist and antagonist muscles.[22] The ordered firing of motor units on the cellular level, in synchrony with the actions of the muscles of the body on the macro level, lays the foundation for purposeful movement. The ability of a torso muscle to contract and stabilize the trunk while a seemingly unassociated limb muscle contracts to produce a movement is an example of this. Without the coordinated contraction of the torso muscle group, the action carried out by the lower limb muscle group would probably be off balance, inefficient, and not purposeful. Rehabilitating a specific part of a lower limb actually encompasses a much broader scope of training than merely focusing on the isolated injured area.

Stability is the component of skill that allows for the use of agonist and antagonist muscle groups to maintain balance over the center of gravity. Much of the training for balance is done in positions of "off balance" so that the body can more easily accommodate when challenged from a position of "on" balance to one of "off" balance. An example of this is the tossing and catching of a weighted ball while standing on a balance board such as a BAPS (biomechanical ankle platform system, CAMP, Jackson, Michigan).

Force production concepts are familiar to most people. Weight training to improve strength, sprinting to decrease race time, and repetitive jumping to improve vertical leap are examples of force production training techniques. In the gym force production is translated to bench pressing for improving pectoralis strength, or knee extension exercises to improve quadriceps strength.

Force absorption directly relates to the ability of the antagonist muscle groups to control the action of the agonist groups. Consider the fact that if it were not for the ability of the shoulder decelerators to slow down a ball player's overhand pitch, the upper extremity would propel in a forward direction unchecked except by the anatomic limits of the shoulder's bone, ligament, muscle, and skin—a highly inefficient technique and detrimental to the athlete. There has been a significant deficit in training for force absorption in many rehabilitation protocols, and much of our training is now focused in this area.

In our discussion we will survey select disabilities of the lower limb and offer guidelines for the management of each. The components of skill will be incorporated into each strategy when appropriate.

FOOT AND ANKLE

Often the foot and ankle complex serves as the first line of contact between the environment and the body, so an athlete's ankle is one of the most frequently injured joints.[23,58] The basic function of the ankle and subtalar joint complex has been likened to a universal joint.[34] The interaction of these two joints allows for both static and dynamic support of the ankle while each serves to accommodate for a deficiency in the other. A practitioner should evaluate each of them separately when developing a rehabilitation program. Too often an athlete injures his/her ankle and is told, "Just ice and rest it and it will be OK." We must not assume that all ankle sprains are minor and will simply "get better." Twenty-five to 40% of people with ankle sprains have chronic disability and instability.[5] This kind of injury is most common in runners.[5,18] It is rare to treat an athlete who has never sustained an ankle sprain at one time or another.

In general, most injuries to the ankle follow acute trauma, but up to 30% of injuries are related to overuse.[18] Overuse injuries often are more difficult to treat because the associated anatomy usually is more negatively affected and the psyche of the athlete does not allow enough down time to recoup. One of the most challenging athletes to treat is a dedicated runner. It is important for the clinician to be inventive and imaginative when choreographing a treatment plan for this group. The so-called "runner's high" is a strong force that resists keeping a runner off his/her feet.

The rehabilitation strategies for treating foot and ankle disabilities largely overlap. In common to most is a period of rest, ice, compression, and elevation (RICE). The specifics of each of these have been described in the chapter on spine rehabilitation. One difference in treating the ankle and foot is the length of time for the period of rest. In treating the foot and ankle complex for a sprain or strain, a protracted period of relative rest may be required before the patient returns to aggressive weight bearing. Since the foot and ankle are under constant stress in the gait cycle, two weeks is probably a conservative guide to restricting "normal" activities and protecting this complex. However, weight bearing, for even the most severe sprains, may be beneficial because it can actually reduce inflammation and decrease pain. Even the most minor sprains and strains take approximately six weeks to heal, and this must be considered when deciding on the appropriate time for relative rest. It is a good idea to keep the foot and ankle protected with a supportive device, at least throughout this early healing phase.

Rehabilitation of the foot and ankle is essentially the same regardless of complaint. The basic problems are strains (Achilles tendon, posterior tibial tendon, extensor hallucis longus tendon), sprains (anterior and posterior talofibular ligament, calcaneofibular ligament, deltoid ligament), hyperpronation syndrome, plantar fasciitis, peroneal tendon dislocation, heel pain (plantar fasciitis, retrocalcaneal bursitis, tendo-Achilles bursitis), seronegative spondyloarthropathies (bone tumor, tarsal tunnel syndrome, calcaneal disorders, sciatica), turf toe, and fractures. A generalized rehabilitation program for foot and ankle disorders will be offered after a brief description of specific recommendations for some.

Sprains are classified as grades I to III, as indicated in Tables 30-1 and 30-2.[3,5,34] Generally, a mild sprain is grade I and a severe sprain grade III. Grade I usually connotes a mild tear of ligamentous structures with minimal pain and disability. Grade III signifies a relatively unstable structure (for example, greater than 3 mm side-to-side anterior displacement on anterior drawer test, or greater than 10 degrees talar tilt on stress radiography for anterior talofibular ligament sprain) with significant pain and disability. Weight bearing for all three phases is guided by pain and swelling. As soon as the patient is able to bear weight, and when swelling has subsided, progress toward full weight bearing can begin. Ankle support should continue for at least three to four weeks after the injury to foster ligamentous healing, including collagen proliferation and maturation. To reduce stress on injured ligaments or muscles, a wedge can be added to footwear. For Achilles tendinitis, a heel wedge can be added. It should be of sufficient height to free the Achilles from gait-cycle stresses. A ⅜-inch felt pad can elevate the heel sufficiently to lessen stress on the Achilles tendon.[31] For posterior tibial tendinitis, a medial wedge can be added. For flexor hallucis tendinitis, a rigid plantar splint is beneficial in limiting motion of the great toe. For acute strains these are worn until symptoms subside, and for chronic strains their use may be more protracted.

Hyperpronation syndrome (dynamic pronation, i.e., the foot that "flattens" as one transfers from heel strike to foot flat in the gait cycle) and plantar fasciitis often are present simultaneously, and the former may indeed cause the latter. Hyperpronation syndrome, which is noted by increased medial drift of the ankle complex (forefoot abduction) on weight bearing, is a relatively common cause of foot and ankle pain. It is not likened to pes planus, or the fixed flat foot. A person with hyperpronation syndrome maintains a medial longitudinal arch, with the foot not in contact with the floor, but tends to lose or flatten this arch when bearing weight. This repetitive motion tends to stretch the plantar surface and produce pain and disability. Knee pain, particu-

Table 30-1. Practical universal classification of sprains/strains

Grade	Symptoms[a]	Signs[a]	Stability	Anatomy[b]
1	pain—0–2 swelling—0–2 disability—0–2	edema—0–2 tenderness—0–2 function loss—0–2	stable	< 20% fibers torn; internal micro damage (micromechanical dissociation) with full continuity
2	pain—3 swelling—3 disability—3	edema—3 tenderness—3 function loss—4 ecchymosis 30%–50%	unstable + solid endpoint	20%–70% fibers torn; mechanical dissociation with partial loss of continuity
3	pain—4 swelling—4 disability—4	edema—4 tenderness—4 function loss—4 ecchymosis 70%–90% palpable mass— strain only palpable gap	unstable + no/mushy endpoint	> 70% fibers torn; total rupture

Note: Pain, tenderness, swelling, edema, and function loss are graded on a 0-to-4 scale with 0 = absent, 1 = minimal, 2 = mild, 3 = moderate, 4 = severe.
[a]Injuries seen during the golden period have no or minimal pain, swelling, ecchymosis, or tenderness.
[b]Sprain: ligament fibers are torn; strain: muscle-tendon unit is torn.
From Birrer RB: Ankle injuries. In Birrer RB, ed, *Sports medicine for the primary care physician,* ed 2, Boca Raton, Fla, 1994, CRC, p 310.

larly of the patellofemoral joint, is sometimes caused by hyperpronation. It is clearly understood that the valgus knee drift that accompanies foot pronation is certainly a factor in patellofemoral syndrome. In addition to stretching the plantar soft tissues, hyperpronation tends to stretch the posterior tibial tendon. The eventual fraying and/or rupture of this tendon can be directly associated with this excess pronation.

The best method for evaluating loss of posterior tibial function is the single heel rise.[28] In this test the patient stands on one leg with the knee extended and rises onto the ball of the foot. A positive test is noted if the patient fails to achieve heel rise or if the heel fails to invert. The failure of heel rise is secondary to the gastrocnemius muscle's inability to flex the foot if the tibialis posterior is malfunctioning and fails to set the heel into a locked, varus position. As will be emphasized later in this chap-

ter, the emphasis in treating plantar fasciitis or plantar surface pain should not be on stretching the plantar soft tissues but rather on strengthening the intrinsic foot muscles. Peroneal tendon subluxation occurs after moderate to severe inversion stress or forceful dorsiflexion tears the peroneal retinaculum. The associated tendons are then free to dislocate from their groove.[2] If this occurs, 5 to 6 weeks of compressive strapping is indicated. After this period, if instability persists, surgical stabilization may be necessary.

Systemic etiologies of heel pain must be considered. An example is Reiter's Syndrome, for which heel pain can be an arthropathy associated with uveitis and urethritis. Treatments are geared toward the primary diagnosis of Reiter's Syndrome, and rehabilitation strategies are focused on improvement in overall functional performance.

Neurologic entities such as S1 radiculopathy, tarsal

Table 30-2. Classification of acute ankle sprains

Grade	Precipitating injury	Findings
I	Stepping off curb; stepping on rock; alighting from vehicle; other low-level activity	Little functional deficit; patient can walk without limping and can hop on ankle; swelling minimal and localized; tenderness localized over ATL; may be isolated partial rupture of ATL
II	Misstep while running; inversion sprain while descending stairs; other higher-level activities	Some functional loss; patient may be unable to hop on ankle and walks with a limp; localized lateral swelling; localized tenderness around ATL and possibly calcaneofibular ligament; possible rupture of ATL and tearing of calcaneofibular ligament
III	Vigorous force during footstrike while ankle is plantar-flexed and internally rotated	Patient prefers crutches to weight bearing; diffuse pain and swelling; usually complete rupture of ATL and calcaneofibular ligament; anterior and lateral laxity

ATL, anterior talofibular ligament
From Baker CL, Todd JL: Intervening in acute ankle sprain and chronic instability, *J Musculo Med* July 1995:54

Table 30-3. Rehabilitation sequence

- Diagnosis
- RICE
- Range of Motion
- Stretch/Flexibility
- Proprioception
- Gait
- Strength
- Functional Performance

Adapted from Nicholas JA, Strizak AM, Veras G: A study of thigh muscle weakness in different pathological states of the lower extremity, *Am J Sports Med* 4(6):241, 1976.

tunnel syndrome (posterior tibial nerve entrapment), deep peroneal nerve entrapment, superficial peroneal nerve entrapment, abductor digiti quinti entrapment, and sural nerve entrapment can be all culprits in heel pain. Eliciting Tinel's sign over various nerves can be helpful if entrapment is suspected. In evaluating heel pain, pay close attention to the distribution of pain and note any associated dermatomal or nerve distribution.

The general algorithm for treating foot and ankle pain is shown in Table 30-3. This model, with minor alterations, is applicable to most rehabilitation programs. The first phase in treating foot and ankle injuries consists of pain reduction and control of swelling. Ice should be used liberally and, in foot and ankle disorders, is helpful beyond the depicted first 24 to 48 hours. In general, after any prolonged activity requiring repeated foot-surface contact, ice should be used liberally to control swelling and decrease pain. Pain and swelling can be further controlled with medications and adjunct modalities.

Analgesics and nonsteroidal anti-inflammatory drugs (NSAIDs) are recommended. Analgesics must be used with caution because they may mask potentially detrimental instabilities or injuries. They should be given so as to take the edge off of high-grade injury pain without masking informational signs or symptoms.

In general, the pain associated with most soft tissue injuries will begin to abate a few days after the injury. If pain persists or progresses, the insult may be more serious than initially thought. For instance, a presumed grade II to III ankle sprain may actually be a subtle fracture. Although x-rays should be routine for many injuries, they are not always taken. A good clinician is aware of subtle changes and lack of progress that alerts him/her to reevaluate an injury.

NSAIDs are useful in reducing edema but must be used with caution because many possess analgesic properties. Modalities such as pulsed ultrasound and electrical stimulation are helpful and should be applied if available. The settings for ultrasound are 1.5 W/cm^2 for approximately seven minutes. This modality can be applied to a submerged limb. In that case the settings are increased to 2.0 W/cm^2 for seven minutes. Under water, there is no direct contact of the ultrasound probe with the skin. A distance of approximately one inch should be maintained during its application. Electrical stimulation is useful for edema and pain control. Its intensity is to patient tolerance and it is not used underwater. Positive pole galvanic current is an electrical modality that is very effective for ankle sprains. Contraindications for ultrasound and electrical stimulation are listed in Tables 32-1 and 32-2.

The next phase of rehabilitation emphasizes range of motion. Early ranging is recommended (1 to 2 days after the injury), beginning with active motion. This

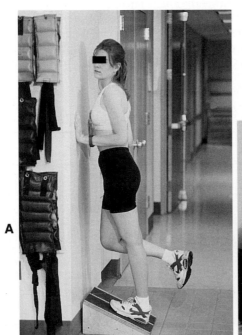

A

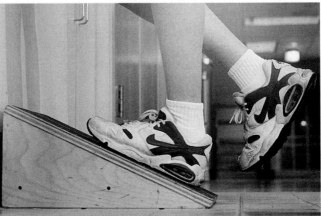

B

Fig. 30-1. Standing calf and Achilles stretch. **A** and **B**, Standing on an incline board or on a flat surface, lean forward, keeping the torso and lower extremity straight. The rear leg tries to maintain heel contact with the ground. Hold this stretch for 20 to 30 seconds. Repeat 10 to 15 trials, 3 to 4 times per day.

allows the patient to guide the amount of early motion attempted. If passive motion is emphasized too early, collagen reorganization may be hindered. Once swelling and pain have diminished, more aggressive passive range of motion should commence. Careful measurements should be made of the uninvolved limb to establish range-of-motion goals for the involved limb. Frequent measurements are made throughout the rehabilitation process to identify ranges that may be lagging. The use of hydrotherapy (cool temperature) allows pain and swelling reduction while increasing range. This can be combined with surgical tubing[52] or muslin. The tubing is placed around the foot and ankle and held with the hands. The patient can then assist in ranging his/her own limb. As pain subsides, the rubber tubing can be used for resistive exercises and in more advanced strengthening techniques. Stretching of the soleus and Achilles tendon is important. These groups are tight in most people and tend to become tighter after injury of the foot and ankle. Fig. 30-1 and Fig. 30-2 depict a standing calf stretch and Achilles stretch. Each of these stretches is done at least 3 or 4 times a day.

During this phase, attention should be paid to the remainder of the musculoskeletal system, particularly the proximal portion of the injured limb. Disabilities of the distal limb often are associated with proximal muscle weakness.[42] The hip abductors have been shown to have a 31% deficit on the involved lower limb side (Table 30-4). This is a significant finding and must be considered in rehabilitation of the limb. This relationship supports the concept that the musculoskeletal system is an interconnected linkage or chain and that when we address any specific region, attention must be payed to the entire system. If we consider all the components of skill training, we can understand

Table 30-4. Average proximal muscle strength deficits in patients with pathologic conditions of the foot and ankle

Affected body part	Affected vs. normal leg deficit
Hip abductors	31%
Hip adductors	30%
Quadriceps	19%
Hamstrings	26%
Total leg strength	26%

Adapted from Nicholas JA, Strizak AM, Veras G: A study of thigh muscle weakness in different pathological states of the lower extremity, *Am J Sports Med* 4(6), 1976, p 241.

why rehabilitation training must involve the entire system.

Proprioception training is important and can be accomplished with the use of a balance board, that is, BAPS (Fig. 30-3). This type of training reeducates the brain as to where a limb is in space, which capacity is often lost after injury. For the proprioceptive reflexes to function properly, the corresponding joints' range of motion and local muscle balance must be restored.[19,21] A balance board allows the foot and ankle to range through a full arc of motion in a controlled fashion.

Strengthening the foot and ankle complex is achieved by a variety of exercises. Heel raises can be done on any raised platform while the body is supported on the forefoot. This can be done standing erect (gastroc-soleus group) or with knees bent (isolates the soleus group) (Fig. 30-4). A series of 10 to 20 repetitions repeated three

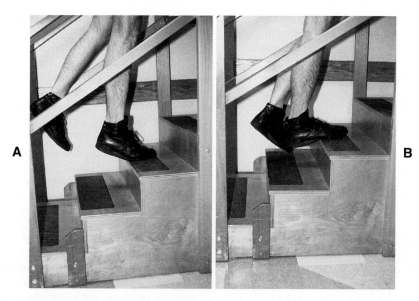

Fig. 30-2. Standing calf and Achilles stretch. **A** and **B,** With the ball of the foot supported on the edge of a step, slowly lower the heel toward the ground. Hold this for 20 to 30 seconds. Repeat 10 to 15 trials, 3 to 4 times per day.

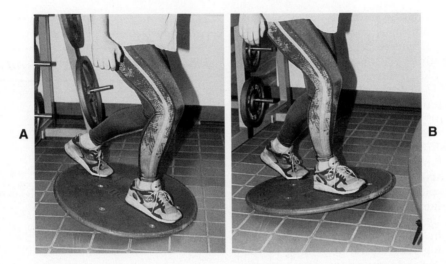

Fig. 30-3. BAPS for proprioception. **A** and **B,** The involved limb is placed onto the BAPS board and goes through a range of motion in all directions while maintaining contact with the board to increase joint position awareness.

to four times is recommended. As a patient begins to master this exercise, he/she is asked to either wear a weighted vest or hold free weights in the hands (Fig. 30-5). These weights should be held close to the body to maintain a stable center of gravity.

Writing the letters of the alphabet using the toes as writing instruments is another efficient way of strengthening the foot and ankle complex. To increase the challenge of this exercise, the patient is instructed to wrap a rubber tubing such as Thera-Band (The Hygenic Corporation, Akron, Ohio) under the ball of the foot and perform the exercises against the resistance of the rubber (Fig. 30-6). The entire alphabet should be attempted and repeated 2 to 3 times.

The mechanics of forward and backward ambulating place direct stresses on the foot and ankle complex. Forward walking invokes a valgus moment at the knee along with pronation of the foot and ankle complex. Conversely, retrowalking causes a varus moment at the knee and supination at the foot-ankle joint. It relates biomechanically to the progression of heel-to-toe mechanics in forward ambulating and toe-to-heel mechanics in retrowalking. This exercise is done in an isotonic fashion with resistance offered by the pulling of a weighted sled (Fig. 30-7). We initially start with a load of ½ body weight and progress as tolerated. The amount of added weight must not be so much as to alter the mechanics of retrowalking. We ask the patient to either strap a belt that is attached to the sled around his/her waist or pull the sled, attached to a cord, with the upper extremities. In both instances, there should be anatomic pelvic tilt and good upper-body posture. The weighted sled is pulled a distance of 10 meters (five to ten times) and this sequence is repeated two to three times.

Plantar roll-bar exercises are another method of strengthening the plantar muscle groups. In this exercise the foot is placed upon a roller (roughly 4 inches in di-

ameter) and the patient is asked to grasp the roller with the plantar muscles in a rocking fashion (Fig. 30-8 on page 472). This is repeated several times and may best be guided by a time frame rather than number of repetitions. For example, the patient should rock over the roller for 5 consecutive minutes.

The Elgin ankle exerciser can be used to increase ankle strength and improve range of motion (Fig. 30-9 on page 473). The patient places her foot and ankle firmly into the device, and weights are added progressively while the patient performs exercise sets. The ankle is ranged to the limits of the motion, that is, the patient achieves maximum dorsiflexion, and then this position is held for 2 seconds before it is returned to neutral. Three sets of ten to twelve repetitions are done (Fig. 30-10 on page 473).

More advanced exercises include off-balance weighted ball tossing. This exercise is not used solely to treat the ankle and foot complex but is a key exercise in addressing the components of skill. The complex task of maintaining postural control on a rocker board while accomplishing upper-extremity acceleration and deceleration training is demonstrated in Fig. 30-11 on pages 474–475. We find this type of multitask challenge very beneficial in our rehabilitation programs. It plays a key role in enhancing proprioception in the ankle and foot complex while challenging the neuromusculoskeletal system.

The final phase of ankle and foot rehabilitation involves improving agility and speed. To accomplish this we incorporate forward, lateral, backward, and multidirectional jogs, shuffles, and sprints. Obstacles are strategically placed to challenge the neuromuscular system to solve problems and efficiently complete the pattern. Typically we start with short distances and increase both distance and repetitions. Most gains are achieved by mixing obstacle patterns and timing their completion. We use box patterns and alternate running around and over them (Fig. 30-12 on page 476). The heights of the boxes are varied to increase the challenge.

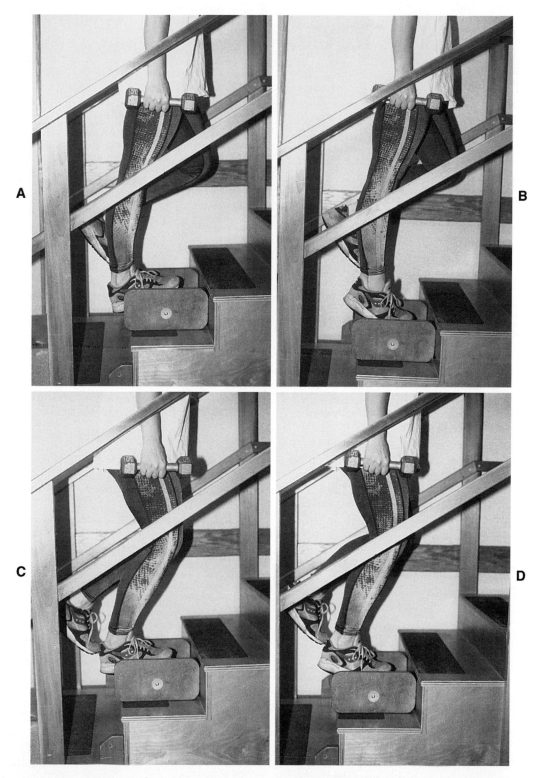

Fig. 30-4. Standing gastrocsoleus strengthening. **A** and **B,** With the ball of the foot supported on the edge of a step, slowly raise the heel upward. Then slowly lower the heel to neutral. Ten repetitions are done per set. Three or four sets should be done 4 times per day. **C** and **D,** Standing flexed knee soleus strengthening. Same as 30-4**A** and **B,** but with a flexed knee (approximately 30° to 45°). This technique isolates the soleus muscle, which is important in closed-chain knee extension (posterior pull on tibia relative to femur).

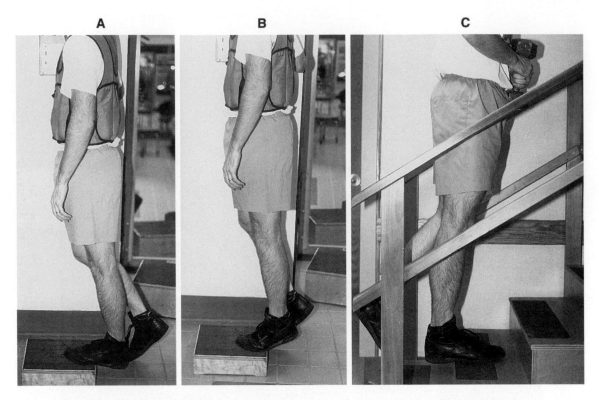

Fig. 30-5. Gastrocsoleus strengthening with weighted vest. **A** and **B,** Progressively add weight to the vest. The proper amount is enough weight so that you must struggle to complete the tenth repetition of the set. The goal is 10 repetitions per set. Three or four sets should be done 4 times per day. **C,** Gastrocsoleus strengthening holding free weights. Same as 30-5**A** and **B** but done holding free weights close to the torso.

The last consideration is footwear. The market is replete with various styles, shapes, contours, heights, and materials of shoe wear. Mann has stated that forces of 2 to 3 times body weight are created at foot-strike during running and jogging.[33] Because it is the first in line to distribute these forces, the ankle and foot complex must be properly protected. The three basic considerations in the construction of athletic footwear are: shock absorption qualities, support of the foot, and comfort to the wearer.[38] Each person may express different needs but all are integral in the management of the ankle and foot.

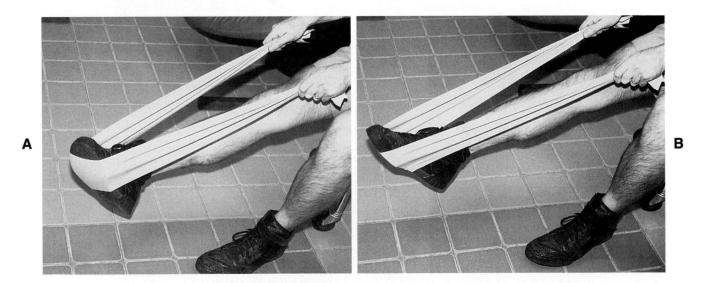

Fig. 30-6. Thera-Band foot/ankle strengthening. **A** and **B,** Placing a Thera-Band around the ball of the foot, write the letters of the alphabet using the foot as the writing tool. The bands are color-coded to give different resistance when stretched. The exercise is performed by repeating the letters of the alphabet several times or reading printed text and copying the letters with the foot-ankle.

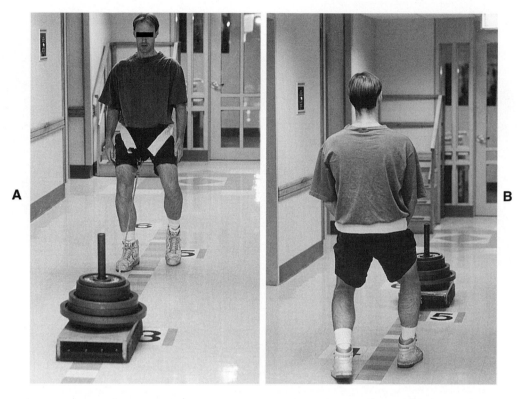

Fig. 30-7. Retrowalking. **A** and **B,** A weighted sled is attached to the body and retrowalking is done in a toe-to-heel pattern. Weights are progressively added to the sled. This exercise unloads the patellofemoral joint by increasing the varus movement at the knee.

The shoe is not evaluated as a whole entity but broken down into two basic areas, the rear foot and the forefoot. Each is evaluated separately and has specific characteristics necessary to provide adequate support. The rear foot must have a snug fit and adequate sole surface area to distribute forces, that is, it must possess as large a purchase as possible. A well-fitted heel counter has been shown to decrease resultant forces at heel-strike.[29] In contrast to the primary role of the rear foot (support and shock absorption), the forefoot's main function is support and sole flexibility. The metatarsophalangeal joint undergoes approximately 25° to 30° of dorsiflexion at toe-off, so the sole must be flexible. If not, there is increased incidence of metatarsal stress fracture and gastrocnemius strain.[38]

The use of orthotics to stabilize ankle-foot mechanics, particularly in conditions such as plantar fasciitis and dynamic pronation, has been written about extensively. A range of simple heel cups (to bolster the calcaneal fat pad), to rigid/semirigid full-length inserts, to inverted cam boots is used. Controversy often arises as to the proper orthotic, but in our experience there is no clear choice between orthotic inserts and cam boots. Patient satisfaction with each is about equal. Clearly, a person with recalcitrant signs and symptoms of plantar fasciitis, who has not responded to conservative care with modalities and medications, deserves a trial with an orthotic.

LEG PAIN

Disorders of the leg are common in sports medicine; their incidence is almost 30%.[11,25,32,46,47] The usual conditions that the clinician should be aware of include shin splints, stress fractures, and strains.

Shin splints are common and historically are associated with any pain in the lower leg related to overuse.[24] Their location is anterior (lateral to the tibia) or posterior (medial to the tibia). When they occur medial to the tibia, they are called medial tibial stress syndrome.[47] That is generally a condition that is specific to inflammation of the musculotendinous units of the leg. Shin splints are biomechanically correlated to forefoot pronation and the subsequent development of overuse syndromes of the lower extremity.[36]

The treatment of shin splints focuses on pain relief, biomechanical corrections, and reinjury prevention. Initially, frequent applications of ice (10 to 15 minutes, 3 to 4 times a day), relative rest (no strenuous stretching or contraction of the involved compartment muscles), NSAIDs, analgesics, and taping are used.[5] Orthotics can be considered early if there is evidence of excessive pronation. After the acute phase (2 to 3 days) modalities such as ultrasound can be applied. This will increase local blood flow and expedite tissue healing. A dosage of 1.0 to 1.5 w/cm^2 is recommended.

The next phases of rehabilitation follow the recommendations described for plantar fasciitis. A minor dif-

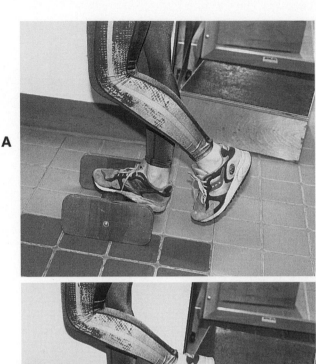

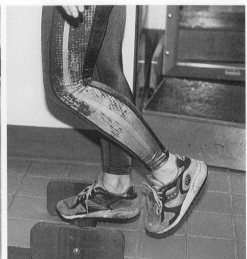

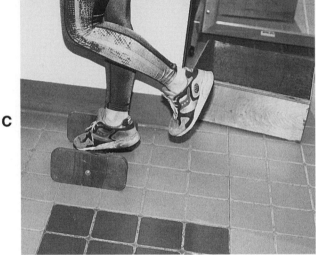

Fig. 30-8. Plantar-roll progressive resistive exercises (PREs). **A, B,** and **C,** While standing, place the foot on a round bar and contract the plantar muscles so as to maintain continuous contact between the foot and the bar. The other leg is flexed and not in contact with the ground. The exercise can be performed by repeating a rocking motion in sets of 30 to 40 repeated 4 to 5 times or, more simply, by repeating the motion for 4 to 5 consecutive minutes. Strengthening of the plantar muscles is important in maintaining upright posture.

ference would be to more closely focus on eccentric muscle action around the medial ankle joint. The eccentric contraction of the medial soleus is largely responsible for controlling subtalar pronation on heel contact. The patient is advised to refrain from all running for at least 2 or 3 weeks and then gradually run toward desired goals over the next 3 or 4 weeks.

Stress fractures are most common in the tibia. Nearly 50% of all stress fractures occur in the tibia.[35] Two differing theories as to the cause of tibial stress fractures somewhat confound the issue of developing rehabilitation strategies, particularly those geared to preventing their occurrence. It is not clear whether muscle weakness or excess contraction causes the fractures. The first theory, proposed by Clement, argues that muscle fatigue reduces the relative shock-absorbing capability of the lower extremities' musculature, predisposing it to fracture.[10] Stanitski and colleagues propose just the opposite.[55] They believe that highly concentrated muscle forces that are repetitively applied to long bones ultimately accumulate to stress fracture.

Once the diagnosis is made, the treatment of stress fractures is essentially rest and pain management. If there is excess pronation, an orthotic should be used. Methods for addressing muscular balance and developing training strategies to prevent future insult are largely undetermined. In general, we focus on stretching the associated inciting musculature and concentrate on cross-friction massage and soft tissue mobilization. Rest is advised for 4 to 6 weeks and return to competitive sports delayed for about 3 months. Weight bearing is allowed as tolerated throughout the healing phase.

If, however, the fracture occurs on the anterior tibial surface (tension side of the bone), there is potential for delayed or nonunion.[53] This phenomenon has been called the "dreaded black line." An x-ray or fluoroscope will reveal a horizontal fracture line transcending the anterior tibial cortex. If there is evidence of nonunion, weight bearing is limited for at least 4 weeks and surgical drilling may be required.

Strains of the leg are fairly common and usually involve the soleus or anterior/posterior tibial tendons. For these isolated instances in the leg, basic conservative treatment is similar to that for any sprain or strain. Ice

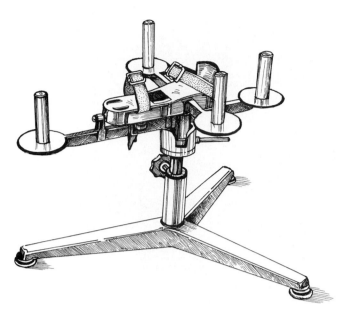

Fig. 30-9. Elgin ankle exerciser. The patient sits and his ankle is placed in the apparatus. Range-of-motion and strengthening exercises are done.

should be applied liberally, rest prescribed for a short period of time, and NSAIDs and analgesics should be given. After pain subsides, a progressive course of stretching and strengthening is indicated. An isolated tear of the proximal portion of the medial gastrocnemius muscle is

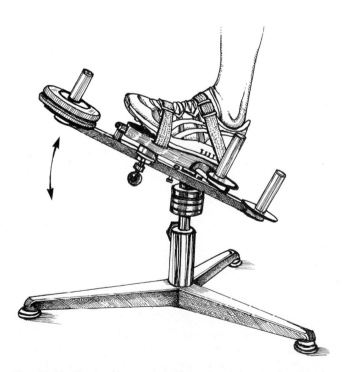

Fig. 30-10. Elgin ankle exerciser. The patient's foot is placed in the apparatus and, against added weight, moved through a complete range of motion and then held for 2 seconds before returning to neutral. Sets of 10 to 12 repetitions are done 3 or 4 times.

termed "tennis leg." As originally described by Powell in 1833, tennis leg was initially thought to be associated with a tear of the plantaris tendon but later was found to be associated with a tear of the medial gastrocnemius.[1,51] Tennis leg typically occurs after a sudden cutting maneuver associated with knee extension and ankle dorsiflexion. Patients feel as though they have received a direct blow to the posterior/proximal part of the leg. On examination, there is often a palpable defect in the region. Treatment includes rest and progressive slow stretching of the leg. We apply a heel lift to unload the gastrocsoleus group during walking. A ⅜- to ½-inch lift is recommended for 2 to 3 weeks.

HIP AND THIGH

Most injuries of the hip and thigh result from overuse or acute trauma. The differential diagnosis of hip pain is rather lengthy and includes disorders such as osteochondritis dissecans, lumbar disk disease, and trochanteric bursitis (see box on page 477).[49] When knee pain is presented, the hip should be examined for the possibility of referred pain. Often the presenting symptom of hip disorders is pain in or about the knee. The hip is pivotal in supporting the upper torso above and transmitting the ground reactive forces from below. For this reason it is particularly vulnerable to injury. Soft tissue injuries including sprains/strains, bursitis, and contusions are all treated conservatively. Degenerative changes of the hip are treated with joint stress reduction or surgery. Neurologic factors must not be forgotten and should be considered in evaluating hip and thigh pathology, especially when there is weakness, atrophy, or progressive radiating pain.

Strains of the hip and thigh usually involve the hip flexors, extensors, adductors, or abductors. The mechanism of injury probably is acute trauma or overuse, and the patient typically has a clear idea of when and how the injury occurred. Injury is often postexertional and the local region very tender. Hip flexor tendinitis is associated with iliopsoas and rectus femoris dysfunction. Isotonic or eccentric overuse is the usual culprit, and rehabilitation strategies are geared to restore flexibility and strength (isotonic and eccentric) to the muscle groups. After a brief period of rest, modalities (ultrasound), and, if warranted, NSAIDs (since the pain associated with acute muscle strain is partly caused by an inflammatory response[30]), the patient should begin active exercise focusing on the groin and anterior thigh muscles. Groin stretching is done in various ways; these are depicted in Fig. 30-13 on page 478. The anterior thigh muscles are addressed similarly, as shown in Fig. 30-14 on page 479. Figs. 30-15 and 30-16 on page 479 show hip extensor and abductor stretches.

Stretches can be made more efficient if the technique of muscle energy is used. If our goal is to increase stretch of the hamstring muscles, we might ask our patient to place his extended lower extremity onto a table as he/she stands alongside (Fig. 30-17 on page 480). The patient then leans forward over his lower limb and achieves stretch on the

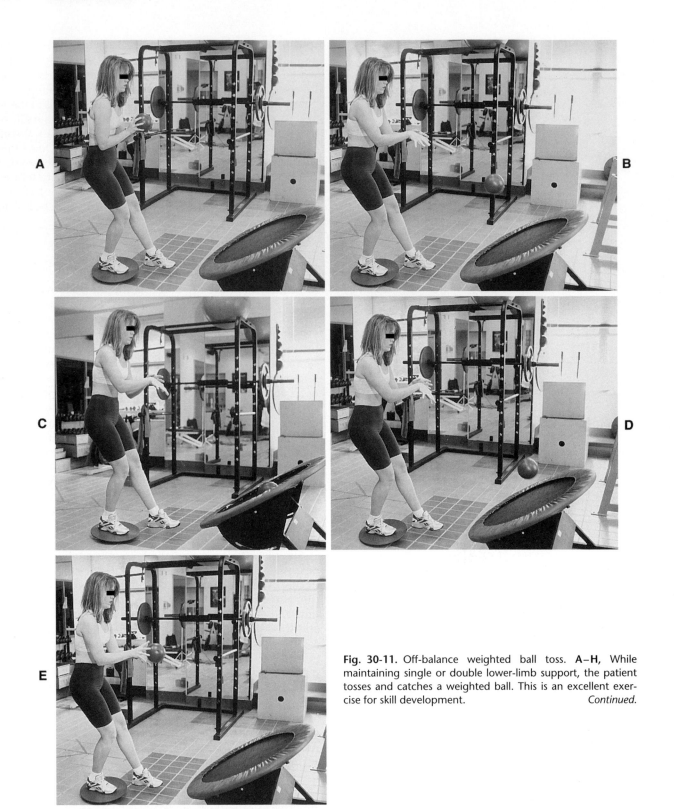

Fig. 30-11. Off-balance weighted ball toss. **A–H,** While maintaining single or double lower-limb support, the patient tosses and catches a weighted ball. This is an excellent exercise for skill development.   *Continued.*

hamstrings. Incorporating the concept of muscle energy can improve stretch while increasing flexibility. Stand next to an examining table and ask your patient to lie down on the table and place his lower limb on your shoulder (Fig. 30-18 on page 480). You should then firmly grasp the patient's distal thigh and ask him to push downward onto your shoulder. The amount of force exerted by the patient is submaximal and the type of contraction is isometric. (I prefer to allow the patient to slightly overpower me, which may avert any sudden exertional stress, with a potential risk of muscle injury or tearing, that a prolonged isometric contraction may have.) The contraction should be held for a count of 5 to 6 seconds. After completion, the degree of straight leg raise is increased by pushing the patient's limb

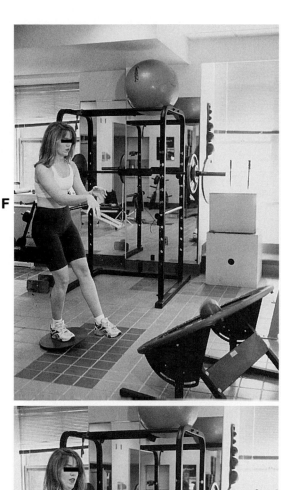

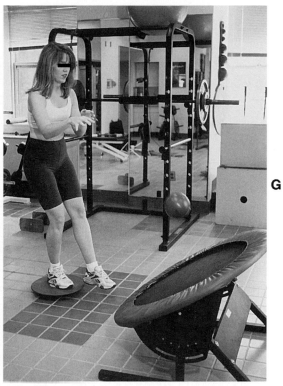

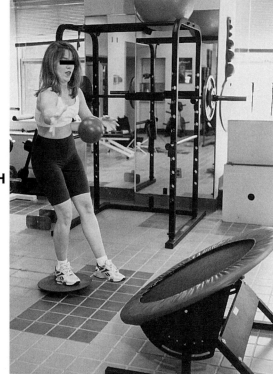

Fig. 30-11, cont'd. For legend see opposite page.

more toward his head. The entire sequence is then repeated two or three times, each time increasing the degree of hip flexion and hamstring stretch. This technique allows for increased flexibility by "fatigue stretching" the target muscle group. The hamstring group fatigues from repeated contraction, allowing greater excursion with less resistance of the muscles. It would not be surprising to find associated trigger points in the setting of strains, and these must be identified and treated.

Strengthening exercises of the hip region are focused on the same groups we discussed for stretching. The emphasis in strengthening is on resistive training.

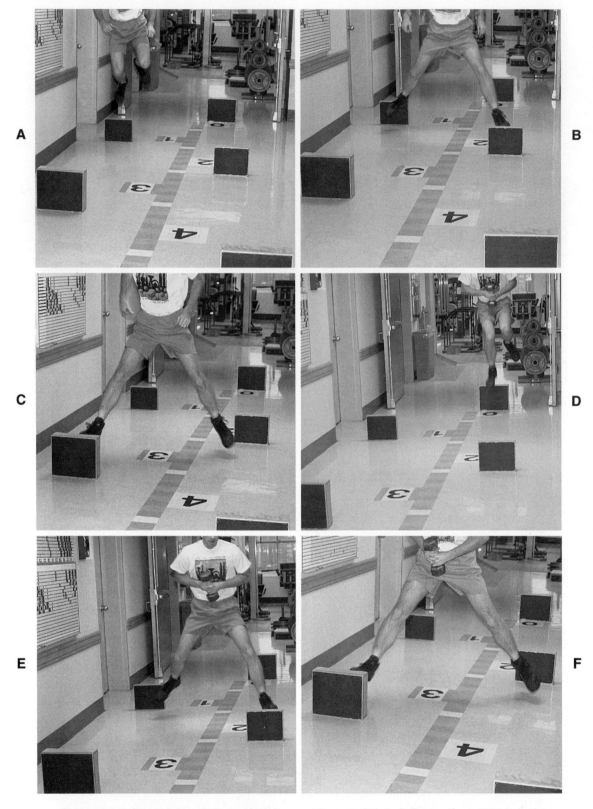

Fig. 30-12. Agility training. **A–F,** An obstacle course is created that challenges the patient in both force acceleration/deceleration, coordination, and balance. As he progresses, timing for completion of the course is monitored. This is an excellent training program for skill development. The pattern of the box layout and the heights of the boxes are alternated on subsequent sessions. **A–C** without hand weights, **D–F** with hand weights.

DIFFERENTIAL DIAGNOSIS OF HIP PAIN IN ATHLETES

Hip dislocation

Hip subluxation with or without acetabulum or labrum injury

Osteochondritis dissecans

Acetabulum or pelvis fracture or stress fracture

Anterior superior iliac spine avulsion

Iliac spine contusion (hip pointer)

Adductor muscle strain

Osteitis pubis

Inguinal hernia

Lateral femoral cutaneous nerve entrapment or injury

Femoral nerve or artery injury

Idiopathic avascular necrosis of the femoral head

Idiopathic chondrolysis

Slipped capital femoral epiphysis

Legg-Calvé-Perthes disease

Metabolic disorders:

Sickle cell disease

Inflammatory disease

Lumbar disk disease

Neoplastic abnormalities of the pelvis, acetabulum, or femur

Piriformis syndrome

Transient synovitis

Snapping hip syndrome

Trochanteric bursitis

From Pearsall AW: Assessing acute hip injury: examination, diagnosis, and triage, *Am J Sports Med* 23(6):40, 1995.

Fig. 30-19 on page 481 illustrates several exercises that strengthen the hip region.

Whereas strains are thought to occur at the musculotendinous junction,[43] contusions can be seen anywhere along the musculotendinous unit. Contusions are best treated with ice and compressive dressings. Gradual return to play is allowed but in the best of all scenarios, healing of a torn muscle (strain) takes a minimum of six weeks. The rehabilitation program for subacute and chronic contusions is similar to that for strains.

Bursitis of the hip, particularly trochanteric bursitis, is fairly common and particularly nagging. It seems rather easy to diagnose but often can be confused with tendinitis of the external hip rotators (or iliotibial band). The insertion of these muscles is onto the greater trochanter, which lies close to the trochanteric bursa. If a course of ice, NSAIDs, and relative rest does not alleviate symptoms, an injection of a steroid and anesthetic into the trochanteric bursa may be helpful (methylprednisolone, 40 mg with 1% lidocaine, 1 to 2 cc).

Degenerative arthritis of the hip is a common, painful disability that progresses with functional loss. Much has been written addressing the impact of joint stresses and the progression or regression of degenerative changes. Joint forces are said to be 2.6 times body weight in single-leg standing and up to 5 times body weight in running.[39] Rehabilitation strategies in treating an arthritic hip are adapted toward pain relief, joint unloading, and improvement of overall function.

Pain relief is mainly achieved with NSAIDs. Be cognizant of the side affects of these medications since patients often take them for a long time. I routinely spot-check liver and kidney chemistries in patients, particularly the elderly and those with multisystem disease, who take NSAIDs for more than 3 or 4 weeks.

Joint unloading may be the key to offering symptomatic relief of degenerative arthritis. The use of an assistance device such as a cane can help. The literature supports using the cane in the contralateral hand to the most symptomatic hip. Pauwels has stated that the use of a cane in the contralateral hand will greatly reduce force on the ipsilateral femoral head.[48] When the body's center of gravity is in front of the second sacral vertebra directly in the center of the pelvis, weight to the lower extremities is equally distributed to each femoral head. This assumption is made if the distance from the body's center to each hip is equidistant, that is, if the lever arms are equal. If a person leans to either side, the center of gravity also shifts to that side, increasing the relative lever arm to the contralateral side and decreasing the lever arm to the ipsilateral side. On the contralateral side, the hip abductor muscles fire to reposition the body's center of gravity toward midline. This generates significant force across the contralateral hip. If a patient uses a cane on the ipsilateral side, contralateral hip abductor firing is reduced and stress decreased across the contralateral hip. The cane creates a force that acts in the same direction as the contralateral hip abductor muscles.[12]

Another mechanism of hip joint stress reduction is a direct result of the force created by the cane. We have stated that when one leans to the ipsilateral side, the contralateral hip abductors fire and create excessive stress across the contralateral hip. However, the effect on the ipsilateral hip is a reduction in joint stress. This is due to both a shorter lever arm on the ipsilateral side and a mechanical advantage whereby the ipsilateral hip abductor muscles fire less because of the relative hip abduction created by the upper torso's leaning over the lower torso. These concepts explain why we recommend use of a cane in the hand opposite the most involved hip, and why a patient has a propensity to lean over the degenerative hip.

Aqua therapy is beneficial in treating degenerative joints because stress across the joints is relieved by the body's buoyancy in water. Resistive exercises can be done with minimal joint compression when a body is submerged. Exercises range from walking in place (which on land can be extremely painful) to flutter-kicking and aerobic conditioning. A practitioner must be careful when preparing an exercise program for a degenerative joint.

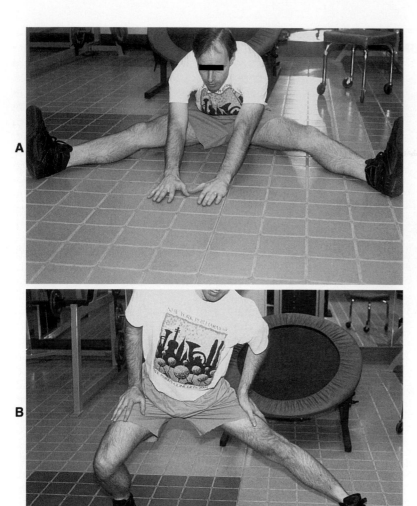

Fig. 30-13. Groin stretch. **A,** Sit with the lower extremities abducted maximally, then lean forward by flexing at the waist. Hold the position for 20 to 30 seconds and repeat several times. **B,** Squat and abduct the lower extremity of the groin to be stretched. Then lean over this limb, place your ipsilateral hand on the waist, and thrust it into adduction. Hold this position for 20 to 30 seconds. It is important not to bounce the area being stretched but to maintain a slow, sustained stretch.

There is a misconception that people with arthritis include those with osteoporosis. While the two often coexist, the rehabilitation and exercise programs for them are quite different. Whereas the patient with degenerative arthritis benefits from the buoyant, stress-reducing effect of water, the osteoporotic patient benefits most from careful loading of the joints, attained by on-land exercises. The deficit in the osteoporotic patient is in the bony matrix, and bone is best strengthened with resistive exercises.

The next consideration in treating the degenerative joint is in ergonomic activity of daily living (ADL) efficiency. Educating patients in proper biomechanical principles often is successful, not so much in pain relief as in increased function. The basic principle is simple. If a patient learns to shorten the effective axial lever arm of each lower extremity, activities of daily living become easier. An example of this is an evaluation of the biomechanics a person uses to arise from a lying-down position. We have viewed and videotaped several patients arising from a prone position. The way a person usually accomplishes this is to thrust the upper torso in front and immediately raise the leg or legs straight. This is followed by a rotational action at the hips and lumbosacral spine, to carry the lower extremities over the bed or exam table. The legs and feet are carried through an arc and are eccentrically controlled by the associated muscles until the feet rest on the floor. The stress across the hips is directly related to the length of the lower extremities and the distance of the distal-most segment from the hip. The accumulated forces across the hip can be significantly reduced when the lower extremities are flexed as a person rises. Also, using the arms and hands to help the upper torso rise increases ergonomic efficiency (Fig. 30-20 on page 482).

KNEE

The knee is one of the largest joints in the body and accounts for one third of sports injuries clinically evaluated.[5] The most common injury seen is tendinitis. This four-bone, three-joint structure is very mobile and has drawn significantly increased attention in sports-related injuries. From simple strains to total joint

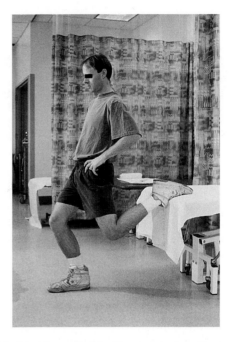

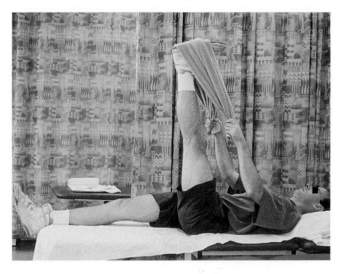

Fig. 30-15. Assisted hip extensor stretch supine (hamstrings). A towel is used to stretch the hamstring group while the patient is lying down.

Fig. 30-14. Quadriceps stretch. Stand and place the back of the foot onto a table behind you. Try not to hyperflex the knee. While maintaining erect posture, perform a posterior pelvic tilt that should. If you are doing the stretch correctly, produce a feeling of stretch on the anterior thigh group. Hold this for 20 to 30 seconds and repeat several times.

arthroplasty, the disabilities affecting the knee present an array of therapeutic options for rehabilitation protocols.

In this section, we will focus specifically on rehabilitation options. Sprains, strains, and tendinitis are common disorders of the knee. The most common injuries affect the anterior/posterior cruciate ligaments, medial/lateral collateral ligaments, capsule, quadriceps, hamstrings, iliotibial band, and patella tendon. The anterior cruciate ligament sprain/tear has become the rehabilitation challenge of the nineties. In the not-too-distant past, it took a year or more for an ACL rehabilitation patient's recovery after surgery. Some doctors today discharge patients in a few months with a green light for athletic participation. The trend to accelerate rehabilitation protocols began with Shelbourne in the eighties.[54] In evaluating noncompliant postoperative patients, he found those who progressed at their own accelerated pace did not as a group suffer adverse effects. Many programs have been developed since with varying rates of progression. Our program has fluctuated between a 4- to 7-month time frame. It is unfortunate, but true, that many patients search for a rehabilitation facility with the promised time frame for completion as a pivotal determining factor. I spend hours counseling patients and trying to redirect their focus. Using our com-

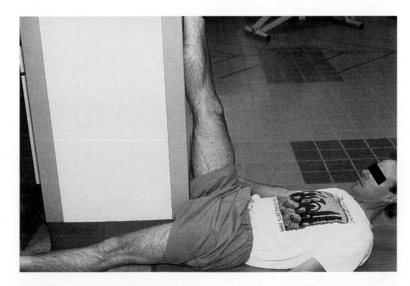

Fig. 30-16. Wall hamstring stretch. This is best done lying on the floor in a doorway. The leg to be stretched is placed on a wall while the other leg may, if needed, be placed in the doorway. This allows the buttocks to approach the wall and affords the opportunity for the greatest stretch of the hamstrings. As the exercise progresses, the limb is placed, little by little, further up the wall by scooting the buttocks closer to the all. Hip abductor stretch technique is depicted in Figure 30-36 on page 505.

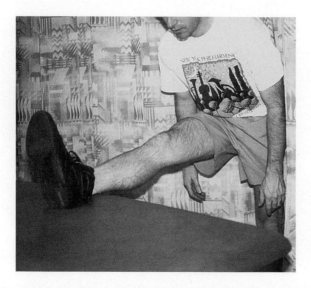

Fig. 30-17. Standing hamstring stretch. The leg to be stretched is placed onto an adjacent table and the hip is slowly flexed. The cervico-thoracic-lumbar spine remains fairly straight during this maneuver. The stretches in Figures 30-15, 30-16, and 30-17 are held for 20 to 30 seconds and repeated several times. Be careful not to hyperextend the knee when doing these stretches. This could lead to patellofemoral symptoms.

ponents of skill as the foundation for our training program, patients are encouraged to concentrate on functional outcomes rather than time frames.

Our postoperative training program is broken into four phases (see box on pages 483–485). Phase I is called Early Functional and incorporates weeks 1 and 2. The emphasis is on pain/edema reduction, gaining functional range of motion, achieving normal gait mechanics, balance control, and independent ambulating. We allow full available range of motion within the first few days after surgery. Weight bearing is as tolerated. Retrowalking while pulling a nonweighted sled is started in the first phase (Fig. 30-21 on page 486). This technique is particularly useful for strengthening the lower extremity while unloading the patellofemoral joint. It causes a supination moment at the subtalar joint while the knee goes into varus.

Phase II is the Progressive Functional and covers weeks 3 through 9. During this phase the post-op brace is usually discontinued. Neuromotor developmental training enters full swing as we prepare for sport-specific training. Progressive resistive training of the quadriceps begins around postoperative week (POW) 5 or 6. We use various modes of resistive training to

Text continued on page 485

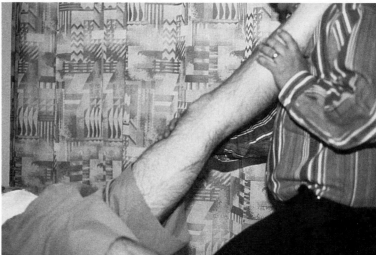

A

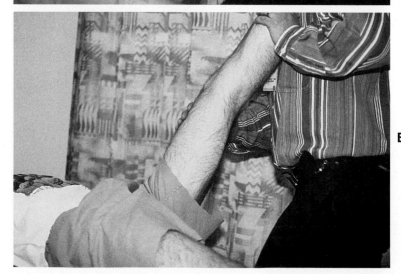

B

Fig. 30-18. Muscle energy hamstring stretch. **A** and **B,** The patient lies down and places an extended leg on the hands and shoulder of the examiner. He/she attempts to hyperextend the hip against resistance offered by the examiner. The contraction is held for 5 seconds and released. The leg is then flexed further by the examiner and the cycle is repeated.

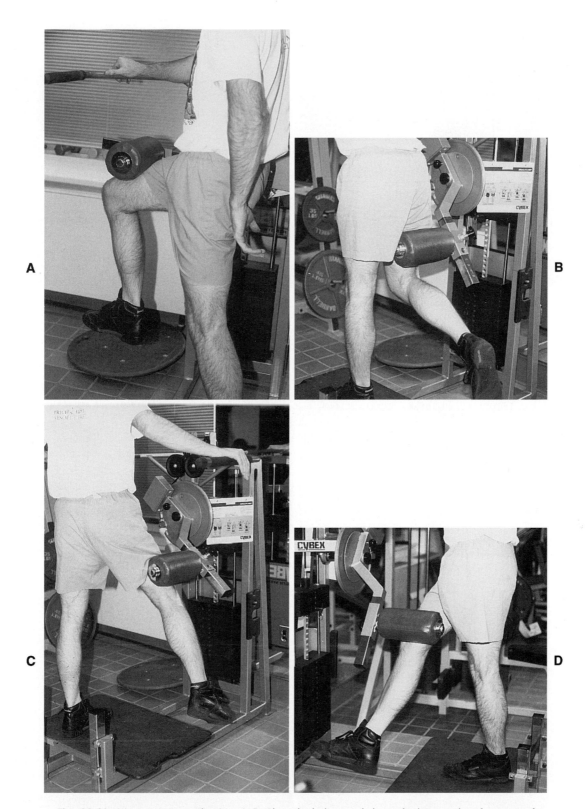

Fig. 30-19. Hip group strengthening. **A–D,** Place the bolster pad above the knee and perform sets of ten repetitions 3 to 4 times. The exercise should be carried through a complete range of motion. To increase stability, the upper limbs can hold onto the support bars. **A,** Hip flexors; **B,** hip extensors; **C,** hip abductors; **D,** hip adductors.

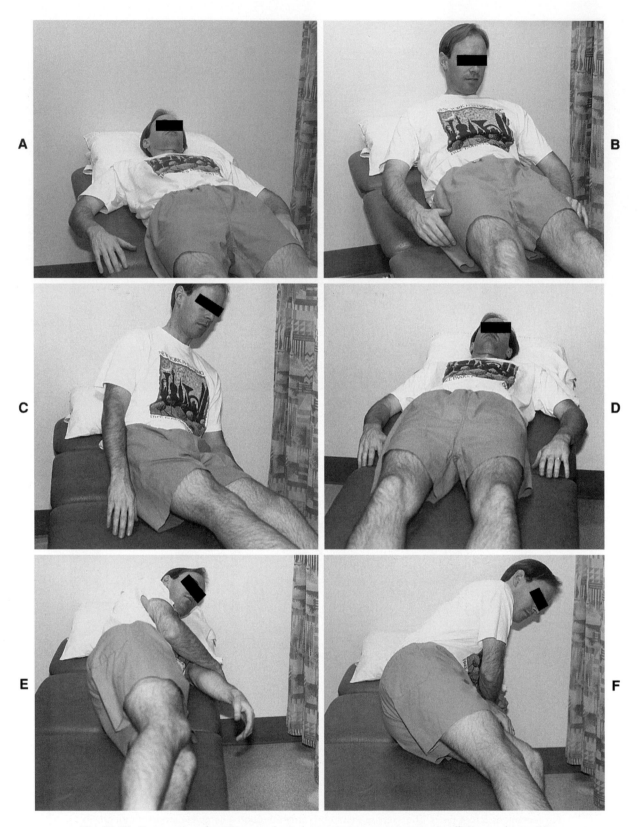

Fig. 30-20. Ergonomics of getting up. **A–C** demonstrates poor ergonomic efficiency when arising from a supine position, as compared to **D–F**, which illustrates a more efficient method. The stress on the low back is decreased in **D–F**.

POST-OP ACL REHABILITATION

Phase I—Early Functional (Weeks 1–2)

Goals:
1) Attaining full (involved knee) extension/flexion
2) Pain/edema reduction
3) Ambulation without assistive device
4) Normal gait-cycle mechanics
5) Early balance control
6) Baseline values for uninvolved limb training program, including 10 rep max testing (leg press), and isokinetics

PO Day 1

Bledsoe 0–60 for ambulation, increased excursion as knee ROM increases (sleep with brace locked in full extension until attaining comfortable extension)

CPM 0–60 or as tolerated started in recovery room, twice/day for 2 hours each session. Continued daily CPM until attaining 90° active knee flexion, increased CPM daily, approximately 10 (more if tolerated)

Ice for 20 minutes every 1-2 hours

Ambulating bearing weight as tolerated with brace on, using axillary crutches

Beginning patella mobilization when drain removed

Electrical stimulation to decrease pain/effusion, and for quadriceps/hamstrings cocontraction

Passive extension 4-5 times/day (Passive knee extension with use of bolster or pillow under ankle)

Heel slides

Supine wall slides with operated limb supported by nonoperated limb

Pain medication

Standing knee extension (soleus, hamstrings, quadriceps)

Gait training

ACL PROTOCOL

PO Day 2

Continuing above as needed

Hamstring isometrics 0–90

Active quadriceps/hamstrings cocontraction (hamstrings by first pushing heel into table followed by pushing knee into table)

Ambulating stairs

Attempting SLR with brace locked at 0 (all directions, may remove brace if good quad control)

Full passive extension

Sitting hip flexion

PO Days 3–7

Continuing above as needed

Retrowalking–Start with no load, progress to pulling weighted sled, increase load in subsequent weeks

Calf raises

BAPS sitting, progress to standing

Multi-hip–to involved limb

Active flexion (full arc), active extension 90°–0° (or as tolerated)

Prone hangs

Quadriceps isometrics at varied degrees of knee flexion

Standing wall slide to 30° knee flexion

Stationary bicycle–start with comfortable seat to promote flexion, most force through nonoperated extremity– increases seat height in subsequent sessions

Teaching home stretching for quadriceps, hamstrings, gastroc

Bilateral standing knee bend 0–30

Bilateral standing balance exercises, i.e., sidestepping, marching, line walking in parallel bars

Forward propulsion of rolling chair using alternating lower extremities

PO Days 8–14

Continuing as above

Resisted knee flexion prone

Full active range of motion

Multi-hip bilateral lower limbs (AP/Lat)

Step-ups without weights (add weights and height gradually)

Continued.

POST-OP ACL REHABILITATION—*cont'd*

Unilateral knee bends (0–30), be aware of patellofemoral signs and symptoms
Unilateral balance standing
Resisted SLR (without brace if good quad control) resistance applied proximal to knee
Beginning (closed-chain) leg press (begin with short arc) and targeted range of motion to increase proprioception
D/C crutches
Multi-hip in all directions

ACL PROTOCOL

Phase II—Progressive Functional (Weeks 3–9)
Goals:　1)　D/C Post-op brace—Begin knee sleeve with patella cut out
　　　　　　2)　Achieving symmetric balance proprioception of bilateral lower limbs
　　　　　　3)　Maximizing neuromotor development of all muscle groups

Weeks 3–4
Continuing as above
D/C post-op brace when knee stable (good quad control), switch to sleeve with patella cut out (when sutures removed)
Progressing to medicine ball toss on weighted stool
Unilateral standing medicine ball toss
Pool activities-FAROM, underwater flutter kicking with knees flexed and motion occuring at hips
Cable column with locked knee or brace in full extension. Must have good quad control. Begin flexion and extension. Progress to abduction/adduction (be more cautious with those patients who have meniscal and MCL/LCL involvement)
Relaxed knee dead lifts
Forward and backward fast walking
Short step closed-chain step machine (low resistance)

Weeks 5–6
Continuing as above
Progressing to PREs for knee extension. Begin with cuff weight for involved leg. Perform this exercise with cuff weight until patient can do at least 20 lbs
Ball toss on rocker board (double support, single support)
Standing cable column (flex, extend, abd, add) with multi-joint motion, BLE (including knee)

Weeks 7–8
Continuing as above
Begin progression of lateral activities: Ski simulator, lateral stepping, lateral shuffles, and slide board
Simulated running using cable column
Crossover stepping; progress to cariocas as tolerated
Modified posterior lunge to 45° flexion, weight on lead leg

ACL PROTOCOL

Weeks 8–10
Continuing as above
Standing bicycle with high resistance
Initiating plyometrics: mini-jumps on leg press at approximately 30% of body weight
Lunges (modified range of motion)

Phase III—Functional (Weeks 10–16)
Goals:　1)　Mastering functional tasks of desired physical activity

Weeks 10–12
Progressing to mini-jumps in the hallway
Initiating depth jumping and hopping as tolerated
Beginning sport-specific activity
Evaluating light jogging

Week 16
Leaping

POST-OP ACL REHABILITATION—*cont'd*

KT 2000, isokinetic evaluation (Repeat isokinetics every month until side to side for quads adequate, i.e., 10%. Hams should be symmetric)

Video analysis of functional performance, i.e., running, jumping

Phase IV—Return to Sport (4–6 months)

4–6 months

Goals:
1) Isokinetic values to exceed baseline uninvolved limb values
2) Normal performance on functional testing
3) Pain alleviation
4) No effusion with sports-specific exercises
5) KT 2000   4 mm side to side
6) Return to sport
7) Adaption to accelerator and decelerator forces and changes of direction
8) Development of power

ACL PROTOCOL

Functional brace if:
KT   5 mm side to side
Pain on sport-specific activity
Patient chooses so

* Throughout program, patients undergo intense, uninvolved lower-extremity and bilateral upper-extremity training program as well

Onset

Performing Cybex evaluation on sound limb
Performing baseline functional testing and periodic 10 rep max testing

Strength Assessment

The patient's maximal lifting capabilities will be assessed in order to assign the optimal training loads necessary to induce maximal strength gains. The patient will determine the most weight that can be safely lifted ten times in a given exercise. This value will be considered his ten repetition maximum (10 RM)

The 10 RM–value represents 75% of a patient's total lifting capacity and is useful in establishing training workloads for specific exercises. This test is currently administered in the following exercises: knee bends, step-ups, leg extensions, stiff-leg dead lifts. The 10 RM–test, however, is appropriate for any exercise involving multiple sets with a distinct number of repetitions

---

maximize efficiency by training the nervous system to solve problems. Knee extensions using ankle weights challenge the system in a different way from performing knee extensions using a cable column (Fig. 30-22). With progressive weight training, our strategy is to impose greater responsibility on the entire body while tasks are attempted. For greater coordination and balance, we ask a patient to stand and balance (single or double support) on a BAPS or rocker board rather than sitting in a chair to perform biceps curls. These techniques, which are the foundation of motor learning, are the forerunners of skill development. Motor learning strategies integrate the afferent, perceptive, and efferent functions of the mind and body that govern posture and movement.[45] Before progressing to Phase III we begin to emphasize force-absorption strategies.

It is well known that we all seem to focus on gaining strength to improve force production—to be able to throw a baseball harder, to kick a football further, to jump higher, and to sprint faster. But when one looks more closely, a few questions surface. Why are there so many knee injuries in basketball players? Why are there so many rotator cuff ailments in baseball pitchers? Why do golfers strain their quadratus lumborum and rhomboid muscles? The common link among all three is the probable mechanism of injury: poor force absorption or inefficient deceleration of the agonist muscle group. McNair, studying landing characteristics in normal and ACL–deficient knees noted that ACL–deficient knees were not adept at force absorption.[37] Our focus is primarily on accepting forces rather than producing them.

Consider the martial art aikido. It isn't unusual for a 95-pound aikido player to accept the challenge of and dominate a 230-pound attacker. Certainly the attacker is larger and may be more powerful, at least for force production, but the aikido player is functionally stronger. He/she summates forces from within with the absorbed forces from the attacker. The aikido player actually uses the strength of an opponent to overpower him/her. By skillfully maneuvering the body, the player can internalize extrinsic forces and put them to productive use. In essence, the aikido player is skilled and masters force absorption. In our training sessions, we try to achieve similar skill. For example, we employ box jumping (Fig. 30-23 on page 489). The focus is not so much the height of ascent achieved but rather the technique of descent. With video analysis, frame-by-frame sequences can be reviewed to identify weakness in landing. This has been extremely helpful and the combination of off-balance and force-absorption training has made the most significant positive impact on our functional testing scores.

The next phase in our rehabilitation program is the Functional (POW 10 to 16) period. Jogging is begun and the focus is on sport-specific activities. This is an extension of the activities from the prior phase. The last phase (IV) begins with POW sixteen and spans approximately 2 months. It involves more advanced techniques of pivoting and leaping. At completion of this phase, the athlete is usually ready to be tested for return to sport. This functional testing is done at about 6 months. There is a series of five variables we evaluate. To test static integrity of the ACL graft, we use KT arthrometry (MEDmetric, San Diego, Calif.) (Fig. 30-24 on page 490). Anterior and posterior excursion of the tibia relative to the femur is measured at 15, 20, or 30 pounds of anterior force at 20 pounds of posterior force. We closely track side-to-side comparisons at 30

pounds. We accept differences of less than 4 mm side to side. Isokinetic testing for peak torque, endurance, and power are evaluated in side-to-side analysis and for comparison of current values to pretraining sound-limb values (patients routinely are tested within the first week of the rehabilitation program for baseline sound-limb values). Speeds of 60° and 180° are employed (Fig. 30-25 on page 491). Noyes Hop Test is performed (Fig. 30-26 on page 491).[44] This is a series of hops including single hop, triple hop, crossover hop, and 6-m hop for time. Eighty-five percent symmetry is acceptable. Currently we use the Modified Cincinnati ACL questionnaire to correlate subjective perceptions. The final challenge is the Hop-N-Stop test (Fig. 30-27 on page 492). This was developed at our training facility and its full description is in publication. The test evaluates force production and absorption while assessing a patient's ability to perform the pivot shift maneuver during a functional activity.

There are certain caveats for possible damage to be aware of during the ACL training program. There is a direct correlation between anterior knee pain (patellofemoral syndrome) and the amount of loaded knee bending performed. If someone squats with a heavy load, and the knee is pushed beyond 55° to 60°, our results show a higher incidence of anterior knee pain. The best take-home message for managing anterior knee pain is to avoid its occurrence. If it does appear, it must be identified and treated early. If not, there likely will be protracted pain. In the acutely painful stage, a short course of anti-inflammatory medication and ice massage

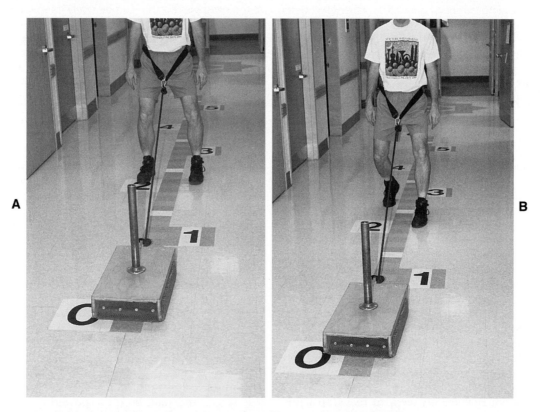

Fig. 30-21. Retrowalking pulling a non-weighted sled. **A** and **B,** Retrowalking is useful to unload the knee and relieve patellofemoral forces while strengthening the lower extremities.

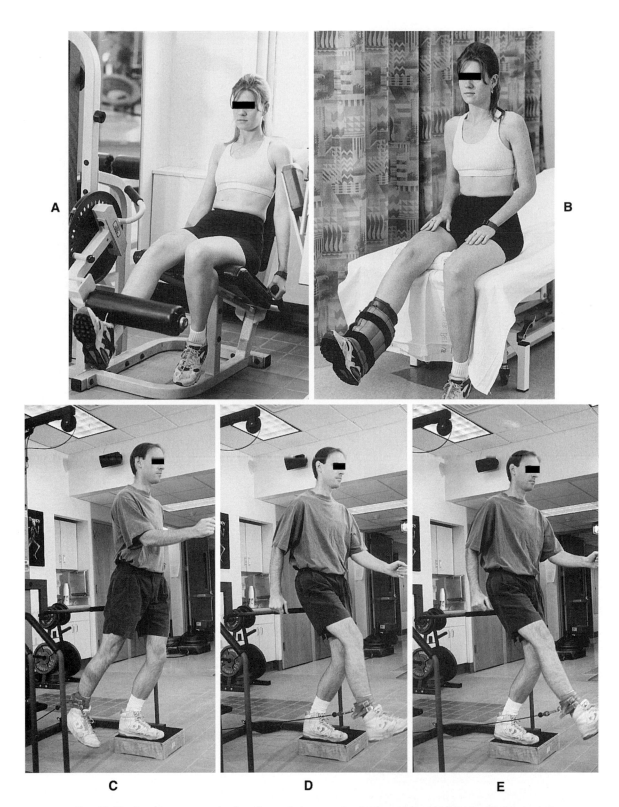

Fig. 30-22. Quadriceps strengthening. Open-chain strengthening is performed when the distal aspect of the exercising limb is not in direct contact with an external source; and closed-chain strengthening is performed when the distal aspect of the exercising limb is in direct contact with an external source. This, a rather confusing issue, is clarified if one thinks in terms of **perpendicular** and **axial** load when speaking of **open-** and **closed-**chain respectively. With the quadriceps, a perpendicular load exercise is one in which the majority of forces passes through (anterior-posterior or posterior-anterior) the tibio-femoral joint. An axial load exercise is one in which the majority of forces passes through (cephalad-caudad or caudad-cephalad) the tibio-femoral joint. If you want to spare undue stress across the ligaments of the knee, axial loading is more appropriate, and when trying to spare undue stress on the articular surfaces of the knee, perpendicular loading is more appropriate. Figs. **A–E** depict open-chain quadriceps exercises and **F–H** depict closed-chain quadriceps exercises. **A,** Seated supported knee extension. **B,** Seated unsupported knee extension (requires more intrinsic balance and coordination than **A**). **C–E,** Standing cable column knee extension (requires more balance and coordination than **A** or **B**).

Continued.

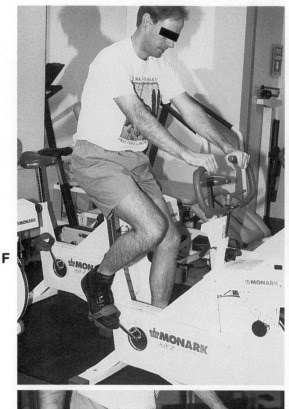

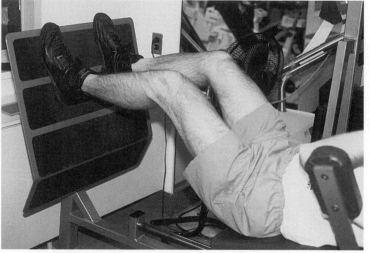

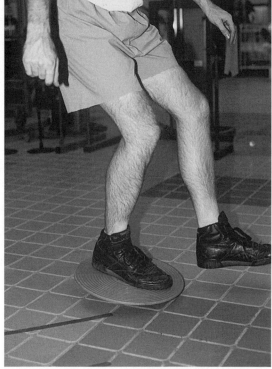

Fig. 30-22, cont'd. **F**, Stationary bicycle. **G**, Leg press (be careful not to hyperflex/extend the knee). **H**, Knee bend. The above should be done in sets of ten repetitions, 4 to 5 times. Be careful not to hyperextend the knee in the above exercises; this could lead to patellofemoral symptoms.

is helpful. Once pain is identified, patients should be instructed to limit the amount of knee flexion during squatting. A patient can continue to add weight but should not bend the knees beyond 55°- to 60°-angle.

Another concern many express is the effect that aggressive training has on the ACL graft. It is commonly thought that excess terminal extension of the involved knee will stretch the graft. Most aggressive rehabilitation programs allow early full active range of motion (FAROM), without specific limitation on terminal extension. Beynnon studied ACL stress by placing a transducer on 12 healthy volunteers' ligaments.[4] He found that certain ranges of motion caused more stress on the ACL than others. Our KT 2000 data, radiographic assessment, and subjective functional scales do not show positive evidence for graft stretching. Data for our current protocol are similar to those when we were limiting terminal extension.

Bracing is an issue that is becoming more controversial. In the recent past a patient with ACL surgery could expect to wear some sort of knee support for most athletic activities. There was a three-phase system: post-op brace, rehabilitation brace, functional brace. (There is a fourth, which is the prophylactic brace, but it is not directly related to the post-operative scheme described here.) More recently, the decision as to whether or not to brace has become less simple. The ultimate usefulness of a knee brace depends on its ability to protect the ligamentous structures.[6] This raises the question of whether a particular knee needs external support, or is it strong

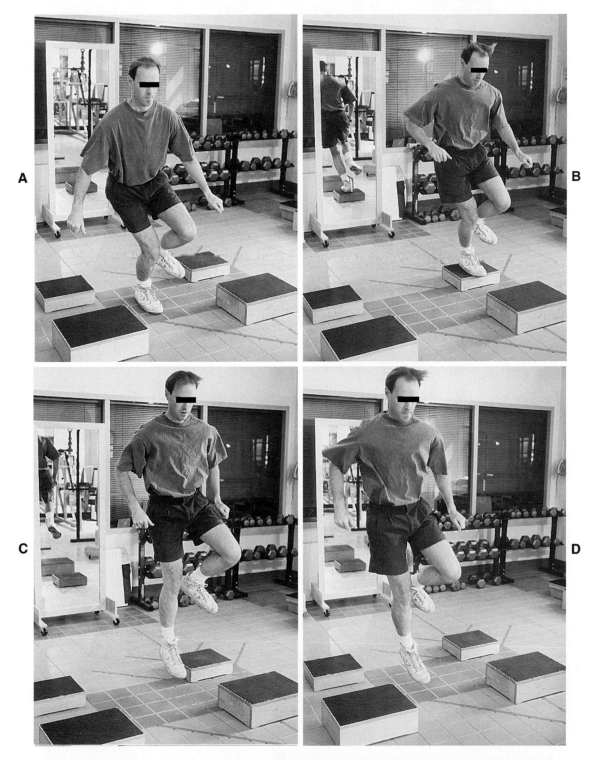

Fig. 30-23. Box jumping. **A–F,** Jumping onto and off of boxes of different heights set in different patterns assists in skill development.   *Continued.*

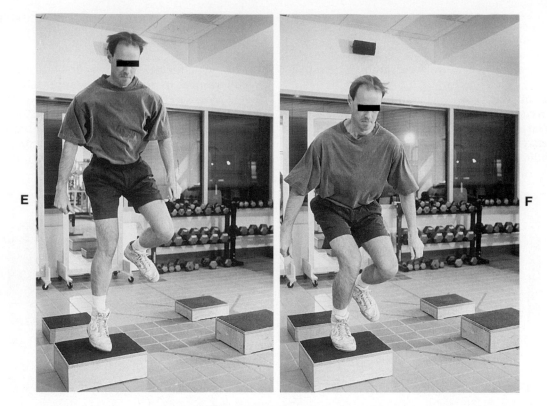

Fig. 30-23, cont'd. For legend see page 489.

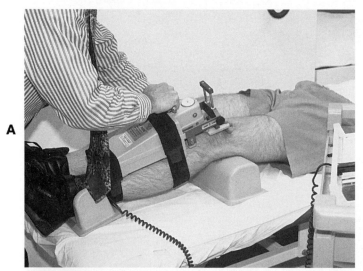

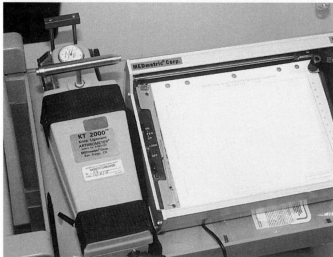

Fig. 30-24. KT 2000 Arthrometer. **A** and **B,** The patient lies down with the distal thigh placed on a bolster. The knee will be flexed approximately 20°. The inferior aspect of the patella should be aligned with the superior aspect of the bolster. The arthrometer is secured to the leg with two Velcro straps. Several trials are then performed measuring anterior and/or posterior excursion of the tibia with reference to the femur. The plotter graph quantifies the excursions that measure millimeters of anterior/posterior movement of the tibia relative to the femur on the x axis and force of anterior/posterior pull or push respectively of the arthrometer on the y axis.

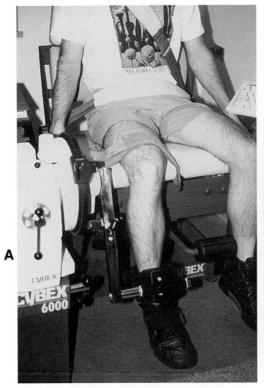

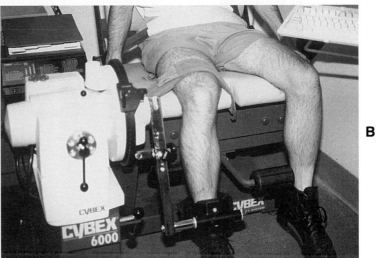

Fig. 30-25. Isokinetic testing. **A** and **B**, Baseline evaluation of sound limb and periodic testing for comparison between limbs serves as a training guide. It is particularly useful for the force-production component of skill training.

enough to safely perform without one? Also, are the limb muscles strong enough to dynamically protect the knee, thereby negating the need for a brace? Tibone and others reported prolonged hamstring firing in the post-surgical (weight-bearing) limb of an ACL–deficient patient. This prolonged firing is natural as the hamstrings work synergistically to stabilize an ACL–deficient knee.[56]

The literature is replete with investigative opinions on bracing. Johnston and Paulos investigated prophylactic lateral knee braces, and their conclusion was that no clear scientific or clinical consensus could be reached regarding the efficacy of these braces.[27] Likewise, rehabilitation and functional braces have shown varied results with tibia-femur shear stress. The notion of brace-related proprioceptive feedback has been reviewed. Although I believe that braces add proprioceptive feedback, there are several opposing opinions.[9,57] In one review, bracing did not alter electromyographic activity nor did it change firing patterns, compared to nonbracing. All muscles showed similar changes in activity, suggesting that bracing did not have proprioceptive influence.

At our center, we prescribe a hinge brace, which is worn for the first 2 to 3 weeks after surgery. Except for a knee sleeve, no other bracing is considered for 5 or 6 months, when we test function. Based on the combined results of these tests we determine the need for bracing. Generally, if KT 2000 scores are less than 4 to 5 mm side to side, and quadriceps and hamstring strengths are within 20% and 10% side to side respectively, no brace is recommended. However, the single most important determinant in applying a brace is patient choice. Even with excellent functional scores, if the patient desires a brace, one should be prescribed. In selecting a brace, a patient may consider some basic points: the brace should be lightweight (14 to

18 ounces), comfortable, nonintrusive on athletic performance, and economically reasonable.

Our conservative (nonsurgical) training program is very similar to the postoperative program. The length of training is shorter (2 to 3 months) since the early phase

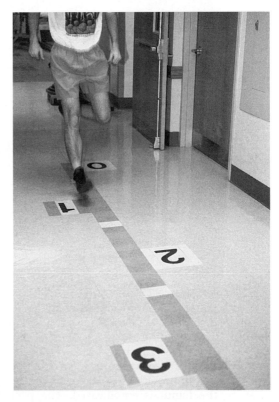

Fig. 30-26. Noyes Hop test.

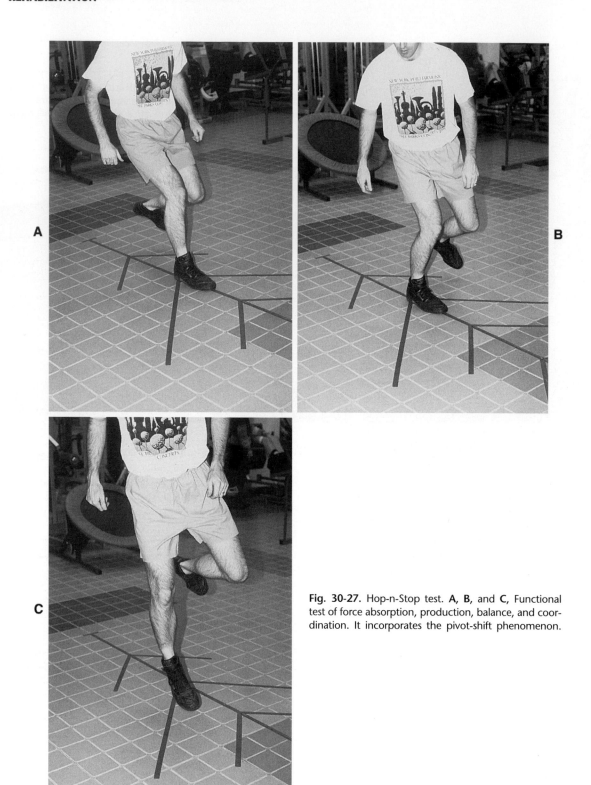

Fig. 30-27. Hop-n-Stop test. **A, B,** and **C,** Functional test of force absorption, production, balance, and coordination. It incorporates the pivot-shift phenomenon.

of the program proceeds more rapidly. Our goals and emphases are essentially the same. One significant difference is in strength training (force production and absorption), in which the hamstrings are a major focus. The dynamic ability of the hamstring group, particularly the lateral, to assist in posterior displacement of the tibia in relation to the femur is emphasized. The posterior cruciate ligament (PCL) rehabilitation program is not as well developed. Many centers have structured protocols,

but the relative number of patients with this injury is significantly less than those with anterior cruciate ligament injuries. The training sequence provides slightly more protection against extrinsic forces in the early stages. Post-op bracing persists for 4 to 6 weeks, with initial settings at minimal (on weight bearing) free motion. We avoid hamstring strengthening (if possible) until about POW 6. Our emphasis is on strengthening the quadriceps, with progression to functional training start-

POSTERIOR CRUCIATE LIGAMENT (PCL) REHABILITATION

Postoperative Day 1
Brace locked at 0
Continuous passive motion 5→60°
Ambulation bearing weight as tolerated with crutches
Ice, elevation
Quadriceps setting, straight leg raise, ankle pumps
Electrical stimulation prn to quadriceps

Postoperative Days 2–7
Brace open for available range of motion
Isometric hip abduction/adduction
Passive knee flexion
Multi-angle quadriceps isometrics
Patellar mobilization
Toe raises (extended knee)
Reverse stool slides

Postoperative Weeks 2–7
Stationary bicycle as tolerated
Balance training
Pool walking
Adding weight to previous exercises
Mini–knee bends (no more than 50°)
Sitting range of motion (POW 3–4)
Hamstring curls (POW 7) with light weights
Fitter (POW 7)

Postoperative Weeks 8–13
Nordic Track
Jogging (POW 12–13)
Step-ups
Step machine—short arc (POW 10–12)

Postoperative Weeks 14–16
Sports-specific training
Light running
Endurance training

Postoperative Weeks 17–6 Months
Agility drills
Running
Plyometrics

Table 30-5. Classification of medial collateral ligament injury at 30 degrees of flexion

First-degree injury	No laxity
	Firm endpoint
Second-degree injury	≤ 5 mm laxity
	Firm endpoint
Third-degree injury	> 5 mm laxity
	Soft endpoint

From Nicholas JA, Hershman EB, editors: *The lower extremity and spine in sports medicine*, ed 2, St Louis, 1995, Mosby–Year Book, p 832.

Table 30-6. Treatment of first-degree medial collateral ligament injuries

Stage I	Ice
	Knee immobilizer
	Full weight-bearing with crutches
	Isometric exercises
Stage II (as pain and swelling subside)	Discontinuing immobilizer
	Discontinuing crutches
	Range-of-motion exercises
	Hip flexor and abductor strengthening
	Closed-chain exercises
	Adduction strengthening with resistance proximal to knee
Stage III (as range of motion returns)	Progressive resistance exercises
	Isokinetic exercise
	Proprioceptive training
	Functional rehabilitation

Thoughout the program, aerobic, well-leg, and upper-body conditioning are continued.
From Nicholas JA, Hershman EB, editors: *The lower extremity and spine in sports medicine*, ed 2, St Louis, 1995, Mosby–Year Book, p 832.

ing at 3 months. The box in the first column illustrates the training progression.

Medial and lateral collateral ligament sprains are usually treated conservatively. Medial collateral ligament sprains are graded I to III. The classification is outlined in Table 30-5. Training for low-grade sprains (I) progresses more quickly than training for high-grade sprains (III). Tables 30-6 and 30-7 outline conservative regimens for medial collateral

Table 30-7. Treatment of second-degree medial collateral ligament injuries

Stage I	Ice
	Compression
	Knee immobilizer
	Partial weight-bearing with crutches
	Isometric exercises
Stage II (as acute symptoms resolve)	Gentle range of motion
	Progression to full weight bearing in brace
	Quadriceps setting
	Straight leg raising
	Closed-chain exercises
	Hip flexor and adductor strengthening
	Hip adduction strengthening with resistance proximal to knee
Stage III (when 90 degrees of flexion is present)	Continuation of range-of-motion program
	Exercise bicycle
	Isokinetic program (high speed)
	Beginning proprioceptive training
Stage IV (when full range of motion is present)	Progessive resistance exercises in flexion
	Isokinetic program (full)
	Exercise bicycle
Stage V (full painless range of motion)	Running in brace
	Functional program (progressive)

Thoughout the program, aerobic, well-leg, and upper-body conditioning are continued.
From Nicholas JA, Hershman EB, editors: *The lower extremity and spine in sports medicine*, ed 2, St Louis, 1995, Mosby–Year Book, p 833.

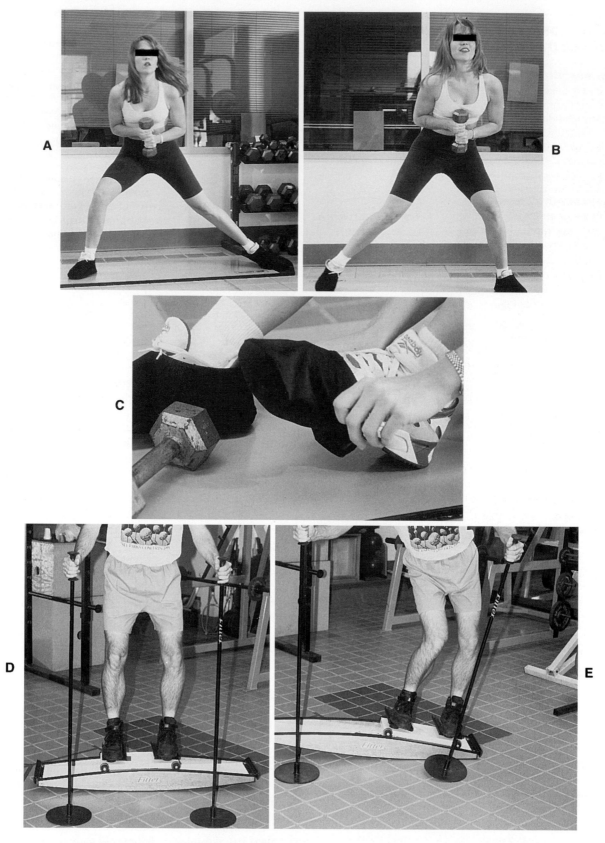

Fig. 30-28. Slide and roller board. **A** and **B,** The slide board is an effective conditioning device that can be combined with upper-body techniques including hand-held weight or ball toss. The boards have various lengths and are easily stored. **C,** Cloth booties are worn to decrease friction while gliding on the board. Treatment sessions are based upon time on board rather than number of slides. **D** and **E,** The roller board is a good device to begin lateral agility training. It offers proprioceptive feedback and strengthens the lower extremities in general.

sprains. Lateral collateral ligament sprains are treated much the same way, with care taken not to gap the lateral joint line. For third degree sprains, surgical intervention is sometimes required, and the length of post-op immobilization varies. Usually a rigid cast is applied for 2 to 3 weeks for the surgically repaired medial collateral ligament.

The menisci are frequently injured. This is understandable considering their role in joint stabilization, shock absorption, and weight bearing. Forty to 60% of the weight transferred across the knee is carried by the menisci. Conservative treatment of diagnosed meniscal tears is somewhat effective. A program design emphasizing open-chain (perpendicular load) and short arc closed-chain (axial load) exercises can dynamically stabilize the knee. Once pain control is achieved and swelling reduced, patients who successfully complete a conservative program are quite satisfied. In addition to closed-chain progressive resistive exercises, functional activities including Nordic Track, slide board, and roller board help to maximize performance (Fig. 30-28).

For postoperative meniscal injuries, the number of meniscal tears currently being treated by repair vs. resection is growing. Long-term follow-up data on outcomes of meniscal repair are unavailable, but a decrease in the high incidence of degenerative changes, which are seen in meniscectomy, is anticipated. It is reported that degenerative changes are seen in the joints after meniscectomy as early as three months after surgery.[13] If meniscal repair proves a successful salvage procedure, the functional benefits will be very rewarding.

Rehabilitation after meniscal repair historically has been a slower process than after meniscectomy, but more aggressive programs now are being advocated (Table 30-8). After meniscectomy, patients are allowed to bear weight as tolerated. Riding a stationary bicycle is encouraged. The liberal application of ice helps to decrease effusion and pain. It is important to let the patient know of potential degenerative changes. Avoidance of excessive impact loading onto the knees is important. Modification of activities like running should be discussed. Swimming is encouraged. Exercises to stretch and strengthen the associated muscles are emphasized.

For the patient undergoing meniscal repair, many advocate a more conservative protocol.[16] This would in-

Table 30-8. Rehabilitation after meniscectomy/repair

Postoperative week 1	Ambulation bearing weight as tolerated Ice prn Range of motion as tolerated Bicycle for range of motion (high seat)
Postoperative weeks 2–4	Short arc closed-chain (axial load) exercise 0–30° Open-chain (perpendicular load) exercises with light weights Bicycle
Postoperative weeks 5–8	Progression to functional exercises and sport-specific exercises

From Nicholas JA, Hershman EB, editors: *The lower extremity and spine in sports medicine*, ed 2, St Louis, 1995, Mosby–Year Book, p 833.

Table 30-9. Meniscal repair

Postoperative weeks 0–6	Partial weight bearing Range of motion 0–90°
Postoperative weeks 6–12	Progression to weight bearing as tolerated Progressive weight training Endurance training Progression to full range of motion

clude limited weight bearing for 4 to 6 weeks after surgery (Table 30-9). Range of motion is also limited for the first 6 weeks. Resistive exercises are delayed until the third month after surgery and returning to competitive sports until 4 or 5 months. The more aggressive rehabilitation program for meniscal repair closely follows the guidelines for meniscectomy. The major difference is the ability of the patient to continue athletic performance, including impact absorption, because of the returned integrity of the meniscus. The details of this program are similar to those of post-op ACL rehabilitation.

Osteoarthritis (OA) of the knee is one of the most frequently occurring musculoskeletal diseases.[40] After the spine and the hip, the knee is the site most often affected.[8] Approximately 10% of persons older than 65 (a greater number of females than males) have symptomatic OA of the knee.[8] Before embarking on a specific rehabilitation program, careful evaluation of the entire musculoskeletal system should be made. Aberrations elsewhere can predispose or directly influence a person to the development of OA. An example is the person who pronates at the subtalar joint. As previously stated, this causes a valgus stress on the knee and loads the lateral compartment. If the patient has heel spurs or plantar fasciitis, anterior knee pain can occur because of increased load onto the quadriceps in avoidance of heel-strike. This predisposes to quadriceps tendinitis and increased anterior joint stress.

A patient's first step in OA treatment is to modify his/her activity and avoid being overweight. Loaded knee flexion extension activities, particularly those with large impact, should be avoided. Occupations that require prolonged squatting are detrimental and are associated with symptomatic OA. Obesity is a precursor to OA of the knee, and weight loss may prevent the development of symptoms.[14] Remember that stress across the joint is a factor of body weight, and forces across the knee range from 1 to 7 times body weight (depending upon the activity, e.g., there are higher forces with running).

Pharmacologic management includes acetaminophen and NSAIDs. There are many NSAIDs to chose from; they are listed in the discussion on spine rehabilitation. Careful attention must be paid to GI, liver, and kidney function when using NSAIDs. A low dosage of tricyclic antidepressants can be used for the management of OA. Patients with OA who complain of prolonged morning stiffness often do not sleep well. These people may sleep and feel better after taking tricyclics.[15] Commonly used preparations include amitriptyline, starting at 25 mg/day and progressing to 75 mg/day. I ask for baseline electrocardiograms on patients with known cardiac arrhythmia or those with compromised cardiac status. Tricyclics can

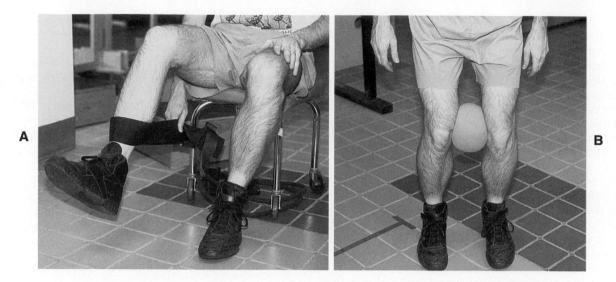

Fig. 30-29. Isometric knee exercise. **A,** A simple belt can be used to effectively isometrically strengthen the periarticular muscles of the knee. The contractions should be held for 3 to 4 seconds and repeated. Patients should be cautioned not to forcibly exhale with mouth and nostrils closed and to limit this exercise if there is a significant cardiac history. **B,** A ball could be squeezed between the knees to effect an isometric contraction.

have untoward effects on the PR interval, and arrhythmia may be induced. The cardiogram is periodically checked throughout the course of administration of the tricyclic. Corticosteroids, taken orally or parenterally, are minimally effective for OA. The route of choice is intraarticular. I use triamcinolone hexacetonide, 20 mg, or methylprednisolone acetate, 40 mg. Care should be taken in administering repeated doses because they may speed the degenerative process.

Exercises to treat OA focus on joint preservation. Initially, isometric exercises are done. These can be supine straight leg raising, or against the fixed resistance of a belt (Fig. 30-29). Isotonic exercises are performed and focused in the pain-free arc. Isokinetic exercises are particularly useful since the speed and direction of motion can be carefully monitored (Fig. 30-30). Exercises must be

done regularly; a minimum of three times a week is required. Daily routines should be considered if time allows. To simplify things, each exercise should have a fixed number of repetitions and consist of three sets. Fig. 30-31 illustrates exercises for OA.

For more advanced cases of OA, total joint arthroplasty may be recommended. This procedure has been one of the most successful joint replacement procedures in terms of morbidity and patient satisfaction. The rehabilitation program after total knee arthroplasty initially focuses on restoring functional range of motion. This is accomplished with hands-on ranging by a therapist along with a continuous passive motion device (CPM) (Fig. 30-32). Benefits of CPM include improved range of motion[26] and earlier independent mobility. The use of electrical stimulation has been shown to improve motion after to-

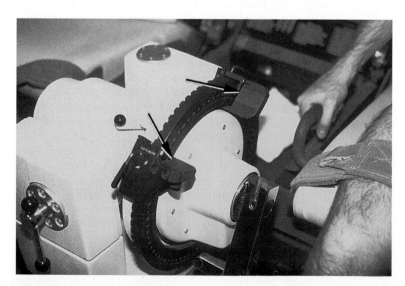

Fig. 30-30. Isokinetics with limited range of motion. After securing a limb into the device, a limited range of motion can be set by adjusting the mechanical blocks as shown on the dynamometer. Specific joint arcs can be protected with this device. For example, if there is pain on knee flexion beyond 60°, limiting the range to less than 60° can avoid the painful arc.

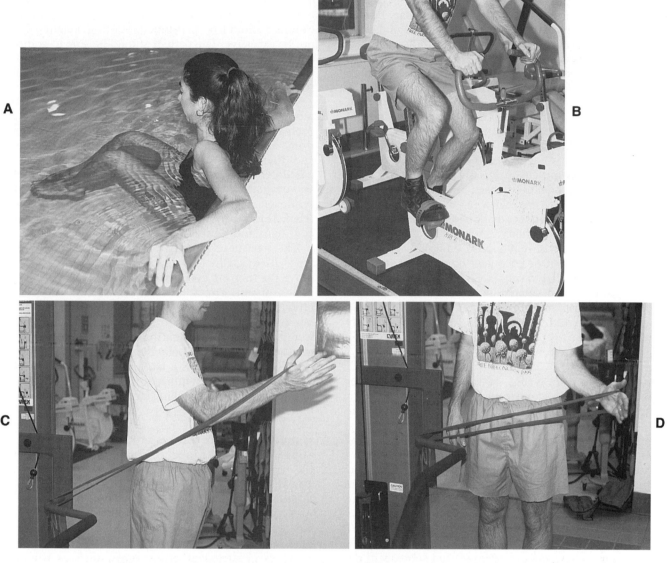

Fig. 30-31. Exercises for osteoarthritis. **A,** Aqua therapy spares the joint surfaces and provides a medium for resistive and aerobic training. It is very effective in treating the arthritic joint. **B,** Riding a stationary bicycle is a good exercise, especially when the degree of knee flexion/extension is kept midrange. This is achieved by raising or lowering the seat height. **C** and **D,** Thera-band exercise can be individualized for different planes of motion. It is easy to use and is available in various degrees of resistance.

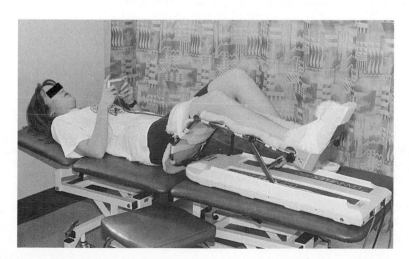

Fig. 30-32. Continuous Passive Motion (CPM). The limb is mechanically ranged at predetermined degrees of motion. CPM assists in attaining increased motion in the involved joint.

tal knee arthroplasty, particularly by decreasing extensor lag.[20] Patients are typically hospitalized for 4 to 7 days and continue their exercises at home. A stationary bicycle is very effective for gaining knee motion and obtaining an aerobic workout. Ambulating is done as tolerated, typically with an assistance device (such as a cane) for a few weeks. There is persistent swelling about the knee, which lasts for approximately 6 months. Patients should be alerted to expect this normal finding. Greatly increased swelling may not be normal. It could signify overuse but may be a sign of infection. Patients should call their surgeon if any significant change occurs, such as sudden loss of motion, fever, drainage, or erythema.

The associated musculature is strengthened the same way as for OA. Guidelines for activity limitation are unclear at this time. A recent review of younger (less than 55 years of age) patients after total knee replacement (TKR) showed their increased ability to tolerate load on the prosthetic knee. We advise patients to limit impact on the postsurgical knee, but we encourage physical activity. Doubles tennis is preferred to singles. Running on solid ground is not recommended. Swimming is encouraged. The patient should expect to feel encouraged sometimes between 6 weeks and 6 months after surgery. The activities severely hindered before surgery can then become feasible.

Tendinitis

Anterior knee pain is one of the most usual musculoskeletal complaints, having a number of possible etiologies. Patella tendinitis and patella femoral syndrome (PFS) are two common diagnoses. Patella tendinitis, jumpers knee,[7] is usually seen in athletic activities requiring forceful eccentric muscle contractions or repeated flexion and extension of the knee.[50] The most common presentation is pain at the inferior pole of the patella. It can also occur at the tibial tubercle and at the superior pole of the patella. Pain is common after physical exercise and when ascending or descending stairs.

The biomechanics of this complex are important to understanding the mechanism of injury and subsequent development of appropriate rehabilitation strategies. The forces on the the patella—the quadriceps tendon above and the patella tendon below—are not equally distributed during muscle contraction.[50] During closed-chain activities (landing from a jump) the ratio of quadriceps tendon tension to patella tendon tension increases with increasing knee flexion; but during open-chain activities (seated knee extension) the ratio of quadriceps tendon tension to patella tendon tension increases with knee extension.[17] When the quadriceps undergoes eccentric contraction, significantly increased force is transmitted to the patella tendon. The treatment of patella tendinitis begins with a brief period of rest, use of ice, ultrasound, and NSAIDs.

Before a patient begins rehabilitative exercises, a general warm-up is recommended. Riding a stationary bicycle for 15 to 20 minutes with low resistance and an elevated seat height is a good way to begin. Stretching the quadriceps and hamstrings is next. Strengthening the associated muscles, particularly the eccentric knee extensors, will best prepare the knee to successfully absorb impact. This can be done through progressive step-downs (Fig. 30-33). The patient should progress to short jumpdowns from varied heights (Fig. 30-34). In addition, lunges, isokinetic quadriceps eccentrics, and hamstring isotonics should be performed. Starting weights should not be excessive. The patient should be able to complete ten repetitions with relative ease. As he/she progresses, the workout weight should be such that the patient struggles to lift it ten times.

Patellofemoral syndrome is probably the most common presentation of anterior knee pain. Much has been written about this syndrome, both its manifestations and treatment. It often remains a diagnostic and therapeutic dilemma. The biomechanics of the patellofemoral joint are constantly being researched and evaluated. The basic understanding in treating this syndrome is that the patellofemoral relationship is altered; this incongruence sets the stage for the associated signs and symptoms.

The treatment paradigm mimics many of those we have discussed in this chapter. The first step is to remove the inciting event, which is achieved with a brief period of rest. The adjunct treatments of ice, NSAIDs, ultrasound, and electrical stimulation are followed. At our center we approach this disorder as if the patella were an object freely floating in the anterior compartment of the knee, desperately searching for a niche to call home. The knee is a large joint and is acted upon by muscles in an asymmetric manner, which lays the foundation for maltracking and malalignment. Rehabilitation entails stretching and strengthening the associated muscles in a way that most closely creates symmetry for force vectors around the patella. At the same time, we try to reduce perpendicular loads across the patellofemoral joint, to salvage the joint surfaces. The training progression is carried out over a 2- to 3-month period.

Fig. 30-35 depicts the techniques used to rehabilitate a patient with patellofemoral syndrome. As with patella tendinitis, patellofemoral syndrome is influenced by the activities occurring at other joints, such as when the subtalar joint pronates and there is an associated valgus moment at the knee. This then increases the Q angle and promotes maltracking. Retrowalking in a toe-to-heel gait causes subtalar supination and results in a varus moment at the knee that acts to decrease the Q angle (and unload the patellofemoral joint). If a person pronates excessively, it is important to consider the use of orthotics. Sleeves and braces are advocated for the knee. There are many braces on the market that manufacturers claim are effective in treating PFS. None stands alone as a clear choice, and research continues to evaluate the role of bracing in PFS. In general, most practitioners attempt to align the patella centrally between the femoral condyles. McConnell taping uses directed taping sequences. These unload the patellofemoral joint during training sessions.

Iliotibial band friction syndrome is a condition that usually manifests itself as pain over the lateral femoral condyle. It is common in runners, especially those who run on uneven terrain. It is thought to occur secondarily to translocation of the iliotibial band (ITB) from an-

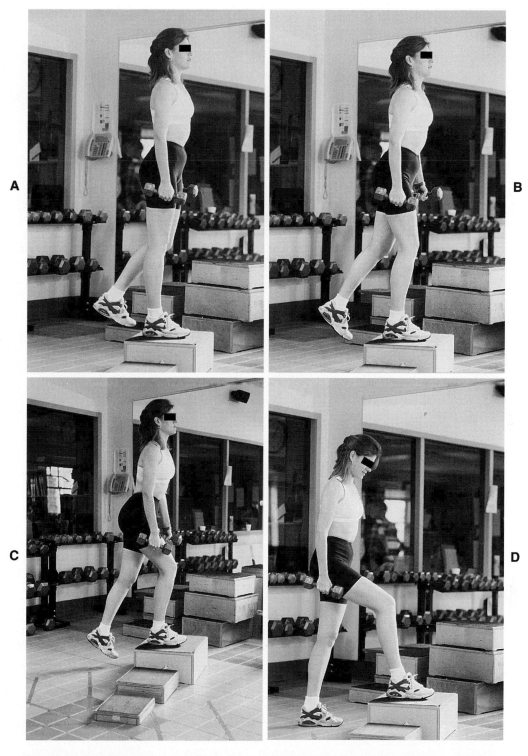

Fig. 30-33. Step-downs. **A–D,** To effectively train the limb to absorb force, controlled step-downs are done. We want to support the weight of the body while progressively increasing velocity. As the patient begins to master the technique, the force of impact is distributed through the muscles in a very synchronous way. Weight can be added to increase the mass that the limbs must support.

terior to posterior as a runner goes from knee extension to knee flexion. It is proximally related to the tensor fascia lata at the fascia of the gluteus maximus. Treatment of this syndrome includes rest, ice, NSAIDs, ultrasound, stretching of the ITB (Fig. 30-36 on page 505), and orthotics if there is concomitant foot and ankle pathology. Normal gait causes internal tibial rotation, which is exaggerated if excess pronation occurs. This exaggerated internal tibial rotation will stretch the ITB across the femoral condyle.

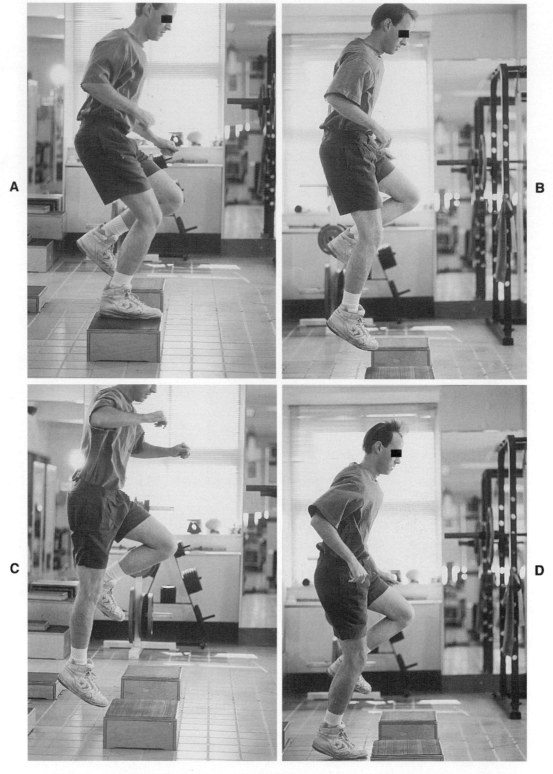

Fig. 30-34. Jump-downs. **A–D,** The progression from step-downs is to jump-downs. The patient jumps to the floor from varied heights and must control the landing by allowing a springing-type motion at the joints to distribute the forces of impact.

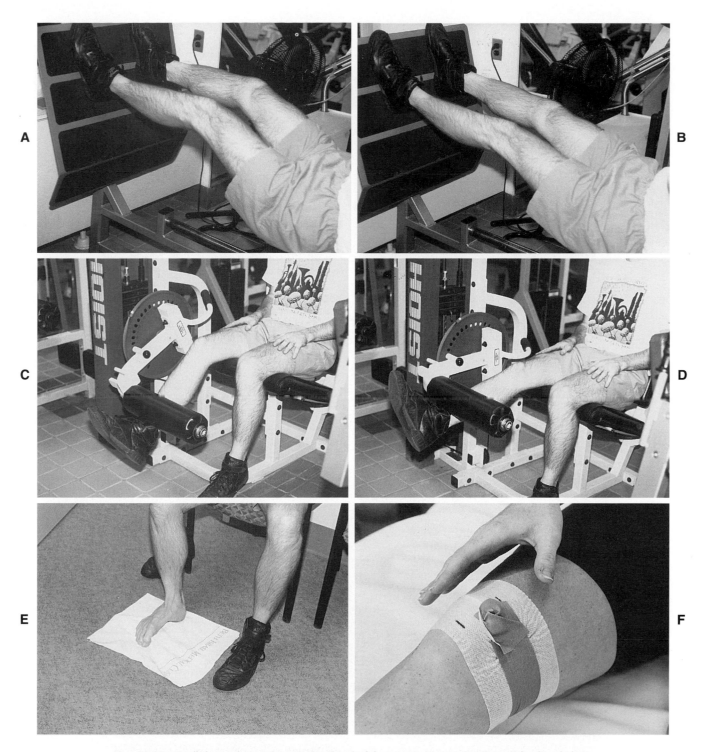

Fig. 30-35. Patellofemoral exercises. **A–N,** Terminal knee extensions—Starting with closed-chain (axial load, **A, B**) in the range of 30° to 0° and progressing to open-chain (perpendicular load, **C, D**), these exercises are effective in strengthening the quadriceps while sparing undo patellofemoral stresses. **E,** Towel grab—to increase supinator strength and prevent excessive subtalar pronation, this is a very effective exercise. The towel is grabbed with the forefoot and attempts are made to pick it up with the toes. **F,** McConnell taping—a technique to realign a maltracking patellar. Tape is applied to the knee, attempting to place the patella in a more congruent position with respect to the femur. Hopefully, the tape will maintain proper contact to allow the patella to track more anatomically.

Continued.

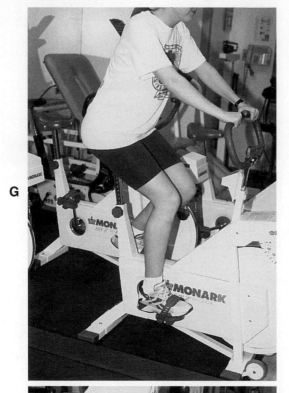

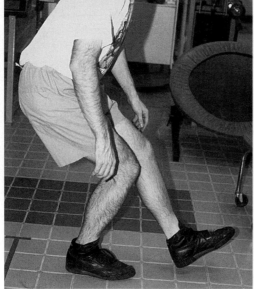

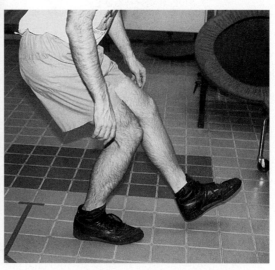

Fig. 30-35, cont'd. G, High seat bicycle—Set seat height to prevent knee flexion beyond 50° to 55°. Pedal resistance should be low. Time exercise to pedal for 20 to 30 minutes 1 to 2 times/day. **H** and **I,** Short-arc knee bends—Standing firmly on a single leg, flex knee to maximum of 50° to 55°. Upright posture must be maintained. Multiple sets are performed. *Continued.*

J K L

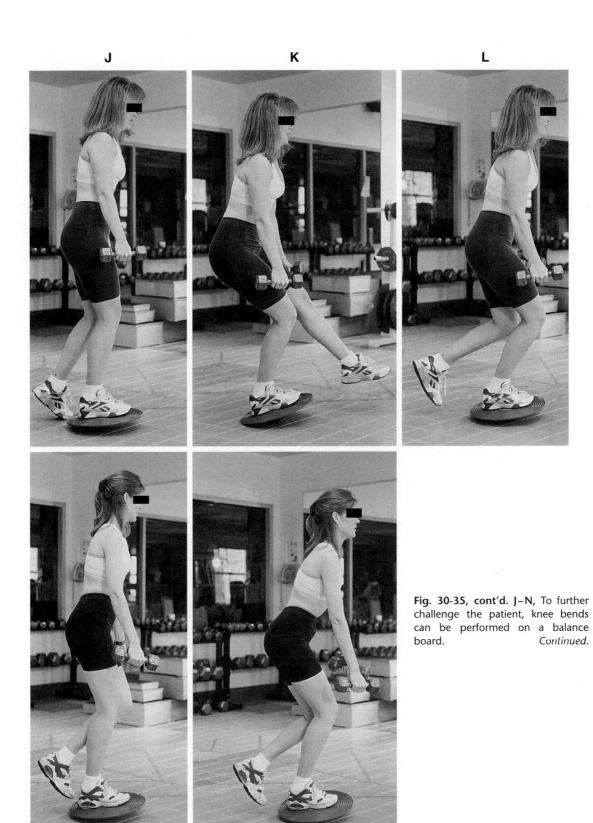

M N

Fig. 30-35, cont'd. J–N, To further challenge the patient, knee bends can be performed on a balance board. *Continued.*

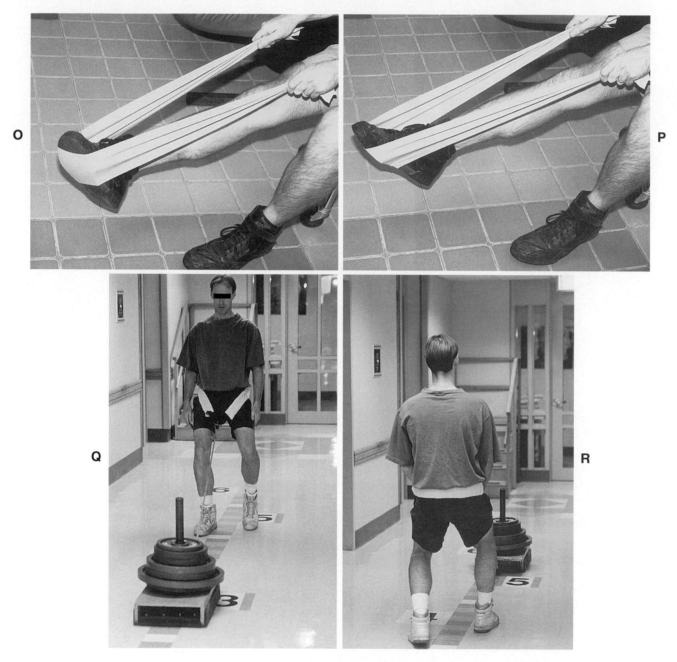

Fig. 30-35, cont'd. O and **P,** Thera-band alphabets—see Fig. 30-6 for description. **Q** and **R,** Retro-walking—see Fig. 30-7 for description.

Continued.

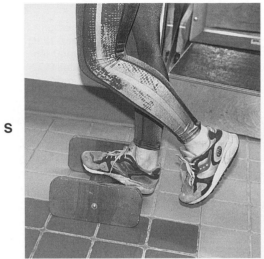

S

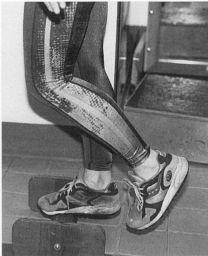

T

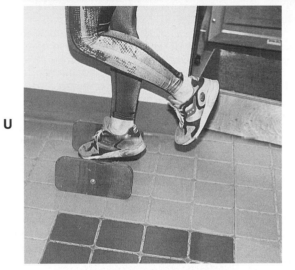

U

Fig. 30-35, cont'd. S,T, and **U,** Plantar roll bar exercises—see Fig. 30-8 for description.

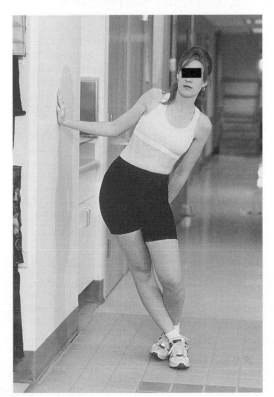

Fig. 30-36. Iliotibial band stretch. The patient stands, and the limb to be stretched is placed across the body in front of the other limb. The ipsilateral hip is then thrust laterally while the foot maintains contact with the ground. This position is held for 30 seconds.

REFERENCES

1. Arner O, Lindholm A: "What is tennis leg?" *Acta Chir Scand* 116:73, 1958.
2. Arnheim DD, Prentice WE: The ankle and lower leg. In Smith JM, ed: *Principles of athletic training*, ed 8, Baltimore, MD, 1993, Mosby-Year Book.
3. Baker CL, Todd JL: Intervening in acute ankle sprain and chronic instability, *J Musculoskeletal Med* 54, July 1995.
4. Beynnon BD, et al: Anterior cruciate ligament strain behavior during rehabilitation exercises in vivo, *Am J Sports Med*, 23:24–34, 1995.
5. Birrer RB: Ankle injuries. In Birrer RB, ed: *Sports medicine for the primary care physician*, ed 2, Boca Raton, Fla, 1994, CRC Press.
6. Black KP, Raasch WG: Knee braces in sports. In Nicholas JA, Hershman EB, eds: *The lower extremity and spine in sports medicine*, ed 2, St. Louis, 1995, Mosby-Year Book.
7. Blazina M, Kerlan R, Jobe F: Jumpers knee, *Orthop Clin North Am* 4:665–678, 1973.
8. Bradley JD: Nonsurgical option for managing osteoarthritis of the knee, *J Musculoskeletal Med* 14-26, August 1994.
9. Branch TP, Hunter R, Donath M: Dynamic EMG analysis of the anterior cruciate deficient legs with and without bracing during cutting, *Am J Sports Med* 17:35, 1989.
10. Clement DB: Tibial stress syndrome in athletes, *Am J Sports Med* 2:81–85, 1974.
11. Devereaux MD, Lachmann SM: Athletes attending a sports injury clinic—A review, *Br J Sports Med* 17(4):137–142, 1983.
12. Edwards G: Contralateral and ipsilateral cane usage by patients with total knee or hip replacement, *Archives of Phys Med Rehab* 67:734, 1986.
13. Fairbank TJ: Knee joint changes after meniscectomy, *J Bone Joint Surg* 30B:664, 1981.
14. Felson DT, Andrews JJ, Naimark A: Obesity and knee osteoarthritis. The Framingham Study. *Annals of Internal Medicine* 109:18–24, 1989.
15. Frank RG, Kashani JH, Parker JC, et al: Antidepressant analgesia in rheumatoid arthritis, *J Rheumatol* 15:1632–1638, 1988.
16. Fu FH, Baratz M: Meniscal injuries. In DeLee JC, Drez D, eds: *Orthopaedic sports medicine, principles and practice*, vol 2, Philadelphia, 1994, WB Saunders.
17. Fulkerson J, Hungerfor D: *Disorder of the patellofemoral joint*, ed 2, Baltimore, Md, 1990, Williams and Wilkins.
18. Garrick JG, Requa RK: The epidemiology of foot and ankle injuries in sports, *Clin Sports Med* 7(1):29–36, 1988.
19. Gary G: Ankle rehabilitation using the ankle disk, *Phys Sports Medicine* 6(6):141, 1978.
20. Gotlin RS, et al: Electrical stimulation effect on extensor lag and length of hospital stay after total knee arthroplasty, *Arch Phys Med Rehabil* 75:957–959, 1994.
21. Grimes DW, Bennion D, Blusk K: Functional foot reconditioning exercises, *Am J Sports Med* 6:194, 1978.
22. Higgins JR: *Human movement: An integrated approach*, St. Louis, 1977, CV Mosby.
23. Jackson DW, Ashley RL, Powell JW: Ankle sprains in young athletes, *Clin Orthop* 101:201–215, 1974.
24. Jackson D, Bailey D: Shin splints in the young athlete a non specific diagnosis, *Phys Sports Med* 3(3):45, 1975.
25. James SD, Bates BT, Osternig LR: Injuries to runners, *Am J Sports Med* 6(2):40–50, 1978.
26. Johnson DP, Eastwood DM: Beneficial effects of continuous passive motion after total condylar knee arthroplasty, *Ann Royal Col Surg Engl* 74:412–416, 1992.
27. Johnston JM, Paulos LE: Prophylactic lateral knee braces, *Med Sci Sports Exerc* 23(7):783–787, 1991.
28. Johnson KA: Tibialis posterior tendon rupture, *Clin Orthop* 177:140–147, 1983.
29. Jorgenson U: Body load in heel strike running: the effects of a firm heel counter, *Am J Sports Med* 18:77, 1990.
30. Kellett J: Acute soft tissue injuries: A review of the literature, *Med Sci Sport Exerc* 18:489–500, 1986.
31. Leach R, Schepsis A: When hind foot pain slows the athlete, *J Musculoskeletal Med* 114, April 1992.
32. Lehman WL Jr: Overuse syndromes in runners, *Am Fam Physician* 29(1):157–161, 1984.
33. Mann, RA: Biomechanics of running. In Mack RP, editor: *American Academy of Orthopaedics Surgeons Symposium on the Foot and Leg in Running Sports*, St. Louis, 1982, CV Mosby.
34. Mann RA: Foot and ankle: Biomechanics of the foot and ankle linkage. In DeLee JC, Drez D, eds: *Orthopaedic sports medicine principles and practice*, Philadelphia, 1994, WB Saunders.
35. Matheson GO, Clement DB, McKenzie DC, et al: Stress fractures in athletes: A study of 320 cases, *Am J Sports Med* 15(1):46–58, 1987.
36. McKenzie DC, Clement DB, Taunton JE: Running shoes, orthotics and injuries, *Sports Med* 2:334–347, 1985.
37. McNair PJ, Marshall RN: Landing characteristics in subjects with normal and anterior cruciate deficient knees, *Arch Phys Med Rehab* 75:584–589, 1994.
38. Micheli LJ, Vorderer TW, Santopietro F, Sohn R: Athletic footwear and modifications in the lower extremity and spine. In Nicholas JA, Hershman EB, eds: *Sports medicine*, ed 2, vol 1, St. Louis, 1995, Mosby-Year Book.
39. Morris J: Biomechanical aspects of the hip joint, *Orthop Clin of North Am* 2:33, 1971.
40. Morrey BF: Primary osteoarthritis of the knee: A step wise management plan, *J Musculoskeletal Med* 79–94, 1992.
41. Mubarak SJ, Gould RN, Lee YF, Schmidt DA, Hargens AR: The medial tibial stress syndrome, a cause of shin splints, *Am J Sports Med* 10(4):201–205, 1982.
42. Nicholas JA, Strizak AM, Veras G: A study of thigh muscle weakness in different pathological states of the lower extremity, *Am J Sports Med* 4(6):241, 1976.
43. Nikolao PK, Ribbeck BM, Glisson RR, et al: The effect of muscle architecture on the biomechanical failure properties of skeletal muscle under passive extension, *Am J Sports Med* 16:7–12, 1988.
44. Noyes FR: The Noyes knee rating system. An International Publication of Cincinnati Sports Medicine Research and Education Foundation. Cincinnati, Oh, 1990, Cincinnati Sports Medicine Center, 1990.
45. Nyland J, Brosky T, Currier D, et al: Review of the afferent neural system of the knee and its contribution to motor learning, *JOSPT* 19(1):2–8, 1994.
46. Orava S, Jormakka E, Hulkko A: Stress fractures in young athletes, *Arch Orthop Trauma Surg* 98:271–274, 1981.
47. Orava S: Stress fractures, *Br J Sports Med* 14:40–44, 1980.
48. Pauwels F: *Der Schenkelhalsbruch ein Mechanisches Problem*, Stuggart, 1935, Ferdinand Enke Verlag.
49. Pearsall AW: Assessing acute hip injury; examination, diagnosis, and triage, *Phys Sports Med* 23(6):40, 1995.
50. Pezzullo DJ, Irrgang JJ, Whitney SL: Patellar tendonitis: Jumpers knee, *J Sports Rehab* 1:56–88, 1992.
51. Powell RW: Lawn tennis leg, *Lancet* 2:44, 1883.
52. Regan K, Underwood L: Surgical tubing for rehabilitating shoulder and ankle, *Phys Sports Med* 9:1, 1981.
53. Rogers R, Lipscomb B: Non union stress fractures of the tibia, *Am J Sports Med* 13:171, 1985.
54. Shelbourne DK: Accelerated rehabilitation after anterior cruciate ligament reconstruction, *JOSPT* 15(6):256–264, 1992.
55. Stanitski C, McMaster J, Scranton P: On the nature of stress fractures, *Am J Sports Med* 6(6):391–396, 1978.
56. Tibone JE, et al: Functional analysis of anterior cruciate ligament instability, *Am J Sports Med* 16:332, 1988.
57. Vailas JC, et al: Dynamic biomechanical effects of functional bracing, *Med Sci Sports Exerc* (Suppl):582, 1989.
58. Vegso JJ, Harmon LE: Non operative management of athletic ankle injuries, *Clin Sports Med* 1:85–97, 1982.

CHAPTER 31

THE UPPER EXTREMITY

Daniel J. Kane
Robert S. Gotlin

The lower extremities' predominant role, as they make the motions of running, skating, and jumping, is to maneuver an athlete's body in the environment. The upper extremities, on the other hand, function to actually manipulate the environment. In most sports, the athlete uses his upper extremity to catch, propel, or guide an object either directly or with an apparatus such as a glove, bat, or racket. In some sports, such as swimming, gymnastics, and pole vaulting, the athlete's upper extremity provides force to move the body. Whereas the lower extremities put the athlete in position to perform a task, the upper extremity accomplishes the task. The muscles, bones, and joints of the shoulders, elbows, wrists, and hands work as a unit to perform the fine manipulative neuromuscular behavior necessary for the athlete's sport.

The shoulder positions the arm and supplies power intrinsically, using the muscles of the shoulder joint complex, and extrinsically, by harvesting the energy generated by the remainder of the athlete's body. The elbow helps to preposition the hand and provide force. The wrist and hand are the final common pathway. They not only transmit forces but grip objects and perform fine manipulation.

An athlete's upper extremity can be injured by either macro- or micro-trauma. Macro-trauma describes impairment from a single event, such as a blow to the arm during a football tackle. Micro-trauma pertains to injuries originating from repetitive movements that result in cumulative pathological conditions. An example of micro-trauma is anterior shoulder instability from repeated overhead throwing motions.

The rehabilitation for macro-trauma is relatively straightforward. The clinician should allow sufficient time for healing and then work on regaining lost range of motion, strength, and skill. The rehabilitation of an athlete with an injury from micro-trauma is more complex. Essentially, the biomechanics of the athlete must be evaluated in order to diagnose the disorder. Thus the capable rehabilitative clinician must not only be familiar with the actions of the athlete's

muscles, but also the nuances and demands of the athlete's sport. Not until the abnormal flexibility, muscular imbalance, or faulty technique leading to poor biomechanics is addressed and corrected is the task of rehabilitation possible.

This chapter focuses on the rehabilitation of the shoulder, elbow, wrist, and hand. To elaborate on the treatment of each injury of the upper extremity is beyond the scope of this text. Instead, a generalized rehabilitation plan is offered and then applied to each major area of the upper extremity (see box on p. 508).

SHOULDER

Joint Mobilization

The focus of an early rehabilitation program for the shoulder emphasizes range of motion rather than strength. Magnusson's conclusions help support the theory that is the basis for this emphasis. He found that professional baseball pitchers actually had weaker arms but greater range of motion than nonpitchers.[32]

There is a time frame for maximal effectiveness in exercises for motion, whereas strengthening exercises are generally effective at most times after an injury. If active exercises begin too soon, muscle soreness can be increased and this pain can limit the recovery of motion. Too much range-of-motion exercise in one sitting can cause muscle fatigue, soreness, and muscle tightening, so can be counterproductive. Multiple therapies for short durations throughout the day, as opposed to one or two longer therapy sessions, are preferred.

After an injury or surgery, a brief period is allowed for inflammation and swelling to subside. Then passive range-of-motion exercises are initiated. To restore motion in the shoulder, Codman's pendulum exercises classically are used early (Fig. 31-1).[11] Before initiating range-of-motion exercises, warming the area, perhaps with hydrocollator packs, is useful. Heat is not used for five days after surgery because it may induce hematoma formation.[37]

GENERAL REHAB STRATEGY

1) Rest
   A) absolute
   B) "actual" rest

2) Mobility—to decrease effects of immobility

3) Range of motion (ROM)
   A) Passive range of motion (PROM)
   B) Continuous passive range of motion
   C) Active assisted range of motion
   D) Active range of motion

4) Strengthening
   A) For stability
   B) For force production
   C) For force absorption

5) Flexibility

6) Coordination/neuromotor control

7) Proprioception

8) Sport-specific exercise

9) Biomechanics

Continuous passive motion (CPM) can be applied to the joints of the upper extremity, as for the knee, to help achieve an increased range of motion (Fig. 31-2). Another type of passive range of motion is termed early passive motion or EPM (Fig. 31-3).[37] In this technique, the patient completely relaxes the arm that has been operated on, like the arm of a "rag doll." Then an experienced clinician elevates the arm in the scapular plane while he/she supports its full weight. The clinician also may exert distraction force on the glenohumeral joint. Unlike Neer's description of EPM with the patient standing, we prefer to have the patient lying down. In this way, once 90° of elevation is obtained, the clinician and patient are assisted by gravity in achieving additional range of motion.

The patient ultimately is in charge of his/her own rehabilitation and is taught active assisted range-of-

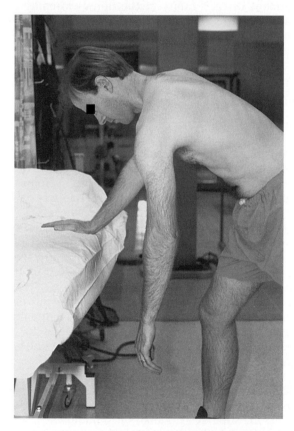

Fig. 31-1. Passive range of motion exercises. Exercises such as Codman's pendulums are effective in restoring early motion and curtailing the occurrence of adhesions. Gravity will distract the glenohumeral joint and allow free motion. A light weight can be held in the hand to foster this effect.

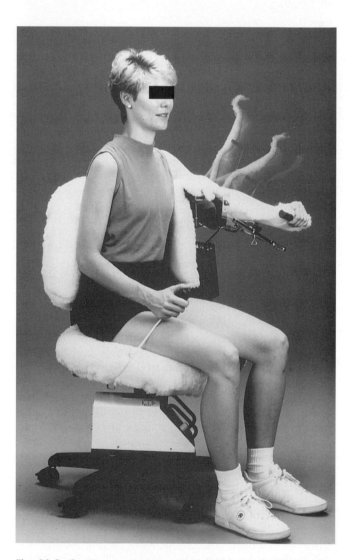

Fig. 31-2. Continuous passive motion (CPM). Mechanical devices such as CPM are useful in increasing range without the need of an assistant or active participation by the patient. The desired speed and range of motion is set and increased as tolerated. Smith and Nephew Richards Shoulder CPM pictured. Manufactured by Kinster. Used with permission.

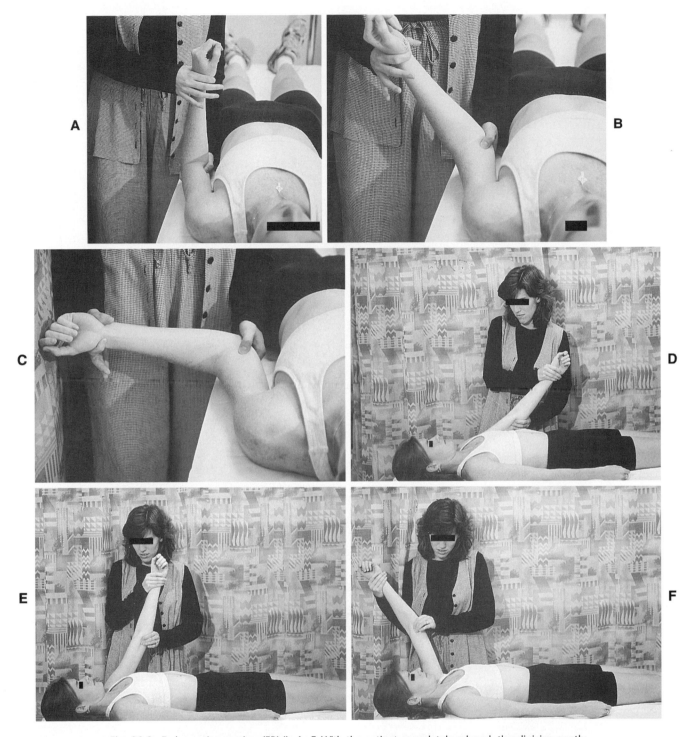

Fig. 31-3. Early passive motion (EPM). **A–F,** With the patient completely relaxed, the clinician gently distracts the glenohumeral joint and glides it through anatomic range of motion (i.e., flexion in the scapular plane). If the patient is lying down, gravity will assist the motion once 90° forward flexion is achieved.

motion exercises. These can be performed with the uninvolved arm alone, or with a cane, T-bar, pulley, or towel (Fig. 31-4). When muscle soreness has dissipated, active range-of-motion exercises can begin. These exercises assist the patient in achieving full range of motion (Fig. 31-5).

At our institution we divide shoulder rehabilitation into phases. In Phase I the patient lies supine and undergoes passive range of motion. Phase II includes active ROM of the shoulder while the patient is supine, and PROM while the patient is sitting or standing. Phase III of the program includes active ROM with the patient in

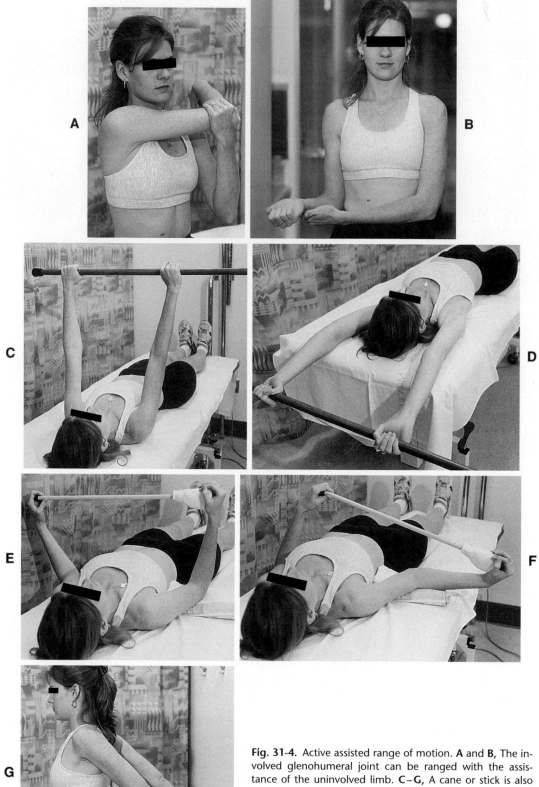

Fig. 31-4. Active assisted range of motion. **A** and **B**, The involved glenohumeral joint can be ranged with the assistance of the uninvolved limb. **C–G**, A cane or stick is also helpful in increasing forward flexion/extension and internal/external rotation.

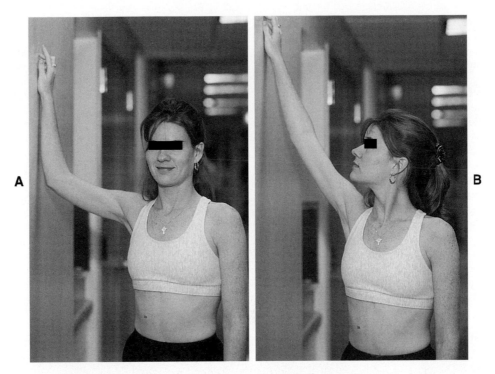

Fig. 31-5. Active range of motion, wall climb. **A** and **B**, On repeated trials, the patient elevates the involved arm by sequentially placing the fingers upward on a wall board, each time trying to raise the arm higher.

the upright position. This phase progresses toward resistive exercise training.

The scapula also must have full range of motion. Any limitation in scapula range of motion must be addressed. The range of motion can be tested by the lateral scapula slide test or the modified scapular slide test.[13,14,30] Motion of the glenohumeral joint is accompanied by motion between the scapula and the thoracic vertebrae. Codman defined this as scapulohumeral rhythm.[11] Elevation of the upper extremity requires both glenohumeral and scapulothoracic motions that move synchronously through a 3:2 ratio of glenohumeral motion versus scapular rotation. Without proper movement of the scapula, glenohumeral motion is limited.

Joint mobilization is effective for lysing adhesions and maintaining or increasing range of motion. Its goal is to restore normal motion to a joint. Early range of motion can prevent the formation of a stiff joint, however, restricted movement of the periarticular tissues is common after an injury or period of immobilization. Once they become stiff, mild joint adhesions can be lysed with mobilization techniques. These maneuvers consist of a group of skilled passive movements applied to improve soft tissue and joint mobility. Joint mobilization is based on a sound knowledge of muscle function, arthrokinematics, and osteokinematics (Fig. 3-6).

The effects of passive movements to an injured joint include:

1. Decreases in wound edema and joint effusion[17]

2. Provision of proprioceptive information to the central nervous system, which in turn may interfere with the transmission of pain[17]
3. Stimulation of mechanoreceptors, which may diminish many types of pain[64]
4. Decreases in complications of immobilization
5. Maintenance of tissue homeostasis[17]
6. Reduction in the restrictions of scar tissue[15]
7. Lengthening of an immature scar[1]
8. Proper orientation of collagen fibers[1]

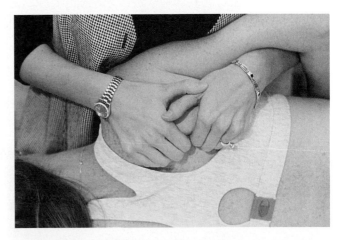

Fig. 31-6. Joint mobilization. For stiff joints, soft tissue adhesions can be broken by skilled passive ranging. This technique also establishes normal congruency between the scapula and thoracic cage.

9. Reestablishment of normal active range of motion
10. Breaking of intracapsular adhesions that may have formed during immobilization
11. Enhancement of collagen fiber glide[1]

Mobilization techniques vary.[33] Closely related types of passive movement to a joint include manipulation, articulations, oscillations, distractions, and thrust techniques.[15] Manipulation is described as "the forceful passive movement of a joint beyond its active limit of motion." Articulation is passive movement applied in a smooth rhythmic fashion to stretch contracted muscles, ligaments, and capsules gradually.[56] Oscillatory technique involves passive movements that can be of small or large amplitude and applied anywhere in the range of motion of a joint, whether the joint surfaces are distracted or compressed. Distraction involves stretching a joint capsule by separating the surfaces of the joint. Thrust techniques are of two basic types. You can employ a high velocity, low amplitude- or a low velocity,

high amplitude–technique. The common goal of these is to free restricted joint motion.

These passive range-of-motion exercises can be delivered by the clinician to help prevent or treat joint limitations. Sometimes manipulation under anesthesia is indicated to break larger adhesions that may have formed during a period of immobilization. This is a more aggressive technique and can be done under general anesthesia or with a brachial plexus block. Some centers use an interscalene brachial plexus block for the manipulation and leave the catheter in the interscalene space. The patient receives anesthesia via the catheter daily for 2 to 4 days as she receives physical therapy, in an effort to retain the motion gained in the operating room.[3]

Closely related to mobilization strategies is the concept of proprioceptive neuromuscular facilitation (PNF) (Fig. 31-7).[31] This is a type of neuromuscular mobilization. In this technique, the patient is instructed to contract an antagonist muscle or group of muscles. Immediately following this contraction, the therapist instructs

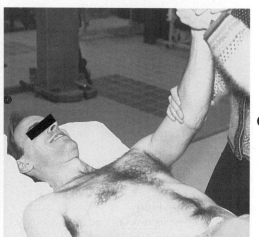

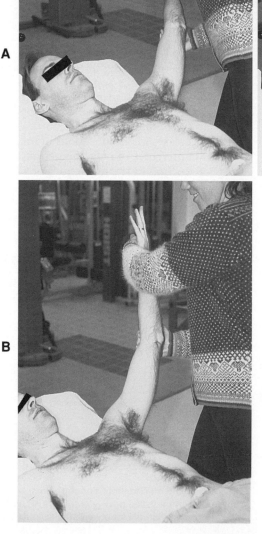

Fig. 31-7. Proprioceptive neuromuscular facilitation. **A, B,** and **C,** In increasing range of motion, the antagonist muscle must not be resistive to the desired movement. Initially, the antagonist muscle is contracted, immediately followed by a contraction of or passive movement of the agonist muscle. The antagonist muscle is refractory during the agonist contraction.

the patient to perform a contraction of the agonist muscle or passively moves the patient's limb in the desired direction, in an effort to increase the range of motion. Theoretically, the preliminary contraction of the range-limiting muscle group (the antagonist) will inhibit its refiring for a short time as it repolarizes. This is called the refractory period. Then the agonist can contract without a cocontraction by the antagonists, via the stretch reflex. Also, while the agonist contracts, the antagonist will be silenced at the spinal level by the principle of reciprocal inhibition. In this way, it is possible to obtain more range of motion in the desired plane. The repeated contractions of the antagonist muscles will fatigue them, reducing their ability to counteract the agonist muscles. This is similar to the theory of muscle energy described in the discussion of spine rehabilitation.

Knott and Voss modified PNF techniques for use around the shoulder.[44] They described four basic diagonal patterns for the shoulder and upper extremity. By facilitating agonist muscles and inhibiting antagonist muscles around the scapula and humerus, dysfunctional movements of the shoulder were eliminated. The result was a more fluent, rhythmic shoulder movement pattern in an effort to obtain full range of motion.

Some patients have difficulty moving their shoulders early in the rehabilitation period. This may be due to pain and anxiety but also could be the result of an inability to contract the muscles around the shoulder effectively. A recent study by Ben-Yishay revealed that pain inhibits shoulder strength.[65] This parallels the findings that neurological inhibition decreases quadriceps function in a painful knee.[16,35,55,63] Therefore it is important that the patient avoid painful positions during rehabilitation.

Hydrotherapy entails placing a patient in a warm pool of water to neck level. It is felt that the buoyancy effect of the water helps decrease pain around the shoulder joint. Also, the resistance offered by the water translates into sensory and proprioceptive feedback. Typically PNF shoulder axis patterns are practiced underwater to help achieve greater range of motion and kinetically correct shoulder movements.[53]

Spencer's techniques use gentle repeated stretching to treat shoulder dysfunction.[44,54] They are especially useful in adhesive capsulitis and other painful shoulder conditions. Since the patient's scapula is stabilized and not permitted to rotate, the arm should not be ranged past 90° of elevation lest an impingement or rotator cuff disorder be aggravated (Fig. 31-8).

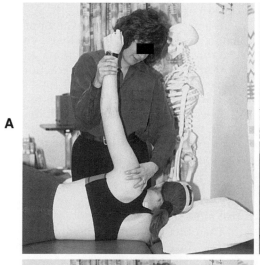
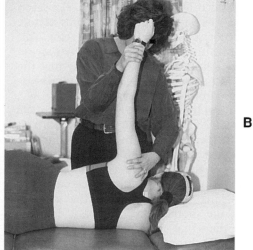
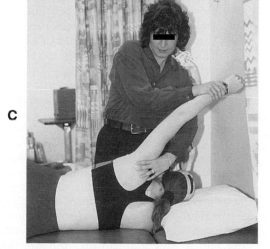

Fig. 31-8. Spencer's techniques. **A, B,** and **C,** A series of passive exercises is performed to increase all motions of the glenohumeral joint.

STRENGTHENING

"History does not long entrust the care of freedom to the weak or timid." D.D. Eisenhower, January 20, 1953 at The Inaugural Address.

Once the patient's range of motion has been sufficiently maximized, rehabilitation focuses on strengthening the shoulder girdle musculature.[9] The shoulder has great freedom of movement, so it is imperative for the muscles around the shoulder to be strong. The muscles of the shoulder girdle have three major functions: stability, force production, and force absorption.

The rotator cuff muscles afford stability of the glenohumeral joint.[59] From a purely structural aspect, the subscapular muscle lies anterior to the glenohumeral joint, thereby helping to prevent subluxation. The same can be said about the teres minor and infraspinatus muscles, posteriorly. The rotator cuff muscles blend with the capsule, and contraction of the muscle produces tension in the capsule and the capsular ligaments. This is referred to as dynamic ligament tension. The biceps brachii also assist with anterior stability, especially in the vulnerable overhead throwing position.[45,46]

The circle concept of stability originally was described for the capsule and ligaments around the glenohumeral joint.[24,48,49,60,62] However, it can be extrapolated to include the muscles of the rotator cuff. The circle concept implies that stability is provided by opposing structures on each side of the joint. For example, the posterior musculature helps prevent anterior subluxation and vice versa. This point is very evident with inferior instability. There are no dynamic inferior stabilizers, therefore we know that the supraspinatus and deltoid muscles are integral in preventing the humeral head from subluxing inferiorly.[7]

Another mechanism by which the rotator cuff muscle affords stability is force coupling. When the rotator cuff muscles contract, they pull the humeral head into the glenoid. This maximizes joint congruity, increases adhesion and cohesion of the joint surfaces, and prevents humeral translation. Any rotator cuff muscle contraction helps center the humeral head within the glenoid, thereby increasing the shoulder's stability. For dynamic stability, it is important that the force couples are properly balanced with synchronized cocontraction to prevent abnormal joint kinematics.

In addition to the rotator cuff, deltoid, and biceps, the scapular stabilizer muscles need to be strengthened.[30,36,42] The glenoid fossa must be positioned correctly to prevent the humeral head from gliding inferiorly. Also, the scapulohumeral rhythm allows the rotator cuff muscles to be set properly, which provides the optimum length tension ratio. If the scapula is unstable, the rotator cuff muscles will not have a strong base of support and will be much less efficient. Therefore it is imperative to strengthen the scapular stabilizers, especially the serratus anterior, trapezius, and the rhomboids (Fig. 31-9).[27] By keeping the glenohumeral joint dynamically stable, we can decrease the likelihood of the development of impingement.

Strong scapular stabilizers, smooth scapulohumeral rhythm, and strong rotator cuff muscles work together in an efficient glenohumeral relationship. When the deltoid contracts, the glenoid fossa acts as a fulcrum and the arm rotates correctly. But when the humeral head depressors are weak, the humeral head does not properly enter the glenoid. Upon contraction of the deltoid, the humeral head migrates superiorly, which narrows the subacromial space and can trigger symptoms of impingement. Smooth scapular motion positions the glenoid properly to maintain an adequate subacromial space. Normal elevation of the acromion is approximately 36° from the neutral position and is achieved in maximum abduction of the arm.[66]

The preceding paragraphs outlined reasons for maximizing the dynamic shoulder stabilizers. This function is essential in providing the foundation for the upper extremities' role in functional performance. Strengthening strategies apply to the use of the arm, forearm, and hand. There are two specific entities, force production and force absorption.

Force production is quite important in sports such as wrestling, weight lifting, and rugby. A larger muscle can produce more tension and therefore produce more force, or torque. However, this does not always translate into better function in other sports. In Wilke's study of professional baseball pitchers, he concluded that there was no significant difference between the dominant and the nondominant throwing arm in internal and external rotator muscle strength.[61] Aldenrink and colleagues reported similar results in their investigation of rotator cuff strength.[2,25]

Where does the force of the upper extremity originate? We must look at the kinetic chain. For activities like throwing a ball or swinging a golf club, force generation is mainly by ground reaction forces and rotational forces of the trunk and hips. These are guided, increased, and directed by the anterior shoulder muscles' working in concentric fashion. Kibler has compared the shoulder to a funnel.[30] The energy generated by the lower extremities and the trunk is transferred to the upper extremities by the smooth integrated movement of the stable shoulder. This helps explain why some Little League baseball pitchers can throw a baseball 90 miles per hour and why golfers can drive a golf ball more than 300 yards.

The other function of the muscles around the shoulder is force absorption. This can refer to the followthrough of a pitcher's arm when the posterior rotator cuff muscles must contract eccentrically to slow down the upper extremity, or it can refer to an offensive lineman's stopping an oncoming rusher with his arms. Typically, force generation requires a concentric muscular contraction, whereas force absorption requires a strong eccentric effort. We also call these muscle groups accelerators and decelerators, or agonists and antagonists. Typically an agonist muscle, or group of muscles, will contract to accelerate a body part, and towards the end of the motion the antagonist muscle or muscles will fire eccentrically to decelerate the body part. When both muscle groups are firing simultaneously, we call it a cocontraction. If there is a great disparity between the force a body can generate and the force it can absorb, injury can ensue. For example, in the throwing motion, the internal rotators contract to help internally rotate the shoulder (along with momentum from the body turn). The

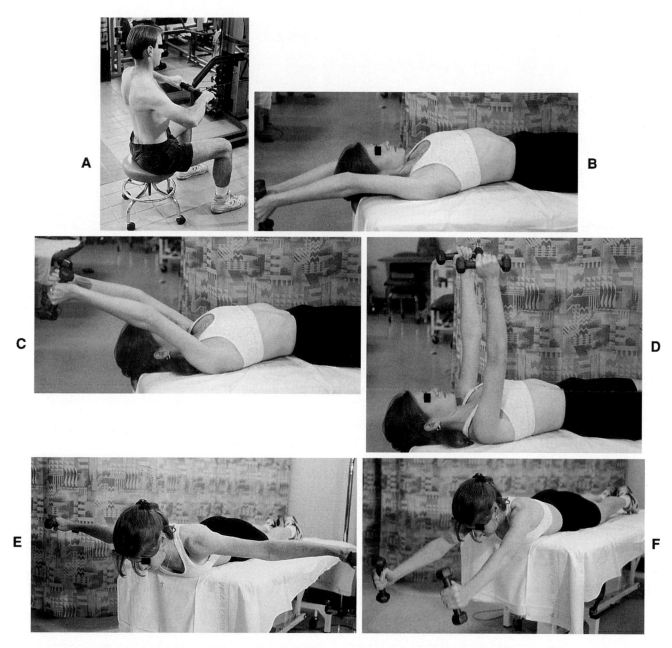

Fig. 31-9. Scapular stabilizer exercises. **A,** Rhomboid progressive resistive exercise. **B–D,** Serratus anterior progressive resistive exercises. **E** and **F,** Trapezius progressive resistive exercises.

external rotators must slow down the shoulder's internal rotation to prevent injury.

There are three basic types of muscle-strengthening exercises: (1) isometrics, (2) isotonics, and (3) isokinetics.

Isometric refers to equal length (Fig. 31-10). During this type of contraction no work is performed. This can be understood when one considers the formula work = force × distance. In an isometric contraction, no net change in muscle length or movement of the body part occurs. Therefore the distance traveled is zero. If work = force × distance, net work must be zero if no distance is traveled. Some clinicians feel that injured joints are inflamed and undue motion can adversely affect them. Isometrics allow for strengthening muscles around a joint

without straining them, so this technique is relatively safe for strengthening muscles around an inflamed joint. Caution must be exercised in performing isometrics when muscles or tendons are injured because high muscle tensions further injure the compromised structures.

Isotonic connotes "equal tension" (Fig. 31-11). In this type of exercise, the load remains constant as the muscle shortens or lengthens. When the muscle shortens, it is termed a concentric contraction, and when the muscle lengthens in a controlled fashion, it is termed eccentric. Note that equal resistance is not offered throughout the full arc of these exercises. Free weights, weight machines, push-ups, pull-ups—all exercise muscle isotonically in both concentric and eccentric fashions.

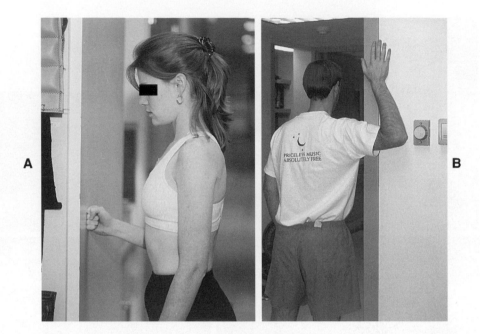

Fig. 31-10. Isometric exercises. **A** and **B,** This is an excellent exercise when you are trying to strengthen an inflamed joint. A wall acts as an excellent resistive force for isometric training of the shoulder complex. Precaution must be taken with isometric exercises in patients with cardiac compromise.

Isokinetic means equal velocity or speed (Fig. 31-12 on page 522). In this type of exercise the speed of the limb does not change, no matter how much load is applied. Therefore there is maximal resistance throughout the range of the exercise. This is not the case with isotonic exercise. Isokinetic exercise can be performed either concentrically or eccentrically.

Most exercises are beneficial, but each one has its limitations. No one type of exercise has proven to be universally superior. All have a place in the strengthening of an athlete.[34]

Another way to differentiate strengthening exercises involves open–kinetic chain versus closed–kinetic chain exercise.[62] In closed–kinetic chain, or CKC exercise, the distal segment of the limb to be exercised is relatively fixed, whereas in open–kinetic chain exercise the distal segment of the limb to be exercised is free to move. An example of closed–kinetic chain exercise is the push-up, whereas an open–kinetic chain would be the biceps curl. The advantage of closed–kinetic chain exercise is the promotion of muscular cocontraction around the joint, the promotion of a more fluent movement pattern, and increased dynamic joint stability (Fig. 31-13 on page 522).

We prefer to use the terms axial and perpendicular load when describing these concepts. Axial load is likened to closed–kinetic chain, and perpendicular load is likened to open–kinetic chain exercises. For descriptive purposes, a closed–kinetic chain exercise (axial load) is one that produces force across a joint line, whereas an open–kinetic chain exercise (perpendicular load) produces force tangent to or along a joint line. For example, if a person does a push-up, an axial load is generated across the elbow joint as she elevates her body from the floor. If someone does a biceps curl, the predominant

force is tangent to the elbow joint, and this produces a perpendicular load through the elbow.

There are combined versus isolated movement patterns. Exercises can be performed that concentrate on one individual muscle or on a movement pattern (Fig. 31-14 on page 523).[58] For instance, the triceps surae muscles can be exercised alone with resisted elbow extension (the scapular stabilizers also are firing to stabilize the origin of the long head of the triceps) or as part of a movement pattern such as the military press. Both types of exercises are beneficial. The weak link in a movement pattern should be strengthened individually so that the stronger muscles in that pattern do not mask the deficit. Gross movements should be exercised first during a workout. It would be counterproductive to fatigue a muscle that is already the weak link in a movement pattern with a single muscle exercise. When the gross movement is required there would be even greater substitution, and abnormal movement patterns might ensue.

Strength is different from endurance. A muscle can be trained for each. Muscle strength is the maximum force a muscle or group of muscles can exert against resistance. Muscle endurance is the ability to perform repeated contractions of the muscle or muscle groups over an extended period before fatiguing. These elements of physical conditioning are related, so exercises to increase muscle strength may also increase endurance, and vice versa. The principle of overload states that increases in strength occur when muscles are exercised at or near their maximal strength. To increase endurance, exercises at or near maximum repetitions must be done. Classically, to increase strength we use resistance exercises with high loads and low repetitions, and to increase endurance we use low loads at high rep-

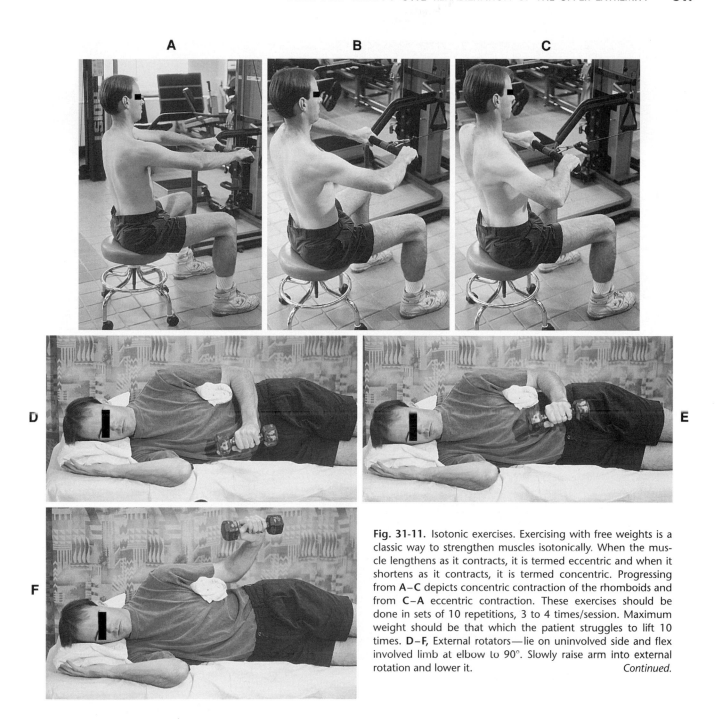

Fig. 31-11. Isotonic exercises. Exercising with free weights is a classic way to strengthen muscles isotonically. When the muscle lengthens as it contracts, it is termed eccentric and when it shortens as it contracts, it is termed concentric. Progressing from **A–C** depicts concentric contraction of the rhomboids and from **C–A** eccentric contraction. These exercises should be done in sets of 10 repetitions, 3 to 4 times/session. Maximum weight should be that which the patient struggles to lift 10 times. **D–F,** External rotators—lie on uninvolved side and flex involved limb at elbow to 90°. Slowly raise arm into external rotation and lower it. *Continued.*

etitions. The muscle group will adapt to stresses, so it is imperative that the clinician know the goals of the athlete. To prescribe only endurance-type exercises to a power lifter would be a disservice, as would the prescription of only strengthening exercises to a tennis player who must compete for several hours. A balanced program incorporating strength and endurance training is recommended.

Power

Power = force ÷ time. It denotes a muscle's or a group of muscles' ability to exert a high amount of force in the shortest amount of time. It is sometimes referred to

as explosive strength. Plyometric exercise is concerned with developing power (Fig. 31-15 on page 524). Plyometric exercise involves rapid loading of a muscle followed by a powerful muscle contraction. Plyometrics consist of three phases:

1. Eccentric phase—the muscle is being stretched
2. Amortization phase—the time between eccentric stretch and concentric contraction
3. Concentric phase—the forceful contraction of the agonist

This eccentric and concentric coupling is also known as stretch shortening. It makes use of the stretch reflex of

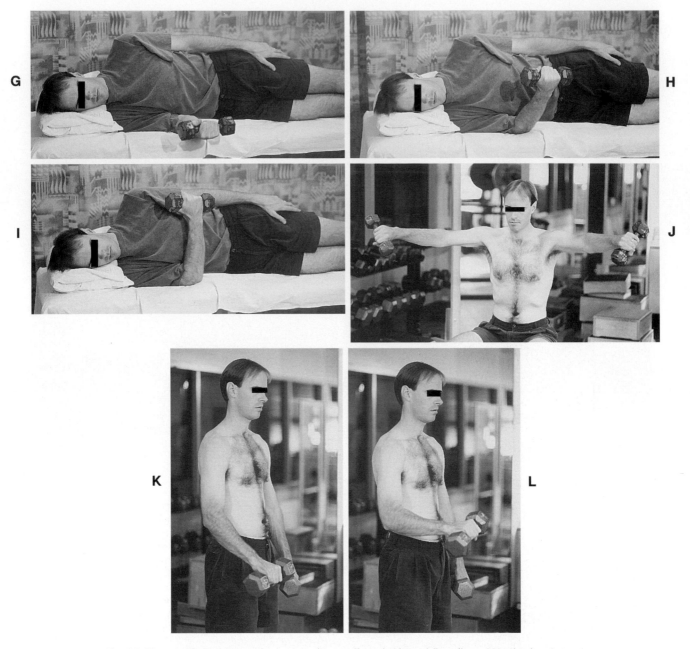

Fig. 31-11, cont'd. G–I, Internal rotators—lie on affected side and flex elbow 90°. Slowly raise arm into internal rotation and lower it. **J,** Supraspinatus—sit on a stool with upper extremities extended. Horizontally rotate the upper extremities approximately 30° anterior in the frontal plane and pronate the forearms. Then lower and raise the upper extremities in the scapular plane, not to rise above eye level. A weight is held in the hands. Starting weight should be that which can be lowered and raised ten times with moderate difficulty. **K** and **L,** Brachioradialis, brachialis—stand with elbows slightly flexed. Forearms are pronated with weights held in each hand. Slowly flex and extend the elbow.
Continued.

the muscle tendon unit. Simply put, the stretch reflex involves the proprioceptors of the body including the muscle spindle, the Golgi tendon organ, and the joint capsule and ligamentous receptors. When the sensory end-organs are stimulated via a stretch of the muscle, they will activate and transmit an afferent impulse to the spinal cord. This afferent impulse can be either facilitory, from the muscle spindle, or inhibitory, from the Golgi tendon organ. After synapse in the spinal cord, the efferent alphamotor neuron will activate the agonist muscle. The total time of this reflex is 0.3 to 0.5 ms. In addition to the stretch reflex, the recoil action of the soft tissues adds to the power of the agonist contraction. During the eccentric phase, soft tissues are stretched, and at the cessation of the stretch these tissues must return to their original form. Newton's principles state that energy is

Text continued on p. 523.

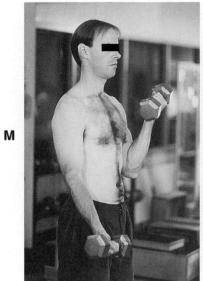

M

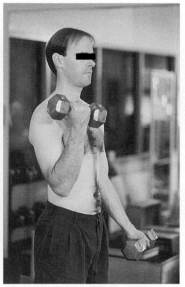

N

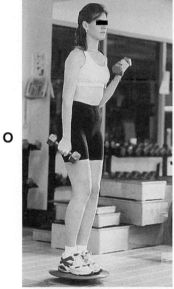

O

Fig. 31-11, cont'd. M and **N,** Biceps—stand with elbows slightly flexed. Forearms are supinated with weights held in each hand. Slowly flex and extend at the elbow. **O,** Biceps curl on balance board—to add complexity to the biceps strengthening, you can maintain balance on a balance board while performing the exercise. This adds complexity and challenges the nervous system to devise strategies to successfully achieve the task. **P** and **Q,** Shoulder shrug (levator scapulae and trapezius)—stand with upper extremities extended. Shrug shoulder against resistance supplied by hand-held weights. *Continued.*

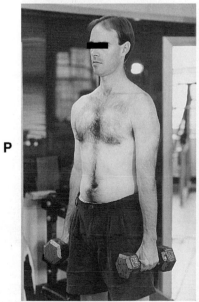

P

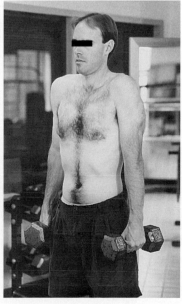

Q

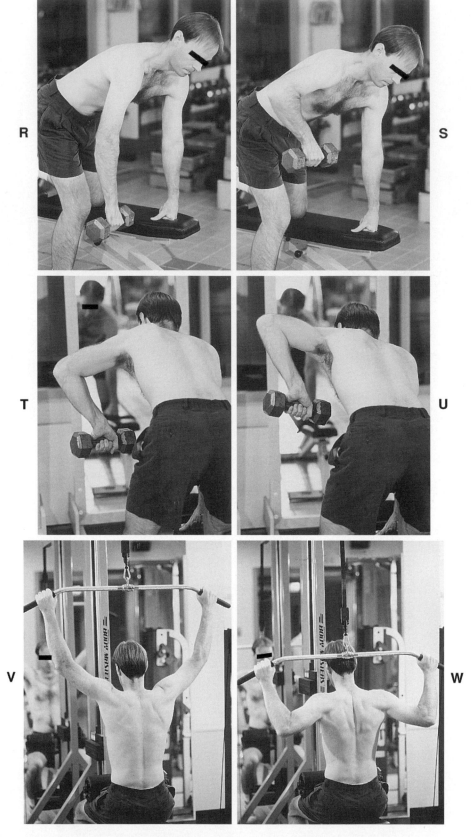

Fig. 31-11, cont'd. R–U, Rows (deltoids, rhomboids, levator scapulae and trapezius)—standing with hips flexed approximately 45°, place unaffected upper extremity on support (table or bench). While holding hand weights, extend the shoulder, maintaining flexion at the elbow. **V** and **W,** Lattisimus dorsi—sitting facing the weight stack, place upper extremities on the weight bar. Slowly lower the bar to the shoulders and then return to starting point.

Continued.

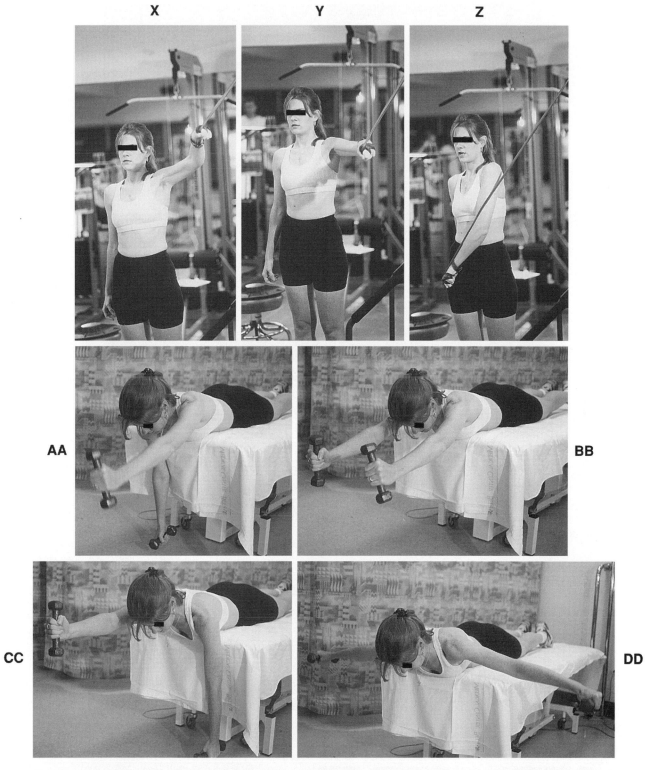

Fig. 31-11, cont'd. X–Z, Shoulder adductors (pectorals)—stand with upper extremity attached to cable column. Slowly pull cable across body maintaining extension at elbow. **AA–CC,** Prone trapezius, deltoids, and levator scapulae—lie prone with head over edge of table. Forward-flex upper extremities while holding hand weights. Alternate raising and lowering each upper extremity. **DD,** Prone deltoids and trapezius—lie prone with head over edge of table. Abduct upper extremities while holding hand weights.

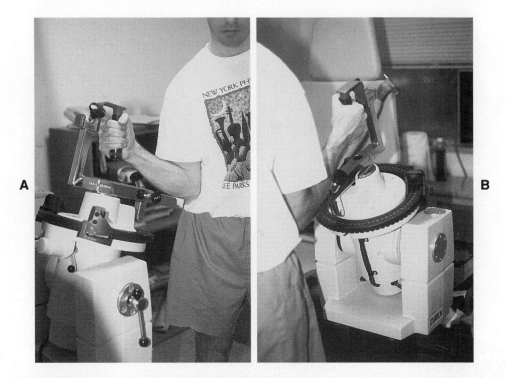

Fig. 31-12. Isokinetic exercises. **A** and **B,** This form of exercise is speed-dependent and gives maximum resistance throughout the range of motion. The limb is usually secured in the equipment, so this is a very good controlled-motion exercise. The movement of the limb will be guided by the range of the machine; this is thought to be a very safe exercise.

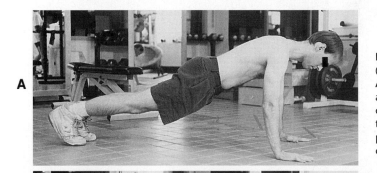

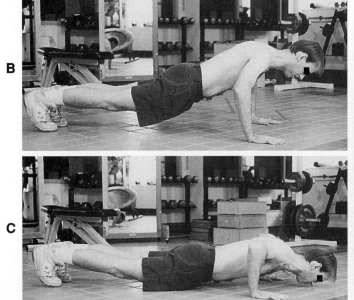

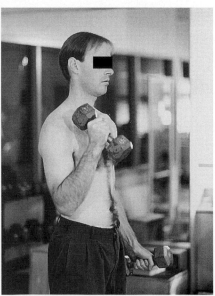

Fig. 31-13. Closed (axial load)–and open (perpendicular load)–kinetic chain exercises. **A–C,** When forces are primarily generated across a joint, the exercise is predominantly closed (axial load) chain. **D,** If the forces are tangent to the joint, the exercise is open (perpendicular load) chain. The push-up is closed chain and the biceps curl open chain.

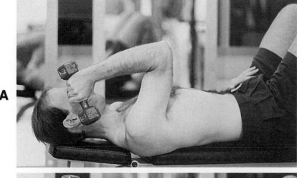

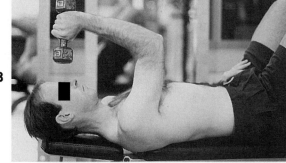

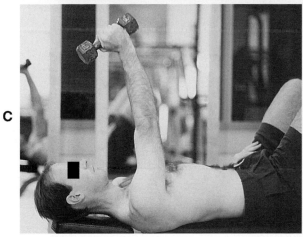

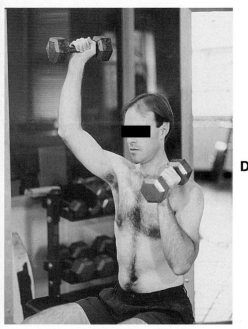

Fig. 31-14. Combined versus isolated strengthening exercises. A muscle such as the triceps can be strengthened in an isolated fashion as in **A–C**. In **D** the triceps is strengthened in combination with other muscles, such as in the military press. Ten repetitions repeated 3 or 4 times is recommended. The ideal weight is that which the individual must struggle to successfully lift 10 times.

neither gained nor lost and each action produces an equal and opposite reaction. The energy needed to stretch the soft tissues is stored in those tissues and then transferred and used as elastic dynamic energy to aide the concentric contraction of the agonist.

Force generation of the agonist is highest in plyometrics when the eccentric stretch is rapid and of short range and the period of amortization is minimal. Plyometric exercise attempts to train the neuromuscular system to use the added force supplied by the myotactic reflex and the elastic recoil of the soft tissues. Plyometrics should be employed only after the limb has been strengthened by conventional exercises. Bench jumping is a good example of plyometrics for the lower extremity, whereas traditionally, medicine balls have been used for the upper extremity. As an athlete catches the medicine ball, the momentum of the ball causes an eccentric contraction of the agonist muscles and the athlete quickly tosses the ball away. This can be done with the assistance of a trainer or a trampoline.

Flexibility

Certainly, the shoulder, with its constant mobility, needs to be flexible. In the throwing athlete, flexibility of the internal rotators and external rotators is particularly important. Arthrokinematically, tight posterior musculature can cause anterior translation and superior migration of the humerus during the throwing motion. This can lead to anterior instability. Paradoxically, tightness of the anterior shoulder muscles also can create an anterior subluxating force by altering the thrower's proper biomechanics. Therefore stretching the anterior and posterior shoulder musculature is important (Fig. 31-16).[43]

Coordination/Neuromotor Control

Once range of motion and strengthening have been addressed, attention can be shifted to coordination and neuromotor control. The movement of an upper limb is not an isolated event. For instance, throwing a baseball involves harvesting energy of the ground reaction and supplementing it via concentric, eccentric, and isometric

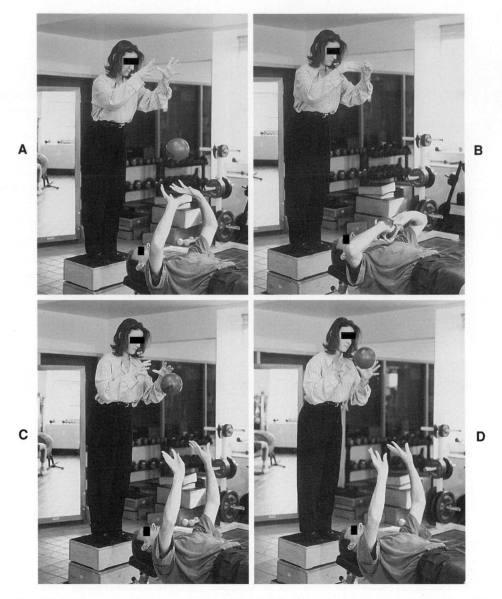

Fig. 31-15. Plyometrics. This sequence demonstrates the initial eccentric preload (**A, B**) followed by the concentric contraction of the agonist group (**C, D**) for the triceps.

contractions, of alternating force and duration, of muscles in the feet, leg, pelvis, trunk, shoulder, arm, forearm, and hand. Once the ball is trajected, the body must slow down and stop, and this requires another pattern of muscular activity. Coordination is the ordered control of the timing, amplitude, and duration of the neuromuscular firing patterns. Coordination requires that the athlete:

1. Know what he or she wants to do
2. Have a neuromotor plan to accomplish his or her goal
3. Be aware of where the body parts are in space (proprioception) and at what speed they are moving (kinesthesia)
4. Know the force, both linear and rotational, his or her muscles can produce and absorb
5. Know the mechanical properties of the object he or she wishes to throw, catch, manipulate, or have manipulated

Proprioneuromuscular facilitation exercises (PNF) assist patients in gaining awareness of their body. Closed–kinetic chain exercises are multijoint activities that assist the athlete in gaining insight into the relationships between different body parts. Sport-specific exercises and practices are a prime way to gain coordination and skill. By performing a task repetitively, the central nervous system may generate patterns, or perfect engrams that will enable the athlete to perform a task most efficiently. To increase coordination, we often employ an exercise with multiple tasks. For instance, we will ask an athlete to stand on a BAPS board or slide along a slide board while catching and throwing a medicine ball. As the athlete performs multiple tasks, he/she

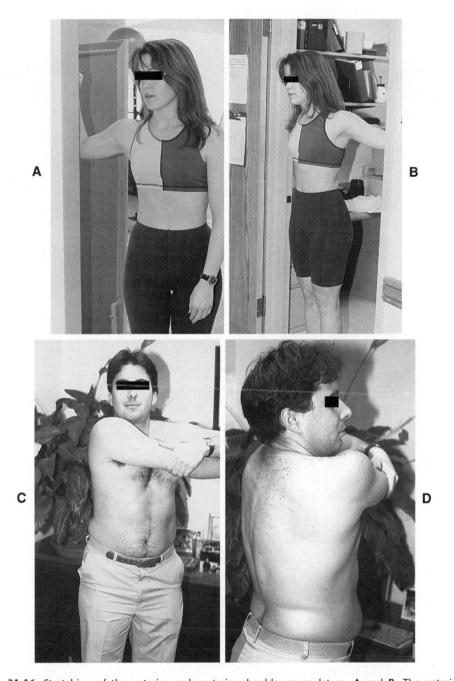

Fig. 31-16. Stretching of the anterior and posterior shoulder musculature. **A** and **B,** The anterior musculature is stretched to allow increased range of motion and improved flexibility. **C** and **D,** Likewise, the posterior shoulder musculature is stretched. Both of these groups are passively stretched by holding the elongated position for 30 seconds, or we can incorporate muscle-energy techniques, as previously described, to focus particularly on flexibility. If you wish to increase flexibility of the shoulder flexors, the shoulder extensors must be fatigued. This is done with serial 5-second contractions of the shoulder extensors, bringing the shoulder into increased flexion after each one. This promotes improved anterior shoulder flexibility.

must develop strategies to coordinate the complex patterns required to achieve a goal. This will assist him/her in achieving maximal skill (Fig. 31-17).

Proprioception

As stated earlier, shoulder stability is provided by static factors, including the bony architecture, the glenoid labrum, low intraarticular pressure, joint surface adhesion, the joint capsule and ligamentous structures, and dynamic structures including the muscles around the glenohumeral joint and the periscapular region. [6,7,10,39-41,52]

Since the peri glenohumeral muscles contract as the humerus nears end-range, the body must have an awareness as to where the humerus is in relation to the glen-

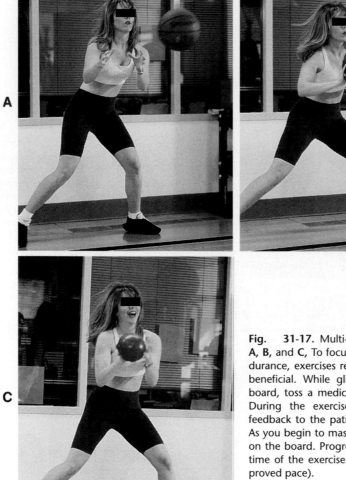

Fig. 31-17. Multi-task rehab exercises. **A, B,** and **C,** To focus on coordination and endurance, exercises requiring multiple tasks are beneficial. While gliding laterally on a slide board, toss a medicine ball or weighted ball. During the exercise, the clinician provides feedback to the patient on proper technique. As you begin to master this drill, increase time on the board. Progress is guided by increased time of the exercise (with a consistent or improved pace).

oid. This is termed joint position sense. The knowledge that the limb is moving is termed kinesthesia. Proprioception encompasses both joint position sense and kinesthesia.

Sensory feedback from the shoulder to the central nervous system is important for dynamic stability of the shoulder.[4,5,8,18,23,57] The sensory end-organs are found in the muscles and tendons around a joint[50] and in the capsule and ligaments.[50] Afferent impulses will increase when the shoulder nears end-range, then presumably efferent messages are sent to the muscles to reverse the motion of the humerus. This postural change as a response to proprioceptive input is termed neuromuscular control.

Research suggests that diminished proprioception is associated with shoulder instability,[50] therefore shoulder rehabilitation must address proprioception. Proprioneuromuscular facilitation (PNF) exercises, closed–kinetic

chain exercises, and plyometric exercises all encourage the patient to appreciate afferent proprioceptive input and develop motor patterns to prevent instability.

Rhythmic stabilization exercises also assist in proprioceptive awareness.[13] In these exercises, the shoulder is placed in a position vulnerable to anterior subluxation, that is, 90° of humeral abduction with 90° of external rotation. A force is applied to the patient's arm to increase the instability, and the patient must counteract that force. With repetition, the patient's proprioception will increase and he/she will better be able to make neuromuscular adjustments (Fig. 31-18).

The scapulothoracic joint is also involved in movement of the shoulder. An athlete should appreciate the motion of the scapula to perfect smooth glenohumeral movements.

Therapeutic intervention for the most common ailments of the shoulder region (rotator cuff tendinitis, im-

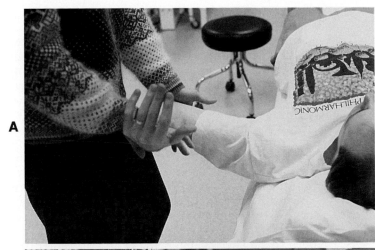

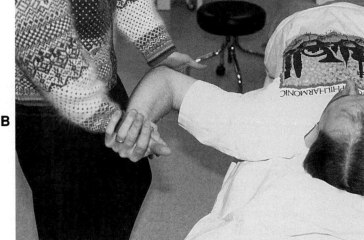

Fig. 31-18. Rhythmic stabilization exercises. **A** and **B,** The patient's shoulder is placed in a vulnerable position, i.e., apprehension, then a gentle destabilizing force is applied by the examiner. The patient must counteract this force to prevent subluxation. The examiner is trying to translocate the humeral head anteriorly while the patient is trying to stabilize it and prevent this action. This exercise assists in developing proprioceptive input to the joint.

pingement, and instability) includes a short period of rest. A few days usually will suffice. This can be in conjunction with medications such as nonsteroidal anti-inflammatories. People with allergies to these preparations or GI sensitivity are cautioned as to their use. Ice massage or heating modalities are useful, and the choice is largely one of patient preference. The basic guidelines of ice for the first 24 hours followed by intermittent heat can be followed. Range-of-motion and strengthening exercises are employed.

The initial phase of the rehabilitation emphasizes restoration of maximal range of motion. Care must be taken to remain in the pain-free range of motion and gently progress to overhead exercises as guided by pain. It is most useful to begin these range-of-motion exercises with the patient supine and progress to sitting and standing. The use of pulleys and sticks can assist in obtaining adequate range of motion (Fig. 31-19). For rotator cuff tears and shoulder instabilities that have been corrected surgically, progressive resistive exercises do not begin until about the tenth to twelfth week after surgery.

The use of injection for rotator cuff tendinitis/bursitis is common. After a positive impingement test, a steroid preparation such as methylprednisolone (40 mg) can be injected into the subacromial bursa. If this is somewhat successful, it may be repeated in about 1 to 2 weeks. The patient should be warned that there may be some transient discomfort in the region of the injection. This is usually alleviated with one or two doses of a pain killer or anti-inflammatory medicine.

THE ELBOW

The elbow joint assists in positioning the hand, in production of force, and in force absorption. A common disorder of the elbow is lateral epicondylitis. This is usually an overuse injury that results in microscopic or macroscopic tears in the extensor aponeurosis, most frequently at the origin of the extensor carpi radialis brevis muscle (ECRB). It is characterized by painful inflammation in the area of the extensor musculature origin. It is aggravated by forceful wrist extension, forearm supination, or passive wrist flexion with forearm pronation. Because the ECRB inserts into the base of the third metacarpal, resisted extension of this digit also may cause elbow discomfort secondary to injury.

By following the hierarchy outlined in box on p. 508 we can properly rehabilitate elbow overuse injury. Initially, rest is indicated, with nonsteroidal anti-inflamma-

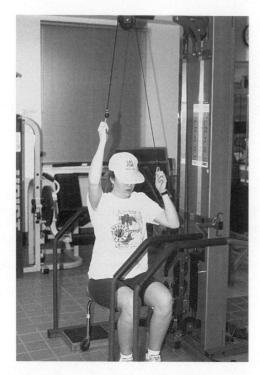

Fig. 31-19. Overhead pulleys to increase range of motion. Pulleys are useful in increasing range of motion. The uninvolved limb pulls the involved limb through a range of motion. This exercise has been stated to be passive to the injured limb but in reality there is active involvement on the part of the injured limb.

tory drugs and proper modalities such as ultrasound with or without cortisone phonophoresis. The liberal use of ice in the acute phase is recommended. For more resistant cases, local steroid injections around the enthesis have been helpful. If these are given, patients must be carefully instructed to rest the arm for approximately one week.

We can use the concept of relative rest by fitting the patient with a lateral forearm counterforce brace.[22,51] This brace is worn over the forearm extensor musculature and acts as a fulcrum to prevent excessive strain on the origin of the wrist extensors (Fig. 31-20). The use of the brace allows an athlete to move his elbow sooner and therefore decrease the deleterious effects of immobility. We also prescribe a cock-up wrist splint to stabilize the wrist extensors. Flexibility of the wrist and finger extensors plays a role in the development of tennis elbow syndrome. Therefore, a proper stretching program should begin when pain in the area has sufficiently decreased (Fig. 31-21).

A weak muscle is likely to fatigue and be injured. Therefore strengthening of the wrist and finger extensors, forearm supinators, and, to a lesser extent, all the other muscles of the upper extremities is required. Special attention should be given to the posterior musculature of the shoulder. Injury of these muscles is a good example of the failure of a muscle complex to absorb force. In this case, force is represented by a moving tennis ball's being struck by a moving tennis racket head. A

strengthening program should include exercises for improving both strength and endurance.

Lateral epicondylitis rehabilitation requires knowledge of the epidemiology of the disease and the proper biomechanics of a tennis swing, specifically the one-handed backhand stroke. It has been shown that improper technique can lead to tennis elbow. Kelly, revealed that all of the patients with tennis elbow in their study had at least two of four deviations from proper stroke mechanics.[29] Improper stroke mechanics include: (1) leading elbow with the olecranon pointing toward the net and the shoulder elevated and in internal rotation, (2) wrist flexion in the early phases with an abrupt change to extension, (3) exaggerated wrist pronation, and (4) ball impact on the lower portion of the racket. Schnatz and Steiner concluded that a late backhand stroke and off-center contact of a racket are the two basic stresses that lead to tennis elbow.[47]

Studies with electromyography (EMG) and cinematography analysis revealed that injured players had significantly greater activity in the wrist extensors and pronator teres muscles during ball impact and followthrough than noninjured players.[29] It has been found that decreasing the tension of the racket strings and changing to a larger racket grip helps reduce some of the stresses placed on the extensor origin.[12,19]

The treatment of tennis elbow is therefore incomplete until the clinician treats the presenting condition and advises the patient as to how to avoid the ailment in the future. If the player cannot adjust their swing, they may have to go to a two-handed backhand or slice backhand, both of which require less stress on the wrist extensors. Please note that a proper one-handed backhand places as much stress on the wrist extensors as the two-handed backhand.[20] No differences were found in EMG activity of the wrist extensors between the single-handed and double-handed backhand ground strokes in a study involving elite noninjured tennis players.[20]

Medial epicondylitis, or golfer's elbow, is caused by overload of the wrist flexors and pronators of the arm. The common flexor tendon of the flexor carpi ulnaris, flexor carpi radialis, and palmaris longus becomes inflamed. The overload can be due to either increased duration of muscle activity, increased force, or both. Nirschl postulated that repetitive strains are cumulative and lead to disruption of the muscle-tendon unit.[38] Glazebrook and colleagues, using EMG analysis, found that golfers with medial epicondylitis had a higher mean flexor musculature activity during address and swing phase than did asymptomatic golfers.[21] A player may be trying to exert too much wrist snap to the tennis serve or golf swing.

Often the problem may be an unstable shoulder with inability to transfer energy through the shoulder joint. The player compensates for this lack of force generation in the shoulder by trying to produce force at the elbow and wrist; overloading these muscles causes injury. Treatment is similar to that for lateral epicondylitis but with attention to the wrist flexor musculature. This time a

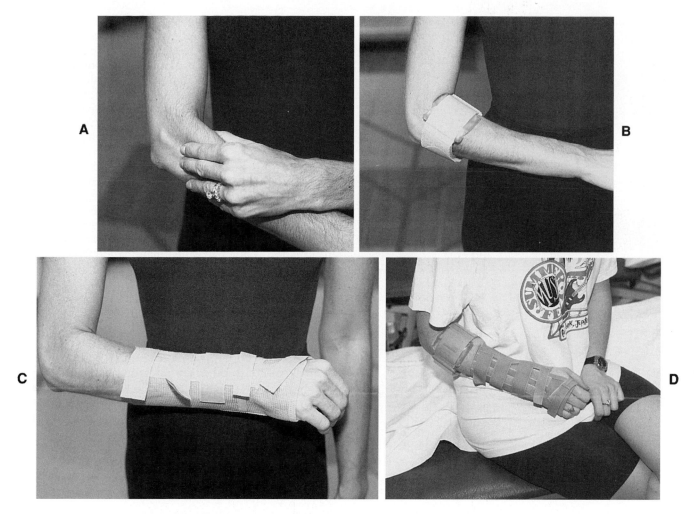

Fig. 31-20. Lateral forearm counterforce brace (lateral epicondylitis). **A,** To locate the best place to apply the brace, flex the elbow and point the thumb superiorly. Grab the lateral forearm muscles with your thumb and index finger. This area, directly below the elbow, is the site the brace should contact. **B,** The brace, in place, acts to unload the forearm muscles closest to the brace and substitutes a new origin for the muscle (beneath the brace). **C** and **D,** A cock-up splint stabilizes the wrist, which is important because the muscles involved cross this region.

medial forearm counterforce brace is employed. The forearm brace decreases EMG duration and muscle activity in the service and backhand drive of tennis players.[21] Stretching the wrist flexors and pronator teres and strengthening these muscles is paramount. Attention to the shoulder musculature, especially the anterior muscles, is recommended. A wider golf-club grip also may help alleviate symptoms.

WRIST AND HAND

The wrist and hand are the final common pathway for all movements of the upper extremity. Their role may be to provide a powerful grip to an apparatus such as a bat or an oar, or to perform more skillful maneuvers requiring fine manual dexterity, such as pitching a ball. The wrist and hand also may aid in power generation. For this reason, the proper rehabilitation of a wrist or hand injury is essential. Again, we can use box on p. 508 as a guide to rehabilitation.

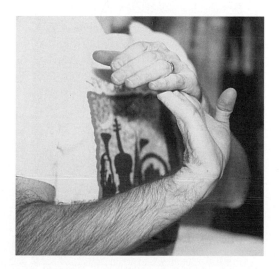

Fig. 31-21. Stretching the digits and wrist. As the muscles are rested and pain is subsiding, it is important to stretch the associated soft tissues to prevent adhesions and stiff joints.

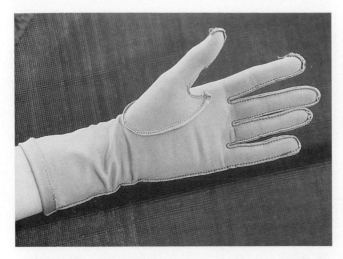

Fig. 31-22. Compressive garments for edema of the hand/wrist. Application of compressive garment for edema of the hand and wrist. It should have a snug fit and not cause paraesthesias in the distal digits. It should be worn as much as possible.

After an injury, rest is recommended. Fractures, injuries of the ligaments, and tendon tears are immobilized. More rigid casts are preferred to over-the-counter splints. It is prudent to only immobilize the injured wrist and to allow the non-injured hand to carry out its function. This will decrease the deleterious effects of immobility in the intact areas of the hand.

Once movement is allowed, obtaining full range of motion is the primary goal. Active and passive range of motion should be measured separately. Passive range of motion typically is restricted by joint effusions or capsular tightening. Active range of motion, on the other hand, requires excursion of the tendon and may be limited by tendon rupture, inflammation, or constriction of the tendon sheath. A hand goniometer should be used to monitor progress. A large discrepancy between active and passive range of motion may indicate a muscle, tendon, or nerve injury.

Edema in the hand can severely limit range of motion and be quite painful (Fig. 31-22). It can be measured by using volume displacement of water, with a volumetric container. Treatment of edema involves keeping the hand elevated, retrograde massage, and the application of a pressure device. Active range of motion should not be painful. If it is, there may be inflammation. Edema results and ultimately decreases range of motion and prolongs the rehabilitation process. Overzealous rehabilitation sessions may be harmful, so we prefer short but frequent therapy sessions.

After the patient achieves full range of motion, strengthening can begin (Figs. 31-23 and 31-24). This should be of both the fine and gross types. A simple tennis ball or sponge can be used to increase grip strength. Therapeutic putty allows the clinician to titrate the resistance. Some devices can strengthen digits individually. A dynamometer allows the grip strength to be monitored. Keep in mind that the strength generated on the ulnar side of the wrist does indeed represent strength. This is in contrast to the strength that is generated on the radial aspect. That is a precision-type of strength.

A   **B**   **C**

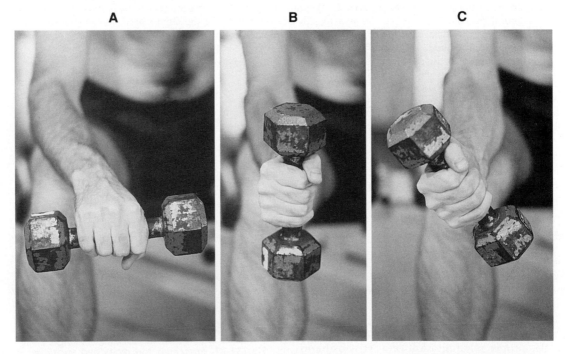

Fig. 31-23. Strengthening of the wrist/digits. **A–C,** Forearm supinator strengthening, **D** and **E,** wrist extensor strengthening.
Continued.

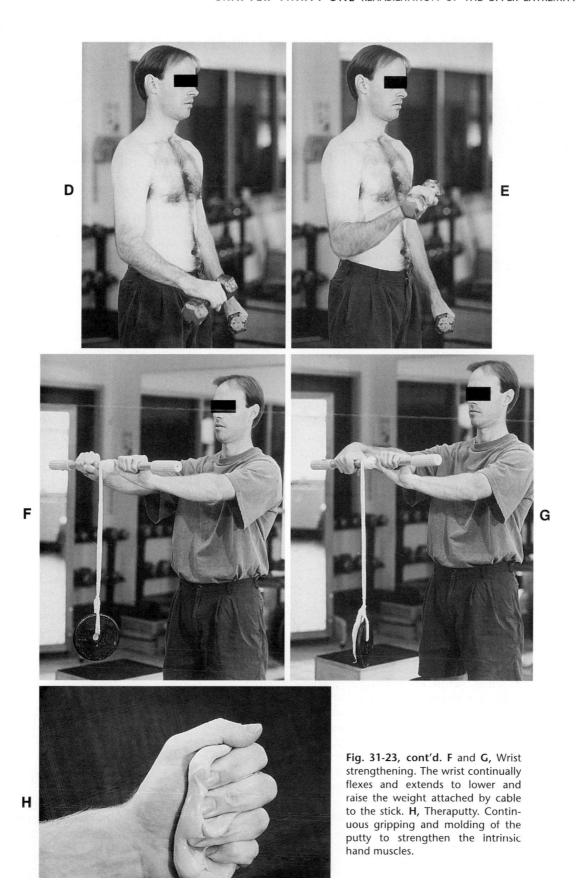

Fig. 31-23, cont'd. F and **G,** Wrist strengthening. The wrist continually flexes and extends to lower and raise the weight attached by cable to the stick. **H,** Theraputty. Continuous gripping and molding of the putty to strengthen the intrinsic hand muscles.

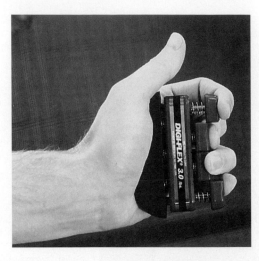

Fig. 31-24. Dynamometer for grip strength. A device that measures grip strength. The trainee grabs the handle and squeezes it with as much force as possible. The dial on the dynamometer records the strength.

Coordination and Neuromotor Control

The long finger flexors are four times as strong as the wrist extensors. When the fingers flex, the wrist will flex unless acted on by the wrist extensors. The cocontraction is necessary for a powerful grip. Therefore, the strengthening of both wrist flexors and wrist extensors should be emphasized. The need for coordination of the hand is evident since the hand carries out fine motor movements. There are numerous dexterity drills to promote coordination of the hand.

Proprioception

Sensory feedback from the fingers is crucial to the athlete in almost all sporting endeavors. Edema in the hand interferes with the sensory end-organs and therefore must be addressed.

Carpal tunnel syndrome is a common ailment affecting the wrist joint, and conservative treatments sometimes prove helpful. One must try to identify the disorder's etiology, if possible, before embarking on a cure. The list of possibilities is lengthy and includes arthritis, pregnancy, diabetes, and hypothyroidism. We try bracing with a neutral alignment cock-up splint, which is worn as much as possible. Also, manual techniques can be tried. The goal of these is to open up the region of the carpal tunnel to decompress it. This can be attempted by opposing the thumb and fifth digit in a repeating series. Vitamin B_6, starting with 50 mg po qhs and increasing to 100 mg po qhs is also prescribed. Injection with a steroid preparation such as methylprednisone is indicated when all else fails. If symptoms persist, refer the patient for surgical opinion.

REFERENCES

1. Akeson WH, Amiel D, Woo SL-Y: Immobility affects on synovial joints. The pathomechanics of joint contracture, *Biorheology* 17:95, 1980.
2. Aldenrink G, Kuck D: Isokinetic shoulder strength of high school and college-aged pitchers, *JOSPT* 7:163–172, 1986.
3. Anthony R, Brown MB: Regional and intermittent anesthesia. Presented at the seminar, Current concepts in shoulder rehabilitation, Columbia-Presbyterian Medical Center, New York, Saturday, October 29, 1994.
4. Bassett RW, Browne AO, Morrey BS, An KN: Glenohumeral muscle forces and moment mechanics in a position of shoulder instability, *J Biomech* 23:405–415, 1990.
5. Blasier R, Carpenter J, Huston L: Shoulder proprioception: Effect of joint laxity, joint position and direction of motion, *Ortho Review* 23(1):45–50, 1994.
6. Blasier RB, Guldberg RE, Rothman EG: Anterior shoulder stability: Contributions of rotator cuff forces and the capsular ligaments in a cadaver model, *J Shoulder Elbow Surg* 1(3):140–150, 1992.
7. Bowen MK, Warren RF: Ligamentous control of shoulder stability based on selective cutting and static translation experiments, *Clin Sports Med* 10:757, 1991.
8. Buchwald JS: Exteroceptive reflexes and movement, *Am J Phys Med* 46:121, 1967.
9. Burkhead W, Rockwood C: Treatment of instability of the shoulder with an exercise program *JBJS* 74A:890–896, 1992.
10. Cain PR, Mutschler TA, Fu FH, Lee SK: Anterior stability of the glenohumeral joint: A dynamic model, *Am J Sports Med* 15(2):144–148, 1987.
11. Codman EA: *The shoulder*. Boston, 1934, Thomas Todd.
12. Coonrad R, Hooper R: Tennis elbow: its course, natural history, conservative and surgical management, *JBJS* 55A: 1177–1182, 1973.
13. Davies G, Dickoff-Hoffman D: Neuromuscular testing and rehabilitation of the shoulder complex, *JOSPT* 18:449–458, 1993.
14. Davies GJ, Heidersceit B, Jones B: Isokinetic testing of scapula-thoracic protraction/retraction and correlation to a modified lateral scapular slide test. Unpublished research, University of Wisconsin-LaCrosse, 1992–1993.
15. Donatelli RA: Mobilization of the shoulder. In *Physical therapy of the shoulder*, ed 2, New York, 1991, Churchill Livingstone.
16. Fahrer H, Rentsch HV, Gerber WJ: Effusion and reflex inhibition of the quadriceps, *JBJS* 70B:635–638, 1988.
17. Frank C, Akeson, WH, Woo S, et al: Physiology and therapeutic value of passive joint motion, *Clin Orthop* 185:135, 1984.
18. Freeman MAR, Wyke B: The innervation of the knee joint. An anatomical and histological study in the cat, *J Anat* 101:505, 1967.
19. Gardner R: Tennis elbow: Diagnosis, pathology, and treatment, *Clin Orthop* 72:248–253, 1970.
20. Giangarra LE, Jobe FW, Perry J: Electromyographic and cinematographic analysis of elbow function in tennis players using single and double handed back hand strokes, *Am J Sports Med* 21(3):394–399, 1993.
21. Glazebrook MA: Medial epicondylitis. An electromyographic analysis and an investigation of intervention strategies, *Am J Sports Med* 22(5), 1994.
22. Groppel JL, Nirschl RP: A mechanical and electromyographical analysis of the effects of various joint counterforce braces on the tennis player, *Am J Sports Med* 14:195–200, 1986.
23. Hall LA, McCloskey DI: Detections of movements imposed on finger, elbow and shoulder joint, *J Physiol* 335:519–533, 1983.
24. Hawkins RJ: Basic science and clinical application in the athlete's shoulder, *Clin Sports Med* 10:4, 1991.
25. Ivey FM: Isokinetic testing of shoulder strength: normal values, *APMR* 66, 1985.

26. Jobe F, Moynes D: Delineation of diagnostic criteria and a rehabilitation program for rotator cuff injuries, *AJSM* 10:336–339, 1982.

27. Jobe F, Moynes D, Brewster D: Rehabilitation of shoulder joint instabilities, *Orthop Clin N Am* 18:473–482, 1987.

28. Kamkar A, Irrgang J, Whitney S: Nonoperative management of secondary shoulder impingement syndrome. *JOSPT* 5:211–224, 1993.

29. Kelley JD, et al: Electromyographic and cinematographic analysis of elbow function in tennis players with lateral epicondylitis, *Am J Sports Med* 22(3), 1994.

30. Kibler WB: Role of the scapula in the overhead throwing motion, *Cont Orthop* 22:525–532, 1991.

31. Knott M, Voss DE: *Proprioceptive neuromuscular facilitation,* New York, 1968, Harper and Row.

32. Magnusson S, Gleim G, Nicholas J: Shoulder weakness in professional baseball pitchers, *Med Sci Sports Exerc* 5–9, 1994.

33. Maitland GD: *Peripheral manipulation,* London, 1970, Butterworth.

34. Mont M, Mathur S, et al: Isokinetic concentric versus eccentric training of shoulder rotators with functional evaluation of performance enhancement in elite tennis players, *AJSM* 22:513–517, 1994.

35. Morrissey MC: Reflex inhibition of the thigh muscles in knee injury: causes and treatment, *Sports Med* 263–276, 1989.

36. Mosely J, Jobe F, et al: EMG analysis of the scapular muscles during a shoulder rehabilitation program. *AJSM* 20:128–134, 1992.

37. Neer CS II: *Shoulder reconstruction,* Philadelphia, 1990, WB Saunders.

38. Nirschl R: Soft tissue injuries about the elbow, *Clin Sports Med* 5:637–652, 1986.

39. Ovensen J, Nielsen S: Anterior and posterior shoulder instability: A cadaver study, *Acta Orthop Scand* 57:324–327, 1986.

40. Ovensen J, Nielsen S: Posterior instability of the shoulder: A cadaver study, *Acta Orthop Scand* 57:436–439, 1986.

41. Ovensen J, Nielsen S: Stability of the shoulder joint. Cadaver study of stabilizing structures, *Acta Orthop Scand* 56:149–151, 1985.

42. Paine R, Voight M: The role of the scapula, *JOSPT* 18:386–391, 1993.

43. Pappas A, Zawacki R, McCarthy C: Rehabilitation of the pitching shoulder, *AJSM* 12:223–235, 1985.

44. Patriqin DA: The evolution of osteopathic manipulative technique: the Spencer technique, *JAOA* 92, 1992.

45. Pollock RG, Bigliani LU, Flatow EL, et al: The mechanical properties of the inferior glenohumeral ligament, *Orthop Trans* 14:259, 1990.

46. Rodosky M, Harner C, Fu F: The role of the long head of the biceps muscle and superior glenoid labrum in anterior stability of the shoulder, *Am J Sports Med* 22:121–130, 1994.

47. Schantz P, Steiner C. Tennis elbow: A biomechanical and therapeutic approach, *JAOA* 93, 1993.

48. Schwartz RE, O'Brien SJ, Warren RF: Capsular restraints to anterior-posterior motion of the abducted shoulder. A biomechanical study, *Orthop Trans* 17:727, 1988.

49. Silliman J, Hawkins R: Current concepts and recent advances in the athlete's shoulder, *Clin Sports Med* 10:693–705, 1991.

50. Smith RL, Brunolli J: Shoulder kinesthesia after anterior glenohumeral joint dislocation, *Phys Ther* 69(2):106–112, 1989.

51. Snyder-Macklin L, Epler M: Effect of standard and aircast tennis elbow bands on integrated electromyography of forearm extensor musculature proximal to the bands, *Am J Sports Med* 17:278–281, 1989.

52. Soslowsky LJ, Flatow EL, Bigliani LU, et al: Quantitation of in situ contact areas at the glenohumeral joint: A biomechanical study, *J Orthop Res* 10:524–534, 1992.

53. Speer K, Wickiewicz T, et al: A role for hydrotherapy in shoulder rehabilitation, *AJSM* 21:850–853, 1991.

54. Spencer H: Shoulder technique *JAOA* 15, 1916.

55. Spencer JD, Keith CH, Alexander IJ: Knee joint effusion and quadriceps reflex inhibition in man, *Arch Phys Med Rehab* 65:171–177, 1984.

56. Stoddard A: *Manual of osteopathic technique,* London, Hutchinson Medical Publishers, 1959.

57. Ticker JB, Bigliani LU, Soslowsky LJ, et al: Biomechanical properties of the inferior glenohumeral ligament: A study of fast and slow strain rates. Presented at the Tenth Anniversary Annual Meeting of the American Shoulder and Elbow Surgeons, Seattle, Washington, September 4–7, 1991.

58. Townsend H, Jobe F, Pink M, Perry J: Electromyographic analysis of the glenohumeral muscles during a baseball rehabilitation program, *AJSM* 19:264–271, 1991.

59. Turkel SJ, Panio MW, Marshall JL, Girgis F: Stabilizing mechanisms preventing anterior dislocation of the glenohumeral joint, *JBJS* 63A:1208–1217, 1981.

60. Warren RF, Kornblatt IB, Marchand R: Static factors affecting posterior shoulder stability, *Orthop Trans* 8:89, 1984.

61. Wilk K, Andrews J, et al. The strength characteristics of internal and external rotator muscles in professional baseball pitchers, *AJSM* 21:61–66, 1993.

62. Wilk K, Arrigo C: Current concepts in the rehabilitation of the athletic shoulder, *JOSPT* 18:365–378, 1993.

63. Wood L, Ferrell WR, Baxendale RH: Pressures in normal and acutely distended human knee joints and effects on maximal voluntary contractions, *QJ Exo Physiol* 73:305–314, 1988.

64. Wyke BD: The neurology of joints, *Ann R Coll Surg Engl* 41:25, 1966.

65. Yishay AB, Zuckerman JD, Gallagher M, Cuomo F: Pain inhibitor of shoulder strength in patients with impingement syndrome, *Orthopedics* 17:685–688, 1994.

66. Poppin NK, Walker PS: Normal and abnormal motion of the shoulder. *JBJS* 58A:195–201, 1976.

CHAPTER 32

THE SPINE

Robert S. Gotlin
Michael A. Palmer

Low back pain and neck pain are two of the leading causes of functional disability in adults under age 45.[1] The annual medical costs of treating back pain in the United States are estimated to be 18 to 25 billion dollars.[25,58] Often referred to by patients as vague discomfort, rather than with "textbook" descriptives, spine pain challenges the practitioner both diagnostically and therapeutically. He/she must be able to see the "forest through the trees" and evaluate the whole person housing the spine, not just an isolated segment.

Understanding the static anatomy and fundamental physiology of the spine's many interrelated segments is important but not always sufficient to accurately diagnose its disability. This is particularly true since 50% of individuals with low back disabilities have no objective findings.[46,65] A thorough appreciation of functional anatomy, muscle dynamics, principles of force production and absorption, and the chemical environment surrounding the spine is essential in treating spine-related disabilities. Many health care professionals routinely treat disorders originating from within or about the 33 bony segments composing the spine. Although perspectives and insights for diagnosing and treating these patients are varied, practitioners should have the common goal of decreasing pain and increasing functional ability. Accomplishing this would satisfy most of the people with spine-related pain.

The field of spine rehabilitation has experienced great strides in therapeutic interventions as technology has advanced. In the past, patients were treated only with passive modalities such as heat and ultrasound. Today patients are exercised back into good health. Rehabilitation strategies are most effective when they are customized to a person's needs. The rehabilitation program should accommodate an individual's lifestyle, needs, training time, and occupation.[61] Although protocol-type treatment algorithms clearly outline progression in a step-by-step structured format, they are inappropriate for many patients. They are useful as generalized therapies and basic guidelines, but practitioners should make every effort to customize and individualize rehabilitation programs.

OVERVIEW

It is only when one has arrived clearly at a working diagnosis of a spinal disorder that treatment strategies can be implemented. Since a patient typically describes pain as the primary symptom, uncovering the pain generator is essential. This critical step is not easily made. Sources of pain are varied, including bone, soft tissue, and nerve. Facet pain has a rather sudden onset, is usually of short duration, is localized in the back (and/or buttock), and is aggravated by extension movements. Disk pain has more of a gradual onset, is long-lasting, is primarily localized in the back, and is aggravated by flexion. Nerve root pain is acute or chronic in onset, intermediate in duration, localizes to an extremity, and is relieved with flexion.[29] Of course, there are many other pain sources and it is as much a challenge to identify the etiology of dysfunction as it is to develop a treatment paradigm. You should keep an open mind when treating spine-related pain since there is often significant overlap in the presentation of pain from different sources.

In this chapter, treatment options for the common afflictions generally seen in the private practitioner's office are discussed.

MUSCLE STRAIN/LIGAMENTOUS SPRAIN

Strain/sprain occurs when a person overstretches a muscle or ligament. It is a problem that almost everyone is sure to experience at one time or another, most commonly affecting joints undergoing undue stress or muscles subject to overuse. Considering that the back is composed of such a large mass of soft tissue, you might wonder why this injury is so common. The answer may lie in the fact that it is not always the amount of stretch that induces injury, but rather the velocity or direction of tension development. This is one of the principles by which an automobile air bag activates. You are certainly happy when the air bag inflates as the result of a high-speed collision. But you are rather curious as to why the bag inflates if your automobile merely taps an object in the direction of travel.

This occurs because the angle of impact is sufficient to engage the air bag device even though the car is traveling slowly. Strains and sprains can occur through a similar mechanism.

It is very common to injure your back performing maneuvers that, on the surface, are rather harmless. The reason may be lack of the body's accommodation for an action by the driving force of movement, the nervous system. It is the function of muscles to move bones, but it is the nervous system that directs muscle activity. To better understand this, we must understand the concepts defined in "motor learning."[31] This foundation is integral to the thorough knowledge of just how we move. The coordinated motor neurons, firing in frequency, duration, and amplitude, choreograph the movement patterns of our musculoskeletal system. Movements require an adaptation for both force production and force absorption. Otherwise, our motions all would be of the acceleration type without ability to decelerate. We can clearly appreciate this phenomenon when we consider the act of bending forward at the waist. If it were not for the ability of our thoraco/lumbar extensor muscles to control this gravity-assisted motion of lumbosacral flexion, as we carry our upper torso toward the ground we would flex in an accelerating manner until our head hit the floor. Obviously, this does not happen, because of the ability of the thoraco/lumbar extensor muscles to decelerate the flexion motion, preventing our upper torso from thrusting toward the floor. The coordinated effort is under direct control of our central nervous system.

Treatment of the acute strain/sprain is similar to treatment of other body regions, with slight modification. We must remember that most strains/sprains take 4 to 6 weeks to heal and any significant challenge to the area of injury during that time may be detrimental. RICE (rest, ice, compression, and elevation) is often very helpful in the acute stage. Rest should be brief, most often no more than a day or so.

Restoration of mobility is essential and seems to expedite the healing process. Ice can be applied for 10 to 20 minutes (unless the region is excessively erythematous or hypoesthetic) three to four times a day. There is always the question of whether ice or heat is more appropriate. The adage that ice is best for the first 24 to 48 hours and heat for the time after can be followed. Ice and heat, however, seem to offer equal benefit in most spine-related strain/sprain injuries no matter when applied. In a select group of patients I recently surveyed (200) there was almost a 50/50 distribution in the efficacy of cold versus heat in those with strains/sprains, regardless of chronicity. Either can be applied for 10 to 20 minutes directly over the involved area. Care should be taken, however, not to freeze or burn the area treated.

Compression is typically achieved by bracing, usually using a soft Velcro-type support. It adds stability during the healing phase but should not be a substitute for muscle stabilization. Often compressive wraps become substitutes for training and actually promote future instability. This probably is due to abdominal weakness that results from wearing a support brace for prolonged periods of time. Although commonly used for extremity strains/sprains, elevation is not typically part of the treatment of strains/sprains in the spine.

Adjunct modalities such as ultrasound and electrical stimulation are useful. Ultrasound can be applied over the paraspinal muscles at 1.5 to 2.0 W/cm^2 for 7 to 10 minutes (Fig. 32-1). Two settings may be applied, pulsed or continuous. Pulsed acts via mechanical "pumping" and assists in edema reduction by improving drainage from the region. Continuous acts as a deep-heating modality and is most focused at the muscle-bone interface. In general, the higher the pulse rate, the more heat production; and the lower the pulse rate, the greater the mechanical pumping effect.

The indications and contraindications for the use

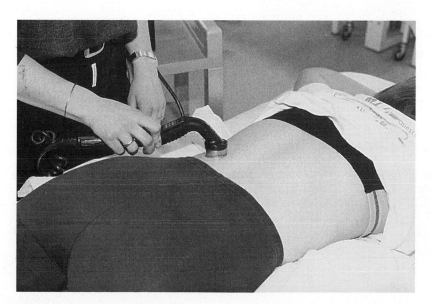

Fig. 32-1. Ultrasound. A deep-heating modality on continuous setting and a mechanical pumping modality on pulsed setting, this is a very effective adjunct therapy in the treatment of musculoskeletal ailments.

Table 32-1. Ultrasound

Indications	muscle spasm
	scar tissue
	warts
Contraindications	over: growing epiphysis, pregnant uterus, bony prominences, ailments of the testes
	in presence of pacemakers
	in areas of sensory loss
	near metallic implants, orthopedic cement, or healing fractures

From Kahn J: *Principles and practice of electrotherapy*, New York, 1987, Churchill Livingstone.

of ultrasound are listed in Table 32-1.[37] Electrical current in the form of electrical stimulation can be used to achieve physiologic effects on muscle and body fluid regulation (Fig. 32-2). A common mode of electrical stimulation is galvanic stimulation, which can be of the positive or negative pole. Typically, the positive pole is used in the acute injury phase and the negative pole is used in the chronic injury setting. Positive is helpful in reducing pain and swelling (acute) whereas negative increases blood flow (chronic) and cleanses the region. The indications and contraindications for the use of electrical stimulation are listed in Table 32-2.[37]

In addition to modalities, progressive range-of-motion and general limbering exercises should be initiated early in the treatment. These could include supine knee-to-chest and standing toe-touching and side-bending. Nonsteroidal anti-inflammatory or muscle relaxant medications may be beneficial if medically tolerable. Muscle relaxants used for a brief period can assist in increasing mobility once a definitive diagnosis is established, but they should not be overly sedating. Adjunct passive treatments can be used, as with other ailments, to improve motion and decrease pain.

Massage therapy, which has both reflex and mechanical actions, is effective in reducing muscle hypertonicity and increasing venous return. Also, soft tissue adhesions can be broken up with strategies such as friction massage. In this technique the direction of massage is perpendicular or parallel to the muscle fibers, and it helps to increase muscle efficiency.

The next phase in treating strains/sprains includes regaining flexibility. Up to this point we have focused on pain relief and adjunct therapy to help regain range of motion. Flexibility is an entity I like to define as "the ease of motion." I am not as concerned about a patient's available range of motion as I am about how difficult it is to achieve that motion. There are several strategies that are efficacious for improving flexibility. Proprioceptive neuromuscular facilitation (PNF)[63] and muscle energy techniques are two that are extremely helpful. PNF techniques employ the active contraction of an antagonist muscle, to be immediately followed by a contraction of the related agonist muscle. The active contraction of the agonist muscle is improved secondarily to the antagonist muscle's being in a refractory period, therefore unable to fire and resist the direction of contraction of the agonist. Muscle energy technique will be discussed in the following section of the text.

The final stage of healing involves strengthening. This begins once pain is under control, maximum functional range of motion is restored, and flexibility is achieved. It should encompass all associated muscles, particularly those involved in spinal stabilization as described under "lumbar stabilization."

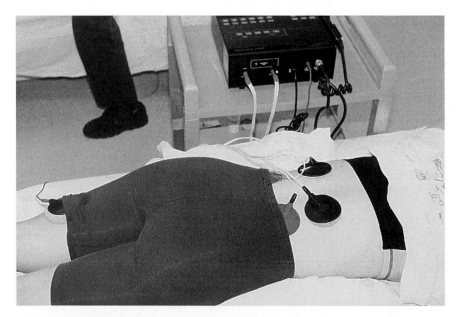

Fig. 32-2. Electrical stimulation. Electrical current is effective in regulating body-fluid flow and in muscle relaxation and contraction. A dispersive pad is used and placed at a site distant to the active pads or applicator.

Table 32-2. Electrical stimulation

Indications	muscles that need to be relaxed
	muscles that need contracting, simulating active exercise
	lack of endorphin production
	impaired circulation because of lack of pumping action of muscles
	waste products that need clearing away by reticuloendothelial response
Contraindications	over fresh fractures, to avoid unwanted motion
	active hemorrhage
	phlebitis
	demand-type pacemaker

From Kahn J: *Principles and practice of electrotherapy,* New York, 1987, Churchill Livingstone.

INTERVERTEBRAL DISK DISEASE/MYOFASCIAL PAIN

Intervertebral disk disease actually represents a broad array of associated musculoskeletal aberrations that fall under many different titles. Bulging disk, protruding disk, herniated disk, somatic dysfunction, lesion, malalignment, and myofascial pain are all associated ailments. Depending on the treating health care professional's background, what seems very clear to him/her may not seem so to you and me, and vice versa. Many authors make a clear distinction between disk disease and myofascial pain, but as it relates to the spine, this distinction is difficult to delineate. In this section, an overview of rehabilitation techniques used to conservatively treat musculoskeletal disorders directly related to the spine is presented. Because turf wars are common among health care practitioners who treat disorders of the spine, it is up to you, the clinician, to determine areas of expertise when applying these theories. The success of conservative treatment is well known, and the need for more aggressive surgical intervention is available but not often necessary. As we enter the twenty-first century, most of the surgery performed might soon be unfashionable and replaced by less invasive procedures with a stronger emphasis on and confidence in rehabilitation.[61]

A key element in rehabilitation of the spine is exercise training, which is achieved by gaining adequate control of the dynamic spine forces. Active participation by the patient is essential, and a goal-oriented approach is important. Two factors seem most pressing when a person suffers physical disability: pain control and ability to increase functional performance. Attaining either of these may be enough for some patients, whereas others must attain both. In general, if a patient can be in control of his/her disability rather than the disability being in control of him/her, the therapeutic intervention undertaken can be considered successful.

As with all rehabilitation programs, goal-setting is essential. Spinal disk disease is often painful and physically disabling, and you must clearly establish individualized goals when embarking on the road to optimal health. Pain control is the first concern when treating disk-related disease, and the mainstay of pain control is NSAIDs.[54] Saal proposes avoidance of narcotics, muscle relaxants, and sleep hypnotics for the reasons outlined in Table 32-3.[54] It is my belief, however, that muscle relaxants and narcotics are effective when used for acute, well-identified pain flares. All medications carry the risk of harm, particularly when overused or abused. Patients must be educated about the proper indications and usage for medicines. Particular cautions should be taken with muscle relaxants since their mechanism of action is often through the central nervous system. The sedating and "mind-altering" effects of these can interfere with a patient's mental status. Limited use of them is suggested.

In addition to pain medications, passive modalities such as traction, manual techniques, deep heating modalities, and injection treatments can be used. Traction is helpful in both the cervical and lumbar regions. It aids in soft tissue relaxation and intervertebral disk space winding. There is controversy as to whether, as traditionally applied, traction actually widens the intervertebral disk space, since it is well recognized that the force required for intervertebral distraction is quite large. With this in mind, the following recommendations may be clinically useful. For the cervical spine, try to gradually increase weight up to the target value. Colachis and Strohm have shown that 30 pounds of traction with a slightly flexed cervical spine (24 degrees) can cause vertebral separation.[16] Others have suggested that a minimum of 25 pounds is needed to have vertebral separation.[36]

When receiving cervical spine traction, the patient's head should be slightly flexed and comfortably relaxed. If you are using an automated traction device, be sure your patient has an emergency cutoff switch (one that deactivates the traction toward zero pounds) or access to disengage the device manually. Treatment sessions should be for 20 to 30 minutes and can be done two or three times a week. Colachis and Strohm

Table 32-3. Medication check list

Medication	Indications and use
Nonsteroidal anti-inflammatory drugs	Useful for anti-inflammatory action and analgesia
Narcotic analgesics	To be avoided because of endorphin blockade and addictive potential
Muscle relaxants	To be avoided because of their central nervous system sedative effects
Sleep hypnotics	To be avoided because of their central nervous system depressive effects
Tricyclic antidepressants	Useful to promote sleep and decrease serotonergic pain stimuli

From Saal J, Dillingham M: Nonoperative treatment and rehabilitation of disk, facet, and soft tissue injuries. In Nicholas J and Hershman E, editors, *The lower extremity in spine and sport medicine,* ed 2, St Louis, 1995, Mosby–Year Book.

suggest that the optimum time for vertebral separation is 25 minutes.[17]

In the lumbar spine, our target poundage is 60% to 65% of body weight. This type of traction is best done with the patient lying down and with the same emergency parameters and duration of treatment as for the cervical spine. Traction can be applied in a continuous manner or intermittently. The decision as to which to use depends largely on patient comfort. Geiringer indicates that both physician and patient preference is most important in deciding between intermittent and continuous traction.[26] When applied intermittently, on/off times can vary. I prefer brief slow-ramping times, 10 to 15 seconds on and 5 to 7 seconds off. Be aware that the onset of traction may invoke discomfort rather than alleviate it. Individuals with spinal stenosis and disk disease may actually complain of more, rather than less, pain. The reason for this may be root irritation from column lengthening.

If a patient wishes to use a "home traction device," there are several considerations. First, the most popular of these devices are those that contain water-fillable pouches with an over-the-door suspension apparatus (Fig. 32-3). Second, remember to instruct your patient to face the frame (typically a door) from which the unit is suspended. This traction device too is accompanied by a slight flexion of the cervical spine. Finally, make sure your patient follows all directions carefully. Strict attention must be paid to the amount of water/pounds applied to the spine. Home cervical traction units do not typically allow a patient to apply too much weight because the water (or sometimes sand) container will allow only safe amounts of substance to be added. This is usually 20 to 25 pounds maximum. This, however, may not be enough external weight to achieve sufficient traction. When you consider that part of the applied external weight is negated by the inherent weight of the patient's head (typically 10 to 13 pounds), the resultant net traction force is not enough to promote intervertebral lengthening. For example, if the water bag is filled with 25 pounds of water, and you subtract 10 pounds for the weight of the head, the net traction force is only 15 pounds.

It is important to emphasize to patients that careful application of home cervical traction is paramount. Patients often think, "If some is good then more is better." This certainly is not the case, and patients must be reminded to follow recommended guidelines and not be overzealous. Not doing so could lead to significant complications. Contraindications and relative contraindications do exist for the use of traction. These are outlined in Table 32-4.[21] Manual techniques are very helpful in cervical, thoracic, and lumbosacral disk disease. They are particularly useful in treating restrictions of motion, particularly those caused by hypomobility of related joints.

Although mentioned here under the category of disk disease, manual therapies are used in treatments of various musculoskeletal disorders. There are several types of manual interventions, ranging from soft tissue–to forceful bony thrusting–techniques (Fig. 32-4).

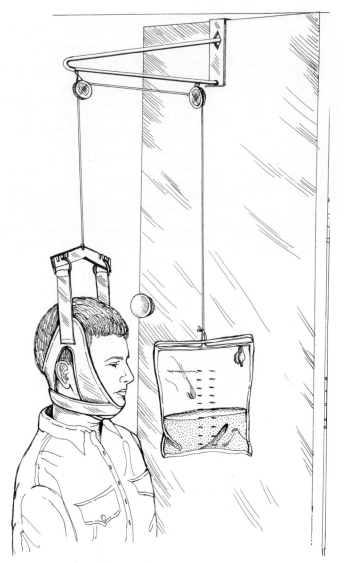

Fig. 32-3. Cervical spine traction. Home traction devices are somewhat useful in treating cervical spine pathology, but caution must be used when applying the device (see text).

Table 32-4. Traction

Indications	pain
	vertebral separation/disk herniation
	muscle hypertonicity
	nerve root decompression
	disk and facets that need unloading
Contraindications	malignancy
	sepsis
	vascular compromise
	unstable spine
Precautions	inflammatory arthropathy, aortic aneurysm, pregnancy, hiatal hernia, vertigo

From Esses, 1995.
From Greenman PE: *Principles of manual medicine,* Baltimore, 1989, Williams and Wilkins.

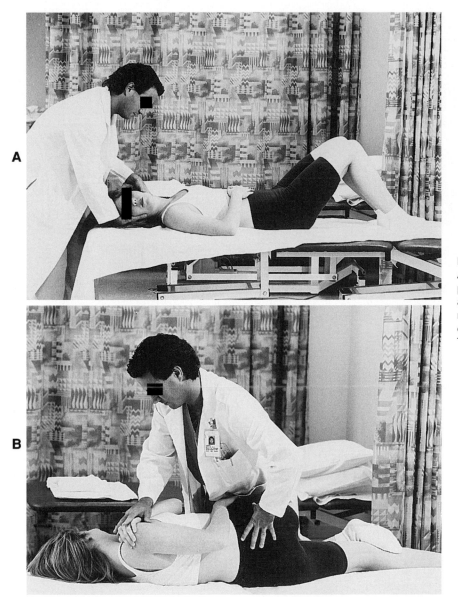

Fig. 32-4. Manipulation-thrusting technique. **A** and **B,** After taking the associated joint to its physiologic limit, a gentle high velocity, low amplitude thrust is administered. Before any manipulative procedure, a complete knowledge of contraindications must be known (see Table 32-5).

An example of soft tissue intervention is muscle energy (Fig. 32-5). In this strategy the focus is to relax a hypertonic motion–restricting muscle, to allow freedom of movement in the opposite direction of the restrictive muscle's action. As an example, if you try to extend your lumbosacral spine but find yourself unable to, the reason may be tight abdominal muscles. If the abdominals are not relaxed or do not offer pliability, they will inhibit movement in the opposite direction (extension).

To overcome stiff abdominal muscles, muscle energy techniques can be applied. In this instance, trying to extend the lumbosacral spine will be resisted by the tight abdominals, so stretching the abdominals is impractical. To achieve the desired effect of lumbosacral extension, we attempt to contract the abdominal muscles, usually for a count of 5 to 6 seconds, against resistance (isometric) and then passively extend the lumbosacral spine.

The isometric contractions of the abdominals hopefully induce muscle fatigue. Then the abdominals no longer act hypertonically to resist the extension movement. The exercise is repeated several times, each time increasing the amount of lumbosacral extension. This is a very effective technique to increase flexibility and relax muscles.

Practitioners use and claim success for many other manual techniques, such as craniosacral, counterstrain, and myofascial release. Craniosacral technique was introduced by William G. Sutherland in about 1940. The foundation of his therapy lies in the consistent architecture of the skull's sutures, which maintain mobility during health. When a person is traumatized or ill, this normal mobility is interrupted and restrictions of motion occur. Because the skull is connected to the sacrum by the meninges, restrictions of motion in one will directly influence the other. Hence the name *craniosacral.*

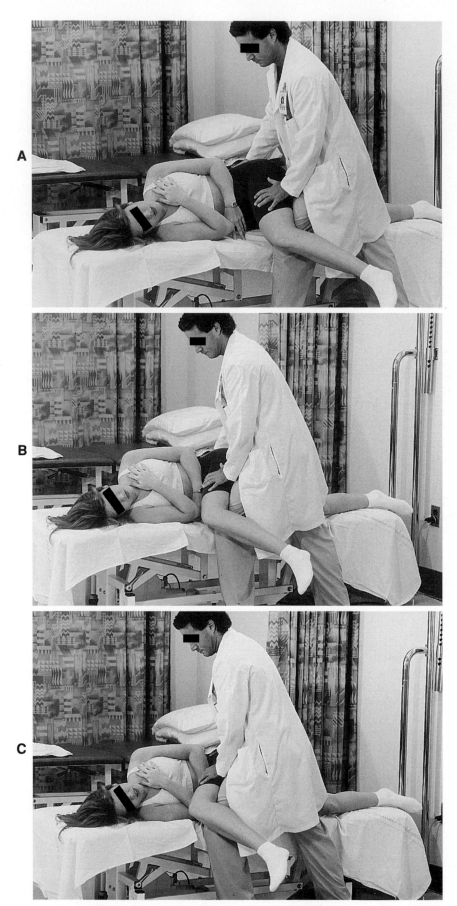

Fig. 32-5. Muscle energy technique. **A, B,** and **C,** Through a series of repetitive contractions of a hypertonic muscle, increased freedom of movement in the opposite direction can be achieved. If the lumbosacral extensors are hypertonic, a series of repeated contractions of these muscles can lead to relaxation and increased freedom of motion in the opposite direction, i.e., lumbosacral flexion.

Craniosacral technique involves manual pressures exerted onto various key bony regions to unrestrict mobility. There is a growing number of clinicians who deliver craniosacral therapy. Its indications in musculoskeletal treatments are rather broad and range from simple joint stiffness to complex soft tissue restrictions.

Counterstrain technique was formally introduced by Lawrence H. Jones in his text entitled *Strain and Counterstrain*.[35] It is believed that spinal pathology has a consistent coinciding muscular reference area that is tender to palpation. These so-called tender spots, when localized, are the monitoring areas for the success of this technique. When a clinician confidently palpates such a tender spot, he/she positions the patient's body in such a way that the tender region under the palpating finger no longer produces discomfort. This position is held for about 90 seconds and the body part is then slowly returned to the pretreatment habitus. Often the pain and discomfort the patient was experiencing in this tender spot no longer exists (Fig. 32-6).

Myofascial release involves massage-like stretching of soft tissue structures. Its goal is to elongate restricted muscles and soft tissue regions. Although similar, it is not massage therapy. If muscles are restricting motion and muscle energy technique is being used, myofascial release technique is an excellent adjunct. Bony techniques fall under several names. These include adjustment, manipulation, mobilization, and "cracking." Historically, the chiropractic (DC) profession uses the term "adjustment," osteopathic (DO) physicians "manipulate" the bony segments, and physical therapists (PT) "mobilize" the joints. In recent years allopathic (MD) physicians are more frequently making use of this alternative approach for musculoskeletal disorders.

It is no longer uncommon for physicians to refer patients to practitioners with expertise in manual medicine. Manipulation aims at correcting functional impairment rather than treating pathology. It attempts to restore natural play between body parts so that they can resume normal functioning.[14] Techniques vary from very gentle stretching maneuvers to high-velocity thrusting techniques. There are two commonly accepted thrusting techniques. The first is high velocity, low amplitude technique. This is a quick thrust applied to a bony structure to overcome a restrictive soft tissue barrier. The second is low velocity, high amplitude technique, which implies a slow movement but with force carried over a longer distance.

Several studies have investigated the efficacy of spinal manual medicine. For patients with low back pain in whom manipulation is not contraindicated, chiropractic treatment almost certainly confers worthwhile, long-lasting benefit compared to hospital outpatient management.[41] In comparing spinal mobilization (nonrotational) to spinal manipulation/adjustment, Hadler and others found significant improvement in the manipulation/adjustment group.[28] On December 4, 1994, the U.S. Agency for Health Care Policy and Research proposed federal guidelines for the treatment of low back pain. In its report, manipulation/adjustments were endorsed and encouraged as a treatment of choice. It should be noted that this recommendation was not inclusive for those with radiculopathy.[1] Also, after one month of unsuccessful manipulation further diagnostic work-up is indicated. Before performing spinal manipulation/adjustment, I do a series of muscle energy therapies to ease the application of thrusting techniques. In this manner, the muscles in the region to be manipulated are more flexible. Contraindications to manipulation/adjustments do exist and are noted in Table 32-5.[28,34] Two other approaches in the treatment of intervertebral disk disease are McKenzie extension exercises and lumbar stabilization.

Lumbar stabilization, as proposed by Saal and others, has gained considerable popularity in the management of disk disease.[16] Their notion is that a well-thought-out and scientifically based program could result in successful conservative treatment for herniated disks. The basic premise of stabilization theory requires a thorough understanding of spinal/vertebral forces and their relationship to biomechanical motion. Attainment of what is described as "neutral" spine helps to minimize extraneous forces upon the spine and associated soft tissues. Neutral spine is that anterior-posterior, medial-lateral, superior-inferior alignment whereby the net forces transmitted through the spine are balanced by increasing the purchase of the vertebral segments. The increased surface area allows for more evenly distributed forces. When the overall contact areas are increased, the force per unit–area is decreased. This can be accomplished, for example, by pelvic tilts.

One could appreciate this maneuver if attempting the following. While standing, try to thrust the superior border of your iliac crests posteriorly, then tighten your abdominal muscles and squeeze your buttocks together. This maneuver will relax the lumbosacral paraspinal region, and there is usually a feeling of pressure relief if the technique is done correctly. Once a patient can attain and maintain this posture, a fully structured and monitored exercise program can be developed. The exercises are performed with the pelvis in "neutral spine," which assists in maximizing ergonomic efficiency and acts to protect the spinal structures (Fig. 32-7 on page 544).

In the cervical spine, the natural lordotic curve does not promote optimal bony contact. To begin training, we must establish the position of optimal function (POF). This can take place with slight occipito-atlanto flexion. It is only when the patient feels comfortable with postural adaptations that the appropriate exercise program can begin.

For the lumbar spine, our goal is to train the abdominal, lumbosacral extensor, and buttock muscles while maintaining neutral spine. For the cervical spine we focus on the posterior cervical paraspinal muscles and the scapula stabilizers (particularly the serratus anterior and rhomboids) to help stabilize the spine. The program has several different phases, each with a further progression of exercises. The ultimate goal is relative freedom from pain with increased mobility. The box on p. 543 depicts the treatment phases for lumbar stabilization.[55]

Akin to the stabilization techniques described above, the McKenzie technique of postural control and vertebral stabilization has gained much popular-

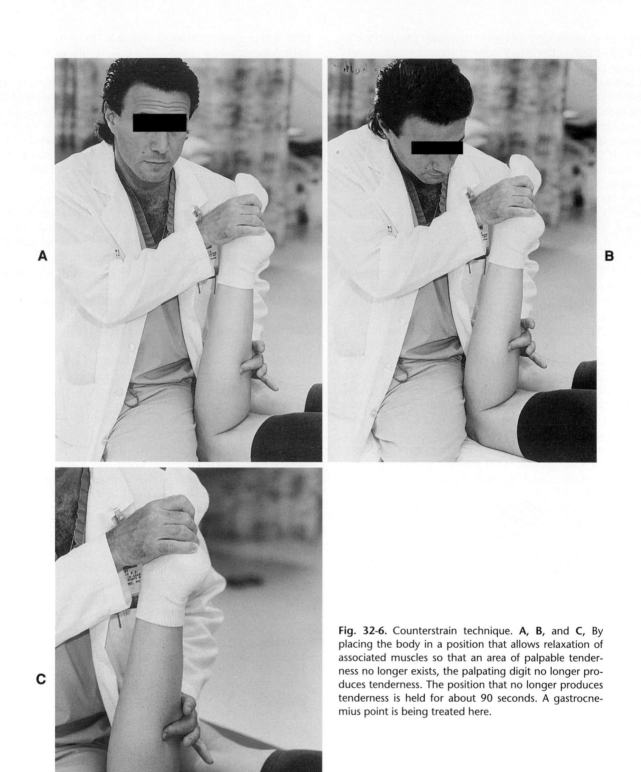

Fig. 32-6. Counterstrain technique. **A, B,** and **C,** By placing the body in a position that allows relaxation of associated muscles so that an area of palpable tenderness no longer exists, the palpating digit no longer produces tenderness. The position that no longer produces tenderness is held for about 90 seconds. A gastrocnemius point is being treated here.

TREATMENT PHASES

Pain Control
Back first aid

Trial of extension exercises

Trial of traction

Basic stabilization exercise training

NSAIDs

Non-narcotic analgesics

Corticosteroids
Oral
Epidural injection
Selective nerve root injection
Facet injection

Exercise Training
Soft tissue flexibility
Hamstring musculotendinous unit
Quadriceps musculotendinous unit
Iliopsoas musculotendinous unit
Gastroc-soleus musculotendinous unit
External and internal hip rotators

Joint Mobility
Lumbar spine segmental mobility

Hip range of motion

Thoracic segmental mobility

Stabilization Program
Finding neutral position

Sitting stabilization

Prone gluteal squeezes

Supine pelvic bracing

Bridging progression
Basic position
One leg raised
Stepping
Balance on gym ball

Quadriped
With alternating arm and leg movement

Kneeling Stabilization
Double knee

Single knee

Lunges
Wall slide quadriceps strengthening
Position transition with postural control

Abdominal Program
Curl-ups

Dead bugs

Diagonal curl-ups

Diagonal curl-ups on incline board

Straight leg lowering

Gym Program
Latissimus pull-downs

Angled leg press

Lunges

Hyperextension bench

General upper body strengthening exercises

Pulley exercises to stress postural control

Aerobic Program
Progressive walking

Swimming

Stationary bicycling

Cross-country ski machine

Running
Initially supervised on a treadmill

From Saal JA, Saal JS: Nonoperative treatment of herniated lumbar intervertebral disk with radiculopathy: An outcome study, Spine 14(4), 1989.

ity.[40] As proposed by Robin McKenzie, a physiotherapist from New Zealand, this technique emphasizes extension-type movements to counteract one's slumped biomechanically inefficient posture. Its exercise sequence focuses on restricted versus pathologic movement. An example of this is when a patient has difficulty extending his/her lumbosacral spine in a sitting position. Is this due to tight abdominal muscles or posterior spinal pathology that inhibits the extension movement?

Table 32-5. Manipulation

Indications	joint restrictions
	joint immobility
	nerve root compression
	psychological stress
Contraindications	unstable spine
	cauda equina syndrome
	systemic anticoagulation
	rheumatoid arthritis
	vertebral insufficiency
	vertebral malignancy
	myelopathy
	advanced spondylosis
	spondyloarthropathies
	osteoporosis
	osteomalacia

From Janse J: History of the development of chiropractic concepts: chiropractic terminology. In Goldstein M, editor, *The research status of spinal manipulation*, NINCDE Monograph No 5, DHEW Pub No (NIH) 76-998, 1975.

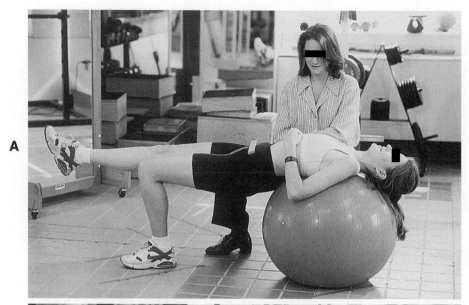

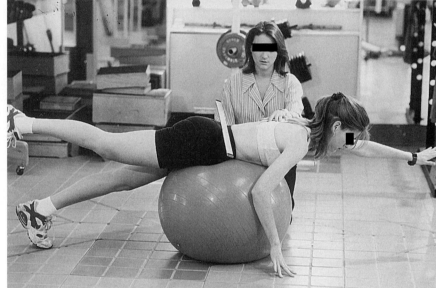

Fig. 32-7. Stabilization in neutral spine. **A, B** While maintaining neutral spine, a series of exercises are performed. The maintenance of neutral spine is essential during these exercises. A stick or pole can be placed across the lumbar spine to monitor stable pelvic tilt during these exercises.

TENS (transcutaneous electrical nerve stimulation) is a modality used to reduce pain. It produces a strong but comfortable current that is thought to provide analgesic effects in the applied areas. The current is delivered from a beeper-like device into small surface pads that are attached to the unit with fine wire (Fig. 32-8). Its efficacy is controversial, so it is merely mentioned here as an alternative modality to reduce pain. In a recent study evaluating the efficacy of TENS and exercise for chronic low back pain, results did not show evidence for more effective pain relief with TENS.[19] In general, we do think a trial of TENS is worthwhile for patients who do not obtain pain relief from more conventional interventions.

Deep-heating modalities are effective for both subjective and physiologic effects. The application of warm packs or ultrasound makes most people subjectively feel better. This may be a placebo effect or related to muscle re-

laxation. Physiologically, heat increases blood flow, which subsequently increases the body's local metabolic rate. This, in turn, allows a cleansing of metabolic byproducts and accelerates the rate of healing. Heating packs are commercially available in several varieties. Some are operated electrically (dry heat), others have heat-retaining gels (moist heat) (Fig. 32-9). The gel packs are moistened by placing them in hot water to allow the gel to absorb the heat. The pack is then placed over the area to be treated, but we recommend placing a layer or two of toweling between the moist pack and the skin's surface. The packs tend to get rather warm and could inadvertently cause a superficial burn on the skin. Patients should be instructed to remove the packs if they feel uncomfortable.

The health care provider should periodically check with the patient to make sure that he/she is comfortable. Total treatment time should be 10 to 20 minutes. The

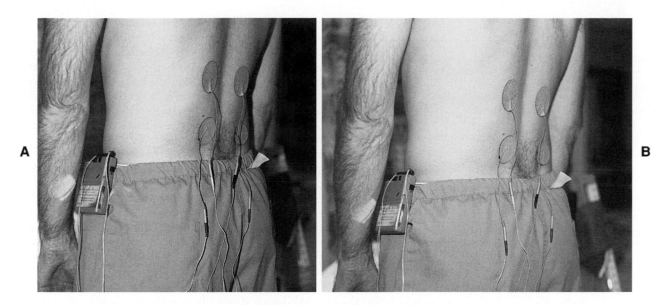

Fig. 32-8. Transcutaneous electrical nerve stimulation (TENS). **A** and **B**, Electrodes are placed at key sites of pain referral to control transmission of aberrant sensation. The unit is regulated by control dials to increase/decrease intensity and frequency of impulse transmission.

true physiologic effects of this heating modality are often questioned, since heating pads (moist or dry) only penetrate the superficial subcutaneous layers. To achieve deeper heating effects, ultrasound can be used. The indications and contraindications of heat are listed in Table 32-6.[21]

Injection techniques are gaining popularity in the treatment of musculoskeletal injuries. In some instances injections are diagnostic. Other times they are used as adjunct treatments, and occasionally they are curative. A variety of approaches is used. These include paraverte-

bral nerve blocks, selective nerve root blocks, epidurals, trigger-point injections, facet blocks, and sacroiliac injections. Injection techniques such as facet joint and epidural injections are examples of invasive nonsurgical approaches to specific anatomic diagnoses and treatments.[8] The use of injection therapy allows for directed, rapid control of pain generators. Because disk herniations and facet injuries have distinct pain referral zones, injections can be administered specifically to the corresponding generator zone. The pain referral pattern associated with disk herniations follows dermatomal maps,

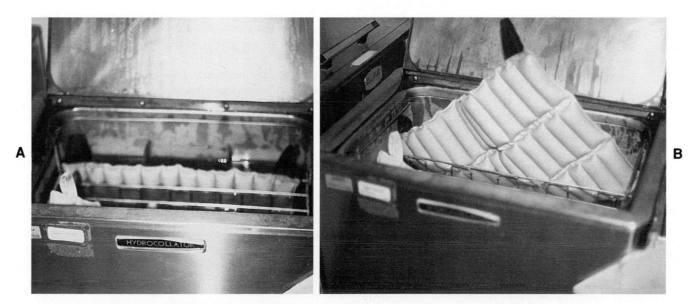

Fig. 32-9. Heating packs. **A** and **B**, Heating devices are useful to reduce musculoskeletal pain and ease muscle hypertonicity. They are usually applied in the chronic setting of injury but are not restricted to this use only. Application is for 10 to 20 minutes and frequent checks are made to assure comfort (i.e., that the packs are not too hot).

Table 32-6. Heat

Indications	pain and muscle spasm
	need for range-of-motion improvement
	pain
	lowered metabolic rate
Contraindications	anesthetic area
	obtunded patient
	over: gonads, gravid uterus
	malignancy
	hemorrhagic diathesis
	area of poor vascularity

Adapted from Michlovitz SL: *Thermal agents in rehabilitation,* Philadelphia, 1986, FA Davis.
Adapted from Esses SI: *Textbook of spinal disorders,* Philadelphia, 1995, Lippincott.

and that of facet joints follows a corresponding blueprint.[3] If you can localize the pain-producing level with an injection of lidocaine, a follow-up injection with a steroid preparation may prove effective in decreasing pain. This may allow earlier return to normal activity.

The biggest dilemma in delivering facet-joint injections is clearly defining facet-joint syndrome. To date, there is no clear-cut definition, and most clinicians simply describe it in those who respond to facet-joint injection. In one series, a response to injection was seen in 50% to 60% of patients, which was lasting in only 20% to 30% at 6 months.[39] Delivery of these injections usually requires a radiology suite since they are administered under fluoroscopic guidance. Initially a dye or contrast material is injected to identify the area of injury. This injection often provokes discomfort. Once identified, the area can be infiltrated with a steroid/anesthetic preparation.

Many theories exist regarding the etiology of referred pain. Certainly, direct mechanical pressure on root fibers will produce pain. Recent studies suggest an alternate pain generator. An inflammatory enzyme known as phospholipase A_2 is reportedly liberated at the time of disk herniation. This results in an intense neural inflammatory reaction that causes pain and axonal damage to the spinal nerve root.[51,52,53] It is for this reason that epidural steroid injections in the setting of disk herniation may be beneficial. They can be given to a selective root or in the vicinity of the spinal cord. In the past, selective nerve root blocks have been performed with anesthetic agents alone to assist in specific localization of a disorder. Studies are currently underway to evaluate the therapeutic efficacy of adding a steroid to the solution.[38,62,68] To date, studies have not revealed whether observable improvements from injections result from the particular steroid medication, injection volume, or the diluent used.[4,22]

Several controlled studies have failed to document the effect of epidural steroids in patients with documented lumbosacral nerve root compression.[50,60] Commonly used steroid solutions include hydrocortisone, 25 mg,[11] dexamethasone 8 mg,[10] and methylprednisolone 80 to 120 mg.[2,30] Some of the more common anesthetic agents used are 1% procaine, 5 ml, and 0.25% to 0.50% bupivacaine 5 to 10 cc.[5,12] The literature clearly depicts the great diversity of techniques for administering epidural steroids. These can range from choice of medication, concomitant physical therapy, needle localization (blind-stick or fluoroscope-guided), follow-up schedule, and frequency of injections. It is clear why the variance in outcomes is so great. Randomized, double-blind studies have used blind-injection techniques. This technique has been reported to approach a 25% misplacement rate in needle insertion.[8] In general, epidural steroids are good interventions in treating disk disease/myofascial pain, particularly with or after conservative therapy.

Complications and contraindications do exist for the use of epidural steroids, and the clinician must be aware of these.[9] They are outlined in Table 32-7. Local infection and/or arachnoiditis is a rare complication. It should be understood that after receiving an epidural steroid injection, the adrenal axis may be suppressed for 2 to 3 weeks.[33]

Although it usually is accurate to discuss intervertebral disk disease and myofascial pain as the same entity, they certainly can exist independently. Myofascial pain is not always synonymous with intervertebral disk disease and is often an isolated entity. There are several clearly defined syndromes that manifest themselves as myofascial pain, including piriformis syndrome, quadratus lumborum syndrome, and iliopsoas myofascial dysfunction.

It is a most difficult task for a practitioner to determine the etiology of pain in the region of the buttocks. Certainly radiculopathy can refer pain to the buttocks, particularly L5 radiculitis. Arthritic conditions of the hip, spine, or pelvis can also produce discomfort in the buttock. Visceral pain of pelvic origin can be a culprit. The quality, duration, and temporal patterns of the pain may differ, and it is confusing to try to delineate the specific etiology of buttock/low back pain.

Piriformis syndrome is a well-recognized but often ignored syndrome with very characteristic findings. Buttock tenderness and pain is usually the chief complaint of patients with this syndrome, particularly in the region of the greater trochanter, specifically in the vicinity of the insertion of the external hip rotator muscles. These areas that are tender to palpation are commonly called trigger points (to be discussed in detail below). Freiberg's

Table 32-7. Epidural injections

Indications	pain
	inflammation
Contraindications	in area of congenital anomaly or previous surgery
	if steriods may unmask an infection
	hemorrhagic diathesis
	local infection
	medicine allergy (to solution being injected)

From Bogduk N, Aprill C, Derby R: Epidural steroid injections. In White AH, Schofferman JA, Goldstein M, editors, *Spine care diagnosis and conservative treatment,* vol 1, St Louis, 1995, Mosby–Year Book.

sign (pain reproduced on passive internal rotation of the extended thigh), Pace's sign (pain and/or weakness noted on resisted external rotation of the extended thigh), posterior/lateral rectal pain on digital exam, and tenderness to palpation directly over the piriformis muscle are all characteristic.[24,47] This malady is best treated with techniques such as muscle energy, sacroiliac manipulation, and injections. Because piriformis syndrome is often a diagnosis of exclusion, a thorough neurologic exam must be done to rule out a concomitant pathologic condition.

The writings of Travell and Simons clearly define a disease of hyperirritable soft tissue foci located in the skeletal muscle or its associated fascia.[64] These foci are called "trig-

ger points" and are soft tissue regions that are very tender to palpation. Inherent to these is a distinct pain-referral pattern when they are stimulated (Fig. 32-10). The muscle that harbors a trigger point contains taut fibers in the form of a palpable band that tightens and shortens the muscle.[64] This taut band refers pain when tension is placed on it. The treatment for trigger points usually consists of injection with a solution of anesthetic, commonly 1% lidocaine (without epinephrine), in a volume of 5 to 10 cc. When you inject the trigger point the typical response is a "jump sign." The area will twitch upon needle insertion, which is a good indication that the needle is in the correct location. Once the needle is positioned, it is gently moved in a short range back and forth several

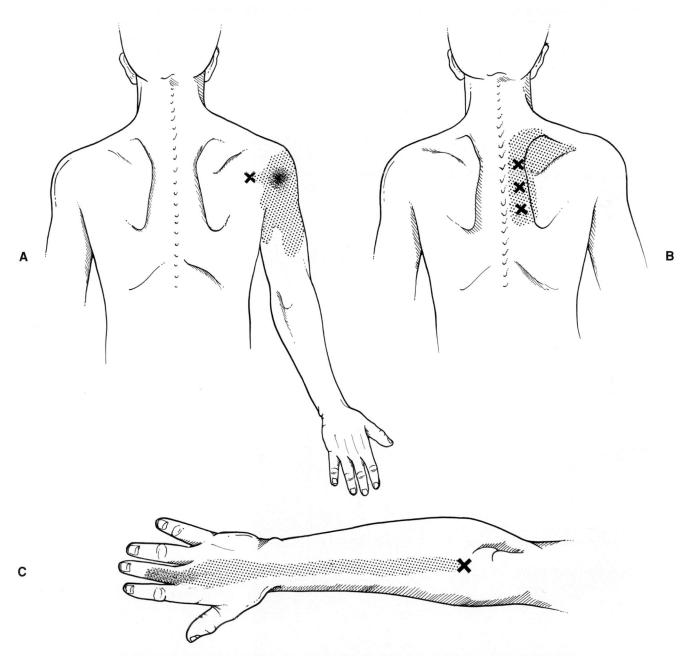

Fig. 32-10. Trigger points/myofascial pain. Map of trigger points and associated pain referral zones. **A,** Teses minor; **B,** Rhomboid; **C,** Digit extensors. Trigger points noted by the X and pain referral zone by the shaded area.

times to assist in breaking up the trigger foci. Response to this technique is very positive when you precisely localize a specific trigger point to be injected. The injections can be repeated several times over a few weeks. Skin preparation before injection should follow basic aseptic technique guidelines. It is not uncommon to feel transient soreness several hours after the injections, and patients should be made aware of this. A steroid solution can be added to the injection solution. If this is done, you should limit the frequency of injections (with steroid) to not more than three in 4 to 6 months.

Along with trigger point injections, other treatments such as Spray and Stretch are useful. In this technique, Ethyl Chloride or Fluori-Methane spray is used to assist muscle flexibility. This spray is rather cold when applied to the skin and assists in briefly desensitizing the region sprayed. This allows slow sustained stretch to be applied to the muscles below the sprayed sites. The spray is aimed at the area of the body where muscles are irritated; and while you spray in the same direction as the muscle fibers, the patient stretches the muscles.

Another muscle commonly implicated in, but rarely identified when discussing, myofascial pain is the quadratus lumborum. It is a well recognized source of low back and buttock pain but only when the examiner knows to look for it. This quadrangular-shaped muscle lies beneath the erector spinae muscle group and functions as a lateral flexor/extensor of the lumbar spine, elevator of the pelvis, and depressor of the twelfth rib.[70] One must specifically palpate this muscle when examining a patient. To best identify its painful trigger point areas, the practitioner should place the patient lying on the side with his/her knees flexed in the fetal position. The neck should be comfortably tucked onto the chest, and the patient should take slow, deep breaths. The examiner then gently palpates, with pads of several digits, the region between the erector spinae and the ribs on the raised side of the patient's torso. Palpating with several digits increases the purchase of skin contact so as not to tense the muscles of the patient's back by examining in a probing fashion (Fig. 32-11). If trigger points are present in this muscle, they will be palpated easily with

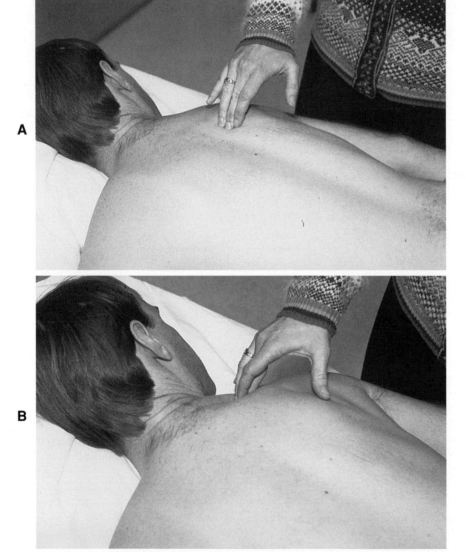

Fig. 32-11. Palpatory technique for trigger points. **A** and **B**, With the pads of 1–2 digits, deep palpation in the direction of muscle fibers reveals "taut" bands. When isolating such, there is a sensation of discomfort.

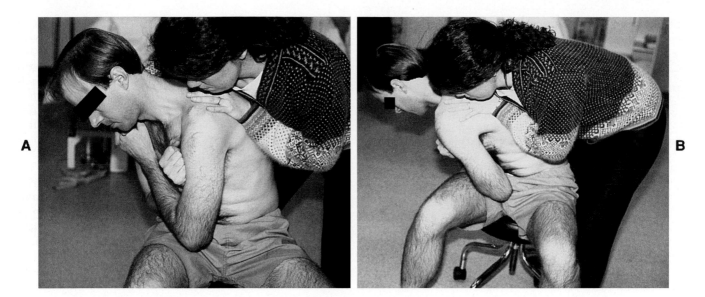

Fig. 32-12. Muscle energy techniques for quadratus lumborum strain. **A** and **B**, With the patient sitting comfortably and both feet firmly on the ground, the examiner leans over the patient's thoracic spine and passively sidebends/rotates the torso in the direction of the strain. The patient is then instructed to upright the torso to neutral against resistance applied by the examiner's chest. This isometric contraction technique is held for approximately 5 seconds. The resistance is then released and the patient is laterally flexed passively and rotated further to the involved side. The entire process is then repeated. A series of 4 to 5 contraction sets are done. Typically, the same series is done to the opposite side.

this technique. Muscle energy techniques should be directed at relieving these painful areas and should prove very effective.

A particularly useful manual technique is performed with the patient sitting comfortably in a chair with their feet firmly on the ground. The patient then crosses their arms across the chest and the examiner, standing behind the patient, leans onto the patient's upper back with their chest (Fig. 32-12). The patient will tilt further toward one side little by little, each time going through a series of isometric contractions back toward midline, against resistance from the examiner. This is repeated several times before performing the same exercise on the opposite side. It can be repeated two or three times on each side. Flexibility/stretching exercise is also useful and includes lateral trunk-bending and toe-touching. Injections are warranted in conjunction with or after failed conservative approaches. These would be administered as described above for myofascial pain.

The iliopsoas muscle is said to be a treatable cause of "failed" low back syndrome.[32] This ventral spinal muscle functions as a hip flexor and is thought to be tightened in certain pathologic conditions of the low back. Ingber proposes a "dry" needling technique whereby a 30-gauge, 2.5-inch needle is slowly inserted into the iliopsoas muscle in an attempt to relax the tightened fibers.[32] In this technique, no solution is injected into the trigger point. After the injection, a series of lumbosacral extension exercises is performed by the patient to stretch out the previously tightened region.

Acupuncture is an alternative injection technique that is rapidly gaining a strong following in the Western world. This ancient Chinese therapy has been practiced for more than 2500 years. It is indicated for pain relief and disease cure. Its followers believe its results occur by restoring the balance between yin (blood) and yang (spirit). These energies flow within the body along fourteen channels or meridians.[42] There are 361 sites (acupuncture points), which, when stimulated by pressure or needle insertion, stimulate innate processes within the body. Researchers argue that acupuncture is a form of neuromodulation. Two theories are proposed. The needles used in acupuncture may stimulate large sensory afferent fibers and suppress pain perception. Or the needle insertion can act as a noxious stimulus and induce intrinsic production of opiate-like substances to control pain.[70]

It has been shown that a significant similarity exists between myofascial trigger points and acupuncture sites.[43] The sensation generated by the use of an acupuncture needle resembles the dull ache often reported by a patient after a trigger point has been injected. Acupuncture can aid in reducing muscle hypertonicity and trigger point sensitivity. Also, it is useful in controlling radicular pain by increasing endorphin levels within the central nervous system.[54] It seems that regardless of the substance injected, the result is likely to be pain relief. The trigger points of myofascial injection may indeed be the same as areas of needle insertion associated with acupuncture.[66] Trigger point therapy is very effective in the management of myofascial pain, and clinicians should be familiar with its application.

The above disorders are conservatively managed with manual techniques and injection therapies. Table 32-8

Table 32-8. Advanced pain control methods

Clinical presentation	Treatment techniques
Persistent radicular pain	Selective epidural cortisone injection
	Epidural cortisone injection
	Acupuncture
Facet joint synovitis and capsular pain	Facet joint cortisone injection
Muscle hypertonicity and trigger point sensitivity	Trigger point injection with local anesthetic
	Acupuncture
Cervicogenic headaches	Acupuncture
	Facet joint injection to symptomatic and relevant joints

From Saal J, Dillingham M: Nonoperative treatment and rehabilitation of disk, facet, and soft tissue injuries. In Nicholas J and Hershman E, editors, *The lower extremity in spine and sport medicine*, ed 2, St Louis, 1995, Mosby–Year Book.

reviews various injection techniques used for advanced pain control.[54]

SPONDYLOLISTHESIS

The classification of spondylolisthesis as described by Witse, Newman, and McNab, includes six categories:[69]

Type I. Congenital/Dysplastic
Type II. Isthmic
Type III. Degenerative
Type IV. Traumatic
Type V. Pathologic
Type VI. Postsurgical

The most common levels of occurrence are L5-S1 (congenital and isthmic) and L4-5 (degenerative). The grading of spondylolisthesis is from low Grade I through high Grade V. These grades are determined by the degree of anterior (anterolisthesis) or posterior (posterolisthesis) movement of the superior vertebrae in reference to the inferior vertebrae. A slip of up to 25% of the width of the inferior endplate by the superior vertebrae is Grade I. 25% to 50% slippage is Grade II; 50% to 75%, Grade III; 75% to 100%, Grade IV; and when the superior vertebrae slip entirely off of the inferior vertebrae (spondyloptosis), Grade V. Conservative treatment of this disorder is useful in low-grade slips (Grades I and II). This includes lumbosacral flexion exercises, lumbar stabilization, and bracing. I have found that flexion exercises are not as successful in patients with spondylolisthesis who have increased slippage as seen by flexion views radiographically. This subtle sign of instability may exaggerate pain even though the lumbosacral flexion moment tends to unload the painful articular facets. Young people with Grade I spondylolisthesis have a 78%–success rate in terms of symptom resolution when treated conservatively. Treatment should include the use of a modified Boston brace (worn full-time for six months and then weaned over the subsequent six months).[49]

Often adult patients do rather well with lumbosacral corsets with or without stays. Stabilization exercises with a flexion bias should be emphasized, because they have been shown to achieve better results in patients with spondylolisthesis.[54] Bracing is most successful when it promotes lumbar flexion and decreases the inherent lordosis. The braces that accomplish this are usually bulky, and many patients reject them. Also the time commitment for wearing the brace is lengthy and involves most hours of the day. Low-profile designs are preferable but may not be successful in symptomatic relief.

To evaluate the efficacy of exercise protocols addressing the symptoms of spondylolisthesis, one study evaluated 48 patients with Grade I slippage.[59] A comparison of lumbar flexion versus extension exercises was done. Flexion exercises consisted of abdominal strengthening, pelvic tilting, and chest-to-thigh positioning. Extension exercises consisted of prone lumbar and hip extension. At a three-year followup, 19% of the flexion group had moderate or severe pain as compared with 67% in the extension group. Also, 24% of the flexion group were unable to return to work compared to 61% in the extension group. In our experience, flexion exercises that include pelvic tilting in conjunction with lumbar flexion seem to give symptomatic pain relief. This may be due to unloading of the pars region, which may be the prime pain generator. There have been less successful results with lumbar extension exercises.

Muscle energy technique is also beneficial in this setting when the lumbosacral paraspinal muscles are treated. Through serial contractions, fatigue of the lumbar extensors can assist in unloading the posterior elements. Williams's flexion exercises help to unload the lumbar paraspinal region and also strengthen the abdominal muscles. This series of exercises includes single and double knee-to-chest, straight leg raising, and sit-ups. It is recommended that any exercise program be performed at least three times a week and about 30 minutes per session be set aside to complete that day's exercises.

STENOSIS/SPONDYLOSIS

Stenosis and spondylosis (degenerative arthritis) are afflictions everyone fears, especially with advancing age. It must be stated clearly, however, that developing arthritis is not an automatic component of aging. Many elderly people are amazingly free of arthritis, and, on the contrary, many younger people are very arthritic. The key to treating arthritis is to clearly diagnose and understand the ongoing pathophysiology. Simply stated, if we are discussing a purely degenerative process, the location of the changes can guide our therapy efforts. If there is a predominance of anterior degenerative changes, our goals are to unload this area by promoting extension exercises. Alternatively, if there is a predominance of posterior changes, our goals are to unload this area and we promote flexion exercises. The addition of modalities such as warm packs, ultrasound, and electrical stimulation (applications discussed in a previous section) along with techniques such as muscle energy and soft tissue massage offer symptomatic relief.

Table 32-9. Nonsteroidal antiinflammatory drugs: dosing suggestion

Generic name	Brand name	Starting dose	Maximum dose
Short half-life			
Aspirin		650 mg q6h	4000–6000 mg
Flurbiprofen	Ansaid	50 mg q6h	3000 mg
Ibuprofen	Motrin	400 mg q6h	4200 mg
Ketoprofen	Orudis	50 mg q6–8h	300 mg
Intermediate half-life			
Choline salicylate	Trilisate	1500 mg once, then 1000 mg bid	4000 mg
Diflunisal	Dolobid	1000 mg once, then 500 mg bid	1500 mg
Diclofenac	Voltaren	50 mg q6–8h	225 mg
Etodolac	Lodine	400 mg once, then 200 mg q8h to 300 mg q12h	1200 mg
Nabumetone	Relafen	500 to 750 mg bid	2000 mg
Naproxen	Naprosyn, others	375 mg q8–12h	1250 mg
Sulindac	Clinoril	100 mg q12h	400 mg
Long half-life			
Piroxicam	Feldene	20 mg q24h	40 mg

From Schofferman JA: Use of medication for pain of spinal origin. In White AH, Schofferman JA, Goldstein M, editors, *Spinal care diagnosis and conservative treatment*, vol 1, St Louis, 1995, Mosby–Year Book.

Narcotics and nonsteroidal medications are used also (see Table 32-9).[56] Recently we began using individualized videotaping in treating arthritis. This allows us to generate feedback of a patient's biomechanical efficiency, which greatly assists in establishing specific training programs. A patient is initially videotaped performing activities of daily living. There is no coaching or prompting during this session. A standard video camera is sufficient to capture the maneuvers patients frequently perform, and analysis may be done on any standard tape-playing machine (Fig. 32-13). The purpose of the video is to capture the efficiencies and inefficiencies of the biomechanical actions associated with selected tasks. When they review the videotape, the patients usually are amazed. They don't believe they do it "that way." The ergonomic flaws of motion are easily seen.

The most consistent inefficient pattern occurs when a person tries to rise from a lying-down position. Most people "lurch" forward and thrust their bodies to achieve a sitting posture. This, as seen by videotape, is an ergonomically inefficient maneuver. Our goal is to make patients aware of this and, through exercise sessions, correct the inefficiencies. To accomplish this, we revideotape the same tasks with guidance and prompting. The clinician and patient review both the "before" and the "after" actions and try to reinforce proper biomechanics. A series of exercises is then customized to specifically address the needs of the patient in improving ergonomic efficiency. This process is repeated on several follow-up visits to remind the patient of proper techniques. The results of this intervention have been rewarding. Although we are not addressing any specific pain generator or symptom focus, the overall ability of the patient to do more and walk further is viewed by many as successful treatment.

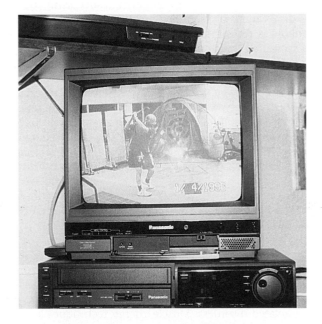

Fig. 32-13. Video analysis. Ergonomic efficiency is evaluated by videotape to isolate particular deficiencies. These deficiencies are reviewed with the patient and serve as an excellent mechanism of biofeedback. Adjustments for deficiencies are easily accomplished when patients are directly involved in viewing the inefficiencies.

SACROILIAC DYSFUNCTION

A common cause of pain, often described as low back pain, actually arises from dysfunction of the sacroiliac joint. This often-forgotten joint probably plays a significant role in the low back pain–scenario. Sacroiliac pathology has been underestimated as a cause of back or sciatic-type pain.[6,18,20,45,57] Very often patients complaining of low back pain point to the posterior superior iliac spine. Sacroiliac pain has been shown to occur in the groin as well as the buttock and posterior proximal thigh.[23]

There has been debate for several years as to the role of the sacroiliac joint as a pain generator. The increased interest in sacroiliac pain may be due to advances in spinal imaging techniques, which assist physicians in eliminating pathologic conditions of the disks or canals.[49] Also, evidence does support motion in this unique synovial joint.[67] Treatments for dysfunction of this joint include manual techniques, injection, stabilization, prolotherapy, and muscle energy. Manual medicine has been used by a variety of practitioners offering a myriad of techniques. All have the common goal of restoring normal mechanics to the region. Cassidy and associates reported 90% success in the manipulation of the sacroiliac region.[13]

When provocative injections (usually fluoroscopically guided) reproduce similar pain, infusion of the joint with a combination of water-soluble steroid and anesthetic agent may be effective.[6] In one series, 72 patients underwent sacroiliac (SI) joint injection and achieved 81%–successful pain relief at 9 months.[7] Stabilization of the sacroiliac joint is also somewhat successful. Use of one of a variety of sacroiliac belts that are commercially available is recommended. Another technique for treating sacroiliac dysfunction aims to stabilize the joint. By injecting a proliferant solution (one that is said to proliferate collagen-like tissue), unstable joints can be stabilized. Prolotherapy is a technique whereby a hypertonic solution is injected into an area of ligament or tendon insertion onto a bony structure. This agent is said to promote proliferation of collagen-like tissue that acts to stabilize a hypermobile joint. There are two commonly used proliferants. The first consists of 4 ml D50, 2 ml 2% lidocaine, and 6 ml of bacteriostatic water. The second consists of 2.5% phenol, 25% glucose, 25% glycerin, and pyrogen-free water. This solution is then diluted 50% with 0.5% lidocaine. A 0.5 to 0.75 ml–solution is injected at each site.[48]

The clinician should be very familiar with the technique of prolotherapy before attempting it, and readings beyond the scope of this text are recommended. Proponents claim very successful results for this technique with spine-related disorders. Muscle energy techniques are useful in treating sacroiliac dysfunction. They act to relax the lumbosacral extensor muscles and to promote symmetric sacroiliac motion. When the physical examination of the sacroiliac joint suggests decreased motion on forward-bending tests, muscle energy techniques are geared toward freeing the restricted joint. To assess sacroiliac motion, the patient stands with his feet comfortably separated. The examiner then places her thumbs under the posterior and superior iliac spines while the other digits circle the respective iliac crests. The patient is then instructed to bend forward at the waist while the clinician monitors the posterior superior iliac spines for motion. The side that tends to rise superiorly on the forward-bend is thought to be the side of pathology. This is a general guide to establishing the side of sacroiliac dysfunction. It is only a screen, and a complete sacroiliac examination should be done before initiating specific therapies.

SCOLIOSIS

The conservative treatment of scoliosis stresses postural corrections of deformities so as to limit visceral compromise. There are many schools of thought as to the most appropriate timing for and application of conservative versus surgical intervention in scoliosis. A general guideline is to attempt conservative exercises for curves less than 20°, bracing for curves between 20° and 40°, and surgical intervention for curves greater than 40°. Exercises should be of the lateral-bending rotational type. The direction of strengthening should promote reduction of the scoliotic curve. If bracing is warranted, body jacket–type orthoses are required, and these must be worn for 23 hours a day. An example of such is the Milwaukee brace.

AQUATIC THERAPY

Aquatic therapy is an excellent way of applying various exercises with significant joint load reduction. For the arthritic patient, range-of-motion exercises that are more difficult on dry land become an option. From an aerobic perspective, an excellent workout, that spares the joints at the same time, is feasible with water resistance. A detailed regimen of aquatherapy as proposed by Cirullo describes a complete stabilization program that unloads the spine and minimizes post-exercise edema.[15] Patient compliance often is better than with conventional land exercises. The indications for aquatherapy are varied but can be individualized to many musculoskeletal diagnoses.

CONCLUSION

Although treating spinal dysfunction is challenging and can be rewarding, a clinician must not overlook the possibility of associated ailments that produce bony pain but actually represent more serious diseases. Beware of metastatic disease in considering the management of all spinal pain.

REFERENCES

1. US Department of Health and Human Services: Acute low back problems in adults, Clinical Practice Guidelines, Washington, DC, 1994, Agency for Health Care Policy and Research (AHCPR).
2. Andersen KH, Mosdal C: Epidural application of corticosteroids in low back pain and sciatica, *Acta Neurochir* 87:52, 1987.
3. April C, Dwyer A, Bogduk N: Cervical zygapophyseal joint pain patterns. A clinical evaluation, *Spine* 15(6):458, 1990.
4. Benzon HT: Epidural steroid injection for low back pain and lumbosacral radiculopathy, *Pain* 24:277–295, 1986.
5. Berman AT, Garbarinbo JL, Fisher SM, Bosacco SJ: The effects of epidural injection of local anesthetics and corticosteroids on patients with lumbosacral pain, *Clin Orthop* 188:144, 1984.

6. Bernard TN Jr, Kirkaldy-Willis WH: Recognizing specific characteristics of nonspecific low back pain, *Clin Orthop Rel Res* 217:266–280, 1987.

7. Bernard TN, Cassidy JD: The sacroiliac joint syndrome. Pathophysiology, diagnosis, and management. In Frymoyer JW (ed): *The Adult Spine: Principles and Practice*, New York, 1991, Raven Press.

8. Biewen PC: Injection therapy for treatment of low back pain, *J Back Musculoskeletal Rehab* 1(3):17–28, 1991.

9. Bogduk N, April C, Derby R: Epidural steroid injections. In White AH, Schofferman JA, Goldstein M (eds): *Spine care diagnosis and conservative treatment*, 1:327–328, 1995. St. Louis: Mosby-Year Book.

10. Bullard JR, Houghton FM: Epidural treatment of acute herniated nucleus pulposis, *Anesth Analge Curr Res* 56:862, 1977.

11. Burn JMB, Langdon L: Lumbar epidural injection for the treatment of chronic sciatica, *Rheum Phys Med* 10:368, 1970.

12. Bush K, Hillier SA: Controlled study of caudal epidural injections of triamcinolone plus procaine for the management of intractable sciatica, *Spine* 16:572, 1991.

13. Cassidy JD, Kirkaldy-Willis WH, MacGregor M: Spinal manipulation for the treatment of chronic low back and leg pain. An observational study. In Burger AA, Greenman PE, (eds): *Empirical approaches to the validation of spinal manipulation*, Springfield, lll, Charles C. Thomas.

14. Chila AG, Jeffries RR, Levin SM: Is manipulation for your practice? *Patient Care* 77–92, May 1990.

15. Cirullo JA: *Orthopaedic physical therapy clinics of North America*, Philadelphia, WB Saunders.

16. Colachis SC, Strohm BR: Cervical traction: relationship of traction time to a varied tractive force with constant angle of pull, *Arch Phys Med Rehab* 46:815–819, 1965.

17. Colachis SC, Strohm BR: Effect of duration on intermittent cervical traction on vertebral separation, *Arch Phys Med Rehab* 47:353–359, 1966.

18. Dawn WJ: The sacroiliac joint: an underappreciated pain generator, *Am J Orthop* 24(6):475, 1995.

19. Deyo RA, Walsh NE, Martin DC, Schoenfeld LS, Ramamurthy S: A controlled trial of transcutaneous electrical nerve stimulation (TENS) and exercises for chronic low back pain, *N Eng J Med* 322(23):1627–1637, 1990.

20. Don Tigny RL: Function and pathomechanics of the sacroiliac joint. A review, *Phys Ther* 65(1):35–44, 1985.

21. Esses SI: *Textbook of spinal disorders*, Philadelphia, 1995, JB Lippincott.

22. Evans W: Intrasacral epidural injection in the treatment of sciatica, *Lancet* 2:1225–1227, 1930.

23. Fortin JD, Dwyer AP, West S: Sacroiliac joint: pain referral maps in proceedings of the North American Spine Society, Boston paper No. 78, Boston, 1992.

24. Freiberg AH, Vinckle TH: Sciatica and the sacroiliac joint, *J Bone Joint Surg* 16:126–136, 1934.

25. Frymoyer JW, Cats Baril WL: An overview of the incidence and costs of low back pain. *Orthop Clin N Am* 22:263, 1991.

26. Geiringer SR, Kincaid BK, Rechtien JS: Traction, manipulation, and massage. In DeLisa JA (ed): *Rehabilitation Medicine Principles and Practice*, Philadelphia, 1988, JB Lippincott.

27. Greenman PE: *Principles of manual medicine*, Baltimore, MD, 1989, Williams and Wilkins.

28. Hadler NM, Curtis P, Gillings DB: A benefit of spinal manipulation as adjunctive therapy for low back pain: A stratified controlled study, *Spine*, 12(7):703–706, 1987.

29. Hall H: Examination of the patient with low back pain, *Bull Rheum Diseases* 33(4), 1983.

30. Hickey RF: Outpatient epidural steroid injections for low back pain and lumbosacral radiculopathy, *N Zeal Med J* 100:594, 1987.

31. Higgins JR: *Human movement: An intergrated approach*, St. Louis, 1977, Mosby-Year Book.

32. Ingber RS: Iliopsoas myofascial dysfunction: a treatable cause of "failed" low back syndrome, *Arch Phys Med Rehab* 70:382–384, 1989.

33. Jacobs S, Pullan PT, Potter JM, Shenfield GM: Adrenal suppression following extradural steroids, *Anesthesia* 38:953, 1983.

34. Janse J: History of the development of chiropractic concepts: chiropractic terminology. In Goldstein M (ed): *The research status of spinal manipulation*. Goldstein M (ed): NINCDC Monograph No. 5 DHEW publication No. (NIH) 76–998, 1975.

35. Jones LJ: *Strain and Counterstrain*, Colorado Springs, Co, 1981, American Academy of Osteopathy.

36. Judovich BD: Herniated cervical disk; a new form of traction therapy, *Am J Surg* 84:646–56, 1952.

37. Kahn J: *Principles and practice of electrotherapy*, New York, 1987, Churchill Livingstone.

38. KiKuchi S, Have M, Nishqyama K, Ito T: Anatomic and clinical studies of radicular symptoms, *Spine* 9:23–30, 1984.

39. Lewinnek GE, Warfield LA: Facet degeneration as a cause of low back pain, *Clin Orthops* 213:216–222, 1986.

40. McKenzie R: Treat your own neck. *Spinal Publication*, 1983, Waikanae, New Zealand Ltd.

41. Meade TW, Dyers S, Browne W, Townsend J, Frank AO: Low back pain of mechanical origin: randomized comparison of chiropractic and hospital outpatient treatment, *Brit Med J* 300(6737):1431–1436, 1990.

42. Melzak R: Acupuncture and related forms of folk medicine. In Wall PD, Melzak R (eds): *Textbook of Pain*, New York, 1984, Churchill Livingston.

43. Melzak R, Stillwell DM, Fox ET: Trigger points and acupuncture points for pain: correlation and implications, *Pain* 3:3–23, 1977.

44. Michlovitz SL: *Thermal agents in rehabilitation*, Philadelphia, 1986, FA Davis.

45. Mooney V: Understanding, examining for, and treating sacroiliac pain, *J Musculoskeletal Med* 37–49, July 1993.

46. Nachemson A: Work for all, *Clin Orth Rel Res* 179:77–82, 1983.

47. Pace JB, Nagle D: Piriformis syndrome, *West J Med* 124:435–439, 1976.

48. Reeves KD: Technique of prolotherapy. In Lennard TA (ed): *Physiatric procedures in clinical practice*, St. Louis, 1995, Mosby-Year Book.

49. Reynolds JB, Slosar PJ: Spondylolisthesis: isthmic, congenital, traumatic, and post surgical. Spine Care. In White AH, Schofferman JA, (eds): *Diagnosis and conservative treatment* 1:1285, St. Louis, 1995, Mosby-Year Book.

50. Rosen CD, Kahanovitz N, Bernstein R, Viola K: A retrospective analysis of the efficacy of epidural steroid injections, *Clin Orthop* 228:270–272, 1988.

51. Saal JS: The role of inflammation in the lumbar spine. In *Physical medicine and rehabilitation: State of the art reviews. neck and back pain*, vol 4. Philadelphia, 1990, Hanley & Belfus.

52. Saal JS: High levels of inflammatory phospholipase activity in lumbar disc herniations, *Spine* 15(7):674, 1990.

53. Saal JS: *Human disc PLA2 induces neural injury: A histomorphic study*. Poster presentation at the Annual Meeting of Orthopaedic Research Society. San Francisco, Calif, 1993.

54. Saal J, Dillingham M: Nonoperative treatment and rehabilitation of disk, facet, and soft tissue injuries. In Nicholas J,

Hershman E.(eds): *The lower extremity in spine and sport medicine,* ed 2, St Louis, 1995, Mosby-Year Book.

55. Saal JA, Saal JS: Nonoperative treatment of herniated lumbar intervertebral disc with radiculopathy: An outcome study, *Spine* 14 (4):435, 1989.

56. Schofferman JA: Use of medication for pain of spinal origin. In White AH, Schofferman JA, (eds): *Spinal care diagnosis and conservative treatment* 1:519, St. Louis, 1995, Mosby-Year Book.

57. Schuchmann JA, Cannon CL: Sacroiliac strain syndrome: diagnosis and treatment, *Texas Med* 82:33-36, 1986.

58. Shekelle P, et al: Comparing the costs between provider types of episodes of back pain care, *Spine* 20:221–227, 1995.

59. Sinaki M, Lutness MP, Ilstrup DM, Chu CP, Gramse RR: Lumbar spondylolisthesis: A retrospective comparison and three year follow-up of two conservative treatment programs, *Arch Phys Med Rehab,* 70:594–598, 1989.

60. Snoek W, Weber H, Jorgensen B: Double blind evaluation of extradural methylprednisone for herniated discs, *Acta Orthop Scand* 48:635–637, 1977.

61. Sweeny T, et al: Cervicothoracic muscular stabilization techniques. In *Physical medicine and rehabilitation: State of the art reviews,* 4(2):335, Philadephia,1990, Hanley & Belfus.

62. Takeshi T, Kouzaburou F, Kuramachi E: Selective lumbosacral radiculopathy and block, *Spine* 5:68–77, 1980.

63. Tanigawa MC: Comparison of the hold relax procedure in passive mobilization on increasing muscle length, *Phys Ther* 32:725–735, 1972.

64. Travell J, Simons D: Low back pain, *Post Graduate Medicine,* Part I vol 73:2, 1983.

65. Vallfors B: Acute, sub-acute, and chronic low back pain: clinical symptoms, abstenteeism, and working environment, *Scand J Rehab Med* 11:1–98, 1985.

66. Walsh, et al: Treatment of the patient with chronic pain. In DeLisa J (ed): *Rehabilitation medicine: principles and practice,* Philadelphia, 1993, JB Lippincott.

67. Weisl H: The movements of the sacroiliac joints, *Acta Anatomica* 23:80–91, 1955.

68. White AM: Injection techniques for the diagnosis and treatment of low back pain. *Orthop Clin N Am* 14:553–567, 1983.

69. Witse LL, Newman PH, McNab I: Classification of spondylolysis and spondylolisthesis, *Clin Orthop* 117:23, 1976.

70. Zohn DA: The quadratus lumborum: An unrecognized source of back pain, clinical and thermographic aspects, *Orthop Rev* XIV(3): 163, 1985.

OTHER FACTORS AND PERSPECTIVES

CHAPTER 33

NUTRITION

Jacqueline R. Berning

Athletes who eagerly accept high-technology workouts and equipment need also to recognize the importance of diet in enhancing performance quickly, easily, and dramatically. Indeed, no amount of motivation, training, or natural ability will ensure success without proper fuel for the engine. Yet despite the wealth of knowledge regarding nutrition and the specific metabolic needs of the human body in training, not all athletes, coaches, or even dietitians and physicians have bridged the gap between laboratory and clinical research and the practical application of these findings. In today's athletic world of digitizing and rapid rehabilitation, the concern is not only on improving performance but also on using diet and nutrition to maintain an athlete's long-term health for the prevention of injury and illness.

DIETARY HABITS OF ATHLETES

To understand the food consumption habits of athletes, we need to look at the general population. Athletes may be winning Gold Medals and breaking world records, but many have the same dietary habits as their sedentary counterparts. In general, many eat too much fat and protein at the expense of carbohydrates and fiber. Numerous surveys have shown that the food consumption practices of both male and female athletes are proportionally very similar to the national averages, except for total kilocalorie intake. Recent surveys[3,43] of elite adolescent swimmers revealed that, like other typical Americans, they consumed more fat than carbohydrates in their diets. Furthermore, when they were given a nutrition knowledge test, they did very well on basic nutrition knowledge (of the four food groups) but poorly when it came to choosing foods that were high in a specific nutrient. For example, when swimmers were asked to name a nutritious carbohydrate, in a multiple-choice format, 62% chose an apple, but 38% chose French fries. When asked which food is a good source of protein, 63% chose the correct answer of chicken, but 37% chose oatmeal.

In another survey,[9] of competitive swimmers ages 13 to 20, several misconceptions were reported. For example, over half of them believed that everyone should take supplements, that vitamin E improves performance, B complex vitamins provide energy, and milk consumed the day of competition impairs performance. In a study[36] of male track, baseball, and football teams, only 28% could define glycogen loading, 69% did not know which foods were good sources of carbohydrates, and 54% did not know the major functions of vitamins. A nutrition knowledge questionnaire completed by adolescent gymnasts showed that over 50% of the girls could not define the term "complex carbohydrate" and did not know that carbohydrates were an important source of energy for exercise.[30] Instead, 75% of the girls erroneously believed that protein was the best source of energy.

Volleyball players had difficulty with questions on food sources of quality protein and vitamin C, and good sources of energy, carbohydrate loading, and caloric requirements for training.[33] However, they were knowledgeable about the importance of eating a wide variety of foods, vitamin supplements, and the differences between plant oils and animal fats. These findings suggest that most athletes are unable to select the proper balance of foods necessary for the energy demands of their sports. If athletes cannot make informed food choices, they cannot be expected to select a proper diet that is required for peak performance.

Dietary Recommendations for Athletes

An athlete's energy and nutrient requirements vary with weight, height, age, sex, and metabolic rate, and on the type, intensity, frequency, and duration of training. The emotional and physical stress of training and competition, combined with hectic travel schedules, also affects intake. As a result, adequate calories and essential nutrients must be planned carefully to meet nutritional requirements for training and health. Depending upon the training regimen, athletes need to consume at least 50%, but ideally 60% to 70% of their total calories from carbo-

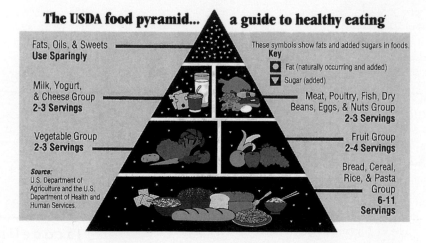

TRAINING DIET BASED OFF THE FOOD GUIDE PYRAMID

	2800 CALORIES	3300 CALORIES
MILK	4 OR MORE	4 OR MORE
MEAT	3 OR MORE	3 OR MORE
VEGE	6 OR MORE	8 OR MORE
FRUIT	4 OR MORE	6 OR MORE
GRAIN	16 OR MORE	18 OR MORE

Fig. 33-1. Food Guide Pyramid.

hydrate. The remaining calories should be obtained from protein (10% to 15%) and fat (20% to 30%). Calories and nutrients should come from a wide variety of foods on a daily basis. The food guide pyramid is an excellent nutrition education tool to teach athletes how to make wise food choices. The food guide pyramid, along with the number of recommended daily servings, is presented in Fig. 33-1.

CARBOHYDRATES—FUEL FOR EXERCISE

Carbohydrates provide fuel for the exercising muscles as well as the central nervous system. The use of carbohydrates by the skeletal muscles of the body depends on the availability of endogenous energy sources and on the intensity and duration of exercise.

Carbohydrate Oxidation

Intensity and duration of exercise have opposite effects on carbohydrate utilization. The portion of energy coming from carbohydrate oxidation increases with the intensity of exercise, whereas it progressively decreases when exercise is prolonged (Fig. 33-2). Training status also can influence the composition of the fuel being oxidized. Indeed, the proportion of carbohydrate being burned is lower in exercise-trained than in untrained individuals at rest.[42] Endurance training increases the ca-

pacity of the aerobic pathway in the mitochondria to break down fat for energy. When more fat is burned, less muscle glycogen is used. This glycogen-sparing effect of fat utilization is advantageous during prolonged exercise because muscle glycogen depletion limits performance.

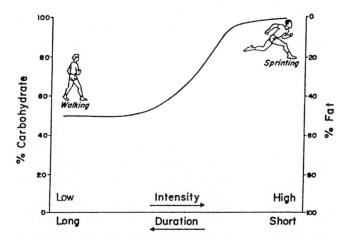

Fig. 33-2. As exercise intensity increases and duration decreases, the prominent food fuel shifts toward carbohydrates. (From Matthew and Fox: *Sports physiology*, Philadelphia, 1979, WB Saunders).

Endurance training also increases the capacity of the muscles to store glycogen. Thus endurance training confers a dual performance advantage: the muscle glycogen stores are higher at the onset of exercise, and the athlete depletes them at a slower rate.

Diet composition also can significantly affect the mixture of fuel being oxidized during exercise. If the diet is high in carbohydrate, the athlete will use more glycogen as fuel. Although the goal is to increase the availability of fat as fuel through endurance training, this does not mean that athletes should eat a high-fat diet. Even the leanest athletes store more fat than they will ever need during exercise.

A high-fat diet compromises carbohydrate intake, which lowers muscle glycogen stores and reduces the ability of an athlete to sustain high-intensity exercise.[37] Low muscle glycogen stores can also limit endurance. Thus the ideal diet to ensure optimal muscle glycogen stores supplies less than 30% of total calories as fat and 60% to 70% as carbohydrates.

CARBOHYDRATES AND TRAINING

During endurance exercise that exceeds 90 minutes, such as marathon running, muscle glycogen stores become progressively lower. When they drop to critically low levels, high-intensity exercise cannot be maintained. In practical terms, the athlete is exhausted and must either stop exercising or drastically reduce his pace. Glycogen depletion may be a gradual process, occurring over repeated days of heavy training, in which muscle glycogen breakdown exceeds its replacement. This can happen as well during high-intensity exercise that is repeated several times during competition or training. For example, a distance runner who averages 10 miles a day but doesn't take the time to consume enough carbohydrates in his diet, or the swimmer who completes several interval sets at above her maximal oxygen consumption can both deplete glycogen stores rapidly.

Training Glycogen Depletion

Costill[11] compared glycogen synthesis on a 40% carbohydrate diet to that on a 70% carbohydrate diet during repeated days of 2-hour workouts. On the low-carbohydrate diet, the muscle glycogen stores dropped lower with each successive day of training. After several days of the diet and exercise regimen, the athletes had low muscle glycogen stores and could not exercise at even a moderate intensity. The high carbohydrate diet provided nearly maximal repletion of the muscle glycogen stores after the strenuous training. The high carbohydrate diet provided the athletes with muscle glycogen values that remained above 100 mmol/kg, and they were able to continue the heavy training (Fig. 33-3). This study suggests that athletes who fail to consume enough carbohydrates on a daily basis while training will possibly decrease endurance as well as exercise performance.

It is suggested that athletes in heavy training should consume a carbohydrate intake of 7 to 10 grams per kilogram of body weight per day to help prevent daily carbohydrate depletion.

Types of Carbohydrate

The type of carbohydrate is another nutritional factor that has been considered to potentially affect carbohydrate metabolism. Unfortunately, research has not provided clear guidance as to the issue. One study by Costill et al.[13] compared the effects of simple- and complex-carbohydrate consumption during a 48-hour period after a glycogen-depleting exercise. During the first 24 hours, no differences were found in muscle glycogen synthesis between the two types of carbohydrates; however, at 48 hours the complex carbohydrates resulted in significantly greater muscle glycogen synthesis than the simple carbohydrates. Recently, Keins et al.[27] reported that increases in muscle glycogen content were significantly greater during the first 6 hours after exercise following the intake of simple rather than complex carbohydrates,

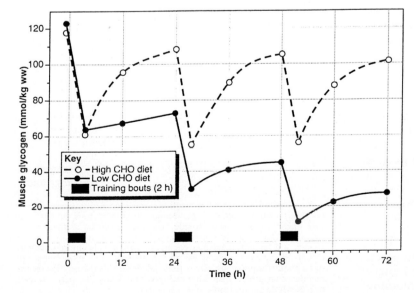

Fig. 33-3. Muscle glycogen gradually declines when daily running is undertaken while consuming a low-carbohydrate diet. A high-carbohydrate diet allows for daily recovery of muscle glycogen.[11]

GLYCEMIC INDEX OF VARIOUS FOODS

High glycemic foods (above 85)
Honey, corn syrup

Bagels, white bread

Cornflakes

Raisins

Potato (baked, boiled, or mashed)

Sweet corn

Moderate glycemic foods (60 to 85)
Spaghetti, macaroni

Oatmeal

Bananas, grapes, oranges

Rice

Yams

Baked beans

Low glycemic foods (less than 60)
Apples, applesauce

Cherries, dates, figs, peaches, pears, plums

Kidney beans, chick peas, green peas, navy beans, red lentils

Whole milk, skim milk, plain yogurt

and that plasma insulin levels were greater following the intake of simple carbohydrates.

Glycemic Index

Coyle[14] and Hargreaves[21] have suggested that part of this conflict over which type of carbohydrate is better may be cleared up if the carbohydrate is considered to be based on its physiologic reaction in the body rather than its structure. They have suggested that carbohydrate foods should be classified according to glycemic index. Glycemic index represents the ratio of the area under the blood glucose curve resulting from the ingestion of a given quantity of carbohydrate food and the area under the glucose curve resulting from the ingestion of the same quantity of white bread.[26] Coyle and Hargreaves recommend that carbohydrates with a moderate to high glycemic index should be consumed after exercise. Indeed, preliminary work by Burke et al.[5] has demonstrated that a diet based on high glycemic index carbohydrate foods promoted greater glycogen storage in 24 hours of recovery after strenuous exercise than an equal amount of carbohydrate eaten in the form of low glycemic index foods. The box above lists foods that are carbohydrate-rich and their respective glycemic indexes.

CARBOHYDRATE INTAKE BEFORE, DURING, AND AFTER EXERCISE

Preexercise Meal

The preevent or pretraining meal serves two purposes. These include keeping the athlete from feeling hungry before and during the exercise bout, and maintaining optimal levels of blood glucose for the exercising muscles during training and competition.

Athletes often train early in the morning without eating. This overnight fast lowers liver glycogen stores and can impair performance, particularly if the exercise regimen involves endurance training.

Carbohydrate feedings before exercise can help restore suboptimal liver glycogen stores, which may be called upon during prolonged training and competition. While allowing for personal preferences and psychological factors, the preevent meal should be high in carbohydrates, nongreasy, and readily digested. High-fat, high-protein foods such as steaks, hamburgers, eggs, and hot dogs should be avoided or limited in the preevent meal because fat slows gastric emptying time. Exercising with a full stomach also may cause indigestion, nausea, and possibly vomiting.

How much carbohydrate should the athlete consume in the precompetition meal? Current research suggests that 1 to 4 grams of carbohydrate per kilogram of body weight should be consumed 1 to 4 hours before exercise.[35] To avoid gastrointestinal distress, the carbohydrate content of the meal should be reduced according to how long before exercise it is consumed. For example, it is suggested that 4 hours before the event the athlete consume 4 grams of carbohydrates

Table 33-1. Examples of preevent meals and recommended carbohydrate intake based upon body weight and length of time before competition

Body weight	Carbohydrate intake	Foods to meet recommendation
120 lbs (54.5 kg)	54 grams (1 hour before the event)	2 slices of toast Jam-1 tbsp 8 oz skim milk
	163 grams (3 hours before the event)	2 slices of toast Jam-2 tbsp 8 oz nonfat yogurt ¼ cup Grapenuts 8 oz orange juice
190 lbs (86.4 kg)	86 grams (1 hour before the event)	2 slices of toast Jam-1 tbsp 8 oz skim milk 8 oz orange juice
	259 grams (3 hours before the event)	2 English muffins Jam-3 tbsp 2 c oatmeal Honey-1 tbsp 1 banana 8 oz skim milk 8 oz orange juice

Fatty foods such as potato chips, doughnuts, french fries, and pastries take longer to digest and provide little energy during racing. Protein foods that are likely to contain high amounts of fat (peanut butter, cheese, and high-fat meats like bacon and ribs) are also more slowly digested. Eating foods high in fat and protein and low in carbohydrate can actually diminish athletic performance. For this reason, it is recommended that athletes eat high-carbohydrate foods like pasta, cereals, bagels, whole grains, fruits, and vegetables.

per kilogram of body weight, whereas 1 hour before the competition the athlete would consume 1 gram of carbohydrate per kilogram of body weight. Table 33-1 lists food examples for preevent meals.

Consuming Sugar Before Exercise

Fifteen years ago, Costill et al.[12] suggested that preexercise glucose intake could be associated with hypoglycemia and increased muscle glycogen utilization during exercise. A recent study[22] contradicts this earlier finding. Cyclists consumed 75 grams of glucose or water 45 minutes before cycling to exhaustion. Although the sugar feedings caused high blood insulin and low blood glucose levels, there were no differences in the exercise time to exhaustion between the two trials. Does this mean that endurance athletes should load up on soft drinks and candy before their events? Comparison of the results of the old and new studies suggest that individuals differ in susceptibility to a lowering of blood glucose during exercise. The physiologic and biochemical basis for this difference has not been determined. At this time, therefore, athletes should be advised that consuming sugar 30 to 45 minutes before exercise could harm their performance if they are sensitive to a lowering of their blood glucose levels.

Carbohydrate Intake During Exercise

Carbohydrate feedings during endurance exercise lasting longer that 60 minutes may enhance endurance by providing glucose for the muscles to use when their glycogen stores have dropped to low levels.

The liver generally supplies glucose to maintain blood sugar levels for proper functioning of the central nervous system. As the muscles run out of glycogen, they will begin to take up some of the blood glucose, placing a drain on the liver glycogen stores. The longer the exercise session, the greater the utilization of blood glucose by the muscles for energy (Fig. 33-4). Although supplies of blood glucose can be drawn from liver glycogen, muscle glycogen stays in the muscle and cannot provide glucose for the blood. When the liver glycogen is depleted, blood glucose drops. A few athletes will experience central nervous symptoms typical of hypoglycemia (dizziness, nausea, confusion, and partial blackout), but most will note local muscular fatigue and will have to reduce their exercise intensity.

The improved performance associated with carbohydrate feedings probably results from the maintenance of blood glucose levels. The dietary carbohydrate supplies glucose for the muscles at a time when their glycogen stores are diminished. Thus, carbohydrate utilization (and therefore ATP production) can continue at a high rate, and endurance is enhanced.

Fatigue is not prevented by carbohydrate feeding; it is simply delayed. During the final portions of exercise, when muscle glycogen is low and athletes rely on blood glucose for energy, their muscles feel heavy and they must concentrate to maintain exercise at intensities that are ordinarily not stressful when muscle glycogen stores are filled.

How much carbohydrate should an athlete consume during exercise to improve endurance? The available evi-

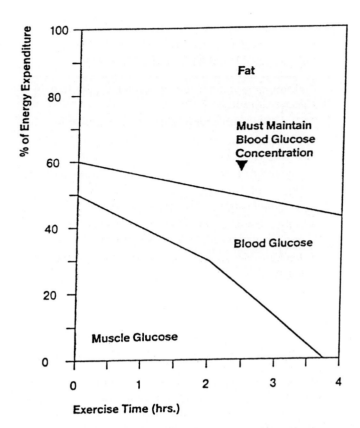

Fig. 33-4. Sources of energy during prolonged cycling at 70% of maximal oxygen uptake. It is important to maintain blood glucose for prolonged exercise because it becomes the primary source of carbohydrate around the 2- to 2½-hour mark. (From Coyle EF: Carbohydrates and athletic performance.

dence suggests that athletes should take in 25 to 30 grams of carbohydrate every 30 minutes.[16,15] This amount can be obtained through either carbohydrate-rich foods or fluids. Drinking 8 ounces of a sports drink containing 6% to 7%, carbohydrate every 15 minutes provides this amount of carbohydrate and also aids in hydration.

Carbohydrates After Exercise

On an average, only 5% of the muscle glycogen used during exercise is resynthesized each hour following exercise. Accordingly, at least 20 hours are required for complete restoration after exhaustive exercise, provided approximately 600 grams of carbohydrate are consumed. Recently Ivy et al.[25] studied glycogen repletion following exercise. When 2 grams of carbohydrate per kilogram was consumed immediately after exercise, muscle glycogen synthesis was 15 mmol/kg. When the carbohydrate feeding was delayed for 2 hours after exercise, muscle glycogen synthesis was cut by 66% to 5 mmol/kg. By 4 hours after exercise, total muscle glycogen synthesis for the delayed feeding was still 45% slower than for the feeding given immediately after exercise.

This means that delaying carbohydrate intake for too long after exercise will reduce muscle glycogen and that

FOODS THAT CONTAIN 100 GRAMS OF CARBOHYDRATE AND PROTEIN

Consumption of the following foods increases muscle glycogen synthesis:

- One bagel with peanut butter and ⅔ cup raisins
- One cup of low-fat yogurt, one banana, and a cup of orange juice
- One turkey sandwich on whole-wheat bread with a cup of applesauce
- Spaghetti with meat sauce and garlic bread
- Eight ounces of skim milk, one apple, one orange, two slices of bread, and three pancakes
- Twelve ounces of a carbohydrate-loading drink and a bagel

glycogen resynthesis can be elevated when carbohydrates are consumed immediately after exercise. The current recommendations are to consume around 100 grams of carbohydrate within a 30-minute window post-exercise to maximize muscle glycogen synthesis. Many athletes find it difficult to consume food immediately after exercise. Usually when body or core temperature is elevated, appetite is depressed and it becomes difficult to consume carbohydrate-rich foods. Many athletes find it easier and simpler to drink their carbohydrates than to eat them. A sports drink rich in carbohydrates after a hard practice will not only provide the necessary carbohydrates for glycogen synthesis but also help with hydration.

Within the last several years Zawadski and colleagues[45] have followed up on the Ivy study and have found that not only does consuming carbohydrates immediately after exercise help restore muscle glycogen stores faster, but adding protein with the 100 grams of carbohydrate will increase the glycogen resynthesis rate. It appears that this amount of protein with the 100 grams of carbohydrate illicits a greater insulin response and therefore activates glycogen synthase, the enzyme responsible for glycogen storage. The box above lists some examples of foods that contain about 100 grams of carbohydrate and protein that could be used immediately after exercise.

PROTEIN

Proteins are a group of structural and regulatory molecules, each made up of a specific combination of 20 different amino acids. Eight of these amino acids cannot be synthesized in the body and therefore must be supplied by the diet if body proteins are to be synthesized. Generally, dietary intake of most athletes exceeds even the highest recommendation.

Because protein, especially the branched-chain amino acid leucine, is used as a metabolic fuel during exercise,

much controversy surrounds the need for protein in exercising individuals.[6,29] There are now sufficient data to suggest that protein requirements do vary with the type and intensity of exercise performed and the total energy consumed.

Protein Needs for Endurance Athletes

Early work by Yoshimura[44] and Gontzea[20] illustrated a fall in nitrogen balance in response to beginning a moderate endurance exercise program, suggesting an increased need for protein under these conditions. However, this decline corrected itself within two weeks of the start of exercise without dietary intervention. Butterfield and Calloway[8] confirmed the transient nature of the decline in nitrogen balance with initiation of an exercise program like those proposed in programs to improve health and fitness. They found that nitrogen balance was more positive after the adaptation than before, suggesting that the protein intake requirement for nitrogen equilibrium in individuals performing moderate endurance exercise may actually be lower than that of the sedentary population, provided energy intake is adequate.

More recent work suggests that individuals who exercise at a higher intensity have protein needs that might be greater.[41,31] Meredith[31] has conducted a classic nitrogen balance regression assessment of trained male runners exercising daily at 75% of their Vo_2max and has estimated protein requirements of 0.94g/kg/bw/day.

Protein need in exercise is dependent on energy intake. Butterfield[7] demonstrated that feeding as much as 2 grams of protein/kg/bw/day to men running 5 or 10 miles a day at 65% to 75% of their Vo_2max is insufficient to maintain nitrogen balance when energy intake is inadequate by as little as 100 kcal/day. This points out the important role that calories play in sparing protein. Protein will be used as an energy source if calories are insufficient.

Protein Needs for Resistance Exercise

For body builders or individuals who are interested in increasing body mass, the mythology of increased protein needs is rampant. Weight lifters consume anywhere from 1.2 to 3.4 grams of protein/kg/bw/day. Most of this protein is in the form of supplements. The basis for this practice is word of mouth and traditions that have not been substantiated by scientific studies. The traditional thinking among body builders and weight lifters is that the more protein consumed, the bigger the muscles.

Since 1991 sufficient data have accumulated to allow division of the study of protein needs with resistance exercise into two areas: the need for maintenance (minimum protein required to accomplish nitrogen equilibrium) and the need for increasing lean tissue (positive nitrogen balance).

Tarnopolsky[40] showed that experienced body builders could maintain nitrogen equilibrium on intakes similar to those required by sedentary controls. However, the high protein intakes used to generate their regression lines may have resulted in overestimation of protein requirements.

Requirements for maintenance of nitrogen balance under circumstances of beginning a resistance exercise program may depend on the intensity of the exercise performed. Tarnopolsky[41] has estimated protein requirements in young novice male body builders exercising 6 days a week for 1.5 hours a day to be 1.5 grams/kg/bw/day. Energy intake is not reported in Tarnopolsky's paper. Hickson[24] found no change in nitrogen excretion with the initiation of a program of 30 minutes of lifting 3 times a week at an intensity of about 50% of maximum capacity when subjects were consuming 0.8 grams of protein/kg/bw/day, the RDA for protein for adults.

Recently, Butterfield and colleagues (in press) have attempted to establish the relevance of added protein in the accretion of lean tissue in recreational weight lifters. They found that when energy intake exceeded need by 400 kcal, increasing nitrogen intake from requirement (mean = 10 g n/day) to 1.5 times requirement (mean = 15 g n/day) had no significant effect on nitrogen retention. Any improvement in nitrogen balance seen with increased energy and protein intake was explained by the energy contribution of the protein.

Nutritional Implications

If protein need for exercising people is slightly more than that for sedentary individuals, the usual protein intake of the population will more than meet these needs. Reports of food intake in athletes and nonathletes consistently indicate that protein represents from 12% to 20% of total energy intake, or 1.2 to 2 g protein/gk/bw/day. The exception to the rule is small active women who consume a low-energy intake in conjunction with an exercise or training program. These women may consume close to the RDA for protein, but if the data of Butterfield are correct, this value in conjunction with the restricted energy intake may be inadequate to maintain lean mass.

Consuming more protein than the body can use should be avoided. When athletes consume diets that are high in protein, they compromise their carbohydrate status and therefore may affect their ability to train and compete at peak performance. The National Research Council also points out that protein foods often are also high in fat; consumption of excess protein creates difficulty in maintaining a low-fat diet. In addition, the hypercalciuric effect of high protein diets is still considered by some a significant factor in calcium balance, and until the controversy is settled a conservative approach is advised.

Amino Acid Supplementation

Protein or amino acid supplementation in the form of powders or pills is not necessary and should be discouraged. Taking large amounts of protein or amino acid supplements can lead to dehydration, loss of urinary calcium, weight gain, and stress on the kidney and liver.[38] Taking amino acids singly or in combination, such as arginine and lysine, may interfere with the absorption of certain essential amino acids.[38] An additional concern is that substituting amino acid supplements for food may cause deficiencies of other nutrients found in protein-rich foods, such as iron, niacin, and thiamine. Athletes and coaches need to realize that amino acid supplements taken in large doses have not been tested in human subjects and no margin of safety is available. It is important for the health professional to develop a strategy to effectively approach and discuss supplement use with both athletes and coaches.[2]

FAT

Even though maximal performance is impossible without muscle glycogen, fat also provides energy for exercise. Fat is the most concentrated source of food energy and supplies more than twice as many calories (9 kcal/gm) by weight as protein (4 kcal/g) or carbohydrate (4 kcal/g). Fat provides essential fatty acids, which are necessary for cell membranes, skin, hormones, and transporting fat-soluble vitamins. The body has total glycogen stores (both muscle and liver) that equal about 2500 calories, whereas each pound of body fat supplies 3500 calories. This means that an athlete weighing 74 kg (163 pounds) with 10% body fat has 16.3 pounds of fat, which equals 57,000 calories.

Fat is the major, if not most important, fuel for light to moderate intensity exercise. Although fat is a valuable metabolic fuel for muscle activity during longer-term aerobic exercise, and performs many important functions in the body, no attempt should be made to consume more fat. In addition, athletes that consume a high-fat diet typically consume fewer calories from carbohydrates. Recently, Simonsen and his colleagues[37] had elite rowers consume either 40% of their calories from fat or 20% of their calories from fat and then compared the two diets on power output and speed. Afterward, they performed muscle biopsies and found that the rowers who consumed the low-fat, high-carbohydrate diet had more muscle glycogen. Rowers on the high-fat, low-carbohydrate diet had moderate levels of muscle glycogen and actually were able to complete the workout sets. However, when it came to power output and faster speeds, the athletes who consumed the lower-fat, higher-carbohydrate diets had significantly more power and speed. This has important implications for athletes in muscular endurance sports that require a burst of power, such as rowing, swimming, gymnastics, figure skating, judo, boxing, or any sport in which some energy will need to be generated by the anaerobic pathway. Following a low-fat, high-carbohydrate diet is also important for health reasons, because a high-fat diet has been associated with cardiovascular disease, obesity, diabetes, and some kinds of cancer.[28]

Types of Fat

Fats are categorized as either saturated or unsaturated (including monounsaturated and polyunsaturated) because they have differing chemical structures and, as a result, different effects on bodily function and health. Saturated fats are solid at room temperature, are derived mainly from animal sources, and tend to raise blood levels of cholesterol. Unsaturated fats are liquid at room temperature, found mainly in plant sources, and tend to decrease blood cholesterol. Palm and coconut oil are exceptions. They are un-

Table 33-2. Fat substitutions

Instead of:	Try:
* Whole milk	Skim milk
* Cheddar, Jack, or Swiss cheese	Part-skim mozzarella, string, or low-fat cottage cheese, other cheese that contains less than 5 grams of fat per ounce
* Ice cream	Ice milk or low-fat/nonfat frozen yogurt
* Butter or margarine	Jam, yogurt, ricotta cheese, light or nonfat cream cheese
* Sour cream	Low-fat yogurt, light sour cream, blender-whipped cottage cheese dressing
* Bacon	Canadian bacon or bacon bits
* Ground beef	Extra lean ground beef or ground turkey
* Fried chicken	Baked chicken without the skin
* Doughnuts and pastries, breads	Bagels, whole-grain homemade breads, muffins, and quick breads
* Apple pie	Baked or raw apples
* Chocolate candy or bars	Jelly beans, hard candy, licorice
* Cookies, cakes, brownies	Vanilla wafers, ginger snaps, graham crackers, fig bars

saturated fats and are liquid at room temperature; however, they tend to raise blood levels of cholesterol.

Athletes need to recognize the many sources of hidden fat in foods. Fat is present, but not separately visible, in dairy products such as cheese, ice cream, and whole milk, and in bakery items, granola bars, french fries, avocados, chips, nuts, and many highly processed foods. The other dietary sources are more clearly visible, such as margarine, butter, mayonnaise, salad dressing, oil, and meats with high marbling of fat.

It is recommended that athletes should consume 20% to 30% of their calories from fat. Aside from decreasing overall calories, limiting consumption of dietary fat is the first step towards losing excess body fat. Doing so eliminates excess calories but not nutrients. Suggestions for reducing fat intake are listed in Table 33-2.

VITAMINS AND MINERALS

Vitamins and minerals are food components that serve as coenzymes in the metabolic reactions that release energy, transport and consume oxygen, and maintain cell integrity. Because of these important functions, their use as ergogenic aids has been highly touted, although there is little scientific evidence to document their effect. The need for these food components in exercise has been reviewed recently by Haymes[23] and Clarkson,[10] with the consensus that unless an individual is deficient in a given nutrient, supplementation with that nutrient does not have a major effect on performance.

Nutrients at Risk

Nutrients at risk in the athletic population are similar to those of concern for the general population. In other words, just because you are an athlete does not mean that you need special amounts of any vitamin or mineral. The nutrients that are of concern for the general population and athletes include folate, vitamin B_6, calcium, and zinc. Because many women athletes are also vegetarians, iron and, perhaps, vitamin B_{12} may be of specific concern to them. Components that protect against free radical attack will be discussed.

Free Radicals and Exercise

Exercise is thought to increase the production of superoxide radicals consequent to the increased rate of oxygen utilization in the mitochondria.[17] The nutrients involved in these complex reactions include vitamins C, E, and A as beta-carotene (which acts as an antioxidant), and zinc, copper, manganese (which occur as various forms of superoxide dismutase), iron as a catalase, and selenium as glutathione peroxidase.[1]

Although the research data for exercising humans still remain controversial, several investigators conclude that the increased superoxide radical production that accompanies repeated bouts of exercise is adequately buffered by shifts in the existing systems and results in no deleterious permanent changes.

Vitamin Supplementation

Because athletes often are looking for an edge, something that will give them an advantage, many turn to supplements in the form of pills, powders, and magical elixirs in an effort to make the body perform at its best. Unfortunately, many self-claimed "experts" are eager to convince athletes that their products will improve athletic performance by improving muscle contractions, preventing weight gain, enhancing strength, or supplying energy—just to name a few. These "experts" may insist that athletes' fatigue and muscle soreness are due to a vitamin or mineral deficiency. In fact, when there is a nutritional reason for fatigue, it is usually a lack of calories and/or carbohydrates.

Vitamins can be divided into two groups—water soluble and fat soluble. Vitamins A, D, E, and K are soluble in fat, whereas vitamin C and the B complex vitamins are soluble in water. Table 33-3 lists all of the vitamins, their physiologic functions, and major food sources.

Fat-soluble vitamins are stored in body fat, principally in the liver. Excess accumulation of fat-soluble vitamins, particularly vitamins A and D, can produce serious toxic effects. Although excess of most water-soluble vitamins is typically excreted, some may pose toxicity problems, particularly if they are taken at a pharmacologic level. Large amounts of niacin, for example, can cause burning or tingling, a skin rash, nausea, and diarrhea.[38] High doses of niacin also interfere with fat mobilization and increase glycogen depletion.[38] Vitamin B_6 can cause nervous sys-

Table 33-3. Vitamins

Vitamin	Main function	Good sources
A	Maintenance of skin, bone growth, vision, teeth	Eggs, cheese, margarine, milk, carrots, broccoli, squash, spinach
D	Bone growth and maintenance of bones	Milk, egg yolk, tuna, salmon
E	Prevents oxidation of polyunsaturated fats	Vegetable oils, whole-grain cereal, bread, dried beans, green leafy vegetables
K	Blood clotting	Cabbage, green leafy vegetables, milk
Thiamine B_1	Energy-releasing reactions	Pork, ham, oysters, breads, cereals, pasta, green peas
Riboflavin B_2	Energy-releasing reactions	Milk, meat, cereals, pasta, mushrooms, dark green vegetables
Niacin	Energy-releasing reactions	Poultry, meat, tuna, cereal, pasta, bread, nuts, legumes
Pyridoxine B_6	Metabolism of fats, proteins, formation of red blood cells	Cereals, bread, spinach, avocados, green beans, bananas
Cobalamin B_{12}	Formation of red blood cells, functioning of nervous system	Meat, fish, eggs, milk
Folacin	Assists in forming proteins, formation of red blood cells	Dark green leafy vegetables, wheat germ
Pantothenic acid	Metabolism of proteins, carbohydrates, fats, formation of hormones	Bread, cereals, nuts, eggs, dark green vegetables
Biotin	Formation of fatty acids, energy-releasing reactions	Egg yolk, leafy green vegetables
C	Maintenance of bones, teeth, blood vessels, collagen	Citrus fruits, tomato, strawberries, melon, green pepper, potato

tem damage when taken at high doses. In 1983 seven women consumed more than 2000 mg of B_6 in supplement form for 2 months because they had been told that this amount would help them cure the edema associated with premenstrual syndrome (PMS). The women developed numbness in their feet, then lost sensation in their hands, then became unable to work. They may have suffered irreversible nerve damage. At last report, although the symptoms had been clearing up after withdrawal from the supplements, they had not completely disappeared.

Athletes need to understand that more is not always better. The National Academy of Sciences has established recommended dietary allowances (RDAs) for vitamins and minerals as a guide for determining nutritional needs.[32] The RDA is the daily amount of a nutrient recommended for practically all healthy individuals, in promoting optimal health. It is not a minimal amount needed to prevent disease symptoms—a large margin of safety is added in. Even though it has been shown that a severely inadequate intake of certain vitamins can impair performance, it is unusual for an athlete to have such deficiencies. Even marginal deficiencies do not appear to markedly affect the ability to exercise efficiently.

Minerals

Minerals perform a variety of functions in the body. Whereas some are used to build tissue, such as calcium and phosphorus for bones and teeth, others are important components of hormones, such as iodine in thyroxine. Iron is critical for the formation of hemoglobin, which carries oxygen within the red blood cells. Minerals also are important for regulation of muscle contractions and body fluids, conduction of nerve impulses, and regulation of normal heart rhythm.

Minerals are divided into two groups. The first is referred to as macrominerals, and they are needed in amounts of from 100 mg to 1 g. These include calcium, phosphorus, magnesium, sodium, potassium, chloride, and sulfur. The others fall under the category of trace minerals: copper, iodine, zinc, cobalt, fluoride, and selenium. Food sources and the physiologic functions for each mineral are listed in Table 33-4.

Iron

The iron status of athletes, particularly female athletes, is of concern because occurrence of low serum iron (ferritin, iron, and hematocrit) has been observed.[39] Reasons for these low levels may be due to inadequate dietary intake, low bioavailability of iron, or high rates of iron loss.[39] Females are at an increased risk for iron deficiency not only because of increased physiologic need, but because of sometimes lower caloric intakes. In addition, many athletes, particularly females, are vegetarians. In one report, 43% of the female distance runners studied were modified vegetarians and consumed less than 200 grams of meat per week.[4]

Although dietary intake of iron is tied to caloric intake, iron absorption depends upon the bioavailability of the iron. Meats contain heme-iron, which is highly bioavailable and, therefore, a more adsorbable source of iron. Heme-iron also enhances the absorption of the non–heme-iron found in plant foods such as leafy greens, legumes, cereals, whole grains, and enriched breads. Combining these foods with a source of vitamin C can significantly enhance the absorption of iron—for example, orange juice with an iron-enriched cereal, or pasta in combination with broccoli, tomatoes, and green peppers.

Table 33-4. Minerals

Mineral	Main function	Good sources
Calcium	Formation of bones, teeth, nerve impulses, blood clotting	Cheese, sardines, dark green vegetables, clams, milk
Phosphorus	Formation of bones, teeth, acid-base balance	Milk, cheese, meat, fish, poultry, nuts, grains
Magnesium	Activation of enzymes, protein synthesis	Nuts, meats, milk, whole-grain cereal, green leafy vegetables
Sodium	Acid-base balance, body water balance, nerve function	Most foods except fruit
Potassium	Acid-base balance reactions, body water balance, nerve function	Meat, milk, many fruits, cereals, vegetables, legumes
Chloride	Gastric juice formation, acid-base balance	Table salt, seafood, milk, meat, eggs
Sulfur	Component of tissue, cartilage	Protein foods
Iron	Component of hemoglobin and enzymes	Meats, legumes, eggs, grains, dark green vegetables
Zinc	Component of enzymes, digestion	Milk, shellfish, wheat bran
Iodine	Component of thyroid hormone	Fish, dairy products, vegetables, iodized salt
Copper	Component of enzymes, digestion	Shellfish, grains, cherries, legumes, poultry, oysters, nuts
Manganese	Component of enzymes, fat synthesis	Greens, blueberries, grains, legumes, fruit
Fluoride	Maintenance of bone, teeth	Water, seafood, rice, soybeans, spinach, onions, lettuce
Chromium	Glucose and energy metabolism	Fats, meats, clams, cereals
Selenium	Functions with Vitamin E	Fish, poultry, meats, grains, milk, vegetables

Regular monitoring of iron levels in athletes, including biochemical evaluations and dietary assessments, is recommended to ensure optimal performance.

CALCIUM

Osteoporosis is a major health concern, especially for women. Although the disease has been regarded as an elderly women's problem, young females, especially those who have had interrupted menstrual function, may be at risk for decreased bone mass. Although there is still much to be discovered about the cause of osteoporosis, three major risk factors have been identified: hormonal status, particularly estrogen deficiency; calcium consumption; and physical activity.

Bone mass is attained until the age of 35 to 40 years; however, peak bone mass is obtained between the ages of 14 and 24. The amount of bone mass a woman has by age 35 strongly influences her susceptibility to fractures in later years. Therefore it is important that young women consume calcium throughout the peak bone-mass years and through early adulthood.

The National Institute of Health (NIH) recommends that premenopausal adult women consume 1000 mg of calcium per day. Postmenopausal women who are not on estrogen should consume 1500 mg of calcium per day. Although calcium levels have been recommended for women, the Health and Nutrition Examination Survey (HANES) found that 50% of all females age 15 and over consume less than 75% of the RDA of 1200 mg, and that three quarters of women over 35 consume less than the RDA of 800 mg.

Athletic Amenorrhea

Some women who exercise strenuously stop menstruating, a condition known as athletic amenorrhea. It is associated with many factors, such as nutritional inadequacy, physical stress, energy drain, and acute and chronic hormonal alterations.[34]

Although the specific cause of athletic amenorrhea is unknown and may vary among women, it appears to coincide with decreased estrogen production. Because estrogen deficiency is an important risk factor for the development of osteoporosis, amenorrhea may predispose female athletes to early-onset osteoporosis and fractures. Spinal bone mass has been found to be lower in amenorrheic women runners than in eumenorrheic women runners.[18] Especially disturbing is the fact that further follow-up of these women indicated that bone mineral density remained well below the average for their age group four years after the resumption of normal menses.[19]

Women with athletic amenorrhea should consult a physician to rule out any serious medical problems, and all amenorrheic women should be consuming 1500 mg of calcium per day.

After consultation with a physician, several strategies may be recommended to promote the resumption of menses. These include estrogen replacement therapy, weight gain, diet modification, and reduced training.

Regardless of menstrual history, most female athletes need to increase their calcium intake to meet the RDA for calcium. Low fat and nonfat dairy products, such as nonfat and low fat milk, yogurt, cottage cheese, and other low-fat cheeses, are excellent sources of dietary calcium.

CONCLUSION

Nutrition plays a critical role in athletic performance, and sponsors of organized sport programs need to realize that if they educate their athletes to make wise food choices, the chances of optimal athletic performance increase. Athletes, parents, coaches, and sports medicine professionals should not fall prey to nutrition misinformation and fads just because they have had no formal training in nutrition. Using a qualified sports nutritionist as part of a sports medicine program will help athletes compete at their best.

REFERENCES

1. Benedich A: Exercise and free radicals effect of antioxidant vitamins, *Med Sport Sci* 32:59–78, 1991.
2. Berning JR: The facts and fallacies of sports nutrition: how athletes can evaluate nutrition claims. In Berning JR, Steen SN, eds: *Sports nutrition for the nineties: the health professional's handbook*, Gaithersberg, MD, 1991, Aspen Publishers.
3. Berning JR, Troup JP, VanHandel PJ, et al: The nutritional habits of young adolescent swimmers, *Int J Sport Nut* 1:3, 240–248, 1991.
4. Brooks SM, Sanborn CF, Albrecht BH, Wagner WW: Diet in athletic amenorrhea, *Lancet* 1:559, 1984.
5. Burke LM, Collier GR, Hargreaves M: Muscle glycogen storage following prolonged exercise: effect of glycemic index of carbohydrate feeding, *J Appl Physiol* 75:1019–1023, 1993.
6. Butterfield GE: Amino acids and high protein diets. In Lamb DR, Williams MH, eds: *Perspectives in exercise science and sports medicine*, vol 4, *Ergogenic enhancement of performance in exercise and sport*, Ann Arbor, 1991, Brown and Benchmark.
7. Butterfield GE: Whole body protein utilization in humans, *Med Sci Sports Exerc* 19:S157–S165, 1987.
8. Butterfield GE, Calloway DH: Physical activity improves protein utilization in young men, *Brit J Nutr* 51:171–184, 1984.
9. Campbell ML, McFadyen KL: Nutritional knowledge, beliefs and dietary practices of competitive swimmers, *Can Home Econom J* 34:47, 1984.
10. Clarkson PM: Vitamins and trace minerals. In Lamb DR, Williams MH, eds: *Perspectives in exercise science and sports medicine*, vol 4, *Ergogenic enhancement of performance in exercise and sport*, Ann Arbor, 1991, Brown and Benchmark.
11. Costill DL, Bowers K, Branam G, Sparks K: Muscle glycogen utilization during prolonged exercise on successive days, *J Appl Physiol* 31:834–838, 1977.
12. Costill DL, Coyle EF, Dalsky G, et al: Effects of elevated plasma FFA and insulin on muscle glycogen usage during exercise, *J Appl Physiol* 43:695–699, 1977.
13. Costill DL, Sherman WM, Fink WJ, et al: The role of dietary carbohydrate in muscle glycogen resynthesis after strenuous running, *Am J Clin Nutr* 34:1831–1836, 1981.
14. Coyle EF: Timing and method of increased carbohydrate intake to cope with heavy training, competition, and recovery, *J Sport Sci* 9:29–52, 1991.
15. Coyle EF, Coggan AR, Hemmert MK, Ivy JL: Muscle glycogen utilization during prolonged strenuous exercise when fed carbohydrate, *J Appl Physiol* 61:165–172, 1986.
16. Coyle EF, Hagberg JM, Hurley BF, et al: Carbohydrate feeding during prolonged strenuous exercise can delay fatigue, *J Appl Physiol* 55:230–235, 1983.
17. Davies KJA, Quinantilla AT, Brooks GA, Packer L: Free radical and tissue damage produced by exercise, *Biochem Biophs Res Comm* 107:1198–1205, 1982.
18. Drinkwater BL, Nilson K, Chestnut CH: Bone mineral content of amenorrheic and eumenorrheic athletes, *N Eng J Med* 311:277–281, 1984.
19. Drinkwater BL, Nilson K, Ott S, Chestnut CH: Bone mineral density after resumption of menses in amenorrheic athletes, *JAMA* 256:380–382, 1986.
20. Gontzea I, Sutzesco P, Dumtrache S: The influence of muscular activity on nitrogen balance and on the need of man for protein, *Nutr Reports Internat* 10:35–43, 1974.
21. Hargreaves M: Carbohydrate and exercise, *J Sport Sci* 9:17–28, 1991.
22. Hargreaves M, Costill DL, Fink WJ, et al: Effect of pre-exercise carbohydrate feedings on endurance cycling performance, *Med Sci Sports Exerc* 19:33–36, 1987.
23. Haymes EM: Vitamin and mineral supplementation to athletes, *Int J Sport Med* 1:146–169, 1991.
24. Hickson JF, Wolinsky I, Divarnik JM: Repeated days of body building exercise do not enhance urinary excretions from untrained young adult males, *Nutr Res* 10:723–730, 1990.
25. Ivy JL, Datz AL, Cutler CL, et al: Muscle glycogen synthesis after exercise effect of time of carbohydrate ingestion, *J Appl Physiol* 64:1480–1485, 1988.
26. Jenkins DJA, Woolever JMS, Thorne MJ, et al: The relationship between glycemic response, digestibility and factors influencing the dietary habits of diabetics, *Am J Clin Nutr* 40:1175–1192, 1989.
27. Kiens B, Raben AB, Valeur AK, Richter EA: Benefit of dietary simple carbohydrates on the early post exercise muscle glycogen repletion in athletes, *Med Sci Sports Exerc* 22(S4):88, 1990.
28. Krause ME, Mahan CK: *Food Nutrition and Diet Therapy*, ed 7, Philadelphia 1984, Saunders.
29. Lemon PWR: Protein and amino acid needs of the strength athlete, *Int J Sport Nutr* 1:127–145, 1991.
30. Loosli AR, Benson J, Gillien DM, Bourdet K: Nutrition habits and knowledge in competitive adolescent female gymnasts, *Phys and Sports Med* 14:118, 1986.
31. Meredith CN, Zachin MJ, Fontera WR, Evan WJ: Dietary protein requirements and body protein metabolism in endurance trained men, *J Appl Physiol* 66:2850–2856, 1981.
32. National Research Council: Recommended Dietary Allowances, ed 10, Washington, DC, 1990, National Academy Press.
33. Perron M, Endres J: Knowledge, attitudes and dietary practices of female athletes, *J Am Diet Assoc* 85:573, 1985.
34. Sanborn CF, Albrech BH, Wagner WW: Athletic amenorrhea, lack of association with body fat, *Med Sci Sports Exerc* 19:207–212, 1987.
35. Sherman WM, Brodowicz G, Wright DA, et al: Effects of 4-hour pre-exercise carbohydrate feedings on cycling performance, *Med Sci Sports Exerc* 12:598–604, 1989.
36. Shoaf LR, McClellan PD, Birskovich KA: Nutrition knowledge, interests and information sources of male athletes, *J Nutr Education* 18:243, 1986.
37. Simonsen JC, Sherman WM, Lamb DL, Dernbach AR, et al: Dietary carbohydrate, muscle glycogen, and power output during rowing training, *J Appl Physiol* 70:4, 1500–1505, 1991.
38. Slavin J: Protein needs for athletes. In JR Berning, Steen SN, eds: *Sports nutrition for the nineties: the health professional's handbook*, Gaithersberg, MD, 1991, Aspen Publisher.
39. Synder AC, Dvorak LL, Roepke JB: Influence of dietary iron on measures of iron status among female runners, *Med Sci Sports Exerc* 21:7–10, 1989.
40. Tarnopolsky MA, Lemon PWR, Macdougall JD, Atkinson SA: Effect of body building exercise on protein requirements, *Can J Sports Sci* 15:225, 1991.
41. Tarnopolsky MA, MacDougall JD, Atkinson SA: Influence of protein intake and training status on nitrogen balance and lean body mass, *J Appl Physiol* 64:187–193, 1988.
42. Tremblay A, Fontaine E, Nadeau A: Contribution of post-exercise increment in glucose storage to variations in glucose-induced thermogenesis in endurance athletes, *Can J Physiol Pharmacol* 63:1165–1169, 1985.
43. Van Handel PJ, Cells KA, Bradley PW, Troup JP: Nutritional status of elite swimmers, *J Swim Res* 1:27–31, 1984.
44. Yoshimura H: Adult protein requirements, *Fed Proc* 20:103–110, 1961.
45. Zawadski KM, Yaspelkis BB, Ivy JL: Carbohydrate-protein complex increases the rate of muscle glycogen storage after exercise, *J Appl Physiol* 72(5):1854–1859, 1992.

CHAPTER 34

FLUID BALANCE

Gilbert B. Cushner
Fred D. Cushner

In 490 B.C. the Greeks were victorious at the Battle of Marathon. To deliver the historic news, a soldier in full armor ran 22 miles to Sparta, only to collapse and die after delivering his important message.[70] Fortunately, the role of the messenger has been replaced by more modern methods of communication, and a new emphasis on fluid balance and hydration has developed in this era of triathlons and "iron man" competitions.

The need for fluid replacement in competitive athletes, to help maximize performance and reduce the incidence of heat-associated disorders, has only been emphasized in the last 25 years. Even in the early 1950s, it was common dogma that "to run a complete marathon without any fluid replacement was regarded as the ultimate aim of most runners."[71] A 1969 paper by Wyndham and Strydom[99] stimulated modern interest in fluid replacement during exercise. The writers found correlation between the degree of dehydration and rectal temperature and deduced that avoidance of dehydration might prevent heat injury during exercise. This interest, in turn, has produced an enormous commercial outpouring of sports drinks promoted as being superior to water replacement alone.

In this chapter, the pathophysiology of temperature regulation and dehydration is reviewed and exercise-associated medical disorders are discussed. At the end of this chapter, specific recommendations for fluid, electrolyte, and carbohydrate replacement before, during, and after exercise are given.

THERMOREGULATION

Approximately 70% to 80% of energy generated by the working muscle is released as heat.[65,89] As oxygen consumption increases, heat generation also increases, and thermal regulation is needed to control the increased heat production. Unlike lizards and other creatures that rely upon the sun's heat to raise their body temperatures to a level that allows for physical activity, humans are warm-blooded animals (homeotherms) and require a relatively constant internal body temperature that is usually in excess of the ambient temperature.[65] As reviewed by Sawka,[83] core temperatures may become elevated from 0.1 to 0.4 degrees for each percent decrease in body weight under a variety of conditions. Without the body's intact heat loss mechanism, a 1% centigrade–increase in body temperature could take place every 5 minutes, with death occurring within 20 minutes.[13] With mild to moderate ambient temperatures, conduction, convection, and radiation may be sufficient; but when the environmental temperature is higher than the skin temperature, or in the competing athlete, the most critical thermoregulatory mechanism remains the evaporation of sweat.

Thermoregulation is monitored by thermoreceptors in the skin and body core and then regulated by the hypothalamus. This is a fragile regulatory center, one in which even minor dehydration adversely affects the hypothalamus function. Cohen et al.[17] concluded that even a deficiency as low as 1.2% could lead to thermoregulatory dysfunction. Man's thermoregulatory function can best be studied by example. Let us examine the "Gatorade Iron Man World Championship Triathlon," an event that includes a 2.4-mile swim, followed by a 112-mile bicycle ride, and ending in a full marathon run of 26.2 miles. According to Santi and Gonzales,[86]

> A triathlon typically starts with a morning swim. In cold water, heat loss is rapid, but the response is partially offset by the intense muscular activity. The participants emerge from the water and begin the bicycle stage, perhaps along a winding coastal highway, alternating exposure to sun and shade, wind and calm, was well as the air flow created by the speed of their own motion. As the morning progresses, the sun rises higher in the sky, increasing both air temperature and solar radiation. As the ground heats, wind movement, directed as up-and-down slow breezes, and more gentle winds change in strength and direction. Along the coast, the air tends to be humid, limiting the cooling value of body sweat. At the end of the cycle ride, the participants begin a marathon, generally running on more level terrain under the afternoon sun as air

temperatures reach their daily maximum. In the warmer air, away from the ocean's moisture, sweat evaporates more readily, allowing more heat to be lost. For the slower participants, the sunlight wanes at sunset and they will continue their run into the night, either benefiting from the absence of direct sunlight and cooler air temperatures, or becoming chilled due to the combination of colder air and radiant heat loss.

This passage summarizes the four mechanisms of heat transfer that are produced during athletic activity. These include conduction, such as the conduction of heat to the surrounding cooler water, and convective cooling, which occurs during the bicycle portion of the event. Solar radiation takes place during the entire event, and the most critical thermoregulatory mechanism remains the evaporation of sweat.

SWEATING AND DEHYDRATION

As monitored by the anterior hypothalamus, increases in core temperature that exceed the set point result in stimulation of sympathetic cholinergic nerves that stimulate the 2 to 4 million sweat glands in the human skin to produce sweat.[85] Also, skin blood flow accelerates because of raised skin temperature and as a result of central sympathetic control. This helps increase heat loss through sweat evaporation.

Human sweat is a hypotonic solution with an osmolality of between 80 and 185 mosm/L. For comparison, normal plasma osmolality is 302 mosm/L. During heavy sweating, observed water loss is greater than electrolyte loss. Therefore the greatest need is to replace the body's water loss rather than to replace the electrolytes.[20]

The sweat rate is proportional to not only the rate of energy expanded but also the rate of work performed. White et al.[97] evaluated the effect of competition on body fluid losses. With 2½ hours of activity in relatively mild conditions, the average body weight loss was found to be 3.25%. Sweat rate during exercise is influenced by multiple factors (see box below) including acclimation, hydration, aerobic fitness, and clothing of the athlete. External factors include temperature, humidity, and air velocity. The sweating athlete can produce up to 1.8 liters of sweat and can dissipate all the exercise-gener-

ated heat. The sweat rate, however, on occasion can rise as high as 2 to 3 L/hr.[7,21] The highest sweating rate reported in the literature was 2.7 L/hr, measured for Alberto Salazar during the 1984 Olympic marathon.[7]

As dehydration occurs, the sweat rate decreases or stays the same.[71] A rise in serum osmolality and serum sodium correlates with the rise in esophageal temperature[64] and may be the stimulation for any reduction in sweating that occurs at high levels of dehydration.[55] The highest sweat rate takes place during prolonged, high-intensity exercise in the heat. Therefore sweating is a vital thermoregulatory response that occurs at the expense of both intra- and extracellular compartments. If intake cannot keep pace with losses, dehydration will occur. Dehydration will definitely limit the capacity for work and the health of athletes. A practical example would be the finish of a 1984 women's marathon, when Gabrielle Anderson-Scheris staggered her way around to the final lap showing signs of hyperthermia and dehydration.[65] Dehydration has been shown to result in decreases in anaerobic capacity, muscle endurance, maximal aerobic power, and physical work capacity.[84] The effects are not limited to physical measurements since the ability to do mental tasks is also impaired.[37]

PHYSIOLOGIC RESPONSE TO DEHYDRATION

The body responds to dehydration in a variety of ways, some of which are positive and protect the physiologic homeostasis, whereas others have a deleterious effect on the organism. Primary changes include gastrointestinal, cardiovascular, and hormonal adaptation (see box below).

FACTORS AFFECTING THE SWEAT RATE IN ATHLETES

Aerobic fitness

Hydration status

Environmental temperature and humidity

Air velocity

Radiant heat load

Type of clothing

Intensity of exercise

GASTROINTESTINAL, CARDIOVASCULAR, AND HORMONAL RESPONSES TO DEHYDRATION

Gastrointestinal Changes
1) Decreased gastric emptying
2) Increased intestinal absorption

Cardiovascular Changes
1) Restoration of plasma volume by fluid movement
2) Decreased stroke volume
3) Increased heart rate
4) Decreased central blood volume
5) Decreased central venous pressure
6) Decreased cardiac filling pressure
7) Decreased cardiac output
8) Decreased splanchnic & renal blood flow

Hormonal Changes
1) Increased vasopressin
2) Increased renin, angiotensin II, and aldosterone activity

Gastrointestinal Changes

Dehydration decreases gastric emptying,[68] impeding the rate of rehydration. In contrast, intestinal resorption probably increases with a declining blood volume.[88] Symptoms related to diminished gastric emptying include nausea, bloatedness, and a general gastrointestinal distress.[79]

Cardiovascular Changes

The plasma volume falls when exercise is initiated, influenced by the type, the intensity, and the posture adopted.[26] With a fall in plasma volume, plasma osmolality increases[32] as well as plasma viscosity.[94] This is aggravated by fluid loss until fluid movement from the intracellular space and glycogen breakdown[84] tends to restore it. As to be expected with a fall in plasma volume, there is a decreased central blood volume,[84] decreased central venous pressure,[52] and decreased cardiac output. Blood flow is redistributed from inactive tissues (e.g., digestive organs, liver, and kidney, into the central blood volume).[82] In spite of the decreased renal blood flow, no change in renal function is observed with dehydration in less than 4% of body weight.[46,47] Heart rate also increases with dehydration,[4,14,39,62,90] and stroke volume is reduced. However, if fluid intake prevents dehydration, cardiac output and stroke volume do not fall,[40] and heart rate remains elevated. This suggests that dehydration is not the only cause of exercise-induced tachycardia.

Hormonal Changes

During prolonged exercise, plasma concentrations of the fluid and electrolyte-regulating hormones increase, specifically, vasopressin, renin, and aldosterone.[5,11,33,95] Vasopressin secretion from the posterior pituitary gland can be influenced by plasma osmolality, blood volume, and various chemical mediators, all of which operate in the dehydrated state. A plasma osmolality of 280 mmol/kg is considered to be the threshold level at which osmoreceptors trigger vasopressin release.[81] Even in the presence of decreased plasma osmolality, a decrease in effective circulating blood volume will cause vasopressin release. Baroreceptors are located in many areas of the circulatory system, but the left atrial receptor seems to be the most important, responding to smaller changes in volume than its arterial counterpart.[91] The renin-angiotensin system described earlier also participates in vasopressin release with angiotensin II having a stimulatory role.[93] Vasopressin increases the water permeability of collecting ducts, resulting in water absorption and producing a maximally concentrated urine.

Renin is a proteolytic enzyme stored and synthesized in the juxtaglomerular apparatus in the wall of afferent glomerular renal arteriolae. Renin is secreted in response to decreased renal perfusion, increased plasma osmolality, and hypovolemic stimulation of beta-adrenergic neurons.[31] The enzyme cleaves to angiotensinogen (renin substrate), an α_2-globulin synthesized in the liver to produce the decapeptide angiotensin I. Angiotensin I is rapidly split by the angiotensin enzyme in the lungs and other tissues to form the octapeptide angiotensin II. As already described, angiotensin II stimulates vasopressin release and causes an increase in aldosterone secretion. Potassium release by the active muscle fibers also stimulates release of this mineralocorticoid hormone. Aldosterone promotes active sodium absorption and excretion of potassium in its major target organs (kidney, colon, and salivary glands). Although these changes begin early in exercise by the movement of up to 13 percent of fluid into muscle, they continue to operate as sweat-induced fluid loss persists, conserving water and sodium.

RISK FACTORS FOR HEAT-INDUCED ILLNESSES

Although dehydration secondary to sweating is the most important factor in heat-induced illness, there are other conditions that may play a significant role. These include obesity, age, previous heat injury, hypertension, and a variety of drugs (Table 34-1). Deserving special mention are diuretics. Diuretic use, although discouraged, is currently practiced by athletes, not only to weigh in at an appropriate level for sports such as wrestling and boxing, but also in attempts to conceal illegal drug or substance use during urine testing. Diuretics are currently banned by the National Collegiate Athletic Association (NCAA) as well as the International Olympic Committee Medical Commission. Diuretic use is dangerous not only because of dehydration effect, but also because of secondary electrolyte imbalances such as hypokalemia and hypomagnesemia. Not only can the fluid loss from diuretics cause a larger loss of plasma volume than that caused by voluntary exercise, it is usually accompanied by potassium and magnesium losses of a far greater magnitude than we observe with exercise. In conjunction with self-induced vomiting or laxative abuse, the potential for an electrolyte imbalance is accentuated.

For many reasons, obesity can be a significant risk factor. Much of this increased risk is secondary to the obese athlete's being unable to tolerate heat was well as thinner athletes. The specific heat of adipose tissue, compared to lean body mass, leads to an increased heat production. Thermoregulation in the obese patient is also decreased secondarily to altered sweating and decreased sweat gland production.[89] Other risk factors include age. Children appear to be at increased risk because of a less effective thermoregulatory system.[89] Prior heat stroke also can be a risk factor for heat-induced illness.

Table 34-1. The mechanism of action of various drugs on the thermoregulatory system

Drug	Mechanism
Thyroid hormone (excess)	Excessive heat production
Amphetamines	Excessive heat production
Haloperidol	Decreased thirst
Antihistamines	Decreased sweating
Phenothiazines	Decreased sweating
Diuretics	Sodium and fluid loss
Beta-blockers	Decreased sweating
Benztropine mesylate	Decreased sweating

ENVIRONMENTAL RISK FACTORS FOR HEAT-INDUCED ILLNESSES

Not only is an athlete's thermoregulation mechanism important, but environmental factors play a role in the development of heat-induced injuries. Ambient temperature, humidity, air velocity, and radiating heat sources are important in determining conditions that may prove harmful to the athlete. Although these factors may be announced by the local weather services, they may be different at the actual athletic site. Therefore, measurements should be made before the starting of the event to accurately predict the risk of heat-induced illnesses.

To evaluate temperature, humidity, air movement, and radiating heat, the wet-globe temperature (WBGT) is calculated as noted below:

$$WBGT = (0.1 \times \text{ambient dry-bulb temperature}) + (0.2 \times \text{black-globe temperature}) + (0.7 \times \text{wet-bulb temperature})$$

The black globe (a black toilet-tank float with a thermometer inside) measures the radiant heat while the wet bulb, minus the dry bulb, measures relative humidity when both bulbs are exposed to similar air movement. As can be seen from the above formula, 70% of the WBGT comes from the humidity level. A relative humidity of 60% or greater indicates that sweat evaporation will occur only if significant air movement is present. If a wet bulb temperature is greater than 75° F (24° C), rest periods every 30 minutes are advised; and at wet bulb temperatures over 76° F (24.4° C) only light exercise should be performed.[89]

A WBGT below 65° F (18° C) indicates a low risk, while temperatures of 74° to 82° F (23° to 28° C) constitute a high risk.[89] No activities should be performed with a WBGT value greater than 90.

By monitoring the relative humidity as well as the WBGT, modifications in sporting events can be made to decrease the relative risk to participating athletes.

EXERCISE-ASSOCIATED ILLNESSES

The incidence of heat-related illnesses is unknown. Many of the incidents occur and are treated with simple hydration, whereas the more catastrophic illnesses make local newspaper headlines. In this section we will discuss both heat and dehydration–induced illnesses (muscle cramps, exertional heat injury, heat exhaustion, and heat stroke) and those associated illnesses in which dehydration probably does not play a role (exercise-associated collapse {EAC} and hyponatremia).

Muscle Cramps

Muscle cramps, although often painful, are the most benign of the injuries described as heat-induced injuries. These cramps occur in the large muscle groups such as the hamstrings or gastrocnemius muscles.[1] This cramping is thought to be secondary to an impaired circulation in the exercising muscle. Because only a few muscle bundles are involved at a time, the pain is noted to "wander" as different muscle bundles are affected. This circulation defect is thought to be secondary to dehydration. A decrease in serum sodium and chloride also may be associated with the development of muscle cramps.

Treatment of muscle cramps begins with prevention. Attention to hydration before, during, and after an athletic event decreases the incidence of muscle cramps. Proper conditioning and heat acclimatization also serve to prevent the onset of muscle cramps. If these muscle cramps develop, the exercise should be stopped and oral hydration initiated. The athlete should be placed in a supine position to increase blood flow to the muscles involved. Massage of the affected muscle groups also may help to relieve symptoms, and improved conditioning may serve to decrease the occurrence of a repeat episode of cramping.

Exertional Heat Injury, Heat Exhaustion, and Heat Stroke

Exertional heat injury is really heat exhaustion in the setting of athletic competition. These conditions are a continuing spectrum culminating in the severe, and often fatal, heat stroke. Heat exhaustion can occur in any athlete who participates in activities that lead to profuse sweat loss. This sweat loss can occur during the activity itself or during time spent exposed to sunlight; an example is the shot-putter on a track-and-field team who has only short periods of sustained athletic activity but is exposed to the elements during the day's events. Heat exhaustion is the most common form of heat intolerance noted.

Symptoms of heat exhaustion include nausea, headache, ataxia, dizziness, and muscle weakness.[24] Rectal temperature may rise as the body's thermoregulatory system fails to compensate for the increased heat production. Cutaneous flushing with profuse sweating may be noted. An elevated temperature as high as 104 degrees may be present.

The focus of treatment for heat exhaustion is rehydration as well as reduction of the body's temperature. The athlete first should be moved away from direct sunlight into a shady area. This will help to reduce the body temperature. Placing ice bags in the area of the great vessels also serves to decrease the body's temperature. Toweling dry the athlete as well as fanning her may be helpful. Rectal temperature should be monitored for a rapidly rising core temperature—an early indication of heat stroke. Treatment of heat exhaustion includes hydration of the athlete. This should be performed as early as possible. Fluids can be given via the oral route, with a goal of 1 to 2 L over a 2- to 4-hour period.[89] Intravenous fluids should be initiated if the patient is unconscious or otherwise unable to tolerate oral hydration. Hydration should continue until preathletic body weight is obtained and polyuria is present. Once heat exhaustion occurs, a high recurrence rate can be noted. Sensay[87] studied military reservists and noted an 8.5%–hospital readmission rate 2 to 3 days after the initial heat illness event.

Water is the first fluid choice provided to the athlete with heat exhaustion. Controversy does exist as to the benefit of adding glucose to the rehydration fluid.[59,77]

Glucose may be of value if glycogen storage in the muscles and liver is felt to be depleted.

Heat Stroke

Heat stroke is the second most common cause of death in the athlete. Although many animals will decrease their running and activity levels as body temperatures increase, humans in a quest for victory will often ignore these natural protective mechanisms. As the body temperature rises above 106° F, heat stroke is said to occur. The presenting symptom of heat stroke is hypovolemic shock in the setting of a markedly elevated core temperature. Profuse sweating may be present,[41] and neurologic symptoms such as irritability, aggression, and delirium may occur. Heat stroke is a medical emergency with a mortality rate estimated to be 50% to 70%.[6] It is not the degree of hyperthermia but rather the duration of sustained hyperpyrexia and unconsciousness that is the most important prognostic factor for heat stroke. Because a shortened length of hyperpyrexia is critical, an early diagnosis and treatment are urgent. Misdiagnosis may be made, including that for encephalitis, meningitis, dysentery, hepatitis, malaria, epilepsy, and conversion reaction,[10,49] leading to a delay in treatment. Therefore, a high index of suspicion must be maintained for any athlete who collapses during physical activity. Measurement of rectal temperature may aid in the early diagnosis of this condition.

Treatment of heat stroke begins with the cooling of the patient. As for the patient with heat exhaustion, the athlete is moved to a shaded area, and ice bags are placed near the great vessels. Fanning and massage are initiated to aid in the lowering of the core temperature.[6] Although immersion in ice water may induce a sudden drop in the body's core temperature,[16] it also causes vasoconstriction. Vasoconstriction and shivering have a negative effect on subsequent heat loss. Hubbard and others[45] have used niacin to help counteract vasoconstriction that occurs with ice immersion, but the use of niacin remains experimental at this time.

Rehydration and cardiac support should be provided early. Blood pressure should be monitored, as should urine output, and a catheter should be placed as needed. Beta-adrenergic drugs may be needed to increase cardiac output, but alpha-adrenergic drugs should not be used since they may hamper skin perfusion and, therefore, hamper heat transfer. Hospital monitoring for 24 to 36 hours is recommended, to observe for complications associated with heat stroke. Individual system, as well as multisystem, involvement may occur as a result of heat stroke. In 10% to 35% of patients, acute renal tubular necrosis may develop.[50] Liver involvement such as lobular necrosis and marked cholestasis[51] also can occur. In a study by Senay,[87] 40 out of 42 patients readmitted for heat exhaustion had an increased SGOT level. This may be a marker for the severity of heat injury, but further experimentation needs to be done. A malabsorption syndrome may develop if the gastrointestinal tract has an ischemic event at the time of the heat stroke.

EXERCISE-ASSOCIATED DISEASES WITHOUT DEHYDRATION

Exercise-Associated Collapse

For a long period of time, runners who were thought to have suffered from dehydration were treated with IV fluids.[2,29,42–44,56,58,75,98] Recent studies have shown that collapsing runners are not more likely to be hyperthermic or dehydrated than their noncollapsing peers.[72,73,80] In fact, IV fluids seem to retard recovery.[30] Noakes[71] has proposed a postural hypotension caused by fluid displacement to the muscles of the lower extremities as a most likely cause. Rational therapy, therefore, would include elevation of the pelvis and legs, and this has been proven to be effective.[38]

HYPONATREMIA. With the exception of one case reported in a marathon runner,[67] all reports of symptomatic hyponatremia have occurred in endurance athletes participating in triathlon or ultramarathon events.[34,44,74] A variety of neurologic symptoms has been reported, including convulsions and comma. Serum sodium is less than 125 mEq/L, and normal to increased blood volumes are compatible with the observation that these athletes have had excessive fluid intake, rather than increased sodium losses.

Noakes[71] has postulated three possible etiologies that operate in combination to cause hyponatremia. The syndrome of inappropriate antidiuretic hormone (SIADH) may be present, with expanded blood volume failing to shut off ADH secretion but appropriately shutting off aldosterone. The latter is associated with increased urinary sodium loss, contributing to the hyponatremia state.

A second possible cause is a disturbed regulation of the extracellular volume, so that the normal relationship between the volume and its sodium chloride content is lost; and, possibly, a third space phenomenon of sodium moving into the unabsorbed fluid in the large bowel may contribute. Since most athletes are "reluctant" drinkers and more prone to develop voluntary dehydration, the "avid" drinkers are a small subset who may develop hyponatremia if associated with over 6 hours of fluid replacement exceeding 1.3 L/hr.[71]

Prevention of Heat Illnesses

As for any disease process, the best form of treatment for heat illness is prevention. Because of increased awareness of exertion-induced injuries, as well as more formal sports medicine education, the importance of proper hydration in the athlete is being stressed. It is now common knowledge that water breaks are not to be considered "a sign of weakness" for the training athlete.[53]

Hydration is the first line of prevention against heat-induced injuries. Proper hydration begins before the start of a sports event. The athlete should be well hydrated at the beginning of the competition. During the event, hydration should be stressed despite the absence of thirst. A subjective feeling of thirst occurs only after 2% to 3% of body weight is lost. At this point athletic performance is already impaired.[89] Because athletes will not voluntarily replace all fluids lost,[10] the guidelines of 12 oz of fluid for every 20 minutes of exercise should be followed. The sweat rate is proportional to body mass.[17] Fluid requirements for a middle linebacker will be much different from those of a female gymnast. Because some sports (soccer, rugby) have only one break, at halftime, the intermission is not long enough for adequate replenishment of fluids. Coaches should agree before the start of the game to divide the game into quarters, thereby providing proper rehydration time during extreme weather conditions.

As a guide to fluid replacement after exercise, athletes can provide a rough estimate by weighing themselves nude before the event and then following the event. One pound of weight loss equals approximately one pint of fluid that needs to be replenished after exercise.[89]

Proper clothing is essential for the prevention of heat-induced illnesses. In heat and humidity, uniforms should be lightweight, with as much skin exposure as possible, to facilitate perspiration. Sports such as soccer and rugby, which are played in both the cool and warmer months, should have heavier- and lighter-weight uniforms to accommodate the extremes of temperatures present at game time during both seasons. Football players should remove their helmets when on the sidelines to facilitate heat dissipation. Of course, running in sauna suits or multiple sweatshirts to "make weight" is a dangerous practice that should be discouraged.

Proper conditioning as well as acclimatization to local weather conditions are other factors that can reduce the incidence of heat-associated illnesses. It is well known that both training and acclimatization will confer some protection against heat illness. Although, adaptation is most marked when conditioning is carried out in the heat, some benefit will also be achieved at moderate temperatures. Training expands the blood volume, contributing to better cardiac output. Physiologic changes with acclimatization include increased skin blood flow at a given core temperature, increased sweat protection, decreased rate of glycogen utilization, and more dilute sweat production.[89] In the adult, maximal sweat acclimatization can be achieved in 8 to 12 days with as little as 30 minutes of intense exercise daily. Despite optimal heat acclimatization, no athlete can develop complete immunity to heat illness.[89] Adequate hydration is still essential to minimize the risk of exercise-associated dehydration illnesses.

SPECIFIC RECOMMENDATIONS FOR FLUID, CARBOHYDRATE, AND ELECTROLYTE REPLACEMENT

Sports drinks have become big business in the world of athletics today. Millions of dollars are spent in advertising each year on such products. Corporate institutions, such as Pepsi (All Sport) and Coca Cola (Powerade), have introduced their versions of sports drinks to compete with the long-standing Gatorade Corporation. The question remains: do these products offer an advantage over just plain cold water? We will evaluate this question, and guidelines to fluid replacement for specific athletic events will also be detailed.

Table 34-2. Composition of various sports drinks

Beverage (8 oz)	CHO (g)	Na (mg)	K (mg)
Gatorade	14	110	30
"Powerade"	19	55	30
"All Sport"	22	55	55
Coca Cola	13	16.3	0
Water	0	trace	trace

All sports drinks are not created equal. Table 34-2 shows the contents of several popular sports drinks as provided by their nutritional labels. Formulation is different not only in their sodium content but also in their carbohydrate content. Therefore, caloric amounts also may be varied for these drinks. Johnson et al.[48] evaluated several sports drinks and found no difference between the various formulations and their abilities to prevent dehydration or electrolyte imbalance. There was no difference noted in sweating or athletic performance. Johnson[48] and other authors[97] concluded that the sports products may be beneficial according to their palatability, thereby encouraging a more, or less, voluntary oral hydration.

As suggested by Gisolfi and Duchman,[36] choice of replacement fluids depends on the intensity and the length of the event. We have divided our discussion into short events (less than 1 hour), intermediate events (1 to 3 hours), and prolonged events (in excess of 3 hours). In Table 34-3, the choice of fluid replacement and the need for carbohydrate/electrolyte replacement are summarized for all three types of events.

Short Events (Less Than 1 Hour)

Short events include team sports such as cycling as well as essentially all track events. Sports in these categories have an intensity level between 75% and 100% Vo_2max. Preexercise hydration for this sports category depends on the intensity of the exercise expected and the state of hydration of the athlete. Either no fluids are necessary or the use of 300 to 500 cc of a 6% to 10%–carbohydrate solution is deemed appropriate. The latter is required so as to avoid glycogen depletion in a highly intense athletic event. Otherwise, water only would be appropriate to ensure that the patient enters the event hydrated.

During events there is rationale for replacing all fluids to attenuate any rise in core temperature. In contrast to other species, only humans develop voluntary dehydration when given free access to fluid during exercise.[3,9,15,28,92] A significant dehydration (2% of body fluid loss) occurs before thirst is perceived, resulting in voluntary dehydration with exercise. A water deficiency of 3% reduces maximum aerobic power in a temperate climate. In hotter environments, 2% will show some reduction. We suggest that, for fluid replacement, approximately one half of the sweat rate, which is 500 to 1000 cc in most athletes, should be replaced. Gastric volume does play a role in gastric emptying. The larger the volume, the greater the gastric emptying rate, up to 600 cc.[23]

Table 34-3. Guidelines for fluid hydration for mild, moderate, and severe activity levels

	1 hour	**1–3 hours**	**Over 3 hours**
Exercise intensity	75%–100% Vo_2 maximum	60%–90% Vo_2 maximum	30%–70% Vo_2 maximum
Events	teamsports, some cycling events, most track events	soccer, marathon	ultramarathon, triathlon
Formula			
Preevent	30–50g CHO or H_2O	H_2O	H_2O
During exercise	H_2O	Na + = 10–20 mEq Cl − = 10–20 mEq CHO–6%–8%	Na + = 20–30 mEq Cl − = 20–30 mEq CHO–6%–8%
Fluid volume			
Preevent	300–500 cc	300–500 cc	300–500 cc
During exercise	500–1000 cc	500–1000 cc/hr will meet CHO need 800–1600 cc/hr will meet fluid need	500–1000 cc/hr will meet CHO fluid requirements of most
Rationale			
Preevent	CHO—only for events that produce glycogen depletion in less than 1 hour	H_2O—to encourage fat metabolism (see text) and combat dehydration	H_2O—to encourage fat metabolism (see text) and combat dehydration
During exercise	H_2O—to prevent rise in core temperature	CHO—to replete glycogen stores Fluid—to prevent rise in core temperature Na +, Cl − will promote CHO & fluid absorption and enhance palatability	CHO—to replete glycogen stores Fluid—to prevent rise in core temperature Na +, Cl − will promote CHO & fluid absorption, enhance palatability, & prevent hyponatremia

Cool liquids were preferred at one time because of enhanced gastric emptying, but more recent studies have cast doubt upon the importance of liquid temperature.[63] In a similar vein, there is probably no effect from carbonation, although earlier studies suggested that increased emptying[63] was present with carbonated fluids.

Is there any need to add carbohydrate or salt to sports drinks during exercise lasting less than 1 hour? Sweat is hypotonic, and using a 3 L/hr–sweat rate, no more than 120 mg of sodium loss will occur within 1 hour. As calculated by Gisolfi and Duchmann,[36] a serum sodium would exceed 136 mEq/L after 1 hour of exercise. Therefore, no use of sodium is necessary in short events except to increase the palatability of the beverage and perhaps facilitate fluid absorption,[36] although the latter is not substantiated.[66,96]

The evidence for glucose replacement is unclear. There is documentation by earlier authors of the possibility of delayed gastric emptying related to carbohydrate concentration, but this has not been substantiated in more recent studies.[27] No carbohydrate should be added in short exercise. Heat[76] and high-intensity exercises[23] also delay emptying. Glucose polymers have been studied to see if, in theory, the decreased osmolality for the same carbohydrate content causes increased fluid and substrate to reach the small intestine. The results have been variable,[63] but polymer has been found to empty more slowly. Fructose should be avoided because of increased GI problems.[61]

In summary, the use of electrolyte and carbohydrate solutions offers no improvement in plasma volume or electrolyte concentrations for short-event competition. The question of whether they might perhaps improve performance is equivocal.

Intermediate Events of 1 to 3 Hours' Duration

Intermediate-length events (soccer games, rugby games, as well as marathons) take place for the majority of well-trained athletes. An exercise intensity of 65 to 90 Vo_2max is achieved in this sports category.

Preevent hydration for this class of athletic events would include 300 to 500 cc of water, to ensure adequate hydration at the start of competition. Early in the event fat metabolism should be promoted, and the inclusion of carbohydrated drinks might cause increased carbohydrate metabolism and glycogen deposition, leading to premature fatigue.[36] In contrast to the short events, longer events can result in hypoglycemia, hypovolemia, hyperthermia, dehydration, and glycogen depletion.[25,38,78] There is no question that adequate fluid replacement is necessary in events that last for 1 to 3 hours. Between 800 and 1600 cc of fluid, including carbohydrate, can definitely enhance performances, since glycogen stores are reduced.[57,60] Is sodium necessary in these events? The answer is probably "No." The sodium level would probably rise to 130 mEq/L, or even a little higher, since some fluid enters the cells.

Potassium Replacement

Potassium ranges from 1 to 15 mEq/L in sweat and does not increase with the sweat rate.[19] Some data suggest that there are significant losses,[8,54] but this is not supported.[18] On the other hand, potassium facilitates rehydration of the intracellular fluid (ICF) compartment,[12,69] and glucose causes secretion of potassium in the liver. Therefore, to prevent any potential losses, 3 to 5 mEq/L of potassium should be included in a sports drink for an extended event.

Magnesium Replacement

The likelihood of hypomagnesemia secondary to magnesium losses in sweat is an unlikely phenomenon.[89] Maximum losses based on a concentration of 0.02 to 0.05 mmol/L will result in only a 1% decrease in total body content.[22] Magnesium should be replaced for the average daily intake of 10 to 15 mmol/L/day. As emphasized before, magnesium and potassium losses are more accentuated when athletes have used diuretics.

Fluid Replacement During Recovery

The goals of fluid replacement during recovery should be storage of glycogen and restoration of fluid and sodium balance. Appropriate solutions should contain 40 mEq/L of sodium, with the fluid rate adjusted to replace losses and supply 25 to 50 g of carbohydrates every 2 hours.

SUMMARY

The body often has adapted to a variety of conditions to avoid elevations in temperature during exercise, particularly in hot environments. However, elevations in core temperatures can have severe consequences, and failed defense mechanisms can result in deadly dehydration if appropriate fluid and electrolyte needs are not addressed during competition. The need for fluid replacement and, on occasion, carbohydrate and electrolyte replacement, has been summarized in this chapter. It varies, of course, with the intensity and the duration of the exercise plan. A number of exercise-induced illnesses can be prevented, or at least appropriately treated, if the sports physician is aware of the consequences and the possibilities. The need for a comprehensive approach to fluid and electrolyte balance in competitive athletes has been emphasized only in the last 25 years and the approach probably will become better developed over the next decade.

REFERENCES

1. Adams WC, Fox RH, Fry AJ, McDonald IC: Thermoregulation during marathon running in cool, moderate, and hot environments, *J Appl Physiol* 38:1030–1037, 1975.
2. Adner MM, Scarlet JJ, Casey J, et al: The Boston Marathon Medical Care Team: Ten years of experience, *Phys Sports Med* 16:99–106, 1988.
3. Adolph EF: Measurement of water drinking in dogs, *Am J Physiol* 125:75–86, 1939.
4. Adolph EF: *Physiology of man in the desert*, New York, 1947, Interscience Publishers.
5. Altenkirch HU, Gerzer R, Kirsch KA, et al: Effect of prolonged physical exercise on fluid regulating hormones, *Eur J Appl Physiol* 61:209–213, 1990.
6. Appenzeller O, Atkinson R: *Sports medicine: Fitness; training; injuries*, Baltimore, 1981, Urban and Schwarzenberg.
7. Armstrong LE, Hubbard RW, Jones BH, Daniels JT: Preparing Alberto Salazar for the heat of the 1984 Olympic Marathon, *Phys Sports med* 3:73–81, 1986.
8. Armstrong LE, Hubbard RW, Szlyk PC, et al: Voluntary dehydration and electrolyte losses during prolonged exercise in the heat, *Aviat Space Environ Med* 56:765, 1985.
9. Arnauld E, duPont J: Vasopressin release and firing of supraoptic neurosecreting neurones during drinking in the dehydrated monkey, *Pflugers Arch* 394:195–201, 1982.
10. Bar-Or O, Dotan R, Inbar O, et al: Voluntary hypohydration in 10–12 year old boys, *J Appl Physiol; Respir Environ Exerc Physiol* 48:104–108, 1980.
11. Brandenberger G, Condas V, Follenius M, Kahn KM: The influence of the initial state of hydration on endocrine response to exercise in the heat, *Eur J Appl Physiol* 58:674–679, 1989.
12. Brigs AP, Koechig I: Some changes in the composition of blood due to the injection of insulin, *J Biol Chem* 58:721–730, 1923.
13. Brotherhood JR: The nutritional stresses consequent to thermoregulation in athletes, Proceeding of the Nutrition Society of Australia 6:123–125, 1981.
14. Candas V, Libert JP, Brandenberger G: Thermal and circulatory responses during prolonged exercise at different levels of hydration, *J Physiol (Paris)* 83:11–18, 1988.
15. Choshniak I, Wittenberg C, Saham D: Rehydrating Bedouin goats with saline: rumen and kidney function, *Physiol Zool* 60:373–378, 1987.
16. Clowes GHA Jr, O'Donnell TF Jr: Heat stroke, *N Engl J Med* 291:564, 1974.
17. Cohen I, Mitchell D, Seider R, et al: The effect of water deficit on body temperature during rugby, *S Afr Med J* 60:11–14, 1981.
18. Costill DL: Muscle metabolism and electrolyte balance during heat acclimation, *Acta Physiol Scand* 128:111, 1986.
19. Dostill DL: Sweating: its composition and effects on body fluids. In Milvey P, editor: *The marathon physiologic, medical, epidemiological, and psychological studies*, 1977, NY Academy of Science.
20. Costill DL: Water and electrolyte requirements during exercise, *Clin Sports Med* 3(3):639–648, 1984.
21. Costill DL, Cote E, Fink W: Muscle water and electrolytes following varied levels of dehydration in man, *J Appl Physiol* 40:6–11, 1976.
22. Costill DL, Miller JM: Nutrition for endurance sport: carbohydrate and fluid balance, *Int J Sports Med* 1:2–14, 1980.
23. Costill DL, Saltin B: Factors limiting gastric emptying during rest and exercise, *J Appl Physiol* 37:679–683, 1974.
24. Costrini AM, Pitt HA, Gustafson AB, et al: Cardiovascular and metabolic manifestations of heat stroke and severe heat exhaustion, *Am J Med* 66:296–302, 1979.
25. Coyle EF, Coggan AR, Hemmert MK, Ivy SL: Muscle glycogen utilization during prolonged strenuous exercise when fed carbohydrates, *J Appl Physiol* 61:165–172, 1986.
26. Coyle EF, Hamilton M: Fluid replacement during exercise: effects on physiologic homeostasis and performance. In Gisolfi CV, Lamb DR, editors: *Perspectives in exercise science and sports medicine* vol 3, *Fluid homeostasis during exercise*, Indianapolis, 1990, Benchmark Press.
27. Davis JM, Lamb DR, Burgess WA, et al: Accumulation of deuterium oxide in body fluids after ingestion of D_2O labelled beverages, *J Appl Physiol* 63:2060–2066, 1987.

28. Dill DB: Physiologic effects of hot climates and great heights. *Life, heat and altitude,* Cambridge, 1938, Harvard University Press.

29. Eichner ER: Sacred cows and straw men, *Phys Sports Med* 19:24, 1991.

30. Ellis D, Verdile V, Heller M, et al: The effectiveness of the addition of intravenous hydration of oral hydration in post-marathon patients, *Med Sci Sports Exerc* 22 (Suppl) S101, 1990.

31. Fitzsimons JT: *The physiology of thirst and sodium appetite,* New York 1979, Cambridge University Press.

32. Fortney SM, Wenger CB, Bove JR, Nadel ER: Effect of hyperosmolality on control of blood flow and sweating, *J Appl Physiol* 57:1688–1695, 1984.

33. Freund BJ, Claybaugh JR, Hashiro GM, et al: Exaggerated ANF responses to exercise in middle-aged vs. young runners, *J Appl Physiol* 71:2518–2527, 1991.

34. Frizzell RT, Lang GH, Lowance DC, Latham SR: Hyponatremia and ultra marathon running, *JAMA* 255:772, 1986.

35. Gisolfi CV, Copping JR: Thermal effects of prolonged treadmill exercise in the heat, *Med Sci Sports* 6:108–113, 1974.

36. Gisolfi CV, Duchman, SM: Guidelines for optimal replacement beverages for different athletic events, *Med Sci Sports Exerc* 24 (6):679–687, 1992.

37. Gopinathan PM, Pichan G, Sharma VM: Role of dehydration in heat-stress induced variation in mental performance, *Arch Environ Health* 43:15–17, 1988.

38. Gough KJ: Why marathon runners collapse (letter), *S Afr Med J* 30:461, 1991.

39 Greenleaf JE, Castle BL: Exercise temperature regulation in man during hypohydration and hyperhydration, *J Appl Physiol* 30:847–853, 1971.

40. Hamilton MC, Gonzalez-Alonso J, Montain S, Coyle EF: Fluid replacement and glucose infusion during exercise cardiovascular drift, *J Appl Physiol* 71:871–877, 1991.

41. Hart LE, Egier BP, Shimizv AG: Exertional heat stroke: the runner's nemesis, *Can Med Assoc* 122:1144–1150, 1980.

42. Hiller WDB: Current and future research: Report on the Ross Symposium on Medical Coverage of Endurance Athletic Events, Columbus, Oh, 1987, Ross Laboratories.

43. Hiller WDB, O'Toole ML, Laird RH: Hyponatremia and ultra marathons (letter), *JAMA* 256:213, 1986.

44. Hiller WDB, O'Toole ML, Fortess EE, et al: Medical and physiologic considerations in triathalons, *Amer J Sports Med* 15:164,167, 1987.

45. Hubbard RW, Armstrong LE, Young AJ: Rapid hypothermia subsequent to oral nicotinic acid ingestion and immersion in warm (30 degrees C) water (letter), *Am J Emerg Med* 6:316–317, 1988.

46. Irving RA, Noakes TD, Burger SC, et al: Plasma volume and renal function during and after ultramarathon running, *Med Sci Sports Exerc* 22:581–587, 1990.

47. Irving RA, Noakes TD, Raine RI, Van Zyl-Smit R: Transient oliguria with renal tubular dysfunction after a 90 km running race, *Med Sci Sports Exerc* 22:756–761, 1990.

48. Johnson HL, Nelson RA, Consolazio CF: Effects of electrolyte and nutrient solutions on performance and metabolic balance, *Med Sci Exerc* 20(1):26–33, 1988.

49. Keren G, Shonfeld Y, Sohar E: Prevention of damage by sport activity in hot climates, *J Sports Med* 20:452–459, 1980.

50. Kew MC, Abrahams C, Seftel HC: Chronic interstitial nephritis as a consequence of heat stroke, *Q J Med* 39:189, 1970.

51. Kew MC, Berson I, et al: Liver damage in heat stroke, *Am J Med* 49:192, 1970.

52. Kirsch KA, Von Amelin AH, Wicke HJ: Fluid control mechanisms after exercise dehydration, *Eur J Appl Physiol* 47:191–196, 1981.

53. Knochel JP: Dog days and siriasis: How to kill a football player, *JAMA* 233(6):513–515, 1975.

54. Knochel JP, Dotin LN, Hamburger RJ: Pathophysiology of intense physical conditioning in a hot climate, *J Clin Invest* 51:242–255, 1972.

55. Ladell WSS: The effects of water and salt intake upon the performance of men working in hot and humid environments, *J Physiol* 127:11–46, 1955.

56. Laird RH: Medical complications during the ironman triathlon world championship 1981–1984, *Ann Sports Med* 3:113–116, 1987.

57. Lamb DR, Brodowicz GR: Optimal use of fluids of varying formulations to minimize exercise induced disturbances in homeostasis, *Sports Med* 3:247–274, 1986.

58. Lind RH: The western states 100 mile run, Report on the Ross Symposium on Medical Coverage of Endurance Athletic Events, Columbus, Oh, 1987, Ross Laboratories.

59. Mallard D, Owen KC, Kregel P, et al: Exercise physiology and medicine: Effects in ingesting carbohydrate beverages during exercise in heat. In The year book of sports medicine, *Exerc Med Sci Sports* 18:568–575, 1986.

60. Maughan R: Carbohydrate-electrolyte solutions during prolonged exercise. In Lamb DR, Williams MH, editors: *Perspectives in exercise science and sports medicine, ergogenics: Enhancement of performance in exercise and sport,* Indianapolis, 1991, Benchmark Press. pp. 35–85.

61. Maughan RJ, et al: Fluid replacement in sport and exercise–a consensus statement, *Br J Sports Med* 27:34–35, 1993.

62. Maughan RJ, Fenn CE, Gleeson M, Leiper JB: Metabolic and circulatory responses to the ingestion of glucose polymer and glucose/electrolyte solutions during exercise in man, *Eur J Appl Physiol* 56:356–362, 1987.

63. Maughan RJ, Noakes TD: Fluid replacement and exercise stress: A brief review of studies on fluid replacement and some guidelines for the athlete, *Sports Med* 12:16–31, 1991.

64. Montain SJ, Coyle EF: The influence of graded dehydration on hyperthermia and cardiovascular drift during exercise, *J Appl Physiol* 73:1340–1350, 1992.

65. Murray R: Nutrition for the marathon and other endurance sports: environmental stress and dehydration, *Med and Science in Sports and Exerc* 24 (9 Suppl):319–323, 1992.

66. Murray R: The effects of consuming carbohydrate-electrolyte beverages on gastric emptying and fluid absorption during and following exercise, *Sports Med* 4:322–351, 1987.

67. Nelson PB, Robinson AG, Kapoor W, Rinaldo J: Hyponatremia in a marathon runner, *Phys Sports Med* 16(10):78, 1988.

68. Neufer PD, Young AJ, Sawka MN: Gastric emptying during exercise: effects of heat stress and hypodehydration, *Eur J. Appl Physiol* 58:433–439, 1989.

69. Nielsen B, Sjogaard G, Ugelvig J, et al: Fluid balance in exercise dehydration and rehydration with different glucose-electrolyte drinks, *Eur J Appl Physiol* 55:318–25, 1986.

70. Noakes TD: Exercise-induced heat injury in South Africa, *S Afr Med J* 47:1968–1972, 1973.

71. Noakes TD: Fluid replacement during exercise, *Exerc Sport Sci Rev 1993* 21:297–330.

72. Noakes TD: Sacred cows revisited, *Phys Sports Med* 19:49, 1991.

73. Noakes TD, Berlinski N, Solomon E, Weight LM: Collapsed runners: blood biochemical change after IV fluid therapy, *Phys Sports Med* 19:70–81, 1991.

74. Noakes TD, Goodwin W, Rayner BL, et al: Water intoxica-

tion: a possible complication during endurance exercise, *Med Sci Sports Exerc* 17:370, 1985.

75. Novak D: Ironman Canada Triathlon Championship: Medical coverage of an ultra distance event, Report on the Ross Symposium on Medical Coverage of Endurance Athletic Events, Columbus, Oh, 1987, Ross Laboratories.

76. Owen MD, Kregel KC, Wall PT, Gisolfi CV: Effects of ingesting carbohydrate beverages during exercise in the heat, *Med Sci Sports Exerc* 18:568–575, 1986.

77. Pinorka RW, Robinson S, Gay UL, Manalis RS: Preacclimatization of men to heat by training, *J Appl Physiol* 20:379–389, 1965.

78. Pugh LG, Corbett JL, Johnson RH: Rectal temperatures, weight losses and sweat rates in marathon running, *J Appl Physiol* 23:347–352, 1967.

79. Rehrer NJ, Beckers EF, Brouns F, et al: Effects of dehydration on gastric emptying and gastrointestinal distress while running. *Med Sci Sports Exerc* 22:790–795, 1990.

80. Roberts WO: Exercise-associated collapse in endurance events: a classification system, *Phys Sports Med* 117:49–59, 1989.

81. Robertson GL, Berl T: Water metabolism. In Bremer BM, Rector FC Jr, editors: *The kidney*, ed 3, Philadelphia 1986, W.B. Saunders.

82. Rowell LB: Human cardiovascular adjustments to exercise and thermal stress, *Physiol Rev* 54:75–159, 1974.

83. Sawka MN: Physiologic consequences of hypohydration: exercise performance and thermoregulation, *Med Sci Sports Exerc* 24:657–670, 1992.

84. Sawka MN, Pandolf KB: Effects of body water loss on physiologic function and exercise performance. In Gisolfi CV, Lamb DR, editors: *Perspectives in exercise science and sports medicine*, vol 3, *Fluid homeostasis during exercise*, Indianapolis, 1990, Benchmark Press.

85. Sawka MN, Wenger CB: Physiologic responses to acute exercise-heat stress. In Pandolf KB, Sawka MN, Gonzolez RR, editors: *Human performance physiology and environmental medicine at terrestrial extremes*, Indianapolis, 1988, Benchmark Press.

86. Schultz SG, Curran PF: Coupled transport of sodium and organic solutes, *Physiol Rev* 50:637–718, 1970.

87. Senay LC: Effects of exercise in the heat on body fluid distribution, *Med Sci Sports Exerc* 11:42–48, 1979.

88. Sjovall H, Abrahamsson H, Westlander G, et al: Intestinal fluid and electrolyte transport in man during reduced circulating blood volume, *Gut* 27:913–918, 1986.

89. Squire DL: Heat illness–fluid and electrolyte issues for pediatric and adolescent athletes, *Ped Clin N Am* 37:1085–1109, 1990.

90. Strydom NB, Benade AJS, Van Rensburg AJ: The state of hydration and the physiologic responses of men during work in the heat, *Aust J Sports Med* 7:28–33, 1975.

91. Sved AF: Central neural pathways in baroceptor control of vasopressin secretion. In Schrier, RW, editor: *Vasopressin*, New York, 1985, Raven.

92. Thrasher TN, Nistal-Herrera JF, Keil LC, Ramsay DJ: Satiety and inhibition of vasopressin secretion and drinking in dehydrated dogs, *Am J Physiol* 240:E394–E401, 1981.

93. Usberti M, Federico S, Cianciaruso B and others: Effects of angiotensin II on plasma ADH, PGE_2 synthesis and water excretion in normal man, *Am J Physiol* 248:F254–F259, 1985.

94. Vanderwalle H, Lacombe C, Lelievre JC Poirot C: Blood viscosity after a 1-h submaximal exercise with and without drinking, *Int J Sports Med* 9:104–107, 1988.

95. Wade CE, Freund BJ: Hormonal control of blood volumes during and following exercise. In Gisolfi CV, Lamb DR, editors: *Perspectives in exercise science and sports medicine*, vol 3, *Fluid homeostatis during exercise*, Indianapolis, 1990, Benchmark Press.

96. Wheller KB, Banwell JG: Intestinal water and electrolyte flux of glucose-polymer electrolyte solutions, *Med Sci Sports Exerc* 18:436–439, 1986.

97. White J, Ford MA: The hydration and electrolyte maintenance properties of an experimental sports drink, *Br J Sports Med* 17(1):51–58, 1983.

98. Winslow EBJ: The Chicago Marathon, Report on the Ross Symposium on Medical Coverage of Endurance Athletic Events. Columbus, Oh, 1987, Ross Laboratories.

99. Wyndham CH, Strydom NB: The danger of an inadequate water intake during marathon running, *S Afr Med J* 43:893–896, 1969.

CHAPTER 35

SUBSTANCE ABUSE

Dennis J. Gleason

Substance abuse among athletes is a major concern for medical personnel. To review the major aspects of this issue, this chapter is divided into four sections: attitudes and influences resulting in substance abuse among athletes; "roid rage"; symptoms of substance abuse in athletes; and substance abuse prevention.

ATTITUDES AND INFLUENCES

There is tremendous interest in athletics in the United States today, and, some may argue, an overemphasis on "winning at all costs," not only in collegiate and professional sports but also at the high school and grade school levels. Pressures exist among athletes to "do whatever it takes" to win. Consequently, there is interest among some athletes in investigating drugs that may enhance performance. Recent reports of Olympic athletes banned from international competition as a result of failing routine drug tests confirm the fact that there are strong influences upon athletes to find ways to use drugs to enhance performance. Many athletes believe the reports that certain drugs may increase athletic performance by as much as 15% and consider their use in spite of known long-term health hazards.[4] In summary, both cultural and competitive pressures certainly can influence athletes and contribute to the problem of substance abuse in sports medicine today.

"ROID RAGE"

One of the most common substances being abused by athletes is anabolic steroids. These chemical derivatives of testosterone are used medically in the treatment of some blood disorders, cancers, and other illnesses.[1] Anabolic steroids also contribute to the increase of muscle mass, which improves strength and power.[2] For this reason, there is considerable interest in them as performance-enhancing drugs.

The long-term side effects of anabolic steroids include liver cancer, prostate cancer, and abnormal sperm production.[2] These long-term side effects are frequently overlooked by the athlete whose primary goal is short-term increase in muscle mass. Other side effects of anabolic steroids include severe acne, hair loss, atrophy of the testicles, and increased moodiness.[4] One of the most serious side effects of the steroids, especially in younger athletes, is sudden outbursts of aggressive and violent behavior, frequently referred to as "roid rage." Anabolic steroids do increase muscle mass relatively quickly but, at higher doses, certainly contribute to the development of psychologic changes.[2,4] Aggressive behavior may manifest itself in the classroom as discipline problems since the young athlete is unable to control these outbursts even off the playing field. Such behavior is a warning sign of substance abuse and will be addressed in the next section of this chapter. A videotape entitled "The Downfall of Sports and Drugs," produced by the National Parents Resource Institute for Drug Education, offers a dramatic example of the signs and symptoms of "roid rage."[3]

SYMPTOMS AND WHEN TO MAKE A REFERRAL

The symptoms of substance abuse in the athlete often are subtle, therefore it is sometimes difficult to establish the diagnosis. It is important for medical personnel, athletic coaches, and trainers to be familiar with subtle signs of substance abuse because often a younger athlete will be more inclined to discuss problems with these professionals than with his parents.

One major sign of substance abuse is wide mood swings, including both elation and depression. These are illustrated graphically in Fig. 35-1. The straight line represents the stresses of normal daily living, including the pressures placed upon athletes by their peers, schoolwork, teachers, and parents. The higher and lower curves represent larger stresses and unusual occurrences in the

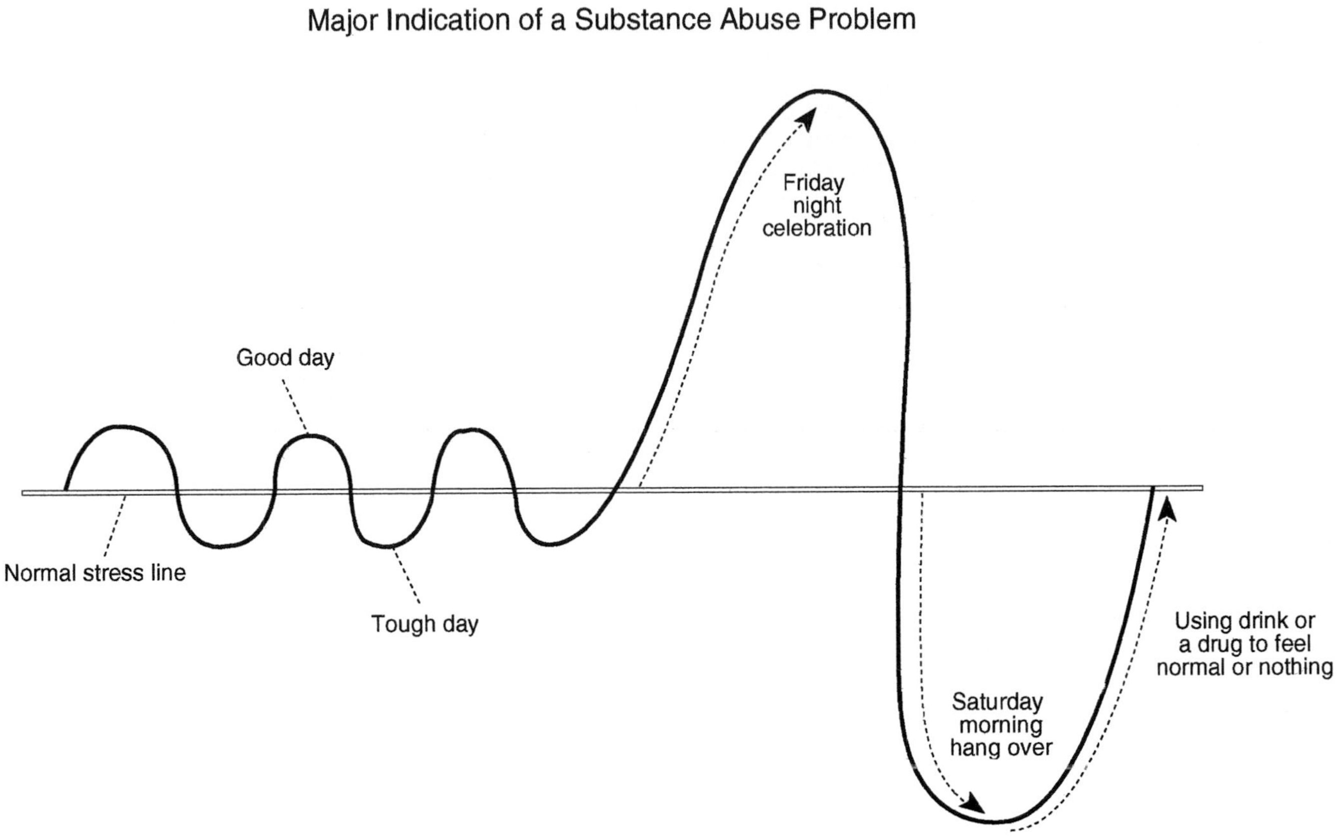

Major Indication of a Substance Abuse Problem

Fig. 35-1. The normal mood swings of everyday activities and the excessive mood swings that may be indicative of substance abuse.

athlete's life. Wide variations in mood may be an indication of substance abuse. Poor performance in academic work and inability to maintain commitments in school or part-time employment are early warning signs of possible substance abuse. In addition to a student's missing classes or practices and a drop in his grades, other signs of substance abuse may include changes in groups of friends, withdrawal and secretiveness, unfinished schoolwork, and excessive lateness for school or sporting events. As soon as they recognize these signs and symptoms, the school and/or medical personnel should consider referral of the athlete to an appropriate mental health expert.

Once the suspicion of substance abuse is raised, appropriate referral for treatment is mandatory. In a school or university setting, there often are programs established by the administrations that may include a guidance counselor to offer the first step of an appropriate referral for substance abuse. If the suspicion is raised by a trainer or team physician, this avenue of referral would be the first logical step. Many educational facilities have policies and procedures in place that review in student handbooks the appropriate mechanism for making such a referral. Outside the academic realm, sources of referral include the local chapters of Alcoholics Anonymous or the National Substance Abuse Council. These agencies have a wide variety of services available to both adults

and students and provide counseling and intervention programs. The essential step for the primary care medical provider is to recognize the possibility of substance abuse and make an appropriate referral to a medical professional who is capable of treating the problem.

PREVENTION

Perhaps the most important step in the prevention of substance abuse among athletes is to recognize that it does exist. Hence the most important strategy is education. Administration, coaches, and parents should address the possibilities of substance abuse in both preseason gatherings and team meetings for school-age athletes. Specifically, parents need to be educated and involved in the process. Among athletes at the collegiate and professional levels, addressing the issues of substance abuse must be done in open team-level forums.

Team sports should have specific team policies regarding substance abuse among team members. Again, the most important aspect is an open discussion of the possibilities of substance abuse. One strategy for decreasing the opportunity for substance abuse can be for parent or booster club groups to provide post game parties for athletes and their families in a safe, controlled environment, so that they can celebrate without excesses of drugs or alcohol.

Probably the most effective program for the prevention of substance abuse is a clear statement, reemphasized periodically, of team policies regarding substance abuse. These policies are to be adhered to not only by the team members but by the coaching staff as well, since coaches and trainers often are positive role models for student athletes.

CONCLUSION

The best program for prevention of substance abuse among athletes is an open and direct discussion of the problems and tendencies that lead to drug abuse, a consistent review of policies and procedures, and an understanding by the team members that drug and alcohol abuse simply will not be tolerated. For athletes in whom substance abuse is suspected, early referral to an appropriate medical professional is essential for successful treatment.

REFERENCES

1. Dolan EF Jr: *Drugs in Sports,* New York, 1986, Franklin Watts.
2. Lukas SE: *Steroids,* Springfield, NJ, 1994, Enslow Publishers.
3. National Parents Resource Institute for Drug Education: *The downfall of sports and drugs,* Capitol Heights, MO, 1988, National Audiovisual Center (videotape).
4. Yesalis CE: *Anabolic steroids in sports and exercise,* Champaign, Ill, 1993, Human Kinetics.

CHAPTER 36

INFECTIOUS DISEASES

David C. Helfgott

Exercise has an integral role in the maintenance of our society's health and well-being. Mainly because of the salutary effects of exercise on the cardiovascular system, as well as its role in weight reduction and enhancing muscle strength and tone, athletes are considered "healthier" than the population who do not exercise. Also, participation in athletics requires a degree of strength and endurance that persons with acute and chronic diseases do not typically possess. However, acute infections are common in everyday life to both the healthy and the sick. Therefore issues such as susceptibility to infection during exercise training and the effects of acute infection on training and physical performance are of special concern to the athlete. Athletes also are exposed to certain contagious diseases simply by their close proximity to each other. Infections may be transmitted via skin contact, respiratory secretions, and other body fluids. The fear of contracting contagious diseases and minimizing the risk of doing so also are important issues to athletes.

EFFECTS OF EXERCISE ON IMMUNE CELLS AND MEDIATORS

Several studies examining the effects of exercise and athletic training on the body's natural defenses against infection have been performed. These investigations mostly focus on changes in the number and function of the cells and mediators of the immune system. In assessing the conclusions from these studies, it is important to note that the subjects are mostly males and that their level of fitness within and across studies varies greatly. In addition, the intensity and duration of the exercises employed vary significantly across studies.

Polymorphonuclear leukocyte concentration rises immediately after exercise.[1,17,21,22,34,52,56,59,65] This increase is short-lived; granulocyte numbers return to baseline values within 45 minutes.[17,52] Foster et al demonstrated that the less fit the participant and the more intense the exer-

cise, the higher the degree of granulocyte increase.[22] Two to four hours after intense exercise, there is a second rise in the concentration of polymorphonuclear leukocytes.[31,52] The increase in granulocyte concentration has been attributed to several factors, including hemoconcentration, catecholamine release resulting in demargination of leukocytes, and cortisol release resulting in demargination and subsequent delayed remargination of white blood cells.[58] However, a few studies refute the premise that granulocyte concentrations increase after exercise. Hanson and Flaherty[32] reported no change in granulocytes in athletes after a 13–km run, and Gray et al noted no change in this leukocyte subset after anaerobic exercise.[27]

In addition to number, granulocyte function after exercise has been studied. Schaefer et al demonstrated that elastase, a product of polymorphonuclear leukocyte degranulation, increased 16% in male subjects after a 2000–m jog and increased almost four-fold after a 10,000–m jog.[56] Lewicki et al found that neutrophil adherence and bactericidal activity decreased in well-trained cyclists but not in untrained males after maximal exercise.[43] In addition, resting measurements of neutrophil adherence were lower in trained than in untrained subjects, and the phagocytic activity of neutrophils increased after exercise in untrained males but did not change after exercise in the well-trained cyclists.[43]

Many studies demonstrate that total lymphocytes increase immediately after exercise,[1,5,17,18,27,34,52,59,67] but other studies report absolute numbers of lymphocytes unchanged[20,33,65] or decreased[16,31] when measured after exercise. Analysis of lymphocyte subpopulations reveals similar discrepancies among published reports. Most demonstrate numbers of B lymphocytes increasing after exercise,[5,27,34,40,62,67] though others refute this.[17,33] Similarly, numbers of T lymphocytes appear to mostly increase,[5,17,27,32,34,40,52,67] however, as a percentage of total lymphocytes, they appear to decrease.[17,27,40,67] Natural killer (NK) cells, another lymphocyte subset, seem to have an important role in recognizing malignant cells, as well as in antiviral immunity,[51] and there are conflicting data regarding changes in their number after exercise. Deuster et al described an increase in NK cell number, and as a percentage of total lymphocytes, after maximal treadmill exercise;[17] and Hoffman-Goetz demonstrated that after significant exercise the number of NK cells rises, then falls to below baseline within 2 hours and returns to baseline within 24 hours.[37] However, Haq et al measured a decrease in the concentration of NK cells, and as a percentage of total lymphocytes, in subjects after a 42–km marathon.[33]

Studies of lymphocyte function are equally inconclusive. Lymphocyte transformation in response to antigenic stimulation *in vitro* has been shown to decrease[21,34] and increase[56,59] after exercise. Cytokines, the mediators released from mononuclear leukocytes that affect a myriad of metabolic and immune functions, have been measured after exercise. Serum "endogenous pyrogen" (interleukin-1 plus other inflammatory cytokines) activity increased immediately after moderate bicycle exercise,[10] and interleukin-1 activity after antigenic stimulation of peripheral blood mononuclear cells *in vitro* increased in marathon runners after a race.[65] The effect of exercise on other cytokines also has been studied.[30] NK cell activity was found to decrease after maximal exercise and remain depressed compared to baseline for almost one day.[7]

Serum immunoglobulins appear to change little after exercise,[19] however, several groups have noted changes in secretory IgA concentrations in saliva with training as well as after exercise. Tomasi et al found that salivary IgA levels in United States National cross-country skiers were lower than in controls and that marathon skiing lowered their salivary IgA levels even more.[63] In well-trained cyclists, there was no difference in salivary IgA levels compared to controls; however, these levels significantly fell after two hours of cycling.[44]

EFFECTS OF EXERCISE ON SUSCEPTIBILITY TO INFECTION

Despite well-documented, albeit sometimes contradictory, alterations in immune mechanisms with exercise and training, the correlation between these changes and susceptibility to infection is unclear. The transient perturbations in immune cell number and function that occur immediately after exercise and return to baseline within hours are unlikely to have long-term clinical consequences. However, whether or not one's "resistance" to infection can be affected for a short time by exercise, and whether or not conditioning results in more chronic changes in resting state immunity, remain open to investigation.

In a study of the incidence of upper respiratory tract infections in marathoners, one third of the runners reported such symptoms within two weeks after a race, compared with 15% of age-matched controls.[49] The symptoms lasted more than three days in 80% of the marathoners, however, these symptoms were self-reported and were not documented by medical personnel. Nieman[47] studied marathoners during training for the Los Angeles marathon and found that those who ran at least 60 miles weekly reported twice as many upper respiratory tract infections as those who ran less than 20 miles a week. Compared to the runners who did not run in the marathon but were similarly trained, those that completed the marathon reported six times as many upper respiratory tract infections. On the other hand, Nieman[48] had previously reported a trend toward fewer infectious episodes in runners training for a half-marathon compared to runners training for shorter 5-km or 10-km races. The stress of training and competition may contribute to susceptibility to infection, since persons with greater psychologic stress have been shown to be more likely to develop upper respiratory tract infections when challenged with intranasal aerosolized virus.[14]

There are other data to suggest that athletes may have increased susceptibility to infection and that exercise may worsen active viral infection. In several college outbreaks of viral meningitis (which occurs most frequently in autumn), the attack rate for the college football team was much higher than the general student attack rate.[45] In two of these outbreaks, although several athletes required hospitalization, there were no hospitalizations in the infected nonathletes. In one outbreak, the longer the athletes continued heavy exercise, the longer they remained symptomatic. In a poliomyelitis outbreak at a boarding school in 1973, all of the infected students were athletes.[66]

Ongoing physical activity despite acute illness also has been reported to exacerbate the course of poliomyelitis in several studies,[38,54,55] and monkeys exercised during incubation for poliomyelitis developed worse paralysis than did nonexercised animals.[42] Similarly, murine studies demonstrated that coxsackievirus myocarditis was more severe and was associated with increased mortality in exercised versus nonexercised mice.[25,39,50,62] With regard to bacterial infections studied, Cannon and Kluger showed that exercise training improved the survival rate in rats subsequently infected with *Salmonella typhimurium*,[11] but Friman and colleagues demonstrated that rats with tularemia fared worse if they were subsequently exercised.[24]

EFFECTS OF INFECTION ON ATHLETIC PERFORMANCE

Several studies demonstrate that infection decreases athletic performance capacity. Subjects experimentally infected with plasma from a patient harboring the virus that causes sandfly fever had diminished muscle strength and exercise endurance during fever.[15] Similar observations have been made during pyrogen-induced fever[28] and malaria in humans.[36] Friman's group[23] tested muscle strength in patients with viral diseases just after illness, as well as in healthy controls who were put to bed rest for one week and then similarly tested. Muscle strength was significantly decreased after illness compared to strength 4 months later in the subjects, whereas no change was seen in the control group between initial and subsequent testing. Bengtsson[2] also demonstrated that exercise capacity was diminished during convalescence from acute infection.

INFECTIONS COMMON IN ATHLETES

Transmission of contagious diseases is facilitated in athletes by their contact with each other and the environment (dirt, locker room floors, swimming pools) in the course of training and competition, as well as by teammates sharing beverages and towels. Most of the infections that are more common to athletes than the nonathletic population are therefore dermatologic; however, isolated outbreaks of systemic illnesses among teammates have been reported.

There have been several outbreaks of viral meningitis on college campuses, between August and October, which have involved a disproportionate number of football players.[45] Sharing water from common cups or a water bucket was documented as a cause of increased transmission among football players at two of the campuses, and, presumably, similar factors and close contact among teammates facilitated viral transmission in the other teams. At the College of the Holy Cross, 93% of the football team became infected with viral hepatitis in 1969.[46] This outbreak, which involved only football players, was linked to an infected water supply used to irrigate the practice field and provide drinking water at the field.

Swimmer's Ear (Otitis Externa)

Otitis externa is a common infection involving the external auditory canal, which results from exposure to fresh water or swimming pools. Repeated exposure may result in desquamation of the epithelium of the external ear canal, with subsequent infection of this abnormal skin. Symptoms and signs include itching in the ear, pain in the ear exacerbated by pulling on the pinna, and redness and swelling, sometimes with purulence, involving the external canal. The most common organism that causes this infection is *Pseudomonas aeruginosa*, although other bacteria may be etiologic. Treatment should be with topical antibiotic drops, which include neomycin and polymyxin B; systemic antibiotics usually are unnecessary.

Impetigo

Impetigo is a bacterial infection of the epidermis caused by *Streptococcus pyogenes* and much less commonly by *Staphylococcus aureus*, which presents itself as vesiculopustular lesions that rupture and form thick, yellow crusts.[61] This infection is easily communicable and is transmitted in swimming pools, by direct contact, and by sharing towels and athletic equipment. Swimmers and wrestlers are therefore especially susceptible.[3] Diagnosis is made by gram stain and/or culture of the vesicle fluid or base of a crusted lesion. Treatment should be with an anti-Streptococcal systemic antibiotic such as penicillin, clindamycin, or erythromycin, which is superior to topical treatment for this infection. In rare cases acute glomerulonephritis may occur secondary to impetigo. Athletes should not participate in sports activities until the lesions have completely healed.

Folliculitis

Folliculitis is characterized by small, erythematous papulopustular lesions originating within hair follicles. *Staphylococcus aureus* is usually the etiologic organism, however folliculitis from swimming pools, whirlpools, and hot tubs is caused by *Pseudomonas aeruginosa*. Outbreaks from these exposures occur when pH and chlorine levels are inadequate. Swimming pools should be maintained at a pH of 7.2 to 8.2 with chlorine levels at 0.4 to 1.0 mg/L; and hot tubs should have chlorine levels of 2.0 to 5.0 mg/L to prevent outbreaks of pseudomonas folliculitis.[41] Antibiotics are usually unnecessary because the folliculitis is typically self-limited.

Furunculosis

Furuncles are abscesses caused by *Staphylococcus aureus* that arise at the site of hair follicles, usually preceded by folliculitis. A furuncle begins as a tender, erythematous nodule that becomes fluctuant and usually spontaneously drains purulent material.[61] Sometimes clinical drainage is necessary, but usually the application of warm soaks results in spontaneous drainage. If a surrounding cellulitis is present, systemic antibiotic therapy with an anti-Staphylococcal penicillin, clindamycin, or erythromycin should be used. Some individuals develop recurrent furunculosis for unknown reasons; attempts at control and prevention with multiple systemic and topical antibiotics as well as meticulous skin and clothing care have had limited success. An outbreak of furunculosis occurred among basketball and football players at a Kentucky high school in 1986–1987; the risk of infection was higher in players who had a skin injury and in players who had skin exposure to other players with furuncles.[60]

Herpes Gladiatorum (Herpes Simplex)

Herpes simplex is a viral infection transmitted by direct contact with infected skin lesions, which occur as vesicles on an erythematous base. Herpes simplex typically appears on the face and genitalia, however lesions can occur anywhere that affected skin is contacted. Several days after vesicle formation the lesions break and become crusted, before disappearing in about a week. Herpes gladiatorum describes this infection in wrestlers, since they are the athletes most commonly affected by herpes simplex virus because of the constant skin contact between competitors. The initial infection may be associated with fever, malaise, and headache. Recurrences can be triggered by physical or emotional stress. Diagnosis is made by recognizing the clusters of typical lesions and by the revealing of multinucleated giant cells by Tzanck preparation of the base of a lesion. Although the lesions are self-limited, treatment with acyclovir can shorten the time of viral shedding and of visible lesions by a day or two. For individuals with frequent recurrences, prophylaxis with acyclovir (400 mg twice daily) has been demonstrated to significantly decrease their number of outbreaks.[53] Athletes with herpes simplex infection should not participate in contact sports while lesions are present.

Molluscum Contagiosum

Molluscum contagiosum is a viral infection transmitted by skin-to-skin or fomite-to-skin contact.[3] The characteristic lesions are multiple flesh-colored umbilicated papules that are most commonly found on the trunk, thigh, or groin areas. Characteristic appearance or skin biopsy is required for diagnosis; the lesions will resolve spontaneously, but treatment is accomplished by curettage or destruction of the skin lesions. Athletes with these lesions should not participate in contact sports.

Cutaneous Warts

Warts are hyperkeratotic papules of the epithelium caused by papillomaviruses. Athletes are more susceptible to warts because these viruses are more likely to invade at sites of calluses.[57] Plantar warts occur on the plantar aspect of the feet, and pressure causes the lesions to be flatter than common warts. Common warts are exophytic and occur mostly on the hands and fingers.[6] The virus is inoculated via direct skin contact or via fomites such as floors and equipment. The incubation period from exposure to development of a cutaneous wart is about 6 months.[57] Although spontaneous resolution of warts typically occurs, they can be present for years.

Superficial Fungal Infections

Superficial fungal infections of the skin are usually caused by the dermatophytes *Trichophyton rubrum* and *Trichophyton mentagrophytes*. These organisms are the etiologic agents in athlete's foot (tinea pedis) and jock itch (tinea cruris), which are the most common dermatophytoses of athletes. Infection is facilitated by increased moisture from sweat in these areas and is acquired on locker room floors and from towels and clothing harboring the fungus. Infection can spread from foot to groin as a person towels off or dresses. Tinea pedis has pruritic and sometimes painful scaling or blisters, usually in the webs of the toes, and can lead to onychomycosis (nail tinea). Tinea cruris occurs in the groin and on the upper thighs and produces pruritic, erythematous, scaling patches. Treatment is with topical antifungal agents; terbinafine twice daily for one week is probably the most efficacious.[4] Prevention is most effective and consists of using only clean, dry towels and clothing, protective footwear in the locker room, and putting on socks before underclothing and trousers. Onychomycosis is extremely difficult to treat, requiring a prolonged course of systemic antifungal therapy. The imidazoles, fluconazole and itraconazole, recently have been proven to be relatively safe and effective in treating onychomycosis, however hepatic toxicity may limit their use in some patients.

Other fungi also may cause dermatophytoses in athletes. Ringworm, or tinea corporis, is characterized by annular erythematous lesions mostly on the back, shoulders, and neck,[57] and is caused by *T. rubrum, T. mentagrophytes*, or *T. tonsurans*. Tinea corporis gladiatorum refers to this infection in wrestlers, in whom several outbreaks have been documented.[13] Tinea versicolor occurs typically on the torso and arms of swimmers and is caused by *Malassezia furfur*. The lesions are lightly colored scaling patches that are generally nonpruritic and are treated with 2% selenium sulfide.[3]

THE SPECIAL CASE OF HUMAN IMMUNODEFICIENCY VIRUS

Recent disclosures by several professional athletes that tested positive for human immunodeficiency virus (HIV) have attracted significant attention to issues surrounding the HIV-positive athlete. Athletes have repeated physical contact with teammates and opponents and may sustain a bleeding laceration in the course of competition. Fear of HIV infection has fueled an ongoing debate as to the usefulness and ethical propriety of mandatory HIV testing of athletes.[9]

HIV is transmitted via infected blood and blood products, by sexual exposure, and by perinatal transmission. There has been no documentation that the virus is transmitted by sweat or saliva. In evaluating the risk of HIV transmission for health care workers after occupational exposure, studies support a transmission rate of 0.2% to 0.5% after percutaneous injuries with contaminated devices.[26] For any individual worker, the risk of acquiring HIV after such an injury appears to be related to the volume of blood exposure and the depth of the injury.[12] The risk of transmission to health care workers with mucocutaneous exposure to HIV may be half that of percutaneous injuries, and there have been no reported HIV conversions in health care workers with only intact skin exposure.[35] The likelihood of hepatitis B or C transmission after percutaneous injury is 10 to 100 times as likely as is HIV transmission.[26] Extrapolating these data to possible exposure of an athlete to the blood from an HIV-infected athlete, the likelihood of HIV transmission would seem to be anywhere between 0 and 0.25%. The prevalence of HIV infection in the population depends upon the population studied, but prevalence rates in applicants to the U.S. military between 1985 and 1989 was 0.13%.[8]

Athletes would seem to have a much greater risk of acquiring HIV off the playing venue than on it. Despite this, a report of HIV transmission presumed to be the result of a sports injury has been reported.[64] In this particular case there was bloody wound contact between an HIV-positive and an HIV-negative (one year previously) athlete in a soccer match, and no other explanation could be found to account for the HIV-negative athlete's seroconversion. Prudence dictates that any athlete who suffers a bleeding injury should be removed from competition until the bleeding stops and the wound is appropriately covered.

PREVENTION OF INFECTION IN ATHLETES

Some simple guidelines can minimize the risk of infection in athletes in the course of training and strenuous exercise. Since it is unclear how exercise-caused alterations in immune mechanisms affect the risk of clinical infection, the usual recommendations such as good nutrition, adequate sleep, and efforts to minimize stress may help to reduce the risk of infection. It *is* clear that acute infection compromises athletic performance, and that certain infections may be exacerbated by strenuous exercise; therefore it is wise to avoid such exercise and athletic competition during an acute infection.

Athletes can acquire communicable diseases from each other and the environment. Avoidance of sharing beverages, athletic equipment, and towels, attention to good foot care, and enforcing nonparticipation in contact sports by athletes with communicable skin diseases can minimize transmission of these infections.

Immunizations are important in preventing communicable diseases. After the initial childhood diphtheria-pertussis-tetanus series, diphtheria-tetanus boosters should be administered routinely every ten years, but if a person suffers a wound involving potentially contaminated soil or debris, a tetanus toxoid booster should be given if it has not been administered within five years.[29] Two measles-mumps-rubella vaccinations are required since about 5% of recipients will not respond to the first measles vaccination.[29] The second vaccine is not always given at the recommended 4 to 6 years of age, so athletes should have proof of two vaccinations or evidence of measles immunity. Since they are in such close contact with one another, and because influenza would severely hamper their athletic performance, athletes who participate in winter sports may choose to receive annual influenza vaccinations.

REFERENCES

1. Ahlborg B, Ahlborg G: Exercise leukocytosis with and without beta-adrenergic blockade, *Acta Med Scand* 187:241–246, 1970.
2. Bengtsson E: Working capacity and exercise electrocardiogram in convalescents after acute infectious diseases without cardiac complications, *Acta Med Scand* 154:359–373, 1956.
3. Bergfeld WF: Dermatologic problems in athletes, *Primary Care* 11:151–160, 1984.
4. Bergstresser PR, Elewski B, Hanifin J, et al: Topical terbinafine and clotrimazole in interdigital tinea pedis: A multicenter comparison of cure and relapse rates with 1- and 4-week treatment regimens, *J Am Acad Dermatol* 28:648–651, 1993.
5. Bieger WP, Weiss M, Michel G, Weicker H: Exercise-induced monocytosis and modulation of monocyte function, *Int J Sports Med* 1:30–36, 1980.
6. Bonnez W, Reichman RC: Papillomaviruses. In Mandell GL, Bennett JE, Dolin R, eds: Principles and practice of infectious diseases, ed 4, New York, 1995, Churchill Livingstone.
7. Brahmi Z, Thomas JE, Park M, et al: The effect of acute exercise on natural killer-cell activity of trained and sedentary human subjects, *J Clin Immunol* 5:321–328, 1985.
8. Brundage JF, Burke DS, Gardner LI, et al: Tracking the spread of the HIV infection epidemic among young adults in the United States: Results of the first four years of screening among civilian applicants for U.S. military service, *J Acquir Immune Defic Syndr* 3:1168–1180, 1990.
9. Calabrese LH, Haupt HA, Hartman L: HIV and sports: What is the risk? *Phys Sports Med* 21:173–180, 1993.
10. Cannon JG, Kluger MJ: Endogenous pyrogen activity in human plasma after exercise, *Science* 220:617–619, 1983.
11. Cannon JG, Kluger MJ: Exercise enhances survival rate in mice infected with *Salmonella typhimurium, Proc Soc Exp Biol Med* 175:518–521, 1984.
12. Case-control study of HIV seroconversion in health-care workers after percutaneous exposure to HIV-infected blood: France, United Kingdom, and United States, January 1988-August 1994, *MMWR* 44:929–933, 1995.
13. Cohen BA, Schmidt C: Tineal gladiatorum. *N Engl J Med* 327:820, 1992.
14. Cohen S., Tyrrell DAJ, Smith AP: Psychological stress and susceptibility to the common cold, *N Engl J Med* 325:606–612, 1991.
15. Daniels WL, Sharp DS, Wright JE, et al: Effects of virus infection on physical performance in man, *Military Med* 150:8–14, 1985.
16. Davidson RJL, Robertson JD, Maughan RJ: Haematological changes due to triathalon competition, *Br J Sports Med* 12:159–161, 1986.
17. Deuster PA, Curiale AM, Cowan ML, Finkelman FD: Exercise-induced changes in populations of peripheral blood mononuclear cells, *Med Sci Sports Exer* 20:276–280, 1988.
18. Edwards AJ, Bacon TH, Elms CA, et al: Changes in the populations of lymphoid cells in human peripheral blood following physical exercise, *Clin Exp Immunol* 58:420–427, 1984.
19. Eichner ER: Infection, immunity, and exercise: what to tell patients? *Phys Sports Med* 21:125–135, 1993.
20. Eskola J, Ruuskanen E, Soppi E, et al: Effect of sports stress on lymphocyte transformation and antibody formation, *Clin Exp Immunol* 32:339–345, 1978.
21. Eskola J, Soppi E, Viljanen K, et al: Effect of sport stress on lymphocyte transformation and antibody formation, *Clin Exp Immunol* 32:339–345, 1978.
22. Foster NK, Martyn JB, Rangno RE, et al: Leukocytosis of exercise: role of cardiac output and catecholamines, *J Appl Physiol* 61:2218–2223, 1986.
23. Friman G: Effect of acute infectious disease on isometric muscle strength, *Scand J Clin Lab Invest* 37:303–308, 1977.
24. Friman G, Ilback N-G, Beisel WR, Crawford DJ: Effects of strenuous exercise on *Francisella tularensis* in rats, *J Infec Dis* 5:706–714, 1982.
25. Gatmaitan BG, Chason JL, Lerner AM: Augmentation of the virulence of murine coxsackievirus B-3 myocardiopathy by exercise, *J Exp Med* 131:1121–1136, 1970.
26. Gerberding JL: Management of occupational exposures to blood-borne viruses, *N Engl J Med* 332:444–451, 1995.
27. Gray AB, Smart YC, Telford RD, et al: Anaerobic exercise causes transient changes in leukocyte subsets and IL-2R expression, *Med Sci Sports Exer* 24:1332–1338, 1992.
28. Grimby G: Exercise in man during pyrogen-induced fever, *Scand J Clin Lab Invest* (suppl 67) 14:1–112, 1962.
29. American College of Physicians: Guide for adult immunization, ed 3, Philadelphia, 1994, ACP.
30. Haahr PM, Pedersen BK, Fomsgaard A, et al: Effect of physical exercise on in vitro production of interleukin-1, interleukin-6, tumor necrosis factor-alpha, interleukin-2, and interferon gamma, *Int J Sports Med* 12:223–227, 1991.
31. Hansen JB, Wilsgard L, Osterud B: Biphasic changes in leukocytes induced by strenuous exercise, *Eur J Appl Physiol* 62:157–161, 1991.
32. Hanson PG, Flaherty DK: Immunological responses to training in conditioned runners, *Clin Sci* 60:225–228, 1981.
33. Haq A, Al-Hussein K, Lee J, Al-Seidairy S: Changes in peripheral blood lymphocyte subsets associated with marathon running, *Med Sci Sports Exer* 25:186–190, 1993.
34. Hedfors E, Holm G, Ohnell B: Variations of blood lymphocytes during work studied by cell surface markers, DNA synthesis and cytotoxicity, *Clin Exp Immunol* 24:328–335, 1976.

35. Henderson DK, Fahey BJ, Willy M, et al: Risk for occupational transmission of human immunodeficiency virus type 1 (HIV-1) associated with clinical exposures: a prospective evaluation, *Ann Intern Med* 113:740–746, 1990.

36. Henschel A, Taylor HL, Keys A: Experimental malaria in man. I. Physical deterioration and recovery, *J Clin Invest* 29:52–59, 1950.

37. Hoffman-Goetz L, Simpson JR, Cipp N, et al: Lymphocyte subset responses to repeated submaximal exercise in men, *J Appl Physiol* 68:1069–1074, 1990.

38. Horstmann DM: Acute poliomyelitis: relation of physical activity at the time of onset to the course of the disease, *J Amer Med Assoc* 142:236–241, 1950.

39. Ilback N-G, Fohlman J, Friman G: Exercise in Coxsackie B3 myocarditis: effects on heart lymphocyte subpopulations and the inflammatory reaction, *Am Heart J* 117:1298–1302, 1989.

40. Keast D, Cameron K, Morton AR: Exercise and the immune response, *Sports Med* 5:248–267, 1988.

41. Kramer MH, Herwaldt BL, Craun GF, et al: Surveillance for waterborne-disease outbreaks: United States, 1993–1994, *MMWR* 45(SS-1)1–30, 1996.

42. Levinson SO, Milzer A, Lewin P: *Am J Hygiene* 42:204–213, 1945.

43. Lewicki R, Tchorzewski H, Denys A, et al: Effect of physical exercise on some parameters of immunity in conditioned sportsmen, *Int J Sports Med* 8:309–314, 1987.

44. Mackinnon LT, Chick TW, Van As A, et al: Decreased secretory immunoglobulins following intense endurance exercise, *Sports Training Med Rehab* 1:290–218, 1989.

45. Moore M, Baron RC, Filstein MR, et al: Aseptic meningitis and high school football players: 1978 and 1980, *J Amer Med Assoc* 249:2039–2042, 1983.

46. Morse LJ, Bryan JA, Hurley JP, et al: The Holy Cross college football team hepatitis outbreak, *J Amer Med Assoc* 219:706–708, 1972.

47. Nieman DC, Johanssen LM, Lee JW, et al: Infectious episodes in runners before and after the Los Angeles Marathon, *J Sports Med Phys Fitness* 30:316–328, 1990.

48. Nieman DC, Johanssen LM, Lee JW: Infectious episodes in runners before and after a roadrace, *J Sports Med Phys Fitness* 29:289–296, 1989.

49. Peters EM, Bateman ED: Ultramarathon running and upper respiratory tract infections: an epidemiological survey, *S Afr Med J* 64:582–584, 1983.

50. Reyes MP, Lerner AM: Interferon and neutralizing antibody in sera of exercised mice with coxsackie B-3 myocarditis, *Proc Soc Exp Biol Med* 151:333–338, 1976.

51. Ritz J: The role of natural killer cells in immune surveillance, *N Engl J Med* 320:1748–1749, 1989.

52. Robertson AJ, Ramesar CRB, Potts RC, et al: The effect of strenuous physical exercise on circulating blood lymphocytes and serum cortisol levels, *J Clin Lab Immunol* 5:53–57, 1981.

53. Rooney JF, Straus SE, Mannix ML, et al: Oral acyclovir to suppress frequently recurrent herpes labialis: A double blind, placebo-controlled trial, *Ann Intern Med* 118: 268–272, 1993.

54. Russell WR: Paralytic poliomyelitis: the early symptoms and the effect of physical activity on the course of the disease. *Br Med J* 1:465–471, 1949.

55. Russell WR: The pre-paralytic stage and the effect of physical activity on the severity of paralysis, *Br Med J* 2:1023–1029, 1947.

56. Schaefer RM, Kokot K, Heidland A, Plass R: Jogger's leukocytes (letter), *New Engl J Med* 316:223–224, 1987.

57. Sevier TL: Infectious disease in athletes, *Med Clin N Amer* 78:389–412, 1994.

58. Simon HB: The immunology of exercise: a brief review, *J Amer Med Assoc* 252:2735–2738, 1984.

59. Soppi E, Varjo P, Eskola J, et al: Effect of strenuous physical stress on circulating lymphocyte number and function before and after training, *J Clin Lab Immunol* 8:43–46, 1982.

60. Sosin DM, Gunn RA, Ford WL, et al: An outbreak of furunculosis among high school athletes, *Am J Sports Med* 17:828–832, 1989.

61. Swartz MN: Cellulitis and subcutaneous tissue infections. In Mandell GL, Bennett JE, Dolin R, eds: Principles and practice of infectious diseases, ed 4, New York, 1995, Churchill Livingstone.

62. Tilles JG, Elson SH, Shaka JA, et al: Effects of exercise on coxsackie A-9 myocarditis in adult mice, *Proc Soc Exp Biol Med* 117:777–778, 1964.

63. Tomasi TB, Trudeau FB, Czerwinski D, et al: Immune parameters in athletes before and after strenuous exercise, *J Clin Immunol* 2:173–178, 1982.

64. Torre D, Sampietro C, Ferraro G, et al: Transmission of HIV-1 infection during sports injury (letter), *Lancet* 335:1105, 1990.

65. Weight LM, Alexander D, Jacobs P: Strenuous exercise: analagous to the acute phase response? *Clin Sci* 81:677–683, 1991.

66. Weinstein L: Poliomyelitis—a persistent problem, *N Engl J Med* 288:370–372, 1973.

67. Yu DTY, Clements J, Pearson CM: Effect of corticosteroids on exercise-induced lymphocytosis, *Clin Exp Immunol* 28:326–331, 1977.

CHAPTER 37

SPORTS PSYCHOLOGY

Ulla Kristiina Laakso

RECOGNITION OF THE PROBLEM

Comprehensive medical care for athletic patients today must incorporate the psychologic as well as the physical aspects of management. Approaching the patient and athlete as a whole has given rise to an entirely new field called "Sports Psychology." Although the field has experienced a tremendous growth in the past 15 years, it is still afforded little attention in the standard psychiatry and psychology textbooks and even in the sports medicine texts. The fact that people are concerned about their psychologic as well as their physical well-being is reflected in the veritable explosion of self-help, fitness, and self-improvement books and manuals, along with the appearance of workshops, seminars, and various support organizations. In fact, the need to "keep fit" has spawned an entirely new kind of social interaction. Social lives often revolve around various sports, recreational, and fitness activities. The rapidly growing phenomenon of health and fitness clubs, running clubs, biking and skiing clubs, and other sports-related social groups has, in turn, had a ripple effect in the economy in terms of fitness gear, clothing, and other related paraphernalia. Sports-related injuries that cause absence from work also have an impact on the economic environment.

Coaches, trainers, and teachers all have become increasingly familiar with the importance of psychologic training of athletes to enhance their performances and maximize their achievements. Virtually all professional, and many college, teams routinely employ the services of a sports psychologist for consultation on a regular basis. Most players have some familiarity with specific psychologic techniques and strategies to enhance their performances. These are various forms of "psyching up" for a particular event. They range from forms of ritualistic behavior such as wearing the same "lucky" pair of socks, to a more logical type of behavior like eating a specific kind of meal before performing. Beneath the surface of these fairly benign mannerisms and activities one finds that these actions are well rooted in the field of sports psychology.

Coaches have been using psychologic motivation for decades, for example, in the use of "pep talks." This type of psychologic motivation is used to enable athletes to increase their concentration, enhance their reflexes, and focus their attention. It also helps to alleviate and displace anxiety and nervousness prior to the sporting event. It helps to put the athlete in the proper mood for participation and optimizes his performance. The coaching staff and players use psychologic techniques such as self-talk, imagery, and cognitive restructuring. These same motivators that enhance athletic performance can be adapted and applied to the rehabilitation process following an injury.

It may be conceded that most athletes who are injured, including recreational and elite professionals, may recover without any need for formal psychologic intervention. However, as the stakes for achievement in sports grow higher and higher in terms of social implication and commercial worth, every avenue must be pursued to ensure satisfactory clinical outcomes. Even an orthopedic surgeon performing reconstructive hip and knee arthroplasty is often asked by more active patients whether or not they may continue their jogging, tennis, and even skiing or bowling after their reconstructive surgery. Although these may not be primary medical concerns, the patients still want to preserve as highly active a lifestyle as possible.

THE SPORTS, HEALTH, AND FITNESS EXPLOSION

Decades of epidemiologic research on how lifestyle factors affect the morbidity of chronic illnesses paved the way to the current exercise and fitness boom. Work begun in the 1950s at the American Health Foundation and by fitness pioneers such as Nathan Pritikin at the Pritikin Longevity Institute led to more public awareness of the benefits of physical fitness. It emphasized the benefits of regular exercise on cardiovascular disease, weight reduction, cancer, and even in lowering cholesterol. Exercise became an important adjunct to smoking cessation and therefore has had a role in the prevention of smoking-related cancers. Exercise also has had a beneficial effect on diabetic patients and those with arthritis and other diseases.

The benefits of exercise affect not only our physical being but also our mental and emotional state. Today every kind of stress reduction program invariably includes some form of exercise. These range from vigorous running to simple meditation, yoga, and breathing exercises. Because there are more people exercising, there has been an increase in sports-related injuries. This has caused an acute awareness of how to prevent these injuries, in the form of adequate warm-up and significant physical, mental, and academic preparation for a sport.

Exercise stimulates secretion of naturally produced hormones called endorphins that have a euphoric effect at moderate levels. Oversecretion has been implicated in so-called exercise addiction, in which the act of exercise itself becomes the dominant part of a person's life. In the same way that the primary care physician has always been the traditional person to whom the family could go for advice, the practitioner has once again become the storehouse for information on this very important part of patients' lives. This physician often is called upon to give recommendations for exercise planning, injury prevention, weight reduction, and for an overall program of physical fitness including the physiologic and psychologic aspects. To this end, the practitioner must be prepared to intervene psychologically on the patients' behalf. The injured recreational athlete, like the professional one, may require a flexible, safe, and alternative exercise plan while he is recovering, to boost his morale and provide continuity in his exercise regime. This is euphemistically referred to as "something for his head." Although the physician's main attention may be on treating the injury, the discontinuation of exercise routines can have a significant negative consequence for the patient's emotional and psychologic condition.

The field of sports psychology has become a subdiscipline of the broader field of psychology and has evolved into an academic discipline as well. Through the ever-growing body of publications and conferences, information reaches a wide and varied audience. There has been a rapid proliferation of books dealing with the subject of Sports Psychology. "Performance enhancement" as it applies to different sports is the main focus of these books. Sports psychologists have correlated certain personality traits with varying degrees of athletic success and motivation. Also, certain character features have been shown to be not compatible with sustained satisfactory athletic performance. There are personality traits that are likely to cause an undesirable amount of anxiety and even lead to depression. This, of course, has a negative impact upon athletic performance. Psychology reveals a direct relationship between mental health and sports performance. We now know that a number of mental skills and cognitive functions can be trained like motor skills. Programs in this specific area are already in place at all levels of competitive sports, including professional teams, college and high school teams, and in Olympic and international competition.

The core area of performance enhancement is anxiety management using cognitive skills. A variety of mental phenomena influence athletic performances. These include arousal, attention, concentration, imagery, and altered states of consciousness. Cognitive skills training uses techniques such as self-talk, thought stopping, mental rehearsal, and imagery. There is an emphasis on the holistic approach to this subject, an example of which is the program developed by the Performance Enhancement Center at the Military Academy at West Point. Various psychologic instruments have been used to measure emotional states and their relationship to athletic performance. Tests such as the Sports Competitive Anxiety Test (SCAT) have found wide acceptance among sports psychology researchers.[21] Anxiety and stress management techniques have employed performance curves related to confidence, stress, and even arousal. In these "inverted U" theories, optimal performance is found at moderate levels of confidence, stress, and arousal. On the other hand, performance is relatively impaired by either too little or too much of these emotions. A variety of techniques stem from this concept, including progressive muscle relaxation, biofeedback, and autogenic training.

THE ROLE OF THE PRIMARY CARE PHYSICIAN

The Good Listener

The benefits of having a "good listener" to hear our troubles and difficulties at times are well known. Primary care physicians should try to develop an empathetic style of listening and communicating with athletes, especially at the time of an injury. The physician needs to carefully screen every statement made by the athlete when he is describing his ailment or injuries, paying attention to the specific language that the patient is using. A determination must be made as to whether the patient is exaggerating or perhaps even minimizing his symptoms. It is not uncommon for the high-performance athlete to want to trivialize his injury "for the good of the team." On the other hand, some athletes might exaggerate the injury for secondary gain, reflecting perhaps a fear of performance or some other psychologic entity. The physician must determine whether or not the patient's description and language is appropriate and whether the emotions associated with the injury are in the expected range.

Interviewing Techniques

Evaluating the athlete's psychologic profile requires some specific skills and techniques. Not only must the physician be an empathetic listener, but body language and eye contact must convey the message that the practitioner is interested in whatever the athlete is going to share with him or her. It is strongly recommended that this encounter be conducted with the physician sitting down, a comfortable distance away from the patient. It has been clearly shown that the patient perceives the interview as lasting longer and being more thorough if the physician is sitting down rather than standing up. It also is important to have as much privacy as possible. Exploration of psychologic issues is a delicate matter. It should not be conducted in a public environment.

The physician needs to convey to the patient that he can be trusted with sensitive psychologic material and that it will not be shared unless the patient consents. Appropriate body language helps facilitate the conveyance of this message. Even a simple nodding of the head or a neutral comment such as "I understand," or "that is normal," can ingratiate the physician to the patient and facilitate communication. This will further enhance the likelihood of the patient's opening up with his true feelings. If the patient perceives the feedback or body language as even mildly critical or judgmental, it is likely to cause him disappointment and thereby shut down the communication between them. It is recommended that the physician ask open-ended questions that cannot be answered merely with a "yes" or a "no." This allows the athlete to reveal more, and it fosters a rapport between the patient and the physician. Using the patient's own words to reframe responses, comments, and questions has proven to be a valuable technique. It reassures the patient that he has indeed been heard.

It must be remembered that many athletes are perfectionists and therefore they may regard their health situations very negatively and pessimistically. When explaining the nature of an injury to his patient, the physician certainly must be honest with the patient but also he should be careful not to take away the hope of recovery when at all possible. To this end, it is helpful to emphasize and reemphasize the treatment possibilities and the progress that the patient has made so far. The injured athlete is likely to welcome the physician's knowledge about some of the psychologic techniques available. The athlete may be hesitant to ask about relaxation training, biofeedback, or meditation if he perceives his physician as being closed-minded. Often the injured athlete welcomes an adjunct therapy from outside the traditional medical venue. Such techniques, when used individually or in combinations, enhance athletic performance and improve the rehabilitation process.

INJURY: PSYCHOLOGIC IMPLICATION AND ATHLETE'S PERCEPTION

Following a serious injury, athletes will typically experience three phases of reaction. During the initial phase the athlete is likely to express *denial and disbelief*. Denial may be so strong that the athlete is ready to continue to play despite warnings that his injury may worsen. Disbelief may cause the injured patient to seek several professional opinions.

During the second phase the patient exhibits a variety of *negative emotions*. Those likely to surface include anger, anxiety, frustration, depressed mood, insomnia, poor concentration, and disruption of usual activities. These psychologic reactions slow treatment and rehabilitation. The athlete's anxiety and frustration often is more difficult to deal with than the actual injury. During this phase, the physician needs a great deal of patience. The athlete's frustration may impair his ability to listen to professional advice.

The third phase includes *acceptance and adaptation*. During this phase, the injured athlete comes to terms with his injury and its consequences. The physician can help the patient to adjust to the new medical information and find reasons for hope and optimism. Helping the athlete to reach this phase is important in reducing the length of the rehabilitation and recuperation process. Some of the patient's previous activities may be resumed and some goals may be revised. Some of the goals may have to be given up. The physician is required to show compassion, support, and helpfulness.

THE ATHLETE'S PERCEPTION OF INJURY

The primary care physician working with injured athletes will witness a variety of reactions to injuries. Sometimes, an athlete may exhibit lack of concern, indifference, or even detachment to his injury. Further exploration of these observations may show that he is actually relieved at being excused from competitive activities because he fears that his poor performance or losing might result in embarrassment. He also may welcome having the "safe" excuse for further suboptimal performances.

Another athlete may totally catastrophize his injury. He may feel that all is lost, and he may hold rigidly to one single explanation for his injury. There may be paranoid thoughts expressed towards training practices, coaches, team leadership, or even another player. The primary care physician needs to be aware of his kind of maladaptive reaction and poor insight to the injury at hand. If the athlete is unable to view his injury from a more flexible perspective, his psychologic state will be a road block to recovery and rehabilitation. The athlete may decide that his recovery may be "exactly the same" as that of a fellow athlete whose recovery has been suboptimal.

The primary care physician needs to remember that a whole host of other factors influences the rehabilitation process. Medical issues include whether or not the doctor is perceived as open and helpful. The patient may mask pain and physical symptoms. Marital problems and other social problems, as well as low expectation of support from others and lack of religious faith, appear to influence the rehabilitation process. Patients with a history of psychologic problems and a high anxiety level are more likely to have impaired recovery.[19,20] Low ego strengths lead to poor coping skills at the time of injury. These coping skills are put under considerable demands. Patients with a history of substance and alcohol abuse predictably have problems in recovery. The athlete with more concerns of all kinds is vulnerable to slow rehabilitation. Athletes may perceive injury as a punishment or they may read special meaning into the injury. Parental views of health, injury, and overall coping in life can influence, on an unconscious level, the athlete's coping mechanisms.[7]

There is a wide range of ways that athletes can cope with illness and injury. In order to cope effectively with stress, one must make a conscious effort to do so and must seek and obtain help from others. Important parts of the coping mechanism are the ego's unconscious adaptive mechanisms. These include altruism, humor, suppression, anticipation, and sublimation. They are called mature defenses. A less mature defense, such as denial, is also common in severe circumstances.

WARNING SIGNS OF PSYCHOLOGIC IMPAIRMENT

As in the general population, the athlete's signs of psychologic impairment and disturbance can be quite subtle. Often the athlete and his family, as well as his coach and the training staff, may have little suspicion. The skilled observer, however, can sort out some of the cardinal warning signs of psychologic illness, which can respond to intervention. Common types of psychologic disturbances include depression, anxiety, manic-depressive illness, panic disorder, and obsessive-compulsive disorder. It is not uncommon for patients and athletes so affected to question whether or not these symptoms represent "weakness" in their will and character. The physician can help to reassure the patient that these conditions are not rare.

Depression

The physician can assure the athlete that depression can affect anyone at any time, including children and adolescents. Depression can have multiple causes, including genetic patterns. Tendency to have mood disorders does run in families. Illnesses, infections, some medications, and substance abuse also can cause depression.[7] The social and work settings, with interpersonal conflicts, can prompt depressive symptoms. Certainly, personality traits may increase the likelihood of depression. These include being highly self-critical and seeing things as "black or white" or "either-or." Also, individuals that tend to be dependent or passive seem to be more prone to depression.[7]

The physician may observe a wide range of symptoms, including physical complaints for which no physical cause is found. The athlete may complain of sleep disturbances including insomnia, hypersomnia, or early morning awakening with inability to fall back to sleep. There may be complaints of chronic fatigue and lack of usual energy. The athlete may tell about unexplained backaches, headaches, or similar pains. There may be reports of digestive upsets including nausea, indigestion, stomach pain, constipation, or diarrhea. Other symptoms of depression include changes in attitude and behavior. The athlete, his coaching staff, or the physician may observe slowed-down behavior, poor grooming and dress, neglected responsibilities, and irritability. He may report loss of appetite or the opposite, an increased appetite with significant weight gain. He may not be able to concentrate. The athlete may report different emotions and changed perceptions including feelings of emptiness, emotional flatness, or feeling "blue" or "down in the dumps." The patient is likely to report inability to find pleasure in his usual activities. He may experience complete loss of, or a diminished, sexual desire, as well as feelings of hopelessness and helplessness. Feelings of guilt, exaggerated self-blame, and sad ruminations with loss of self-esteem are further symptoms of de-

pression. Preoccupation with death, suicidal thoughts, and suicidal gestures or threats are clear signals of depression.

There are three main types of depression, which sometimes occur in combination. *Dysthymia* is a milder form of depression. It may last for years, so that a person may have forgotten any different mood state. He may describe his "introverted" mood even as a part of his personality. This type of chronic mild depression will prevent the person's achieving his or her full potential. Sometimes a more severe form of depression can be superimposed on dysthymia and then it is called *double depression.* The third, *major depression,* commonly starts rather suddenly, precipitated by a crisis, a change, or a loss. Symptoms usually are severe enough to interfere with work or social functioning. This type of depression may last for a few months or become chronic, lasting even years. A person may have repeated episodes of major depression during his lifetime. The phenomenon of repeated episodes is actually more common than a single episode.

TREATMENT. For depression, as for most illnesses, early intervention works best. Combinations of different methods may be the approach of choice. Psychotherapy, the traditional talking therapy, still remains an important part of the treatment, but alone it may not be adequate so it is often supplemented with drug therapy. The goal of psychotherapy is to understand underlying causes and to map out depressive patterns of thinking. The cognitive-behavioral theorists led by Aaron Beck[13] explain that the depressed person has cognitive dysfunctions regarding himself, others, and the future. For example, a depressed person is likely to view himself as worthless, inadequate, and undesirable. Others, as well as the world in general, are seen as negative, demanding, and defeating. Consequently, the depressed person expects failure and, therefore, punishment. The future is viewed as a continuation of deprivation, suffering, and inevitable failure. Psychotherapy addresses these cognitive-depressive errors and goes further in providing support and help in finding solutions.

Pharmacologic agents most commonly used today in the treatment of depression include fluoxetine (Prozac), sertraline (Zoloft), paroxetine (Paxil), bupropion (Wellbutrin), venlafaxine HCL (Effexor), and nefazodone HCL (Serzone). The older antidepressant classes, which include tricyclic and heterocyclic antidepressants and MAO inhibitors, are less often used by primary care physicians because of their various and complex side effects.

Anxiety Disorders

Although anxiety may be used as a term in the general sense, it actually includes many specific disorders, including generalized anxiety disorder, anxiety disorders caused by general medical conditions, acute stress disorder, panic disorder (with or without agoraphobia), specific phobia, social phobia, obsessive-compulsive disorder, posttraumatic stress disorder, and substance-induced anxiety disorder.

The patient reports anxiety and worry, which he may

have difficulty in controlling. He is likely to complain of restlessness, feeling "on edge," being easily fatigued, feeling irritable, and difficulty in concentrating. He may report muscle tension and sleep disturbances. In acute stress disorder, a person has been exposed to a traumatic event in which he may have experienced or witnessed an episode that involved a serious injury or he himself may have been threatened by death or serious injury. The person's response involves intense fear, helplessness, and horror. This is followed by a subjective sense of numbness—detachment or absence of emotional responsiveness. There may be feelings of "being in a daze," feelings of derealization and depersonalization, and inability to recall important aspects of the trauma. The traumatic event is re-experienced in recurrent images, thoughts, dreams, illusions, flashbacks, and a sense of reliving the experience when reminded of it. There is an avoidance of stimuli that remind the patient of the trauma. Anxiety symptoms as well as hypervigilance and exaggerated startle response are part of the clinical picture. When the symptoms last longer than four weeks, the disorder is called posttraumatic stress disorder.

TREATMENT. Before making a diagnosis of generalized anxiety disorder, a physician needs to rule out medical diagnoses and evaluate the patient for other possible psychiatric conditions. One must of course exclude the normal anxiety state so common before engaging in athletic competition or artistic performance. Antianxiety medications including benzodiazepines can be prescribed on an as-needed basis. They also can be given as a standing dose for a period of time while other psychotherapeutic approaches are implemented. However, physicians need to keep in mind that benzodiazepines may impair alertness and thus negatively affect athletic performance. Buspirone (Buspar) is a nonbenzodiazepine antianxiety drug with a delayed onset of action. It may be a better choice for athletes because it does not share the problems of the benzodiazepines including drowsiness and the possible development of physical dependency during longer periods of use. Beta-adrenergic blocking agents such as propranolol (Inderal) have been used successfully to treat peripheral symptoms of anxiety including rapid heartbeat and tremor. These have been especially effective for performing artists.

Acute stress disorder and posttraumatic stress disorder usually are treated with antidepressant medications. These include serotonin uptake inhibitors like fluoxetine (Prozac) and sertraline (Zoloft), as well as paroxetine (Paxil), bupropion (Wellbutrin), venlafaxine HCL (Effexor), and nefazodone HCL (Serzone). Therapeutic success has been reported with clonidine (Catapres). Sometimes antipsychotic medications like risperidone (Risperdal) or haloperidol (Haldol) are required in the beginning of treatment for a short period of time. Other effective medications include the tricyclics imipramine (Tofranil) and amitriptyline (Elavil), as well as the monoamine oxidase inhibitor phenelzine (Nardil). These drugs should be given only by an experienced psychopharmacologist under close supervision. Drug interactions and serious, even fatal, side effects have been reported and observed with MAO inhibitors.

Within the broad category of anxiety disorders lies the phobic conditions, including social phobias and specific-object phobias. The treatment of phobias can be behavioral as well as pharmacologic. In the behavioral technique called systematic desensitization, the patient is exposed to the anxiety-provoking stimuli, starting from the least frightening and proceeding to the most frightening. Furthermore, a relaxation technique is taught to be practiced when the patient confronts anxiety-causing stimuli. In another technique called flooding, the patient is exposed to the phobic stimulus either in actuality or through imagination for as long as he can tolerate the fear or as long as it takes not to feel the fear any longer. Stage fright has been successfully treated with beta-adrenergic antagonists such as propranolol (Inderal). These agents are usually simpler to use than phenelzine (Nardil). The potentially serious side effects of Nardil have been mentioned above.

Manic-Depressive Illness (Bipolar I Disorder)

Manic-depressive illness is characterized by prominent mood swings, mania and depression, interspersed with normal moods. Symptoms of the "highs" include feelings of exaggerated competence, very much increased energy, and hyperactivity. The patient may report no need for sleep and reduced appetite. There are likely to be racing thoughts, rapid speech, irritability, grandiose feelings, and lack of good judgment often leading to recklessness in different areas of behavior. The length of these different phases can be variable. Obviously, this disorder must be differentiated from the normal elation of victory and the also-normal sadness and frustration of athletic defeat. Manic-depressive illness may occur in more subtle forms. Once diagnosed, it is best treated by a mental health specialist familiar with the range of mood stabilizers and anti-depressant medications.

Bipolar I disorder is likely to run in families, and it appears to be equally common in men and women.[7] The first episode appearing in men is usually a manic episode, whereas in women the first episode is more likely to be a major depressive episode. This disorder is a recurrent disorder and nearly all individuals (more than 90%) who experience a manic episode will have more episodes in the future. Also, the intervals between episodes tend to become shorter with time.

Another form of cyclical mood disorders is bipolar II disorder, which is characterized by recurrent major depressive episodes with milder hypomanic episodes. It also has been shown to have a clear familial pattern of inheritance. Cyclothymic disorder is a chronic cyclical mood disturbance that includes episodes of hypomania and mild depression. People with these cyclical mood disorders feel as if they are on an emotional roller coaster. At one moment they feel on top of the world, with overconfidence and multiple plans, yet during the depressive periods they feel worthless and hopeless, with little interest in the future.

TREATMENT. Lithium remains the prototypical drug for bipolar disorder. However, other mood stabilizers are available including carbamazepine (Tegretol), valproic acid (Depakene), clonazepam (Klonopin), verapamil (Calan), and clonidine (Catapres).

Successful treatment of cyclical mood disorders requires the detailed exploration of the patient's psychiatric history, proper medical workup, good knowledge of psychopharmacology, and ongoing monitoring for potential side effects. Certain mood stabilizers, such as lithium, require ongoing blood level monitoring on a routine basis. Overall, the treatment of bipolar disorders is more complicated than that of depression. Often physicians need to combine several psychotropic drugs to obtain a satisfactory result. Other biologic treatments include electroconvulsive therapy (ECT), light therapy, and manipulation of sleep cycles.

Panic Disorder

In panic disorder the essential features are unexpected panic attacks followed by persistent worries of having another attack. The patient reports palpitations, pounding heart, sweating, trembling, or shaking. There may be a sensation of shortness of breath or a feeling of smothering or choking, accompanied by chest pain or discomfort, nausea, abdominal distress, dizziness, unsteadiness, and lightheadedness. There may be feelings of unreality or feelings of being detached from oneself. Fear of losing control or "going crazy" or fear of dying are the symptoms that are likely to bring the patient to an emergency room or to seek immediate medical attention. Panic disorders may be accompanied by "agoraphobia," in which the patient avoids being in places or situations from which egress or escape may be difficult or embarrassing, or in which help may not be available. These locations and situations typically include being outside the home alone, being in a crowd, on a bridge, or traveling in a bus, train, or car. This disorder commonly leads the patient to seek multiple medical consultations, including visits to the emergency room, cardiologists, pulmonary specialists, and gastroenterologists. Despite repeated assurance and many medical tests, the patient is likely to remain uncertain and frightened. Panic disorder may occur infrequently or up to several times a day. It may occur as either a full-blown panic attack or as a "limited-symptom" attack.

Panic disorder has been known to evolve into a major depressive episode and even to suicide ideation.[5] Athletes commonly experience "panic" before an upcoming sporting event, but these episodes are usually short-lived and disappear once the competition has begun.

TREATMENT. The principal treatment approach to panic disorder is pharmacologic. Serotonin uptake inhibitors, for example fluoxetine (Prozac), starting in small doses, has become a common treatment. Tricyclic antidepressants (TCAs) and monoamine oxidase inhibitors (MAOIs) have also been shown to be effective. The benzodiazepine alprazolam (Xanax) in sufficient and in multiple daily doses is effective treatment. Most psychopharmacologists prefer using benzodiazepines only in the initial phase of treatment until the antidepressant medications take effect. It must be stressed that because of the variable reactions of patients to the initial drug dosage and because of serious drug interactions and side effects, the primary care physician might consider referral to a specialist once the diagnosis of panic disorder is made.

Obsessive-Compulsive Disorder (OCD)

Obsessive-compulsive disorder was previously thought to be rather rare. However, recent community studies have estimated a lifetime prevalence of approximately 2.5%.[7] This is a disorder that is likely to cause embarrassment and shame. The patient usually tries to hide or camouflage his unwanted and senseless behaviors. The essential features of obsessive-compulsive disorder are recurrent obsessions or compulsions that cause marked distress and significant impairment. Obsessions are recurrent and persistent thoughts, impulses, or images that are experienced at some time during the disturbance. They are intrusive and inappropriate and cause anxiety and distress. These are not simply excessive worries about real-life problems. The patient attempts to ignore or neutralize the impulses with some other thoughts or actions. He recognizes that the obsessional thoughts, impulses, or images are a product of his own mind. Compulsions are repetitive behaviors (for example, hand washing, tapping, ritualistic touching) or mental acts (for example, praying, counting, repeating words silently) that the person feels driven to perform in response to an obsession or according to a rule that must be applied rigidly. These behaviors or mental acts are aimed at preventing or reducing distress or preventing some dreaded event or situation. This type of behavior can be seen in a mild form with various types of ritualistic behavior in sports, for example, wearing the same pair of socks during a successful period of competition, or the ritualistic movements before batting the ball in baseball or shooting a free throw in basketball. In this context the behaviors should not be considered senseless, but rather a means of increasing concentration on the athletic task at hand. These behaviors, of course, require no treatment.

Obsessive-compulsive patients may demonstrate biologic abnormalities in an electroencephalogram (EEG), sleep EEG, computed tomography of the brain (CT scan), and neuroendocrine studies.[16] These abnormalities may be found in the left hemisphere. Some of the neurologic abnormalities are similar to those found in depression.

TREATMENT. The most common treatment approach today to obsessive-compulsive disorder is the combination of behavioral therapy with effective psychopharmacologic agents. The drug clomipramine (Anafranil) was the first truly effective agent in the treatment of OCD. Newer agents include serotonin uptake inhibitors such as fluoxetine (Prozac) and fluvoxamine (Luvox). The serotonin uptake inhibitors have surpassed clomipramine in popularity because of their more favorable side-effect profile. Behavioral techniques can be effective, however they require a high degree of motivation and are quite time consuming.

SPECIAL CIRCUMSTANCES

The Child Athlete

The injured child athlete requires special attention. Serious competitive child athletes often miss many conventional childhood activities. Emotional and physical challenges of the relentless training routine are likely to take their toll. Peer relationships are particularly important during childhood in the development of healthy self-esteem, and the child athlete commonly feels isolated and lonely. Rebellion against strict athletic discipline surfaces from time to time. The child athlete may be reminded of significant family sacrifices and of the big changes in family life caused by his rigorous training routines and travel requirements. A child's athletic career may require temporary parental separation and consequently cause feelings of guilt. He is constantly reminded of high stakes, including potential future financial rewards. Child athletes also may be reminded of the financial sacrifices and investment by his parents in his present and future athletic career.

When dealing with the injured child athlete, the physician often is called upon to treat the emotional consequences to the entire family. At times, parents may disagree with each other about the treatment recommendations and proposed rehabilitation plan, and the injury can lead to a true family crisis. In these instances, the rehabilitation process can be enhanced by consultation with an experienced child therapist or family therapy counselor. Rehabilitation of the child athlete requires perseverance and always some form of family counseling. Overanxious and overinvolved parents may, at times, impair the rehabilitation process and confuse decision making. A child whose parents are only living for their child's achievements and victories is bound to feel anger and resentment. These emotions can lead to feelings of guilt if the athlete thinks he is not living up to parental expectations. His harsh training may be experienced as physical punishment and as a demand to please others. There is always a danger of ambitious parents projecting their own values onto the athletic youngster. Parents may need to be reminded that their child's chronological age may not reflect his psychologic readiness to take on adult pressures.

The Female Athlete

The successful female athlete by necessity must have characteristics that traditionally have been considered masculine. These include intense determination to win, aggressiveness, and competitiveness that often encompass the "killer instinct." The male athlete's masculinity is fortified by winning, whereas the female athlete is likely to feel torn between athletic achievement and societal expectations of femininity. Frequently the female athlete experiences depression while struggling with these conflicting issues. Some gender traits, like emotionality, may be cultural, while others, like aggression, may have a biological basis. Some studies have looked into the relationship between the female athlete and the onset of menstrual function.[22] Menarche in the United States occurs at an average of 12.5 to 12.8 years of age. Studies of elite competitive athletes and dancers have shown a clear delay in menarche of up to two or more years.[16] The cause of this is multifactorial. The onset of menarche is dependent upon the maturation of the hypothalamus-pituitary-ovarian axis. Furthermore, a minimum requirement of body fat is needed for the onset of menarche. It appears that 17% body fat is a minimum

prerequisite. If a rigorous training regimen decreases the percentage of body fat to below a critical level, menarche may be delayed. Another important factor in delaying menarche seems to be the impaired nutritional state prompted by repeated dieting and starvation efforts starting at an early age. It is obvious that rigorous athletic training may have a profound effect on body systems.

Although eating disorders are generally associated with females, more recent knowledge shows a significant involvement of males as well. Given the rigors of training and the need to be at "optimal" body weight for strength and endurance, the athlete, male or female, is at high risk for these disorders. The intense preoccupation with weight in our culture affects as many as 5% to 10% of adolescent girls and young women.[15] These figures are far higher in the athletic population.

For many young people, dieting and excessive exercising becomes a way of coping with life and a distraction from the stress with which they cannot cope. Our western culture emphasizes *thinness* as a virtue. This is reflected in our fashions and in our advertising. Many women, and increasing numbers of men, consequently feel that thinness is the outward manifestation of overall success in life. The need for thinness among athletes, especially figure skaters, gymnasts, and ballet dancers, increases their risk for eating disorders.

ANOREXIA NERVOSA (ANOREXIA). Biologic factors have been implicated in the syndrome of anorexia.[10] Researchers believe that severe dieting leads to emotional stress and also to various hormonal imbalances present in anorexia. It is felt, however, that these may be the result of anorexia rather than the cause of it. A number of psychologic factors have been associated with anorexia. Fear of growing up and fear of adult responsibilities often are seen at the root of the problem. The goal of being "the best" is shared by many people with eating disorders as well as by athletes. It is agreed that food is not the central issue, however, anorectics feel that control over food intake represents control over various aspects of their lives. Eating disorders become a way to express control over life, which may seem to be out of control.

Often this disorder is seen as rebellion against parental standards that may be too high. Typically, anorexic patients have not had major problems before adolescence. The patient is often described as a model child with good behavior at home and at school. Usually dieting begins with a change such as puberty or leaving home for school or college. Dieting makes the patient feel good about herself, and it creates a feeling of control in a changing environment. Little by little, food and fat phobia becomes the most important thing in life.

Often exhausting exercise is added. There may be rigid rules regarding exercise schedule and intensity. Food intake may be contingent upon having completed a self-imposed daily exercise regimen.

BULIMIA NERVOSA (BULIMIA). Bulimia nervosa is characterized by binge eating and purging. During a binge, a person may consume large quantities of food in a short period of time. The purging part of bulimia is getting rid of the food consumed during a binge. This includes self-induced vomiting, periods of starvation, severe diets, the use of laxatives, diuretics, and vigorous exercise. Typically, people with bulimia are young women for whom weight, dieting, and food in general are extremely important. They are usually of normal weight but harbor a distorted image of their bodies. They are likely to be perfectionists like anorectics and they are usually also high achievers.[9,12,24] Bulimic women are overly concerned about their looks and body weight and about being accepted by their peers. They feel out of control with eating and emotionally insecure and lonely. They usually lack confidence and have low self-esteem. Commonly, they feel inadequate in their relationships. A person with bulimia uses food to cope with conflicting emotions. Often the binge-purge cycle starts with diet as a means to improve self-esteem. Dieting, however, is likely to lead to craving for rich, highly caloric foods. This is likely to cause overeating as a response to attempts to starve. Overeating also is used to alleviate anxiety, anger, frustrations, loneliness, and a variety of complicating emotions. Guilt and fear following binges and purging are discovered as an ideal solution against gaining weight. Soon a person is feeling out of control and locked in a vicious binge-purge cycle. Often substance abuse and depression accompany bulimia nervosa.[17]

Increasing numbers of bulimics fall into a category of *exercise* bulimics. In this category, rigorous and rigid exercise has replaced purging. There is a preoccupation with maintenance of frequently exaggerated exercise routines. Social pursuits and relationships become secondary to exercise. Often exercise bulimics describe a feeling that they are "addicted" to exercise and that they feel out of control if they are prevented from exercising or have to cut short a planned exercise routine. This represents a pathological entity that, on the surface, is difficult to distinguish from the "dedicated exercise enthusiast." A red flag should rise when the patient displays inordinate resistance to discontinuing her exercise regimen while an injury heals. If the patient appears highly agitated, anxious, and irrational when given medical advice to suspend exercise even after repeated explanations, the diagnosis of exercise bulimia should be considered.

People with eating disorders suffer several hormonal consequences. Anorectics can suffer from impaired menstruation, or even complete lack of menstruation (amenorrhea). This has serious consequences in the patient's hormonal status, thereby leading to osteoporosis, abnormally low body temperature, anemia, and even cardiac arrhythmias.[14,23] Repeated binging and purging can cause erosion of dental enamel, esophagitis, and even gastric rupture. Depression is a very common consequence of eating disorders. The feeling of poor control over weight and the sensation of hunger often lead to hopelessness, helplessness and despair. The treating physician must be vigilant for these depressive symptoms. Suicidal ideation is an issue among the eating-disorder population.

To say that the treatment of eating disorders is difficult would be an understatement. Because eating disorders are often chronic serious illnesses, it is advisable to seek help or second opinions from mental health professionals specializing in the treatment of eating disorders. Hospitalization of a patient is usually reserved for immediately life-threatening consequences of anorexia or bulimia or active suicidal preoccupations. The younger the patient, the more important is the need for family therapy, to bring about a successful outcome. The mortality rate of eating disorders may exceed 10% because of medical complications and suicides.[7]

Suicidal ideation always warrants psychiatric referral. Complex psychologic factors have been found to contribute to the development of eating disorders, including family enmeshment, rigidity, overprotectiveness, inability to express emotions, and overemphasis on achievements in life. Although advances in psychopharmacology have added to the drug armamentarium of treating depression and urges to binge and purge, individual psychotherapy combined with family therapy remains the cornerstone of the treatment of eating disorders. Early intervention with a specialist is recommended to improve clinical outcomes. Sadly, many adolescents with eating disorders have harbored symptoms for several years before coming for treatment, and denial of the problem is quite common in families of such a patient. Problems centering around food and eating can appear from generation to generation in families.[11]

DRUGS, SUBSTANCE ABUSE, AND THE ATHLETE

The athlete, like any other member of society, is subject to the temptations and weaknesses that we all face everyday. The athlete may feel especially pressured because his performance is constantly being judged and evaluated. In addition to being subject to the influence of alcohol and "recreational" drugs, the athlete may become interested in drugs that can enhance his athletic performance, such as anabolic steroids and stimulants. Drug use and substance abuse by athletes, in its worst form, has led to fatalities caused by either the ordinary type of "overdose" or unique medical conditions such as coronary artery spasm, ventricular arrhythmia, myocardial infarctions, and sudden death syndrome. Certain drugs also can precipitate seizures as well as cerebrovascular accidents. The widespread use of drugs has led to random and routine checking during athletic sporting events.

Cocaine

The initial effect of cocaine is usually pleasurable. It produces a feeling of well-being and increased self-confidence. There is also a sense of being more energetic and more alert. The psychologic effects of cocaine include euphoria, increased libido, enhanced vigor, feelings of grandiosity, aggression, and manic excitement. These qualities have led athletes to use it in the competitive setting for performance enhancement. It has been reported that up to 18% of high school athletes have used cocaine at least once.[4] The use of this drug among elite female athletes is reported at up to 3%,[8] and it has been implicated as one of the most popularly used illegal drugs in the National Football League.

Cocaine use and abuse has become an increasingly common and serious problem in the United States. The alkaloid drug found in the leaves of the coca plant is readily available and can be purchased in an inexpensive form called "crack" cocaine. This highly concentrated chemically reconstituted cocaine is extremely addictive. It is commonly smoked and its effects are felt in less than ten seconds. Cocaine stimulates the central nervous system. It dilates the pupils and elevates the heart rate, blood pressure, respiratory rate, and body temperature. Cocaine abuse can lead to several organic syndromes including intoxication, withdrawal, delirium, and delusional disorders. Inhalation of cocaine on a chronic basis can cause serious ulceration of the mucous membranes of the nasal passages. Cocaine intoxication is likely to result in paranoid ideations, increased libido, ringing in the ears, and bizarre syndromes of behavior such as organizing common objects into pairs.[7] Disorientation and violent behavior are seen in states of delirium. Another unusual phenomenon, called formication, can occur, leading a person to believe that insects or animals are crawling under his skin. Cocaine is appealing for athletes because of its initial pleasurable effect and the production of a feeling of well-being and increased self-confidence with a sense of being more alert and energetic.

Alcohol

Athletes are no more immune to the appeal of alcohol than is the general population of the United States. Approximately three quarters of adult Americans consume some form of alcohol on a regular basis.[3] It remains the main substance abused by teenagers. It is not surprising that alcohol use has been reported by up to 88% of the athletic population.[1] The physician must maintain a high index of suspicion for alcohol abuse. It is extremely difficult to detect, especially when an athlete's performance is not impaired. It should be remembered that alcohol experimentation begins at an early age. The use of alcohol is attractive to adolescents and teenagers because it creates feelings of independence and rebellion, causing excitement for them and helping in their quest to overcome nervousness.

Alcohol abuse can lead to various chemical presentations including intoxication, idiosyncratic intoxication, uncomplicated alcohol withdrawal, withdrawal delirium, hallucinations, amnestic disorder, and even dementia. These syndromes present unique characteristic symptoms and diagnostic criteria.

In alcohol intoxication we may see familiar adaptational behavioral changes, including disinhibition, aggression, labile moods, poor judgment, and impairments in occupational or social functioning. All of these characteristics may be accompanied by slurred speech, lack of coordination, unsteady gait, nystagmus, and flushed facies. In uncomplicated alcohol withdrawal, there is a coarse tremor of the hands, tongue, or eyelids. This follows cessation or reduction of heavy and prolonged consumption. Further signs include nausea or vomiting, weakness and malaise, tachycardia, sweating, and increased blood pressure. There is anxiety, irritability and perhaps transient hallucinations or illusions, insomnia, and headaches. The

more serious clinical picture is alcohol withdrawal delirium, more commonly known as delirium tremens (DTs). The syndrome includes delirium, autonomic hyperactivity, visual or tactile hallucinations, sensory disturbances, lethargy, and hyperexcitability.[7] It usually follows within seven days after a person stops or reduces the alcohol intake. This serious condition requires symptomatic treatment, hydration, bed rest and benzodiazepines such as chlordiazepoxide (Librium). In alcohol hallucinosis, the patient develops auditory or visual hallucinations usually within 48 hours after cessation or reduction of heavy drinking. These persistent and vivid hallucinations occur in a clear sensorium. This disorder can occur in any age group in people who are dependent upon alcohol.

Marijuana

Marijuana is one of the oldest drugs, used throughout centuries as an intoxicant as well as a medical adjunct. This drug is called by its various slang names including pot, grass, smoke, reefer, weed, tea, and Mary Jane. The drug itself comes from the hemp plant *Cannabis sativa*, containing over 400 chemical substances. The cannabis is primarily responsible for the mind-altering properties of marijuana. Its major psychoactive component is tetrahydrocannabinol, known as THC. Cannabis can be smoked in a pipe, rolled into a cigarette as a tobacco-like mixture, or even eaten, as in a baked cookie. Marijuana affects the cardiovascular as well as the central nervous system. In low doses, it can temporarily relieve tension, boredom, or depression and produce a feeling of relaxation and well-being as well as sleepiness. In higher doses, it leads to impairment of short-term memory, altered state of time, and distortions in sensorium. There also may be loss of balance and difficulties in following a logical thought process. When marijuana is used in high doses, it can lead to unpleasant feelings of anxiety, panic reactions, and paranoia. There is also a loss of insight, and psychotic symptoms with hallucinations and delusions may occur. When habitual users stop using the drug, they are likely to experience anxiety and depression as withdrawal phenomena.

Marijuana poses a particular hazard to the young athlete because it interferes with normal maturation and the process of growing up. Youngsters involved with marijuana are likely to have a limited range of interests and show apathy and indifference in their pursuits of athletic goals. An athlete who is at one time enthusiastic about his sport but then rapidly becomes apathetic should be evaluated for the possibility of marijuana use. Although marijuana is frequently considered rather innocuous, it has been implicated as possibly leading to exposure to a variety of drugs, each stronger and "better." Research has shown that marijuana smoke contains large amounts of carcinogens.[13] Reportedly, 36% of athletes have experimented with this drug and an estimated 3% use it on a regular basis.[37]

Anabolic Steroids

These drugs, developed in the 1930s, are compounds related to the male sex hormone testosterone. The enticement of taking steroids for athletes is that they induce a rapid increase in muscle mass, bulk, and strength. The perils of steroid use in sports are now well publicized and should be quite familiar to players, trainers, coaches, and administrators. The psychologic effects for both sexes include aggressive behavior, personality changes, combativeness, mood swings, depression, and even psychoses. The use of anabolic steroids has been universally banned and prohibited in competitive sports except for the treatment of specific diseases. Detoxification or withdrawal after long-term steroid use may be quite difficult medically and psychologically.

If substance abuse in any form is suspected or confirmed, a thorough psychiatric evaluation is indicated. There are many psychiatric conditions that predispose the patient to substance abuse since unpleasant mood states are easily medicated with alcohol or drugs. Early intervention is crucial, before the athlete and his performance suffer or he has adopted further well-entrenched drug habits.

REFERRAL TO A MENTAL HEALTH SPECIALIST: ABSOLUTE INDICATIONS

The athlete's career can be severely curtailed or impaired by untreated emotional problems. The pressure of vigorous training, demanding competition, and constant judging and evaluating can prompt any preexisting emotional problem to the surface. A number of emotional problems may warrant referral immediately to a mental health professional or at least a consultation or second opinion.

Severe depression or a depression that has not adequately responded to the prescribed antidepressant treatment regimen requires psychiatric referral. The same applies to panic disorder and obsessive-compulsive disorder. The latter two disorders usually respond very well to medications; however, the patient needs a practitioner with firm expertise and familiarity with these conditions and the drugs that are used to treat them. Untreated cases will lead to loss of athletic careers and may even cause suicidal preoccupation.

Suicidal ideations always warrant psychiatric referral. Most suicide victims suffer from mental illness, mood disorders, alcoholism, or drug abuse. Suicide is more common among males than females. Risk factors for suicide include depression and bipolar disorders, as well as schizophrenia, anxiety disorders, alcoholism, drug abuse, personality disorders, and also serious physical illnesses. Suicide is much more common in patients who have previously attempted it.[2]

Psychosis is another absolute indication for referral. In the psychotic state, the patient commonly expresses paranoid ideation and delusions, and many have hallucinatory experiences. This state can be dangerous and may eventually lead to violent behavior, homicide, or suicide. This requires immediate specialized professional treatment. Substance abuse is also an absolute indication for referral to a specialist in that field or a mental health specialist.

Patients must be referred to a mental health specialist if the initial treatment plan proposed and implemented by the primary care physician has not successfully treated the problem. Lack of response to a medication regimen is also an indication for referral. When in doubt, a second opinion to determine whether or not a mental disorder is present is always warranted. Needless to say, if a patient or a family member requests a mental health evaluation, it should be considered quite seriously.

Another situation in which referral to a mental health specialist is essential is when a devastating, potentially career-ending injury occurs to an elite athlete. In these situations early intervention will help the athlete put his injury in perspective and allow him to prepare for the future.

It should also be remembered that in today's health care society, especially within the guidelines of managed care, the "mental health specialist" can be a physician, psychologist, psychiatric nurse, or social worker.

SUPPORT GROUPS

Patients with psychiatric diagnoses, such as substance abuse, anorexia, bulimia, depression, obsessive-compulsive disorder, and others, can benefit from interaction with peers who share the same diagnosis. Once the diagnosis is established, in addition to the routine psychologic care given to a patient, referral to an appropriate support group should be made. To obtain the most up-to-date pertinent information on these support groups, inquiries should be made to the local branch of the American Psychiatric Association or the American Psychological Association.

SUMMARY

The primary care physician treating athletes and sports injuries should remember three important steps in maintaining proper mental health: (1) preventive vigilance, (2) early diagnosis, and (3) early intervention. Implementing these recommendations will enhance successful clinical outcomes.

REFERENCES

1. Anderson WA, McKeag DB: *The substance use and abuse habits of college student athletes,* Mission, Kan, 1995, NCAA.
2. Beck H, Resnick LP, Letieri DJ, eds: *The prediction of suicide,* Bowie, Md, 1974, Charles Press.
3. Calahan D, Cisin IH, Crossley HM: *American drinking practices: A national survey of behavior and attitudes,* Monograph No. 6, New Brunswick, NJ, 1969, Rutgers University Center of Alcohol Studies.
4. Clement DB: Drug use survey: Results and conclusions, *Phys Sports Med* 11(9):64-67, 1983.
5. Conyell W, Noyes R Jr, Howe JD: Mortality among outpatients with anxiety disorders, *Am J Psychiatry* 143:508-510, 1983.
6. Dale E, Gerlach D, Willhote A: Menstrual dysfunction in distance runners, *Obstet and Gynecol* 54:47, 1979.
7. *Diagnostic and statistical manual of mental disorders,* ed 4 (*DSM-IV*), Washington, DC, 1994, American Psychiatric Association.
8. Duda M: Female athletes: Targets for drug abuse, *Phys Sports Med* 14:142-146, 1986.
9. Fairborn CG: A cognitive behavioral approach to the treatment of bulimia, *Psychological Medicine* 11:707-711, 1988.

10. Fava M, Copeland PM, Schweigher V, Herzog DB: Neurochemical abnormalities of anorexia nervosa and bulimia nervosa, *Am J Psychiatry* 146(9):963-971, 1989.
11. Garshon ES, et al: Anorexia nervosa and major affective disorders associated in families (preliminary report). In Guze SR, Earls FJ, Barnett JE, eds: *Childhood psychopathology and development,* New York, 1983, Raven Press.
12. Garver DM, Garfinkel PE, Schwartz D, Thompson M: Cultural expectation of thinness in women, *Psychological Reports* 47:483-491, 1980.
13. Grinspon L: Marijuana, *The Harvard Medical School Mental Health Letter* 4(5), 1987.
14. Halmi KA, Falk JR: Common psychological changes in anorexia nervosa, *Intl J of Eating Dis* 1:16-27, 1981.
15. Brownell KD, Foreyt JP: *Handbook of eating disorders,* New York, 1986, Basic Books.
16. Jennke MA: Obsessive compulsive disorder, *Comp Psych* 24:99, 1983.
17. Johnson C, Larson R: Bulimia: An analysis of moods and behavior, *Psychosomatic Medicine* 44:341-351, 1982.
18. Kaplan HI, Sadock BJ: *Comprehensive textbook of psychiatry,* ed 5, vol 1, Baltimore, Md, 1989, Williams and Wilkins.
19. Kerr G, Cairns L: The relationship of selected psychosocial factors to athletic injury occurrence, *J Sport Ex Phys* 10(2):167-173, 1988.
20. Kerr G, Fowley B: The relationship between psychological factors and sports injuries, *Sports Med* 6, 1988.
21. Martens R: Sport competition anxiety test, Champaign, Ill, 1977, Human Kinetics.
22. Menstrual changes in athletes: A round table, *Phys Sports Med* 9(11):99-112, 1981.
23. Silverman JA: Anorexia nervosa: Clinical and metabolic observations, *Intl J of Eating Disorders* 2:159-166, 1983.
24. Vigersy RA: *Anorexia Nervosa,* New York, 1977, Raven Press.

BIBLIOGRAPHY

Anderson WA, Albrect RR, McKeag DB, et al: A national survey of alcohol and drug use by college athletes, *Phys Sports Med* 19 (2):91-104, 1991.

Anthony J: Psychologic aspects of exercise, *Clin Sports Medicine* 10:171-180, 1991.

Ashe AR: *A hard road to glory,* New York, 1988, Warner Books.

Athletic training and sports medicine, ed 2, Rosemont, Ill, 1991, American Academy of Orthopaedic Surgeons.

Birrer R, ed., *Sports medicine for the primary care physician,* ed 2, Boca Raton, Fla, 1994, CBC Press.

Borgen JS, Corbin CB: Eating disorders among female athletes, *Phys Sports Med* 15(2):19, 1987.

Clark K, Parr R, eds: *Evaluation and management of eating disorders: Anorexia, bulimia and obesity,* Champaign, Ill, 1988, Life Enhancement Publications.

Diagnostic and statistical manual of mental disorders, ed 4, (*DSM-IV*), Washington, DC. 1994, American Psychiatric Association.

Dick RW: Eating disorders in NCAA athletes, *Athletic Training* 26:136, 1991.

Haupt HA: Drugs in athletes, *Clin Sports Med* 8(3)561-582, 1989.

Jonas AP, Sickles PT, Lombardo JA: Substance Abuse, *Clinic Sports Med* April, 1992.

Kaplan HI, Sodock BJ, eds: Comprehensive handbook of psychiatry, ed 5, Baltimore, MD, 1989, Williams and Wilkins.

Kuipers H, Kazer H: Overtraining in elite athletes, *Sports Med* 6:79-92, 1988.

Loucks AB, Vartukaitis J, Cameran JL, and others: The reproductive system and exercise in women, *Med Sci Sports Exerc* 24(65):S288-S293, 1992.

Lynch GA: Athletic injuries and the practicing sports psychologist: Practical guidelines for assisting athletes, *Sports Psychologist* 2:161-1678, 1988.

Marks IM: *Fears, phobias and rituals,* Oxford, 1987, Oxford University Press.

Mellion MB: *Sports medicine secrets,* Philadelphia, 1994, Hanley and Belfus.

Micheli LJ: Sports wise: An essential guide for young athletes, parents and coaches, Boston, 1990, Houghton Mifflin.

Olgilvie BC: The child athlete: Psychological implications of participation in sport, *Am Acad Polit Soc Sci* 445:47-58, 1979.

Paglin JS: Anxiety and sports performance, *Exerc Sports Sci Rev* 1992, 20:243-274.

Raglin JS: Exercise and mental health: Beneficial and detrimental effects, *Sports Med* 9(6):323-329, 1990.

Shanegold MM, Mirkin G, eds: *Women and exercise: Physiology and sports medicine,* Philadelphia, 1988, F.A. Davis.

Silva JM, Weinberg RS: *Psychological foundation of sports,* Champaign, Ill, 1984, Human Kinetics.

Sinoll FL, Smith RE: Psychology of the young athlete—stress related maladies and remedial approaches, *Ped Clinics North Am* 37:1021-1046, 1990.

Smith AM, Scotts G, Wiese DM: The psychological effects of sports injuries, *Sports Med* 9(6):352-369.

Tutko T, Tosi U: *Sports psychiatry,* New York, 1976, Tacher/Pedigree Books.

Weinberg RS: *The mental advantage,* Champaign, Ill, 1988, Leisure Press.

Wells C: *Women, sports and performance,* Champaign, Ill, 1991, Human Kinetics.

Wichmann S, Markin DR: Exercise excess: Treating patients addicted to fitness, *Phys Sports Med* 20:193-200, 1992.

Wiese DM, Weiss MR: Psychological rehabilitation and physical injury: Implications for the sports medicine team, *Sports Psychology,* 1:318-330, 1987.

Williams JM: *Applied sports psychology—personal growth to peak performance,* ed 2, 1993, Mayfield.

Walker SH: *Winning: The psychology of competition,* New York, 1986, WW Norton.

CHAPTER 38

SPORT FOR THE ATHLETE WITH A PHYSICAL DISABILITY

Michael S. Ferrara
Kenneth J. Richter
Susan M. Kaschalk

Sport opportunities for athletes with disabilities have been increasing every year. The nature and type of injuries that occur to these athletes are not as widely known as are those for athletes without disabilities. The purpose of this chapter is to inform the reader of sporting opportunities available, specific medical concerns, and typical injury patterns among athletes with physical and sensory disabilities.

Sport is of immense therapeutic value; its object is to optimize physical and psychologic equilibrium for the enjoyment of daily life.[20] An estimated 2 to 3 million athletes with physical and mental disabilities are involved annually in athletic competition within the United States.[4,11] A large number of people with disabilities also are involved in recreational and leisure sports. The range of activities for athletes with disabilities includes a variety of recreational and competitive activities. Sporting opportunities are available even for those with the most involved disabilities.

BENEFITS OF SPORT

Knowledgeable physicians realize the need for physical activity for disabled people.[7] They recognize that persons with disabilities can successfully participate and compete in a wide range of recreational and competitive pursuits, from bocci to swimming to marathons. Sometimes a person with a disability can participate with his able-bodied peers in interscholastic and intercollegiate activities. Depending on the activity, slight modification may be needed in equipment for the person to participate. On the other hand, unique sporting events such as goal ball for the blind have been established and are increasing (Fig. 38-1).

Active participation in sports is generally associated with positive outcomes for people with disabilities.[49,50] It has been reported that involvement in competitive sports has a beneficial impact on disabled athletes' social interactions at home, helps them make friends, and improves their physical coordination, strength, endurance, and self-confidence.[25]

SCOPE OF SPORTS FOR THE DISABLED

The sports movement for athletes with disabilities started with military programs after World War II. The large number of injured veterans used sport and related activities for rehabilitation. By the 1970s, involvement in sports grew to the extent that exercise and fitness programs were available to most people with disabilities. The Amateur Sports Act of 1978 detailed the rights for United States amateur athletes, including athletes with disabilities. This law was a major step forward in legitimizing sports for the disabled.

In 1979, the United States Olympic Committee (USOC) formed a category (Group E) under its authority for athletes with disabilities. The category now comprises Wheelchair Sports, USA (WSUSA); the American Athletic Association for the Deaf (AAAD); the United States Cerebral Palsy Athletic Association (USCPAA); the Special Olympics International (SOI); Disabled Sports USA (DSUSA); the Dwarf Athletic Association of America (DAAA); and the United States Association for Blind Athletes (USABA). There also are two organizations that serve a large number of athletes but are not members of the USOC. They are the National Wheelchair Basketball Association (NWBA) and the United States Les Autres Sports Association (USLASA). The box on p. 599 lists the addresses for each organization.

Currently, the USOC Group E category has been re-

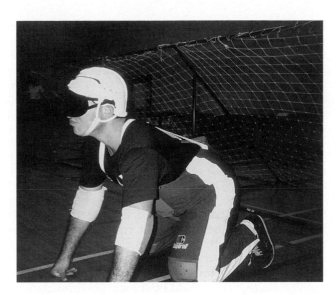

Fig. 38-1. Athlete with a visual impairment playing golf ball.

SPORT ORGANIZATIONS FOR ATHLETES WITH DISABILITIES

American Athlete Association for the Deaf (AAAD)
1052 Darling Street
Odgen, UT 84403

Disabled Sports USA (DSUSA)
1145 19th Street NW
Suite 717
Washington, DC 20036

Dwarf Athletic Association of America (DAAA)
3725 West Holmes
Lansing, MI 48910

National Wheelchair Basketball Association (NWBA)
1100 Elythe Boulevard
Charlotte, NC 28203

Special Olympics International (SOI)
1350 New York Avenue NW
Suite 500
Washington, DC 20005

United States Association for Blind Athletes (USABA)
33 North Institute Street
Brown Hall, Suite 015
Colorado Springs, CO 80903

United States Cerebral Palsy Athletic Association (USCPAA)
200 Harrison Avenue
Newport, RI 02840

United States Les Autres Sports Association (USLASA)
1101 Post Oak Boulevard
Suite 9–486
Houston, TX 77056

Wheelchair Sports, U.S.A. (WSUSA)
3595 E Fountain Boulevard
Suite L–1
Colorado Springs, CO 80910

named the Disabled in Sports Organizations (DSO). The Committee on Sports for the Disabled (COSD) was developed by the USOC for all DSOs. The membership of the committee includes two individuals from each organization and one of each must be disabled. At least 20% of the COSD membership must comprise active athletes. The AAAD, WSUSA, DSUSA, USABA, USCPAA, DAAA, and SOI are current members of the COSD.

The international sports movement for the disabled moved toward cross-disability, or integrated, competition in 1992 with the formation of the International Paralympic Committee (IPC). The current philosophy of the IPC is cross-disability, or sport-specific, competition, although there are concerns with this approach.[46] It would allow athletes with all types of disabilities to compete against each other in major competitions, that is, World Championships and Paralympics. The 1992 Paralympics in Barcelona, Spain, was the largest sports event for athletes with disabilities, with almost 4000 competitors and 1.4 million spectators. The Paralympics, which has become the second largest multisport event in the world (second only to the summer Olympics), were held in Atlanta, Georgia, in 1996 shortly after the conclusion of the Olympic Games (Fig. 38-2).

PHYSICIAN CONCERNS

Physicians sometimes fail to promote sport as a life option for people with disabilities because they lack awareness of sport opportunities available. There is a broad spectrum of sport options, ranging from casual recreational events to elite sports such as the Paralympics. Having a disability, even a severe disability, does not prevent a person from being an athlete even on the world class, elite level.

Opportunities for competition are available through various classification schemes.[48] Classification has long been an acceptable practice in the sports world for the able-bodied, with systems of gender, weight, age, and performance. Classification in sport is even more essential for the disabled.[48] Although there are some controversies regarding classification,[29,46] it should provide athletes with disabilities an equitable starting point for athletic competition. It should not be assumed that an individual with an above-the-knee amputation cannot be a world class high jumper, or a person with spastic athetoid quadriplegia caused by cerebral palsy cannot be a world class swimmer.

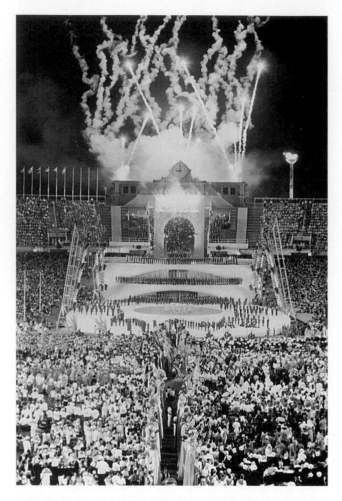

Fig. 38-2. Opening ceremonies, Paralympics, Barcelona, 1992.

Frequently, we have observed problems with precompetition evaluation. Physicians may make one of two mistakes. They may assume that sport for athletes with a disability cannot be very rigorous or risky, therefore anyone can compete. The other error is assuming that athletes with a disability are so fragile that any competition should be prohibited. Sports physicians must evaluate potential athletes objectively and fairly to accurately apprise them of any potential risks yet not needlessly prevent them from participating. To do this effectively requires knowledge both of sport medicine and of the specific disability that an individual may have.

PHARMACOLOGIC CONCERNS

It is not unusual for athletes with disabilities to use prescribed medications as muscle relaxants or for asthma, seizures, hyperactivity, and other conditions. Physicians and involved allied medical personnel should be aware of the indications, contraindications, side effects, and synergistic effect of using multiple medications.

Some athletes may be using antiseizure medicines that are known to have significant cognitive effects and to decrease the attention span of the athlete.[43] There are three drugs commonly used to control seizures. They can

be placed on a continuum based on the severity of their side effects, which range from mild to potentially severe.[43] The usual medications for seizures include phenobarbital, phenytoin, and carbamazepine; and, to a lesser extent, valproic acid is now being used. Carbamazepine may be the preferred medication for disabled athletes,[43] since it may have the fewest side effects and should not adversely affect athletes' performance.

It is very important to stress compliance with a medication's prescribed dosage. Athletes, particularly those involved in national or international travel, may have their usual schedules disrupted and therefore forget to take a medication. An athlete needs to keep a proper blood level of his drug to maintain desired affects. He should keep the medicine always available, for example, by carrying it on his person while traveling, so that a dose is not missed. Do not adjust or change medications before major competitions or events. This may upset the equilibrium that the athlete has obtained with a particular medication. If a drug must be changed, monitor blood levels and look for physical changes or side effects, such as nystagmus and ataxia with the antiseizure drugs, that may occur from the new medicine.

Physicians need to be aware of an important principle when treating athletes with seizures. In aerobic athletic activities the incidence of seizures usually decreases.[43] As a person exercises aerobically, he/she tends to develop a metabolic acidosis, which can be (incompletely) compensated for only by hyperventilation. This results in a lower hydrogen ion concentration (pH), which tends to stabilize neuromembranes (Fig. 38-3). There are few cases in which an athlete experiences seizure activity during sporting events. If there is a question about seizures occurring, it is possible to do a stress test with EEG to see if there is any seizure activity.[36]

Exercise and Seizures

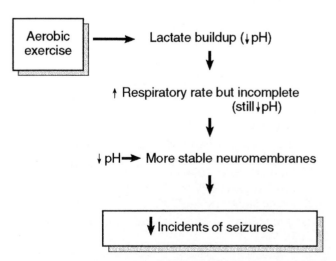

Fig. 38-3. Algorithm of relationship between exercise and incidence of seizure.

A physician evaluating an athlete with seizures for competition may need to be made aware of the impact seizures could have, not only on the athlete but also on fellow competitors. For example, if a cyclist has a seizure while riding in the peloton in a mountain road race, it could cause serious injuries to nearby riders. However, if the athlete is in good seizure control, there is not a high risk. Keep in perspective that physicians are always making this kind of judgment as to whether or not people with seizures can drive a car, which with good control is legally permitted in every state.

With most antiseizure medications there is some cognitive dysfunction. Therefore the athlete will often need to have more time to focus their attention before an athletic competition. The athlete and coach need to be advised of this so that they can incorporate appropriate mental preparation strategies.

TEMPERATURE REGULATION

Exposure to heat and cold may provide unique challenges for athletes with disabilities.[3,41] Some athletes may not be able to tolerate normal environmental conditions as well as can athletes without disabilities. This intolerance is due to decrease in sensory awareness, sympathetic nervous system dysfunction, and a deficient body mechanism for warming and cooling.[1] The problem typically affects the athlete with spinal cord injury, but it also may be prevalent in athletes with disabilities such as cerebral palsy, obesity, and Down syndrome.[39]

HEAT INTOLERANCE

Athletes with spinal cord injuries tend to be more susceptible to heat injuries. Quadriplegics and those with a spinal cord lesion above the eighth thoracic level are particularly vulnerable to heat stress.[8,13,51] These athletes do not sweat or have effective vasodilation below the level of the spinal cord injury, thus there is no effective mechanism for body cooling. Specific drugs (tranquilizers, diuretics, alcohol, sympathomimetics, anticholinergics, and thyroid replacement drugs) may predispose the athlete to problems with heat.[15] Further, athletes with high blood pressure, diabetes, and sweat gland dysfunction may have an increased incidence of heat illness.[39]

Prevention

Given the probability of heat illness for athletes with disabilities, prevention is a major issue. Limit practice and competitive sessions when the temperature is greater than 85°F and the humidity is higher than 70%. High temperature and humidity will not allow efficient cooling of the body through heat dissipation and normal sweating.[3]

All athletes should be encouraged to drink plenty of fluids. The disabled athlete should hydrate the body as much as possible before any event and should consume 1 to 2 cups of water every 10 to 15 minutes during competition or training.[13] Athletes who use a wheelchair should be encouraged to attach a water bottle to the wheelchair while training.

Pay particular attention to athletes with a swallowing disorder. This is sometimes manifested by drooling in an upper motor neuron–type of condition such as cerebral palsy. These athletes may not only have a difficult time taking in fluid, but may also have a significant fluid loss from the saliva. They need to be counseled to drink frequently before they sense any problem, use swallowing strategies, and to monitor the volume and color of their urine output.

The use of shade, light clothing, and hats is recommended. Sunscreens should be applied whenever the athlete will be exposed to the sun for prolonged periods. The athlete with a spinal cord injury may be at an increased risk for sunburn because of decreased sensory awareness.[47] Special attention should be paid to athletes who will be required to remain in the sun for a long time. They should be encouraged to move to a shaded and cooler area before and after competition. Meet organizers should provide tents and other shade to which the athletes can escape from the sun.

HYPOTHERMIA

An athlete's ability to tolerate the cold is based on several factors: level of fitness, percent of body fat, and environmental conditions such as the wind chill factor and wetness. Normal mechanisms for heat production by the body, such as shivering, goose-bump production, and circulatory shunting, may not take place in athletes with a spinal injury. Air temperature around 50° F may produce problems for athletes with quadriplegia.[13,14] However, in water, which has a much higher specific heat, a temperature much below 90° F may be problematic to a quadriplegic. Athletes having prolonged exposure require careful monitoring.[31]

Prevention

Physicians and other allied medical personnel should investigate the athlete's medical history before he participates in winter sports. Prior episodes of hypothermia may predispose the athlete to further problems in a cold environment. Also, certain medications or medical conditions may predispose the athlete to temperature regulation problems in the cold.[31]

Athletes should be encouraged to wear appropriate clothing in cold weather. Cotton and other fabrics that absorb moisture are advised for the inner layers of clothing. Additional layers should be added or deleted to maintain proper body heat. Hats should be worn since a large amount of heat is lost through the head.

All wet clothing should be removed immediately after the exercise session. This will eliminate postexercise chilling. Careful attention should be given to those athletes with communicative or cognitive disorders who may not be able to relate symptoms of hypothermia. Special awareness of environmental conditions also should be considered.

AUTONOMIC DYSREFLEXIA

Autonomic disreflexia (AD) is a condition seen in athletes with a spinal injury at the T6 level or higher with involvement of the splanchnic nerves.[16] The splanchnic nerves control peripheral vascular resistance, which is the primary determinant of blood pressure. AD is a massive sympathetic discharge of the splanchnic nerves with resultant hypertension. There may be a corresponding bradycardia as the baroreceptors cause an increase in vagal output, which can affect the heart rate but is not effective in lowering the blood pressure.[16] The usual cause of AD in over 90% of cases is a distended bladder; in approximately 9%, it is a distended bowel; and other causes can be anything from ingrown toenails to appendicitis, or anything that particularly causes a sacral input.[44]

It appears that AD may be a performance-enhancing technique called "boosting." Athletes with high-level spinal injuries deliberately induce autonomic dysreflexia, which has been shown in the laboratory to improve performance.[6] Athletes need to be cautioned about the risk and dangers,[52] which include death. This technique is banned by the IPC.

Prevention

The chief prevention strategy for autonomic dysreflexia is to make sure that the athlete's bladder and rectum are emptied before he begins physical activity.

Recognition

The symptoms of AD may include sudden hypertension, bradycardia, increased sweating, severe headache, and goose flesh. However, athletes with quadriplegia may not demonstrate bradycardia because of their injured sympathetic nervous system.[16]

Treatment

When autonomic dysreflexia occurs, the athlete should be placed in an upright position to take advantage of orthostatic changes, then the bladder should be drained and, if necessary, the bowel emptied carefully, using lidocaine gel as a lubricant. Approximately 99% of cases are relieved with this treatment. Caution must be used when interpreting the blood pressure because it normally will be low in quadriplegics, with systolic blood pressure less than 100 mm/Hg. The use of drug therapy is rarely indicated. When it is rarely needed, acute antihypertensive agents can be administered; however, one must be careful of rebound/hypotension.

INJURY PATTERNS AMONG ATHLETES WITH DISABILITIES

Several authors[5,28,32] characterized the common injuries suffered by athletes with disabilities. They listed abrasions, contusions, strains, and carpal tunnel syndrome, and described methods for the prevention and care of these injuries.

Health care providers should realize that injuries are to be expected in sports and should be addressed promptly and appropriately. Practitioners should evaluate, treat, and rehabilitate disabled athletes as they would any well-conditioned athlete. An injury may mean a decrease in training and conditioning level, thus a reduction in motivation. The goal of the physician should be to restore strength and function as quickly and safely as possible so that the athlete can resume activity.

GENERAL INJURY INVESTIGATIONS

Sports for the disabled have been considered to place the athlete with a disability at an increased risk of injury.[23] However, researchers have provided documentation for the theory that the percentage of injuries is no higher than for athletes without disabilities.[4,18,30,45] This theory is further substantiated by the Athletes with Disabilities Injury Registry (ADIR), an epidemiologic investigation that determined an injury rate of 7.23 injuries per 1000 athlete exposures for 12 months (Ferrara-unpublished data). This injury rate is within the normative values reported in literature for athletes without disabilities.

Typically, medical professionals treat problems such as minor illnesses, dehydration, and sprains and strains at major competitions for disabled athletes. Richter[45] found that the majority of injuries to athletes with cerebral palsy at the 1988 Paralympics were minor and acute in nature. The shoulder, low back, and knee were the most common injury locations. At the 1990 World Championships and Games for the Disabled held in Assen, Holland, illnesses were the most common injury reported to the US medical staff. Illnesses are not unexpected considering the drastic environmental, diet, stress, and sleep pattern changes that occur from international travel and competition.

In 1989, a cross-disability retrospective injury survey was administered to athletes from the WSUSA, USABA, and USCPAA. For the WSUSA athletes, the highest percentage of injuries were in the upper extremity, with the shoulder accounting for 40% of the total injuries, as seen in Fig. 38-4. The USABA athlete had a high percentage of injuries in the shoulder and leg/ankle complex, as presented in Fig. 38-5. The shoulder, hand/finger, knee, and leg/ankle were the most frequently involved body locations for the USCPAA athlete, as shown in Fig. 38-6. Each disability manifests itself with different effects and demands on the body. Accordingly, a specific injury prevention program, as opposed to a general program, needs to be designed for each organization.

In the following sections, common injuries that are specific to each type of disability are described. Prevention strategies and common methods for the treatment of these injuries will be presented.

WHEELCHAIR ATHLETES

Athletes with disabilities experience injuries that are specific to the demands and risks of their sports. Track, road racing, and basketball have the potential for the highest incidence of injuries. Curtis and Dillon[11] found a relationship between injuries and the number of hours trained per week and age of wheelchair athletes. The participants in the 21- to 30-year-old age group suffered the highest number of injuries of any age group. Ferrara and Davis[18] found that 50% of the injuries in an athletic wheelchair population were strains and muscular injuries of the upper extremity.

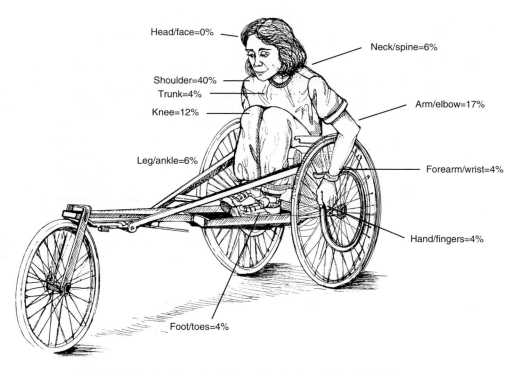

Fig. 38-4. Injury incidence in athlete with spinal cord injury/wheelchair user.

Hand and Finger Injuries

Hand and finger injuries are not uncommon in wheelchair athletes. Since the hands are used continuously for propulsion, blisters of the fingers and thumbs may develop. Thick calluses may form over the first and second digits and the palm of the hand from the repetitive contact with the hand rim. However, the elbow and upper arm are also frequent places where blisters occur.

A wheelchair design change of a drop in the seat height to allow for a lower center of gravity may contribute to more injuries. This decreased seat height places the elbow and upper arm in contact with the wheel, where a friction burn may occur. Blisters of the fingers and hand are a potential problem for infection and painful fissures. Further, fractures of the metacarpal bones and phalanges are possible from falls and colli-

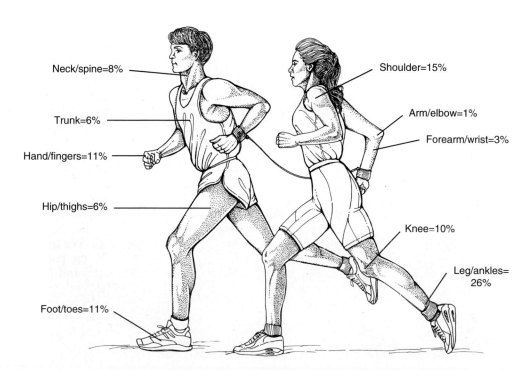

Fig. 38-5. Injury incidence in athlete with a visual impairment.

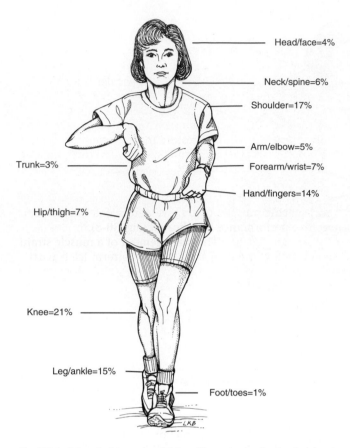

Head/face=4%

Neck/spine=6%

Shoulder=17%

Arm/elbow=5%

Forearm/wrist=7%

Hand/fingers=14%

Trunk=3%

Hip/thigh=7%

Knee=21%

Leg/ankle=15%

Foot/toes=1%

LKB

Fig. 38-6. Injury incidence in athlete with cerebral palsy (ambulatory).

sions with other wheelchairs. Thumb fractures may occur if the digit slips off of the hand rim and gets caught in the spokes of the wheel. Basketball and other such contact activities place the athlete at risk of fracture.

PREVENTION. Prevention of blisters is a matter of protective devices and proper use of the wheelchair. Many wheelchair athletes use specially designed gloves with protective taping in the region of high friction at the point of contact with the hand rim (Fig. 38-7). They also may place protective pads (knee pads, socks, etc.) in the elbow and upper arm region to reduce the potential of injury from the wheel.

The hands and other high-friction areas should be cleaned frequently and calluses filed to reduce skin layers. For any athlete who appears to have numbness and tingling in the hand and fingers, carpal tunnel syndrome should be considered. This can be diagnosed by electromyography (EMG) and mild cases treated with neutral wrist splints.

Shoulder Injuries

Wheelchair propulsion is characterized as a forceful and repetitive motion applied to the hand rim. Researchers have estimated that for some athletes, the hand is in contact with the hand rim for 270°.[19] This repeated stress is on the athlete's anterior chest and shoulder muscles. The use of the arm to propel the wheelchair requires repetitive motion by the shoulder, elbow, and wrists. The rotator cuff may develop overuse injuries such as impingement and painful arch syndrome, as well as bicipital tendinitis.

PREVENTION. Many shoulder injuries could be prevented through the use of strength and flexibility exercises and a carefully monitored training program. The posterior musculature, especially the external rotators and scapular adductors, needs to be strengthened.

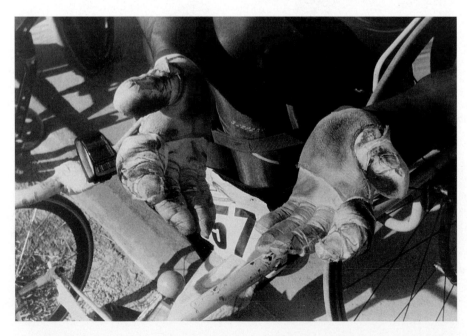

Fig. 38-7. An example of the wear and tear on hands and gloves of a wheelchair athlete.

This will help to achieve a balance with the often-overdeveloped anterior shoulder musculature.[6] A static flexibility program for all ranges of motion of the shoulder should be instituted, particularly for the anterior muscles and the rotator cuff. Careful monitoring of the training program and alteration of activity could reduce the number and incidence of chronic shoulder injuries.

MANAGEMENT. Treatment of chronic and acute shoulder injuries should follow conventional treatment patterns. Ice, rest, and nonsteroidal anti-inflammatory medications are particularly effective. To maintain cardiovascular fitness of the athlete, alternative exercise should be prescribed.

AMPUTEE ATHLETES

Stump Problems

The athlete who has an amputation is subject to the same injuries and stress as the athlete without a disability. Additionally, the amputee may be subject to irritations and stress at the junction with the prosthetic device. This problem particularly occurs with lower-limb prostheses. It is characterized by redness and irritation at the prosthesis-skin interface.

PREVENTION. The athlete normally knows when a skin irritation or breakdown from the stump is beginning. These problems can be prevented by a proper fit and maintenance of the prosthetic device. Protective padding at the end of the prosthesis or friction-eliminating material such as NuSkin® over irritated areas may aid in the healing process. An excessively loose or tight fit will increase the stress at the junction.

Various materials have been used between the skin and the socket to reduce the stress from vigorous athletic activity. The materials have included gels, soft fabrics, and foam padding. Advances in prosthetic design, development, and fit have reduced the number of prosthesis-related problems. The new knee prosthetic device allows for a truer knee range of motion and less rotational stress, plus the added feature of a plantar flexion to absorb the forces transmitted from the ground during heel strike.

MANAGEMENT. Protective padding of the end of the prosthesis and cleansing at the irritated area aids the healing process for a stump injury. In advanced cases, the athlete may have to temporarily discontinue use of the prosthesis and reduce athletic participation.

INJURIES TO ATHLETES WITH CEREBRAL PALSY

Muscle Strains and Miscellaneous Conditions

There are varying degrees of cerebral palsy that range from severe to barely perceptible spasticity. Muscular problems can be caused by the influence of spasticity on the muscle. Many individuals with cerebral palsy have had Achilles tendon surgery and hamstring surgery to allow for a greater degree of range of motion. This surgical intervention may cause a decrease in the active muscle units for a muscular contraction, hence an imbalance between the agonist and antagonist muscles may exist.

Seizures are an infrequent problem during sports for individuals with cerebral palsy. Richter[43] stated that 1 out of 87 athletes with cerebral palsy had a minor seizure incident at the 1988 Paralympic Games.

PREVENTION. Prevention of muscular injuries is facilitated by flexibility and strength training programs. It is important that the physician who is treating the athlete with cerebral palsy work with the available range of motion to maintain and restore motion that may be lost because of contractures and spasticity. Proprioceptive neuromuscular facilitation (PNF) stretching appears to be particularly effective when used in conjunction with static stretching programs. Further, strength training of sport-specific muscles to achieve a muscular balance and improve performance is indicated (Fig. 38-8).[33]

MANAGEMENT. The management of a muscle strain should follow the typical treatment pattern. Ice is particularly helpful, not only because of its anti-inflammatory properties, but also because prolonged use may decrease spastic tone.[10] Stretching must be slow and steady because quick movements will trigger the muscle spindles, causing a reflex shortening. The stretch must be comfortable enough to be held for at least thirty seconds, but preferably for over two minutes.[55] Key areas of spastic tightness include the shoulder internal rotators, hip flexors, and ankle plantar flexors. If anti-inflammatory medication is prescribed, the physician should be aware of possible drug interactions with antiseizure drugs or other medicine that the athlete may be taking.

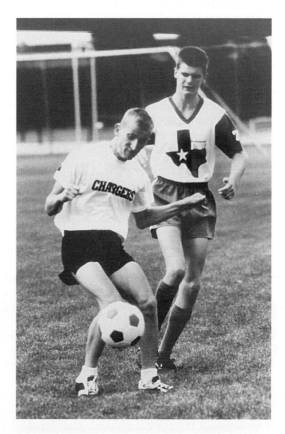

Fig. 38-8. Athletes with cerebral palsy playing soccer.

Falls

Falls usually are seen in the USCPAA Class V (diplegic) and Class VI (athetoid) competitions. Although not a common problem leading to injury, falls from a loss of balance and coordination may occur. However, most athletes are able to catch and brace themselves for a fall, thus reducing the severity of the injury.

INJURIES TO ATHLETES WHO ARE VISUALLY IMPAIRED

Barrier Problems

The athlete with a visual impairment may not have visual cues in relation to road surface and condition as well as various barriers such as walls, curbs, and other competing athletes. Many events, such as track and tandem cycling, employ a guide runner to assist the athletes who are visually impaired.

Lower Extremity Injuries

The athlete with a visual impairment tends to have a higher proportion of lower-extremity injuries. Ferrara[17] found that 26% of the injuries were to the leg/ankle, 11% to the foot/toes, and 10% to the knee. This could be due to improper training techniques and overuse mechanisms.

There also are biomechanical considerations that can contribute to the increased percentage of lower-extremity injuries. Changes in stepping frequency, stride length, prolonged stance time, and excessive braking and acceleration forces have been documented.[17] The athlete with a visual impairment may expend more energy when performing the same tasks as the athlete without a visual impairment; therefore, the athlete is more likely to fatigue quickly. A higher incidence of overuse of the lower extremity may result.

PREVENTION. Monitoring the training program to eliminate overuse is extremely important. Other considerations for prevention involve the selection of a matched (physiologically and biomechanically) guide runner to maintain an even pace and stride length. The inappropriate selection of the guide runner could hinder the training of an athlete with a visual impairment. Training periodization should be instituted to allow for recovery time and decrease the potential for injury.

SPECIAL OLYMPIANS

Special Olympics International provides athletic competition for athletes with mental impairment and offers a number of sporting opportunities including track, field, ice skating, gymnastics, floor hockey, and skiing. There is a heightened awareness of athletes with Down syndrome, the most recognizable form of mental retardation because of the physical appearance of people with this disability. However, orthopedic problems that particularly afflict athletes with Down syndrome may not be familiar to medical personnel. The typical medical problems include pes planus, patellar instability, and atlantoaxial instability.[24]

Cervical Spine Instability

In 1983, Special Olympics International issued a directive to all medical personnel, coaches, parents, and athletes restricting participation of athletes with Down syndrome until they had received medical examinations for atlantoaxial instability. The sudden concern was due to a finding of collagen and ligamentous laxity in a number of athletes. Researchers have estimated a prevalence of 10% to 20%[9,12,22,35] for cervical spine instability. The ligament laxity and bony abnormality can be completely asymptomatic, or it can result in a variety of symptoms including weakness of the extremity, neck pain, and deterioration of ambulatory skills.

PREVENTION. The Special Olympics general rules now restrict participation by these athletes in activities that could produce "hyperextension, hyperflexion, or direct pressure on the upper spine."[35] Radiographic evidence demonstrating normal atlantoaxial stability and no bony abnormalities must be presented for the athlete to be allowed to participate without any sport restrictions. Permanent sport restrictions are placed on athletes who demonstrate positive radiographic evidence.

DIAGNOSIS. Atlantoaxial instability is detected by radiographic findings in conjunction with a physical examination. Radiographic examination should include the anterior/posterior, lateral, flexion/extension, and odontoid views of the spine. Longitudinal radiographic examinations should be performed to detect any changes in spinal stability.

MANAGEMENT. There are several treatment options available to those with spinal instability. Obviously, the restriction of activities that would increase the risk of spinal injury is indicated. Those activities that result in axial loading, hyperflexion, or hyperextension mechanisms are contraindicated. Spinal fusions may be performed to stabilize the joint in persons with symptomatic dislocations.

MULTIPLE SCLEROSIS

Multiple sclerosis is an upper motor neuron lesion of fluctuating clinical presentation. It has an often-unpredictable clinical course. It is important for athletes with multiple sclerosis to not become overfatigued and particularly to not increase core body temperature, both of which may lead to an exacerbation of the condition.[37] Swimming is a good sport for people with MS because the relatively cool water temperature with its high specific heat (skin temperature is usually 91°F) tends to cool the athlete and prevent a rise in body core temperature. In particular, these athletes need to be counseled to not participate in sports during hot weather, which could be very detrimental to them.

ASTHMA

Asthma is a common disorder; over 15% of the US Olympic Team in Los Angeles has asthma or exercise-induced asthma (EIA).[40,53] Athletes can deal with asthma by avoiding times of high pollution, such as during the heat of the day when the ozone level is up and traffic pollution may be higher. They should warm up slowly for long periods of time, such as 15 minutes, gradually increasing the workload. This permits bronchial dilation to occur. It helps to exercise in humid air. Dry, cold air tends to increase the likelihood of bronchial spasm. Swimming is often an excellent exercise for asthmatics.

The inhalation of long-acting bronchodilators such as salbuterol is very effective for an acute bronchial spasm. For chronic asthma the use of anti-inflammatories such as inhaled steroids or nedocromil sodium are often effective. Elite athletes using prescribed inhaled steroids need to notify the USOC.

DIABETES

Physicians have been aware for years of the positive benefits of exercise for diabetics. Exercise has been a key component to proper management of diabetic care, along with proper diet and regularly scheduled medication.[21] Physicians should be aware of complications and risks that can occur when diabetics exercise. One of the frequent complications for insulin-dependent diabetic athletes is hypoglycemia.[42]

A hypoglycemia attack may occur because too much insulin is present or not enough calories have been taken in. Most frequently, hypoglycemia is the result of escalated absorption of insulin that has been injected into an active muscle. This is especially true when short-acting insulin is being used. The best injection sites are the buttocks and abdomen.[21] Insulin requirements can change. Insulin may need to be decreased one to two units and/or carbohydrate intake may need to be increased by 10 to 15 grams of additional carbohydrates for every half-hour of exercise.[34] For prolonged activity, 5 to 20 grams of carbohydrates should be consumed for every 20 minutes of activity. The diabetic should be encouraged to eat approximately 30 to 60 minutes before beginning an exercise program. Blood sugar should be monitored before, as well as after, the completion of an exercise bout since exercise can lower blood sugar levels for 24 to 48 hours following an exercise session.

If hypoglycemia occurs during exercise, the athlete should ingest a high-glucose drink or food and perhaps discontinue the activity.[21] The athlete should be encouraged to always carry glucose and proper identification during exercise and, if blood sugars are unstable, not to exercise alone.

Another complication occurring with diabetes is hyperglycemia. If blood sugars are over 250 mg/dL the athlete should monitor for presence of ketones.[54] If ketones are present, exercise should be postponed. Diabetic patients should be encouraged to wear proper footwear and practice good foot hygiene. Often it is helpful to alternate footwear, that is, have several pairs of good shoes, to redistribute pressure points. Injuries to the foot, such as blisters or infection, should be treated immediately. Diabetics should avoid prolonged isometrics or heavy resistance exercises that increase blood pressure if retinopathy is present.[21] Physicians should be aware that the diabetic athlete who is on beta-blockers may be unable to experience the symptoms of hypoglycemia and/or angina. It also should be noted that exercise in excess heat may lead to problems from dehydration, which must be rigorously prevented.[34]

OBESITY

A high level of success is noted for obese people who follow an exercise regimen that increases caloric expenditure when joined with a diet program that decreases caloric intake.[2,27] Appropriate types of exercise for obese people include walking, recumbent cycling, using a stair climber or rowing machine, and water exercise. Exercise at a low intensity may be an effective technique in decreasing fat stores. At lower intensity levels the lipid mobilizing system provides energy, but the carbohydrate system functions during intense exercise. After intense exercise there is a lipid to carbohydrate shift, but the obese athlete may have difficulty performing at an intense level. The more conditioned the athlete, the more the athlete can mobilize the fat stores. The obese person's goal in getting involved in an exercise program is to increase caloric expenditure. This decreases such problems as joint and orthopedic trauma. Because of the buoyancy of water, exercise in water is often a good choice for conditioning, but not for weight loss, when compared to land exercises.[38]

Although more intense exercise may have more health benefits,[26] physicians should encourage sedentary individuals that the greatest health benefit may actually be for people who go from no exercise to any form of exercise.

A special thanks to Marie Laidler.

REFERENCES

1. American Academy of Orthopedic Surgeons: *Athletic training and sports medicine*, ed 2, Parkridge Ill, 1991, The Academy.
2. Bennett WI: Beyond overeating, NEJM 332:673–674, 1995.
3. Benzinger TH: Heat regulation: Homeostasis of central temperature in man, *Physiol Rev* 671–759, 1969.
4. Birrer RB: The Special Olympics: An injury overview, *Phys and Sports Med* 12:95-97, 1985.
5. Bloomquist LE: Injuries to athletes with physical disabilities: Prevention implications, *Phys and Sports Med* 14:97–10, 1986.
6. Burnham R, Wheeler G, Bhambhani Y, et al: Intentional induction of autonomic dysreflexia among quadriplegic athletes for performance enhancement: Efficacy, safety, and mechanism of action, *Clin J Sport Med* 4:1–10, 1994.
7. Clark MW: Competitive sports for the disabled, *Am J Sports Med* 8:366–369, 1980.
8. Colachis SC III, Otis SM: Thermal regulation and fever in SCI, *Am J PM&R* 74(2):114–119, 1995.
9. Committee on Sports Medicine: Atlanto-axial instability in Downs Syndrome, *Orthop Clin North Am* 74:152–154, 1984.
10. Corcos DM, Gottlieb GL, Penn RD, et al: Movement deficits caused by hyperexcitable stretch reflexes in spastic humans, *Brain* 109:1043–1058, 1986.
11. Curtis KA, Dillon DA: Survey of wheelchair athletic injuries: Common patterns and prevention, *Paraplegia* 23:170–175, 1985.
12. Diamond LS, Lynne KD, Sigman B: Orthopedic disorders in patients with Down's syndrome, *Orthop Clin North Am* 12:57–71, 1981.
13. Downey JA, Chiodi HP, Darling RC: Central temperature regulation in the spinal man, *J Appl Physiol* 22:91–94, 1967.
14. Downey JA, Miller JM, Darling RC: Thermoregulatory re-

sponses to deep and superficial cooling in spinal man, *J Appl Physiol* 27:209–212, 1969.

15. Downey RJ, Downey JA, Newhouse E, et al: Hyperthermia in a quadriplegic: Evidence for a peripheral action of haloperidol in malignant neuroleptic syndrome, *Chest* 101:1728–1730, 1992.

16. Erickson RP: Autonomic hyperreflexia: Pathophysiology and medical management, *Arch Phys Med Rehabil* 61: 431–440, October, 1980.

17. Ferrara MS, et al: The injury experience of the competitive athlete with a disability: prevention implications, *Medicine and Science in Sports and Exercise* 24(2):184–188, 1992.

18. Ferrara MS, Davis R: Injuries to elite wheelchair athletes, *Paraplegia* 28:335–341, 1990.

19. Gehlsen GM, Davis RW, Bahmonde R: Intermittent velocity and wheelchair performance characteristics. *APAQ* 7: 219–230, 1990.

20. Guttmann L: The importance of sport and recreation for the physically handicapped. In Leon AS, Amundson G, editors, Proceedings of the First International Conference on Lifestyle and Health, Minneapolis, 1979.

21. Horton ES: Role and management of exercise in diabetes mellitus, *Diabetes Care* 11(2):201–211, 1988.

22. Hreidarsson S, Magram G, Singer H: Symptomatic atlantoaxial dislocation in Down Syndrome, *Pediatrics* 69: 568–571, 1982.

23. Huberman G: Organized sports activities with cerebral palsy, *Adoles Rehabil Lit* 37:103–106, 1976.

24. Hudson PB. Preparticipation screening of Special Olympics Athletes, *Phys Sports Med* 16:97–104, 1988.

25. Kleiber DA, et al: Involvement with special recreation associations: Perceived impacts in early adulthood, *Ther Rec J* 24:32–44, 1990.

26. Lee I, Hsieh C, Paffenbarger RS Jr: Exercise intensity and longevity in men, *JAMA* 273:1179–1184, April 19, 1995.

27. Leibel RL, Rosenbaum M, Hirsch J: Changes in energy expenditure resulting from altered body weight, *NEJM* 332: 621–628, 1995.

28. Magnus BC: Sports injuries, the disabled athlete, and the athletic trainer, *Ath Train* 22:305–310, 1987.

29. McCann C: Medical classification: Art, science, or instinct? *Sport'n Spokes* 5:12–14, 1980.

30. McCormick DP: Injuries in handicapped alpine ski racers, *Phys Sports Med* 13:93–97, 1985.

31. Menard MR, Hahn G: Acute and chronic hypothermia in a man with spinal cord injury: Environmental and pharmacologic causes, *Arch Phys Med Rehabil* 72:421–424, 1991.

32. Modorski JB, Curtis, KA: Wheelchair sports medicine, *Am J Sports Med* 12:128–132, 1984.

33. Mushett CA, Wyeth DO, Richter, KJ: Cerebral palsy, traumatic brain injury, and stroke. In Goldberg B, editor: *Sports and exercise for children with chronic health conditions,* Champaign Ill, 1995, Human Kinetics.

34. Nathan DM, Madnek SF, Delahanty L: Programming pre-exercise snacks to prevent post-exercise hypoglycemia in intensively treated insulin-dependent diabetics, *Ann Intern Med* 102(4):483–486, 1985.

35. Official Special Olympics Summer Sports Rules, No 6: Participation by individuals with Downs Syndrome who suffer from the atlantoaxial dislocation condition, Washington D.C., 1992, revised 1995.

36. Ogunytmi A, et al: Seizures induced by exercise, *Neurology* 38:633–634, 1988.

37. Olgiati R, Jacquet J, di Prampero PE: Energy cost of walking and exertional dyspnea in multiple sclerosis, *Am Rev Respir Dis* 134:1005–1010, 1986

38. Pate RR, et al: *Guidelines for exercise testing and prescription: ACSM,* ed 4, Philadelphia, 1991, Lea & Febiger.

39. Pickering GW: The vasomotor regulation of heat loss from the human skin in relation to external temperature, *Heart* 115–135, 1932.

40. Pierson WE, Voy RO: Exercise-induced bronchospasm in the XXIII Summer Olympic games, *NE & Reg Allergy Pro* 9(3):209–13, May-June, 1988.

41. Randall WC, et al: Central peripheral factors in dynamic thermoregulation, *J Appl Physiol* 18:61–64, 1963.

42. Richter EA, Ruderman NB, Schneider SH: Diabetes and exercise, *Am J Med* 70:201, 1981.

43. Richter KJ: Seizures in athletes, *J Osteo Sports Med* 3:19–23, 1989.

44. Richter KJ: Hypertensive crisis—autonomic hyperreflexia. Letter to the editor, *NEJM* 994, April 4, 1991.

45. Richter KJ, et al: Injuries in world class cerebral palsy athletes of the 1988 Seoul, Korea Paralympics, *J Osteo Sports Med* 15–18, October, 1991.

46. Richter KJ, et al: Integrated swimming classification: A faulted system. *APAQ* 9:5–13, 1992.

47. Secondorf R, Randall WC: Thermal reflex sweating in normal and paraplegic man, *J Appl Physiol* 16:796–800, 1961.

48. Sherrill C, Adams-Mushett C, Jones JA: Classification and other issues in sports for the blind, cerebral palsied, les autres, and amputee athlete. In Sherrill C, editor: *Sports and disabled athletes* Champaign Ill, 1986, Human Kinetics.

49. Sherrill C, Hinson M, Gench B, et al: Self-concepts of disabled youth athletes, *Perceptual and motor skills* 70: 1093–1098, 1990.

50. Sherrill C, Rainbolt W: Self actualization profiles of male able-bodied and Cerebral Palsied athletes, *APAQ* 5(2): 108–119, 1988.

51. Simon E: Temperature regulation: The spinal cord as a site of extrahypothalamic thermoregulatory functions, *Rev Physiol Biochem Pharmacol* 71:1–76, 1974.

52. Steadward, et al: Vista '93, Edmonton, Alberta, Canada, 1993, Rick Hansen Centre; 242–247.

53. Voy RO: US Olympic committee experience with exercise-induced bronchospasm, 1984, *Med & Sci Sport & Ex* 18(3): 328–30, June 1986.

54. Wilberg-Henriksson H: Exercise and diabetes mellitus, *Exerc Sport Sci Rev* 20:339–368, 1992.

55. Wolf SE: Morphological and functional considerations for therapeutic exercises. In Basmajian JV, editor: *Therapeutic Exercise,* ed 4, Baltimore, 1984, Williams & Wilkins.

CHAPTER 39

MEDICOLEGAL ISSUES

Andrew H. Patterson

Liability issues have been a constant concern to all health care professionals since the late 1960s, when there was a steady and dramatic increase in the frequency of liability claims and in the severity of their results. This increase in legal action affected not only physicians and others providing health care but also manufacturers of sports equipment. Indeed, some companies chose to close their doors rather than try to continue to function in a climate in which liability costs had risen so precipitously.

The issues of professional liability and the obvious inequities of our current system have been well covered in other forums. The extensive statistics compiled by the Physician Insurers Association of America (PIAA) and the Medical Liability Mutual Insurance Company (MLMIC), the physician-owned New York company, do not present a clear picture of the sources of professional liability in sports medicine. However, there do seem to be common elements in liability suits that occur with regularity. The health care professional's awareness of these factors will help avoid litigation, the ideal goal, or at least help make lawsuits easier to defend.

PATIENT ANGER

A serious, unexpected injury that, in the best of hands, may lead to a poor result can generate considerable anger on the part of a patient or the patient's family. There have been a number of cases in which a physician was sued only after litigation against the person responsible for the injury failed or yielded limited results.

Anger over an injury sustained in a sports event may be directed toward the opposing players, coaches, or even the officials. The organization sponsoring the event or the facility in which it took place can also become the object of hostility. Physicians and trainers should be careful not to say anything that might inflame a potentially volatile situation. One ill-advised comment about an individual or organization can come back to haunt the person who made it. The physician's responsibility is to render the best possible medical care; under no circumstances should he make a comment that can reinforce or fuel anger. The result of a careless statement may well have the unanticipated effect of turning the patient's anger against the physician.

Furthermore, the physician should never be tempted to give legal advice. If asked for advice regarding a prospective lawsuit, he should respond that he is not qualified to give such advice and will not do so.

COMMUNICATION AND FOLLOW-UP

Because of the nature of sports medicine and marked variations in the quality of care immediately available at an athletic event, communication is extremely important. Typically, a patient injured on the athletic field receives emergency care at the site, further care in an emergency room setting, and definitive care from a private physician in the appropriate specialty.

A lack of communication among the caregivers may lead to a preventable disaster. Better communication might well have saved the leg of a 13-year-old boy injured on the playing field. The boy underwent "a reduction of a dislocated knee" on the field. The real injury, a completely displaced fracture of the distal proximal tibial epiphysis, was not diagnosed until it was too late. First a splint and later a full cast masked the fracture, which was perfectly reduced. A laceration of the popliteal artery was diagnosed too late to salvage a viable extremity. Even though either diagnosis should have raised real concern regarding an arterial injury, it is clear from a review of this case that more direct communication would have been extremely valuable.

Individuals involved in primary care of athletes should try to arrange to have their findings transmitted at least to the next-level caregiver. This is especially important when the injury is serious. Obviously, this sharing of information is relatively simple in small towns but more difficult in large cities. One suggested solution is to require that the sponsoring entity of the sporting event obtain a legible and reasonably complete record of any initial findings and tentative diagnoses. This record could then be supplied to the physician rendering subsequent care.

DEALING WITH COACHES, FAMILIES, AND ATHLETES

In an ideal world a physician would be responsible only to his individual patient. In the real world, however, coaches, trainers, parents, or other family members may well become involved. Furthermore, the amount of potential outside interference can vary greatly with the level of competition. The overwhelming majority of coaches would rather rest a player than risk further injury, but a small number will insist that an athlete "play hurt." This attitude of stoicism is unfortunately reinforced when the news media praise professional athletes who play despite significant injuries. Although such an attitude may be appropriate at the professional level, it should never be allowed when youngsters at or below high school level are involved.

The desire to win can be carried much too far. One of my patients was a 12-year-old pitcher who could not extend his arm beyond 40 degrees. When I suggested that he stop pitching, his parents stormed out of the office, pulling their son along. A physician has no control over this kind of behavior. It is important, however, to remember that the physician's first duty is to the patient, and that caution is frequently the best approach to treatment. Trainers and coaches can help reinforce treatment plans, especially since they often know the young athlete better than the physician. However, they should not be permitted to override the physician's judgment if the risk of a more serious injury exists. The physician who allows emotional appeals and demands from others to overrule his carefully thought-out treatment decision may very well find himself defending a lawsuit.

EMERGENCY CARE AND EQUIPMENT

Financial considerations always limit the availability of both emergency equipment and transportation, especially at lower levels of competition. Even though serious injuries occur rarely, it is important for physicians who provide primary care at sports events to insist upon a reasonable plan to secure care for a seriously injured athlete. At a high school football game I attended, a player with a devastating knee injury (that required extensive surgery) lay on the sidelines through halftime and the entire second half. Although he had an excellent recovery, the initial management of this injury was far from ideal. The covering physician must also keep in mind the fact that adequate primary care and prompt, safe transportation can be life-saving in a few cases. A balance between providing maximum care for a seriously injured athlete and the practical considerations of having sophisticated equipment on hand at all times will probably never be found. Despite this, it is the responsibility of the covering physician (who is, after all, the ultimate patient advocate) to insist upon the best compromise possible. Certainly, everything that can be provided at a reasonable cost should be available. If an injury is aggravated by inadequate primary care, the physician will probably be caught in the crossfire of a future lawsuit.

EVALUATION OF THE SPORTS FACILITY

It is highly unlikely that any physician can ever influence the design or choice of the facility provided for an athletic event. The physician can, however, identify conditions within the facility that increase the risk of serious injury by simply conducting a brief tour during the warm up period before the event. The physician should consider the placement of sideline benches, which can usually be changed easily. Control of players on the sidelines not only will reduce the possibility of injury, but may very well reduce the incidence of fights and personal fouls. Immovable barriers and other obstructions near or adjacent to a playing field or indoor court should be carefully marked and well padded. Although physicians should not be sued because of inadequate physical facilities, a primary physician should make every effort to identify potential problem areas and to suggest reasonable corrections that will prevent injuries. The investment of a few minutes of time in reviewing safety conditions can pay great dividends.

CHAPTER 40

LEGAL ISSUES IN SPORTS MEDICINE

David L. Herbert

A variety of major legal concerns face those who provide primary medical care services for athletes.

The legal system is frequently called upon to resolve a variety of sports medicine issues related to preparticipation examinations of athletes, clearance- or return-to-play decisions, training and conditioning of athletes, mismatching of athletes, examination, diagnosis, treatment, and rehabilitation of athletes, drug testing, compliance with the bloodborne pathogen rule, and many other issues. These issues are continually examined in publications that report on relevant practice developments and in actual case filings and decisions.[2]

Although one chapter cannot provide a discussion of all of these concerns,[1] a close examination of one selected sports medicine issue should be of benefit to those in primary care.

During the last 10 to 15 years, the practice of medicine has been inundated by the development and publication of practice guidelines for various medical care providers. These guidelines, often referred to as "standards," "consensus statements," or "parameters of practice," have been developed by a number of professional associations, various governmental agencies, and many respected authorities. At last count, there were more than 20,000 of these statements.[3]

Despite the proliferation of statements, many medical care practitioners have resisted this movement. A number of providers have even criticized the trend as mandating that physicians provide medical care according to a "cookbook-type recipe" that allows little room for implementing the "art" of medicine.[4] Notwithstanding criticism of the trend, efforts to standardize medical care have increased exponentially. Because of efforts to standardize care, reduce the likelihood of untoward events, minimize claims and suits, lower costs, limit defensive medical care practices, and provide clear benchmarks for expected care, standardization will continue.

Even if this approach to medical care practice is a form of cookbook-type medicine, providers should remember, as others have stated, that every great chef (and every competent physician) starts with some recipe that is enhanced by personalized attention and the blending of various spices that add to the final product.[5] Although enhancements in medicine may be based upon "intelligent reasoning and clinical intuition"[5] rather than spices, there must be some basic protocol available to care givers. Otherwise, there will be nothing to enhance through individualized care.

In this regard, sports medicine is not different from other branches of medicine. To date, nearly 100 sports medicine standards or guidelines statements have been developed and published by a number of respected professional associations.[6] These include standards dealing with preparticipation examinations,[7] the management of sports-related concessions,[8] and the treatment of HIV-infected athletes through compliance with the bloodborne pathogen standard.[9]

Like other health care practitioners, sports medicine physicians must be aware of relevant standards statements and use them to enhance their care of athlete-patients. However, it may be that many practitioners in sports medicine, like their counterparts in other practice areas, do not know or fully appreciate the benefits of practice parameters in their own practices. Based upon recent research findings as well as actual litigation filings, providers may run certain medicolegal risks in addition to creating unnecessary risks for their patients if such practitioners do not heed these standards statements.

In the litigation following the 1990 death of Loyola Marymount University star basketball player Hank Gathers, certain of his heirs cited the 16th Bethesda Conference guidelines[10] in challenging the courtside care that was provided to Gathers following his collapse during a nationally televised basketball game.[11] The plaintiffs contended in their detailed, 52-page complaint against, among others, Gathers' sports medicine physicians, that Gathers, who was suffering from hypertrophic cardiomyopathy, was not properly treated and that he died as a consequence of negligent care. The lawsuit, which sought $32.5 million in damages, was settled for a substantial amount.[12] The suit did, however, represent one of the first times that practice guidelines were actually cited in court filings to allege negligence in the care of a patient. More recently, the 26th Bethesda Conference guidelines[13] were cited by Northwestern University, in litigation related to the exclusion of an athlete from participation,[14] to support rather than to challenge a sports medicine care decision.

It is clear, even from these two high-profile cases, that standards statements can have an impact in the medical-legal arena even at the onset of litigation and long before experts are deposed. Standards statements may be used either as a sword, to attack sports medicine care, or as a shield, to protect against an attack. The application of standards as a weapon (an inculpatory device) or as a shield (an exculpatory device) may not, however, be available to practitioners who do not know or understand the standards and the potential use of those standards.

In an effort to determine if and how practice parameters are used in the medicolegal setting, researchers from three respected institutions recently surveyed almost 1000 attorneys who pursue medical malpractice claims on behalf of patients. They also reviewed over 250 malpractice claim files from two medical malpractice insurance carriers.[15] Their summary and analysis of this information sought to determine how practice guidelines are used in claims and litigation, for what purposes, and with what results. Interestingly, the researchers determined that, although attorneys and malpractice insurers currently make only moderate use of standards statements, it appears, at least to the plaintiffs' bar, that the use of statements is increasing. The researchers also determined that statements are used more often to challenge the care rendered to patients than to defend care rendered. The researchers noted, however, that when a provider followed and cited a practice guideline to support specific care, plaintiffs' attorneys were less likely to pursue malpractice claims or lawsuits on behalf of their clients.

As a corollary to the foregoing findings, there is both an upside and a downside to the development, publication, and dissemination of practice guidelines. If physicians use standards statements in their care of athlete-patients and support the care provided with standards statements, they may insulate themselves from litigation, and even claims, alleging substandard care. If, however, sports medicine care givers ignore standards or do not use them to improve patient care, harm will result to patients and physicians alike. The sword will harm both patient and physician, to the detriment of sports medicine and the medical profession as a whole. Sports medicine practitioners should concentrate on using standards statements as a shield to protect against their use as a sword.

REFERENCES

1. For a more comprehensive examination of essentially all sports medicine, medico-legal related issues see Herbert: *Legal Aspects of Sports Medicine,* ed 2, Canton, Ohio, 1995, PRC Publishing.
2. See *The Sports Medicine Standards and Malpractice Reporter,* a quarterly newsletter examining legal, professional, and standards issues related to sports medicine care published by PRC Publishing, of Canton, Ohio.
3. *Healthcare Standards Directory,* Plymouth Meeting, PA, 1993, ECRI.
4. Herbert D: Practice guidelines take center court, How to Limit Liability, *The Physician and Sportsmedicine* 24(3): 81–83, March 1996.
5. Roberts: Practice Guidelines, A Positive Perspective, *The Physician and Sportsmedicine* 24(3):86, March 1996.
6. Herbert D: *The Sports Medicine Standards Book,* Canton, Ohio, 1992, suppl 1993, Professional Reports.
7. Smith, Kovan, Rich, et al: *Preparticipation Physical Evaluation,* ed 2, Minneapolis, MN, 1997, American Academy of Family Physicians, American Academy of Pediatrics, American Medical Society for Sports Medicine, American Orthopaedic Society for Sports Medicine, American Osteopathic Academy of Sports Medicine.
8. Colorado Medical Society: *Guidelines for the Management of Concussion in Sports,* Colorado Medical Society, Sports Medicine Committee.
9. American Academy of Pediatrics: Policy statement; human immunodeficiency virus [acquired immunodeficiency syndrome (AIDS) virus] in the athletic setting, *AAP News* 6:18, 1991.
10. Mitchell JH, Maron BJ, Epstein SE: 16th Bethesda Conference: cardiovascular abnormalities in the athlete; recommendations regarding eligibility for competition, *J Am Coll Cardiol* 6(6):1186–1232, 1986.
11. Herbert: The death of Hank Gathers: An examination of the legal issues, *The Sports Medicine Standards and Malpractice Reporter* 2(3):45, 46–47, 1990.
12. Gathers Case Resolved, *The Sports Medicine Standards and Malpractice Reporter* 4(2):27, 1992.
13. The 26th Bethesda Conference: Recommendations for determining eligibility for competition in athletes with cardiovascular abnormalities, *Med and Sci in Sports and Exercise,* S227–S283, 1994.
14. *Knapp v. Northwestern University,* et al, Case No. 95–C–6454 (N.D. Ill., E.D., filed 1995). The defendants' answer to the plaintiff's complaint.
15. Hyams, Brandenburg, Lipsitz, et al: Practice guidelines and malpractice litigation: A two way street, *Ann Intern Med* 122(6):450–455, 1995.

INDEX

A

AAHPERD: *see* American Alliance of Health, Physical Education, and Recreation
Abdominal examination, before sports participation, 68
Abdominal injury, on-field emergencies, 82
Abdominal pain, 40
  irritable bowel syndrome and, 40
  psychogenic, 41
Abrasions, eye, 120
Accessory meniscofemoral ligaments, 336
Acetabulum, hip dislocation and, 328
Achilles bursitis, 392
Achilles tendinitis, 392
Achilles tendon, ruptures, 393
Acneiform lesions, 107
Acromial fractures, 236
Acromioclavicular separations, 238
Action potential, 8
Adductor canal syndrome, 318
Adductor muscle injuries, 314
Adhesive capsulitis, 234
  management, 235
  pathomechanics, 234
Adolescents, females, anorexia nervosa and bulimia, 43
Adrenergic stimulants, 30
Advanced Trauma Life Support guidelines, craniofacial injuries and, 129
Aerobic exercise, 26
Albuterol, 30
Alcohol use, 595
Alupent, 30
Alveolar process fracture, 161
Alveolar socket, comminution of, 161
Amenorrhea
  athletic, 566
  estrogenic, 89
  secondary, risk factors associated with, 89
American Alliance of Health, Physical Education, and Recreation, history of, 3
American College of Sports Medicine, recommendations for muscular strengthening and endurance exercises, 5
American Orthopaedic Society for Sports Medicine (AOSSM), 6
Amino acid supplementation, 563
Amnesia, posttraumatic, head injury and, 35
Amoxicillin, rickettsial diseases and, 109

Amputee athletes, 605
Anabolic steroids
  abuse, 595
  abuse of, 578
Anaphylaxis
  exercise-induced, 33
  on-field, management of, 82
Anemia
  sports hematuria and, 48
  wound healing and, 101
Anger, patient, 609
Angioedema
  exercise-induced, 33
  exercise-induced anaphylaxis and, 33
Angioplasty, 4
Ankle
  fractures/dislocations, 400, 406
  injuries, 386–409
  instability, 389
  nerve entrapment syndrome, 406
  overuse injuries, 397
  pediatric athletes, 426
  rehabilitation, 464
  stress fractures, 399
  syndesmotic ligament injuries, 391
  tendon abnormalities, 392
Anorexia nervosa, 43, 593
Antalgic gait, iliopectineal bursitis and, 316
Anterior cruciate ligament, 336
  evaluation of, 344
  injury, female athletes, 93
Anterior cruciate ligament tears, 354
Anticipatory phase, 19
Antifungal medications, 109
Anxiety, psychogenic abdominal pain and, 41
Anxiety disorders, 590
Aortic valvular disease, congenital, 24
Aortic regurgitation, 24
AOSSM: *see* American Orthopaedic Society for Sports Medicine
Apnea, sleep, 34
Applanation tonometry, 118
Aquatic therapy, 552
Aqueous humor, 115
Arcuate ligament instability, 279
Arthrography, wrist, 272
Arthrosis, 283
Articular cartilage, senior athletes and, 5

Asthma, 29
  drug treatment, 30
  emergent therapy, 31
  medical history checklist, 31
Athletes
  cardiovascular screening, 20
  dietary habits, 557
  disabled, 4
  female: *see* Women in sports
  perception of injury, 589
  preparticipation physical examination, 61
Athlete's foot, 109, 408
Athletes with disabilities
  amputees, 605
  injury patterns, 602
    wheelchair-bound, 602
Athletic training, evolution of, 3
Aurilianus, postoperative exercise programs and, 3
Autonomic dysreflexia, athletes with disabilities, 601
Avascular necrosis
  carpal bones, 284
  hip dislocations, 329
  hip fracture and, 319
  Legg-Calvé-Perthes disease and, 331
Avulsion fractures, 320
Axonal injury, diffuse, brain damage and, 36

B

Back injury, 210
Back pain
  injury and, 210
  pediatric athletes, 445
Bacterial colonization, wound healing and, 100
Bacterial infections, 105–109
Baseball, disabled athletes and, 4
Baseball league, female, during the 1940s, 4
Basketball, disabled athletes and, 4
Benchwarmer's bursitis, 316
Beta-blocker medications, mitral valve prolapse and, 23
Bicycling
  elderly athletes participation in, 5
  head injury and, 35
  history of female participation in, 4
  urethral injury, 55
Binocular diplopia, 126
Bipolar I disorder, 590
Bladder contusion, 55
Bladder injury, 53
  diagnosis of, 53
  mechanism of, 53
Bladder rupture
  blunt trauma and, 53
  extraperitoneal, treatment, 55
Blisters, trauma and, 104
Blood
  cooling functions, 18
  heat transport, 18
Blood chemistry tests, preparticipation physical
  examination and, 69

Blood poisoning, 107
Blood pressure, high, exercise effects on, 5
Blood supply, heart function and, 18
Blunt trauma, renal injury and, 49
Boxing, head injury prevention and, 37
Brachial plexus, 186–200
  injury, 195
Bradycardia, endurance training and, 20
Brain
  edema, 36
    malignant, 36
  thermoregulatory centers in, 19
Brain damage
  primary, 35
  secondary, 36
Breathing, dyspnea and, 26
Brethaire, 30
Bronchospasm, exercise-induced, 32
  exercise testing for, 32
  therapy for, 32
Bulimia, 43, 593
Bunions, 409
Burns, superficial, 131
Bursitis
  knee, 369
  olecranon, 246
  pelvis, hip, and thigh, 316
  subacromial, 231

C

Calcium metabolism, disorder, myocardial cells of left
      ventricle, 22
Calcium requirements, 566
Callouses, 104
1988 Canadian Paralympics, 4
Candida albicans infection, 109
Capillaries, plasma flow from, 19
Capital femoral epiphysis, slipped, 330
Capitate fracture, 281
Carbohydrate intake, 560
Carbohydrate oxidation, 558
Carbohydrate replacement, 573
Carbohydrate requirements, athletes, 558
Carbohydrates, types of, 559
Cardiac abnormalities, congenital, screening for, 21
Cardiac anomalies, 24
Cardiac index, 18
Cardiac monitoring, on-field emergencies and, 77
Cardiac output
  circulatory function and, 28
  definition of, 18
Cardiac stress testing, 24
Cardiomyopathy
  dilated, 23
  hypertrophic, 21
    ECG and, 24
Cardiopulmonary arrest, on-field emergencies, 74
Cardiopulmonary resuscitation, on-field, 74
Cardiovascular morbidity/mortality, 4
Cardiovascular screening, athletes, 20

Cardiovascular system
  endurance training and, 20
  functions of, 18
  messenger function, 18
Carpal bone fracture, 279
Carpal bones, 265
Carpal ligaments, 267
Carpal tunnel, anatomy, 269
Carpal tunnel syndrome, 282
Carpometacarpal bossing, 283
Carpometacarpal joint, 292
  sprain, 296
Cartilage fractures, knee, 336
Catecholamine mediation, 18
Catecholamine surge, 18
Cauliflower ear, 104
CBC, preparticipation physical examination and, 69
Cell diameter, 8
Cellulitis, 106
Central extensor tendon rupture, 288
Central nervous system (CNS)
  craniofacial injuries and, 129
  selective motor unit recruitment and, 11
Cerebral palsy
  athletes with, injury patterns, 605
  injury patterns of athletes with, 4
Cervical cord neurapraxia, 197
Cervical fractures, unstable, 194
Cervical injuries, 165
Cervical spine, 186–200
  catastrophic injury, 193
  emergency management, 186
  evaluation, pediatric athletes, 441
  immobilization on the field, 36
  injuries, prevention of, 192
  protection, on-field emergencies and, 77
Cervical sprain syndrome, 197
Cervical subluxation, 193
Chemical injuries, eye, 122
Chemotherapeutic agents, wound healing and, 102
Chest pain, 22, 28
  causes of, 28
  gastrointestinal symptoms and, 397
Chest radiograph, 29
Chicago Cubs, female league, 4
Cholinergic urticaria, 33
Chondromalacia, 283, 366
Choroid, 115
Ciliary body, 115
Circulation, on-field emergencies and, 77
Circulatory function, 28–29
Clavicle
  fractures, 236
  injuries, pediatric athletes, 439
  overuse injuries, pediatric athletes, 439
Closed kinetic chain exercises, posterior cruciate
    ligament injuries, 361
Closed reduction, metacarpal fractures, 303
Clubbing, 27
  causes of, 27
CNS: *see* Central nervous system

Cocaine abuse, 594
Coccyx fractures, 320
Cognition, exercise effects on, 5
CO_2 laser excision, plantar warts, 112
Collateral ligament, 293
  injuries, knee, 351
  knee, 337
    evaluation of, 342
Commotio, 123
Commotio cordis, 23
Compartment syndrome
  acute
    diagnosing, 376
    management of, 377
  ankle and foot, 406
  chronic exertional, 377
  leg, 375
    pathophysiology of, 375
Competitive sports, women and, 4
Computed tomography (CT), pulmonary function and,
    29
Concussion, 35
  cerebral, dental injuries and, 167
  postconcussive syndrome, 36
Conditioning, 5
Conditioning program, 6
  senior athletes and, 5
Conditioning techniques, 6
Conduction velocity, nerve cells and, 8
Congenital disorders, complex, 22
Congenital problems/disorders, preparticipation physical
    examination and, 62
Conjunctiva, 115
Conjunctival injuries, 120
Contact, on-field emergencies and, 75
Contraction, maximal volitional, 10
Contractions: *see* specific type
Contusions
  brain damage and, 36
  pelvis, hip, and thigh, 312
Cornea, foreign body removal, 121
Corneal injury, 120
  ruptured globe, 125
Corns, 104
Coronary artery bypass grafting, 4
Coronary artery disease, 22
  exercise-related decrease in, 4
Coronoid process fractures, 261
Corporeal bodies, penile trauma and, 58
Cough, causes of, 28
Cramping, 40
Craniofacial injuries, physical evaluation, 140–147
Craniofacial injury, 129–147
Craniomaxillofacial region, 129
Crown fractures, 150
Crown-root fractures, 150
Cryotherapy, 456
Cubital tunnel syndrome, 254
Curettage, molluscum contagiosum, 112
Cutaneous erythema, exercise-induced anaphylaxis and,
    33

Cutaneous warts, 584
Cyanosis, 27
Cycling, elderly participation in, 5
Cystogram, bladder injury, 53

D

Debridement, wound management and, 99
Deceleration forces, renal injury and, 49
Deep tendon reflexes, lower extremity, 208
Defibrillation, 74
Dehydration
  physiologic response to, 569
  prevalence in athletes with cerebral palsy, 4
  sports hematuria and, 48
  sweating and, 569
Dental first aid, 172
Dental injury, 149–172
  assessment of, 171
Dental screening, 149
Dental sports trauma readiness, 171
Dentoalveolar injuries, 131
Depression, 590
  exercise effects on, 5
Dermatitis, contact, 113
Dermatologic conditions, 104–114
Dermatophyte, 109
Developmental problems/disorders, preparticipation
    physical examination and, 62
Diabetes mellitus
  athletes with, 607
  wound healing and, 101
Diarrhea, 41
  traveler's, 41
Diastolic properties, abnormal, 20
Diathermy, 455
Diet, therapeutic, history of, 3
Dietary habits, athletes, 557
Dietary recommendations, athletes, 557
Disabled athletes, injury patterns, 4
Distal biceps tendon avulsion, 245
Distal clavicle osteolysis, 235
Distal humerus fractures, 258
Distal radial epiphysis stress fracture, 277
Distal radius fractures, 281
Distal triceps tendon avulsion, 246
Doppler echocardiography, 25
Doppler wave techniques, during echo-stress testing, 25
Down syndrome, cervical stability and, pediatric
    athletes, 445
Doxycycline, rickettsial diseases and, 109
Dynamic exercise, 25
Dyspnea, 26
  causes of, 27
  types of, 27

E

Ear cartilage, cauliflower ear, 104
Ear problems, 175
Eating disorders, 43
  menstrual dysfunction and, 89

Ecchymosis, bladder injury and, 53
ECG: *see* Electrocardiogram
Echocardiography
  cardiac screening and, 25
  hypertrophic cardiomyopathy and, 21
Echo stress testing, 22
Ecthyma, 105
Efferent systems, muscle activity and, 13
Ejection fraction, 18
Elbow, 242–262
  anatomy of, 242
  dislocation, 256–257
  fractures, 257
  fractures/dislocations, pediatric athletes, 436
  injury
      pediatric athletes, 436
      rehabilitation, 527
  lateral epicondylitis, 244
  neuropathies, 251–256
  overuse injuries, 243
      pediatric athletes, 437
  tendinopathies, 244–246
  tennis elbow, 244
  throwing injuries, 248
Elderly
  sports and, 4
  United States Masters Swimming Association and, 5
Electrical stimulation, 458
Electrocardiogram (ECG), cardiac screening and, 24
Electrolyte replacement, 573
Electromyography, integrated, 13
Electromyography (EMG), nervous system activity and, 12
Emergencies
  evaluation of potential for, 74
  on-field, 74–84
Emergency care, medicolegal issues, 610
Emergency personnel, equipment, and transportation,
    on-field emergencies, 74
EMG: *see* Electromyography
EMG activity, muscle tension and, 14
Emotional considerations, genital injury and, 56–58
Emotional disturbance, exercise effects on, 5
Endorphins, 5
Endurance, senior athletes and, 5
Endurance training
  carbohydrates and, 559
  and the heart, 20
Epidural hematoma, 36
Epilepsy, posttraumatic, 36
Epinephrine, 18, 30
Erosions, trauma and, 104
Escherichia coli, traveler's diarrhea and, 41
Estrogen, chronic unopposed, ovulatory oligomenorrhea
    and, 89
Excitatory potentials, motor units, 8
Exercise: *see also* specific types
  asthma and, 29
  cardiac benefits of, 26
  heart and, 18
  volume status, 19
Exercise-associated illness, 571

Exercise classification, general, 25
Exercise physiology, 8
Exercise speed, isokinetic torque and, 15
Extensor carpi ulnaris, 274
    dislocation, 277
Extensor mechanism, knee, evaluation of, 340
Extensor pollicis longus tendinitis, 274
External oblique muscle tears, 314
Eye, anatomy of, 115
Eye injury, 115–128
    chemical, 122
    common, diagnosis and treatment, 120–127
    examination after, 115
    eye examination kit contents, 127
    foreign bodies, 121
    orbital bone fractures, 126
    periorbital injury, 127
    prevention of, 127
    ruptured globe, 125

F

Facet dislocation, 194
Facial skeletal fractures, 131
Facial skeleton injuries, 130
Fast twitch fibers: *see also* entries under Motor unit
    area and ratio changes, 14
Fat, 563
    types of, 563
Fatigue, motor unit resistance to, 8
Female Athletic Triad, 89
Femoral neck stress fractures, 326
Femur, 306
Femur injuries, pediatric athletes, 417
Fenoterol, 30
Fibrillation, on-field defibrillation, 74
Fibrous nodules, 105
Fibula, stress fractures, 379
Finger fractures, 301
Finger proprioception, 532
Firing behavior, isometric and isotonic contractions and, 12
Fitness explosion, 587
Fixed body position, motoneuron pool activity during, 11
Flexibility
    aging influence on, 5
    definition of, 5
Flexor carpi radialis, 274
Flexor carpi ulnaris, 274
Flexor hallucis brevis, 396
Flexor hallucis longus, 396
Flexor profundus avulsion, 289
Fluid balance, 568–575
Fluidotherapy, 454
Follicular papules, 107
Folliculitis, 107, 583
Food ingestion, exercise-induced anaphylaxis and, 33
Foot
    fractures and dislocations, 400
    injury, 386–409
        pediatric athletes, 426

Foot—cont'd
    nerve entrapment syndrome, 406
    overuse injuries, 397
    overuse injury of, female athletes, 93
    rehabilitation, 464
    stress fractures, 399
    tendon abnormalities, 392
Football, head injury and, 35
Footwear, pediatric athletes, 415
Force
    modulation, 9
    motor-unit activity and, 12
Forearm, 242–262
    fractures of, 257
    neuropathies, 251–256
    throwing injuries, 248
Forefoot abnormalities, 409
Fractures
    extremity, on-field, 83
    prevalence in wheelchair-bound athletes, 4
Free posture position, motoneuron pool activity during, 11
Free radicals, exercise and, 564
Frontal bone fractures, 140
Frontal sinus fractures, physical examination, 146
Frostbite, 105
Fungal infections, 109
    superficial, 584
    widespread, 110
Furunculosis, 583

G

Galen, first team physician, 3
Ganglion cyst, 283
Gastric emptying, 40
Gastrocnemius, medial head tear, 382
Gastroesophageal reflux, 39
    treatment of symptoms, 40
Gastrointestinal bleeding, 42
    evaluation and treatment, 42
Gastrointestinal problems, nonsteroidal anti-inflammatory drugs and, 43
Gastrointestinal system
    overview, 39
    trauma and, 39
Genital injury, males, 56–59
Genitourinary examination, before sports participation, 68
Genitourinary injury, 46–59
Genitourinary system, hematuria and, 46
Gerota's fascia, 49
Gingival mucosa injuries, 162
Gladiators, injury treatment, 3
Glasgow Coma Scale, neurologic assessment on the field, 36
Glaucoma, 118
Glenohumeral dislocation, 238
Glenohumeral instability, 232
    conservative management, 233
    history and examination specifics, 233

Glenohumeral instability—cont'd
  operative management, 234
  orthopedic referral indications, 234
  pathomechanics of, 233
Glenoid fractures, 236
Gluteal muscles, 306
Gluteus maximus, 306
Gluteus medius, 306
  injury, 314
Gluteus minimus, 306
Glycemic index, 560
Glycogen depletion, during training, 559
Golfing, elderly athletes participation in, 5
Goose foot, 307
Gram negative rods, 109
Grass lime, eye injury and, 122
Greater trochanter, bursitis, 316
Griseofulvin, fungal infections and, 110
Gris-PEG, fungal infections and, 110
Groin, Legg-Calvé-Perthes disease and, 331
Groin pain, osteitis pubis and, 317
Growth factors, wound healing and, 102
Growth plate, hip fracture and, 319
Growth spurts, 415
Guyon's canal, 269
Gymnastics
  physical education and, 3
  urethral injury, 55

H

Hair, green discoloration, contact dermatitis and,
  113
Hallux rigidus, 409
Hallux valgus, 409
Hamate body fracture, 280
Hamstring muscle, 307
  injury, 313
  ischial apophysis avulsion fractures and, 323
Hand, 287–304
  fractures/dislocations, pediatric athletes, 433
  injury
    collateral ligaments, 297
    fingers, 296
    fractures, 301–303
    knuckle, 297
    pediatric athletes, 433
    rehabilitation, 529
  ligament injuries, 292
  muscle/tendon injuries, 287–292
  overuse injuries, pediatric athletes, 435
  sprain, 292
Haptoglobin, 48
Head injury
  classification and pathology of, 35
  evaluation and treatment on the field, 36
  prevention of, 37
  return to athletic activity after, 37
  sport-related, epidemiology of, 35
Health care reform, injured athletes and, 6
Heart

Heart—cont'd
  attack, exercise effects on, 5
  block, endurance training and, 20
  diastolic abnormalities, 21
  disorders, 22
  endurance training and, 20
  exercise benefits, 26
  functions of, 18
  myocardial oxygen consumption, 18
Heartburn, 39
Heat acclimatization, physiologic adjustments during,
  20
Heat exhaustion, exertional, 571
Heat illness
  on-field emergencies, 82
  prevention of, 572
Heat-induced illness
  environmental risk factors, 571
  risk factors for, 570
Heat injury, exertional, 571
Heat intolerance, athletes with disabilities, 601
Heat stroke, exertional, 571
Heat treatment, 454
Helicobacter pylori
  chronic active antral gastritis and, 44
  treatment regimens for, 44
Helmet, polycarbonate, 193
Hematochezia, 42
Hematocrit determination, preparticipation physical
  examination and, 69
Hematoma
  pelvic, bladder injury and, 55
  subungual, trauma-induced, 104
Hematuria
  nonexercise-associated, 48
  renal injury and, 49
  sports-related, 46
Hemodynamic changes, during exercise, 25
Hemoglobin, preparticipation physical examination and,
  69
Hemoglobinuria, march, 48
Henneman's size principle, 10
  synchronization and, 11
Herodicus, first sports physician, 3
Herpes gladiatorum, 583
Herpes simplex, 111, 583
Herpes zoster, 111
Hindfoot fractures/dislocations, 404
Hip, 306–334
  acetabular labral tears, 333
  anatomy of, 306
  bursitis, 316
  dislocations, 328
    avascular necrosis, 329
  external rotators of, 307
  fracture, neurologic examination and, 328
  fractures, 319
  history and physical examination, 309
  injury
    pediatric athletes, 416
    rehabilitation, 473

Hip—cont'd
  Legg-Calvé-Perthes disease, 331
  muscle injuries, 313–314
  myositis ossificans traumatica, 314
  pain
    acetabular labral tears, 333
    iliopectineal bursitis and, 316
  snapping hip syndrome, 317
  soft tissue injuries, 312–313
  transient synovitis of, 333
Hitchcock, Jr., Edward, 3
Holter monitoring, mitral valve prolapse and, 23
Hormones, cardiovascular system and, 18
Horseback riding
  head injury and, 35
  urethral injury, 55
Human immunodeficiency virus, 111, 584
Human papilloma virus, 111
Humerus fractures
  pediatric athletes, 437
  proximal, 235
Hydrocollator packs, 454
Hyperextension, knee dislocations and, 362
Hyperhidrosis, 409
Hypertrophy
  muscle, strength development and, 13
  muscular, 13
  selective, 14
Hyponatremia, 572
Hypothermia, athletes with disabilities, 601
Hypoxemia, oxygen delivery and, 19
Hypoxia, 27

I

IEMG: *see* Electromyography, integrated
Iliac crest avulsion fractures, 321
Iliac spine
  anterior inferior fractures, 323
  anterior superior fractures, 323
Iliopectineal region, bursitis, 316
Iliopsoas, 307
Iliopsoas injuries, 314
Iliotibial band friction syndrome, 369
Imidazoles, dermatophyte infections and, 109
Immobilization, 449
  splinting, 450
Immune cells, exercise effects on, 581
Immune mediators, exercise effects on, 581
Impetigo, 105, 583
Impotence, urethral injury and, 56
Infection
  effects on athletic performance, 582
  prevalence in athletes with cerebral palsy, 4
  prevention in athletes, 584
  susceptibility, exercise effects on, 582
  wound healing and, 101
Infectious agents, skin problems and, 105
Infectious diseases, 581–585
Injury patterns, 4
Intellectual acuity, exercise effects on, 5

Intercollegiate athletics, 3
  NCAA and, 3
Interphalangeal joint
  dislocations, 296
  distal, injuries, 301
  proximal, injuries, 299
Intersection syndrome, 274
Intervertebral disc, 203
Intervertebral disc disease, rehabilitation, 537
Intervertebral disc injury, 200
Intracerebral hematoma, 36
Intracranial pressure, 36
Intravenous pyelography, renal injury and, 52
Iris, 115
Iritis, 122
Iron, 565
Irritable bowel syndrome, 40
Ischemia, abdominal stitch and, 40
Ischial apophysis avulsion fractures, 323
Ischial tuberosity, bursitis, 316
Isokinetic torque, exercise speed effects, 15
Isometric contractions
  firing behavior, 12
  maximal motor-unit recruitment and, 12
  submaximal, motoneuron pool activity during, 11
Isoproterenol, 30
Isotonic contractions
  firing behavior, 12
  maximal motor-unit recruitment and, 12
Itraconzole, fungal infections and, 110

J

Jammed finger, pediatric athletes, 434
Jaw fracture, 161
Jock itch, 109
Jogger's nail, 408
Jogger's testicles, 58
Jogging, elderly athletes participation in, 5
Joint, range of motion, 5
Jumper's knee, 367
Jump training, fast twitch/slow twitch area ratio, 14

K

Kawasaki's disease, 22
Ketoconazole, fungal infections and, 110
Kidney
  horseshoe, 49
  sports-related injury, 48–52
Knee
  anatomy of, 336–339
  bursitis, 367
  clinical evaluation, 339
  collateral ligaments, 337
  dislocation, on-field, 82
  dislocations, 362
  extension strength, isometric, 13
  injury, 336–372
    female athletes, 90
    imaging studies, 346
    pediatric athletes, 417
    rehabilitation, 478

Knee—cont'd
intraarticular pathology, MRI analysis, 349
joint compartments, 336
ligament injury, female athletes, 92
ligamentous injuries, 351
meniscal injuries, 350
overuse injuries, pediatric athletes, 420
palpation, 339
physical evaluation, 339
tendonitis, 367
valgus, female athletes, 91

L

Laboratory tests, preparticipation physical examination and, 69
Laceration, eye, 120
Lachman test, posterior, 349
Lactose intolerance, 42
Laryngeal fracture, on-field emergencies and, 77
Larynx, penetrating trauma, 184
Lateral compression injuries, 250
Lateral epicondylitis, 244
Leg
anatomy of, 376
compartment syndrome, pathophysiology of, 375
injury, 375–383
lower, pediatric athletes, 423
pain, rehabilitation for, 471
Legal issues, in sports medicine, 611–612
Legg-Calvé-Perthes disease, 331
pediatric athletes, 415
Leg-length discrepancy, hip fracture and, 319
Lesser toe deformities, 409
Lifestyle changes, middle-age and elderly, 5
Life support
advanced, 74
basic, 74
Ligament of Humphrey, 336
Ligament of Wrisberg, 336
Limb pacing, control of, 15
Limbus, 115
Little League elbow, 437
Little League shoulder, 438
Liver chemistry, elevated, 44
Lower extremity
anatomic malalignment, 415
bone fractures, pediatric athletes, 413
growth cartilage, pediatric athletes, 414
injury
physical examination, pediatric athletes, 418
risk factors, pediatric athletes, 414
treatment, pediatric athletes, 420
innervation, 208
joint injuries, pediatric athletes, 413
muscle-tendon imbalance, pediatric athletes, 415
muscle/tendon injuries, pediatric athletes, 414
overuse injuries, pediatric athletes, 413
pediatric athletes, 413–431
rehabilitation, 463–505
trauma, pediatric athletes, 413

Lumbar spine, 202–218
anatomy of, 202
biomechanics, 206
clinical evaluation, 206
evaluation, pediatric athletes, 442
ligaments, 204
muscles, 204
neural structures, 205
osseous conditions, 213
vascular supply, 206
vertebrae, 202
Lunate dislocation, 282
Lungs, function of, 26–34
Lunotriquetral instability, 277
Lunotriquetral ligament injury, 277
Lyme borreliosis, 108
Lympangitis, 107
Lymphatic drainage and, 19

M

Macula, 115
Magnetic resonance imaging (MRI), pulmonary function and, 29
Mallet finger, pediatric athletes, 434
Mandible fracture, 161
physical examination, 142
Mandibular fracture, 131
Manic-depressive illness, 590
Marfan syndrome, 22
Marijuana abuse, 595
Mass: *see* Muscle mass
Massage, 452
Maxilla fracture, 161
Maxillary fracture, 135
physical examination, 144
Maximal volitional contraction, 10
Medial collateral ligament, 242
Medial epicondylitis, 245
Medial tension injuries, 248
Medial tibial stress syndrome, 377
pathophysiology, 379
presentation, evaluation, and diagnosis, 377
Median nerve entrapment, 251
Medical history, preparticipation physical examination and, 65
Medicolegal issues, 609–610
Melanoma, malignant, 114
Melena, 42
Meniscus, evaluation, 341
Menstrual dysfunction, 87
eating disorders, 89
Mental acuity, exercise effects on, 5
Mental disabilities, sports participation and, 4
Mental health specialist, referral to, 596
Mental status examination, on the field, 37
Metacarpal fractures
management, 303
pediatric athletes, 434
Metacarpophalangeal joint, 293, 297
dorsal capsule, 293

Metaproterenol, 30
Metatarsalgia, 409
Metatarsal fractures, 404
Metatarsophalangeal dislocations, 404
Metatarsophalangeal joint instability, 399
Methylxanthines, 30
Midfoot fractures/dislocations, 404
Midsystolic click, 23
Miliaria, 107
Milo, Olympic wrestler, 3
Mineral requirements, 565
Mitral valve prolapse, 23
Molluscum contagiosum, 112, 584
Morphologic adaptation, neural drive and, 13
Morton's neuroma, 406
Motoneuron pools, activity of, 11
Motor axon diameter, 8
Motor neuron, muscle cell and, 8
Motor unit, 8
    activation
        extent of, 11
        factors influencing, 11
    continuously firing long interval, 12
    discharges from, 10
    excitatory potentials, 8
    fast-fatigable (FF), 8
    fast-fatiguable, muscle fibers, 9
    fast-fatigue resistant (FR), 8
    fast twitch, 8
        maximal volitional contraction and, 10
    intermittently firing short interval, 12
    recruitment, 9
        force levels and, 12
        selective, by CNS, 11
        strategies, 9
    resistance to fatigue, 8
    signal transmission characteristics, 8
    slow-fatigue resistant (S), 8
    slow twitch, 8
    synchronization, 10
Mouthguard
    considerations, 164
    ethylene vinyl acetate, 165
Mouth protector
    considerations, 164
    construction, 168
Movement, nature of, 11
Multiple sclerosis, 606
Muscle, essential role of, 8
Muscle contractile capability, 12
Muscle contraction, gradation of, 9
Muscle cramps, 571
Muscle fiber breakdown, after exercise, 48
Muscle fibers
    fast twitch, myosin-ATPase levels, 9
    slow twitch, myosin-ATPase levels, 9
Muscle force, directional programming, 16
Muscle force output
    dynamic control of, 10
    governing, 10
Muscle growth, selective hypertrophy, 14

Muscle light attachments, 118
Muscle mass, increases in, 13
Muscle strengthening, electrical stimulation, 458
Muscle tension
    EMG amplitude and, 12
    graded, recruitment strategies and, 10
Muscle tone, increases in, 13
Muscular activity, nervous system and, 8
Musculoskeletal examination, before sports
        participation, 68
Myalgia, pelvic floor, 333
Mycelex, 110
Myelin, 8
Myocardial biopsy specimens, 21
Myocardial oxygen consumption, 18
Myocarditis, 22
Myofascial pain, rehabilitation, 537
Myofibrillar disarray, 21
Myoglobinuria, exercise, 48
Myosin-ATPase activity, isokinetic training and, 14
Myosin-ATPase levels, muscle fibers, 9
Myositis ossificans traumatica, 314

N

Nasal congestion, 183
Nasal fractures, 139
Nasal problems, 180
Nasoethmoid fractures, 139
    physical examination, 146
National Collegiate Athletic Association, history of, 3
National Football Head and Neck Injury Registry, 35
National Institute of Allergy and Infectious Disease,
        asthma and allergies statistics, 29
Nausea, 40
NCAA: *see* National Collegiate Athletic Association
Neck injuries, 184
Neoplasms, sun exposure and, 114
Nerve entrapment syndromes, foot and ankle, 406
Nerve root injury, 195
Nervous system, muscular activity coordination, 8
Neural drive, morphologic adaptation and, 13
Neural hormones, 18
Neural learning, 13
Neurologic assessment, on the field after head injury, 36
Neurologic examination, on-field emergencies, 78
Neurologic impairment, sport-related head injury and, 35
Neurologic injuries, physical examination, 142
Neuromuscular system
    muscle activity amplitude control, 9
    tension rate of change, 9
Neurons
    fast twitch, excitatory threshold, 9
    slow twitch, excitatory threshold, 9
Neuropathy
    central, rickettsial diseases and, 109
    elbow and forearm, 251–256
Neurophysiology, muscle physiology and, 8
Nizoral, fungal infections and, 110
Nonsteroidal anti-inflammatory drugs, gastrointestinal
        problems and, 43

Nonsteroidal anti-inflammatory medications, 6
Norepinephrine, 18
Nose problems, 175
Nutrition, 557–566
Nutritional status, wound healing and, 101

O

Obesity, athletes with, 607
Obsessive-compulsive disorder, 592
Olecranon bursitis, 246
Olecranon fractures, 260
Oligomenorrhea, risk factors associated with, 89
Olympic games, ancient, 3
On-field emergencies
   abdominal injury, 82
   anaphylaxis, 82
   assessment, 76
   athlete injured but moving under own power, 82
   athlete down from contact and moving, 81
   athlete down on field without contact, 81
   cervical spine injuries, 186
   emergency personnel, equipment, and transportation, 74
   extremity fractures, 83
   heat illness, 82
   injury patterns, 75
   knee dislocation, 83
   player conscious and breathing but not moving, 79
   player unconscious and not breathing, 76
   player unconscious but breathing, 78
   spinal cord injury, 186
Onychomycosis, 408
Ophthalmologic injuries, physical examination, 142
Ophthalmoscope, 115
Optic nerve, 115
   damage, 117, 123
Oral first aid, 172
Oral mucosa injuries, 162
Oral screening, 149
Orbital bone fracture, 126
Oribasius of Pergamum, 3
Orthopnea, 27
Osgood-Schlatter apophysitis, 370
Osteitis pubis, 317
Osteochondral defects, knee, 336
Osteochondritis dissecans, 250, 371
   pediatric athletes, 415, 420
Osteoporosis
   female athletes, 89
   senior athletes and, 5
Otorhinolaryngology, 175–184
   general principles of, 175
Overextension, 287
Overload injuries, extension, 250
Overstretch injury, flexor profundus, 289
Overuse injuries
   ankle and foot, 397
   elbow, pediatric athletes, 437
   female athletes, 89
   knee, pediatric athletes, 420
   wrist, 272

Ovulatory oligomenorrhea, 89
Oxygenation
   local tissue, wound healing and, 101
   pulse oximetry and, 29
Oxygen delivery, vascular system and, 19

P

Pain control, electrical stimulation, 458
Pain killers, serotonins and endorphins, 5
Palmar soft tissue, 269
Panic disorder, 592
Paraffin baths, 455
Parasympathetic discharge, 18
Paratenonitis, 392
Paresthesias, burning, 197
Paroxysmal nocturnal dyspnea, 27
Passive motion, continuous, 454
Patella, evaluation of, 340
Patella subluxation/dislocation, 364
Patella tendon, extensor mechanism disruptions, 367
Patellofemoral joint injuries, 364
Patellofemoral stress, female athletes, 92
Patellofemoral stress syndrome, female athletes, 90
Patellofemoral syndrome, 366
Pediatric athletes, 413
Pelvic floor myalgia, 333
Pelvic injuries, pediatric athletes, 416
Pelvis, 306–334
   anatomy of, 306
   bursitis, 316
   fractures, 318
   gynecoid, knee valgus development and, 92
   history and physical examination, 309
   muscle injuries, 313–314
   myositis ossificans traumatica, 314
   soft tissue injuries, 312–313
   stress fractures, 325
Penetrating trauma, renal injury and, 49
Penile injury/trauma, 58
Perilunate dislocation, 282
Perineal trauma, 58
Perineum, straddle injury, 55
Periodontal tissue injuries, 157–161
   displacement injuries, 157
   nondisplacement injuries, 157
Periostitis, reactive, osteitis pubis and, 317
Peripheral nerve injuries, 239
Peripheral vascular responses, 18
Peroneal dislocation, 394
Peroneal rupture, 393
Peroneal subluxation, 394
Peroneal tendinitis, 393
pes anserinus, 307
Phalangeal fractures, 402
   pediatric athletes, 434
Pharmacotherapy, asthma, 30
Photodermatitis, 113
Phototoxic reactions, 113
Physical activity, elderly participation in, 4
Physical capabilities, sports medicine and, 3

Physical disabilities
   athletes with, 598–607
   sports participation
      pharmacologic concerns, 600
      physician concerns, 599
   sports participation and, 4
Physical education
   history of, 3
   promotion of, 3
Physical examination
   preparticipation, 61–72
   screening, frequency of, 63
Physical fitness, health and, 3
Pisiform fracture, 280
Pitching motion, injuries, 248
Plantar warts, 111, 408
Platypnea, 27
Postconcussive syndrome, 36
Posterior cruciate ligament, 336
   evaluation of, 346
   injuries, 357
      closed kinetic chain exercises, 361
      reconstruction, 362
Postoperative exercise programs, history of, 3
Power, definition of, 13
Power training exercise, 13
   neuromuscular system selective recruitment and, 14
Precordium, commotio cordis and, 23
Preparticipation Physical Evaluation, joint statement, 69
Preparticipation physical examination
   clearance for participation in sports, 69
   cost effectiveness, 62
   frequency of, 63
   goals of, 62
   laboratory tests and procedures, 69
   medical history and, 65
   methodology of, 63
   office-based, 63
   outcome studies, 61
   overview of, 61
   standardization, 70
   state requirements for, 62
   station examination, 63
   timing of, 65
President's Council on Physical Fitness, history of, 3
Primary care physician
   injured athletes and, 6
   interviewing techniques, 588
   sports psychology and, 588
Progressive resistance exercise, 5
   history of, 3
Pronator syndrome, 251
Proparacaine, eye examination and, 118
Prostate gland, high riding, urethral injury and, 56
Protein requirements
   endurance athletes, 562
   resistance exercise, 562
Pruritis, exercise-induced anaphylaxis and, 33
Pseudocysts, testicular injury and, 58
Pseudomonas organisms, folliculitis and, 107

Psychological problems, mental health specialist referral, 596
Psychologic disturbance, exercise effects on, 5
Psychologic factors, lower extremity injury, pediatric athletes, 415
Psychologic impairment, warning signs of, 590
Psychologic well-being, exercise effects on, 5
Psychology
   female athletes, 593
   pediatric athletes, 592
   sports, 587–596
Puberty, female athletes, 89
Pubic rami, stress fractures, 325
Pulmonary disease, chronic obstructive, 34
Pulmonary embolism, 34
Pulse oximetry, 29
Pupil reactivity, after trauma, 116

Q

Quadriceps femoris injuries, 314
Quadriceps femoris muscles, 307
Quadriceps tendon, extensor mechanism disruptions, 367
Quadriplegia, transient, 197

R

Racquet player's pisiform, 283
Radial head fractures, 259
Radial nerve entrapment, 253
Radial shaft fractures, 261
Radial tunnel syndrome, 253
Radiography, wrist, 272
Radionuclide studies, 25
Radioulnar dislocation, 282
Radius
   force transmission between hand and forearm, 270
   fractures, pediatric athletes, 435
Range of motion exercises, fractures and, 303
Recruitment strategy, force modulation and, 9
Rehabilitation
   lower extremity, 463–505
   techniques, 449–460
      immobilization, 449
Renal cysts, 49
Renal failure, sports hematuria and, 48
Renal injury, 48–52
   signs and symptoms of, 51
Renal ischemia, sports hematuria and, 48
Renal pedicle injury, 49
Respiratory system, function of, 26–34
Respiratory tract, disabled athletes, 4
Retina, posterior, examination of, 119
Retinal detachment, 118, 123
Retinal hemorrhage, 118
Retinal injury, 123
Retinal swelling, 123
Retinal tears, 123
Retrobulbar hemorrhage, 118
Rickettsial disease, 108
Rock climbing, elderly athletes participation in, 5

Roid rage, 578
Root fractures, 155
Rotator cuff disorders, 230
    conservative management, 232
    operative management, 232
    pathomechanics, 231
Rotator cuff tear, 237
Runners, long distance, gastrointestinal bleeding and, 42

S

Sacroiliac dysfunction, rehabilitation for, 551
Sacroiliac joint pain, 333
Salmeterol, 30
Saltatory conduction, 8
Sartorius muscle, 307
    anterior superior iliac spine avulsion fracture, 323
Scalp wound, evaluation and treatment on the field, 36
Scaphoid bone fracture, 279
Scapholunate instability, 277
Scapholunate ligament injury, 277
Scapular body fractures, 236
Scar tissue, 99
Schiotz tonometer, 118
Scholastic sports, preparticipation physical examination,
        state guidelines, 62
Sclera, 115
Scleral injury, 120
    ruptured globe, 125
Scoliosis, rehabilitation for, 552
Scrapes, trauma and, 104
Scrotal trauma, 58
Second Impact Syndrome, 36
Sedentary men, cardiovascular screening, 20
Self-concept, exercise effects on, 5
Serotonins, 5
Sesamoid bursitis, 399
Sesamoid fractures, 404
Sesamoiditis, 399
Shin splint rehabilitation, 471
Shin splint syndrome, 377
Shortening, motor-unit activity and, 12
Shoulder, 220–240
    anatomic and biomechanical concerns, 220
    articular anatomy, 221
    assessment of, 222
    biomechanics, 222
    bony anatomy, 220
    diagnostic modalities, 228
    evaluation, history obtaining, 223
    first aid, 222
    flexibility, 523
    fractures/dislocations, pediatric athletes, 437
    impingement syndrome, pediatric athletes, 439
    injury
        disabled athletes, 4
        rehabilitation, 507
    joint mobilization, 507
    muscular anatomy, 221
    overuse injuries, pediatric athletes, 438
    painful, evaluation of, 222

Shoulder—cont'd
    physical examination, 224
    proprioception, 525
    radiographic anatomy, 222
    rotator cuff disorders, 230
    strengthening, 514
Signal transmission, motor units and, 8
Sinus-related symptoms, 33
Size principle, synchronization and, 11
Skeletal injuries, 131
Skin cancer, 114
Skin problems
    infectious agents and, 105
    trauma-induced, 104
Skull fracture, 36
Slow twitch fibers: *see also* entries under Motor unit
    area and ratio changes, 14
Smoking, wound healing and, 101
Snapping hip syndrome, 317, 333
Soft tissue contusions, immobilization, 449
Soft tissue edema, 130
Soft tissue injury, 129, 131
    pelvis, hip, and thigh, 312–313
    physical examination, 142
    thoracic/lumbar spine, 210
Spear tackler's spine, 194
Special Olympics, 606
Spinal cord, 186–200
    emergency management, 186
Spinal cord injury
    catastrophic, 193
    prevention of, 192
Spinal cord resuscitation, 194
Spinal deformity, 217
Spinal disc degeneration, senior athletes and, 5
Spineboard, 186
Spine injuries
    pediatric athletes, 441–445
    physical evaluation and radiography, pediatric
        athletes, 441
    rehabilitation, 534
Splinting, 450
Spondylolisthesis, 214
    rehabilitation for, 550
Spondylolysis, 214
Spondylosis, rehabilitation for, 550
Sporonox, fungal infections and, 110
Sport performance, female athletes, 86
Sports medicine
    communication and follow-up, 609
    evolution of, 3
    female athletes and, 4
    growth of, 6
    history of, 3
    legal issues in, 611–612
    physicians, disabled athletes and, 4
    rehabilitation and, 8
Sprain
    ankle, 389
        recurrent, 391
    hand, 292

Sprain—cont'd
   first degree, 292
      second degree, 292
   spinal, rehabilitation, 534
   stretching and conditioning techniques and, 6
Squat exercises, strength development and, 13
Static exercise, 25
Stenosis, rehabilitation for, 550
Steroid administration, wound healing and, 101
Strain
   hand
      first degree, 287
         second degree, 287
   spinal, rehabilitation, 534
   stretching and conditioning techniques and,
      6
Strength
   definition of, 13
   developing, exercise, 13
   development, 12
      muscle hypertrophy and, 13
   improvement
      exercise speed and, 15
      maximal volitional contraction increase and,
         13
   task-specific, 16
   training
      history of, 3
      recommendations for, 15
Stress fractures
   female athletes, 90
   fibula, 379
   lower extremity, rehabilitation, 472
   tibia, 379
Stress levels, exercise effects on, 5
Stretching techniques, 6
Stroke volume, 18
   arterial pressure and, 19
   heart rate changes and, 19
   supine exercise and, 19
   subarachnoid hematoma, 36
Subconjunctival hemorrhage, 120
Subdural hematoma, 36
Substance abuse, 594
   prevention, 579
   symptoms of, 578
Substance abuse, 578–580
Sunscreens, photodermatitis and, 113
Supine exercise, stroke volumes and, 19
Support groups, 596
Supraorbital rim fractures, physical examination,
      146
Sweating, dehydration and, 569
Swimmer's ear, 583
Swimming, disabled athletes and, 4
Swinging flashlight test, 117
Sympathetic discharge, 18
Synchronization, motor unit, 11
Syncope, 21
Synovial plica, 370
Synovitis, transient, of hip, 333

T

Tachycardia, 21
Talon noir, 104
Team physician, history of in America, 3
Team physicians, concept of, 6
Team sports, history of female participation, 4
Teeth, injuries to, 150–157
Temperature regulation, 19
   athletes with disabilities, 601
Tendinitis
   extensor pollicis longus, 274
   flexor carpi radialis, 274
   flexor carpi ulnaris, 274
   knee, rehabilitation, 498
Tendonitis, patella, 367
Tennis
   elbow, 244
   elderly athletes participation in, 5
   senior athletes participation in, 5
   toenail, 408
Tenosynovitis, overuse, 274
Tension development
   rate of, 14
   time course of, 14
Terbutaline, 30
Terminal extensor tendon rupture, 288
Testes, physiology of, 58
Testicular trauma, 58
Therapeutic exercise, history of, 3
Therapeutic modalities, 449–460
   continuous passive motion, 454
   cryotherapy, 456
   diathermy, 455
   electrical stimulation, 458
   fluidotherapy, 454
   heat treatment, 454
   hydrocollator packs, 454
   massage, 452
   mechanical, 452
   paraffin baths, 455
   in rehabilitation, 454
   stretching, 452
   thermotherapy, 454
   traction, 452
   ultrasound, 456
   whirlpool, 454
Thermoregulation, 568
Thermoregulatory centers in brain, 19
Thermotherapy, 454
Thigh, 306–334
   adductor canal syndrome, 318
   anatomy of, 306
   bone, 306
   bursitis, 316
   history and physical examination, 309
   injury
      pediatric athletes, 417
      rehabilitation, 473
   muscle injuries, 313–314
   myositis ossificans traumatica, 314

Thigh—cont'd
quadriceps femoris muscles, 307
soft tissue injuries, 312–313
Thoracic spine, 202–218
anatomy of, 202
biomechanics, 206
clinical evaluation, 206
evaluation, pediatric athletes, 442
ligaments, 204
muscles, 204
neural structures, 205
osseous conditions, 213
vascular supply, 206
vertebrae, 202
Throat problems, 175
Throwing injuries, elbow and forearm, 248
Thumb, 292
fracture, 301
Tibia, stress fractures, 379
Tibial growth plate, Osgood-Schlatter apophysitis and, 370
Tibial rupture, posterior, 395
Tibial tendinitis, posterior, 395
Tibial tendon, anterior, 396
Tibial tendon dislocation, posterior, 396
Tibial tendon subluxation, posterior, 396
Tibiofibular joint dislocations, proximal, 371
Tinea corporis, 110
Tinea pedis, 109
Title IX of Educational Amendments, 86
history of, 4
Toenails
blue, 408
fungal infections, 408
ingrown, 408
Tone: see Muscle tone
Total lung capacity, 28
Traction, 452
Training programs, integrated EMG and, 13
Trauma, skin problems caused by, 104
Treadmill stress test, 24
Triangular fibrocartilage complex, 267, 279
Tripopnea, 27
Triquetrum fracture, 280
Turf toe, 404
Twitch tension, 9

U

Ulna fractures, pediatric athletes, 435
Ulnar artery injury, 282
Ulnar collateral ligament, 242
Ulnar impaction syndrome, 277
Ulnar nerve entrapment, 254
Ulnar shaft fractures, 261
Ulnar styloid fracture, 281
Ulnar tunnel syndrome, 282
Ultrasound, 456
Ultrasound examination, genital injury, 58
United States Masters Swimming Association, 5
United States Tennis Association, elderly athletes
participation in, 5

Upper extremity injuries
pediatric athletes, 433
rehabilitation, 507–532
Ureteral injury, 52
Ureteropelvis junction obstructions, 49
Urethral catheter drainage, urethral injury in females, 56
Urethral injury, 55
diagnosing, 56
Urethrogram, retrograde, 56
Urinary retention, prevalence in athletes with cerebral
palsy, 4
Urticaria, exercise-induced anaphylaxis and, 33

V

Valgus stress testing, 353
Varus stress testing, 353
Vascular system, functions of, 18
Vasoconstriction, 19
Velocity, motor-unit activity and, 12
Ventilation, on-field emergencies and, 77
Ventilatory function, measurement of, 28
Ventricle, left, hypertrophic cardiomyopathy and, 21
Ventricular dysplasia, right, 23
Ventricular function, diastolic properties of, 20
Ventricular tachycardia, on-field defibrillation, 74
Verrucae, 111
Vertebrae, thoracic and lumbar, 202
Viral infections, 111–112
Vision
checking after trauma, 116
peripheral
confrontation technique for checking, 117
retinal detachment and, 124
Visual impairment, athletes with, injury patterns, 606
Vital capacity, 28
forced, 28
Vitamin supplementation, 564
Vitreous hemorrhage, 118
Vitreous humor, 115
Vitreous injury, 123
Volar plate dislocations, 295
Volar plate tears, 297
Volar wrist splint, carpometacarpal joint sprain, 296
Volume status, in exercise, 19
Vomiting, 40

W

Warts, 111
Whirlpool therapy, 454
Winter sports, urethral injury, 55
Women in sports, 86–95
anatomic and physiologic characteristics, 86
conditioning, 89
history of, 4
history of acceptance into sports, 4
injury rates and types, 90–94
menstrual dysfunction, 87
nutritional concerns, 89
overuse injuries, 89
psychologic concerns, 94–95
Title IX and, 4

Women's Suffrage Movement, 4
Wound healing, 99–103
    anemia and, 101
    chemotherapeutic agents and, 102
    diabetes mellitus and, 101
    factors affecting, 101–103
    growth factors and, 102
    infection and, 101
    inflammatory phase, 99
    local tissue oxygenation, 101
    nutritional status and, 101
    phases of, 99
    proliferative phase, 99
    smoking and, 101
    steroid administration and, 101
Wrist, 265–286
    anatomy of, 265–270
    biomechanics, 270–271
    carpal bones, 265
    classification of injury, 272
    dorsal nerves, 269
    dorsal soft tissue, 267
    evaluation of, 271–272
    first dorsal compartment, 273
    fractures/dislocations, pediatric athletes, 435
    imaging, 272
    immediate management, 272

Wrist—cont'd
    injury, rehabilitation, 529
    intersection syndrome, 274
    kinematics, 270
    kinetics, 270
    ligaments, 274–275
    load-bearing injury, 276
    overuse injuries, 272
        pediatric athletes, 435
    pain, dorsal, 277
    physical examination, 271
    tendons, 273–274
    trauma
        bones, 279–280
        cartilage, 281–282
        contusion, 282
        ligaments, 277
        neurologic, 282–283
        tendons, 277
        vascular, 282

Y

Yeast infections, 109

Z

Zygoma fractures, 135
    physical examination, 145